The Complete Directory
for
Pediatric Disorders

2015/16
Eighth Edition

The Complete Directory
for
Pediatric Disoders

- Disorder Descriptions
- Body Systems Descriptions
- National & State Associations
- Libraries & Resource Centers
- Support Groups & Hotlines
- Books & Periodicals
- Research Centers
- Web Sites

A SEDGWICK PRESS Book

Grey House
Publishing

PUBLISHER: Leslie Mackenzie
EDITORIAL DIRECTOR: Laura Mars

PRODUCTION MANAGER & COMPOSITION: Kristen Thatcher
MARKETING DIRECTOR: Jessica Moody

A Sedgewick Press Book
Grey House Publishing, Inc.
4919 Route 22
Amenia, NY 12501
518.789.8700
FAX 845.373.6390
www.greyhouse.com
e-mail: books@greyhouse.com

Complete directory for pediatric disorders – 8th ed. (2015)-
    v.; 27.5 cm.
    Includes index.

1. Pediatric–Directories. 2. Children–Diseases–Treatment–Directories. 3. Pediatrics–Periodicals. 4. Children–Diseases–Treatments–Periodicals. 5. Pediatrics–United States–Directory. 6. Child Health Services–United States–Directory. 7. Information Services–United States–Directory. 8. Self-Help Groups–United States–Directory. I. Grey House Publishing, Inc. II. Title: Directory for pediatric disorders.

RJ61.C728
618.92

ISBN: 978-1-61925-551-7
ISSN: 1537-7180

Table of Contents

Table of Contents

Table of Contents

Table of Contents

Introduction

This eighth edition of *The Complete Directory for Pediatric Disorders* provides current, understandable medical information, resources and support services for 213 pediatric disorders. A repeat winner of the National Health Information Awards "Honoring the Nation's Best Consumer Health Information Programs and Materials," this reference work provides vital information for afflicted children and their support network, including family, friends, and medical professionals.

Praise for previous editions:

> *"The strength of this source is in the information referral portion for each entry: the wide range of resources and organizations presented that can assist with additional information and support."*
> —ARBA

> *"...thousands of resources are provided covering a diverse range of services... All entries offer resource descriptions, as well as full contact information. Three indexes assist readers in locating specific information..."*
> —Against the Grain

> *"...It will be particularly useful for libraries serving parents of young children and youth, and for medical professionals working in the pediatrics field...the information is comprehensive and current."*
> —Choice

The disorders and issues covered in this directory have been determined to be most prevalent in the pediatric population, ages 0-18. They include both physical and mental conditions, and range from cancer to nightmares.

Violence by Children and Teenagers is a **NEW** chapter in this edition. Criminal behavior by children and teenagers doubled since the 1980s, and this content addresses cause and treatment.

The front matter for *The Complete Directory for Pediatric Disorders* includes:
- Two glossaries. The first is a guide to medical terminology that provides important navigational tips and more than 200 commonly used medical prefixes, roots and suffixes to help readers decipher terms they may encounter in the disorder descriptions or in other resources they are using. The second glossary includes medical acronyms, especially as they relate to vaccines.
- Guidelines for Obtaining Additional Information and Research. These guidelines assist parents and caregivers who are interested in obtaining more information on such diverse topics as physicians who specialize in certain pediatric disorders, accredited hospitals, approved drugs or medical devices for certain pediatric conditions, or current clinical trials that are investigating possible new therapies for particular diseases.
- A valuable list of Disorders by Biologic System.
- An article titled *The Health Impact of Childhood Bullying Can Last a Lifetime*, which explains the long-term effects that bullying can have on an individual.

This reference work includes 8,837 listings. Each listing has updated contact data – address, phone, fax, web site, e-mail – and helpful descriptions. You will find 6,366 fax numbers, 5,955 e-mail addresses, 7,898 web sites and 14,325 key executives – 6,945 more data points than the last edition.

This Directory is a one-stop resource, enabling professionals and the families they serve to obtain immediate, important information from one comprehensive source. It is organized in the following six sections:

Section I – Disorders

This section includes 213 major disorder chapters that comprise more than 266 specific disorders, diseases, or conditions. They are arranged in alphabetical order, from Achondroplasia to Wilson Disease. Each chapter begins with an extensive description, written in understandable language. The descriptions in this eighth edition have been reviewed by medical professionals to include the most up-to-date methods of diagnoses and treatment. Each description includes: Disorder name and synonyms; Primary symptoms; Physical findings; Related Disorders; Cause: Body system affected; Standard treatment.

Following each description are *disorder-specific resources*, including Associations, Federal and State Agencies, Support Groups, Libraries, Resource Centers, Research Centers, Web sites, Media Resources and Camps. The more prevalent a disorder is, the more resources there are available.

The Complete Directory for Pediatric Disorders also includes care centers, medical organizations, and advocacy groups that offer extended information on a great variety of conditions. These combined resources offer the most comprehensive coverage available of the most prevalent pediatric disorders being diagnosed in pediatrician's offices around the country.

Section II – General Resources

This section includes 1,014 resources, including Government Agencies, National Associations, State Agencies, Support Groups, Newsletters, Books, Magazines, Camps and Wish Foundations. These may not be limited to a specific disorder, but offer information and support for categories of disorders.

Users will find resources on not only physical pediatric disorders, but also on mental and emotional conditions that affect our younger population. There are also resources that deal with multi-disorder conditions.

Section III – The Human Body

This educational element is comprised of 14 detailed descriptions of body systems or medical categories. This section is designed to provide a comprehensive overview of the human body, enabling the user to broaden his or her understanding of how a particular disorder affects a specific body system(s) and further, how it may relate to the body as a whole. It includes twelve specific body systems, from Cardiovascular to Urologic, plus two additional chapters: Human Cells and Child Growth & Development.

Section IV – Indexes

The Complete Directory for Pediatric Disorders contains three indexes to help readers access the information from several places:

- **Entry Index** is an alphabetical listing of all entry names.
- **Geographic Index** groups listings by state.
- **Disorder & Related Term Index** is an alphabetical list of pediatric disorders, condition names, synonyms, and related disorders.

The Complete Directory for Pediatric Disorders is available for subscription online at http://gold.greyhouse.com, for even faster, easier access to this vast array of information. With a subscription, users can search by disorder, keyword, geographic area, bodily system, and much more. Visit the site or call (800) 562-2139 to set up a free trial of the Online Database.

Glossary

A Concise Guide to Medical Terminology

This Guide is designed to help the reader decipher some unfamiliar terms used in the disorder descriptions. It is helpful to divide medical terms into their basic elements: prefix, root, and suffix. Following these examples are 249 commonly used medical prefixes, roots, and suffixes - over a dozen more than last edition.

Example 1: The medical term *microcephaly* is a combination of "micr(o)," meaning small, and "cephal(o)," which means head. Therefore, microcephaly denotes an abnormally small head. In contrast, "macr(o)" means large. Thus, *macrocephaly* indicates an unusually large head.

Example 2: The word *polydactyly* includes "poly," meaning much or many, and "dactyl," which refers to fingers or toes. Thus, the medical term *polydactyly* means the presence of extra fingers or toes. Accordingly, because "brachy" means short, the word *brachydactyly* indicates abnormally short fingers or toes.

Example 3: The term *myositis* is a combination of "my(o)," which denotes muscle, and "itis," meaning inflammation. Therefore, *myositis* means muscle inflammation. When "cardi(o)," meaning heart, is added, forming the term *myocarditis,* the meaning becomes inflammation of heart muscle.

Medical Prefixes, Roots, and Suffixes

A . . . . absence of, without	cent. . . . . one hundred
Ab . . . . away from	centr(o). . . . . . . center
Acou . . . . hear	cephal(o) . . . . . head
aden(o). . . . . . . gland	cerebr(o). . . . . . brain
-algia . . . . pain	cervic . . . . neck
all(o). . . . . other, different	chole. . . . . bile
andr(o) . . . . man	chondr(o) . . . . . cartilage
angi(o) . . . . vessel	circum . . . . around
ankyl(o) . . . . . . bent, crooked	-coele . . . . body/organ cavity
ante. . . . . before	contra . . . . against, counter
anti . . . . against, counter	cost(o) . . . . rib
arteri(o) . . . . . . artery	crani(o). . . . . . . skull
arthr(o). . . . . . . joint	cry(o) . . . . cold
audio . . . . hearing, sound	crypt(o) . . . . . . conceal, hide
auri. . . . . ear	cyan . . . . blue
aut(o) . . . . self	cyst(o) . . . . bladder
bacteri(o) . . . . . bacteria	cyt(o) . . . . cell
bio . . . . life	de . . . . away from, down
blast(o). . . . . . . bud, early embryonic budding	dent(o) . . . . tooth
-blast . . . . formative cell, germinal layer	dermat(o) . . . . . skin
blephar(o). . . . . eyelid	di . . . . two
brachi(o). . . . . . arm	dia . . . . apart, through
brachy . . . . short	digit . . . . finger or toe
brady . . . . slow	dipl(o) . . . . double
bronch(o) . . . . . bronchi	dors(o) . . . . back
bucc(o). . . . . . . cheek	dys . . . . abnormal, bad
carcin(o). . . . . . cancer	ect(o) . . . . outside, out of place
cardi(o). . . . . . . heart	-emia . . . . blood
-cele . . . . hernia, protrusion, tumor	en . . . . in, on

Glossary

end(o)......... inside, within

enter(o)....... intestine

epi .... above, upon

erythr(o)....... red

eso .... inside, within

esthesi(o) ...... feel, perceive

eu............ normal, well

ex .... away from, outside

extra.......... beyond, in addition, outside of

flav(o) .... yellow

galact(o)....... milk

gastr(o)........ stomach

gen(o)......... gene or reproduction

gloss(o) .... tongue

glyc(o) .... sweet

gnath(o) .... jaw

gram.......... draw, record, write

graph(o) .... record, write

gynec(o)....... woman

hemat(o)...... blood

hemi.......... half

hepat(o) .... liver

hex........... six

hidr(o) .... sweat

hist(o)........ tissue

hom(o)....... common, same

hydr(o)....... water

hyper .... above, beyond, excessive

hypn(o) .... sleep

hyp(o) .... below, deficient, low

hyster(o)....... uterus

iatr(o)......... physician

idi(o) .... distinct, separate

ili(o)......... intestines

inter .... among, between

intra .... inside, within

ischi(o)........ hip

-itis .... inflammation

kary(o) .... nucleus

kilo........... one thousand

kinet(o)....... move

labio.......... lips

lact(o)........ milk

lapar(o)....... flank, loin

laryng(o) ...... larynx

latero .... side

leuc(o) .... white

leuk(o) .... white

lien(o)........ spleen

lingu(o) .... tongue

lip(o) .... fat

lith(o)........ stone

lymph(o) ..... water

macr(o)........ large

mal.......... abnormal, bad

malac(o)...... soft

mamm(o) ..... breast

mast(o)....... breast

medi.......... middle

mega......... great, large

megal(o)...... great, large

melan(o)...... black

mening(o)..... membrane

mes(o) .... middle

meta .... after, beyond

metr(o)....... uterus

micr(o)....... small

mill(i)........ one thousand

mon(o) .... only, single, sole

morph(o) ..... form, shape, structure

myel(o)....... marrow

my(o) .... muscle

myx(o) .... mucus

narc(o)....... stupor

nas(o)........ nose

necr(o) .... corpse, death

neo .... new

nephr(o)...... kidney

neur(o) .... nerve

noci .... pain

noso .... disease

ocul(o) .... eye

odont(o) ...... tooth

-odyn(o)...... distress, pain

olig(o) .... deficient, few, little

-oma neoplasm.. tumor

omphal(o)..... navel

onc(o)........ mass, tumor

onych(o)...... nail

oo........... egg

ophthalm(o) .... eye

orchi(o) ...... testicle

oro .... mouth

-osis .... process, disease from

osse(o) .... bone

oste(o) .... bone

ot(o) . . . . ear

ovari(o) . . . . ovary

oxy . . . . sharp

pachy . . . . thick

pan . . . . whole, all

para . . . . beside, beyond, resembling

path(o) . . . . disease

ped(o) . . . . child

pen . . . . around

penia . . . . abnormal reduction, deficiency

pent(a) . . . . five

per . . . . through

phag(o) . . . . consume, eat

pharmaco . . . . . . drug, medicine

pharyng(o) . . . . . throat

phleb(o) . . . . vein

phon(o) . . . . sound

phot(o) . . . . light

physi(o) . . . . natural, physical

pil(o) . . . . hair

-plasia . . . . development, formation

platy . . . . broad, flat

pleur(o) . . . . rib, side

-pnea . . . . breathing

pneumat(o) . . . . . air, breathing

pneum(o) . . . . . . air, breath, lung

pod(o) . . . . foot

poly . . . . many, much

post . . . . after, behind

pre . . . . before, in front of

pro . . . . before, in front of

proct(o) . . . . rectum

pseud(o) . . . . false

psych(o) . . . . mind

pulmon(o) . . . . . lung

pyel(o) . . . . pelvis

pyr(o) . . . . fire, heat

quadri . . . . four

rachi(o) . . . . spine

radio . . . . radiation

re . . . . again, back

ren(o) . . . . kidneys

retr(o) . . . . backward, behind

rheo . . . . flow

rhin(o) . . . . nose

sangui . . . . blood

sarc(o) . . . . flesh

scler(o) . . . . hard

-scope . . . . instrument for examining

semi . . . . half

sial(o) . . . . saliva

somat(o) . . . . . . body

somn(i) . . . . sleep

spasm(o) . . . . . . spasm

spermat(o) . . . . seed

splen(o) . . . . . . spleen

spondyl(o) . . . . . vertebra

spor(o) . . . . spore

steat(o) . . . . fat

sten(o) . . . . compressed, narrow

stomat(o) . . . . mouth, opening

sub . . . . below, near, under

super . . . . above, beyond, excessive

syn . . . . together, with

tachy . . . . fast, rapid

tel(o) . . . . end

tetra . . . . four

therm(o) . . . . . . heat

thorac(o) . . . . . . chest

thromb(o) . . . . . clot

-tome . . . . instrument for cutting

tox(o) . . . . poison

trans . . . . through, across

traumat(o) . . . . wound

tri . . . . three

trich(o) . . . . hair

troph(o) . . . . . . food, nourishment

-uria . . . . urine

vas(o) . . . . vessel

vertebr(o) . . . . . vertebrae

vesic(o) . . . . bladder or blister

xanth(o) . . . . . . yellow

xen(o) . . . . foreign, different

xer(o) . . . . dry

zyg(o) . . . . junction, union

GLOSSARY OF ACRONYMS

Note: Compound acronyms denote vaccine combinations.
'DTPHibHepIPV', for example, denotes DTP, Hib, HepB and IPV vaccines combined.

AMC	advanced market commitment
aP	acellular pertussis vaccine
BCG	bacille Calmette-Guérin (vaccine against tuberculosis)
CBAW	childbearing-aged women; refers to ages 15-45 unless otherwise noted
Dip	diphtheria toxoid vaccine
DT	diphtheria toxoid
DTaP	diphtheria and tetanus toxoid with acellular pertussis vaccine
DTP	diphtheria and tetanus toxoid with pertussis vaccine
DTP1	first dose of diphtheria and tetanus toxoid with pertussis vaccine
DTP3	third dose of diphtheria and tetanus toxoid with pertussis vaccine
DTwP	diphtheria and tetanus toxoid with whole-cell pertussis vaccine
EPI	Expanded Programme on Immunization
GAVI	Global Alliance for Vaccines and Immunisation
GNI	gross national income (US)
H1N1	monovalent vaccine against the 2009 influenza A (H1N1) virus
HepA	hepatitis A vaccine
HepB	hepatitis B vaccine
HepB3	third dose of hepatitis B vaccine
HFRS	hemorrhagic fever with renal syndrome (hantavirus) vaccine
Hib	Haemophilus infl uenzae type b vaccine
Hib3	third dose of Haemophilus influenzae type b vaccine
HPV	human papilloma virus vaccine
IPV	inactivated polio vaccine
JE	Japanese encephalitis
MCV	measles-containing vaccine
MCV2	second dose of measles-containing vaccine
MenA	meningococcal A vaccine; this monovalent vaccine protects against meningitis serogroup A

Glossary of Acronyms

MenAC	meningococcal AC vaccine; this bivalent vaccine protects against meningitis serogroups A and C
MenACW	meningococcal ACWY vaccine; this quadrivalent vaccine protects against meningitis serogroups A, C and W-135
MenACWY	meningococcal ACWY vaccine; this quadrivalent vaccine protects against meningitis serogroups A, C, Y and W-135
MenBC	meningococcal BC vaccine; this bivalent vaccine protects against meningitis serogroups B and C
MenC	meningococcal C vaccine; this monovalent vaccine protects against meningitis serogroup C
MenC_conj	meningococcal C conjugate vaccine
MM	measles and mumps vaccine
MMR	measles-mumps-rubella vaccine
MMRV	measles-mumps-rubella-varicella vaccine
MR	measles and rubella vaccine
OPV	oral polio vaccine
PAB	protected at birth against tetanus
Pneumo_conj	pneumococcal conjugate vaccine
Pneumo_ps	pneumococcal polisaccharide vaccine
Pol3	third dose of poliomyelitis vaccine
PPP	purchasing power parity
Pw	whole-cell pertussis vaccine
TBE	tick-borne encephalitis vaccine
TBD	to be determined
Td	tetanus toxoid with reduced amount of diphtheria toxoid
Tdap	tetanus toxoid vaccine (full dose) with acellular pertussis vaccine (reduced dose)
TT	tetanus toxoid

Source: http://www.unicef.org and www.who.int

Guidelines for Obtaining Additional Information and Resources

Many parents and caregivers are interested in obtaining information regarding *physicians* who specialize in certain pediatric disorders, accredited *hospitals, approved drugs or medical devices* for certain pediatric conditions, or current *clinical trials* that are investigating possible new therapies for particular diseases. In addition, some individuals may wish to have access to medical journal articles and other medical literature that may be available on their child's disorder, disease, or condition. Following are several tips that may be shared with parents and caregivers in their efforts to obtain such information and resources.

Disease-Specific Resources: Many of the disease-specific resources in this *Directory* maintain listings of physicians who are experts in a particular pediatric disorder. They may also offer information on accredited hospitals with appropriate specialty departments. In addition, many may provide information on standard therapies for certain pediatric conditions and ongoing clinical trials that are investigating possible new therapies. Some of these organizations, such as certain national voluntary health associations (NVHAs) or support groups, function as patient registries, working closely with expert physicians, researchers, and university medical centers specializing in specific pediatric disorders.

Online "Physician Finder" Services: Several professional medical associations provide searchable databases on the Internet as a public service for individuals who wish to obtain information on physicians.

Example: The *American Medical Association (AMA) Physician Select* database provides information on licensed physicians in the United States, including credential data that has been verified by medical schools, residency training programs, certifying and licensing boards, and accrediting agencies. AMA Physician Select enables online visitors to search for physicians by name, medical specialty, or geographic location. This online service is located at http://www.webapps.ama-assn.org/doctorfinder.

Example: The *American Board of Medical Specialties (ABMS) Public Education Program* offers an online physician locator and information service. This service, which lists all physicians certified by ABMS Member Boards, allows online visitors to verify board certification status, specialty, and location of physicians who are certified by one or more of the ABMS Member Boards. The ABMS also provides the *Certified/Doctor Locator Service,* which lists physicians certified by ABMS Member Boards who have subscribed to the service. Such listings include board certification(s), address, telephone number, and hospital affiliation(s). These online services may be accessed at www.abms.org.

Example: The U.S. federal government has an online service known as *healthfinder*® that serves as a Web portal or directory for those who are interested in locating current, high quality health information and resources on the Internet. The site is located at www.healthfinder.gov.

Hospital Accreditation: Individuals who are interested in learning about a particular medical facility's accreditation status may consider contacting the *Joint Commission,* which is the the United States' leading health care quality evaluator and accredits approximately 15,000 health care facilities, organizations, and programs. Accreditation is recognized as a *"Gold Seal of Approval"* indicating that the hospital meets certain standards of performance and is committed to meeting state-of-the-art performance expectations. The Joint Commission offers an online service known as *Quality Check* that enables online visitors to obtain information about an organization's accreditation, such as how it was rated during its most recent quality report. This service is located at www.qualitycheck.org. Callers may also receive information concerning a hospital's accreditation status by calling the Joint Commission, at (630) 792-5800 or visiting www.jointcommission.org.

Hospital Public Information Lines and Web Sites: Many hospitals are creating and strongly promoting special public information lines. Such help lines are often publicized within local or regional newspapers and in the introductory sections of local phone books. In addition, many hospitals are creating Web sites that: offer information on their services and programs; link to sites offered by different departments or facilities; discuss ongoing research; provide searchable physician directories; publish newsletters, various reports, press releases, and other materials; and offer a variety of additional information. These Web sites may be located by visiting various search engines and using the name of the facility as a search term. (For more information, see *Search Engines* below.)

Academic Hospitals: If children have been diagnosed with a chronic, difficult-to-treat, or relatively uncommon disorder or if they remain undiagnosed after visits to several primary care or specialist pediatricians, parents or other caregivers may wish to consider taking their children to a major academic medical center. Generally, such teaching hospitals use state-of-the-art testing techniques, have comprehensive evaluation centers, and follow multidisciplinary approaches to diagnosis and treatment. In addition, such centers are often affiliated with medical schools where clinical research is conducted.

Food and Drug Administration: Individuals who are interested in learning more about approved drug therapies or medical devices for certain pediatric disorders may wish to contact the *U. S. Food and Drug Administration (FDA)*. The FDA is the U.S. agency that enforces federal regulations to prevent the sale and distribution of dangerous or impure substances, such as unsafe foods, impure cosmetics, or unsafe or ineffective drugs or medical devices. For example, according to the FDA Modernization Act of 1997, one of the agency's primary objectives is "to promote the public health by promptly and efficiently reviewing clinical research and taking appropriate action on the marketing of regulated products in a timely manner." The agency is a branch of the U.S. Department of Health and Human Services. The FDA's Web site provides: FAQs (Frequently Asked Questions) areas; Consumer Drug Information Sheets; information on new and generic drug approvals, medical device product approvals, and drug labeling changes; health advisories; and access to MedWatch, the FDA's *Safety Information and Adverse Event Reporting Program*. MedWatch enables consumers and health care professionals to report adverse reactions to approved medical products directly to the FDA and/or the manufacturers. The primary purpose of MedWatch is to ensure the rapid identification of potential health hazards associated with approved medical products and the prompt communication of safety information to the health care and medical communities. The FDA's Web site is located at www.fda.gov/medwatch. The agency's address follows:

FDA
10903 New Hampshire Ave.
Silver Spring, MD 20993-0002
Toll-free: (888) INFO-FDA or (888) 463-6332

Clinical Research: A clinical protocol is a scientific study that evaluates the safety or effectiveness (efficacy) of a particular drug therapy or medical device in humans. Clinical studies enable researchers and physicians to determine new and more effective ways to prevent, diagnose, manage, and treat disease. Medications and treatments that are found to be safe and effective during laboratory and animal testing must then prove safe and effective in humans before they are approved for use by the general public. Participation in clinical studies may only occur if individuals volunteer and are fully informed and understanding of both the potential benefits and risks of such participation ("informed consent"). Participants may voluntarily leave a clinical study at any time.

Research on new drugs, which are known as *investigational new drug applications* or *INDS,* is conducted in three phases:

Phase I Study - The main objective of a Phase I study is to establish the *safety* of the investigational new drug. Such studies:

• may take several months

• typically involve a relatively small number of participants who are healthy volunteers

• are designed to evaluate the INDs biologic activities in the human body (e.g., absorption, metabolism, etc.) and its potential side effects as drug dosages are raised

Phase II Study - The purpose of a Phase II study is to establish the *safety and efficacy* of the investigational new drug in treating a specific disease. Such studies:
• may take from several months to a few years

• may include a relatively small number or up to several hundred patients

• usually involve randomized, double-blind trials. During such studies, one group of participants receives the drug (experimental group) and the other group is given a harmless, unmedicated substance (placebo) or a standard, well-established therapy (control group). The information concerning which patients are included in which group is hidden from both the patients and the researchers.

Phase III Study - The purpose of a Phase III study is to evaluate the overall *safety, efficacy, possible adverse effects, and benefits* of the investigational new drug in a large number of patients and to compare such therapy with the use of well-established treatments or with an untreated disease course. Such studies:
• may last for several years

• may involve hundreds or thousands of patients

• may include research teams from multiple national or international clinical centers

• typically involve randomized, double-blind trials

If an investigational new drug application successfully completes Phase III studies, the drug's sponsor may request FDA approval for marketing to the public, which is known as a *New Drug Approval* (NDA). In some cases, additional clinical research may be conducted:

Phase IV Study – The purpose of a Phase IV study may be to:
• monitor the drug's long-term efficacy

• compare the drug with other medications that have been available for longer periods

As mentioned above, disease-specific organizations and registries, support groups, and online services may serve as essential sources of information concerning clinical studies for a particular disease. There are also several additional, more general resources that promote and provide information on clinical trials:

Example: The *Warren Grant Magnuson Clinical Center,* which is part of the National Institutes of Health (NIH), is a federally funded biomedical research hospital. The Clinical Center was designed to support studies conducted by the NIH. Only individuals with conditions or disorders under NIH investigation are admitted for treatment, and all patients must be referred by their physicians. The Clinical Center's Web site includes a clinical research database that enables online visitors to search for current research studies by certain predefined parameters, such as primary disease category, or specific diagnosis, symptom, sign, or other keywords. The Clinical Center's Web site is located at www.cc.nih.gov and its Protocol Database may be accessed at http://clinicalstudies.info.nih.gov. The Clinical Center's address follows:

Department of Health and Human Services
Public Health Service
National Institutes of Health (NIH)
Warren G. Magnuson Clinical Center
Patient Recruitment and Referral Center
9000 Rockville Pike
Bethesda, MD 20892
Toll-free: (800) 411-1222

E-mail: prpl@mail.cc.nih.gov

Example: *CenterWatch, Inc.* provides a *Clinical Trials Listing Service*™ on its Web site for patients and research professionals. The site provides listings of over 7 ,000 national and international clinical trials that are searchable by geographic region and therapeutic area. Interested individuals may also sign up for CenterWatch's confidential *Patient Notification Service,* which provides notification via e-mail of future clinical trial postings in a certain therapeutic area. CenterWatch's Clinical Trials Service also provides: a listing of NIH-funded clinical research programs that are currently being conducted at the NIH's Warren Grant Magnuson Clinical Center; a general explanation of clinical trials, profiles of clinical research centers; listings of medications recently approved by the FDA; and linkage to health-related sites for patients and patient advocates. The Clinical Trials Listing Service™ is located at www.centerwatch.com. CenterWatch's address follows:

CenterWatch, Inc.
100 North Washington St., Ste. 301
Boston, MA 02114
Phone: (617) 948-5100
Fax: (617) 948-5101
Toll-Free: 866-219-3440
E-Mail: customerservice@centerwatch.com

Example: The *National Cancer Institute (NCI)* offers an online service known as *CancerNet*™ that provides information for patients and family members, health professionals, and researchers. The site offers: information on current clinical trials; summaries on cancer prevention, screening, treatment, and supportive care; cancer fact sheets; and linkage to the *Physician Data Query* or *PDQ® Cancer Information Service,* the NCI's cancer database. PDQ contains a registry of open and closed cancer clinical trials as well as directories of organizations, physicians, and genetic counselors who provide cancer care. CancerNet™ also provides access to *cancerTrials,* a clinical trials information center, and *CANCERLIT®,* a bibliographic database. CancerNet™ is located at http://cancer.gov. The NCI also offers a Cancer Information Service (CIS) for callers Monday through Friday from 9 a.m. to 4:30 p.m., Eastern Standard Time. The CIS may be reached at (800) 422-6237. Individuals with hearing impairment who have TTY equipment may call (800) 332-8615.

Example: *OncoLink* is an online resource on the Internet that is affiliated with the University of Pennsylvania Medical Center and the University of Pennsylvania Cancer Center. The site provides: information on cancer clinical trials; symptom management; personal experiences and psychosocial support; cancer causes, prevention, and screening; FAQs (frequently asked questions); financial issues for cancer patients; and additional topics. The site is located at www.oncolink.upenn.edu.

Search Engines. If individuals are interested in locating a particular organization's Web site but do not have its address or wish to determine what online services may be available in a certain subject area, Internet search engines are an essential resource. Search engines enable online visitors to conduct general or targeted searches for information within their areas of interest and appropriate to their needs. In addition to searching for and providing direct linkage to certain Web sites, many search engines enable users to search for e-mail discussion groups (listservs), UseNet newsgroups, FAQs (frequently asked questions), or other tools. Following is a sample listing of some of the search engines available on the Web:

Altavista: www.altavista.com
Dogpile: www.dogpile.com
Excite: www.excite.com
HotBot: www.hotbot.com
Lycos: www.lycos.com
Metacrawler: www.metacrawler.com
Snap.com: www.snap.com

Yahoo: www.yahoo.com

General Medical and Professional Association Sites: Some individuals may be interested in visiting medical sites that offer general information on disease and health issues. In addition, many professional medical associations and societies have Web sites that provide access to patient and professional information, press releases, journals, clinical updates, and other areas that may be helpful to those interested in pediatric disorder topics. Following is a brief listing of such sites:

American Academy of Family Physicians: www.aafp.org
American Academy of Pediatrics: www.aap.org
American Medical Association: www.ama-assn.org
MyOptumHealth: www.myoptumhealth.com
Johns Hopkins Health Information: www.hopkinshospital.org/health_info
Mayo Clinic Health Information: www.mayoclinic.com
Medical Matrix: www.medmatrix.org/reg/login.asp
Medscape: www.medscape.com
US Pharmacopeia (information on medications): www.usp.org

Medical Journal Articles. Individuals who are interested in accessing abstracts summarizing medical journal articles may visit the National Library of Medicine's (NLM's) *PubMed.* The PubMed search service provides free access to the approximately 17 million medical journal citations within NLM's *MEDLINE.* MEDLINE is essentially the online version of *Index Medicus,* a monthly subject/author guide to articles in thousands of medical journals. Online visitors to PubMed may conduct searches for medical journal citations and abstracts by journal title and date, author, and topic. In addition to providing access to selected journal abstracts, PubMed offers links to participating online journals and enables registered users to order full-text articles for a fee. (If individuals are interested in accessing other medical journal sites, such online journals may often be located by using various search engines.) PubMed may be accessed at www.pubmed.gov. In addition, several general medical sites provide access to PubMed and enable users to order full-text journal articles for a fee.

Online Mendelian Inheritance in Man (OMIM). Individuals who wish to access comprehensive and timely medical information on genetic disorders may be interested in visiting OMIM™ or *Online Mendelian Inheritance in Man,* a database of genetic disorders and human genes. This searchable database, which is written and edited by Dr. Victor A. McKusick and colleagues at Johns Hopkins University and other locations, was developed for the Web by the National Center for Biotechnology Information (NCBI). OMIM™ contains entries on genetic diseases, clinical synopses, links to relevant MEDLINE citations, and more. OMIM™ is located at www.ncbi.nlm.nih.gov/omim/.

Disorders by Biologic System Affected

Cardiovascular Disorders; see also *Cardiovascular System*, page 1007.
Aortic Stenosis
Arrhythmias
Atrial Septal Defects
Coarctation of the Aorta
Hypertrophic Cardiomyopathy
Hypoplastic Left Heart Syndrome (HLHS)
Kawasaki Disease
Marfan Syndrome
Noonan's Syndrome
Patent Ductus Arteriosus
Pulmonary Hypertension
Pulmonary Valve Stenosis
Syncope
Tetralogy of Fallot
Transposition of the Great Arteries
Ventricular Septal Defects
Williams Syndrome

Connective Tissue Disorders; see also *Cells*, page 1009.
Childhood Dermatomyositis
Ehlers-Danlos Syndrome
Sarcoidosis
Scleroderma

Dental Disorders; see also *Digestive System*, page 1015.
Dental Conditions
Ectodermal Dysplasia
Microdontia

Dermatologic Disorders; see also *Dermatologic System*, page 1013.
Albinism
Alopecia Areata
Burn Injuries
Childhood Dermatomyositis
Cleft Life and Cleft Palate
Ectodermal Dysplasia
Eczema
Epidermolysis Bullosa
Hemangiomas and Lymphangiomas
Icthyosis
Keloids
Neurofibromatosis
Pemphigus
Photosensitivity
Pityriasis Rosea
Tuberous Sclerosis
Psoriasis

Telangiectasia
Urticaria

Developmental, Behavioral and Psychiatric Disorders; see also *Growth and Development*, page 1021.
Asperger Syndrome
Attention Deficit Hyperactivity Disorder
Autistic Disorder
Bipolar Disorder
Childhood Schizophrenia
Conduct Disorder
Depression
Eating Disorders
Encopresis
Lead Poisoning
Learning Disability, Reading Disability Dyslexia
Mental Retardation
Migraine Headaches
Nightmares
Night Terrors
Nocturnal Enuresis
Obesity
Obsessive-Compulsive Disorder
Oppositional Defiant Behavior
Passive-Aggressive Behavior
Phobias
Physical and Sexual Abuse
PICA
Post-Traumatic Stress Disorder
Sleepwalking
Stuttering
Thumbsucking
Violence by Children & Teenagers

Endocrinologic Disorders; see also *Endocrine System*, page 1018.
Congenital Adrenal Hyperplasia
Cushing's Syndrome
Diabetes Mellitus
Growth Hormone Deficiency
Hypothyroidism
McCune-Albright Syndrome
Obesity
Prader-Willi Syndrome
Precocious Puberty

Gastrointestinal Disorders; see also *Digestive System*, page 1015.
Acute Gastrointestinal Infections
Alpha-1-Antitrypsin Deficiency
Anorectal Malformations
Biliary Atresia

Celiac Disease
Colic
Congenital Diaphragmatic Hernia
Crohn's Disease
Encopresis
Esophageal Atresia
Galactosemia
Hepatitis
Hirschsprung Disease
Milk Protein Allergy and Lactose Intolerance
Omphalocele
Pyloric Stenosis
Ulcerative Colitis
Wilson's Disease

Genetic/Chromosomal/Syndrome/Metabolic Disorders; see also *Growth and Development*,
page 1021.
Achondroplasia
Albinism
Alpha-1-Antitrypsin Deficiency
Asperger Syndrome
Congenital Cataracts
Cornelia de Lange Syndrome
DiGeorge Syndrome
Down Syndrome
Familial Dysautonomia
Fetal Alcohol Syndrome
Fragile X Syndrome
Galactosemia
Gaucher's Disease
Hereditary Fructose Intolerance
Homocystinuria
Klinefelter Syndrome
Klipple-Feil Syndrome
Leukodystrophies
Maple Syrup Urine Disease
Marfan Syndrome
McCune-Albright Syndrome
Mucolipidoses
Mucopolysaccharidoses
Noonan's Syndrome
Osteogenesis Imperfecta
Phenylketonuria
Polydactyly
Prader-Willi Syndrome
Tay-Sachs Disease
Trisomy 18 Syndrome
Trisomy 13 Syndrome
Turner Syndrome
Williams Syndrome

Disorders by Biologic System Affected

Hematologic and Oncologic Disorders; see also *Hematologic System*, page 1024.
Acute Lymphoblastic Leukemia
Acute Myeloid Leukemia
Ewing's Sarcoma
Hemolytic Disease of the Newborn
Hemophilia
Histiocytosis
Hodgkins Disease
Neuroblastoma
Neutropenia
Non-Hodgkins Lymphoma
Porphyria
Protein C Deficiency
Retinoblastoma
Sickle Cell Disease
Thalasemias
Thrombocytopenias
Wilm's Tumor

Immunologic and Rheumatologic Disorders; see also *Immune System*, page 1026.
Alopecia Areata
DiGeorge Syndrome
HIV Infection
Juvenile Rheumatoid Arthritis
Kawasaki Disease
Subacute Sclerosing Panencephalitis (SSPE)
Systemic Lupus Erythematosus

Infectious Diseases; see also *Immune System*, page 1026.
Acute Gastrointestinal Infections
Conjunctivitis
Cytomegalovirus
Erythema Infectiosum
HIV Infection
Hepatitis
Herpes Simplex
Lyme Disease
Meningitis
Neonatal Herpes Simplex
Otitis Media
Pinworm
Pityriasis Rosea
Pneumonia
Preventable Childhood Infections
Respiratory Syncytial Virus
Toxoplasmosis
Tuberculosis

Neonatal and Infant Disorders; see also *Growth and Development*, page 1021.
Apnea of Prematurity
Bronchopulmonary Dysplasia
Colic
Congenital Dysplasia of the Hip
Hemolytic Disease of the Newborn
Interventricular Hemorrhage
Kernicterus
Neonatal Herpes Simplex
Neonatal Jaundice
Omphalocele
Prematurity
Respiratory Distress Syndrome of the Newborn
Retinopathy of Prematurity
Sudden Infant Death Syndrome

Neurologic Disorders; see also *Nervous System*, page 1029.
Anencephaly
Arnold-Chiari Malformation
Asperger Syndrome
Ataxia
Autistic Disorder
Brain Tumors
Bell's Palsy
Cerebral Palsy
Chorea
Dyslexia
Dystonia
Encephalocele
Erb's Palsy
Familial Dysautonomia
Guillain-Barre Syndrome
Head Injuries
Hearing Impairment/Deafness
Hydrocephalus
Interventricular Hemorrhage
Lead Poisoning
Leukodystrophies
Lissencephaly
Macrocephaly
Meningitis
Mental Retardation
Microcephaly
Muscular Dystrophies
Narcolepsy
Nystagmus
Ptosis
Seizures
Speech Impairment
Spina Bifida

Spinal Muscular Atrophies
Strabismus
Stuttering
Subacute Sclerosing Panencephalitis (SSPE)
Tics
Tourette Syndrome
Tuberous Sclerosis

Ophthalmologic Disorders; see also *Sensory Organs*, page 1037.
Aniridia
Congenital Cataracts
Congenital Glaucoma
Conjunctivitis
Lazy Eye
Nystagmus
Ptosis
Refraction Disturbances
Retinitis Pigmentosa
Retinoblastoma
Retinopathy of Prematurity
Strabismus

Orthopedic and Muscle Disorders; see also *Musculoskeletal System*, page 1028.
Achondroplasia
Ankylosing Spondylitis
Arthorogryposis Multiplex Congenita
Cerebral Palsy
Charcot-Marie-Tooth Disease
Childhood Dermatomyositis
Cleft Lip and Cleft Palate
Clubfoot
Congenital Dysplasia of the Hip
Craniosynostosis
Dystonia
Ewing's Sarcoma
Legg-Calve-Perthes Disease
Marfan Syndrome
Muscular Dystrophies
Neurofibromatosis
Osteogenesis Imperfecta
Polydactyly
Scoliosis
Spina Bifida
Spinal Muscular Atrophies
Strabismus
Syndactyly

Renal and Urologic Disorders; see also *Urologic System*, page 1039.
Cryptorchidism
Nephrotic Syndrome
Nocturnal Enuresis

Respiratory Disorders; see also *Respiratory System*, page 1035.
Alpha-1-Antitrypsin Deficiency
Apnea of Prematurity
Asthma
Bronchopulmonary Dysplasia
Congenital Diaphragmatic Hernia
Cystic Fibrosis
Pneumonia
Pulmonary Hypertension
Respiratory Distress Syndrome of the Newborn
Respiratory Syncytial Virus Infection
Rhinitis
Sleep Apnea
Tuberculosis

THE CONVERSATION

The health impact of childhood bullying can last a lifetime

Louise Arseneault, Institute of Psychiatry at King's College London

It is still not clear how the experience of being bullied in childhood translates into long-lasting health problems. A new US study has found that victims of bullying have high levels of a protein in their bloodstream that is associated with fighting off an infection – even into early adulthood. This finding may help understand further the association between childhood bullying victimisation and poor health outcomes later.

Research has consistently shown that young victims of bullying show difficulties including symptoms of anxiety, depression and also conduct problems and psychotic symptoms. These problems related to children's mental health can persist even after the bullying has stopped, sometimes up until mid-life.

There are some hypotheses that bullying victimisation is a form of "toxic stress" that can have an impact on physiological responses to childhood adversity. In turn, these responses may help explain why some victims develop health problems.

Mental and physical health problems are often related and although young children are generally healthy, research has started to show that bullied children tend to become adults with health problems.

One such mechanism is the inflammatory response, measured by the release in the bloodstream of a protein called C-reactive protein (CRP). High levels of CRP is a generic response that indicates that the body is either fighting an infectious agent, reacting to an injury or responding to a chronic condition such as arthritis. Research has shown that CRP can also be elevated among people who experienced maltreatment by an adult in their childhood. This suggests that the body reacts in a similar way to "toxic stress" as it does to an infection.

Bullying as a 'toxic stress'

Knowing that bullying is associated with high levels of CRP is important for two reasons. First, it would provide further support that childhood bullying victimisation should be considered as a toxic stress alongside other forms of abuse including child maltreatment. Second, this would provide a novel lead for identifying new targets for various types of interventions aimed at reducing problems related to the experience of being bullied in childhood.

The new findings from the longitudinal Great Smoky Mountains Study of 1,420 children in the US has looked at CRP levels in children involved in bullying as victims, bullies and bully-victims (participants who both bully others and were also bullied). The authors, led by William E. Copeland at Duke University Medical Center, tested whether study participants who were bullied between the age of nine and 16 showed high levels of CRP in adolescence, and also later in early adulthood.

Their results indicate that the participants who experienced several exposures to bullying had higher levels of CRP compared to participants who were not involved in bullying – either as victims, bullies or bully-victims.
These associations remained even after taking into account the participants' prior CRP level and variables associated with CRP levels such as body mass index, medication and alcohol use. They also took into account variables linked to being involved in bullying, including maltreatment, family dysfunction, and anxiety disorders.

Lasting into early adulthood

The authors then looked at CRP levels as the study participants entered adulthood. They observed a similar pattern of findings: victims of bullying had higher levels of CRP compared to those who were not involved in bullying. Furthermore, participants who were repeatedly bullied showed the highest levels of CRP.

Surprisingly, participants who bullied others showed the lowest levels of CRP in early adulthood amongst all four groups of children examined in this study. These associations also remained after the researcher controlled for prior CRP, variables associated with CRP levels and variables associated with being involved in bullying.

We already know from previous research that being bullied in childhood "gets under the skin" and can influence other mechanisms in the body involved in the physiological responses to stress, such as the hypothalamic-pituitary-adrenal axis. For example, bullied children show a blunted level of cortisol response – a hormone released under stress – when exposed to stress in a laboratory experiment.

A study of identical twin pairs where one twin had been bullied but the other not has shown that while non-bullied twins had a normal increase of cortisol after experiencing a social stress laboratory, their bullied co-twins showed a blunted response. And the more severe and frequent the bullying, the lower the cortisol response.

The new Duke research on the inflammatory process adds to a growing body of evidence that demonstrates that we need to move away from the perception that bullying is harmless and part of normal growing up. Instead, bullying should be considered as another form of toxic stress with potentially profound effects on mental and physical health. These effects have been repeatedly observed in childhood and increasingly so in adolescence and in adulthood too.

Arseneault, Louise. "The Health Impact of Childhood Bullying Can Last a Lifetime." *The Conversation*. The Conversation, 12 May 2014. Web. 20 Apr. 2015. <https://theconversation.com/the-health-impact-of-childhood-bullying-can-last-a-lifetime-26541>.

Description

1 **ACHONDROPLASIA**
Synonyms: Chondrodystrophy, Fetal Rickets
Involves the following Biologic System(s):
Genetic/Chromosomal/Syndrome/Metabolic Disorders, Orthopedic and Muscle Disorders

Achondroplasia is a disorder of the skeletal system that occurs in about one of every 20,000 newborn infants. It belongs to a group of disorders known as chondrodystrophies. These disorders involve a disturbance in the cartilage at the ends of the body's long bones (arms and legs). In Achondroplasia, this disturbance interferes with the conversion of cartilage into bone in the regions known as epiphyses, where these bones normally grow in length. This occurs in infancy and childhood, preventing the bones from growing normally and resulting in shortened limbs and a short stature. Achondroplasia does not affect intelligence.

Achondroplasia is caused by a defect in a single, specific gene that permits the body to make a protein known as fibroblast growth factor-3 (FGF3). Normally, FGF3 limits bone growth, and a decline in the production of this protein is what permits growth during childhood and adolescence. The genetic defect in Achondroplasia, however, causes the body to continue to produce FGF3, leading to an excess of this protein that sharply limits growth. Genetically, Achondroplasia is called an autosomal dominant disorder, because the defective FGF3 gene needs to be inherited from only one parent for Achondroplasia to be present.

Symptoms and characteristic findings include a disproportionately large head with a protruding and prominent forehead (frontal bossing); a flattened nasal bridge; an underdeveloped upper jaw and prominent lower jaw (prognothism); a well-developed but shortened trunk; and short, bowed arms and legs. The upper portions of the arms and legs are proportionately shorter than the lower parts of these limbs, and the elbows may have a limited range of motion. Usually, the fingers and toes are also short, with a V-shaped gap between the third and fourth fingers, and the hands are relatively wide. As children with Achondroplasia grow, their pelvis tilts forward, resulting in a pronounced spinal curvature known as lumbar lordosis, that causes prominence of the abdomen and buttocks. Other effects of Achondroplasia can include is made from physical examination and findings on X-ray images of the skeleton. Identification of this condition early in life facilitates family and medical planning for treatment and care.

Complications associated with Achondroplasia may include dental problems such as malocclusion, in which the upper and lower teeth do not meet in the proper alignment, and chronic and severe middle ear infections (otitis media) that can result in a loss of conductive hearing. Potentially life-threatening complications include temporary cessations of breathing during sleep, known as sleep apnea, caused by obstruction of the airways by the craniofacial abnormalities in Achondroplasia, and/or from compression of the spinal cord at the point where the cord passes from the spine into the skull. Additionally, this may obstruct the normal flow of cerebrospinal fluid (CSF) between the brain and spinal cord, resulting in hydrocephalus, a condition in which the cerebrospinal fluid collects in and around the brain, with potentially life-threatening effects.

Treatment with human growth hormone (HGH) is often used to improve growth and height in persons with Achondroplasia, and the availability of recombinant human growth hormone, or somatotropin, has revolutionized the treatment of short stature. Surgical lengthening of the limbs can produce improvement in some patients. Other treatment is directed at preventing or correcting complications of the condition. Monitoring head growth during infancy to insure normal growth limits is effective for detecting hydrocephalus. Physiotherapy, dental treatment and orthopedic appliances such as braces can correct or prevent a number of the complications caused by Achondroplasia. Appropriate counseling can provide emotional and psychological support to persons with the condition and their family members.

Government Agencies

2 **NIH/National Institute of Arthritis and Musculoskeletal and Skin Diseases**
1 AMS Circle
Bethesda, MD 20892
301-495-4484
877-226-4267
Fax: 301-718-6366
TTY: 301-565-2966
e-mail: niamsinfo@mail.nih.gov
www.niams.nih.gov

The mission of the NIAMS, a part of the NIH, is to support research into the causes, treatment and prevention of arthritis and musculosketal and skin diseases, the training of basic and clinical scientists to carry out this research, and the dissemination of information on research progress in these diseases.
Stephen I Katz MD PhD, Director
Robert H Carter MD, Deputy Director
Gahan Breithaupt, Assoc Dir. Management & Operations

3 **NIH/National Institute of Environmental Health Sciences (NIEHS)**
111 T.W. Alexander Drive
Durham, NC 27709
919-541-3345
Fax: 301-480-2978
e-mail: webcenter@niehs.nih.gov.
www.niehs.nih.gov

NIEHS reduces the burden of human illness and dysfunction from environmental causes by defining how environmental exposures, genetics and age interact to affect an individual's health.
Linda S Birnbaum, PhD, Director
Richard Woychik, PhD, Deputy Director
Joellen M. Austin, M.P.Aff., M.S.M., Associate Director for Management

4 **NIH/National Institute on Drug Abuse (NIDA)**
6001 Executive Boulevard/Room 5213
Bethesda, MD 20892
301-443-1124
Fax: 301-443-7397
e-mail: information@nida.nih.gov
www.drugabuse.gov

NIDA leads the nation in bringing the power of science to bear on drug abuse and addiction through support and conduct of research across all disciplines and rapid and effective dissemination of results of that research to improve drug abuse and addiction prevention and treatment.
Nora D. Volkow MD, Director
Glenda Conroy, CPA, MBA, Associate Director for Management
Susan Weiss, Ph.D., Associate Director

National Associations & Support Groups

5   American Academy of Pediatrics
141 Northwest Point Boulevard
Elk Grove Village, IL 60007
847-434-4000
800-433-9016
Fax: 847-434-8000
www.aap.org

The American Academy of Pediatrics and its member pediatricians are committed to the attainment of optimal physical, mental and social health and well-being for all infants, children, adolescents, and young adults.

Sandra Hassink, MD, FAAP, President

6   Human Growth Foundation
997 Glen Cove Avenue, Suite 5
Glen Head, NY 11545
516-671-4041
800-451-6434
Fax: 516-671-4055
e-mail: hgf1@hgfound.org
www.hgfound.org

A voluntary, nonprofit organization whose mission is to help children and adults with disorders of growth and growth hormones through research, education, support and advocacy. The foundation is dedicated to helping medical science to better understand the process of growth. It is composed of concerned parents and friends of children and adults with growth problems; and interested health professionals.

Pisit Pitukcheewanont MD, President/Executive Committee Board
Patricia D Costa, Executive Director
Emily Germain Lee, MD, Vice President/Executive Committee

7   Little People of America
250 El Camino Real, Suite 201
Tustin, CA 92780
714-368-3689
888-572-2001
Fax: 714-368-3367
e-mail: info@lpaonline.org
www.lpaonline.org

A nonprofit organization that provides support and information to people of short stature and their families.

Gary Arnold, President
Jason Rasa, Vice President, Finance
Jon North, Vice President of Programs

8   MAGIC Foundation: Major Aspects of Growth in Children
6645 W North Avenue
Oak Park, IL 60302
708-383-0808
800-362-4423
Fax: 708-383-0899
e-mail: ContactUs@magicfoundation.org
www.magicfoundation.org

A national nonprofit organization providing support and education regarding growth disorders in children and related adult disorders. Provides educational information, networking, a national conference, a kids' program and an extensive medical library.

10,000 members

Rich Buckley, Chairman
Ken Dickard, Vice Chairman
Teresa Tucker, Director at Large

Libraries & Resource Centers

9   NIH/National Library of Medicine (NLM)
8600 Rockville Pike
Bethesda, MD 20894
301-594-5983
888-346-3656
Fax: 301-402-1384
TDD: 800-735-2258
e-mail: custserv@nlm.nih.gov
www.nlm.nih.gov

NLM collects, organizes and makes available biomedical science information to scientists, health professionals and the public. The library's databases, including PubMed/Medline and MedlinePlus, are used extensively around the world. NLM conducts and supports research in biometric communications; creates information resources for molecular biology, biotechnology, toxicology, and environmental health; and provides grant support for training, medical library resources, and biomedical informatics.

Donald Lindberg, Director
Betsy Humphreys, Deputy Director
Paul Kiehl, Deputy Executive Director

Conferences

10   Adult GHD Educational Convention
Magic Foundation
6645 W North Avenue
Oak Park, IL 60302
708-383-0808
800-362-4423
Fax: 708-383-0899
e-mail: contactus@magicfoundation.org
www.magicfoundation.org

An educational program for adults who are affected with Growth Hormone Deficiency and/or other endocrine disorders.
June

Dianne Kremidas, Executive Director
Rich Buckley, Chairman
Mary Andrews, Chief Executive Officer

11   LPA National Conference
Little People of America
250 El Camino Real, Suite 201
Tustin, CA 92780
714-368-3689
888-572-2001
Fax: 714-368-3367
e-mail: info@lpaonline.org
www.lpaonline.org

July

Joanna Campbell, Executive Director
Gary Arnold, President
Bill Bradford, Senior Vice President

Web Sites

12   Achondroplasia UK
52 Vernham Grove
Odd down, Bath, Avon, BA2 2   e-mail: admin@achondroplasia.co.uk
www.achondroplasia.co.uk

Offers information on health supervision for children of all ages, divided into the following growth stages: newborn; infancy; early childhood; late childhood; and adolescence to early adulthood.

13   Human Growth Foundation
997 Glen Cove Ave., Suite 5
Gglen Head, NY 11545
800-451-6434
Fax: 516-671-4055
e-mail: hgf1@hgfound.org
www.hgfound.org

The Human Growth Foundation is a voluntary, non-profit organization whose mission is to help children and adults with disorders of growth and growth horomone through research, education, support, and advocacy.

Pisit Pitukcheewanont, MD, President
Patricia D. Costa, Executive Director
Emily Y. Germain-Lee, MD, Vice President

14   Little People of America
250 El Camino Real, Suite 211
Tustin, CA 92780
714-368-3689
888-LPA-2001
Fax: 714-368-3367
e-mail: info@lpaonline.org
www.lpaonline.org

Offers resources pertaining to dwarfism and Little People of
America, medical data, instructions on how to join an e-mail discussion group, and links to numerous other dwarfism-related
sites.

Gary Arnold, President
Joanna Campbell, Executive Director
April Brazier, Senior Vice President

15   MAGIC Foundation: Major Aspects of Growth in Children
6645 W. North Avenue
Oak Park, IL 60302   708-383-0808
                                                  800-362-4423
                       e-mail: ContactUs@magicfoundation.org
                                          www.magicfoundation.org

Provides educational information regarding growth disorders.

Rich Buckley, Chairman
Mary Andrews, Chief Executive Officer
Dianne Kremidas, Executive Director

16   Medical College of Wisconsin
8701 Watertown Plank Road
Milwaukee, WI 53226   414-955-8296
                                                  www.mcw.edu

A private, academic institution dedicated to leadership and excellence in education, research, patient care, and service.

John R. Raymond, Sr., MD, President/ CEO
Joseph E. Kerschner, MD, Dean/ EVP
Ravi Misra, PhD, Dean/ Professor of Biochemistry

17   Online Mendelian Inheritance in Man
National Library of Medicine, Building 38A
Bethesda, MD 20894   888-346-3656
                                      e-mail: info@ncbi.nlm.nih.gov
                                               www.ncbi.nlm.nih.gov

This database is a catalog of human genes and genetic disorders.

Christine E. Seidman, M.D., Chair
David J. Lipman, M.D., Executive Secretary

18   Restricted Growth Association
www.rgaonline.org.uk

Provides medical advice, welfare and counseling services with the
support of Regional Coordinators, and offers contact with others
and the sharing of helpful information through an information
magazine, advisory booklets, meetings, social events and
conventions.

Pamphlets

19   Achondroplasia
Human Growth Foundation
977 Glen Cove Avenue, Suite 5
Glen Head, NY 11545   516-671-4041
                                                 800-451-6434

Signs, causes, and prevention of achondroplasia.

Description

20   ACUTE GASTROINTESTINAL INFECTIONS
Covers these related disorders: Acute infectious diarrhea, Gastroenteritis
Involves the following Biologic System(s):
Gastrointestinal Disorders, Infectious Disorders

Acute gastrointestinal infections are conditions of the gastrointestinal tract caused by various microorganisms such as certain bacteria, viruses, and parasites (more common outside the U.S.) and are usually characterized by diarrhea and vomiting. Such microorganisms may be transmitted through fecal-oral contamination or contamination of food or water. Bacterial gastrointestinal infection may result from the release of toxins by bacteria or by bacterial growth inside or outside the walls of the intestines. Viral infection by gastroenteritis viruses, especially the rotavirus, is a major source of diarrhea-causing infection in the U.S. Although infectious gastroenteritis often resolves on its own, some patients experience acute or prolonged symptoms that may require treatment, as well as identification of the causative agent.

Symptoms and findings associated with infectious gastroenteritis depend upon the cause of the infection and the age and general health of the patient. The most common manifestation of infection is watery or bloody diarrhea that usually appears suddenly and lasts from a few days to two weeks or longer. Other symptoms may include nausea, vomiting, loss of appetite, and abdominal cramping or distress. Infants and those with compromised immune systems are at risk for potentially severe illness. Diarrhea and vomiting in infants younger than six months, and severe episodes in any child, may result in a potentially life-threatening and excessive fluid loss (dehydration) as well as the loss of essential substances, known as electrolytes, in the fluid portion of the blood (e.g., sodium, potassium, and calcium). Symptoms associated with dehydration may include fever, thirst, less-than-average urinary output, dry mouth, and poor feeding. In addition, severely dehydrated infants and children may become weak, listless, or sleepy and their eyes may have a sunken, dry appearance. Bacteria associated with gastroenteritis sometimes cause infection outside the gastrointestinal tract and may involve the urinary tract, eyes, vaginal areas in females, as well as inflammation of the membranes surrounding the brain and spinal cord (meningitis), the liver (hepatitis), the lungs (pneumonia), the bone and bone marrow (osteomyelitis), and other tissues. In addition, certain food-borne or water-borne infections caused by bacterial or other toxins may produce severe, sudden, and potentially life-threatening symptoms including neurologic involvement such as numbness and paralysis.

Acute infectious diarrhea symptoms are similar to those associated with infectious gastroenteritis. In addition, a temporary inability to properly digest milk may result from damage to the mucosal lining of the small intestine.

Prevention of some types of infectious gastroenteritis may include vaccination against certain infectious diseases when traveling to countries in which these illnesses are widespread. In addition, care in handling and preparing foods may help to alleviate certain types of food-borne illness. Treatment for both infectious gastroenteritis and acute infectious diarrhea is first directed toward the replacement of body fluids and electrolytes through oral preparations or, in the case of more severe dehydration, intravenously. Once dehydration is corrected, breast-feeding, or feeding with lactose-free formula, gradually followed by regular formula, may resume. If indicated, identification of the cause may then be established through evaluation of family history including recent travels, foods eaten, other similar family illness as well as physical examination and testing of stool specimens. Although some cases of acute infectious diarrhea will resolve spontaneously, other treatment may be directed at the underlying cause. Bacterial infections may be treated with appropriate antibiotics. Prevention of this potentially severe condition may often be accomplished by attention to good hygienics such as frequent hand washing, etc. Other treatment is symptomatic and supportive.

Government Agencies

21   NIH/National Institute of Allergy and Infectious Diseases
6610 Rockledge Drive, Room 4017 MSC 6612
Bethesda, MD 20892
301-496-5717
866-284-4107
Fax: 301-402-3573
TDD: 800-877-8339
e-mail: ocposfoffice@niaid.nih.gov
www.niaid.nih.gov

Conducts and supports basic and applied research to better understand, treat, and ultimately prevent infectious, immunologic, and allergic diseases.

Anthony S Fauci MD, Director

National Associations & Support Groups

22   American Academy of Pediatrics
141 Northwest Point Boulevard
Elk Grove Village, IL 60007
847-434-4000
800-433-9016
Fax: 847-434-8000
www.aap.org

The American Academy of Pediatrics and its member pediatricians are committed to the attainment of optimal physical, mental and social health and well-being for all infants, children, adolescents, and young adults.

Sandra Hassink, MD, FAAP, President

23   American College of Gastroenterology
6400 Goldsboro Road Suite 200
Bethesda, MD 20827
301-263-9000
www.gi.org

The American College of Gastroenterology was founded in 1932 to advance the scientific study and medical practice of diseases of the GI tract.

Ronald J. Vender, President
Stephen B. Hanauer, MD Vice President
Harry E Sarles Jr. MD, President-Elect

24   American Gastroenterological Association
4930 Del Ray Avenue
Bethesda, MD 20814
301-654-2055
Fax: 301-654-5920
e-mail: member@gastro.org
www.gastro.org

Society of physicians, surgeons, scientists and other individuals within the healthcare community interested in the functions and disorders of the digestive system.

Loren Laine MD, President
Anil K. Rustgi MD, President Elect
John I. Allen MD, Vice President

25 Digestive Disease National Coalition
507 Capitol Court NE, Suite 200
Washington, DC 20002
202-544-7497
Fax: 202-546-7105
e-mail: ddnc@hmcw.org
www.ddnc.org

Advocacy organization comprised of 22 voluntary and professional societies concerned with the many diseases of the digestive tract and liver.

Diane Paley, Chairperson
James DeGerome, President
Andrew Spiegel, President

26 International Foundation for Functional Gastrointestinal Disorders
700 W. Virginia Suite 201
Milwaukee, WI 53204
414-964-1799
888-964-2001
Fax: 414-964-7176
e-mail: iffgd@iffgd.org
www.iffgd.org

The organization offers responses to those commonly asked questions for families and individuals whose lives have been touched by gastrointestinal disorders.

Nancy J Norton, President
William Norton, Director of Development
Eleanor Cautley, Vice President

27 North American Society for Pediatric Gastroenterology/Hepatology/Nutrition
PO Box 6
Flourtown, PA 19031
215-233-0808
Fax: 215-233-3918
e-mail: naspghan@naspghan.org
www.naspghan.org

Strives to improve the care of infants, children and adolescents with digestive disorders by promoting advances in clinical care of children with chronic abdominal pain, diarrhea, constipation, vomiting, bleeding from the GI tract, inflammatory bowel disease, liver diseases, diseases of the pancreas, poor weight gain and nutritional problems.

Margaret K Stallings, Executive Director
Kate Ho, Associate Director
Dick Colleti, Board of Directors

28 Oley Foundation
214 Hun Memorial, MC-28, Albany Medical Center
Albany, NY 12208
518-262-5079
800-776-6539
Fax: 518-262-5528
e-mail: info@oley.org
www.oley.org

Helping people whose daily survival depends on home intravenous or tube-fed nutrition.

Joan Bishop, Executive Director
Roslyn Dahl, Director, Communications
Felice Austin, Regional Coordinator Program Direct

29 World Health Organization
Avenue Appia 20
CH-1211 Geneva 27,
Switzerland
www.who.int

WHO is the directing and coordinating authority for health within the United Nations system.

Dr Margaret Chan, Director General
Dr.Anarfi Asamoa-Baah, Deputy Director-General
Ala Alwan, Assistant Director General

Libraries & Resource Centers

30 National Digestive Diseases Information Clearinghouse (NDDIC)
31 Center Drive, MSC 2560
Bethesda, MD 20892
301-496-3583
800-891-5389
Fax: 301-907-8906
e-mail: nddic@info.niddk.nih.gov
www.niddk.nih.gov

The National Institute of Diabetes and Digestive and Kidney Diseases conducts and supports research on many of the most serious diseases affecting public health. The Institute supports much of the clinical research on the diseases of internal medicine and related subspecialty fields as well as many basic science disciplines.

Dr. Griffin P. Rodgers, Director
Dr. Gregory G. Germino, Deputy Director
Camille M. Hoover, M.S.W, Executive Officer

Conferences

31 IFFGD Professional Symposia
Int'l Foundation for Functional Gastrointestinal
700 W Virginia Street, #201
Milwaukee, WI 53204
414-964-1799
888-964-2001
Fax: 414-964-7176
e-mail: iffgd@iffgd.org
www.iffgd.org

Aimed at promoting education and awareness among professionals from multiple disciplines who treat gastrointestinal disorders and incontinence.

April

Nancy J Norton, President/Director/Co-Founder
William Norton, Vice President/Director/Co-Founder
Eleanor Cautley, Vice President/Director

32 NASPGHAN Annual Meeting and Postgraduate Course
NASPGHAN
PO Box 6
Flourtown, PA 19031
215-233-0808
Fax: 215-233-3918
e-mail: naspghan@naspghan.org
www.naspghan.org

October

Margaret K Stallings, Executive Director
Athos Bousvaros, MD, President
James Heubi, MD, Secretary-Treasurer

33 Oley Foundation Annual Conference
Oley Foundation
214 Hun Memorial, MC-28, Albany Medical Center
Albany, NY 12208
518-262-5079
800-776-6539
Fax: 518-262-5528
e-mail: info@oley.org
www.oley.org

Helping people whose daily survival depends on home intravenous or tube-fed nutrition.

July

Joan Bishop, Executive Director
Roslyn Dahl, Communications Director
Cathy Harrington, Administrative Assistant

Computer Software

34   Digestive Diseases Self-Education Program (DDSEP 5.0)
American Gastroenterological Association
4930 Del Ray Avenue
Bethesda, MD 20814   301-654-2055
                                          Fax: 301-654-5920
                                   e-mail: member@gastro.org
                                             www.gastro.org

Provides an in-depth review of core topics in gastroenterology
and hepatology. gastroenterologists use this software to assess
and update their knowledge and earn CME credit.

Eugene Chang, MD, Editor
John F Kuemmerle, MD, Associate Editor

Web Sites

35   American Gastroenterological Association
4930 Del Ray Avenue
Bethesda, MD 20814   301-654-2055
                                          Fax: 301-654-5920
                                   e-mail: member@gastro.org
                                             www.gastro.org

Information regarding prevention, treatment and cure of digestive
diseases.

Jessica Duncan, VP, Communications
Ellen Silver, VP, Meetings and Conventions
Lori Marks, PhD, VP, Education and Training

36   Baby Center
163 Freelon Street
San Francisco, CA 94107   www.babycenter.com

The Academy is committed to the attainment of optimal physical,
mental and social health for all infants, children, adolescents, and
young adults. To this end, the members of the Academy dedicate
their efforts and resources.

Colleen Hancock, SVP/ Global COO
Linda J. Murray, SVP/ Global Editor-in-Chief
Clarence Wilhelm, Chief Information Officer

37   Health Research Project (HaRP)
www.harpnet.org

                                    e-mail: harp@kmsgh.org
                                             www.harpnet.org

A program by USAID, the project strives to improve the health
status of infants, children, mothers and families through the development and research of new tools, technologies, policies and
approaches.

38   National Digestive Diseases Information Clearinghouse
9000 Rockville Pike
Bethesda, MD 20892   301-496-3583
                                    www.digestive.niddk.nih.gov

Information regarding digestive and kidney diseases.

Griffin P. Rodgers, M.D., M.A.C.P., Director
Kevin Abbott, Program Director
Kristin Abraham, Program Director

Book Publishers

39   Digestive Diseases Dictionary
Nat'l Digestive Diseases Information Clearinghouse
31 Center Drive, MSC 2560
Bethesda, MD 20892   301-496-3583
                                           800-891-5389
                                          Fax: 301-907-8906
                                 e-mail: nddic@info.niddk.nih.gov
                                             www.niddk.nih.gov

Defines words that are often used when talking or writing about
digestive diseases.

Dr. Griffin P. Rodgers, Director
Dr. Gregory G. Germino, Deputy Director
Janice Balin, Director

40   Digestive Diseases in the United States: Epidemiology and Impact
NDDIC
31 Center Drive, MSC 2560
Bethesda, MD 20892   301-496-3584
                                           800-891-5389
                                          Fax: 301-907-8906
                                 e-mail: nddic@info.niddk.nih.gov
                                             www.niddk.nih.gov

Answers hundreds of questions about the scope and impact of the
major infectious, chronic, and malignant digestive diseases. Provides information about prevalence, incidence, medical care, disability, mortality, and research needs regarding specific digestive
diseases.

800 pages

Dr. Griffin P. Rodgers, Director
Dr. Gregory G. Germino, Deputy Director
Janice Balin, Director

41   Directory of Digestive Diseases Organizations for Professionals
NDDIC
31 Center Drive, MSC 2560
Bethesda, MD 20892   301-496-3585
                                           800-891-5389
                                          Fax: 301-907-8906
                                 e-mail: nddic@info.niddk.nih.gov
                                             www.niddk.nih.gov

Lists organizations that represent health professionals involved in
the study and treatment of digestive disease. The organizations do
not provide medical services or advice.

Dr. Griffin P. Rodgers, Director
Dr. Gregory G. Germino, Deputy Director
Janice Balin, Director

42   What I Need To Know About Hepatitis A
NDDIC
31 Center Drive, MSC 2560
Bethesda, MD 20892   301-496-3586
                                           800-891-5389
                                          Fax: 301-907-8906
                                 e-mail: nddic@info.niddk.nih.gov
                                             www.niddk.nih.gov

Explains the prevention, causes, symptoms, modes of transmission, and treatment of Hepatitis A.

16 pages

Dr. Griffin P. Rodgers, Director
Dr. Gregory G. Germino, Deputy Director
Janice Balin, Director

43   What I Need To Know About Hepatitis B
NDDIC
31 Center Drive, MSC 2560
Bethesda, MD 20892   301-496-3587
                                           800-891-5389
                                          Fax: 301-907-8906
                                 e-mail: nddic@info.niddk.nih.gov
                                             www.niddk.nih.gov

Explains the prevention, causes, symptoms, modes of transmission, and treatment of Hepatitis B.

16 pages

Dr. Griffin P. Rodgers, Director
Dr. Gregory G. Germino, Deputy Director
Janice Balin, Director

44   What I Need To Know About Hepatitis C
NDDIC
31 Center Drive, MSC 2560
Bethesda, MD 20892   301-496-3588
                                           800-891-5389
                                          Fax: 301-907-8906
                                 e-mail: nddic@info.niddk.nih.gov
                                             www.niddk.nih.gov

Explains the prevention, causes, symptoms, modes of transmission, and treatment of Hepatitis C.

16 pages

Dr. Griffin P. Rodgers, Director
Dr. Gregory G. Germino, Deputy Director
Janice Balin, Director

Journals

45 American Journal of Gastroenterology
American College of Gastroenterology
6400 Goldsboro Rd, Ste 200
Bethesda, MD 20817   301-263-9000
                                        gi.org

Publishes scientific papers relevant to the practice of clinical gastroenterology, Features outstanding original research, review articles and consensus papers related to new drugs and therapeutic modalities.

Stephen B. Hanauer, MD, FACG, President
Carol A. Burke, MD, FACG, Vice President
Sunanda V. Kane, MD, MSPH, FACG, Secretary

46 Journal of Pediatric Gastroenterology and Nutrition
Lippincott Williams & Wilkins
Two Commerce Square, 2001 Market Street
Philadelphia, PA 19103   215-521-8300
                                Fax: 215-521-8902
                        www.wolterskluwerhealth.com

Provides a forum for original papers and reviews dealing with nutrition in normal and abnormal functions of the alimentary tract and its associated organs including the salivary glands, pancreas, gallbladder, and liver. Particular emphasis is on development and its relation to infant and childhood nutrition.

Bob Becker, President/ CEO
Susan Yules, Chief Financial Officer
Cathy Wolfe, President/ CEO, Medical Research

Newsletters

47 NASPGHAN News
PO Box 6
Flourtown, PA 19031   215-233-0808
                                Fax: 215-233-3939
                        e-mail: naspghan@naspghan.org
                                www.naspgn.org

Publication of the North American Society for Pediatric Gastroenterolgy, Hepatology and Nutrition, which strives to improve the care of infants, children and adolescents with digestive disorders by promoting advances in clinical care of children with chronic abdominal pain, diarrhea, constipation, vomiting, bleeding from the GI tract, inflammatory bowel disease, liver diseases, diseases of the pancreas, poor weight gain and nutritional problems.

Pamphlets

48 Bleeding in the Digestive Tract
NDDIC
2 Information Way
Bethesda, MD 20892   301-654-3810
                                      800-891-5389
                                Fax: 703-738-4929
                                TTY: 866-569-1162
                        e-mail: nddic@info.niddk.nih.gov
                                www.niddk.nih.gov

Includes information on the causes of bleeding in the digestive tract and how the bleeding is recognized, diagnosed, and treated.

6 pages

Griffin P. Rodgers, M.D., M.A.C.P, Director
Kevin Abbott, Program Director
Kristin Abraham, Program Director

49 Cyclic Vomiting Syndrome
NDDIC
2 Information Way
Bethesda, MD 20892   301-654-3810
                                      800-891-5389
                                Fax: 703-738-4929
                                TTY: 866-569-1162
                        e-mail: nddic@info.niddk.nih.gov
                                www.niddk.nih.gov

Describes the four phases of cyclic vomiting syndrome and the current treatment options available. Outlines the complications associated with the disorder and provides additional resources.

4 pages

Griffin P. Rodgers, M.D., M.A.C.P, Director
Kevin Abbott, Program Director
Kristin Abraham, Program Director

50 Diagnostic Tests
NDDIC
2 Information Way
Bethesda, MD 20892   301-654-3810
                                      800-891-5389
                                Fax: 703-738-4929
                                TTY: 866-569-1162
                        e-mail: nddic@info.niddk.nih.gov
                                www.niddk.nih.gov

Contains patient education fact sheets on seven diagnostic tests for gastrointestinal disorders (Colonoscopy, Sigmoidoscopy, Upper Endoscopy, Lower GI Series, ERCP, Liver Biopsy). Designed to be photocopy masters for health professionals to copy and distribute to patients.

Griffin P. Rodgers, M.D., M.A.C.P, Director
Kevin Abbott, Program Director
Kristin Abraham, Program Director

51 Diarrhea
NDDIC
2 Information Way
Bethesda, MD 20892   301-654-3810
                                      800-891-5389
                                Fax: 703-738-4929
                                TTY: 866-569-1162
                        e-mail: nddic@info.niddk.nih.gov
                                www.niddk.nih.gov

Includes general information on diarrhea and what can cause it. Also provides information about diagnosis, treatment, and prevention.

6 pages

Griffin P. Rodgers, M.D., M.A.C.P, Director
Kevin Abbott, Program Director
Kristin Abraham, Program Director

52 Diverticulosis & Diverticulitis
NDDIC
2 Information Way
Bethesda, MD 20892   301-654-3810
                                      800-891-5389
                                Fax: 703-738-4929
                                TTY: 866-569-1162
                        e-mail: nddic@info.niddk.nih.gov
                                www.niddk.nih.gov

Provides clear definitions of diverticulosis and diverticulitis, along with information on symptoms, causes, complications, and treatments.

6 pages

Griffin P. Rodgers, M.D., M.A.C.P, Director
Kevin Abbott, Program Director
Kristin Abraham, Program Director

53 Facts & Fallacies About Digestive Diseases
NDDIC
2 Information Way
Bethesda, MD 20892   301-654-3810
                                      800-891-5389
                                Fax: 703-738-4929
                                TTY: 866-569-1162
                        e-mail: nddic@info.niddk.nih.gov
                                www.niddk.nih.gov

Provides information about common digestive disorders, including ulcers, inflammatory bowel disease, and constipation, in true/false format.

4 pages

Griffin P. Rodgers, M.D., M.A.C.P, Director
Kevin Abbott, Program Director
Kristin Abraham, Program Director

54 **Gallstones**
NDDIC
2 Information Way
Bethesda, MD 20892

301-654-3810
800-891-5389
Fax: 703-738-4929
TTY: 866-569-1162
e-mail: nddic@info.niddk.nih.gov
www.niddk.nih.gov

Provides general information on gallstones, including what causes them, who is at risk, and how they are diagnosed and treated.

6 pages

Griffin P. Rodgers, M.D., M.A.C.P, Director
Kevin Abbott, Program Director
Kristin Abraham, Program Director

55 **Gas in the Digestive Tract**
NDDIC
2 Information Way
Bethesda, MD 20892

301-654-3810
800-891-5389
Fax: 703-738-4929
TTY: 866-569-1162
e-mail: nddic@info.niddk.nih.gov
www.niddk.nih.gov

Describes what causes gas, discusses the symptoms and the problems they cause, and provides information on treatment.

8 pages

Griffin P. Rodgers, M.D., M.A.C.P, Director
Kevin Abbott, Program Director
Kristin Abraham, Program Director

56 **Gastroesophageal Reflux Disease in Children**
NDDIC
2 Information Way
Bethesda, MD 20892

301-654-3810
800-891-5389
Fax: 703-738-4929
TTY: 866-569-1162
e-mail: nddic@info.niddk.nih.gov
www.niddk.nih.gov

Describes gastroesophageal reflux (GER) in children and adolescents, including information about the causes, symptoms, and diagnosis of this condition, as well as its treatment.

4 pages

Griffin P. Rodgers, M.D., M.A.C.P, Director
Kevin Abbott, Program Director
Kristin Abraham, Program Director

57 **Heart Burn, Hiatal Hernia, and Gastroesophageal Reflux Disease**
NDDIC
2 Information Way
Bethesda, MD 20892

301-654-3810
800-891-5389
Fax: 703-738-4929
TTY: 866-569-1162
e-mail: nddic@info.niddk.nih.gov
www.niddk.nih.gov

Defines gastroesophageal reflux disease (GERD) and describes the role of hiatal hernia. Provides general information on heartburn, as well as treatments for GERD, including surgery.

6 pages

Griffin P. Rodgers, M.D., M.A.C.P, Director
Kevin Abbott, Program Director
Kristin Abraham, Program Director

58 **Hemochromatosis**
NDDIC
2 Information Way
Bethesda, MD 20892

301-654-3810
800-891-5389
Fax: 703-738-4929
TTY: 866-569-1162
e-mail: nddic@info.niddk.nih.gov
www.niddk.nih.gov

Provides information about the causes, risk factors, symptoms, diagnosis, treatment, diagnostic tests for, and current research about hemochromatosis. Includes a list of additional resources.

6 pages

Griffin P. Rodgers, M.D., M.A.C.P, Director
Kevin Abbott, Program Director
Kristin Abraham, Program Director

59 **Irritable Bowel Syndrome**
NDDIC
2 Information Way
Bethesda, MD 20892

301-654-3810
800-891-5389
Fax: 703-738-4929
TTY: 866-569-1162
e-mail: nddic@info.niddk.nih.gov
www.niddk.nih.gov

Describes causes, symptoms, tests to rule out more serious intestinal diseases, and lifestyle and medical approaches to syptom management.

4 pages

Griffin P. Rodgers, M.D., M.A.C.P, Director
Kevin Abbott, Program Director
Kristin Abraham, Program Director

60 **Ulcerative Colitis**
NDDIC
2 Information Way
Bethesda, MD 20892

301-654-3810
800-891-5389
Fax: 703-738-4929
TTY: 866-569-1162
e-mail: nddic@info.niddk.nih.gov
www.niddk.nih.gov

Outlines the symptoms, diagnostic procedures, and risks and benefits of several drugs and kinds of surgery to treat this disease.

6 pages

Griffin P. Rodgers, M.D., M.A.C.P, Director
Kevin Abbott, Program Director
Kristin Abraham, Program Director

61 **Your Digestive System & How it Works**
NDDIC
2 Information Way
Bethesda, MD 20892

301-654-3810
800-891-5389
Fax: 703-738-4929
TTY: 866-569-1162
e-mail: nddic@info.niddk.nih.gov
www.niddk.nih.gov

Providees general information about the organs of the digestive system, the digestive process, and the absorption of nutrients. Includes a list of additional readings.

6 pages

Griffin P. Rodgers, M.D., M.A.C.P, Director
Kevin Abbott, Program Director
Kristin Abraham, Program Director

Description

62   ACUTE LYMPHOBLASTIC LEUKEMIA
Synonyms: Acute lymphocytic leukemia, ALL
Involves the following Biologic System(s):
Hematologic and Oncologic Disorders

Acute lymphoblastic leukemia (ALL) is a malignant disease characterized by excessive production of immature white blood cells known as lymphoblasts. ALL is the most common type of leukemia in children, having a slightly greater incidence, or rate of occurrence, in boys than in girls. Although ALL may develop during adolescence or occasionally in adulthood, it occurs most commonly in children between 3 and 7 years of age. The outcome in childhood ALL is related to a multitude of factors, including age, numbers of lymphoblasts and other blood cells found in the blood and bone marrow, and various genetic factors.

The lymphoblasts involved in ALL are produced in the bone marrow, and normally go on to develop into the white blood cells called lymphocytes, which are primarily responsible for fighting infection. In ALL, these lymphoblasts go through an uncontrolled proliferation that results in their accumulation in huge numbers in the bone marrow, impairing its ability to produce the other types of blood cells that originate in the marrow. The lymphoblasts responsible for ALL also proliferate in organs other than the marrow, particularly the liver, spleen, and lymph nodes.

The lymphoblasts affected by ALL evolve into either of two types of mature lymphocytes. One of these types are T-lymphocytes, which migrate from the bone marrow to the thymus gland in the neck, where they complete their maturation. The second type of lymphocytes, called B-lymphocytes mature entirely within the bone marrow. Because of this difference, ALL itself is divided into two categories — T-cell and B-cell. The technique used for differentiating the two kinds of ALL is known as "immunophenotyping." B-cell ALL is more common than T-cell, which tends to occur more often in boys, after the age of 10 years. Treatment of the two types of ALL may also differ, depending upon age, results of clinical and laboratory tests, and other factors.

All forms of ALL originate from abnormalities in the genetic structure of the cells that give rise to lymphoblasts. These abnormalities include changes in the structure of specific genes, breaks in the chainlike strands of genes known as chromosomes, with the broken parts joining other parts of the same chromosome or to other chromosomes where they do not belong, and other kinds of damage to the chromosomes or genes.

The chromosomal or genetic abnormalities in ALL are responsible for both the uncontrolled proliferation of lymphocytes and a cessation in the development of these cells, preventing them from maturing normally into lymphocytes.

Factors that may increase the risk for developing childhood ALL include Trisomy 21, the chromosomal abnormality responsible for Down syndrome; certain genetic disorders, such as Fanconi's anemia; presence of the aberrant chromosome known as the Philadelphia chromosome, created by the breakage of a specific chromosome and entry of its broken part

into another; exposure to radiation, some drugs used for chemotherapy, and certain chemicals such as benzene.

Many of the symptoms and effects of ALL in children and young adults are related to their uncontrolled proliferation of leukemic cells in the marrow or other organs. Overpopulation of the marrow by the diseased lymphoblasts in ALL may impede the formation of red blood cells, which also develop in the marrow; of the cells known as platelets, which are essential to blood clotting; and of the cells known as granulocytes, that normally team up with lymphocytes to fight off infection. The resulting symptoms typically include pallor, loss of appetite (anorexia), weight loss, and a generalized feeling of ill health (malaise); fatigue and weakness, from decreased numbers of the circulating red blood cells that carry oxygen to the body's tissues (anemia); bleeding from the gums or nose, easy bruising, and the development of small red or purple spots on the skin (petechiae) from decreased levels of the blood platelets responsible for blood clotting; and infection and fever from decreased numbers of mature white blood cells and granulocytes. Other symptoms of ALL may include headache and bone or joint pain. In many cases, effects of ALL include swollen lymph glands and an enlarged spleen (splenomegaly).

The diagnosis of ALL is established by the presence of lymphoblasts in a bone marrow sample obtained through biopsy. Treatment of ALL is directed toward destroying leukemic cells through the use of specific drugs, known as chemotherapy, which is sometimes given together with treatment delivered by high-energy radiation, such as that of X-rays. Treatment of ALL typically involves several stages, or "phases," and may cover a period of many months. The first stage of treatment, known as the "induction phase," is directed at maximum destruction of leukemic cells in the blood and bone marrow. This is commonly followed by what is known as "remission," in which the activity and effects of ALL are markedly reduced. The second phase of treatment, known as the "consolidation phase," is begun during remission and designed to eradicate any residual leukemic cells that may remain anywhere in the body and become reactivated, causing a recurrence or relapse of ALL. The third phase of therapy is known as "maintenance" or "continuation" therapy. The eradication of leukemic cells that have entered the brain, the membranes surrounding the brain and spinal cord (meninges), or the cerebrospinal fluid that surrounds these organs may require direct injection of a chemotherapeutic agent into the cerebrospinal fluid (intrathecal injection). Alternatively, X-ray or other irradiation may be focused on the brain or spinal cord to eliminate residual leukemic cells (intrathecal radiation). In some cases, immature blood cells are taken from the bone marrow of a donor and given to children with ALL to replace cells destroyed by chemotherapy or radiation therapy, with the goal of allowing these immature cells to grow to maturity and restore the patient's production of red and white blood cells and platelets.

Supportive measures in the treatment of ALL may include blood transfusions to alleviate anemia and bleeding irregularities, as well as the administration of antibiotics to treat infections resulting from the white cell abnormalities associated with both ALL and its treatment. Relapse of ALL after successful initial remission therapy usually results from lymphoblasts that have remained in the bone marrow and brain, and may require one or more additional courses of chemotherapy.

Government Agencies

63 **NIH/National Cancer Institute**
6116 Executive Boulevard, Room 3036A
Bethesda, MD 20892
800-422-6237
www.cancer.gov

The National Cancer Institute coordinates the National Cancer Program, which conducts and supports research, training, health information dissemination, and other programs with respect to the cause, diagnosis, prevention, and treatment of cancer, rehabilitation from cancer, and the continuing care of cancer patients and the families of cancer patients.

John E Niederhuber MD, Director

64 **NIH/National Heart, Lung and Blood Institute**
National Institute of Health
31 Center Dr MSC 2486, Bldg 31, Room 5A48
Bethesda, MD 20892
301-592-8573
Fax: 240-629-3246
TTY: 240-629-3255
e-mail: NHLBIinfo@nhlbi.nih.gov
www.nhlbi.nih.gov

Primary responsibility of this organization is the scientific investigation of heart, blood vessel, lung and blood disorders. Oversees research, demonstration, prevention, education, control and training activities in these fields and emphasizes the prevention and control of heart diseases.

Elizabeth G Nabel, MD, Director
Susan Shurin, MD, Deputy Director
Sheila Pohl, Chief of Staff

National Associations & Support Groups

65 **American Academy of Pediatrics**
141 Northwest Point Boulevard
Elk Grove Village, IL 60007
847-434-4000
800-433-9016
Fax: 847-434-8000
www.aap.org

The American Academy of Pediatrics and its member pediatricians are committed to the attainment of optimal physical, mental and social health and well-being for all infants, children, adolescents, and young adults.

Sandra Hassink, MD, FAAP, President

66 **B.A.S.E. Camp Children's Cancer Foundation**
2020 W FAIRBANKS AVE STE 101
Winter Park, FL 32789
407-673-5060
Fax: 407-673-5095
e-mail: email@basecamp.org
www.basecamp.org

Provides a year round base of support for children and families facing the challenge of living with cancer, hemophilia and other blood related illnesses.

Terri Jones, President
Cindy Whitaker, Parent & Program Coordinator
Joyce Lowe, Accounting

67 **Believe In Tomorrow - National Children's Foundation**
6601 Frederick Road, PO Box 21243
Baltimore, MD 21228
410-744-1032
800-933-5470
Fax: 410-744-1984
e-mail: info@believeintomorrow.org
www.believeintomorrow.org

Provides exceptional hospital and retreat housing services to critically ill children and their families.

Brian Morrison, Founder & CEO
Richard E. McCready, Chairman
David Reymann, Vice Chairman

68 **Cancer Fund of America**
2901 Breezewood Lane
Knoxville, TN 37921
865-938-5281
800-578-5284
Fax: 865-938-2968
e-mail: info@cfoa.org
www.cfoa.org

A non-profit organization set up to help cancer patients, hospices, and other non-profit healthcare providers by way of sending products free of charge directly to them

James T Reynolds Sr, CEO

69 **CancerCare**
275 7th Avenue
New York, NY 10001
212-712-6120
800-813-4673
Fax: 212-712-8495
e-mail: info@cancercare.org
www.cancercare.org

Dedicated to providing emotional support, information, and practical help to people with cancer and their loved ones. CancerCare is the oldest, largest, nonprofit agency devoted to offering professional services.

Helen H Miller, CEO
John Rutigliano, Chief Operating Officer
Rosalie Canosa, Program Division Director

70 **Candlelighters Childhood Cancer Foundation**
10920 Connecticut Ave. Suite A
Kensington, MD 20895
301-962-3520
855-858-2226
Fax: 310-962-3521
e-mail: staff@acco.org
www.acco.org

The American Childhood Cancer Organization (ACCO) was founded in 1970 by a group of parents whose children had been diagnosed with cancer. Today, ACCO is one of the largest grass-roots, national organizations dedicated to improving the lives of children and adolescents with cancer and their families.

Naomi Bartley, President
Janine Lynne, Vice President
Ken Phillips, Treasurer

71 **Child Life Council**
11821 Parklawn Dr., Suite 310
Rockville, MD 20852
301-881-7090
800-252-4515
Fax: 301-881-7092
e-mail: CLCadmin@childlife.org
www.childlife.org

Professionals who strive to reduce the impact of stressful or traumatic life events and situations which affect the development, health and well being of infants, children, youth and families. They embrace the value of play as a healing modality while working to enhance the normal growth and development of children through assessment, intervention, prevention, advocacy and education. The council offers publications, annual conferences, professional certification and more.

Diane Hart, President
Amy Bullock Morse, President-Elect
Trish Haneman Cox, Treasurer

72 **Childhood Cancer Canada Foundation**
21 St. Clair Avenue East, Suite 801
Toronto, Ontario,
Canada
416-489-6440
800-363-1062
Fax: 416-489-9812
e-mail: info@childhoodcancer.ca
www.childhoodcancer.ca

Founded in 1987, Childhood Cancer Canada (CCC) is the country's leading Foundation dedicated entirely to the fight against childhood cancer. Through their unique partnership will all of Canada's 17 childhood cancer hospitals and treatment centres, CCC can ensure that children with cancer are exposed to kinder and gentler treatments that will not only cure them but leave them with an improved quality of life into adulthood.

Glenn Fraser, Chair
Megan Davidson, President & CEO
Alan Zimmermann, VP, Operations

73 Children's Blood Foundation
333 E 38th Street, Suite 830
New York, NY 10016   212-297-4336
                                                   Fax: 212-297-4340
                                     e-mail: info@childrenscbf.org
                                              www.childrenscbf.org

The foundation's major emphasis is on blood diseases affecting children: leukemia, thalassemia, hemophilia, sickle cell anemia, platelet disorders, retinoblastoma and cancer.

James B. Bussel MD, Board of Directors
Ronald. J Lervolino, President
Les Lieberman, Chairman

74 Children's Leukemia Association
National Leukemia Research Association
585 Stewart Avenue, Suite 18
Garden City, NY 11530   516-222-1944
                                                   Fax: 516-222-0457
                                  e-mail: info@childrensleukemia.org
                                           www.childrensleukemia.org

A not-for-profit organization dedicated to raising funds to support research efforts towards finding the causes and cure for Leukemia.

Anthony Pasqua, President
Henry Green, Esq., Vice President
William Regina, Secretary/Treasurer

75 Dreams Come True Emery Clinic-Peds
1365 Clfton Road NE
Atlanta, GA 30322   404-778-5000
                                                       800-223-6679
                      e-mail: patient.relations@emoryhealthcare.org
                                             www.emoryhealthcare.org

Serves any child with cancer or chronic blood disease treated at Emory University Homo/Onc Clinic. Dreams submitted by children.

S. Wright Caughman, MD, Chairman
John T. Fox, President/CEO
Robert J. Bachman, CEO

76 Hair Club for Kids: Hair Club for Men
270 Farmington Avenue, Suite 232 (Second Floor)
Farmington, CT 06032   860-674-0202
                                                       888-888-8986
                                                   Fax: 860-676-0805
                            www.hairclub.com/hairclub-for-kids.php

Since 1992, Hair Club has offered free hair restoration services to children who suffer from diseases that lead to hair loss or alopecia. Hair Club for Kids is a non-profit program funded entirely by Hair Club that's available at no charge to children ages 6-17.

Sy Sperling, Founder
Steven Barth, President
Lydia Cassarino, Manager

77 Just In Time
PO Box 27693
Philadelphia, PA 19118   215-247-8777
                                                   Fax: 215-247-0956
                                        e-mail: tome@softhats.com
                                                  www.softhats.com

All cotton headwear for girls and women who have experienced hair loss.

Verlay Platt, President

78 Leukemia & Lymphoma Society
1311 Mamaroneck Avenue, Suite 310
White Plains, NY 10605   914-949-5213
                                                   Fax: 914-949-6691
                                         e-mail: infocenter@lls.org
                                                       www.lls.org

Largest voluntary health organization dedicated to funding blood cancer research, education and patient services.

Timothy S Durst, Chair of the Board
James H Davis Ph.D., Vice Chair
Kenneth Shwartz, Secretary/Treasurer

79 National Bone Marrow Transplant Link
20411 W 12 Mile Road, Suite 108
Southfield, MI 48076   248-358-1886
                                                       800-546-5268
                                                   Fax: 248-358-1889
                                         e-mail: info@nbmtlink.org
                                                   www.nbmtlink.org

The mission of the National Bone Marrow Transplant Link is to help patients, caregivers, and families cope with the social and emotional challenges of bone marrow/stem cell transplant from diagnosis through survivorship by providing vital information and personalized support services.

Myra Jacobs, Founding Director
Barbara Saltz, Program & Administrative Assistant
Cindy Goldman, Patient & Caregiver Support Coordin

80 National Childhood Cancer Foundation
4600 East West Highway, Suite 600
Bethesda, MD 20814   301-718-0042
                                                       800-458-6223
                                                   Fax: 301-718-0047
                                       e-mail: info@curesearch.org
                                                 www.curesearch.org

CureSearch for Children's Cancer is a national non-profit foundation that accelerates the cure for children's cancer by driving innovation, eliminating research barriers and solving the field's most challenging problems.They fight every day to make treatment possible and a cure probable for the 36 children diagnosed with cancer daily.

Stuart Siegal MD, Chair of the Board
Timothy Harmon, Vice Chair
Mary Payne, Treasurer

81 National Coalition for Cancer Survivorship
1010 Wayne Road, Suite 770
Silver Spring, MD 20910   301-650-9127
                                                       888-650-9127
                                                   Fax: 301-565-9670
                                   e-mail: info@canceradvocacy.org
                                              www.canceradvocacy.org

NCCS advocates for quality cancer care for all people touched by cancer and provides tools that empower people to advocate for themselves. Founded by and for cancer survivors, NCCS created the widely accepted definition of survivorship and defines someone as a cancer survivor from the time of diagnosis and for the balance of life.

Michael L Kappel, Chair
Samira K Beckwith, Vice Chair
Barbara Hoffman J.D, Secretary

State Agencies & Support Groups

North Carolina

82 Leukemia & Lymphoma Society-Western NC Chapter
Leukemia & Lymphoma Society
4530 Park Road
Charlotte, NC 28209   704-705-1850
                                                       800-888-9934
                                                   Fax: 704-998-5010
                                                       www.lls.org

The mission of The Leukemia & Lymphoma Society (LLS) is to Cure leukemia, lymphoma, Hodgkin's disease and myeloma, and improve the quality of life of patients and their families.LLS is the world's largest voluntary health agency dedicated to blood cancer. LLS funds lifesaving blood cancer research around the world and provides free information and support services.

Abby Miller, Team In Training
Gwen Tolman, Team In Training,Campaign Manager
Emily Greenfield, Light The Night, Campaign Manager

Ohio

83   Leukemia Society of America - Central Ohio Chapter
Leukemia Society of America
2225 Citygate Drive, Suite E
Columbus, OH 43219   614-476-7194
                                                 800-686-CURE
                                             Fax: 614-476-7189
                              e-mail: timothy.hamburger@lls.org
                                                   www.lls.org

Dedicated to finding cures for leukemia and related cancers and
to improving the quality of life for patients and their families.

Timothy Hamburger, Executive Director
Dan Swisher, Office Manager
Melissa Shawver, Patient Services Manager

84   Leukemia Society of America - Northern Ohio Chapter
Leukemia Society of America
5700 Brecksville Road 3rd Floor
Independence, OH 44131   216-264-5680
                                                 800-589-5721
                                             Fax: 440-617-2879
                                  e-mail: amy.pausche@lls.org
                                                   www.lls.org

Dedicated to finding cures for leukemia and related cancers and
to improving the quality of life for patients and their families.

Amy Pausche, Executive Director
Deborah Kending, Patient Services Manager
Peggy Stephens, Light The Night Walk, Manager

85   Leukemia Society of America - Southern Ohio Chapter
Leukemia Society of America
4370 Glendale Milford Road
Cincinnati, OH 45242   513-698-2828
                                             Fax: 513-351-5386
                                e-mail: michelle.steed@lls.org
                                                   www.lls.org

Dedicated to finding cures for leukemia and related cancers and
to improving the quality of life for patients and their families.
This chapter serves a 22-county geographic area that includes Adams, Brown, Butler, Clermont, Clinton, Darke, Gallia, Greene,
Hamilton, Highland, Jackson, Lawrence, Meigs, Miami, Montgomery, Pike, Preble, Scioto and Warren counties in Ohio and
Boone, Campbell and Kenton counties in Kentucky.

Michelle Steed, Executive Director
Jackie Personett, Patient Services Manager
Tom Carleton, Senior Campaign Manager, Special Ev

Oklahoma

86   The Leukemia & Lymphoma Society
Leukemia & Lymphoma Society
500 N Broadway, Suite 250
Oklahoma City, OK 73102   405-943-8888
                                                 888-828-4572
                                             Fax: 405-945-8355
                                e-mail: sean.simpson@lls.org
                                                   www.lls.org

Our Mission: Cure leukemia, lymphoma, Hodgkin's disease and
myeloma, and improve the quality of life for patients and their
families.

Sean Simpson, Executive Director
Bryn Mecum, Team in Training Campaign Director
Alisia Davis, Patient Services Manager

Oregon

87   Leukemia Society of America - Oregon Chapter
Leukemia Society of America
9320 SW Barbur Boulevard Suite 350
Portland, OR 97219   503-245-9866
                                                 800-466-6572
                                             Fax: 503-245-9865
                                 e-mail: sarah.harris@lls.org
                                                   www.lls.org

Dedicated to finding cures for leukemia and related cancers and
to improving the quality of life for patients and their families.

Sarah Harris, Executive Director
Sue Sumpter, Patient Services Manager
Morgan Tashea, Team In Training Coordinator - Mara

Pennsylvania

**88   Leukemia Society of America - Western Pennsylvania/West
Virginia Chapter**
Leukemia Society of America
E. Carson Street, Ste, 441
Pittsburgh, PA 15219   412-263-2873
                                                 800-726-2873
                                             Fax: 412-395-2888
                              e-mail: christina.massari@lls.org
                                                   www.lls.org

Dedicated to finding cures for leukemia and related cancers and
to improving the quality of life for patients and their families.

Tina Massari, Executive Director
Jeanne Caliguri, Director of Development
Francine Morrison, Patient Services Manager

Tennessee

89   Leukemia & Lymphoma Society, Tennessee Chapter
404 BNA Drive, Suite 102
Nashville, TN 37217   615-331-2980
                                                 800-332-2980
                                             Fax: 615-331-2941
                                  e-mail: jeff.parsley@lls.org
                                                   www.lls.org

To better serve the needs of Tennesseans - offers contribution-funded community services, family support groups, free educational materials and financial assistance for those affected by
leukemia, Hodgkin's disease, myeloma and the lymphomas.

Jeff Parsley, Executive Director
Tricia Ward, Campaign Manager
Kim Patterson, Senior Campaign Director

Texas

90   Leukemia Society of America - North Texas Chapter
Leukemia Society of America
8111 LBJ Freeway, Suite 425
Dallas, TX 75251   972-996-5900
                                                 800-800-6702
                                             Fax: 972-239-0892
                                e-mail: carol.withers@lls.org
                                                   www.lls.org

Dedicated to finding cures for leukemia and related cancers and
to improving the quality of life for patients and their families.

Carol Withers, Office Manager
Stacey Russell, Deputy Executive Director
Jane Beeson, Patient Services Coordinator

91   Leukemia Society of America - South/West Texas Chapter
Leukemia Society of America
431 Isom Road, Suite 125
San Antonio, TX 78216   210-377-1775
                                                 800-683-2458
                                                   www.lls.org

Dedicated to finding cures for leukemia and related cancers and
to improving the quality of life for patients and their families.

Kathleen Griesenbeck, Executive Director
Deborah Barker, Deputy Executive Director
Nicole Bell, Patient Services Coordinator

92   Leukemia Society of America - Texas Gulf Coast Chapter
Leukemia Society of America
5433 Westheimer Suite 300
Houston, TX 77056   713-840-0483
                                             Fax: 281-683-9504
                              e-mail: billiesue.parris@lls.org
                                                   www.lls.org

Dedicated to finding cures for leukemia and related cancers and to improving the quality of life for patients and their families.

Billie Sue Parris, Executive Director
Janie Moore, Deputy Executive Director
Cherry Evans, Patient Services Manager

Virginia

93   Leukemia Society of America - National Capital Area Chapter
Leukemia Society of America
5845 Richmond Highway, Suite 800
Alexandria, VA 22303   703-399-2900
                                          Fax: 703-960-0920
                           e-mail: gabrielle.urquhart@lls.org
                                               www.lls.org

Serves the greater Washington DC metropolitan area, including Northern Virginia, Prince George's and Montgomery counties.

Gabrielle Urquhart, Executive Director
Beth Gorman, Deputy Executive Director
Katherine Goode, Donor Development, Director

Wisconsin

94   Leukemia Society of America - Wisconsin Chapter
Leukemia Society of America
4125 North 124th Street, No A
Brookfield, WI 53005   262-790-4701
                                               800-261-7399
                                          Fax: 262-790-4706
                            e-mail: annmarie.frakes@lls.org
                                               www.lls.org

To serve Wisconsites touched by leukemia, lymphoma, Hodgkin's disease and myeloma.

Ann Marie Frakes, Executive Director
Karen Ropel, Operations Director
Lisa Weisman, Campaign Director, Light The Night

Libraries & Resource Centers

95   Children's National Medical Center
University of South Carolina School of Medicine
111 Michigan Avenue NW
Washington, DC 20010   202-476-5000
                                               888-884-2327
                          e-mail: tbear@childrensnational.org
                                      www.childrensnational.org

Children's National serves as the regional referral center for pediatric emergency, cancer, trauma, cardiac and critical care as well as neonatology, orthopaedic surgery, neurology, and neurosurgery.

Kurt Newman, President and CEO
Mendel Tuchman, Chief Research Officer
Douglas Myers, MBA, CPA, Executive Vice President

Research Centers

96   International Bone Marrow Transplant Registry
Medical College of Wisconsin
9200 W Wisconsin Avenue Suite C5500
Milwaukee, WI 53226   414-805-0700
                                          Fax: 414-805-0714
                            e-mail: contactus@cibmtr.org
                            www.cibmtr.org/pages/index.aspx

CIBMTR collaborates with the global scientific community to advance hematopoietic cell transplantation and cellular therapy research worldwide.

Jeffery Chell MD, Executive Leader
Mary Horowitz MD, Executive Leader
J. Douglas Rizzo MD, MS, Executive Leader

Conferences

97   CLC Annual Conference
Child Life Council
11821 Parklawn Drive, Suite 310
Rockville, MD 20852   301-881-7090
                                               800-252-4515
                                          Fax: 301-881-7092
                            e-mail: clcadmin@childlife.org
                                            www.childlife.org

The premier educational experience for child life professionals. The largest gathering of child life specialists of the year, offers ample opportunities for both formal and informal networking with peers.

1,000 May

Dennis Reynolds, Executive Director
Colleen Maguire, Deputy Director
Wilma Brooks, Director Of Development

Audio Video

98   Coping with Childhood Cancer
Films for the Humanities and Sciences
132 West 31st Street
New York, NY 10001   800-257-5126
                                          Fax: 609-275-0266
                             e-mail: custserv@films.com
                                             www.ffh.films.com

Coping with chronic and perhaps fatal disease and gaining control over their lives is something that childhood cancer victims must learn. This program presents open and honest interviews with five family members of childhood cancer patients. The stress on the family is intense; ofteh, the brothers and sisters of children with cancer or any chronic life-threatening illness are most severely affected emotionally.

28 minutes
ISBN: 1-421320-42-7

99   My Hair's Falling Out...Am I Still Pretty?
Necessary Pictures
7 W 20th Street, Suite 2F
New York, NY 10011   212-675-1809
                                               800-221-3170

Moving film about two children with cancer who are hospital roommates. Using dance, animation and music, the video explores the feelings of the patients, families, and friends while it sensitively informs and educates the viewers about the emotional and physical aspects of childhood cancer. The child with leukemia grows up to become a doctor, while her roommate with a tumor dies. For school-age children and their families. Purchase is $25 for families and $79 for professionals.

22 minutes
ISBN: 0-965083-20-9

Web Sites

100   ALL Kids
www.all-kids.org/

ALL Kids is an Internet mailing list providing support for families and caregivers of children with Acute Lymphoblastic Leukemia.

101   CancerCare
275 Seventh Avenue
New York, NY 10001   800-813-4673
                             e-mail: info@cancercare.org
                                            www.cancercare.org

CancerCare is a national nonprofit, 501(c)(3) organization that provides free, professional support services to anyone affected by cancer: people with cancer, caregivers, children, loved ones, and the bereaved. CancerCare programs - including counseling and support groups, education, financial assistance and practical help - are provided by professional oncology social workers and are completely free of charge.

Patricia J. Goldsmith, Chief Executive Officer
John Rutigliano, Chief Operating Officer
Ellen Miller Sonet, MBA, JD, Chief Strategy & Alliance Officer

102 Children's Cancer Web
www.cancerindex.org/ccw

An independent nonprofit site, established to provide a directory of childhood cancer resources.

103 Leukemia and Lymphoma Society of America
1311 Mamaroneck Avenue, Suite 310
White Plains, NY 10605   914-949-5213
                                          Fax: 914-949-6691
                                          www.leukemia.org

Is the largest voluntary health organization dedicated to funding blood cancer research, education and patient services. The mission is to cure leukemia, lymphoma, Hodgkin's disease and myeloma, and to improve the quality of life of patients and their families.

Louis J. DeGennaro, Ph.D., President/ CEO
Rosemarie Loffredo, CAO/ CFO
Mark Roithmayr, Chief Development Officer

Book Publishers

104 Blood & Circulatory Disorders Sourcebook 2nd Edition
Omnigraphics
PO Box 31-1640
Detroit, MI 48231   800-234-1340
                                          e-mail: info@omnigraphics.com
                                          www.omnigraphics.com

Basic consumer health information on blood and its components, anemias, leukemias, bleeding disorders, and circulatory disorders, including aplastic anemia, thalassemia, sickle-cell disease and hemophilia.

659 pages
ISBN: 0-780817-46-4

105 Childhood Leukemia: A Guide for Families, Friends & Caregivers
O'Reilly & Associates
1005 Gravenstein Highway North
Sebastopol, CA 95472   707-827-7019
                                          800-889-8969
                                          Fax: 707-824-8268
                                          e-mail: orders@oreilly.com
                                          www.oreilly.com

Features a wealth of tools to help parents become strong advocates for their child, detailed and precise medical information, and day-to-day practical advice to help cope with procedures, hospitalization, family and friends, schools, social, emotional and financial issues.

528 pages Softcover
ISBN: 0-596500-15-7

Tim O'Reilly, Founder/CEO

106 Draw Me a Picture
Cancervive
11636 Chayote Street
Los Angeles, CA 90049   310-203-9232
                                          800-486-2873
                                          Fax: 310-471-4618
                                          e-mail: cancervivr@aol.com
                                          www.cancervive.org

A fun coloring book for children with cancer (ages three to six). Marty Bunny talks about how it was when he was in the hospital for cancer and invites readers to draw about their experiences.

107 Having Leukemia Isn't So Bad, of Course, It Wouldn't Be My First Choice
Sargasso Enterprises
18 Ginn Road
Winchester, MA 01890   781-729-9037
                                          Fax: 781-729-2726
                                          e-mail: cak@krumme.com

Personal story of Catherine Krumme, diagnosed with leukemia at age four, relapsed at age seven, finished treatment at age ten. Catherine graduated from college in 1998 and went on to graduate school. The book is a supportive resource for families with cancer, for their friends, and for teachers working with children with health issues.

149 pages Softcover
ISBN: 0-963555-44-8

Ann Combs

108 Kathy's Hats: A Story of Hope
Albert Whitman and Company
250 South Northwest Highway, Suite 320
Park Ridge, IL 60068   847-232-2800
                                          800-255-7675
                                          Fax: 847-581-0039
                                          e-mail: mail@awhitmanco.com
                                          www.awhitmanco.com

A charming book for ages five to ten about chemotherapy and the loss of Kathy's hair.

32 pages Hardcover
ISBN: 0-807541-16-8

Trudy Krisher, Author

109 Let's Talk About Going to the Hospital
Rosen Publishing Group's PowerKids Press
29 E 21st Street
New York, NY 10010   212-777-3017
                                          800-237-9932
                                          Fax: 888-436-4643
                                          e-mail: rosenpub@tribeca.ios.com
                                          www.rosenpublishing.com

If a child has to check into the hospital, chances are he or she is already upset about being ill. Knowing how a hospital functions and what the procedures are, such as when family members can visit, will help in what is already a stressful situation. Grades K-5.

24 pages
ISBN: 0-823950-36-0

110 Pediatric Cancer Sourcebook
Omnigraphics
PO Box 31-1640
Detroit, PA 48231   800-234-1340
                                          Fax: 800-875-1340
                                          e-mail: info@omnigraphics.com
                                          omnigraphics.com

Basic consumer health information about leukemias, brain tumors, sarcomas, lymphomas and other cancers in infants, children and adolescents.

587 pages
ISBN: 0-780802-45-4

111 Surviving Childhood Cancer: A Guide for Families
New Harbinger Publications
5674 Shattuck Avenue
Oakland, CA 94609   510-652-0215
                                          800-748-6273
                                          Fax: 800-652-1613
                                          e-mail: customerservice@newharbinger.com
                                          newharbinger.com

Cancer in a child is an overwhelming experience for a family. This book explains common medical procedures and offers readers practical advice about how to cope with emotions and stress during this time.

1998 232 pages
ISBN: 1-572241-02-0

Magazines

112 Coping with Cancer Magazine
PO Box 682268
Franklin, TN 37068
615-790-2400
Fax: 615-794-0179
e-mail: info@copingmag.com
www.copingmag.com

A bimonthly publication devoted to people whose lives have been touched by cancer.

Paula Chadwell, Vice President

Pamphlets

113 Resource Center for the American Alliance of Cancer - Pain Initiatives
Wisconsin Cancer Pain Initiative
1300 University Avenue, Room 4720
Madison, WI 53706
608-265-4013
Fax: 608-265-4014
e-mail: aacpi@mailplus.wisc.edu
www.aacpi.org

A booklet that helps parents determine if their child is in pain and provides methods to manage the pain. Single copy free. Also available, a Handbook of Cancer Pain Management, 5th edition.

12 pages Paperback

Camps

114 Arizona Camp Sunrise
4550 E Bell Rd, Suite 126
Phoenix, AZ 85032
602-952-7550
Fax: 602-404-1118
e-mail: melissa@azcampsunrise.org
www.azcampsunrise.org

The camp is dedicated to provide an exciting, medically safe camp program for children who have or have had cancer and their siblings.

Melissa Lee, Camp Director

115 Big Sky Kids Cancer Camp
6901 Goldenstein Lane
Bozeman, MT 59715
406-586-1781
Fax: 406-586-5794
e-mail: bigskykids@eaglemount.org
www.eaglemount.org

Provides a positive environment and give children, teens, and their parents emotional support, a sense of normalcy, and a network of friends who share similar experiences.

Mary Peterson, Executive Director

116 Camp Catch-A-Rainbow
American Cancer Society
1755 Abbey Rd
East Lansing, MI 48823
517-332-3300
www.cancer.org

Open to any child who has, or has had, cancer.

117 Camp Fantastic
Special Love
117 Youth Development Court
Winchester, VA 22602
504-667-3774
Fax: 540-667-8144
www.speciallove.org

Nonprofit organization that provides enriching programs for children with cancer, including Camp Fantastic.

118 Camp Sunshine Dreams
PO Box 28232
Fresno, CA 93729
e-mail: contact@campsunshinedreams.org
www.campsunshinedreams.com

Summer camp for children with cancer.

119 Des Moines YMCA Camp
1192 166th Drive
Boone, IA 50036
515-432-7558
Fax: 515-432-7558
e-mail: ycamp@dmymca.org
www.y-camp.org

For boys and girls with cancer, diabetes, asthma, cystic fibrosis, hearing impaired and other disabilities.

Dan Breitbach, Executive Director

120 Okizu Foundation Camps
16 Digital Drive, Suite 130
Novato, CA 94949
415-382-9083
Fax: 415-382-8384
e-mail: info@okizu.org
www.okizu.org

This foundation runs family camp programs for children who have cancer and their families, and for children who have or had a parent with cancer.

Suzie Randall, Executive Director

Description

121 ACUTE MYELOID LEUKEMIA

Synonyms: Acute granulocytic leukemia, Acute myeloblastic leukemia, Acute myelocytic leukemia, Acute myelogenous leukemia, Acute myelomonocytic leukemia, AML

Involves the following Biologic System(s):
Hematologic and Oncologic Disorders

Acute myeloid leukemia (AML) is a malignant disease, or cancer, characterized by excessive production in the bone marrow of the white blood cells called myelocytes, sometimes also known as granulocytes, which are vital in helping the body to combat and prevent infection. Although AML is primarily a disease of adulthood (median age at onset is 60 years), it is responsible for about 20% of all childhood leukemias.

The symptoms and characteristic findings associated with AML result from the accumulation of myelocytes in the bone marrow, eventually impairing the ability of the marrow to produce mature blood cells. In addition, myelocytes are released into the general blood circulation and carried to other organs, where they continue to grow at a rapid rate.

Children and young adults with AML exhibit fatigue, fever, lethargy, headache and bone or joint pain. In older adults, AML tends to have a slow, progressive onset, with lethargy, loss of appetite, and shortness of breath. Other findings may include enlargement of the liver and spleen (hepatosplenomegaly) and swollen lymph glands. Some children with AML may have swollen gums, as well as swelling of the salivary glands, which are located in front of the ears. Other effects of AML can include small leukemic cell tumors (chloromas) that develop under the skin or on the membranes surrounding the brain and spinal cord, and are followed by inflammation of these membranes (meningitis). Most children with AML develop irregularities in the blood, such as an abnormal deficiency in the numbers of circulating red blood cells (anemia) and platelets (thrombocytopenia), although the white blood cell count may range from low to high. Because AML directly affects cells that enable the body to fight off infection, one of its most serious effects is an increased susceptibility to severe, frequent infections.

AML results from mutations in the genes of myeloblasts or myelocytes, or from damage to these genes or chromosomes. This damage distorts the functions of the affected genes in such a way as to cause uncontrolled cell division and a subsequent rapid increase in the numbers of leukemic blood cells. Factors that may increase the risk for developing AML include genetic disorders such as trisomy 21 (the chromosome abnormality responsible for Down syndrome), Bloom syndrome (caused by a gene mutation and marked by small red lesions and sensitivity to light), Fanconi anemia (caused by any of several gene mutations), and certain other inherited disorders. Chemotherapy or radiation for earlier malignancies, as well as exposure to benzene or cigarette smoke, can also increase the risk of developing AML.

The diagnosis of AML is confirmed from a bone marrow sample obtained through biopsy. Treatment of AML is directed initially toward destroying leukemic cells through the use of drugs (chemotherapy) in an initial, induction phase intended to destroy leukemic cells and induce remission. This is followed with a second phase of chemotherapy to destroy any remaining leukemic cells, and by a further, "remission" phase of therapy to ensure lasting destruction of such cells. The chemotherapy used against AML may be given intravenously by infusion into the blood, or by infusion into the spinal canal. In some cases, radiation is directed at the brain and spinal cord to destroy leukemic cells. Chemotherapy or radiation directed at the brain and spinal cord is known as "intrathecal therapy." In some cases, bone marrow from a suitable donor is given to patients with AML to "reconstitute" or restore their capacity to produce normal myelocytes, and better enable them to defend themselves against infection and other effects of the disease.

Because the potent drugs used in chemotherapy also suppress white blood cell production, thus increasing susceptibility to infection, antibiotic therapy is often given to prevent infection. In some patients, transfusions of red blood cells and platelets are given to ease anemia and bleeding irregularities. Greater than 70% of adults younger than 60 achieve complete remission with treatment for AML. For some patients, a bone marrow or cord blood transplant may offer the best chance for a long-term remission.

Government Agencies

122 NIH/National Cancer Institute
BG 9609 MSC 97609609 Medical Center Drive
Bethesda, MD 20892
800-422-6237
www.cancer.gov

The National Cancer Institute coordinates the National Cancer Program, which conducts and supports research, training, health information dissemination, and other programs with respect to the cause, diagnosis, prevention, and treatment of cancer, rehabilitation from cancer, and the continuing care of cancer patients and the families of cancer patients.

Harold E Varmus MD, Director

123 NIH/National Heart, Lung and Blood Institute
National Institute of Health
31 Center Dr MSC 2486, Bldg 31, Room 5A48
Bethesda, MD 20892
301-592-8573
Fax: 240-629-3246
TTY: 240-629-3255
e-mail: nhlbiinfo@nhlbi.nih.gov
www.nhlbi.nih.gov

The National Heart, Lung, and Blood Institute (NHLBI) provides global leadership for a research, training, and education program to promote the prevention and treatment of heart, lung, and blood diseases and enhance the health of all individuals so that they can live longer and more fulfilling lives.

Gary H Gibbons MD, Director
Susan B Shurin, MD, Deputy Director
Nakela Cook MD, Chief of Staff

National Associations & Support Groups

124 American Academy of Pediatrics
141 Northwest Point Boulevard
Elk Grove Village, IL 60007
847-434-4000
800-433-9016
Fax: 847-434-8000
www.aap.org

The American Academy of Pediatrics and its member pediatricians are committed to the attainment of optimal physical, mental and social health and well-being for all infants, children, adolescents, and young adults.

Sandra Hassink, MD, FAAP, President

125 **B.A.S.E. Camp Children's Cancer Foundation**
2020 W FAIRBANKS AVE STE 101
Winter Park, FL 32789   407-673-5060
                                    Fax: 407-673-5095
                              e-mail: email@basecamp.org
                                    www.basecamp.org

Provides a year round base of support for children and families
facing the challenge of living with cancer, hemophilia and other
blood related illnesses.

Terri Jones, President
Cindy Whitaker, Program Coordinator
Joyce Lowe, Accounting

126 **Believe In Tomorrow Children's Foundation**
6601 Frederick Road
Baltimore, MD 21228   410-744-1032
                                          800-933-5470
                                    Fax: 410-744-1984
                         e-mail: info@believeintomorrow.org
                               www.believeintomorrow.org

Provides a variety of special services and programs (such as
beach and mountain retreats or attending Orioles games) to any
child up to 18 years of age who is being treated for cancer. Services are provided free of charge and are available on an ongoing
basis throughout treatment.

Brian Morrison, Founder and CEO
Richard E McCready, Chairman
David Reymann, Vice Chairman

127 **Cancer Fund of America**
2901 Breezewood Lane
Knoxville, TN 37921   865-938-5281
                                          800-578-5284
                                    Fax: 865-938-2968
                                  e-mail: info@cfoa.org
                                        www.cfoa.org

A a non-profit organization set up to help cancer patients, hospices, and other non-profit healthcare providers by way of sending products free of charge directly to them.

James T Reynolds Sr, CEO

128 **CancerCare**
275 7th Avenue
New York, NY 10001   212-712-6120
                                          800-813-4673
                                    Fax: 212-712-8495
                              e-mail: info@cancercare.org
                                     www.cancercare.org

CancerCare provides free, professional support services to individuals, families, caregivers and the bereaved to help them cope
with and manage the emotional and practical challenges of
cancer.

Helen H Miller, CEO
John Rutigliano, Chief Operating Officer
Rosalie Canosa, Program Division Director

129 **Candlelighters Childhood Cancer Foundation**
10920 Connecticut Ave., Suite A
Kensington, MD 20895   301-962-3520
                                          855-858-2226
                                    Fax: 310-962-3521
                                 e-mail: staff@acco.org
                                        www.acco.org

The American Childhood Cancer Organization (ACCO) was
founded in 1970 by a group of parents whose children had been
diagnosed with cancer. Today, ACCO is one of the largest grassroots, national organizations dedicated to improving the lives of
children and adolescents with cancer and their families.

Naomi Bartley, President
Janine Lynne, Vice President
Ken Phillips, Treasurer

130 **Child Life Council**
11821 Parklawn Dr., Suite 310
Rockville, MD 20852   301-881-7090
                                    Fax: 301-881-7092
                            e-mail: CLCadmin@childlife.org
                                     www.childlife.org

Professionals who strive to reduce the impact of stressful or traumatic life events and situations which affect the development,
health and well being of infants, children, youth and families.
They embrace the value of play as a healing modality while working to enhance the normal growth and development of children
through assessment, intervention, prevention, advocacy and education. The council offers publications, annual conferences,
professional certification and more.

Diane Hart, President
Amy Bullock Morse, President-Elect
Trish Haneman Cox, Treasurer

131 **Children's Blood Foundation**
333 E 38th Street, Suite 830
New York, NY 10016   212-297-4336
                                    Fax: 212-297-4340
                            e-mail: info@childrenscbf.org
                                   www.childrenscbf.org

The foundation's major emphasis is on blood diseases affecting
children: leukemia, thalassemia, hemophilia, sickle cell anemia,
platelet disorders, retinoblastoma and cancer.

James B. Bussel MD, Board of Directors
Ronald. J Lervolino, President
Les Lieberman, Chairman

132 **Children's Leukemia Association**
National Leukemia Research Association
585 Stewart Avenue, Suite 18
Garden City, NY 11530   516-222-1944
                                    Fax: 516-222-0457
                         e-mail: info@childrensleukemia.org
                               www.childrensleukemia.org

A not-for-profit organization dedicated to raising funds to support research efforts towards finding the causes and cure for
leukemia.

Anthony Pasqua, President
Henry Green, Esq., Vice President
William Regina, Secretary/Treasurer

133 **Dreams Come True Emery Clinic-Peds**
1365 Clfton Road NE
Atlanta, GA 30322   404-778-5000
                                          800-753-6679
                                   www.emoryhealthcare.org

Serves any child with cancer or chronic blood disease treated at
Emory University Homo/Onc Clinic. Dreams submitted by children.

John T. Fox, President/ CEO
Anne Adams, JD, Chief Compliance Officer
William A. Bornstein, MD, PhD, Chief Quality Officer

134 **Hair Club for Kids: Hair Club for Men**
270 Farmington Avenue, Suite 232 (Second Floor)
Farmington, CT 06032   860-674-0202
                                          800-269-7384
                                    Fax: 860-676-0805
                        www.hairclub.com/hairclub-for-kids.php

Since 1992, Hair Club has offered free hair restoration services to
children who suffer from diseases that lead to hair loss or alopecia. Hair Club for Kids is a non-profit program funded entirely by
Hair Club that's available at no charge to children ages 6-17.

Sy Sperling, Founder
Steven Barth, President
Lydia Cassarino, Manager

135 **ICARE**
4853 Cordell Avenue, Suite 14
Bethesda, MD 20814   301-652-3461
                                          800-422-7361
                                e-mail: contact@icare.org
                                        www.icare.org

The International Care Alliance for Research and Education
(ICARE) is a nonprofit organization which provides high-quality,
focused, user-friendly, cancer information to each patient as well
as their physician on an on-going, and person to person basis.

David Hankins, Chairman; President

136   Just In Time
PO Box 27693
Philadelphia, PA 19118
                                    215-247-8777
                                    Fax: 215-247-0956
                                    e-mail: tome@softhats.com
                                    www.softhats.com

All cotton headwear for girls and women who have experienced hair loss.

Verlay Platt, President

137   Leukemia & Lymphoma Society
1311 Mamaroneck Avenue, Suite 310
White Plains, NY 10605
                                    914-949-5213
                                    Fax: 914-949-6691
                                    e-mail: infocenter@lls.org
                                    www.lls.org

Largest voluntary health organization dedicated to funding blood cancer research, education and patient services.

Timothy S Durst, Chair of the Board
James H Ward, Vice Chair
Kenneth Shwartz, Secretary/Treasurer

138   National Bone Marrow Transplant Link
20441 W 12 Mile Road, Suite 108
Southfield, MI 48076
                                    248-358-1886
                                    800-546-5268
                                    e-mail: info@nbmtlink.org
                                    www.nbmtlink.org

Publications designed to help you understand and deal with the logistics of bone marrow transplantation, finances and medical insurance, information about the National Bone Marrow Transplant Link and its peer support program, and a celebration of BMT survivor stories.

Myra Jacobs, Founding Director
Denise Lillvis, Executive Director
Cindy Goldman, Patient & Caregiver Support Coordin

139   National Coalition for Cancer Survivorship
1010 Wayne Road, Suite 770
Silver Spring, MD 20910
                                    301-650-9127
                                    888-650-9127
                                    Fax: 301-565-9670
                                    e-mail: info@canceradvocacy.org
                                    www.canceradvocacy.org

NCCS advocates for quality cancer care for all people touched by cancer and provides tools that empower people to advocate for themselves. Founded by and for cancer survivors, NCCS created the widely accepted definition of survivorship and defines someone as a cancer survivor from the time of diagnosis and for the balance of life.

Michael L Kappel, Chair
Samira K Beckwith, Vice Chair
Barbara Hoffman J.D, Secretary

State Agencies & Support Groups

New York

140   Leukemia Society of America - Westchester/ Hudson Valley Chapter
Leukemia & Lymphoma Society
1311 Mamaroneck Avenue, Suite 130
White Plains, NY 10605
                                    914-949-5213
                                    Fax: 914-949-6691
                                    e-mail: infocenter@lls.org
                                    www.lls.org

Cure leukemia, lymphoma, Hodgkin's disease and myeloma and improve the quality of life of patients and their families.

Timothy S Durst, Chair of the Board
James H Davis Ph.D., Vice Chair
Kenneth Shwartz, Secretary/Treasurer

141   Leukemia Society of America - Western New York & Finger Lakes Chapter
Leukemia Society of America
1311 Mamaroneck Avenue, Suite 310
White Plains, NY 10605
                                    914-949-5213
                                    800-955-4572
                                    Fax: 914-949-6691
                                    e-mail: infocenter@lls.org
                                    www.lls.org

Dedicated to finding cures for leukemia and related cancers and to improving the quality of life for patients and their families.

Timothy S. Durst, Chair of the Board
James A. Beck, Executive Director
William G. Behnke, Board of Director

North Carolina

142   Leukemia & Lymphoma Society-Western NC Chapter
Leukemia & Lymphoma Society
4530 Park Road Suite 240
Charlotte, NC 28209
                                    704-705-1850
                                    800-888-9934
                                    Fax: 704-998-5010
                                    www.lls.org

Dedicated to finding cures for leukemia and related cancers and to improving the quality of life for patients and their families.

Abby Miller, Team In Training, Campaign Director
Gwen Tolman, Team In Training, Campaign Manager
Emily Greenfield, Light The Night, Campaign Manager

Ohio

143   Leukemia Society of America - Central Ohio Chapter
Leukemia Society of America
2225 Citygate Drive, Suite E
Columbus, OH 43219
                                    614-476-7194
                                    800-686-CURE
                                    Fax: 614-476-7189
                                    e-mail: timothy.hamburger@lls.org
                                    www.lls.org

Dedicated to finding cures for leukemia and related cancers and to improving the quality of life for patients and their families.

Timothy Hamburger, Executive Director
Dan Swisher, Office Manager
Melissa Shawver, Patient Services Manager

144   Leukemia Society of America - Northern Ohio Chapter
Leukemia Society of America
5700 Brecksville Road 3rd Floor
Independence, OH 44131
                                    216-264-5680
                                    800-589-5721
                                    Fax: 440-617-2879
                                    e-mail: amy.pausche@LLS.org
                                    www.lls.org

Dedicated to finding cures for leukemia and related cancers and to improving the quality of life for patients and their families.

Amy Pausche, Executive Director
Deborah Kending, Patient Services Manager
Peggy Stephens, Light The Night Walk, Manager

145   Leukemia Society of America - Southern Ohio Chapter
Leukemia Society of America
4370 Glendale Milford Road
Cincinnati, OH 45242
                                    513-698-2828
                                    Fax: 513-351-5386
                                    e-mail: michelle.steed@lls.org
                                    www.lls.org

Dedicated to finding cures for leukemia and related cancers and to improving the quality of life for patients and their families. This chapter serves a 22-county geographic area that includes Adams, Brown, Butler, Clermont, Clinton, Darke, Gallia, Greene, Hamilton, Highland, Jackson, Lawrence, Meigs, Miami, Montgomery, Pike, Preble, Scioto and Warren counties in Ohio and Boone, Campbell and Kenton counties in Kentucky.

Michelle Steed, Executive Director
Jackie Personett, Patient Services Manager
Tom Carleton, Senior Campaign Manager, Special Ev

Oklahoma

146 The Leukemia & Lymphoma Society
Leukemia & Lymphoma Society
500 N Broadway, Suite 250
Oklahoma City, OK 73102
405-943-8888
888-828-4572
Fax: 405-945-8355
e-mail: sean.simpson@lls.org
www.lls.org

Our Mission: Cure leukemia, lymphoma, Hodgkin's disease and myeloma, and improve the quality of life for patients and their families.

Sean Simpson, Executive Director
Bryn Mecum, Team in Training Campaign Director
Alisia Davis, Patient Services Manager

Oregon

147 Leukemia Society of America - Oregon Chapter
Leukemia Society of America
9320 SW Barbur Boulevard Suite 350
Portland, OR 97219
503-245-9866
800-466-6572
Fax: 503-245-9865
e-mail: sarah.harris@lls.org
www.lls.org

Dedicated to finding cures for leukemia and related cancers and to improving the quality of life for patients and their families.

Sarah Harris, Executive Director
Sue Sumpter, Patient Services Manager
Morgan Tashea, Team In Training Coordinator - Mara

Pennsylvania

148 Leukemia Society of America - Western Pennsylvania/West Virginia Chapter
Leukemia Society of America
E. Carson Street, Ste. 441
Pittsburgh, PA 15219
412-263-2873
800-726-2873
Fax: 412-395-2888
e-mail: christina.massari@lls.org
www.lls.org

Dedicated to finding cures for leukemia and related cancers and to improving the quality of life for patients and their families.

Tina Massari, Executive Director
Jeanne Caliguri, Director of Development
Francine Morrison, Patient Services Manager

Tennessee

149 Leukemia & Lymphoma Society, Tennessee Chapter
404 BNA Drive, Suite 102
Nashville, TN 37217
615-331-2980
800-332-2980
Fax: 615-331-2941
e-mail: jeff.parsley@lls.org
www.lls.org

To better serve the needs of Tennesseans - offers contribution-funded community services, family support groups, free educational materials and financial assistance for those affected by leukemia, Hodgkin's disease, myeloma and the lymphomas.

Jeff Parsley, Executive Director
Tricia Ward, Campaign Manager
Kim Patterson, Senior Campaign Director

Texas

150 Leukemia Society of America - North Texas Chapter
Leukemia Society of America
8111 LBJ Freeway, Suite 425
Dallas, TX 75251
972-996-5900
800-800-6702
Fax: 972-239-0892
e-mail: carol.withers@lls.org
www.lls.org

Dedicated to finding cures for leukemia and related cancers and to improving the quality of life for patients and their families.

Carol Withers, Office Manager
Stacey Russell, Deputy Executive Director
Jane Beeson, Patient Services Coordinator

151 Leukemia Society of America - South/West Texas Chapter
Leukemia Society of America
950 Isom Road
San Antonio, TX 78216
210-377-1775
800-683-2458
www.lls.org

Dedicated to finding cures for leukemia and related cancers and to improving the quality of life for patients and their families.

Kathleen Griesenbeck, Executive Director
Deborah Barker, Deputy Executive Director
Nicole Bell, Patient Services Coordinator

152 Leukemia Society of America - Texas Gulf Coast Chapter
Leukemia Society of America
5433 Westheimer Suite 300
Houston, TX 77056
713-840-0483
Fax: 281-683-9504
e-mail: billiesue.parris@lls.org
www.lls.org

Dedicated to finding cures for leukemia and related cancers and to improving the quality of life for patients and their families.

Billie Sue Parris, Executive Director
Janie Moore, Deputy Executive Director
Cherry Evans, Patient Services Manager

Virginia

153 Leukemia Society of America - National Capital Area Chapter
Leukemia Society of America
5845 Richmond Highway, Suite 800
Alexandria, VA 22303
703-399-2900
Fax: 703-960-0920
e-mail: gabrielle.urquhart@lls.org
www.lls.org

Serves the greater Washington DC metropolitan area, including Northern Virginia, Prince George's and Montgomery counties.

Gabrielle Urquhart, Executive Director
Beth Gorman, Deputy Executive Director
Katherine Goode, Donor Development, Director

Wisconsin

154 Leukemia Society of America - Wisconsin Chapter
Leukemia Society of America
200 S. Executive Drive Suite 203
Brookfield, WI 53005
262-790-4701
800-261-7399
Fax: 262-790-4706
e-mail: annmarie.frakes@lls.org
www.lls.org

To serve Wisconsites touched by leukemia, lymphoma, Hodgkin's disease and myeloma.

Ann Marie Frakes, Executive Director
Karen Ropel, Operations Director
Lisa Weisman, Campaign Director, Light The Night

Libraries & Resource Centers

155 Children's National Medical Center
University of South Carolina School of Medicine
111 Michigan Avenue NW
Washington, DC 20010   202-476-5000
                                              888-884-2327
                        e-mail: tbear@childrensnational.org
                                  www.childrensnational.org

Children's National serves as the regional referral center for pediatric emergency, cancer, trauma, cardiac and critical care as well as neonatology, orthopaedic surgery, neurology, and neurosurgery.

Kurt Newman, MD, President/CEO
Mendel Tuchman, Chief Research Officer
Nellie Robinson, Executive Vice President

Audio Video

156 Coping with Childhood Cancer
Films for the Humanities and Sciences
132 West 31st Street
New York, NY 10001   800-257-5126
                                          Fax: 609-275-0266
                            e-mail: custserv@films.com
                                        www.ffh.films.com

Coping with chronic and perhaps fatal disease and gaining control over their lives is something that childhood cancer victims must learn. This program presents open and honest interviews with five family members of childhood cancer patients. The stress on the family is intense; ofteh, the brothers and sisters of children with cancer or any chronic life-threatening illness are most severely affected emotionally.

28 minutes
ISBN: 1-421320-42-7

Web Sites

157 CancerCare
275 Seventh Avenue
New York, NY 10001   800-813-4673
                            e-mail: info@cancercare.org
                                        www.cancercare.org

CancerCare is a national nonprofit, 501(c)(3) organization that provides free, professional support services to anyone affected by cancer: people with cancer, caregivers, children, loved ones, and the bereaved. CancerCare programs - including counseling and support groups, education, financial assistance and practical help - are provided by professional oncology social workers and are completely free of charge.

Patricia J. Goldsmith, Chief Executive Officer
John Rutigliano, Chief Operating Officer
Ellen Miller Sonet, MBA, JD, Chief Strategy & Alliance Officer

158 Children's Cancer Web
www.cancerindex.org/ccw

An independent nonprofit site, established to provide a directory of childhood cancer resources.

159 Leukemia and Lymphoma Society of America
1311 Mamaroneck Avenue, Suite 310
White Plains, NY 10605   914-949-5213
                                          Fax: 914-949-6691
                                                 www.lls.org

Is the largest voluntary health organization dedicated to funding blood cancer research, education and patient services. The mission is to cure leukemia, lymphoma, Hodgkin's disease and myeloma, and to improve the quality of life of patients and their families.

Louis J. DeGennaro, Ph.D., President/ CEO
Rosemarie Loffredo, CAO/ CFO
Mark Roithmayr, Chief Development Officer

160 Mediconsult
www.mediconsult.com

We are committed to provide excellent and professional services to our business partners. Through a team approach we will develop, provide and continuously improve our knowledge and competency. We work towards the betterment of healthcare delivery systems for the community.

Book Publishers

161 Blood & Circulatory Disorders Sourcebook 2nd Edition
Omnigraphics
PO Box 625
Holmes, PA 19043   800-234-1340
                                          Fax: 800-875-1340
                          e-mail: info@omnigraphics.com
                                      www.omnigraphics.com

Basic consumer health information on blood and its components, anemias, leukemias, bleeding disorders, and circulatory disorders, including aplastic anemia, thalassemia, sickle-cell disease and hemophilia.

659 pages
ISBN: 0-780817-46-4

162 Let's Talk About Going to the Hospital
Rosen Publishing Group's PowerKids Press
29 E 21st Street
New York, NY 10010   212-777-3017
                                              800-237-9932
                                          Fax: 888-436-4643
                        e-mail: rosenpub@tribeca.ios.com
                                   www.rosenpublishing.com

If a child has to check into the hospital, chances are he or she is already upset about being ill. Knowing how a hospital functions and what the procedures are, such as when family members can visit, will help in what is already a stressful situation. Grades K-5.

24 pages
ISBN: 0-823950-36-0

163 Let's Talk About when Kids Have Cancer
Rosen Publishing Group's PowerKids Press
29 E 21st Street
New York, NY 10010   212-777-3017
                                              800-237-9932
                                          Fax: 888-436-4643
                      e-mail: customerservice@rosenpub.com
                                   www.rosenpublishing.com

In a straightforward yet comforting way, this book explains what cancer is, what kinds of treatments surround the disease and how to cope if a child has cancer.

24 pages
ISBN: 0-823951-95-2

164 Pediatric Cancer Sourcebook
Omnigraphics
PO Box 31-1640
Detroit, PA 48231   800-234-1340
                                          Fax: 800-875-1340
                          e-mail: info@omnigraphics.com
                                            omnigraphics.com

Basic consumer health information about leukemias, brain tumors, sarcomas, lymphomas and other cancers in infants, children and adolescents.

587 pages
ISBN: 0-780802-45-4

165 Surviving Childhood Cancer: A Guide for Families
New Harbinger Publications
5674 Shattuck Avenue
Oakland, CA 94609   510-652-0215
                                              800-748-6273
                                          Fax: 800-652-1613
                  e-mail: customerservice@newharbinger.com
                                           newharbinger.com

Cancer in a child is an overwhelming experience for a family. This book explains common medical procedures and offers readers practical advice about how to cope with emotions and stress during this time.

1998 232 pages
ISBN: 1-572241-02-0

Pamphlets

166 Acute Lymphocytic Leukemia
Leukemia and Lymphoma Society
1311 Mamaroneck Avenue, Suite 310
White Plains, NY 10605
                              914-949-5213
                         Fax: 914-949-6691
                               www.lls.org

Information about acute lymphocytic leukemia for patients and their families and a glossary of terms to help readers understand technical terms.

16 pages

Louis J. DeGennaro, Ph.D., President/ CEO
Rosemarie Loffredo, CAO/ CFO
Mark Roithmayr, Chief Development Officer

Camps

167 Arizona Camp Sunrise
4550 E Bell Rd, Suite 126
Phoenix, AZ 85032
                              602-778-7629
                              800-865-1582
                         Fax: 602-404-1118
            e-mail: melissa@azcampsunrise.org
                       www.azcampsunrise.org

The camp is dedicated to provide an exciting, medically safe camp program for children who have or have had cancer and their siblings.

Melissa Lee, Camp Director

168 Camp Catch-A-Rainbow
American Cancer Society
1205 E Saginaw Street
Lansing, MI 48906
                              517-371-2920
                              800-227-2345
             www.cancer.org/camprainbow

Open to any child who has, or has had, cancer.

169 Camp Fantastic
Special Love
117 Youth Development Court
Winchester, VA 22602
                              703-667-3774

Nonprofit organization that provides enriching programs for children with cancer, including Camp Fantastic.

170 Camp Sunshine Dreams
PO Box 28232
Fresno, CA 93729   e-mail: contact@campsunshinedreams.com
                      www.campsunshinedreams.com

Summer camp for children with cancer.

171 Des Moines YMCA Camp
1192 166th Drive
Boone, IA
                              515-432-7558
                         Fax: 515-432-5414
                e-mail: ycamp@dmymca.org
                            www.y-camp.org

For boys and girls with cancer, diabetes, asthma, cystic fibrosis, hearing impaired and other disabilities.

David Sherry, Executive Director
Mike Havlik, Program Director
Alex Kretzinger, Program Director- Summer Camp

172 Okizu Foundation Camps
16 Digital Drive, Suite 130
Novato, CA 94949
                              415-382-9083
                         Fax: 415-382-8384
                    e-mail: info@okizu.org
                             www.okizu.org

This foundation runs family camp programs for children who have cancer and their families, and for children who have or had a parent with cancer.

Suzie Randall, Executive Director
Heather Ferrier, Director of Operations
Beth Dekker, Assistant Camp Director

Description

173   ALBINISM

Covers these related disorders: Tyrosinase negative albinism, Oculocutaneous albinism, Waardenburg syndrome

Involves the following Biologic System(s):

Dermatologic Disorders,
Genetic/Chromosomal/Syndrome/Metabolic Disorders

Albinism refers to a condition that is present at birth (congenital) and results from an inability of the body to produce and distribute the pigment melanin, which normally gives the skin, hair, and eyes their coloration. Albinism occurs in all races and in about one in 20,000 individuals worldwide.

Although there are several types of albinism, and all are caused by genetic defects, two major forms of the condition - tyrosinase-negative, and tyrosinase-positive - have been identified.

Tyrosinase-negative, or type I, albinism is the most severe form of generalized oculocutaneous albinism, or OCA. It results from a genetic defect that reduces or eliminates the activity of tyrosinase, an enzyme essential to the proper metabolism of melanin. Because of the absence of this enzyme, type I is characterized by a complete lack of melanin in the hair, skin, and eyes, resulting in pink or white skin, white hair, and eyes that may appear pink or bluish-gray. Other eye-related or optical irregularities also occur in type I, such as involuntary, flickering-type movements of the eyes (nystagmus), nearsightedness (myopia), and sensitivity or intolerance to bright light (photophobia). OCA type 1 is an autosomal recessive condition, meaning that it develops only when both parents carry the gene responsible for OCA type 1. A variant form of OCA type 1, in which some pigmentation develops in the skin, hair, and eyes with age, occurs in Amish communities in the United States. The optical irregularities in this variant form of OCA type 1 are usually less severe than in the more common form of the condition.

Tyrosinase-positive, or type II OCA is more common and less severe than type I. Rather than being caused by an absence of the enzyme tyrosinase, this type of albinism is thought to result from an inborn error in the transport of the substance known as tyrosinea which the body normally transforms into melanin. Newborns with OCA type II may have little to no melanin at birth, but it may accumulate in their skin, hair, and eyes as these children grow, producing some darkening of skin color during the course of childhood. Moreover, ocular abnormalities present at birth may ease over the course of childhood. Like OCA type I, OCA type II is caused by a genetic defect and is inherited as an autosomal recessive trait. Several variant forms of tyrosinase-positive albinism may be present as a part of several syndromes that affect other organs or systems of the body in addition to its pigmentation. Among these syndromes are Hermansky-Pudlak syndrome, Chediak-Higashi syndrome, and Cross-McKusick-Breen syndrome.

Types of albinism other than OCA types I and II may include ocular albinism that chiefly affects the pigmentation of the eyes and is characterized by photophobia; nystagmus; and decreased visual acuity. The hair and eyes of such persons may

be of lighter than average color, but not excessively so. In what are known as Nettleship-Falls type ocular albinism and Forsius-Eriksson syndrome, ocular albinism may be inherited as a trait, or characteristic, that is associated with or "linked to" the X chromosome, which is inherited from an individual's mother. Ocular albinism may also be inherited as an autosomal dominant trait, in which it results from only a single copy of a defective gene, inherited from either a mother or a father.

Besides these various types of albinism, some individuals may have partial albinism, sometimes called piebaldism, which is characterized by patchy, unpigmented areas of hair or skin. In some individuals this type of albinism may be manifested only by a lock of white hair near the forehead. Piebaldism is inherited as an autosomal dominant trait, and may be part of the condition known as Waardenburg syndrome, which is also characterized by hearing impairment.

Because people with albinism have an increased risk of developing skin cancer from exposure to the sun, protection of their skin is highly important. This may be accomplished with suitable clothing and the use of an appropriate sunscreen of SPF 15 or greater. The deficit in pigmentation of the eyes in albinism may require the use of tinted or dark glasses to reduce light sensitivity. Children with albinism should have early evaluation and treatment for any visual irregularities caused by the condition, to minimize any difficulties at school. Other treatment is symptomatic and supportive.

Government Agencies

174   NIH/National Institute of Child Health and Human Development
31 Center Drive, Building 31 Room 2A32
Bethesda, MD 20892
800-370-2943
Fax: 301-496-1104
TTY: 888-320-6942
e-mail: NICHDInformationResourceCenter@mail.nih.
www.nichd.nih.gov

Established in 1962 by congress, today the institute conducts and supports laboratory research, clinical trials, and epidemiological studies that explore health processes; examines the impact of disabilities, diseases, and variations on the lives of individuals; and sponsors training programs for scientists, health care providers, and researchers to ensure that NICHD research can continue.

Alan E Guttmacher MD, Director
Lisa Kaeser, Program & Public Liaison

National Associations & Support Groups

175   American Academy of Pediatrics
141 Northwest Point Boulevard
Elk Grove Village, IL 60007
847-434-4000
800-433-9016
Fax: 847-434-8000
www.aap.org

The American Academy of Pediatrics and its member pediatricians are committed to the attainment of optimal physical, mental and social health and well-being for all infants, children, adolescents, and young adults.

Sandra Hassink, MD, FAAP, President

176   American Council of the Blind
2200 Wilson Boulevard, Suite 650
Arlington, VA 22201
202-467-5081
800-424-8666
Fax: 703-465-5085
e-mail: info@acb.org
www.acb.org

The council strives to improve the well being of all blind and visually impaired people by serving as a representative national organization of blind people, elevating the social, ecomonic and cultural levels of blind people, improving educational and rehabilitation facilities and opportunities and cooperating with the public and private institutions and organizations concerned with blind services.

Mith Pomerantz, President
Kim Charlson, First Vice President
Brenda Dillon, Second Vice President

177   American Foundation for the Blind
2 Penn Plaza, Suite 1102
New York, NY 10121   212-502-7600
                                            800-232-5463
                                        Fax: 888-545-8331
                                  e-mail: afbinfo@afb.net
                                            www.afb.org

The American Foundation of the Blind, has been eliminating barriers the prevent people who are blind or visually impaired from reaching their potential. AFB is dedicated to addressing the most critical issues of facing this growing population: independent living, literacy, employment, and technology.

Carl R Augusto, President
Paul Schroeder, Vice President
Heidi Kurtz, Programs and Policy Coordinator

178   American School Counselor Association
1101 King Street, Suite 310
Alexandria, VA 22314   703-683-2722
                                            800-306-4722
                                        Fax: 703-997-7572
                            e-mail: asca@schoolcounselor.org
                                   www.schoolcounselor.org

The mission of ASCA is to represent professional school counselors and to promote professionalism and ethical practices.

Richard Wong, Executive Director
Jeff Broderson, Information Technology Admin.
Kathleen M Rakestraw, Director of Communications

179   Genetic Alliance
4301 Connecticut Avenue NW, Suite 404
Washington, DC 20008   202-966-5557
                                            800-336-4363
                                        Fax: 202-966-8553
                             e-mail: info@geneticalliance.org
                                    www.geneticalliance.org

World's leading nonprofit health advocacy organization committed to transforming health through genetics and promoting an environment of openness centered on the health of individuals, families, and communities.

Sharon Terry, President
Lisa Wise, Chief Operating Officer
Tetyana Murza MES, Managing Director

180   Hermansky-Pudlak Syndrome Network
One South Road
Oyster Bay, NY 11771   516-922-3440
                                            800-789-9477
                                        Fax: 516-922-0640
                               e-mail: info@hpsnetwork.org
                                      www.hpsnetwork.org

A volunteer, support group for people and families dealing with Hermansky-Pudlak Syndrome (HPS) and related disorders such as Chediak Higashi Syndrome.

Donna Jean Appell, Founder & President
Heather Kirkwood, VP, Director of Outreach
Richard Appell, Treasurer

181   Natalie's Way Foundation
16 Lyle Court
Staten Island, NY 10306   718-351-0806
                       e-mail: admin@natalieswayfoundation.com
                                       www.ourwebpage.org

Conducts fundraising for research into albinism and children's eye disorders.

Robert Stasi, President
Annette Stasi, VP

182   National Mental Health Consumers' Self-Help Clearinghouse
1211 Chestnut Street, Suite 1207
Philadelphia, PA 19107   215-751-1810
                                            800-553-4539
                                        Fax: 215-636-6312
                               e-mail: info@mhselfhelp.org
                                      www.mhselfhelp.org

The Clearinghouse works to foster peer empowerment through our website, up-to-date news and information announcements, a directory of peer-driven services, electronic and printed publications, training packages, and individual and onsite consultation

Joseph Rogers, Executive Director & Founder
Susan Rogers, Director of Special Projects
Britani Nestel, Program Specialist

183   National Organization for Albinism and Hypopigmentation
PO Box 959
East Hampstead, NH 03826   603-887-2310
                                            800-473-2310
                                        Fax: 800-648-2310
                            e-mail: webmaster@albinism.org
                                        www.albinism.org

NOAH is a volunteer organization for persons and families involved with the condition of albinism. It does not diagnose, treat, or provide genetic counseling. It is involved in self-help, while trying to promote research and education.

Mike McGowan, Executive Director & Founder
Sheila Adamo, Chair
Donna Appell, Vice Chair

184   Positive Exposure
Rick Guidotti
43 E 20th Street, 6th Floor
New York, NY 10003   212-420-1931
                                        Fax: 212-228-0592
                            e-mail: rick@positiveexposure.org
                                     www.rickguidotti.com

Utilizes photography and video interviews to investigate the social and psychological experiences of people with albinism of all ages and ethnocultural heritages. This innovative program challenges the stigma associated with difference, attacks public fears about difference and celebrates the richness of genetic variation.

Rick Guidotti, Founder and Director
Liz Matejka Grossman, Executive Director
Cecilia Burbridge, Administrative Assistant

185   Society for Pediatric Dermatology
8365 Keystone Crossing, Suite 107
Indianapolis, IN 46240   317-202-0224
                                        Fax: 317-205-9841
                               e-mail: spd@hp-assoc.org
                                        www.pedsderm.net

The objective of the Society is to promote, develop and advance education, research and care of skin disease in all pediatric age groups.

Kent Lindeman, Executive Director
Robin Hornung, Dermatologist
Amy Theos, Dermatologist

186   Vision of Children Foundation
4310 Genesee Ave, Suite 101
San Diego, CA 92117   858-560-5181
                                        Fax: 858-560-1926
                      e-mail: frontoffice@visionsource-drsneag.com
                                 www.visionsource-drsneag.com

Provides information, promotes research and assists the families of blind and visually impaired children, including those with ocular albinism, in locating organizations and service providers who can give support.

Gary Sneag, Manager
Vivian L Hardage, Chairman & Co-Founder
Stephanie Durso, Executive Director

Conferences

187 Annual World Symposium on Ocular Albinism
11975 El Camino Real, Suite 104
San Diego, CA 92130   858-314-7917
                                  Fax: 858-314-7920
                     e-mail: info@visionofchildren.org
                              www.visionofchildren.org

The Vision of Children Foundation's team of doctors, scientists and researchers will collaborate on their research efforts in Ocular Albinism.

March

Samuel A Hardage, Chairman & Co-Founder
Vivian L Hardage, Co-Founder
Debora B Farber, Chief Scientific Advisor

188 Genetic Alliance Annual Conference
Genetic Alliance
4301 Connecticut Avenue NW, Suite 404
Washington, DC 20008   202-966-5557
                                       800-336-4363
                                  Fax: 202-966-8553
                       e-mail: info@geneticalliance.org
                              www.geneticalliance.org

Consistently inspirational and enables partnership among all stakeholders: advocates and community leaders, health and industry professionals, policymakers, and academicians.

July

Sharon Terry, President/CEO
Tetyana Murza, Programs/Events Manager

189 Hermansky-Pudlak Syndrome Network Annual Family Conference
One South Road
Oyster Bay, NY 11771   516-922-3440
                                       800-789-9477
                                  Fax: 516-922-4022
                        e-mail: appell@worldnet.att.net
                              www.medhelp.org/web/hpsn.htm

A volunteer, nonprofit, self-help support group for persons and families dealing with the syndrome. Assists in networking families and doctors, maintains a bibliography of materials and promotes research.

Donna Jean Appell, Founder & President

190 NFB National Convention
American Foundation for the Blind
2 Penn Plaza, Suite 1102
New York, NY 10121   212-502-7600; 800-232-5463
                                  Fax: 212-502-7777
                              e-mail: afbinfo@afb.net
                                       www.afb.org

The largest disability conference of its kind.

3000

Carl R Augusto, President/CEO
Paul Schroeder, Vice President
Rick Bozeman, CFO

191 National Organization for Albinism and Hypopigmentation Bi-Annual Conference
PO Box 959
East Hampstead, NH 03826   603-887-2310
                                       800-473-2310
                                  Fax: 800-648-2310
                       e-mail: webmaster@albinism.org
                                       www.albinism.org

NOAH holds a national conference every other year (even years).

192 Society for Pediatric Dermatology Annual Meeting
8365 Keystone Crossing, Suite 107
Indianapolis, IN 46240   317-202-0224; Fax: 317-205-9841
                              e-mail: spd@hp-assoc.com
                                       www.pedsderm.net

Kent Lindeman, Executive Director

Audio Video

193 Assistive Media
400 Maynard Street, Suite 404
Ann Arbor, MI 48104   734-332-0369
                       e-mail: info@assistivemedia.org
                              www.assistivemedia.org/

The mission of Assistive Media is to heighten the educational, cultural, and quality-of-living standard for people with disabilites and help achieve independence and become better integrated within the mainstream of society and community life in general. Assistve Media accomplishes this by providing free-of-charge, copyright-approved, high caliber audio literary works to the world-wide disability community via the internet effectively, inexpensively, and efficiently.

David Henry Erdody, Founder

Web Sites

194 International Albinism Center
www.cbc.umn.edu/iac/

IAC is a team of dedicated research professionals interested in understanding the basis of albinism in humans. We are a munlti-disciplinary group of researchers that include interests in clinical genetics, molecular biology, ophthalmology, dermatology, and biochemistry, all with a central theme of understnading the cause and effect of albinism and other forms of pigment loss in humans.

Newsletters

195 Hermansky-Pudlak Syndrome Network Newsletter
One South Road
Oyster Bay, NY 11771   516-922-3440
                                       800-789-9477
                                  Fax: 516-624-0640
                       e-mail: info@hpsnetwork.org
                                       www.hpsnetwork.org

A volunteer, nonprofit, self-help support group for persons and families dealing with the syndrome. Assists in networking families and doctors, maintains a bibliography of materials and promotes research.

Donna Jean Appell, R.N., Founder/President
Heather Kirkwood, VP/ Director of Outreach
Richard Appell, Treasurer

Camps

196 Camp Discovery
American Academy of Dermatology
930 E Woodfield Road
Schaumburg, IL 60173   847-240-1280
                                       866-503-7546
                                  Fax: 847-240-1859
                        e-mail: jmueller@aad.org
                                       www.campdiscovery.org

A camp for young people with chronic skin conditions. There is no fee and transportation is provided. Three locations: Camp Horizon in Millville, PA, Camp Knutson in Crosslake, MN, and Camp Dermadillo in Burton, TX.

David M Pariser, MD, President
Janine Mueller, Program Coordinator

Description

197 ALOPECIA AREATA

Synonyms: Alopecia circumscripta, Androgenetic alopecia, Pelade

Involves the following Biologic System(s):

Dermatologic Disorders, Immunologic and Rheumatologic Disorders

Alopecia is partial or complete loss of hair (baldness) and may result from genetic factors, aging or local or systemic disease. Alopecia areata is characterized by the sudden, localized loss of patches of scalp hair and other areas of hair growth, such as the eyelashes and eyebrows. These patches are usually well-defined, round or oval in shape, and most often appear on the scalp or beard area. On rare occasions, progression of hair loss may result in the total loss of scalp hair in a condition called alopecia totalis. If the disease progresses to include the total loss of both scalp and body hair, the condition is called alopecia universalis. Another uncommon form of alopecia areata called ophiasis involves the loss of hair in a continuous band around the head. If hair loss associated with alopecia areata is not widespread, the condition is usually reversible, with most patients exhibiting new hair growth within a few months to a year; however, recurrences are quite common. Children who develop this condition at a very young age, patients who experience recurring episodes, and those who have extensive involvement are less likely to experience spontaneous remission. Although this disease occurs most commonly in the adult population, approximately 20 percent of those affected develop the disorder between birth and 20 years of age. This type of hair loss is different than male pattern baldness, an inherited condition.

Although the skin in the area of hair loss may appear unremarkable, microscopic examination may reveal the presence of inflammation. In addition, some individual hairs that appear at the margins of the bald, patchy areas may be easily removed and, upon microscopic examination, reveal a lightly-pigmented, tapered hair shaft that ends in a hair root that is reduced in size (exclamation hairs). Symptoms or characteristic findings sometimes associated with alopecia areata include the development of irregularities such as nail pitting and ridging, allergic or hypersensitivity reactions, and opacities of the lenses of the eye (cataracts). Alopecia areata may also be associated with certain autoimmune diseases such as Addison disease, Hashimoto thyroiditis, vitiligo, and others. In addition, approximately seven percent of children with Trisomy 21 exhibit the symptoms associated with alopecia areata.

The exact cause of alopecia areata is not known; however, approximately 25 percent of those affected are believed to inherit the disease through autosomal dominant transmission. Other suggested causes include autoimmune responses or emotional factors related to stress. Because alopecia areata so often resolves spontaneously, treatment for this disease in young children may simply include ongoing observation. A variety of treatments can be tried. Steroid injections and cream to the scalp have been used for many years. Other medications include minoxidil, irritants (anthralin or topical coal tar), and topical immunotherapy (cyclosporine), each of which are sometimes used in different combinations. The use of hairpieces and other cosmetic considerations may be beneficial to the emotional well-being of children, especially adolescents, with alopecia areata.

National Associations & Support Groups

198 American Academy of Dermatology
PO Box 4014
Schaumburg, IL 60168
866-503-7546
Fax: 847-240-1859
e-mail: MRC@aad.org
www.aad.org

The AAD is the largest, and most representative dermatology group in the United States.

Dirk M. Elston, President
Lisa A. Garner MD, Vice President
Brett M Coldiron MD, President-Elect

199 American Academy of Pediatrics
141 Northwest Point Boulevard
Elk Grove Village, IL 60007
847-434-4000
800-433-9016
Fax: 847-434-8000
www.aap.org

The American Academy of Pediatrics and its member pediatricians are committed to the attainment of optimal physical, mental and social health and well-being for all infants, children, adolescents, and young adults.

Sandra Hassink, MD, FAAP, President

200 American Autoimmune Related Diseases Association, Inc.
22100 Gratiot Avenue
East Detroit, MI 48021
586-776-3900
Fax: 586-776-3903
e-mail: aarda@aarda.org
www.aarda.org

The American Autoimmune Related Diseases Association is dedicated to the eradication of autoimmune diseases and the alleviation of suffering and the socioeconomic impact of autoimmunity through fostering and facilitating collaboration in the areas of education, public awareness, research, and patient services in an effective, ethical and efficient manner.

Betty Diamond MD, Chair
Noel R Rose MD, PhD, Chairman Emeritus

201 American Hair Loss Association
23679 Calabasas Road #682
Calabasas, CA 91301
e-mail: inquire@americanhairloss.org
www.americanhairloss.org

The American Hair Loss Association is committed to educating and improving the lives of all those affected by hair loss. It is their goal to create public awareness of this devastating disease of the spirit, and to legitimize hair loss of all forms in the eyes of our medical community, the media and society as a whole.

202 Children's Alopecia Project
PO Box 6036
Wyomissing, PA 19610
610-468-1011
e-mail: info@childrensalopeciaproject.org
www.childrensalopeciaproject.org

The mission is to help any child in need who is living with hair loss due to all forms of Alopecia.

Betsy Woytovich, Executive Director
Wayne Gehris, President
Christine Cieplinski, Vice President

203 National Alopecia Areata Foundation
14 Mitchell Boulevard
San Rafael, CA 94903
415-472-3780
Fax: 415-472-5343
e-mail: info@naaf.org
www.naaf.org

NAAF supports research to find a cure or acceptable treatment for alopecia areata, supports those with the disease, and educates the public about alopecia areata. NAAF is widely regarded as the largest, most influential and most representative foundation associated with alopecia areata.

Alopecia Areata / Conferences

Maureen McGettigan, Chair
Bob Flint, Chief Financial Officer
Hoy Lanning, Secretary

204   Society for Pediatric Dermatology
8365 Keystone Crossing, Suite 107
Indianapolis, IN 46240
317-202-0224
Fax: 317-205-9841
e-mail: spd@hp-assoc.com
www.pedsderm.net

The objective of the Society is to promote, develop and advance education, research and care of skin disease in all pediatric age groups.

Kent Lindeman, Executive Director
Robin Hornung, Dermatologist
Amy Theos, Dermatologist

Conferences

205   National Alopecia Areata Foundation Annual Conference
National Alopecia Areata Foundation
14 Mitchell Boulevard
San Rafael, CA 94903
415-472-3780
Fax: 415-472-5343
e-mail: info@naaf.org
www.naaf.org

A four day conference for people of all ages who have alopecia areata or care about someone who has alopecia areata. Provides the attendee with the latest medical and research updates, to better understand and manage alopecia areata, and also provides them with a wealth of support.

June

Vicki Kalabokes, President/CEO
Jeanne Rappoport, VP Administration/Meetings

Web Sites

206   Children's Alopecia Project
www.childrensalopeciaproject.org

The mission is to help any child in need who is living with hair loss due to all forms of Alopecia.

Jeff Woytovich, Founder/Director
Betsy Woytovich, Co-Founder
Christine Cieplinski, President

Newsletters

207   Infocus Newsletter
American Autoimmune Related Diseases Associaion
22100 Gratiot Avenue
Eastpointe, MI 48021
586-776-3900
Fax: 586-776-3903
www.aarda.org

The national newsletter of AARDA.

The Rev. Herbert G. Ford, D. Min., Chairman of the Board
Stanley M. Finger, Ph.D., Vice Chairperson
Virginia T. Ladd, President/ Executive Director

208   National Alopecia Areata Foundation Newsletter
National Alopecia Areata Foundation
65 Mitchell Boulevard, Suite 200-B
San Rafael, CA 94903
415-472-3780
Fax: 415-480-1800
e-mail: info@naaf.org
www.naaf.org

NAAF publishes their award winning newsletter four times a year. It is a great resource and is written especially for the alopecia areata community.

Vicki Kalabokes, President/CEO
Jeanne Rappoport, Chief Administrative Officer
Maureen Smith, Chief Development Strategist

Description

209 **ALPHA-1-ANTITRYPSIN DEFICIENCY**
Involves the following Biologic System(s):
Gastrointestinal Disorders,
Genetic/Chromosomal/Syndrome/Metabolic Disorders, Respiratory
Disorders

Alpha-1-antitrypsin (AAT) deficiency is a hereditary metabolic disorder characterized by deficiency of alpha-1-antitrypsin, an enzyme that is produced by the liver and inhibits the actions of other enzymes that break down certain proteins. Deficiency of alpha-1-antitrypsin may result in emphysema, a progressive destructive change in the lungs. In addition, some patients may experience liver disease that is thought to result from abnormal retention of the alpha-1-antitrypsin enzyme in liver cells. Alpha-1-antitrypsin deficiency is caused by certain changes (mutations) of a gene known as Pi (protease inhibitor). Alpha-1-antitrypsin deficiency is typically inherited as an autosomal recessive trait due to inheritance of two deficiency-causing genes (homozygosity).

The specific symptoms associated with alpha-1-antitrypsin deficiency as well as the age of onset vary from patient to patient. Shortly after birth, a small percentage of affected children may develop suppression or cessation of the flow of bile (neonatal cholestasis). Bile, a liquid secreted by the liver, carries waste products away from the liver and assists in the digestion of fats in the small intestine. During the first week of life, affected infants may have yellowish discoloration of the skin, whites of the eyes, and mucous membranes (jaundice); abnormal enlargement of the liver (hepatomegaly); and the presence of unabsorbed fat in the feces. Jaundice often spontaneously resolves within two to four months after birth. Affected infants and children may appear to have no further associated symptoms (asymptomatic), may have chronic liver disease, or, in the most severe cases, may experience scarring of the liver and gradual impairment of liver function (cirrhosis). Older children may develop chronic liver disease or cirrhosis and associated high blood pressure within veins from the spleen and intestines to the liver (portal hypertension). In some patients with portal hypertension, there may be a diversion of portal circulation to veins in the walls of the stomach and esophagus, causing abnormal widening of such blood vessels (esophageal varices). Without treatment, some patients with liver disease may experience potentially life-threatening complications.

In general, AAT deficiency leads to emphysema, progressive degeneration of and destructive changes in the air sacs (alveoli) of the lungs in the fourth decade of life in smokers and a decade later in nonsmokers. (emphysema).

In children with alpha-1-antitrypsin deficiency, the treatment of associated liver disease is primarily symptomatic and supportive. AAT deficiency is the main cause of liver transplantation in children. Preventing or slowing the progression of lung disease is the major goal of AAT deficiency management. No treatment for emphysema has a greater effect on survival than quitting smoking. Other options include prompt, aggressive treatment of respiratory infections and provision of oxygen therapy. Medications are available to improve lung function. In addition, patients should avoid exposure to tobacco smoke, aerosol sprays, and other lung irritants. Alpha-1-antitrypsin enzyme replacement therapy (e.g., prolastin therapy) is also available. Two surgical approaches may help selected patients with AAT deficiency - volume-reduction surgery and lung transplantation.

National Associations & Support Groups

210 **AlphaNet, Inc.**
2937 SW 27 Avenue, Suite 305
Coconut Grove, FL 33133
305-442-1776
800-577-2638
Fax: 305-442-1803
e-mail: info@alphanet.org
www.alphanet.org

Founded to improve the lives of individuals affected by Alpha-1 Antitrypsin Deficiency.AlphaNet provides a wide range of specialized programs and services designed to meet the specific needs of the Alphas it serves.

Robert Barrett, CEO
Robert A. Sandhaus, Medical Director
Janis Berend, Clinical Specialist

211 **American Academy of Pediatrics**
141 Northwest Point Boulevard
Elk Grove Village, IL 60007
847-434-4000
800-433-9016
Fax: 847-434-8000
www.aap.org

The American Academy of Pediatrics and its member pediatricians are committed to the attainment of optimal physical, mental and social health and well-being for all infants, children, adolescents, and young adults.

Sandra Hassink, MD, FAAP, President

212 **American Liver Foundation**
39 Broadway, Suite 2700
New York, NY 10006
212-668-1000
800-465-4837
Fax: 212-483-8179
e-mail: info@liverfoundation.org
www.liverfoundation.org

The American Liver Foundation is the nation's leading nonprofit organization promoting liver health and disease prevention. ALF provides research, education and advocacy for those affected by liver-related diseases, including hepatitis.

Thomas F Nealon III, Chairman of the Board of Directors
Daniel E Weil, Treasurer and Member of the Executi
Carlo Frappolli, Secretary and Member of the Transit

213 **American Lung Association**
1301 Pennsylvania Ave. NW, Suite 800
Washington, DC 20004
202-785-3355
800-548-8252
Fax: 202-452-1805
e-mail: info@alany.org
www.lung.org

The American Lung Association is the leading organization working to save lives by improving lung health and preventing lung disease through Education, Advocacy and Research. With the generous support of the public, we are Fighting for Air.

Don Awerkamp, Ph.D., J.D., Board of Directors
Timothy D. Byrum, MSN, CRNP, Board of Directors
Michael V. Carstens, Board of Directors

214 **Children's Liver Association for Support Services**
25379 Wayne Mills, Suite 143
Valencia, CA 91355
661-263-9099
877-679-8256
Fax: 661-263-9099
e-mail: info@classkids.org
www.classkids.org

CLASS is an all volunteer, nonprofit organization dedicated to serving the emotional, educational and financial needs of families coping with childhood liver disease and transplantation. Our goal is to be both a service to families and a valuable resource for the medical community.

Diane Sumner, President
Ann Whitehead, VP

215 Genetic Alliance
4301 Connecticut Avenue NW Suite 404
Washington, DC 10019
202-966-7955
800-336-4363
Fax: 202-966-8553
e-mail: info@geneticalliance.org
www.geneticalliance.org

World's leading nonprofit health advocacy organization committed to transforming health through genetics and promoting an environment of openness centered on the health of individuals, families, and communities.

Sharon Terry, President
Lisa Wise, Chief Operating Officer
Tetyana Murza MES, Programs and Policy Coordinator

216 March of Dimes Birth Defects Foundation
1275 Mamaroneck Avenue
White Plains, NY 10020
914-997-4488
888-663-4637
Fax: 914-997-4763
e-mail: answers@marchofdimes.com
www.marchofdimes.com

March of Dimes help moms have full-term pregnancies and research the problems that threaten the health of babies.The March of Dimes also acts globally: sharing best practices in perinatal health and helping improve birth outcomes where the needs are the most urgent.

Kenneth A. May, Chair
Jennifer Howse, President & CEO
Alan Fleischman, Medical Director

Conferences

217 Genetic Alliance Annual Conference
Genetic Alliance
4301 Connecticut Avenue NW, Suite 404
Washington, DC 20008
202-966-5557
800-336-4363
Fax: 202-966-8553
e-mail: info@geneticalliance.org
www.geneticalliance.org

Consistently inspirational and enables partnership among all stakeholders: advocates and community leaders, health and industry professionals, policymakers, and academicians.

July

Sharon Terry, President/CEO
Tetyana Murza, Programs/Events Manager

Web Sites

218 Children's Liver Association for Support Services
www.classkids.org

CLASS is an all volunteer, nonprofit organization dedicated to serving the emotional, educational and financial needs of families coping with childhood liver disease and transplantation. Our goal is to be both a service to families and a valuable resource for the medical community.

219 Online Mendelian Inheritance in Man
National Library of Medicine, Building 38A
Bethesda, MD 20894
888-346-3656
e-mail: info@ncbi.nlm.nih.gov
www.ncbi.nlm.nih.gov

This database is a catalog of human genes and genetic disorders.

Christine E. Seidman, M.D., Chair
David J. Lipman, M.D., Executive Secretary

Book Publishers

220 Let's Talk About Going to the Hospital
Rosen Publishing Group's PowerKids Press
29 E 21st Street
New York, NY 10010
212-777-3017
800-237-9932
Fax: 888-436-4643
e-mail: rosenpub@tribeca.ios.com
www.powerkidspress.com

If a child has to check into the hospital, chances are he or she is already upset about being ill. Knowing how a hospital functions and what the procedures are, such as when family members can visit, will help in what is already a stressful situation. Grades K-5.

24 pages
ISBN: 0-823950-36-0

Description

221 ANENCEPHALY

Involves the following Biologic System(s):

Neurologic Disorders

Anencephaly is an abnormality that is present at birth (congenital) and belongs to a group of birth defects known as neural tube defects. This condition is characterized by the absence of a major portion of the brain, skull, and scalp. Approximately one of 1,000 infants is born with anencephaly.

During the early stages of pregnancy, a specialized layer of tissue extends along the back portion of the developing embryo. As the embryo grows, this tissue, known as the neural plate, forms a groove that is bordered by folds. This groove eventually deepens and closes to form the neural tube. Later in development, the neural tube gives rise to tissue that later forms the brain and spinal cord. The neural tube is surrounded and protected by the bones of the back (vertebrae). Failure in this sequence of developmental events results in a neural tube defect.

Anencephaly represents a type of neural tube defect that is incompatible with life. Infants with this disorder are born without a forebrain, the largest part of the brain consisting mainly of the cerebral hemispheres which are responsible for higher level cognition, i.e., thinking. The remaining brain tissue is often exposed - not covered by bone or skin. Infants born with anencephaly are usually blind, deaf, unconscious, and unable to feel pain. Additional physical findings associated with this abnormality include folded ears, incomplete closure of the palate (cleft palate), and congenital heart defects. The cause of anencephaly is unknown, although it is thought to occur as the result of genetic or environmental factors, alone or in combination. Neural tube defects do not follow direct patterns of heredity. However, the theory of a genetic predisposition to anencephaly is supported by the fact that the risk of additional children being born with this defect rises with each pregnancy.

Supplementation with high-dose folic acid, initiated before and given during pregnancy, reduces the risk of neural tube defects to 1%.

Government Agencies

222 NIH/National Institute of Child Health and Human Development
31 Center Drive, Building 31 Room 2A32
Bethesda, MD 10021   800-370-2943
                                       Fax: 301-496-1104
                                       TTY: 888-320-6942
e-mail: NICHDInformationResourceCenter@mail.nih.
                                       www.nichd.nih.gov

Established in 1962 by congress, today the institute conducts and supports laboratory research, clinical trials, and epidemiological studies that explore health processes; examines the impact of disabilities, diseases, and variations on the lives of individuals; and sponsors training programs for scientists, health care providers, and researchers to ensure that NICHD research can continue.

Alan E Guttmacher MD, Director
Lisa Kaeser, Program & Public Liaison

National Associations & Support Groups

223 American Academy of Pediatrics
141 Northwest Point Boulevard
Elk Grove Village, IL 60007   847-434-4000
                                       800-433-9016
                                       Fax: 847-434-8000
                                       www.aap.org

The American Academy of Pediatrics and its member pediatricians are committed to the attainment of optimal physical, mental and social health and well-being for all infants, children, adolescents, and young adults.

Sandra Hassink, MD, FAAP, President

224 Anencephaly Support Foundation
20311 Sienna Pines Ct.
Spring, TX 77379   281-364-9222
                                       888-206-7526
                                       www.anencephaly.net

A nonprofit religious foundation dedicated to serving parents, families and educational communities. Offered are information, personal stories and medical articles regarding the neural tube defect of anencephaly, support and encouragement to parents who have chosen to carry an anencephalic pregnancy to term, and information regarding possible causations, prevention theories, and support group referrals.

225 Birth Defect Research for Children
976 Lake Baldwin Lane, Suite 104
Orlando, FL 10023   407-895-0802
                                       Fax: 407-895-0824
                                       e-mail: staff@birthdefects.org
                                       www.birthdefects.org

Birth Defect Research for Children is a non-profit organization that provides parents and expectant parents with information about birth defects and support services for their children.

Betty Mekdeci, Executive Director

226 Genetic Alliance
4301 Connecticut Avenue NW Suite 404
Washington, DC 10024   202-966-7955
                                       800-336-4363
                                       Fax: 202-966-8553
                                       e-mail: info@geneticalliance.org
                                       www.geneticalliance.org

World's leading nonprofit health advocacy organization committed to transforming health through genetics and promoting an environment of openness centered on the health of individuals, families, and communities.

Sharon Terry, President
Lisa Wise, Chief Operating Officer
Tetyana Murza MES, Programs and Policy Coordinator

227 March of Dimes Birth Defects Foundation
1275 Mamaroneck Avenue
White Plains, NY 10025   914-997-4488
                                       888-663-4637
                                       Fax: 914-997-4763
                                       e-mail: answers@marchofdimes.com
                                       www.marchofdimes.com

March of Dimes help moms have full-term pregnancies and research the problems that threaten the health of babies. The March of Dimes also acts globally: sharing best practices in perinatal health and helping improve birth outcomes where the needs are the most urgent.

Kenneth A. May, Chair
Jennifer Howse, President & CEO
Alan Fleischman, Medical Director

228 National Dissemination Center for Children with Disabilities
1825 Connecticut Avenue NW , Suite 700
Washington, DC 10026   202-884-8200
                                       800-695-0285
                                       Fax: 202-884-8441
                                       e-mail: nichcy@fhi360.org
                                       www.nichcy.org

A national information and referral center for families, educators and other professionals on: disabilities in children and youth; programs and services; IDEA, the nation's special education law; and research-based information on effective practices.

Suzanne Ripley, Executive Director

Conferences

229 Genetic Alliance Annual Conference
Genetic Alliance
4301 Connecticut Avenue NW, Suite 404
Washington, DC 20008

202-966-5557
800-336-4363
Fax: 202-966-8553
e-mail: info@geneticalliance.org
www.geneticalliance.org

Consistently inspirational and enables partnership among all stakeholders: advocates and community leaders, health and industry professionals, policymakers, and academicians.

July

Sharon Terry, President/CEO
Tetyana Murza, Programs/Events Manager

Web Sites

230 Online Mendelian Inheritance in Man
National Library of Medicine, Building 38A
Bethesda, MD 20894

888-346-3656
e-mail: info@ncbi.nlm.nih.gov
www.ncbi.nlm.nih.gov

This database is a catalog of human genes and genetic disorders.

Christine E. Seidman, M.D., Chair
David J. Lipman, M.D., Executive Secretary

231 Rare Genetic Diseases in Children (NYU)
www.med.nyu.edu/rgdc/homenow.htm

We target issues arising from rare genetic diseases affecting children. And to assist in the endeavor to bring knowledge and hope to those for whom there is, at present, so little.

Description

232 ANIRIDIA

Synonym: Hypoplasia of iris

Involves the following Biologic System(s):

Ophthalmologic Disorders

Aniridia is a birth defect characterized by absence of all or a portion of the colored area of the eye (iris). Both eyes are typically affected (bilateral aniridia). The term aniridia may be a misnomer, since an undeveloped (vestigial) portion of the iris is usually present (i.e., apparent upon slit-lamp examination or gonioscopy). The iris is an involuntary circular muscle that is visible through the transparent, front portion of the eye (cornea). When certain fibers in the iris contract, the hole in the center of the iris (pupil) either widens or constricts, allowing in additional or less light.

In some infants with aniridia, the corneas of the eyes are also abnormally small. In addition, many affected infants and children experience loss of transparency of the lenses of the eyes (cataracts) or displacement of the lenses, which are located behind the pupils. Aniridia is often associated with underdevelopment (hypoplasia) of the macula, the central portion of the retina that distinguishes detail in the central field of vision.

Additional eye abnormalities often associated with aniridia include rapid, involuntary movements of the eyes (nystagmus); reduced fields of vision; abnormally increased sensitivity to light (photophobia); and progressively increased fluid pressure within the eyes (glaucoma). In most cases, glaucoma is not apparent during the first month of life (neonatal period).

Depending upon the range and severity of associated eye abnormalities, children with aniridia may have varying levels of visual impairment. However, in most cases, affected children may have visual acuity of approximately 20/200 or even further reductions in vision. The clearness or sharpness of vision (i.e., visual acuity) is typically measured on a scale comparing a patient's vision at 20 feet with that of an unaffected individual with full visual acuity. Thus, a person with 20/200 vision sees at 20 feet what someone with full visual acuity sees at 200 feet.

Aniridia may be an isolated condition or may occur in association with certain syndromes, such as WAGR syndrome, a rare disorder characterized by kidney tumors (Wilms tumor), aniridia, genitourinary anomalies (abnormalities of the reproductive and urinary tracts), due to spontaneous genetic changes (mutations), and retardation. WAGR is inherited as an autosomal dominant trait; in very rare cases, aniridia is inherited as an autosomal recessive trait (e.g., aniridia-cerebellar ataxia-mental deficiency). Medical care for aniridia is directed toward prevention of glaucoma and control of intraocular pressure (fluid pressure inside the eye. Other measures focus on specific problems, such as nystagamus, sensitivity to light (photophobia) and supportive measures, such as removal of cataracts. Visual aids, such as artificial pupil contact lenses, may also be used.

Government Agencies

233 NIH/National Eye Institute
31 Center Drive MSC 2510
Bethesda, MD 10027

301-496-5248
e-mail: 2020@nei.nih.gov
www.nei.nih.gov

Conducts and supports research that helps prevent and treat eye diseases and other disorders of vision. This research leads to sight-saving treatments, reduces visual impairment and blindness, and improves the quality of life for people of all ages. NEI-supported research has advanced our knowledge of how the eye functions in health and disease.

Paul A Sieving M.D., Ph.D., Director

National Associations & Support Groups

234 American Academy of Pediatrics
141 Northwest Point Boulevard
Elk Grove Village, IL 60007

847-434-4000
800-433-9016
Fax: 847-434-8000
www.aap.org

The American Academy of Pediatrics and its member pediatricians are committed to the attainment of optimal physical, mental and social health and well-being for all infants, children, adolescents, and young adults.

Sandra Hassink, MD, FAAP, President

235 Genetic Alliance
4301 Connecticut Avenue NW Suite 404
Washington, DC 10028

202-966-7955
800-336-4363
Fax: 202-966-8553
e-mail: info@geneticalliance.org
www.geneticalliance.org

World's leading nonprofit health advocacy organization committed to transforming health through genetics and promoting an environment of openness centered on the health of individuals, families, and communities.

Sharon Terry, President
Lisa Wise, Chief Operating Officer
Tetyana Murza MES, Programs and Policy Coordinator

236 Lighthouse International
111 E 59 Street
New York, NY 10029

212-821-9200
800-829-0500
Fax: 212-821-9797
TTY: 212-821-9713
e-mail: info@lighthouse.org
www.lighthouse.org

Since 1905, Lighthouse International has led the charge in the fight against vision loss through prevention, treatment and empowerment.

Joseph A Ripp, Chairman
Sarah E Smith, Vice-Chair & Treasurer
Jonathan M Wainwright, Esq, Vice-Chair and Secretary

237 March of Dimes Birth Defects Foundation
1275 Mamaroneck Avenue
White Plains, NY 10030

914-997-4488
888-663-4637
Fax: 914-997-4763
e-mail: answers@marchofdimes.com
www.marchofdimes.com

March of Dimes help moms have full-term pregnancies and research the problems that threaten the health of babies. The March of Dimes also acts globally: sharing best practices in perinatal health and helping improve birth outcomes where the needs are the most urgent.

Kenneth A. May, Chair
Jennifer Howse, President & CEO
Alan Fleischman, Medical Director

238   National Eye Research Foundation
910 Skokie Boulevard, Suite 207A
Northbrook, IL 10031

847-564-4652
800-621-2258
Fax: 847-564-0807
e-mail: info@nerf.org
www.nerf.org

Devoted to the enhancement of care and study of eye related diseases.

Conferences

239   Genetic Alliance Annual Conference
Genetic Alliance
4301 Connecticut Avenue NW, Suite 404
Washington, DC 20008

202-966-5557
800-336-4363
Fax: 202-966-8553
e-mail: info@geneticalliance.org
www.geneticalliance.org

Consistently inspirational and enables partnership among all stakeholders: advocates and community leaders, health and industry professionals, policymakers, and academicians.

July

Sharon Terry, President/CEO
Tetyana Murza, Programs/Events Manager

Web Sites

240   Aniridia Network
22 Cornish House, Adelaide Lane
Sheffield, S3 8B

077-2 8-7 94
e-mail: info@aniridia.org.uk
aniridia.org.uk

We are an international support group which aims to bring people with aniridia closer together as well as providing practical support and information.

241   Aniridia Web Site
22 Cornish House, Adelaide Lane
Sheffield, S3 8B

077-2 8-7 94
e-mail: info@aniridia.org.uk
aniridia.org.uk

The Aniridia Network is an international nonprofit organization dedicated to supporting people with aniridia and their families, increasing awareness of aniridia and improving the quality of information about aniridia around the world.

242   National Association for Visually Handicapped
111 E 59th St
New York, NY 10022

800-284-4422
e-mail: info@lighthouseguild.org
www.lighthouseguild.org

Provides information on large print books, textbooks and educational tools.

243   Online Mendelian Inheritance in Man
National Library of Medicine, Building 38A
Bethesda, MD 20894

888-346-3656
e-mail: info@ncbi.nlm.nih.gov
www.ncbi.nlm.nih.gov

This database is a catalog of human genes and genetic disorders.

Christine E. Seidman, M.D., Chair
David J. Lipman, M.D., Executive Secretary

Book Publishers

244   Children with Visual Impairments: A Parents' Guide
Peytral Publications
PO Box 1162
Minnetonka, MN 55345

952-949-8707
877-739-8725
Fax: 952-906-9777
e-mail: help@peytral.com
www.peytral.com

Covers visual impairments ranging from low vision to total blindness. Offers authoritative information and empathy, parental insight on diagnosis and treatment, orientation and mobility, literacy, legal issues and more. Valuable to parents, educators and support staff.

395 pages

M Cay Holbrook PhD, Editor

245   Let's Talk About Going to the Hospital
Rosen Publishing Group's PowerKids Press
29 E 21st Street
New York, NY 10010

212-777-3017
800-237-9932
Fax: 888-436-4643
e-mail: rosenpub@tribeca.ios.com
www.rosenpublishing.com

If a child has to check into the hospital, chances are he or she is already upset about being ill. Knowing how a hospital functions and what the procedures are, such as when family members can visit, will help in what is already a stressful situation. Grades K-5.

24 pages
ISBN: 0-823950-36-0

Description

246 ANKYLOSING SPONDYLITIS
Synonyms: AS, Marie-Strumpell spondylitis
Involves the following Biologic System(s):
Orthopedic and Muscle Disorders

Ankylosing spondylitis (AS) is a chronic, progressive, inflammatory disease that affects joints of the spine and results in pain, stiffness, and possible loss of spinal mobility. In most patients, the joints between the spine and the hipbones (sacroiliac joints) are affected. In addition, joints in the spinal column of the lower back (lumbosacral spine) and the neck (cervical spine) may be involved to varying degrees. Although the disease usually becomes apparent during young adulthood or middle age, it may also begin during childhood. Males are more commonly affected than females.

In most cases, children initially present with periodic inflammation and discomfort in the joints of the arms and legs (transient peripheral arthritis), particularly the large joints of the legs. Many also experience arthritis in the shoulders, the lower jaw bone (i.e., temporomandibular joints), and the feet. Such inflammation results in swelling, pain, abnormal warmth (erythema), and possible limited movement of affected joints. In children with AS, involvement of the sacroiliac joints may be apparent at the disorder's onset or may develop over several months or years. The different regions of the spine may then be progressively affected, usually beginning in the spinal column of the lower back (lumbar spine) and eventually involving the upper back (thoracic spine) and the cervical spine. Children with the disease experience periodic pain and stiffness that may be alleviated by movement. Many have hip, thigh, and lower back pain that is more severe at night and experience stiffness of affected areas in the mornings. In addition, some children have involvement of the joints that connect the ribs to the spine (costovertebral joints). The resulting inflammation, pain, and stiffness may limit expansion of the chest when taking deep breaths. Disease progression may spontaneously cease at any stage; however, in some cases, all regions of the spine may gradually be affected, potentially resulting in severely impaired spinal mobility.

Other symptoms associated with ankylosing spondylitis include fatigue, low-grade fever, lack of appetite (anorexia), low levels ofred blood cells (anemia), growth retardation, and repeated inflammation of the colored region of the eye (iritis) and its muscle (iridocyclitis). Inflammation of the aorta, the largest artery of the body (aoritis), is a finding that is often seen in adults with ankylosing spondylitis, but is rarely seen in affected children.

Research has shown that approximately 95 percent of affected individuals have a specific human leukocyte antigen or HLA. Antigens are proteins that stimulate the body to produce certain antibodies in response to invading microorganisms or foreign tissues. Most individuals with ankylosing spondylitis have a specific genetically determined HLA known as HLA-B27. The possible role of HLA-B27 in predisposing an individual to the disorder has not been determined. Anklosing spondylitis is thought to be an autosomal dominant disorder. In some cases, individuals with a defective gene for AS may not experience symptoms and findings associated with the

disorder (reduced penetrance). AS is thought to have a higher penetrance among males.

Although HLA-B27 is present in most individuals with ankylosing spondylitis, it is not considered diagnostic for the disorder. AS is typically diagnosed based upon a complete patient and family history, characteristic physical findings, and specialized x-ray techniques. Treatment of children is primarily directed toward relieving pain and ensuring proper posture to help preserve spinal mobility. Certain medications may be prescribed to help alleviate or manage pain (e.g., indomethacin or other nonsteroidal antiinflammatory medications [NSAIDs]). Special exercises may be recommended to help strengthen back muscles and maintain proper posture. In addition, certain lifestyle changes may be suggested, including avoiding thick pillows and using a firm mattress. Additional treatment is usually symptomatic and supportive.

Government Agencies

247 NIH/National Institute of Arthritis and Mu sculoskeletal and Skin Diseases
1AMS Circle
Bethesda, MD 10032
301-402-4484
877-226-4267
Fax: 301-718-6366
TTY: 301-565-2966
TDD: 301-565-2966
e-mail: niamsinfo@mail.nih.gov
www.niams.nih.gov

The mission of the National Institute of Arthritis and Musculoskeletal and Skin Diseases is to support research into the causes, treatment, and prevention of arthritis and musculoskeletal and skin diseases; the training of basic and clinical scientists to carry out this research; and the dissemination of information on research progress in these diseases
Stephen I Katz MD PhD, Director
Robert H Carter MD, Deputy Director
Gahan Breithaupt, Assoc Dir. Management & Operations

National Associations & Support Groups

248 American Academy of Pediatrics
141 Northwest Point Boulevard
Elk Grove Village, IL 60007
847-434-4000
800-433-9016
Fax: 847-434-8000
www.aap.org

The American Academy of Pediatrics and its member pediatricians are committed to the attainment of optimal physical, mental and social health and well-being for all infants, children, adolescents, and young adults.
Sandra Hassink, MD, FAAP, President

249 American Autoimmune Related Diseases Association
22100 Gratiot Avenue
Eastpointe, MI 10033
586-776-3900
800-598-4668
Fax: 586-776-3903
e-mail: aarda@aarda.org
www.aarda.org

The American Autoimmune Related Diseases Association is dedicated to the eradication of autoimmune diseases and the alleviation of suffering and the socioeconomic impact of autoimmunity through fostering and facilitating collaboration in the areas of education, public awareness, research, and patient services in an effective, ethical and efficient manner.
Betty Diamond MD, Chair
Noel R Rose MD, PhD, Chairman Emeritus

250   American Juvenile Arthritis Organization
1330 W. Peachtree Street.; Suite 100
Atlanta, GA 10034

404-237-8771
800-933-7023
Fax: 404-237-8153
TTY: 404-965-7904
e-mail: info.ga@arthritis.org
www.arthritis.org

The Arthritis Foundation is committed to raising awareness and reducing the unacceptable impact of arthritis, a disease which must be taken as seriously as other chronic diseases because of its devastatng consequences.

Daniel T. McGowan, Chair
Rowland W. (Bing) Chang, Vice Chair
Patricia Novak Nelson, Vice Chair

251   Arthritis Foundation
1330 W. Peachtree Street.; Suite 100
Atlanta, GA 10035

404-872-7100
800-568-4045
Fax: 404-872-0457
TTY: 404-965-7904
e-mail: info.ga@arthritis.org
www.arthritis.org

The Arthritis Foundation is committed to raising awareness and reducing the unacceptable impact of arthritis, a disease which must be taken as seriously as other chronic diseases because of its devastatng consequences.

Daniel T. McGowan, Chair
Rowland W. (Bing) Chang, Vice Chair
Patricia Novak Nelson, Vice Chair

252   March of Dimes Birth Defects Foundation
1275 Mamaroneck Avenue
White Plains, NY 10036

914-997-4488
888-663-4637
Fax: 914-997-4763
e-mail: answers@marchofdimes.com
www.marchofdimes.com

March of Dimes help moms have full-term pregnancies and re-search the problems that threaten the health of babies.The March of Dimes also acts globally: sharing best practices in perinatal health and helping improve birth outcomes where the needs are the most urgent.

Kenneth A. May, Chair
Jennifer Howse, President & CEO
Alan Fleischman, Medical Director

253   Spondylitis Association of America
PO Box 5872
Sherman Oaks, CA 10037

818-981-1616
800-777-8189
Fax: 818-892-1611
e-mail: info@spondylitis.org
www.spondylitis.org

Founded in 1983 SAA was the first and remains the largest re-source in the United States for people seeking information on AS and related diseases.

Craig Gimbel DDS, Chair
Charlotte K Howrard, Vice Chair
Leslie Kautz CFA, Treasurer

Web Sites

254   American Autoimmune Related Diseases Association
22100 Gratiot Ave.
Eastpointe, MI 48021

586-776-3900
800-598-4668
Fax: 586-776-3903
www.aarda.org

Dedicated to the eradiction of autoimmune diseases and the alle-viation of suffering and the socio-economic impact of autoimmunity through fostering and facilitating collaboration in the areas of education, public awareness, research and patient ser-vices in an effective, ethical and efficient manner.

Virginia T. Ladd, President/ Executive Director
Patricia Barber, Asst. Director
Eula Hoover, Exec. Assistant/ Newsletter Editor

255   Online Mendelian Inheritance in Man
National Library of Medicine, Building 38A
Bethesda, MD 20894

888-346-3656
e-mail: info@ncbi.nlm.nih.gov
www.ncbi.nlm.nih.gov

This database is a catalog of human genes and genetic disorders.

Christine E. Seidman, M.D., Chair
David J. Lipman, M.D., Executive Secretary

Pamphlets

256   Ankylosing Spondylitis
Arthritis Foundation
1330 W. Peachtree Street, Suite 100
Atlanta, GA 30309

404-872-7100
800-568-4045
Fax: 404-872-0457
www.arthritis.org

An informative pamphlet published by the Arthritis Foundation.

Ann M. Palmer, President/ CEO
Meagan Fulmer, Chief Development Officer
Wayne Guthrie, SPHR, SVP, Staff Operations

Description

257   ANORECTAL MALFORMATIONS

Covers these related disorders: Anal atresia, Anal fistula, Anal stenosis, Ectopic anus, Imperforate anus

Involves the following Biologic System(s):

Gastrointestinal Disorders

Anorectal malformations are a group of birth defects affecting the rectum, the anus, or both. The rectum is the final straight portion of the large intestine that terminates at an external opening known as the anus. Anorectal malformations are birth defects in which the anus and rectum do not develop normally and vary in severity. For example, the anal opening may be in its normal location but may be unusually small or narrow (e.g., anal stenosis or imperforate anus). Some anorectal malformations may not be apparent upon physical examination (e.g., imperforate anus or anal atresia). In infants with imperforate anus, the anal opening is partially or completely closed due to the presence of a thin membrane (i.e., cloacal membrane). In anal atresia, the rectum may end blindly due to absence (atresia) of the anal canal. In addition, in many affected infants, an abnormal channel (fistula) may be present between the rectum and certain other unusual locations. Anorectal malformations affect approximately one in 4,000 newborns.

Most newborns with anorectal malformations experience lower intestinal obstruction within 24 hours after birth due to incomplete passage of meconium, the thick, darkish green material that accumulates in the fetal intestines and forms a newborn's first stool. Newborns normally pass meconium during the first 24 to 48 hours after birth. Affected infants may also have incomplete or infrequent bowel movements or experience difficulty passing stools (constipation) within days or weeks after birth. Associated findings may include rectal bleeding; periodic episodes of diarrhea following constipation and associated abrasions of the skin (e.g., of the perineum and the buttocks); and abnormal enlargement of a segment of the large intestine (megacolon). In affected males with a channel between the rectum and the urinary tract, there can be passage of gas (pneumaturia) and meconium in the urine.

When newborns are diagnosed with anorectal malformations, physicians may consider surgical measures to prevent intestinal or urinary obstruction. Therapies for affected newborns or infants depend upon the nature and location of the anorectal malformation and, in some cases, other associated birth defects that may be present. Treatment measures, which may be conducted during the newborn period or later during infancy, may include surgical correction of anorectal malformations (e.g., anoplasty) and widening (dilatation) of the anal opening or other supportive measures; a colostomy is often needed.

Anorectal malformations are thought to result from abnormalities in the development of the embryonic structures that form the rectum and portions of the urinary tract. In cases in which anorectal malformations occur as isolated findings, such malformations are thought to result from abnormal changes (mutations) of one or several different genes, possibly in association with certain environmental factors (multifactorial). However, familial cases have also been reported that appear to have autosomal dominant, autosomal recessive, X-linked, or multifactorial inheritance. In approximately 50 percent of affected infants, anorectal malformations occur in association with other birth defects or underlying malformation syndromes, such as VACTERL association, a rare disorder that may be characterized by (V)ertebral abnormalities, (A)nal atresia, (C)ardiac defects, (T)racheo(E)sophageal fistula, (R)enal malformations, and (L)imb defects. Therefore, it is essential that newborns diagnosed with anorectal malformations are thoroughly examined and carefully monitored to ensure the detection and appropriate treatment of associated abnormalities.

National Associations & Support Groups

258   American Academy of Pediatrics
141 Northwest Point Boulevard
Elk Grove Village, IL 60007

847-434-4000
800-433-9016
Fax: 847-434-8000
www.aap.org

The American Academy of Pediatrics and its member pediatricians are committed to the attainment of optimal physical, mental and social health and well-being for all infants, children, adolescents, and young adults.

Sandra Hassink, MD, FAAP, President

259   American College of Gastroenterology
6400 Goldsboro Road Suite 200
Bethesda, MD 10038

301-263-9000
www.gi.org

The American College of Gastroenterology was founded in 1932 to advance the scientific study and medical practice of diseases of the GI tract.

Ronald J Vender, President
Stephen B Hanauer MD, Vice President
Harry E Sarles Jr. MD, President-Elect

260   Digestive Disease National Coalition
507 Capitol Court NE, Suite 200
Washington, DC 10039

202-544-7497
Fax: 202-546-7105
e-mail: ddnc@hmcw.org
www.ddnc.org

Advocacy organization comprised of 22 voluntary and professional societies concerned with the many diseases of the digestive tract and liver.

Diane Paley, Chairperson
James DeGerome, President
Andrew Spiegel, Vice-Chairperson

261   International Foundation for Functional Gastrointestinal Disorders
700 W. Virginia St., #201
Milwaukee, WI 10041

414-964-1799
888-964-2001
Fax: 414-964-7176
e-mail: iffgd@iffgd.org
www.iffgd.org

Founded in 1991 by Nancy Norton and William Norton, IFFGD has been working with patients (both adults and children), families, physicians, practitioners, investigators, employers, regulators, and others to broaden understanding about gastrointestinal disorders and support or encourage research.

Nancy J Norton, Founder
William Norton, Co-Founder
Eleanor Cautley, Vice President

262   Intestinal Disease Foundation
1 E Station Square Drive
Pittsburgh, PA 10042

412-261-5888
877-587-9606
Fax: 412-471-2722
e-mail: info@intestinalfoundation.org
www.intestinalfoundation.org

Nonprofit organization whose mission is to improve the quality of life of adults and children affected by chronic digestive illness through information, guidance and support. IDF offers a quarterly newsletter, Intestinal Fortitude, educational seminars, volunteer phone network, and Pittsburgh area support groups.

263 March of Dimes Birth Defects Foundation
1275 Mamaroneck Avenue
White Plains, NY 10043 914-997-4488
888-663-4637
Fax: 914-997-4763
e-mail: answers@marchofdimes.com
www.marchofdimes.com

March of Dimes help moms have full-term pregnancies and research the problems that threaten the health of babies. The March of Dimes also acts globally: sharing best practices in perinatal health and helping improve birth outcomes where the needs are the most urgent.

Kenneth A. May, Chair
Jennifer Howse, President & CEO
Alan Fleischman, Medical Director

264 National Dissemination Center for Children with Disabilities
1825 Connecticut Avenue NW , Suite 700
Washington, DC 10044 202-884-8200
800-695-0285
Fax: 202-884-8441
e-mail: nichcy@fhi360.org
www.nichcy.org

A national information and referral center that provides information on disabilities and disability-related issues for families, educators and other professionals.

Suzanne Ripley, Executive Director

265 North American Society for Pediatric Gastroenterology/Hepatology/Nutrition
PO Box 6
Flourtown, PA 19031 215-233-0808
Fax: 215-233-3918
e-mail: naspghan@naspghan.org
www.naspghan.org

Strives to improve the care of infants, children and adolescents with digestive disorders by promoting advances in clinical care of children with chronic abdominal pain, diarrhea, constipation, vomiting, bleeding from the GI tract, inflammatory bowel disease, liver diseases, diseases of the pancreas, poor weight gain and nutritional problems.

Philip Sherman, President
Margaret K Stallings, Executive Director
Kate Ho, Associate Director

266 Oley Foundation
214 Hun Memorial, MC-28, Albany Medical Center
Albany, NY 12208 518-262-5079
800-776-6539
Fax: 518-262-5528
e-mail: info@oley.org
www.oley.org

Helping people whose daily survival depends on home intravenous or tube-fed nutrition.

Joan Bishop, Executive Director
Roslyn Dahl, Director, Communications & Develop
Felice Austin, Regional Coordinator Program Direct

267 Pull-Thru Network
1705 Wintergreen Parkway
Normal, IL 10045 309-262-0786
e-mail: pullthrunetwork@gmail.com
www.pullthrunetwork.org

Pull-thru Network (PTN) was founded in 1988 and has grown to be one of the largest organizations in the world dedicated to the needs of those born with an anorectal malformation or colon disease and any of the associated diagnoses.

Bonnie McElroy, President
Alberto Pena, Director
Charles Paidas, Chief of Pediatric Surgery

Libraries & Resource Centers

268 National Digestive Diseases Information Clearinghouse
31 Center Drive, MSC 2560
Bethesda, MD 20892 301-496-3583
800-891-5389
Fax: 301-907-8906
e-mail: niddc@info.niddk.nih.gov
www.niddk.nih.gov

The National Institute of Diabetes and Digestive and Kidney Diseases conducts and supports research on many of the most serious diseases affecting public health. The Institute supports much of the clinical research on the diseases of internal medicine and related subspecialty fields as well as many basic science disciplines.

Dr. Griffin P Rodgers, Director
Dr. Gregory G Germino, Deputy Director
Camille M Hoover M.S.W, Executive Officer

Conferences

269 IFFGD Professional Symposia
Int'l Foundation for Functional Gastrointestinal
700 W. Virginia St., #201
Milwaukee, WI 10040 414-964-1799
888-964-2001
Fax: 414-964-7176
e-mail: iffgd@iffgd.org
www.iffgd.org

Founded in 1991 by Nancy Norton and William Norton to help patients (both adults and children), families, physicians, practitioners, investigators, employers, regulators, and others broaden understanding about gastrointestinal disorders and support and encourage research.

April

Nancy J Norton, Founder
William Norton, Co-Founder
Eleanor Cautley, Vice President

270 NASPGHAN Annual Meeting and Postgraduate Course
NASPGHAN
PO Box 6
Flourtown, PA 19031 215-233-0808
Fax: 215-233-3918
e-mail: naspghan@naspghan.org
www.naspghan.org

October

Margaret K Stallings, Executive Director
Athos Bousvaros, MD, President
James Heubi, MD, Secretary-Treasurer

271 Oley Foundation Annual Conference
Oley Foundation
214 Hun Memorial, MC-28, Albany Medical Center
Albany, NY 12208 518-262-5079
800-776-6539
Fax: 518-262-5528
e-mail: info@oley.org
www.oley.org

Helping people whose daily survival depends on home intravenous or tube-fed nutrition.

July

Joan Bishop, Executive Director

272 PTN National Conference
Pull-Thru Network
1705 Wintergreen Parkway
Normal, IL 61761 205-978-2930
e-mail: pullthrunetwork@gmail.com
www.pullthrunetwork.org

July

Bonnie McElroy, President

Web Sites

273 Baby Center
163 Freelon Street
San Francisco, CA 94107   www.babycenter.com

The Academy is committed to the attainment of optimal physical, mental and social health for all infants, children, adolescents, and young adults. To this end, the members of the Academy dedicate their efforts and resources.

Colleen Hancock, SVP/Global COO
Linda J. Murray, SVP/Global Editor-in-Chief
Clarence Wilhelm, Chief Information Officer

274 Health Research Project (HaRP)
www.harpnet.org

e-mail: harp@kmsgh.org
www.harpnet.org

A program by USAID, the project strives to improve the health status of infants, children, mothers and families through the development and research of new tools, technologies, policies and approaches.

275 National Digestive Diseases Information Clearinghouse
www.digestive.niddk.nih.gov

Supports clinical research on the diseases of internal medicine and related subspecialty fields as well as many basic science disciplines.

Journals

276 Journal of Pediatric Gastroenterology and Nutrition (NASPGHAN)
Lippincott Williams & Wilkins
Two Commerce Square, 2001 Market Street
Philadelphia, PA 19103   215-521-8300
Fax: 215-521-8902
www.wolterskluwerhealth.com

Publication of the North American Society for Pediatric Gastroenterolgy, Hepatology and Nutrition, which strives to improve the care of infants, children and adolescents with digestive disorders by promoting advances in clinical care of children with chronic abdominal pain, diarrhea, constipation, vomiting, bleeding from the GI tract, inflammatory bowel disease, liver diseases, diseases of the pancreas, poor weight gain and nutritional problems.

Bob Becker, President/ CEO
Susan Yules, Chief Financial Officer
Cathy Wolfe, President/ CEO, Medical Research

Newsletters

277 NASPGHAN News
PO Box 6
Flourtown, PA 19031   215-233-0808
Fax: 215-233-3918
e-mail: naspghan@naspghan.org
www.naspghan.org

Publication of the North American Society for Pediatric Gastroenterolgy, Hepatology and Nutrition, which strives to improve the care of infants, children and adolescents with digestive disorders by promoting advances in clinical care of children with chronic abdominal pain, diarrhea, constipation, vomiting, bleeding from the GI tract, inflammatory bowel disease, liver diseases, diseases of the pancreas, poor weight gain and nutritional problems.

Carlo Di Lorenzo, MD, President
Michael Narkewicz, MD, Secretary-Treasurer
Margaret K. Stallings, Executive Director

278 PTN News
1705 Wintergreen Parkway
Normal, IL 61761   205-978-2930
e-mail: pullthrunetwork@gmail.com
www.pullthrunetwork.org

Newsletter of the Pull-thru Network, a chapter of the United Ostomy Association and a nonprofit service organization dedicated to the support of children and adults with anorectal malformations.

Quarterly

Pamphlets

279 Anorectal Malformations- A Parent's Guide
1705 Wintergreen Parkway
Normal, IL 61761   205-978-2930
e-mail: pullthrunetwork@gmail.com
www.pullthrunetwork.org

Brochure distributed free to physicians, nurses and hospitals by the Pull-thru Network, a chapter of the United Ostomy Association and a nonprofit service organization dedicated to the support of children and adults with anorectal malformations.

Quarterly

Description

280   AORTIC STENOSIS

Synonym: Aortic stenosis

Involves the following Biologic System(s):

Cardiovascular Disorders

Aortic stenosis is a condition characterized by abnormal narrowing (stenosis) of the aortic valve, through which blood flows from the left ventricle of the heart to the aorta, the major artery of the body. Such stenosis may occur alone, as a sole abnormality, or together with other inborn abnormalities within or outside the heart. Narrowing of the aortic valve prevents the left ventricle from pumping its full load of blood into the aorta and therefore throughout the body. Effects of the diminished blood flow resulting from aortic stenosis include a deficient supply of blood-borne oxygen and nutrients to the body's tissues, including the muscle tissue of the ventricle, damaging these tissues. In an attempt to overcome this reduced blood supply by pumping blood more forcefully through a narrowed or stenotic aortic value and into the aorta, the muscular wall of the left ventricle may gradually thicken (hypertrophy). With its continued effort to pump blood through a stenotic aortic value, the left ventricle can eventually become enlarged and weakened, reducing its ability to pump blood and thereby leaving an increasing volume of residual blood and an increased blood pressure within the heart. Congestive heart failure, in which the heart ultimately becomes unable to pump blood, is a potentially life-threatening effect of aortic valve stenosis.

Normally, the aortic valve consists of three leaflets (cusps) that meet along their outer edges and overlap one another to prevent blood that is in the aorta from pushing back into the heart between heartbeats. These valves open when the heart contracts, permitting the left ventricle to pump blood out of itself and into the aorta. Most cases of aortic stenosis result from abnormalities in the leaflets or cusps of the valve. One such abnormality is an aortic valve that has only a single leaflet rather than the usual three leaflets. Such a monocuspid valve can occur either as an inherited, genetic effect or as the result of fusion of the valve's leaflets with one another. The inborn or congenital abnormality known as a bicuspid aortic valve is characterized by a valve that has only two cusps or leaflets instead of the usual three, and while many such valves work reasonably well, they are more often narrower than the normal aortic valve. Aortic stenosis can also result from genetic or inherited narrowing of the aortic valve, degenerative diseases, and inflammatory diseases that affect the heart, such as rheumatic fever.

Aortic valve stenosis is identified in as many as 15% of patients before the age of 1 year. Among other persons, the condition presents during childhood, adolescence, or adulthood. Congestive heart failure can be a major effect of aortic valve stenosis in newborns. In older children, a heart murmur is often the first indication of such stenosis. Fatigue soon after beginning a physical activity, dizziness, and chest pain may be other indications of aortic valve stenosis in older children.

Symptoms of aortic valve stenosis depend upon the severity of the abnormality. Valve obstruction that occurs in early infancy may be characterized by a weak pulse, a low output of urine difficulty in breathing, enlargement of the heart (cardiomegaly), congestive heart failure, and abnormal accumulation of fluid in the lungs (pulmonary edema). Severe aortic valve stenosis may be life-threatening to infants and older children. Children with less severe aortic stenosis may have no symptoms other than a heart murmur detected during a physical examination, while those with more severe involvement may experience fatigue, dizziness, and chest pain.

Treatment for aortic valve stenosis depends upon the severity of the obstruction. In some cases it is successfully corrected through the procedure known as balloon valvuloplasty, in which a thin, hollow tube (catheter), with a small balloon attached at its tip, is passed into the valve and the balloon is then inflated, increasing the size of the valve opening. The most frequent treatment for aortic satenosis is surgery to repair the valve if possible or to replace it if necessary. During such surgery, a heart bypass machine takes the place of the heart and lungs, oxygenating the patient's blood and pumping it through the body. In the procedure known as valvotomy, the aortic valve is surgically rebuilt so as to allow it to effectively pass blood from the ventricle into the aorta. In the technique known as the Ross procedure, achild's own pulmonary valve, which normally controls the flow of blood from the heart's right ventricle to the lungs, is used to replace a stenotic aortic valve, and is itself then replaced with a surgically implanted pulmonary valve.

Government Agencies

281   NIH/National Heart, Lung and Blood Institu te
National Institute of Health
31 Center Dr MSC 2486, Bldg 31, Room 5A48
Bethesda, MD 10046   301-592-8573
                                           Fax: 240-629-3246
                                           TTY: 240-629-3255
                            e-mail: nhlbiinfo@nhlbi.nih.gov
                                           www.nhlbi.nih.gov

The National Heart, Lung, and Blood Institute (NHLBI) provides global leadership for a research, training, and education program to promote the prevention and treatment of heart, lung, and blood diseases and enhance the health of all individuals so that they can live longer and more fulfilling lives.

Gary H Gibbons MD, Director
Susan Shurin, MD, Deputy Director
Nakela Cook MD, Chief of Staff

**282   NIH/National Institute of Child Health and Human
Development Bethesda, MD 10047**

                                                800-370-2943
                                           Fax: 301-496-1104
                                           TTY: 888-320-6942
        e-mail: NICHDInformationResourceCenter@mail.nih.
                                           www.nichd.nih.gov

Established in 1962 by congress, today the institute conducts and supports laboratory research, clinical trials, and epidemiological studies that explore health processes; examines the impact of disabilities, diseases, and variations on the lives of individuals; and sponsors training programs for scientists, health care providers, and researchers to ensure that NICHD research can continue.

Alan E Guttmacher MD, Director
Lisa Kaeser, Program & Public Liaison

National Associations & Support Groups

283   American Academy of Pediatrics
141 Northwest Point Boulevard
Elk Grove Village, IL 60007   847-434-4000
                                                800-433-9016
                                           Fax: 847-434-8000
                                                www.aap.org

The American Academy of Pediatrics and its member pediatricians are committed to the attainment of optimal physical, mental and social health and well-being for all infants, children, adolescents, and young adults.

Sandra Hassink, MD, FAAP, President

284 American Heart Association
7272 Greenville Avenue
Dallas, TX 10048   214-373-6300
                                                    800-242-8721
                                                Fax: 214-706-1341
                                         e-mail: inquire@amhrt.org
                                          www.heart.org/HEARTORG/

Our mission is to build healthier lives, free of cardiovascular diseases and stroke. That single purpose drives all we do. The need for our work is beyond question

Nancy Brown, CEO
Donna Arnett, President
Suzie Upton, Chief Development Officer

285 Genetic Alliance
4301 Connecticut Avenue NW Suite 404
Washington, DC 10049   202-966-7955
                                                    800-336-4363
                                                Fax: 202-966-8553
                                    e-mail: info@geneticalliance.org
                                          www.geneticalliance.org

World's leading nonprofit health advocacy organization committed to transforming health through genetics and promoting an environment of openness centered on the health of individuals, families, and communities.

Sharon Terry, President
Lisa Wise, Chief Operating Officer
Tetyana Murza MES, Programs and Policy Coordinator

286 March of Dimes Birth Defects Foundation
1275 Mamaroneck Avenue
White Plains, NY 10050   914-997-4488
                                                    888-663-4637
                                                Fax: 914-997-4763
                                  e-mail: answers@marchofdimes.com
                                           www.marchofdimes.com

Partnership of volunteers and professionals dedicates to improving the health of babies by preventing birth defects and infant mortality. Over 100 chapters are located across the country and can be located through the National Office.

Kenneth A. May, Chair
Jennifer Howse, President & CEO
Alan Fleischman, Medical Director

Conferences

287 Genetic Alliance Annual Conference
Genetic Alliance
4301 Connecticut Avenue NW, Suite 404
Washington, DC 20008   202-966-5557
                                                    800-336-4363
                                                Fax: 202-966-8553
                                    e-mail: info@geneticalliance.org
                                          www.geneticalliance.org

Consistently inspirational and enables partnership among all stakeholders: advocates and community leaders, health and industry professionals, policymakers, and academicians.

July

Sharon Terry, President/CEO
Tetyana Murza, Programs/Events Manager

Web Sites

288 Southern Illinois University School of Medicine
PO Box 19639
Springfield, IL 62794   217-545-8000
                                                    800-342-5748
                                              TDD: 217-545-8038
                                  e-mail: admin@siuhealthcare.org
                                       www.siumed.edu/peds/index.htm

Mission is to meet the health care needs of children and their families in Central and Southern Illinois through the provision of high quality, coordinated care of children with acute and chronic heart conditions with inpatient, ambulatory, and community-based programs.

289 Yale University School of Medicine
333 Cedar Street
New Haven, CT 6510   203-432-4771
                                                    medicine.yale.edu

Information on congenital heart conditions, including Aortic Stenosis — symptoms, treatments and support.

Peter Salovey, President of the University
Richard Belitsky, M.D., Deputy Dean for Education
Benjamin Polak, B.A., M.A., Ph.D., Provost of the University

Book Publishers

290 Congenital Disorders Sourcebook
Omnigraphics
PO Box 31-1640
Detroit, PA 48231   800-234-1340
                                                Fax: 800-875-1340
                                   e-mail: info@omnigraphics.com
                                          www.omnigraphics.com

Provides basic consumer health information about the most common types of nonhereditary birth defects and disorders related to prematurity, gestational injuries, congenital infections, and birth complications, including disorders of the heart, brain, gastrointestinal tract, musculoskeletal system, urinary tract, and reproductive system, craniofacial disorders, cerebral palsy, spina bifida, and fetal alcohol syndrome, and detailing the causes, diagnostic tests, and treatments for each.

650 pages
ISBN: 0-780809-45-9

Description

291 **APNEA OF PREMATURITY**

Synonym: Idiopathic apnea of prematurity

Involves the following Biologic System(s):

Neonatal and Infant Disorders, Respiratory Disorders

Apnea is a condition characterized by a temporary cessation of breathing. Newborns may experience episodes of apnea due to several underlying disorders or conditions, including certain respiratory, neurologic, digestive, cardiovascular, metabolic, or infectious diseases. However, in newborns with apnea of prematurity, apneic episodes occur in the absence of identifiable, underlying disorders (idiopathic). The condition primarily affects premature infants who are born before 34 weeks of pregnancy (gestation). In general, the greater the degree of prematurity, the greater the frequency of the condition.

Apnea of prematurity is thought to occur due to immaturity of the region of the brain that controls breathing (respiratory centers of the medulla), causing failed stimulation of respiratory muscles. Resulting episodes of apnea, which are referred to as central apnea, are characterized by an absence of airflow as well as of chest wall movements. Apnea of prematurity may also be caused by obstruction of the upper airways due to improper coordination of the tongue and upper airway muscles, instability of the throat (pharynx), or other factors. Resulting episodes of apnea, known as obstructive apnea, are characterized by absence of airflow but ongoing chest wall movements. Most infants with apnea of prematurity experience both central and obstructive apnea.

With infant apnea, more appropriately called an apparent life-threatening event, initial episodes of apnea typically occur on the second to the seventh day of life. Such episodes are defined as serious if breathing spontaneously ceases for more than 15 to 20 seconds or if they result in decreased levels of oxygen in the blood and associated bluish discoloration of the skin and mucous membranes (cyanosis) and slowing of the heart rate (bradycardia).

The frequency of apnea episodes typically increases during the cycle of sleep that is associated with rapid eye movements (REMs), dreaming, increased levels of brain activity, and involuntary muscle jerks. During REM sleep, infants are more likely to experience abnormal chest wall movements during breathing, such as relaxation of the chest muscles while inhaling rather than exhaling. Abnormal chest wall movements as well as inhibition of muscle tone (particularly of the throat) during REM sleep contribute to the increased frequency of apneic episodes.

Infants at risk for episodes of apnea should be monitored with devices that detect abnormal changes in chest wall movements, heart rate, and respiratory activity. These devices, known as apnea monitors, sound an alarm when spontaneous breathing temporarily ceases. In infants who experience mild, occasional episodes of apnea, supportive measures may be sufficient, such as gentle skin stimulation and massage. In patients with severe, prolonged, and recurrent apnea episodes, treatment should include close monitoring, immediate measures to assist breathing (e.g., bag and maskentilation) and oxygen therapy to ensure sufficient oxygen supply to body tissues. Infants with apnea may be monitored at home which can have a significant impact on caregivers. In general, as the child matures, the cause of the ALTE is diagnosed and treated or spontaneously resolves.

Government Agencies

292 **NIH/National Institute of Child Health and Human Development**

31 Center Drive, Building 31 Room 2A32
Bethesda, MD 10051
800-370-2943
Fax: 301-496-1104
TTY: 888-320-6942
e-mail: NICHDInformationResourceCenter@mail.nih.
www.nichd.nih.gov

Established in 1962 by congress, today the institute conducts and supports laboratory research, clinical trials, and epidemiological studies that explore health processes; examines the impact of disabilities, diseases, and variations on the lives of individuals; and sponsors training programs for scientists, health care providers, and researchers to ensure that NICHD research can continue.

Alan E Guttmacher MD, Director
Lisa Kaeser, Program & Public Liaison

293 **NIH/National Institute of Neurological Dis orders and Stroke (NINDS)**

PO Box 5801
Bethesda, MD 10052
301-496-5751
800-352-9424
Fax: 301-496-0296
TTY: 301-468-5981
www.ninds.nih.gov

Works to reduce the burden of neurological disease by conducting, fostering, coordinating and guiding research on the causes, prevention, diagnosis and treatment of neurological disorders and stroke, while supporting basic research in related scientific areas.

Story C Landis Ph.D., Director
Audrey S Penn M.D., Deputy Director

National Associations & Support Groups

294 **American Academy of Pediatrics**

141 Northwest Point Boulevard
Elk Grove Village, IL 60007
847-434-4000
800-433-9016
Fax: 847-434-8000
www.aap.org

The American Academy of Pediatrics and its member pediatricians are committed to the attainment of optimal physical, mental and social health and well-being for all infants, children, adolescents, and young adults.

Sandra Hassink, MD, FAAP, President

295 **American Sleep Apnea Association**

6856 Eastern Ave, NW #203
Washington, DC 10053
202-293-3650
Fax: 202-293-3656
e-mail: asaa@sleepapnea.org
www.sleepapnea.org

Dedicated to reducing injury, disability and death from sleep apnea and to enhancing the well-being of those affected by this common disorder. They promote education and awareness. Network of voluntary mutual support groups, research, and continuous improvement of care.

Edward Grandi, Executive Director
Rochelle Goldberg, President
Kathe Henke, CFO

296 **National Sleep Foundation**

1522 K Street NW, Suite 500
Washington, DC 10054
202-347-3471
Fax: 202-347-3472
e-mail: nsf@sleepfoundation.org
www.narap.org

Works to improve the quality of life for millions of Americans who suffer from sleep disorders, and to prevent the catastrophic accidents that are related to poor or disordered sleep through research, education and the dissemination of information towards the cause of the Narcolepsy Project. Seeks patients to aid new research project targeting the cause of the disorder.

Richard Gelula, CEO
David Cloud, Executive Vice President
Ronald Sears, Senior Director of Development

Web Sites

297 Apnea of Prematurity
825 Eighth Avenue, 11th Floor
New York, NY 10019   212-301-6700
                        www.emedicine.com/ped/topic1157.htm

Provides information on how to tell if an unborn baby has sleep apnea.

Dharmendra J. Nimavat, MD, FAAP, Author
Ted Rosenkrantz, MD, Chief Editor

Camps

298 VACC Camp
Miami Children's Hospital
3200 SW 60th Court, Suite 203
Miami, FL 33155   305-662-8222
                              Fax: 786-268-1765
                        e-mail: bela.florentin@mch.com
                              www.vacccamp.com

Free, week-long, overnight camp for ventilation assisted children (children needing a tracheotomy ventilator, C-PAP, BiPAP, or oxygen to support breathing) and their families. Gives families a fun oppourtinity to socialize with peers and enjoy activities not readily accessible to technology dependent children.

Moises Simpser, MD, Camp Director
Bela Florentin, Camp Coordinator

Description

299   ARNOLD-CHIARI MALFORMATION

Synonyms: ACM, Arnold-Chiari deformity, Arnold-Chiari syndrome, Chiari malformation

Covers these related disorders: Arnold-Chiari malformation type I, Arnold-Chiari malformation type II

Involves the following Biologic System(s):
Neurologic Disorders

Arnold-Chiari malformation is a developmental abnormality characterized by deformities at the base of the brain that are present at birth (congenital). Such deformities typically include abnormal elongation of a portion of the cerebellum (cerebellar tonsils) and the lowest region of the brain stem (medulla oblongata), resulting in protrusion of these regions through the large opening (foramen magnum) in the base of the skull and into the upper spinal canal (cervical canal). The cerebellum is a region of the brain that plays an essential role in coordinating voluntary movement and maintaining posture and balance. The brain stem, which is the lowest section of the brain and connects it with the spinal cord, helps to relay motor and sensory impulses between other regions of the brain and the spinal cord, and connects with most of the cranial nerves, which conduct impulses involved in such functions as taste, vision, swallowing, and facial expression, as well as movements of the tongue, head, and shoulders. Although the exact cause of Arnold-Chiari malformation is unknown, researchers have suggested that it may result from the interaction of several genes, environmental influences, or both (multifactorial inheritance).

In some affected newborns, Arnold-Chiari malformation occurs in association with myelomeningocele, a developmental abnormality characterized by protrusion (herniation) of a portion of the spinal cord and its protective membranes (meninges) through an abnormal opening in the bone of the spinal column. Arnold-Chiari malformation without a myelomeningocele is termed Arnold-Chiari malformation type I. When it is accompanied by a myelomeningocele, the condition is known as Arnold-Chiari malformation type II. In both types of the condition, the foramen magnum is abnormally large. Additionally, the base of the skull is flattened and may be pushed upward by the upper vertebrae (cervical vertebrae) surrounding the spinal cord.

Infants and children with Arnold-Chiari malformation type II experience progressive hydrocephalus, a condition characterized by the abnormal accumulation of cerebrospinal fluid (CSF) in the brain. This accumulation of CSF, which comes from obstruction of the normal flow of this fluid between the brain and spine, or its impaired absorption results in increased fluid pressure within cavities (ventricles) of the brain. Other findings in Arnold-Chiari malformation type II may include abnormal enlargement of the chambers within the brain that contain its CSF, known as the ventricles, potential enlargement of the head, and other associated symptoms and findings. Some infants with Arnold-Chiari malformation type II may also experience abnormalities due to pressure or damage to lower cranial nerves. Such abnormalities, which vary in range and severity, include uncontrollable twitching (fasciculations) of the tongue, a high-pitched sound upon inhalation (i.e., laryngeal stridor), facial weakness, hearing impairment, lagging of the head (sternomastoid paralysis), or weakness or impaired control of muscles that turn the eyes outward (bilateral abducens palsies). During later childhood, some patients with Arnold-Chiari malformation type II may experience increased stiffness (rigidity), causing restriction of movement (spasticity); abnormalities in walking (abnormal gait); and progressive lack of coordination. During later childhood or adolescence, individuals with this condition may also experience symptoms and findings often associated with Arnold-Chiari malformation type I.

These symptoms may also first occur in adolescence or adulthood rather than in childhood, and often occur without hydrocephalus. Associated symptoms and findings may include recurrent headaches; neck pain; impaired control of voluntary movements (ataxia); or progressive muscle weakness, degeneration (atrophy), spasticity, and potential sensory loss affecting the lower and, in some cases, the upper limbs.

Treatment of Arnold-Chiari malformation depends on the severity of the malformation and associated symptoms and findings. If symptoms are only mild, treatment includes regular monitoring and symptomatic and supportive measures as required, such as the use of medication to relieve pain. However, surgery is the only means of correcting the structural problem in Arnold-Chiari malformation, and is required in more severe cases of this condition. The surgery for Arnold-Chiari malformation is directed at uncrowding the area at the base of the cerebellum where this part of the brain is pushing against the brain stem and spinal cord. This is done by removing a small portion of bone at the base of the skull, and often also by removing a part of the back of the first and occasionally other upper segments of the spinal column (e.g., upper cervical laminectomy).

Government Agencies

300   NIH/National Institute of Child Health and Human Development
31 Center Drive, Building 31 Room 2A32
Bethesda, MD 10055
                                                    800-370-2943
                                            Fax: 301-496-1104
                                            TTY: 888-320-6942
        e-mail: NICHDInformationResourceCenter@mail.nih.
                                                www.nichd.nih.gov

Established in 1962 by congress, today the institute conducts and supports laboratory research, clinical trials, and epidemiological studies that explore health processes; examines the impact of disabilities, diseases, and variations on the lives of individuals; and sponsors training programs for scientists, health care providers, and researchers to ensure that NICHD research can continue.

Alan E Guttmacher MD, Director
Lisa Kaeser, Program & Public Liaison

National Associations & Support Groups

301   American Academy of Pediatrics
141 Northwest Point Boulevard
Elk Grove Village, IL 60007
                                                    847-434-4000
                                                    800-433-9016
                                            Fax: 847-434-8000
                                                    www.aap.org

The American Academy of Pediatrics and its member pediatricians are committed to the attainment of optimal physical, mental and social health and well-being for all infants, children, adolescents, and young adults.

Sandra Hassink, MD, FAAP, President

302   Genetic Alliance
4301 Connecticut Avenue NW
Washington, DC 10056
202-966-7955
800-336-4363
Fax: 202-966-8553
e-mail: info@geneticalliance.org
www.geneticalliance.org

World's leading nonprofit health advocacy organization committed to transforming health through genetics and promoting an environment of openness centered on the health of individuals, families, and communities.

Sharon Terry, President
Lisa Wise, Chief Operating Officer
Tetyana Murza MES, Managing Director

303   March of Dimes Birth Defects Foundation
1275 Mamaroneck Avenue
White Plains, NY 10057
914-997-4488
888-663-4637
Fax: 914-997-4763
e-mail: answers@marchofdimes.com
www.marchofdimes.com

March of Dimes help moms have full-term pregnancies and research the problems that threaten the health of babies.The March of Dimes also acts globally: sharing best practices in perinatal health and helping improve birth outcomes where the needs are the most urgent.

Kenneth A. May, Chair
Jennifer Howse, President & CEO
Alan Fleischman, Medical Director

304   World Arnold-Chiari Malformation Association
31 Newtown Woods Road
Newtown Square, PA 10059
610-353-4737
e-mail: chiari-owner@yahoogroups.com
www.pressenter.com/~wacma/

Staffed by volunteers, we are committed to providing support, current information, and understanding to those affected by the Arnold Chiari malformation and syringomyelia. It is also our goal to raise the awareness of, and educate the medical community as to the complex nature of this disease and how it affects the lives of those who have it.

Bernie Meyer, Manager/Moderator
Ann Hood, Manager/Moderator
Sandi Justin, Manager/Moderator

Conferences

305   Genetic Alliance Annual Conference
Genetic Alliance
4301 Connecticut Avenue NW, Suite 404
Washington, DC 20008
202-966-5557
800-336-4363
Fax: 202-966-8553
e-mail: info@geneticalliance.org
www.geneticalliance.org

Consistently inspirational and enables partnership among all stakeholders: advocates and community leaders, health and industry professionals, policymakers, and academicians.

July

Sharon Terry, President/CEO
Tetyana Murza, Programs/Events Manager

Web Sites

306   National Institute of Health NINDS Information Page
PO Box 5801
Bethesda, MD 20824
301-496-5751
800-352-9424
www.ninds.nih.gov

The mission is to reduce the burden of neurological disease — a burden born by every age group, by every segment of society, by people all over the world.

Walter J. Koroshetz, M.D., Acting Director
Alan L. Willard, Ph.D., Acting Deputy Director
Caroline Lewis, Executive Officer

307   Online Mendelian Inheritance in Man
National Library of Medicine, Building 38A
Bethesda, MD 20894
888-346-3656
e-mail: info@ncbi.nlm.nih.gov
www.ncbi.nlm.nih.gov

This database is a catalog of human genes and genetic disorders.

Christine E. Seidman, M.D., Chair
David J. Lipman, M.D., Executive Secretary

308   Rare Genetic Diseases in Children (NYU)
www.med.nyu.edu/rgdc/homenow.htm

We target issues arising from rare genetic diseases affecting children. And assist in the endeavor to bring knowledge and hope to those for whom there is, at present, so little.

Book Publishers

309   Let's Talk About Going to the Hospital
Rosen Publishing Group's PowerKids Press
29 E 21st Street
New York, NY 10010
212-777-3017
800-237-9932
Fax: 888-436-4643
e-mail: rosenpub@tribeca.ios.com
www.rosenpublishing.com

If a child has to check into the hospital, chances are he or she is already upset about being ill. Knowing how a hospital functions and what the procedures are, such as when family members can visit, will help in what is already a stressful situation. Grades K-5.

24 pages
ISBN: 0-823950-36-0

Description

310 ARRHYTHMIAS

Covers these related disorders: Supraventricular Tachycardia (SVT), Wolff-Parkinson-White Syndrome (WPW)

Involves the following Biologic System(s):

Cardiovascular Disorders

The term arrhythmia refers to an abnormality in the rhythm of the heartbeat. It may take the form of an abnormally slow or abnormally fast heartbeat or another disturbance in heart rhythm. Any such problem can interfere with the ability of the heart to effectively pump blood to the body's organs and tissues. Many such problems can, however, be treated medically, surgically, or in other ways.

Arrhythmias result from disturbances in the electrical conduction system of the heart, also called the cardiac conduction system. This system consists of pathways, made up of specialized tissues that conduct electrical impulses to the muscle cells of the heart, prompting them to contract and pump blood. Within the cardiac conduction system are also several tissue structures known as nodes, which act as pacemakers, coordinating the sequence of muscle contractions by which the heart pumps blood from each of its four chambers into the next chamber and out into the lungs and body. This coordinated pumping begins in the right atrium or upper right chamber of the heart, which collects blood that re-enters the heart after circulating through the body. The muscle tissue of the right atrium then contracts, pumping this blood downward and into the right ventricle, the chamber of the heart that is located immediately below the right atrium. The right ventricle pumps this blood to the lungs, which supply the blood with oxygen and return it to the left atrium of the heart, which pumps this oxygenated blood downward and into the most muscular of the heart's four chambers, the left ventricle. The left ventricle then pumps the oxygenated blood out of itself and into the body by way of the large main artery known as the aorta.

Most of the arrhythmias caused by aberrations in the cardiac conduction system can be detected with the diagnostic procedure known as electrocardiography. In this procedure, small electrodes that sense the electrical impulses that accompany each heartbeat are pasted to the skin at locations on the chest, arms, and legs. The impulses pass into the electrodes and through wires to an instrument that records, on paper or on a computer screen, the visible tracing known as an electrocardiogram (ECG or EKG), which indicates the intensity, rhythm, and other features of the heartbeat.

Normally, the heart contracts at a rate of 60 to 80 beats per minute when the body is at rest, and this rate increases with exercise to meet the body's increased need for oxygen and blood-borne nutrients. An increased heartbeat rate is known as a tachycardia, while a heartbeat that falls below the normal rate is called a bradycardia. In many instances, both tachycardias and bradycardias are temporary, passing events without serious or dangerous effects. Thus, exercise, excitement, and fever can all cause the typically harmless tachycardia known as sinus tachycardia. The most frequent type of medically important tachycardia in infants and children under the age of 12 is known as supraventricular tachycardia (SVT), sometimes also called paroxysmal supraventricular tachycar-

dia (PSVT) or paroxysmal atrial tachycardia (PAT). As its name indicates, this type of tachycardia comes from a disturbance in the cardiac conduction system that originates at some point above the ventricles. It is characterized by a heart rate of more than 220 beats per minute, but is not typically life-threatening. Infants experiencing an instance of SVT may seem restless, have rapid breathing, or be especially sleepy. SVT requires treatment only if it is frequent or its episodes are long-lasting. Treatment of SVT is based on the specific mechanism responsible for the tachycardia and the age of the patient. A variety of medications (anti-arrhythmia agents) are available for controlling SVT.

More potentially serious than SVT is ventricular tachycardia (VT), caused by an aberration in conduction at some point below the atria of the heart. Although it may occur in the absence of any apparent source, VT is most often the result of damage to or an inborn defect in the conduction system or in another component of the heart. If it occurs in the right ventricle, VT can interfere with pumping of blood to the lungs, and in the left ventricle can interfere with pumping of blood through the entire body. One way in which VT may disrupt the heart's pumping of blood is by triggering the condition known as ventricular fibrillation, in which a weak, flaccid pattern of ventricular contraction replaces the normally forceful, coordinated contractions of these chambers of the heart, preventing them from effectively pumping blood.

A cause of serious disturbances in heart rhythm is the condition known as Wolff-Parkinson-White (WPW) syndrome. This results from an aberration in the cardiac conduction system at some point between the atria and ventricles, and can cause the sudden, complete, and life-threatening cessation of heartbeat known as cardiac arrest. In many cases, WPW syndrome shows no outward signs of its existence, and is first identified only on an electrocardiogram. WPW syndrome often responds to medical treatment with drugs. Destruction or ablation of its source within the cardiac conduction system often corrects WPW syndrome. This technique, known as radiofrequency ablation, involves the passage of an electrical current through a catheter and directly into the source of the syndrome. In other instances surgery is often effective in eliminating WPW syndrome.

Also serious is the condition known as complete heart block, which can occur during childhood and even prenatally. This disorder results from a genetic defect or other damage to the cardiac conduction system that interrupts electrical conduction within the heart, interfering with the pumping of blood from the atria into the ventricles. When this happens, a naturally occurring pacemaker within the ventricles sustains their contraction and pumping of blood, but at a reduced heart rate. If this natural process does not restore an adequate heart rate, heart block may be corrected by implantation of an artificial pacemaker.

Another source of interference with normal heart rhythm is sick sinus syndrome. In this condition, the sinus node, one of the natural pacemakers within the cardiac conduction system, is damaged by illness, injury, or accidentally during heart surgery, triggering intermittent episodes of either tachycardia or of the slowed heartbeat rate known as bradycardia. Symptoms of this condition may include fatigue or faintness. The condition can be treated medically, with drugs, and if necessary by implantation of an artificial pacemaker.

National Associations & Support Groups

311 American Academy of Pediatrics
141 Northwest Point Boulevard
Elk Grove Village, IL 60007

847-434-4000
800-433-9016
Fax: 847-434-8000
www.aap.org

The American Academy of Pediatrics and its member pediatricians are committed to the attainment of optimal physical, mental and social health and well-being for all infants, children, adolescents, and young adults.

Sandra Hassink, MD, FAAP, President

312 American College of Cardiology
2400 N Street, NW
Washington, DC 10060

202-375-6000
800-253-4636
Fax: 202-375-7000
e-mail: resource@acc.org
www.cardiosource.org/acc

The mission of the American College of Cardiology is to advocate for quality cardiovascular care, through education, research promotion, development and application of standards and guidelines, and to influence health care policy.

Shalom Jacobovitz, CEO
Patrick T. O' Gara, MD, FACC, President-Elect
Kim Allan Williams, Sr., MD, FACC, Vice President

313 American Heart Association
7272 Greenville Avenue
Dallas, TX 10061

214-373-6300
800-242-8721
Fax: 214-706-1341
e-mail: inquire@amhrt.org
www.heart.org/dallas?

Our mission is to build healthier lives, free of cardiovascular diseases and stroke. That single purpose drives all we do. The need for our work is beyond question

Nancy Brown, CEO
Donna Arnett, President
Suzie Upton, Chief Development Officer

314 Heart Failure Society of America
5425 Wisconsin Avenue - Suite 600
Chevy Chase, MD 10063

301-718-4800
Fax: 301-968-2431
e-mail: info@hfsa.org
www.hfsa.org

The Heart Failure Society of America, Inc. (HFSA) represents the first organized effort by heart failure experts from the Americas to provide a forum for all those interested in heart function, heart failure, and congestive heart failure (CHF) research and patient care.

Thomas Force MD, President
Joann Lindenfield MD, Vice President
Christopher M O'Connor MD, Treasurer

315 Rush Children's Heart Center
1653 W Congress Parkway
Chicago, IL 10064

312-942-5000
888-352-7874
e-mail: contact_rush@rush.edu
www.rush.edu/rumc/page-1099918801842.html

Rush Children's Hospital, part of at Rush University Medical Center in Chicago, Illinois, provides complete clinical services for the diagnosis and treatment of congenital and acquired heart disease in children and young adults.

Larry J Goodman MD, CEO
Richard M Jaffee, Chairman
Susan Crown, Vice Chair

316 Sudden Arrhythmia Death Syndromes Foundati on
508 E South Temple, Suite 202
Salt Lake City, UT 10065

801-531-0937
800-786-7723
Fax: 801-531-0945
e-mail: sads@sads.org
www.sads.org

Our mission is to save the lives and support the families of children and young adults who are genetically predisposed to sudden death due to heart rhythm abnormalities.

Michael J Ackerman MD PhD, Board President
Sunsan Etheridge MD, Board Vice President
Scott Dailard, Board Secretary

Research Centers

317 Cardiovascular Research Foundation
111 East 59th Street
New York, NY 10066

646-434-4500
e-mail: info@crf.org
www.crf.org

A nonprofit organization with a mission to improve the survival and quality of life for people with cardiovascular disease through research and education.

Gary S Mintz MD, CFO
Colette Y Gardner, President
Eric B Woldenberg Esq, Chairman

Conferences

318 HFSA Annual Scientific Meeting
Heart Failure Society of America
2550 University Avenue W
Saint Paul, MN 10062

651-642-1633
Fax: 651-642-1502
e-mail: info@hfsa.org
www.hfsa.org

The Heart Failure Society of America, Inc. (HFSA) represents the first organized effort by heart failure experts from the Americas to provide a forum for all those interested in heart function, heart failure, and congestive heart failure (CHF) research and patient care.

September

Barry M Massie MD, President

Web Sites

319 Heart Center Online
495 East Waterfront Drive Suite 200
Homestead, PA 15120

412-326-0330
www.heartcenteronline.com

The mission of the Heart Center Online is to be the premier cardiovascular specialized health care site on the Internet, to provide cardiovascular patients, their families and site visitors with tools they need to better understand the complex nature of heart-related conditions, treatments and preventive care, and to provide services and applications that deliver value to cardiovascular practices.

320 Rush Children's Heart Center
www.rush.edu

Provides complete clinical services for the diagnosis and treatment of congenital and acquired heart disease in children and young adults.

321 Yale University School of Medicine
333 Cedar Street
New Haven, CT 6510

203-432-4771
medicine.yale.edu

Information on heart conditions, including arrhythmias.

Peter Salovey, President of the University
Richard Belitsky M.D., Deputy Dean for Education
Benjamin Polak, B.A., M.A., Ph.D., Provost of the University

Journals

322   Journal of Cardiac Failure
Cardiac Heart Failure Society of America
6707 Democracy Blvd. Suite 925
Bethesda, MD 20817   301-312-8635
                                                     Fax: 888-213-4417
                                                  e-mail: info@hfsa.org
                                                          www.hfsa.org

Contains review articles on clinical research, basic human studies, animal studies, and bench research with potential clinical applications to heart failure, pathogenesis, etiology, epidemiology,
pathophysiological mechanisms, assessment, prevention and
treatment.

6x year

Michele Blair, CEO
JoAnn Lindenfeld, MD, President
Mandeep R. Mehra, MD, Vice President

323   Texas Heart Institute Journal
Texas Heart Institute
6770 Bertner Avenue
Houston, TX 77030   832-355-3792
                                                     Fax: 832-355-3714
                                          e-mail: webmaster@texasheart.org
                                                 www.texasheartinstitute.org

The purpose of the Texas Heart Institute Journal is to educate,
with emphasis on the dissemination of information to physicians
in practice.

Quaterly

Denton A. Cooley, MD, Founder
L. Maximilian Buja, MD, Chief
C. David Collard, MD, Chief

Newsletters

324   Heart Failure Society Newsletter
6707 Democracy Blvd. Suite 925
Bethesda, MD 20817   301-312-8635
                                                     Fax: 888-213-4417
                                                  e-mail: info@hfsa.org
                                                          www.hfsa.org

Provides information on the society and also on different aspects
of heart failure.

Quaterly

Michele Blair, CEO
JoAnn Lindenfeld, MD, President
Mandeep R. Mehra, MD, Vice President

Description

325 ARTHROGRYPOSIS MULTIPLEX CONGENITA
Synonym: AMC
Covers these related disorders: Amyoplasia
Involves the following Biologic System(s):
Orthopedic and Muscle Disorders

Arthrogryposis multiplex congenita (AMC) refers to a group of disorders present at birth (congenital) that are characterized by limited movement or immobility of multiple joints and partial or complete replacement of involved muscle with fibrous or fatty tissue. Affected joints may be permanently flexed or extended in various fixed postures (joint contractures). Approximately 150 syndromes have been identified that are characterized by the presence of congenital multiple contractures. The most common form of arthrogryposis multiplex congenita is known as amyoplasia. This classic form of AMC affects approximately one in 10,000 newborns.

In newborns with amyoplasia, multiple congenital contractures are present that typically affect the upper and lower extremities. In most newborns who are affected, such contractures include abnormal flexion or extension of the elbows; flexion of the wrists toward either the thumb side or pinky side of the hands(radial or ulnar deviation); cupping of the hands; and internal rotation of the shoulders. Many newborns with amyoplasia also have severe deformities of the feet (clubfoot or talipes equinovarus) in which the heels are turned inward and the soles of the feet are flexed (plantar flexion). Additional musculoskeletal deformities are also typically present including abnormal rigidity of the joints between the bones of the thumbs and other fingers (interphalangeal joints); deformities of the palms of the hands; fixed flexion or extension of the knees; and abnormal flexion, extension, rotation, and possible dislocation of the hips. These abnormalities are usually similar from one side of the body to the other (symmetric). Amyoplasia is also characterized by a susceptibility to bone fractures (i.e., perinatal fractures) and progressive abnormal sideways curvature of the spine (scoliosis) that varies in severity and in age at onset. Most newborns with amyoplasia also have distinctive facial abnormalities including short, upturned (anteverted) nostrils; a rounded face; a slightly small jaw (mild micrognathia); and a benign, reddish, purple growth in the midportion of the face (midline frontal hemangioma). Amyoplasia appears to occur randomly for unknown reasons (sporadically), and the underlying causes of amyoplasia and other forms of AMC are not fully understood.

All newborns with multiple congenital joint contractures should receive a thorough neuromuscular evaluation to help detect, confirm, or rule out potential underlying muscular or neurologic abnormalities. The treatment of infants and children with amyoplasia includes symptomatic and supportive measures. The presence of fractures should be ruled out or confirmed (e.g., with x-ray studies) and treated as necessary (e.g., with appropriate immobilization) before physical therapy is begun. Other treatment measures for congenital contractures and associated abnormalities include physical therapy (e.g., passive range of motion exercises) and splinting of extremities to improve the range of motion; the use of casts or other orthopedic appliances; and possible surgical interventions. In addition, orthopedic appliances may be used to help slow the progression of scoliosis. In most patients with severe scoliosis, surgical measures may also be required.

Government Agencies

326 NIH/National Institute of Arthritis and Musculoskeletal and Skin Diseases
1 AMS Circle
Bethesda, MD 10067

301-402-4484
877-226-4267
Fax: 301-718-6366
TTY: 301-565-2966
TDD: 301-565-2966
e-mail: niamsinfo@mail.nih.gov
www.niams.nih.gov

The mission of the National Institute of Arthritis and Musculoskeletal and Skin Diseases is to support research into the causes, treatment, and prevention of arthritis and musculoskeletal and skin diseases; the training of basic and clinical scientists to carry out this research; and the dissemination of information on research progress in these diseases

Stephen I Katz MD PhD, Director
Robert H Carter MD, Deputy Director
Gahan Breithaupt, Assoc Dir. Management & Operations

National Associations & Support Groups

327 American Academy of Pediatrics
141 Northwest Point Boulevard
Elk Grove Village, IL 60007

847-434-4000
800-433-9016
Fax: 847-434-8000
www.aap.org

The American Academy of Pediatrics and its member pediatricians are committed to the attainment of optimal physical, mental and social health and well-being for all infants, children, adolescents, and young adults.

Sandra Hassink, MD, FAAP, President

328 Genetic Alliance
4301 Connecticut Avenue NW
Washington, DC 10068

202-966-7955
800-336-4363
Fax: 202-966-8553
e-mail: info@geneticalliance.org
www.geneticalliance.org

World's leading nonprofit health advocacy organization committed to transforming health through genetics and promoting an environment of openness centered on the health of individuals, families, and communities.

Sharon Terry, President
Lisa Wise, Chief Operating Officer
Tetyana Murza MES, Managing Director

329 Human Growth Foundation
997 Glen Cove Avenue, Suite 5
Glen Head, NY 10069

516-671-4041
800-451-6434
Fax: 516-671-4055
e-mail: hgf1@hgfound.org
www.hgfound.org

A voluntary, nonprofit organization whose mission is to help children and adults with disorders of growth and growth hormones through research, education, support and advocacy. The foundation is dedicated to helping medical science to better understand the process of growth. It is composed of concerned parents and friends of children and adults with growth problems and interested health professionals.

Patricia D Costa, Executive Director
Earl A. Gershenow, Board of Directors
Emily Germain-Lee MD, Vice President

330 **MAGIC Foundation: Major Aspects of Growth in Children**
6645 W North Avenue
Oak Park, IL 10070   708-383-0808
                                                 800-362-4423
                                                 Fax: 708-383-0899
                                                 e-mail: mary@magicfoundation.org
                                                 www.magicfoundation.org

A national nonprofit organization providing support and education regarding growth disorders in children and related adult disorders. Provides educational information, networking, a national conference, a kids' program and an extensive medical library.

Rich Buckley, Chairman
Kenn Dickard, Vice Chairman
Teresa Tucker, Director at Large

331 **March of Dimes Birth Defects Foundation**
1275 Mamaroneck Avenue
White Plains, NY 10071   914-997-4488
                                                 888-663-4637
                                                 Fax: 914-997-4763
                                                 e-mail: answers@marchofdimes.com
                                                 www.marchofdimes.com

March of Dimes help moms have full-term pregnancies and research the problems that threaten the health of babies.The March of Dimes also acts globally: sharing best practices in perinatal health and helping improve birth outcomes where the needs are the most urgent.

Kenneth A. May, Chair
Jennifer Howse, President & CEO
Alan Fleischman, Medical Director

Conferences

332 **Adult GHD Educational Convention**
Magic Foundation
6645 W North Avenue
Oak Park, IL 60302   708-383-0808
                                                 800-362-4423
                                                 Fax: 708-383-0899
                                                 e-mail: contactus@magicfoundation.org
                                                 www.magicfoundation.org

An educational program for adults who are affected with Growth Hormone Deficiency and/or other endocrine disorders.

June

Rick Buckley, Chairman
Ken Dickard, Vice Chairman
Courtney Lance, Secretary

333 **Genetic Alliance Annual Conference**
Genetic Alliance
4301 Connecticut Avenue NW, Suite 404
Washington, DC 20008   202-966-5557
                                                 800-336-4363
                                                 Fax: 202-966-8553
                                                 e-mail: info@geneticalliance.org
                                                 www.geneticalliance.org

Consistently inspirational and enables partnership among all stakeholders: advocates and community leaders, health and industry professionals, policymakers, and academicians.

July

Sharon Terry, President/CEO
Tetyana Murza, Programs/Events Manager

Web Sites

334 **Online Mendelian Inheritance in Man**
National Library of Medicine, Building 38A
Bethesda, MD 20894   888-346-3656
                                                 e-mail: info@ncbi.nlm.nih.gov
                                                 www.ncbi.nlm.nih.gov

This database is a catalog of human genes and genetic disorders.

Christine E. Seidman, M.D., Chair
David J. Lipman, M.D., Executive Secretary

335 **Wheeless' Textbook of Orthopaedics**
www.wheelessonline.com

Comprehensive, unparalleled, dynamic online medical textbook that is updated daily.

Clifford R. Wheeless, III, M.D., Author

Book Publishers

336 **Let's Talk About Going to the Hospital**
Rosen Publishing Group's PowerKids Press
29 E 21st Street
New York, NY 10010   212-777-3017
                                                 800-237-9932
                                                 Fax: 888-436-4643
                                                 e-mail: rosenpub@tribeca.ios.com
                                                 www.rosenpublishing.com

If a child has to check into the hospital, chances are he or she is already upset about being ill. Knowing how a hospital functions and what the procedures are, such as when family members can visit, will help in what is already a stressful situation. Grades K-5.

24 pages
ISBN: 0-823950-36-0

Description

337 ASPERGER SYNDROME
Involves the following Biologic System(s):
Developmental/Behavioral/Psychiatric Disorders,
Genetic/Chromosomal/Syndrome/Metabolic Disorders, Neurologic
Disorders

Asperger syndrome (AS) is a developmental disorder belonging to the group of neurological conditions known as autism spectrum disorders (ASDs), which are marked by problems in language and communications and confined patterns of thought and behavior. AS usually manifests itself by the age of 3 years, and in some cases may be apparent in infancy through clumsiness and delayed crawling or walking. Children with AS have no difficulty with intelligence or language skills, but may speak in a monotone or in an excessively formal manner or have difficulties with the subtleties of language, such as the slight variations in rhythm and pitch that help to communicate different shades of meaning (prosody). Children with AS also exhibit repetitive or ritualistic behavior; tend to be preoccupied with a single activity or area of personal interest to the exclusion of other activities or interests; have difficulty in their gestures and motor movements, such as those needed for ballplaying or playground activities; and interact poorly with other children of their age group and usually also with adults, manifesting motor symptoms of the syndrome or focusing on their own interests rather than engaging in dialogue. In some cases, AS in children is followed by other psychological problems and symptoms in adolescence and adulthood.

AS occurs in about 2 of every 10,000 children and is more likely to affect boys than girls. Although its precise cause remains unknown, studies suggest that AS stems from aberrations in the structure and function of several regions of the brain, which may come from irregularities in the fetal development and growth of the brain. Recent studies suggest that susceptibility to AS, and the severity with which it affects an individual, may be related to one or more aberrations in a specific group of genes.

The absence of standardized, universally accepted diagnostic criteria for AS has complicated its diagnosis. Currently, several verbal and behavioral procedures are used in diagnostic testing for AS. Because each of these procedures has its own standards, the various procedures can yield different diagnostic results. Moreover, different specialists have different viewpoints about the nature and characteristics of AS, with some considering it a mild form of autism known as high-functioning autism rather than a distinct disorder. In identifying AS, most physicians use a set of criteria based on abnormal eye contact; failure of a child to respond to its name; failure to use gestures to point or indicate an object or item; and a lack of interest in and play with other children of the same age.

The complete examination of a child with suspected AS typically requires a psychologist, psychiatrist, neurologist, and speech therapist, with other professionals called upon as needed. Diagnosis of the syndrome includes testing of intelligence, language and communication skills, motor and other neurologic function, and genetics.

The treatment of AS similarly requires professionals specialized in improving the communications skills, easing the obsessive or repetitive behavioral patterns, and reducing the physical clumsiness of children with the syndrome. This typically involves strengthening the child's interests, actively involving the child in structured activities, and reinforcing socially adaptive behavior through the use of supervised group therapy. Physical and occupational therapy can be used to improve affected childrens' motor skills. Although they usually require these special educational services, children with Asperger syndrome are typically educated in the traditional community setting. If needed, medication can be used to alleviate anxiety and depression in children with AS.

Government Agencies

338 NIH/National Institute of Mental Health
6001 Executive Boulevard, Room 8184, MSC 9663
Bethesda, MD 10072
301-443-4513
866-615-6464
Fax: 301-443-4279
TTY: 301-443-8431
e-mail: nimhinfo@nih.gov
www.nimh.nih.gov

The mission of NIMH is to transform the understanding and treatment of mental illnesses through basic and clinical research, paving the way for prevention, recovery, and cure.
Dr Thomas R Insel, Director

339 NIH/National Institute of Neurological Dis orders and Stroke (NINDS)
PO Box 5801
Bethesda, MD 10073
301-496-5751
800-352-9424
Fax: 301-496-0296
TTY: 301-468-5981
www.ninds.nih.gov

The mission of NINDS is to reduce the burden of neurological disease - a burden borne by every age group, by every segment of society, by people all over the world.
Story C Landis Ph.D., Director
Walter J Koroshetz, Deputy Director
Caroline Lewis, Executive Officer

340 NIH/National Institute on Deafness and Oth er Communication Disorders (NIDCD)
31 Center Drive, MSC 2320
Bethesda, MD 20892
800-241-1044
TTY: 800-241-1055
e-mail: nidcdinfo@nidcd.nih.gov
www.nidcd.nih.gov

Conducts and supports biomedical research and research training on normal mechanisms, as well as diseases and disorders of hearing, balance, smell, taste, voice, speech and language.
Dr James F Battey Jr, Director
Judith A Cooper PhD, Deputy Director
W David Kerr, Executive Officer

National Associations & Support Groups

341 AASCEND
P.O. Box 591011
San Francisco, CA 94159
e-mail: info@aascend.org
www.aascend.org

Adults of all ages on the autism spectrum, their families and friends, academics and professionals in the autism field unite as a community in AASCEND.
Greg Yates, Co-chair

342 AHA Association [Asperger Syndrome and High Functioning Autism Association
PO Box 916
Bethpage, NY 11714
888-918-9198
Fax: 888-918-9198
e-mail: info@ahany.org
www.ahany.org

Serves individuals on the autism spectrum, their families, and the professionals who work with them, providing crucial resources and support as they face challenges, build on their strengths and fulfill their potential.

Pat Schissel, LMSW, President/ Executive Director
Michael A. Buffa, Esq., VP of Board of Directors
Jennifer Feldman, Event Coordinator

343 ASPEN (Asperger Autism SPectrum Education Network)
9 Aspen Circle
Edison, NJ 8820
732-321-0880
e-mail: aspenorg@aol.com
aspennj.org

ASPEN provides families and individuals whose lives are affected by Autism Spectrum Disorders (Asperger Syndrome, Pervasive Developmental Disorder-NOS, High Functioning Autism), and Nonverbal Learning Disabilities with education, support & advocacy.

Lori Shery, President/Executive Director
Rich Meleo, Vice President
Elizabeth Yamashita, Vice President

344 America's Special Kidz
P.O. Box 2098
Woodland Park, NJ 7424
973-521-0433
Fax: 973-341-7423
e-mail: joanne@AmericaSpecialKidz.org
americaspecialkidz.org

America's Special Kidz A.S.K understands the importance of healthy families. With a large population of families with special kids-especially single parents-they serve these struggling families.

345 American Academy of Pediatrics
141 Northwest Point Boulevard
Elk Grove Village, IL 60007
847-434-4000
800-433-9016
Fax: 847-434-8000
www.aap.org

The American Academy of Pediatrics and its member pediatricians are committed to the attainment of optimal physical, mental and social health and well-being for all infants, children, adolescents, and young adults.

Sandra Hassink, MD, FAAP, President

346 American Asperger's Association
1301 Seminole Blvd Suite B-112
Largo, Fl 33770
727-518-7294
e-mail: Knaus@gmail.com
americanaspergers.forumotion.net

The mission of the American Aspergers Association is to initiate, sponsor, support, and promote activities and projects for the care, treatment and education of children and adults afflicted with Autism and Aspergers Syndrome without regard to faith, creed, race, national origin or ethnic background.

Dr. Ronald Knaus, Medical Director/ Founder

347 American Association for Marriage and Family Therapy
112 South Alfred Street
Alexandria, VA 22314
703-838-9808
Fax: 703-838-9805
www.aamft.org

The American Association for Marriage and Family Therapy (AAMFT) is the professional association for the field of marriage and family therapy.

Marvarene Oliver, EdD, President
Tracy Todd, PhD, Executive Director
Chris Michaels, Chief Operations Officer

348 American School Counselor Association
1101 King Street, Suite 310
Alexandria, VA 22314
703-683-2722
800-306-4722
Fax: 703-997-7572
e-mail: asca@schoolcounselor.org
www.schoolcounselor.org

The mission of ASCA is to represent professional school counselors and to promote professionalism and ethical practices.

Richard Wong, Executive Director
Jeff Broderson, Information Technology Admin.
Kathleen M Rakestraw, Director of Communications

349 Asperger Syndrome Education Network (ASPEN)
9 Aspen Circle
Edison, NJ 10075
732-321-0880
e-mail: info@aspennj.org
www.aspennj.org

ASPEN provides families and individuals whose lives are affected by Autism Spectrum Disorders (Asperger Syndrome, Pervasive Developmental Disorder-NOS, High Functioning Autism), and Nonverbal Learning Disabilities.

Lori Shery, President
Rich Meleo, Vice President
Elizabeth Yamashita, Vice President

350 Asperger's Network Support for Well-being Education and Research
12930 30th Ave N
Plymouth, MN 55441
763-227-5059
e-mail: tnamie@aspergersmn.org
www.aspergersmn.org

ANSWER is a group of advocates for improving awareness, research, education and support of individuals and families impacted by Asperger's Syndrome.

Theresa Namie, Executive Director/ Co-Founder
Kathy Hoffman, Chair
James Namie, Treasurer

351 Asperger/Autism Network
51 Water Street, Suite 206
Watertown, MA 2472
617-393-3824
866-597-AANE
Fax: 617-393-3827
e-mail: info@aane.org
www.aane.org

The Asperger/Autism Network (AANE) works with individuals, families, and professionals to help people with Asperger Syndrome and similar autism spectrum profiles build meaningful, connected lives.

Jayne Burke, President
Karen Boyd, Vice President
Stephen Burgay, B.A., J.D., Vice President

352 Aspergers Women's Association
www.aspergerwomen.org

AWA serves to educate the public on issues unique to women and girls on the spectrum, as well as their families.

353 Autism Network International
PO Box 35448
Syracuse, NY 13235
315-476-2462
e-mail: jisincla@syr.edu
www.autreat.com

Supported by individuals who want to make a difference for the sufferers, the foundation provides a variety of support and educational references to inform on the latest changes in the field.

Jim Sinclair, Coordinator
Jame Bordner, List-owners
Sola Shelly, Webmaster

354 Autism Society of America
4340 East-West Way, Suite 350
Bethesda, MD 10077
301-657-0881
800-328-8476
e-mail: info@autism-society.org
www.autism-society.org

The Autism Society, the nation's leading grassroots autism organization, exists to improve the lives of all affected by autism. We do this by increasing public awareness about the day-to-day issues faced by people on the spectrum, advocating for appropriate services for individuals across the lifespan, and providing the latest information regarding treatment, education, research and advocacy.

James Ball, Executive Chair
Ron E Simmons, Vice Chair
Scott Badesch, President & COO

355   Bridges4Kids
www.bridges4kids.org

e-mail: info@bridges4kids.org
www.bridges4kids.org

A non-profit organization providing a comprehensive system of information and referral for parents and professionals seeking help for children from birth through transition to adult life.

Deborah K. Canja, CEO
Jackie D. Igafo-Te'o, Webmaster

356   Center for Autism and Related Disorders
19019 Ventura Blvd., Suite 300
Tarzana, CA 91356   818-345-2345
                                      855-345-2273
                              Fax: 818-758-8015
                            www.centerforautism.com

The Center for Autism and Related Disorders (CARD) uses applied behavior analysis (ABA) in the treatment of autism spectrum disorder.

Doreen Granpeesheh, Founder/ Executive Director

357   Center for Outreach and Services for the Autism Community
500 Horizon Drive, Suite 530
Robbinsville, NJ 10078   609-588-8200
                                      800-428-8476
                              Fax: 609-588-8858
                      e-mail: information@autismnj.org
                                      www.autismnj.org

Autism New Jersey is a nonprofit agency committed to ensuring safe and fulfilling lives for individuals with autism, their families, and the professionals who support them. Through awareness, credible information, education, and public policy initiatives, Autism New Jersey leads the way to lifelong individualized services provided with skill and compassion.

James A Paone II Esq, President
Genare Valiant, Vice President
Mary Jane Weiss PhD, Vice President

358   Families of Adults Afflicted with Asperger's Syndrome
PO Box 514
Centerville, MA 2632   508-790-1930
                          e-mail: faaas@faaas.org
                                      faaas.org

Offers support to the family members of adult individuals with Asperger's Syndrome.

Karen E. Rodman, President/ Founder
Jack Kelley, Events Coordinator
Thomas Rodman, Webmaster/ Docmaster

359   Global and Regional Asperger Syndrome Partnership
419 Lafayette Street
New York, NY 10003   888-474-7277
                              e-mail: info@grasp.org
                                      grasp.org

GRASP works to improve the lives of teens and adults with autism spectrum disorder (ASD). It offers in-school programs to help students with autism learn advocacy skills and improve social skills. Through its website, it educates the public about autism, while also offering free online resources and networking opportunities for individuals with ASD and their families.

360   National Alliance on Mental Illness
3803 N. Fairfax Drive, Suite 100
Arlington, VA 22203   703-524-7600
                                      800-950-6264
                              Fax: 703-524-9094
                          e-mail: info@nami.org
                                      www.nami.org

Grassroots mental health organization dedicated to building better lives for the millions of Americans affected by mental illness. - See more at:
http://www.nami.org/About-NAMI#sthash.IYtjmu5h.dpuf

Jim Payne, J.D., President
David Levy, Chief Financial Officer
Mary Giliberti, J.D., Executive Director

361   National Association of Special Education Teachers
1250 Connecticut Avenue, N.W., Suite 200
Washington, DC 20036   800-754-4421
                              Fax: 800-754-4421
                      e-mail: contactus@naset.org
                                      www.naset.org

A membership organization dedicated solely to meeting the needs of special education teachers and those preparing for the field of special education teaching.

Dr. Roger Pierangelo, Co-Executive Director
Dr. George Giuliani, Co-Executive Director

362   National Autism Association
One Park Avenue, Suite 1
Portsmouth, RI 2871   401-293-5551
                                      877-622-2884
                              Fax: 401-293-5342
                  e-mail: naa@nationalautism.org
                            nationalautismassociation.org

NAA is a parent-run advocacy organization and the leading voice on urgent issues related to severe autism, regressive autism, autism safety, autism abuse, and crisis prevention.

Wendy Fournier, President
Kelly Vanicek, Executive Director
Katie Wright-Hildebrand, Vice President

363   National Institute of Child Health and Human Development
31 Center Drive, Building 31, Room 2A32
Bethesda, MD 20892   800-370-2943
                              Fax: 866-760-5947
                              TTY: 888-320-6942
          e-mail: NICHDInformationResourceCenter@mail.nih.
                                      www.nichd.nih.gov

NICHD conducts and supports laboratory research, clinical trials, and epidemiological studies that explore health processes; examines the impact of disabilities, diseases, and variations on the lives of individuals; and sponsors training programs for scientists, health care providers, and researchers to ensure that NICHD research can continue.

Alan E. Guttmacher, M.D., Director

364   National Institute of Environmental Sciences
P.O. Box 12233, MD K3-16, Research Triangle Park
Research Triangle Park, NC 27709   919-541-1919
                              Fax: 301-480-2978
                      e-mail: webcenter@niehs.nih.gov
                                      www.niehs.nih.gov

The mission of the NIEHS is to discover how the environment affects people in order to promote healthier lives.

Linda S. Birnbaum, Director
Richard Woychik, Ph.D., Deputy Director
Sheila A. Newton, Ph.D., Policy, Planning, and Evaluation

365   National Mental Health Consumers' Self-Help Clearinghouse
1211 Chestnut Street, Suite 1207
Philadelphia, PA 10079   215-751-1810
                                      800-553-4539
                              Fax: 215-636-6312
                      e-mail: info@mhselfhelp.org
                                      www.mhselfhelp.org

The Clearinghouse works to foster peer empowerment through our website, up-to-date news and information announcements, a directory of peer-driven services, electronic and printed publications, training packages, and individual and onsite consultation

Joseph Rogers, Executive Director & Founder
Susan Rogers, Director of Special Projects
Britani Nestel, Program Specialist

366   Oasis at MAAP
PO Box 524
Crown Point, IN 10080   219-662-1311
Fax: 219-682-6372
e-mail: info@aspergersyndrome.org
www.aspergersyndrome.org

MAAP Services is a world wide 501-C-3 non profit organization providing information, networking, referrals and printed materials for families, challenged individuals and professionals concerned with the autism spectrum. Founded in 1984, MAAP Services, adheres to the basic principal that all individuals with autism spectrum challenges have the ability to learn, grow and enjoy a good quality of life.

Susan Moreno, Founder & President
Lara Blanchard, BCBA

367   US Aspergers Association
5364 Ehrlich Rd. #175
Tampa, FL 33624   813-264-0777
Fax: 813-830-7373
e-mail: info@usaspergers.org
usaspergersassn.com

A charitable organization that was created to help those children, adults and their families get the help they need in order to be properly diagnosed with Asperger's Syndrome.

Philip Bernie, President
Nina Bernie, Vice President

368   US Autism & Asperger Association
P.O. Box 532
Draper, UT 84020   888-9AU-ISM
www.usautism.org

US Autism & Asperger Association (USAAA) is a 501(c)(3) non-profit organization for autism and Asperger education, support, and solutions.

Lawrence P. Kaplan, PhD, Chairman/ CEO
Richard Dunie, MPh, MBA, CPA, Secretary/ Treasurer
Phillip C. DeMio, MD, Chief Medical Officer

Conferences

369   ASPEN Annual Fall Conference
Asperger Syndrome Education Network
9 Aspen Circle
Edison, NJ 08820   732-321-0880
e-mail: info@aspennj.org
www.aspennj.org

Practical strategies for teachers and parents of students with autism spectrum disorders for navigating school, home and life

October

Lori Shery, President
Rich Meleo, Vice President
Ann Hiller, Secretary

370   Autism Society National Conference and Exposition
Autism Society of America
4340 East-West Way, Suite 350
Bethesda, MD 20814   301-657-0881
800-328-8476
e-mail: info@autism-society.org
www.autism-society.org

Addresses the range of issues affecting people with autism including early intervention, education, employment, behavior, communication, social skills, biomedical interventions and others, across the entire lifespan.

James Ball, Executive Chair
Ron E Simmons, Vice Chair
Sergio Mariaca, Treasurer

371   Autreat
Autism International Network
PO Box 35448
Syracuse, NY 13235   315-476-2462
e-mail: webmaster@autreat.com
www.autreat.com

A retreat-style conference run by autistic people, for autistic people and friends. Focuses on positive living with autism, not on causes, cures, or ways to make individuals more normal.

August

Jim Sinclair, Coordinator

Audio Video

372   Asperger's Syndrome: Autism and Obsessive Behavior
Films for the Humanities and Sciences
132 West 31st Street
New York, NY 10001   800-257-5126
Fax: 609-275-0266
e-mail: custserv@films.com
www.ffh.films.com

This program profiles the symptoms of Asperger's Syndrome and what sufferers and their families can do to overcome the limitations that it imposes.

28 minutes
ISBN: 1-421387-67-3

373   The Boy Inside
Fanlight Productions
32 Court Street, 21st Floor
Brooklyn, NY 11201   718-488-8900
800-876-1710
Fax: 718-488-8642
e-mail: info@fanlight.com
www.fanlight.com

The harrowing story of the filmaker's son Adam, a 12-year-old with Asperger Syndrome, during a tumultuous year in the life of their family. AS makes Adam's life in seventh grade a minefield, where he finds himself isollated and bullied. As he struggles to find a place for himself, his troublees escalate, both at school and at home. ISBN: DVD: 1-57295-838-3; VHS: 1-57295-449-3

47 minutes DVD or VHS

Web Sites

374   Asperger's Association of New England
51 Water Street, Suite 206
Watertown, MA 2472   617-393-3824
866-597-AANE
Fax: 617-393-3827
e-mail: info@aane.org
www.aane.org

The immediate goal of austistic.org is to build a global database of information and resoures by and for persons on the autistic spectrum.

Jayne Burke, President
Karen Boyd, Vice President
Stephen Burgay, B.A., J.D., Vice President

375   Autism Resources
www.autism-resources.com

Offers information and links regarding the developemental disabilities autism and Asperger's Syndrom.

376   Family Village
www.familyvillage.wisc.edu

A global community that integrates information, resources and communication opportunities on the Internet for persons with cognitive and other disabilities, for their families and for those that provide them services and support.

377 **Online Asperger Syndrome Information and Support**
P.O. Box 524
Crown Point, IN 46308   219-662-1311
e-mail: info@aspergersyndrome.org
www.aspergersyndrome.org

Provides parents, professionals and person with the links they
need to research anything.

378 **University Students with Autism and Asperger's Syndrome
Web Site**
www.users.dircon.co.uk/~cns/

Helps to develop an understanding of the difficulties people with
Asperger Syndrome may face. We also work on a one to one basis
with the student and liase with staff and peers. Help is also given
in setting up support networks such as mentors and providing effective strategies to aid independent learning.

Book Publishers

379 **Asperger Syndrome**

A Klin, F Volkmar, S Sparrow, author

Guilford Publications
72 Spring Street
New York, NY 10012   212-431-9800
800-365-7006
Fax: 212-966-6708
e-mail: info@guilford.com
www.guilford.com

Brings together preeminent scholars and practitioners to offer a
definitive statement of what is currently known about Asperger
syndrome and to highlight promising leads in research and clinical practice. Sifts through the latest developments in theory and
research, discussing key diagnostic and conceptual issues and reviewing what is known about behavioral features and
neurobiology. The effects of Asperger syndrome on social development, learning and communication are examined.
Jan 2000 489 pages
ISBN: 1-572305-34-2

380 **Asperger Syndrome and Your Child: A Parent's Guide**
Autism Society of North Carolina Bookstore
505 Oberlin Road, Suite 230
Raleigh, NC 27605   919-743-0204
800-442-2762
Fax: 919-743-0208
e-mail: books@autismsociety-nc.org
www.autismbookstore.com

Written primarily for parents, this book provides a clinician's
view of Asperger Syndrome.

381 **Asperger Syndrome: A Practical Guide for Teachers**
ADD WareHouse
300 NW 70th Avenue, Suite 102
Plantation, FL 33317   954-792-8100
800-233-9273
Fax: 954-792-8545
e-mail: websales@addwarehouse.com
www.addwarehouse.com

A clear and concise guide to effective classroom practice for
teachers and support assistants working with children with
Asperger Syndrome in school. The authors explain characteristics
of children with Asperger Syndrome, discuss methods of assessment and offer practical strategies for effective classroom
interventions.

90 pages
ISBN: 1-853464-99-6

382 **Asperger Syndrome: Guide for Educators and Parents, Second
Edition**
Pro-Ed
8700 Shoal Creek Boulevard
Austin, TX 78757   512-451-3246
800-897-3202
Fax: 800-397-7633
e-mail: info@proedinc.com
www.proedinc.com

A ground-breaking resource on Asperger Syndrome, this text outlines, in lay terms, the characteristics of the syndrome sometimes
referred to as higher-functioning autism.
215 pages
ISBN: 0-890798-98-2

383 **Asperger's Syndrome: A Guide for Parents and Professionals**
ADD WareHouse
300 NW 70th Avenue, Suite 102
Plantation, FL 33317   954-792-8100
800-233-9273
Fax: 954-792-8545
e-mail: websales@addwarehouse.com
addwarehouse.com

Providing a description and analysis of the unusual characteristics of Asperger's Syndrome, with strategies to reduce those that
are most conspicuous or debilitating. This guide brings together
the most relevant and useful information on all aspects of the
syndrome, from language and social behavior to motor
clumsiness.
240 pages
ISBN: 1-853025-77-1

384 **Autism and Asperger Syndrome**
Autism Society of North Carolina Bookstore
505 Oberlin Road, Suite 230
Raleigh, NC 27605   919-743-0204
800-442-2762
e-mail: info@autismsociety-nc.org
www.austismsociety-nc.org

Chapters include topics such as the relationship of autism and
Asperger Syndrome, living with the syndrome and Asperger Syndrome in adulthood.
247 pages

Beverly Moore, Chairman
Sharon Jeffries-Jones, Vice Chair
Darryl R Marsch, Secretary

385 **Can I Tell You About Asperger Syndrome?: A Guide for
Friends and Family**
Autism Society of North Carolina Bookstore
505 Oberlin Road, Suite 230
Raleigh, NC 27605   919-743-0204
800-442-2762
Fax: 919-743-0208
e-mail: books@autismsociety-nc.org
www.autismbookstore.com

Written for young people so that they can better understand the
challenges faced by a sibling, friend, or classmate who has
Asperger Syndrome. For readers ages 7-15.

386 **Oasis Guide to Asperger Syndrome**
Autism Society of North Carolina Bookstore
505 Oberlin Road, Suite 230
Raleigh, NC 27605   919-743-0204
800-442-2762
Fax: 919-743-0208
e-mail: books@autismsociety-nc.org
www.autismbookstore.com

Combining the most current information about Asperger Syndrome (AS) diagnosis and treatment with hundreds of practical
tips and reosurce listings, this guide is comprehensive in scope.

497 VACC Camp
Miami Children's Hospital
3200 SW 60th Court, Suite 203
Miami, FL 33155
                                    305-662-8222
                                 Fax: 786-268-1765
                         e-mail: bela.florentin@mch.com
                              www.vacccamp.com

Free, week-long, overnight camp for ventilation assisted children
(children needing a tracheotomy ventilator, C-PAP, BiPAP, or oxygen to support breathing) and their families. Gives families a fun
oppourtinity to socialize with peers and enjoy activities not
readily accessible to technology dependent children.

Moises Simpser, MD, Camp Director
Bela Florentin, Camp Coordinator

Description

498 ATAXIA

Involves the following Biologic System(s):

Neurologic Disorders

Ataxia is a neuromuscular condition characterized by an impaired ability to coordinate voluntary movements. The condition is caused by abnormalities of or damage to the region of the brain known as the cerebellum, nerve pathways that transmit messages to and from the cerebellum, or certain regions of the spinal cord. The cerebellum plays an essential role in regulating the maintenance of normal postures, sustaining balance, and producing smooth and coordinated movements. The spinal cord conducts sensory and motor impulses to and from the brain. The symptoms associated with ataxia vary, depending upon the specific regions of the brain that are affected; however, symptoms may often include imbalance and an abnormal staggering manner of walking (gait). Ataxia may be the result of certain infection, malformations of the cerebellum of spinal cord that are present at birth (congenital), head injury, brain tumors, exposure to particular medications, or certain genetic disorders. The primary infectious causes of ataxia during childhood include the formation of pus-filled pockets of infection in the cerebellum (cerebellar abscesses); sudden, severe inflammation of the passages within the inner ear (acute labyrinthitis): or acute cerebellar ataxia. Acute labyrinthitis typically occurs due to middle ear infections and may be characterized by vomiting and a sense that one's body or environment is spinning (vertigo). Acute cerebellar ataxia occurs subsequent to certain viral infections, such as chicken pox, and is thought to result from an abnormal immune response causing inflammation of the brain. Acute cerebellar ataxia typically occurs suddenly and may be characterized by impaired control of voluntary movements of the torso (truncal ataxia) and difficulties sitting or standing; involuntary, rapid eye movements (nystagmus); and severe slurring of speech or an inability to speak. Although the condition typically improves within a few weeks, it sometimes is present for up to two months. Most children have a complete recovery; however, some may have residual speech abnormalities and lack of coordination.

Abnormalities present at birth (congenital) that may cause ataxia include absence of the region of the brain between the two sides or hemispheres of the cerebellum (agensis of cerebellar vermis); protrusion of part of the brain through an opening in the skull (encephalocele); or protrusion of certain, malformed regions of the brain through the opening at the base of the skull (foramen magnum) into the upper spinal canal (Arnold-Chiari malformation). Infants and children with such birth defects develop ataxia due to malformation of or damage to certain regions of the cerebellum.

Ataxia may also be an initial symptom associated with certain brain tumors, including tumors affecting the cerebellum or a particular area of the cerebrum where it joins with the cerebellum (i.e., frontal lobe). In addition, brain tumors known as neuroblastomasmay result in progressive ataxia. Neuroblastomas are solid, malignant tumors that may originate in any part of the sympathetic nervous system, which is that part of the nervous system that regulates certain involuntary activities during times of stress, such as raising blood pressure and increasing the heart rate.

In some children, ataxia may result from the administration of certain drugs, such as anticonvulsant medications, particularly phenytoin. In addition, the condition may be caused by exposure to a household pesticide that is commonly used as a rat poison (thallium).

Ataxia may also occur in association with certain inborn errors of metabolism and is a primary feature of many hereditary degenerative disorders of the brain and spinal cord. These degenerative disorders, which may be referred to as hereditay ataxias, include ataxia-telangiectasia and Friedreich's ataxia.

Ataxia-telangiectasia (AT) is a multisystem disorder that is inherited as an autosomal recessive trait. Affected children typically develop ataxia at approximately two years of age, eventually leading to an inability to walk. Friedreich's ataxia is a genetic disorder that is usually inherited as an autosomal recessive trait. The disorder is characterized by degenerative changes of certain regions of the spinal cord and is categorized as a spinocerebellar ataxia. Children with Friedreich's ataxia typically develop ataxia before age 10. The ataxia is slowly progressive and usually affects the legs and feet more severely than the arms and hands. Patients develop unusual high arching and severe muscle weakness of the feet and progressive difficulties walking, typically resulting in the need of a wheelchair. Additional hereditary spinocerebellar ataxia of childhood, such as Roussy-Levy syndrome, cause symptoms and findings similar to those associated with Friedreich's ataxia. Roussy-Levy syndrome often becomes apparent during infancy and is characterized by loss of joint position sensation (sensory ataxia), causing poorly judged, uncoordinated movements. Such ataxia initially affects the legs, causing difficulty walking, and later progresses to affect the hands. Roussy-Levy syndrome is transmitted as an autosomal dominant trait.

Another group of hereditary disorders, known as the olivopontocerebellar atrophics (OPCAs) are associated with ataxia. These disorders are characterized by progressive degeneration of the cerebellum as well as other areas of the brain. Although associated symptoms of most forms of OPCA become apparent during adolescence or adulthood, one form of the disorder is known to occur during infancy (OPCA of neonatal onset). Symptoms may include severely diminished muscle tone; rapidly progressive ataxia; involuntary, rapid eye movements; episodes of abnormally increased electrical activity in the brain (seizures); failure to grow and gain weight at the expected rate (failure to thrive); abnormalities in the structure and function of heart muscle (hypertrophic cardiomyopathy); and other symptoms and findings. Methods used in the management of ataxia may vary and depend upon the condition's underlying cause, the specific form of ataxia present, and other factors. Such measures are typically symptomatic and supportive.

Government Agencies

499   NIH/National Institute of Neurological Dis orders and Stroke (NINDS)
PO Box 5801
Bethesda, MD 10114

301-496-5751
800-352-9424
Fax: 301-496-0296
TTY: 301-468-5981
www.ninds.nih.gov

The mission of NINDS is to reduce the burden of neurological disease - a burden borne by every age group, by every segment of society, by people all over the world.

Story C Landis Ph.D., Director
Walter J Koroshetz, Deputy Director
Caroline Lewis, Executive Officer

National Associations & Support Groups

500 **American Academy of Pediatrics**
141 Northwest Point Boulevard
Elk Grove Village, IL 60007
847-434-4000
800-433-9016
Fax: 847-434-8000
www.aap.org

The American Academy of Pediatrics and its member pediatricians are committed to the attainment of optimal physical, mental and social health and well-being for all infants, children, adolescents, and young adults.

Sandra Hassink, MD, FAAP, President

501 **National Ataxia Foundation**
2600 Fernbrook Lane N Suite 119
Minneapolis, MN 10115
763-553-0020
Fax: 763-553-0167
e-mail: naf@ataxia.org
www.ataxia.org

The National Ataxia Foundation is dedicated to improving the lives of persons affected by ataxia through support, education, and research.

Harry T Orr PhD, Board of Directors
Michael Parent, Executive Director
William P Sweeney, Treasurer

State Agencies & Support Groups

Alabama

502 **Birmingham Support Group**
National Ataxia Foundation
16 The Oaks Circle
Birmingham, AL 10116
205-987-2883
Fax: 763-553-0167
e-mail: donnelly613b@aol.com
www.ataxia.org

The primary mission is to encourage and support research into Hereditary Ataxia, a group of neurological disorders which are chronic and progressive conditions affecting coordination.

Fred Donnelly, Contact
Becky Donnelly, Contact

Arizona

503 **Arizona Ataxia Support Group**
National Ataxia Foundation
7665 E Placita Luna Preciosa
Tucson, AZ 10117
520-885-8326
Fax: 763-553-0167
e-mail: bbeck15@cox.net
www.ataxia.org/chapters/Tucson/default.aspx

The primary mission is to encourage and support research into Hereditary Ataxia, a group of neurological disorders which are chronic and progressive conditions affecting coordination.

Bart Beck, SG Leader

California

504 **Greater North Valley California Support Group**
4335 Bourdeaux Drive
Oakley, CA 10118
925-625-0738
www.geocites.com/hotsprings/

The primary mission is to encourage and support research into Hereditary Ataxia, a group of neurological disorders which are chronic and progressive conditions affecting coordination.

Debra Kellerman, Contact

505 **Los Angeles Ataxia Support Group**
National Ataxia Foundation
339 W Palmer, Apartment A
Glendale, CA 10119
818-246-5758
Fax: 763-553-0167
e-mail: ccherilynmc@yahoo.com
www.ataxia.org/chapters/losangeles/default.aspx

The primary mission is to encourage and support research into Hereditary Ataxia, a group of neurological disorders which are chronic and progressive conditions affecting coordination.

Sherry McLaughlin, Contact

506 **Northern California Support Group**
National Ataxia Foundation
1980 Saint George Rd
Danville, CA 10120
925-735-7037
Fax: 763-553-0167
e-mail: joanneloveland@gmail.com
www.ataxia.org/chapters/northerncalifornia/default.a

The primary mission is to encourage and support research into Hereditary Ataxia, a group of neurological disorders which are chronic and progressive conditions affecting coordination.

Joanne Loveland, Contact

507 **Orange County Support Group**
National Ataxia Foundation
829 W Gary Ave
Montebello, CA 10121
323-788-7751
Fax: 763-553-0167
e-mail: danieln27@gmail.com
www.ataxia.org/chapters/orangecounty/default.aspx

The primary mission is to encourage and support research into Hereditary Ataxia, a group of neurological disorders which are chronic and progressive conditions affecting coordination.

Daniel Navar, Leader

508 **Pacific Southwest Regional Genetics Group**
2151 Berkeley Way
Berkeley, CA 10122
510-540-2696
Fax: 510-540-2966
www.hgen.pitt.edu/counseling/resources/regional04.ht

Coordinates genetic services; promotes communication among genetic professionals and consumers through network newsletter, meetings, and other events; share resources; and promote education and awareness of genetic disorders,

George C Cunningham, Director

509 **San Diego Support Group**
National Ataxia Foundation
2087 Granite Hills Drive
El Cajon, CA 92019
619-447-3753
Fax: 763-553-0167
e-mail: sdasg@cox.net
www.ataxia.org

The primary mission is to encourage and support research into Hereditary Ataxia, a group of neurological disorders which are chronic and progressive conditions affecting coordination.

Earl McLaughlin, Contact

510 **San Fernando Valley Support Group**
19450 Turtle Ridge Lane
Northridge, CA 10124
818-363-5335
www.ataxia.org

The primary mission is to encourage and support research into Hereditary Ataxia, a group of neurological disorders which are chronic and progressive conditions affecting coordination.

Darneal J Myers, Contact

Colorado

511 Colorado Support Group
National Ataxia Foundation
5902 W Maplewood Drive
Littleton, CO 10125
303-794-6351
Fax: 763-553-0167
e-mail: tom_sathre@acm.org
www.ataxia.org

The primary mission is to encourage and support research into Hereditary Ataxia, a group of neurological disorders which are chronic and progressive conditions affecting coordination.

Donna Sathre, Leader
Tom Sathre, Leader

512 Mountain States Regional Genetics Services Network
4300 Cherry Creek Drive S
Denver, CO 10126
303-692-2423
Fax: 303-782-5576
www.hgen.pitt.edu/counseling/resources/regional04.ht

Coordinates genetic services; promotes communication among genetic professional and consumers through network newsletters, meetings, and other events; share resources; and promote education and awareness of genetic disorders.

George C Cunningham, Director

Florida

513 Broward County Support Group
10603 NW 49th Place
Coral Springs, FL 10127
954-341-8565
Fax: 954-753-6761
e-mail: pathamilto@aol.com
community.insidecentralflorida.com/bcfasg/

The primary mission is to encourage and support research into Hereditary Ataxia, a group of neurological disorders which are chronic and progressive conditions affecting coordination.

Patricia B Hamilton, Contact

514 Clearwater, FL Support Group
2363 Mary Lane
Clearwater, FL 10128
727-799-2852
e-mail: joyous7@mciworld.com
www.ataxia.org

The primary mission is to encourage and support research into Hereditary Ataxia, a group of neurological disorders which are chronic and progressive conditions affecting coordination.

Joyce Robbins, Contact

515 NE Florida Support Group
National Ataxia Foundation
8925 Adams Walk Dr
Jacksonville, FL 10129
904-314-2061
Fax: 763-553-0167
e-mail: coryhannan@hotmail.com
www.ataxia.org

The primary mission is to encourage and support research into Hereditary Ataxia, a group of neurological disorders which are chronic and progressive conditions affecting coordination.

Cory Hannan, Leader

516 Tampa Support Group
National Ataxia Foundation
306 Caloosa Palm St
Son City Center, FL 10130
e-mail: charlie@flataxia1.org
www.ataxia.org

The primary mission is to encourage and support research into Hereditary Ataxia, a group of neurological disorders which are chronic and progressive conditions affecting coordination.

Charlie Kirchner, Contact

Georgia

517 Georgia Ataxia Support Group
National Ataxia Foundation
320 Peters Street, Unit 12
Atlanta, GA 10131
404-822-7451
e-mail: rookssgj@yahoo.com
www.ataxia.org

The primary mission is to encourage and support research into Hereditary Ataxia, a group of neurological disorders which are chronic and progressive conditions affecting coordination.

Greg Rooks, Contact

518 Greater Atlanta Area Support Group
National Ataxia Foundation
320 Peters Street, Unit 12
Atlanta, GA 10132
404-822-7451
e-mail: rookssgj@yahoo.com
www.geocities.com/atlantaataxia

The primary mission is to encourage and support research into Hereditary Ataxia, a group of neurological disorders which are chronic and progressive conditions affecting coordination.

Greg Rooks, Contact

519 Macon Support Group
116 Summerfield Drive
Macon, GA 10133
912-757-9454
e-mail: rookssgj@yahoo.com
www.ataxia.org

The primary mission is to encourage and support research into Hereditary Ataxia, a group of neurological disorders which are chronic and progressive conditions affecting coordination.

Millard H McWhorter III, MD, Contact

520 Southeast Regional Genetics Group
PO Box 1642
Decatur, GA 10134
404-778-8551
Fax: 404-778-8562
e-mail: mlane@sergg.org
www.sergginc.org

SERGG addresses the inequities in genetic service and resources in the region and to expand existing regional capabilities and resources and to develop new regional systems to address these gaps. Another goal is to improve the existing regional communication infrastructure and to facilitate information sharing among providers of genetic services and consumers and to establish collaborative partnerships with other professional organizations.

Hans Andersson, MD, President
Mary Rose Simpson, BS, Secretary/Treasurer

Illinois

521 Chicago, IL Area Ataxia Support Group
National Ataxia Foundation
3400 Wellington Court, #302
Rolling Meadows, IL 10135
847-797-9398
e-mail: caasgz@aol.com
www.ataxia.org

The primary mission is to encourage and support research into Hereditary Ataxia, a group of neurological disorders which are chronic and progressive conditions affecting coordination.

Craig Lisack, Contact

Indiana

522 Central Indiana Support Group
5716 N 225 W
W Lafayette, IN 10136
765-463-3973
Fax: 765-463-3972
e-mail: turtle23@mindspring.com
www.ataxia.org

The primary mission is to encourage and support research into Hereditary Ataxia, a group of neurological disorders which are chronic and progressive conditions affecting coordination.

Judy Marten, Contact

523 NE Indiana Support Group
4522 Shenandoah Circle W
Fort Wayne, IN 10137

219-485-0965
Fax: 763-553-0167
e-mail: naf@ataxia.org
www.ataxia.org

The primary mission is to encourage and support research into Hereditary Ataxia, a group of neurological disorders which are chronic and progressive conditions affecting coordination.

Don & Jenny Roemke, Contact

Louisiana

524 Louisiana Chapter
National Ataxia Foundation
1720 Parker St.
Baton Rouge, LA 10138

985-643-0783
e-mail: louisiananaf@yahoo.com
www.angelfire.com/la/ataxiachapter/

The primary mission is to encourage and support research into Hereditary Ataxia, a group of neurological disorders which are chronic and progressive conditions affecting coordination.

Elizabeth Tanner, Contact

525 Louisiana Support Group
National Ataxia Foundation
1720 Parker St.
Baton Rouge, LA 10139

985-643-0783
Fax: 763-553-0167
e-mail: louisiananaf@yahoo.com
www.angelfire.com/la/ataxiachapter/

The primary mission is to encourage and support research into Hereditary Ataxia, a group of neurological disorders which are chronic and progressive conditions affecting coordination.

Elizabeth Tanner, Contact

Maine

526 Maine Support
National Ataxia Foundation
PO Box 113
Bowdoinham, ME 10140

763-553-0020
Fax: 763-553-0167
e-mail: Kelley3902@myfairpoint.net
www.ataxia.org

The primary mission is to encourage and support research into Hereditary Ataxia, a group of neurological disorders which are chronic and progressive conditions affecting coordination.

Kelly Rollins, Contact

527 New England Regional Genetics Group
PO Box 920288
Needham, MA 10141

781-444-0126
Fax: 781-444-0127
e-mail: mfgnergg@verizon.net
www.nergg.org

To provide a forum for collaboration among genetic professionals, consumers of genetic services and the Public Health Community in New England by Raising awareness about the impact of genetics on health throughout the lifespan and Promoting and facilitating access to genetic services, education and resources

Lisa Demers MS, CGC, President
Marinell Newton, President Elect
Lisa Brailey MD, Service Provider

Maryland

528 Chesapeake Chapter
National Ataxia Foundation
5938 Rossmore Drive
Bethesda, MD 10142

301-530-4989
Fax: 301-530-2480
e-mail: carljlauter@erols.com
www.geocities.com/Hotsprings/Oasis/4988/

The primary mission is to encourage and support research into Hereditary Ataxia, a group of neurological disorders which are chronic and progressive conditions affecting coordination.

Carl J Lauter, President

Massachusetts

529 New England Support Group
National Ataxia Foundation
45 Juliette Street
Andover, MA 10143

978-475-8072
Fax: 763-553-0167
e-mail: naf@ataxia.org
www.ataxia.org

The primary mission is to encourage and support research into Hereditary Ataxia, a group of neurological disorders which are chronic and progressive conditions affecting coordination.

Donna Gorzela, Leader
Richard Gorzela, Leader

Michigan

530 Detroit Michigian Ataxia Support Group
National Ataxia Foundation
20217 Wyoming
Detroit, MI 10144

313-397-7858
Fax: 763-553-0167
e-mail: tinyt48221@yahoo.com
www.ataxia.org

The primary mission is to encourage and support research into Hereditary Ataxia, a group of neurological disorders which are chronic and progressive conditions affecting coordination.

Tany Tunstull, Leader

Minnesota

531 Minneapolis, MN Support Group
National Ataxia Foundation
2549 32nd Avenue S
Minneapolis, MN 10145

612-724-3784
Fax: 763-553-0167
e-mail: schultz.lenore@yahoo.com
www.ataxia.org

The primary mission is to encourage and support research into Hereditary Ataxia, a group of neurological disorders which are chronic and progressive conditions affecting coordination.

Lenore Healey Schultz, Contact

Mississippi

532 Mississippi Chapter
National Ataxia Foundation
PO Box 17005
Hattiesburg, MS 10146

763-553-0020
Fax: 763-553-0167
e-mail: daglio1@bellsouth.net
www.ataxia.org

The primary mission is to encourage and support research into Hereditary Ataxia, a group of neurological disorders which are chronic and progressive conditions affecting coordination.

Camille Daglio, President

Missouri

533 Central Missouri Area Support Group
National Ataxia Foundation
1609 Cocoa Court
Columbia, MO 10147
                                    572-474-7232
                                Fax: 763-553-0167
                    e-mail: rogercooley@localnet.com
                                    www.ataxia.org

The primary mission is to encourage and support research into
Hereditary Ataxia, a group of neurological disorders which are
chronic and progressive conditions affecting coordination.

Roger Colley, Leader

534 Kansas City, Missouri Support Group
National Ataxia Foundation
17700 East 17th Terrace Ct. S #102
Independence, MO 10148
                                    816-257-2428
                                Fax: 763-553-0167
                e-mail: clarkstone9348@sbcglobal.net
            www.ataxia.org/chapters/kansascity/default.aspx

The primary mission is to encourage and support research into
Hereditary Ataxia, a group of neurological disorders which are
chronic and progressive conditions affecting coordination.

Jim Clark, Contact

535 Springfield Area Support Group
12 Jackson St, Apt 811-B
Jefferson City, MO 10149
                        e-mail: drsusie@embarqmail.com
            www.ataxia.org/chapters/strode/default.aspx

The primary mission is to encourage and support research into
Hereditary Ataxia, a group of neurological disorders which are
chronic and progressive conditions affecting coordination.

Susan Strode, PhD, Contact

New York

536 Genetic Network of the Empire State
Laboratory of Human Genetics
Empire State Plaza
Albany, NY 10150
                                    518-474-7148
                                Fax: 518-474-8590
                                    www.sergginc.org

Coordinates genetic services; promotes communication among genetic professionals and consumers through network newsletters,
meetings, and other events; share resources; and promote education and awareness of genetic disorders.

Karen Greendale, Coordinator

537 New York City Area Support Group
National Ataxia Foundation
36 West Redoubt Road
Fishkill, NY 10151
                                    845-897-5632
                    e-mail: vrabsolutely@aol.com
        www.ataxia.org/chapters/valerieruggiero/default.aspx

The primary mission is to encourage and support research into
Hereditary Ataxia, a group of neurological disorders which are
chronic and progressive conditions affecting coordination.

Valerie Ruggiero, Contact

538 New York Support Group
National Ataxia Foundation
423 Church Street
North Syracuse, NY 10152
                                    315-683-9486
                        e-mail: jtarrants@aol.com
        www.ataxia.org/chapters/centralnewyork/default.aspx

Primary mission is to encourage and support research into Hereditary Ataxia, a group of neurological disorders which are chronic
and progressive conditions affecting coordination.

Mary Jane Damiano, Contact

539 Tri-State Support Group
National Ataxia Foundation
Northgate 6C
Bronxville, NY 10153
                                    914-720-2179
                                Fax: 763-553-0167
                    e-mail: markmeghan2@gmail.com
            www.ataxia.org/chapters/tri-state/default.aspx

The primary mission is to encourage and support research into
Hereditary Ataxia, a group of neurological disorders which are
chronic and progressive conditions affecting coordination.

Denise Mitchell, Leader
Mark Mitchell, Contact

Ohio

540 Ohio Support Group
National Ataxia Foundation
7852 Country Court
Mentor, OH 10154
                                    440-255-8284
                        e-mail: wurbanski@oh.rr.com
            www.ataxia.org/chapters/centralohio/default.aspx

The primary mission is to encourage and support research into
Hereditary Ataxia, a group of neurological disorders which are
chronic and progressive conditions affecting coordination.

Cecelia Urbanski, Contact

Oklahoma

541 North Central Oklahoma Support Group
915 Thislewood
Norman, OK 10155
                                    405-447-6085
                    e-mail: czechmarkmhd@yahoo.com
        www.ataxia.org/chapters/Ambassador/default.aspx

The primary mission is to encourage and support research into
Hereditary Ataxia, a group of neurological disorders which are
chronic and progressive conditions affecting coordination.

Mark Dvorak, Contact

Oregon

542 Pacific Northwest Regional Genetics Group
PO Box 574
Portland, OR 10156
                                    503-494-8342
                                Fax: 503-494-4447
                                    www.sergginc.org

Coordinates genetics services; promotes communication among
genetic professional and consumers through network newsletters,
meetings, and other events; share resources; and promote education and awareness of genetic disorders.

Jonathan Zonana, MD, Director

543 Willamette Valley Ataxia Support Group
Albany General Hospital-National Ataxia Foundation
1046 6th Avenue SW
Albany, OR 10157
                                    541-812-4162
                                Fax: 541-812-4614
                    e-mail: istillwell@samhealth.org
            www.ataxia.org/chapters/Willamette/default.aspx

The primary mission is to encourage and support research into
Hereditary Ataxia, a group of neurological disorders which are
chronic and progressive conditions affecting coordination.

Ivy Stilwell, Contact

Pennsylvania

544 Central Pennsylvania Area Support Group
3844 West Linden Street
Allentown, PA 18104
                                    610-395-6905
                        e-mail: rakshys@ptd.net
            www.ataxia.org/chapters/rakshys/default.aspx

The primary mission is to encourage and support research into Hereditary Ataxia, a group of neurological disorders which are chronic and progressive conditions affecting coordination.

Christina Rakshys, Contact

545   Mid-Atlantic Regional Human Genetics Network
260 S Broad Street
Philadelphia, PA 10158
                                                215-456-7910
                                           Fax: 215-456-7911
                                              www.sergginc.org

Coordinates genetics services; promotes communication among genetic professional and consumers through network newsletters, meeting, and other events; share resources; and promote education and awareness of genetic disorders.

Deborah Eunpu, MS, President

546   Southeast Pennsylvania Support Group
National Ataxia Foundation
220 Beechwood Road
Norristown, PA 10159
                                                610-272-1502
                                     e-mail: lizout@aol.com
           www.ataxia.org/chapters/sepennsylvania/default.aspx

The primary mission is to encourage and support research into Hereditary Ataxia, a group of neurological disorders which are chronic and progressive conditions affecting coordination.

Liz Nussear, Contact

South Carolina

547   Carolinas Support Group
National Ataxia Foundation
1305 Cely Road
Easley, SC 10160
                                                864-220-3395
                              e-mail: cecerussell@hotmal.com
              www.ataxia.org/chapters/Carolinas/default.aspx

The primary mission is to encourage and support research into Hereditary Ataxia, a group of neurological disorders which are chronic and progressive conditions affecting coordination.

Cece Russell, Contact

Texas

548   Houston Support Group
National Ataxia Foundation
9405 Hwy 6 South
Houston, TX 10161
                                                281-693-1826
                            e-mail: angelahcloud@aol.com
              www.ataxia.org/chapters/houston/default.aspx

The primary mission is to encourage and support research into Hereditary Ataxia, a group of neurological disorders which are chronic and progressive conditions affecting coordination.

Angela Cloud, Contact

549   North Texas Support Group
National Ataxia Foundation
7 Wentworth Court
Trophy Club, TX 10162
                                                903-785-7058
                           e-mail: cheve11e@sbcglobal.net
            www.ataxia.org/chapters/northtexas/default.aspx

The primary mission is to encourage and support research into Hereditary Ataxia, a group of neurological disorders which are chronic and progressive conditions affecting coordination.

David Henry Jr, Contact

Utah

550   Utah Support Group National Ataxia Foundation
University of Utah - Moran Eye Clinic
65 Mario Copecchi Dr.
Salt Lake City, UT 84132
                                                801-587-3020
                           e-mail: Lisa.ord@hsc.utah.edu
              www.ataxia.org/chapters/Utah/default.aspx

The primary mission is to encourage and support research into Hereditary Ataxia, a group of neurological disorders which are chronic and progressive conditions affecting coordination.

Lisa Ord PhD, Contact

Washington

551   Seattle Area Support Group
National Ataxia Foundation
14104 107th Avenue NE
Kirkland, WA 10164
                                                425-823-6239
                      e-mail: ataxiaseattle@comcast.net
            www.ataxia.org/chapters/Seattle/default.aspx

The primary mission is to encourage and support research into Hereditary Ataxia, a group of neurological disorders which are chronic and progressive conditions affecting coordination.

Milly Lewendon, Contact

Research Centers

552   Ataxia Telangiectasia Children's Project
5300 W. Hillsboro Blvd. Suite 105
Coconut Creek, FL 10165
                                                954-481-6611
                                                800-543-5728
                                           Fax: 954-725-1153
                                      e-mail: info@atcp.org
                                                www.atcp.org

Established in the United States in 1993, the A-T Children's Project is a 501c3 nonprofit organization that raises funds to support and coordinate biomedical research projects, scientific conferences and a clinical center aimed at finding life-improving therapies and a cure for ataxia-telangiectasia (A-T). A-T is a rare, genetic disease that attacks children, causing progressive loss of muscle control, cancer, and immune system problems.

Brad Margus, President
Vicki Margus, Founder

553   Ataxia Telangiectasia Medical Research Foundation
16224 Elisa Place
Encino, CA 91436
                                                818-906-2861
                                           Fax: 818-906-2870
                                     e-mail: atmrf@aol.com
         www.ninds.nih.gov/find_people/voluntary_orgs/volorg1

Private nonprofit organization dedicated to finding a cure for ataxia-telangiectasia.

Story C Landis, PhD, Director
Walter J Koroshetz, MD, Deputy Director
Joellen Harper Austin, Associate Director

554   Ataxia Telangiectasia Project
3002 Enfield Road
Austin, TX 10166
                                                512-472-4892
                         e-mail: A-TProject@austin.rr.com
                                            www.atproject.org

Nonprofit foundation that supports basic scientific research into treatments for neurological deterioration and cancer in children with ataia-telangiectasia.

Conferences

555   National Ataxia Foundation Annual Membersh ip Meeting
National Ataxia Foundation
2600 Fernbrook Lane, Suite 119
Minneapolis, MN 55447
                                                763-553-0020
                                           Fax: 763-553-0167
                                     e-mail: naf@ataxia.org
                                               www.ataxia.org

Brings together NAF members and their families to meet and learn from world leading ataxia researchers and neurologists, but also to build new friendships and reunite with old friends.

Mike Parent, Executive Director

Audio Video

556 Diagnostic Approach to the Dysmorphic Patient
Southeastern Resgional Genetics Group, Inc SERGG
PO Box 1642
Decatur, GA 30031   404-778-8551
                                                         Fax: 404-778-8562
                                                   e-mail: mlane@sergginc.org
                                                         www.sergginc.org

This 2-hour video focuses on learning how to approach, catego-
rize, and conceptualize the patient with multiple congenital anomalies (MCA). Critical terminology is illustrated. Patients are seen
in hospital and clinic settings. Emphasis is placed in prioritizing
clinical features and weighing each feature's value in reaching a
diagnosis. An outline is included with time frames and detailed
explanations of what each statement, definition and
categorization means.

Timothy C. Wood, PhD, President
Mary Rose Simpson, Administrator

557 Pearls of Dysmorphology
Southeastern Resgional Genetics Group, Inc SERGG
PO Box 1642
Decatur, GA 30031   404-778-8551
                                                         Fax: 404-778-8562
                                                   e-mail: mlane@sergginc.org
                                                         www.sergginc.org

This 1 1/2-hour video which contains 87 individual features considered 'pearls' or 'semi-pearls' relative to their value in reaching
or suspecting a specific diagnosis. Many additional features are
commented on as the formal 'pearls' are presented. There is an
exercise at the end of the tape for helping viewers understand
how dysmorphology pearls can be used to prioritize the diagnostic value of individual features. A handout accompanies this tape,
to help make this exercise fun and educational.

Timothy C. Wood, PhD, President
Mary Rose Simpson, Administrator

558 Syndromes Associated with Multiple Congenital Anomalies
Southeastern Resgional Genetics Group, Inc SERGG
PO Box 1642
Decatur, GA 30031   404-778-8551
                                                         Fax: 404-778-8562
                                                   e-mail: mlane@sergginc.org
                                                         www.sergginc.org

This 2-hour video includes 30 of the more common malformation
syndromes within the categories of single gene, chromosomal,
teratogens, associations, and sequences. Each disorder is preceded by a Table of Features and each disorder is shown at different ages and often includes some verbal interaction. The vast
majority of the cases are within the hospital or clinic setting.
There is minimal use of slides.

Timothy C. Wood, PhD, President
Mary Rose Simpson, Administrator

559 Together...There Is Hope
National Ataxia Foundation
2600 Fernbrook Lane, Suite 119
Minneapolis, MN 55447   763-553-0020
                                                         Fax: 763-553-0167
                                                   e-mail: naf@ataxia.org
                                                         www.ataxia.org

A video discussing ataxias genetic patterns of inheritance and the
National Ataxia Foundation and its research efforts.

Charlene Danielson, President
Camille Daglio, Vice-President
William P. Sweeney, Treasurer

Web Sites

560 Gene Clinics
481B Edward H. Ross Drive
Elmwood Park, NJ 7407   888-729-1204
                                                         Fax: 201-212-6457
                                                  e-mail: genetests@genetests.org
                                                         www.geneclinics.org

By providing current, authoritative information on genetic testing
and its use in diagnosis, management, and genetic counseling,
GeneTests promotes the appropriate use of genetic services in patient care and personal decision making.

Roberta A Pagon, Founder
Amar Kamath, Commercial Director
Deb Eunpu, Program Manager

561 Health Answers
410 Horsham Road
Horsham, PA 19044   215-442-9017
                                          e-mail: Michael.tague@healthanswers.com
                                                         www.healthanswers.com

HealthAnswers offers a breadth of services in medical education,
sales force training, patient support solutions, professional promotion and consumer solutions.

Michael Tague, Managing Director

562 International Network of Ataxia Friends
www.internaf.org

Website mailing list which is maintained by volunteers who have
some form of ataxia.

563 National Ataxia Foundation
2600 Fernbrook Lane, Suite 119
Minneapolis, MN 55447   763-553-0020
                                                         Fax: 763-553-0167
                                                   e-mail: naf@ataxia.org
                                                         www.ataxia.org

Information regarding support, education, and research for dominant ataxia, recessive ataxia, and sporatic ataxia.

Charlene Danielson, President
Camille Daglio, Vice-President
William P. Sweeney, Treasurer

Book Publishers

564 A Balancing Act: Living with Spinal Cerebellar Ataxia
8600 Rockville Pike
Bethesda, MD 20894   301-594-5983
                                                             888-346-3656
                                                         Fax: 301-402-1384
                                                         TDD: 800-735-2258
                                                   e-mail: custserv@nlm.nih.gov
                                                         www.nlm.nih.gov

Describes living with Spinocerebellar Ataxia. Available from
Amazon.com only.
ISBN: 1-889826-00-6

Patricia B Hamilton

565 Directory of National Genetic Voluntary Organizations
Genetic Alliance
4301 Connecticut Avenue NW, Suite 404
Washington, DC 20008   202-966-5557
                                                         Fax: 202-966-8553
                                                   e-mail: info@genticalliance.org
                                                         www.genticalliance.orgtm

Lists hundreds of organizations and associations dealing with genetic conditions.

Sharon F. Terry, President/CEO
Natasha Bonhomme, Vice President
Lisa Wise, Chief Operating Officer

566 Hereditary Ataxia: A Guidebook for Managing Speech & Swallowing
National Ataxia Foundation
2600 Fernbrook Lane, Suite 119
Minneapolis, MN 55447
763-553-0020
Fax: 763-553-0167
e-mail: naf@ataxia.org
www.ataxia.org

567 Living with Ataxia
National Ataxia Foundation
2600 Fernbrook Lane, Suite 119
Minneapolis, MN 55447
763-553-0020
Fax: 763-553-0167
e-mail: naf@ataxia.org
www.ataxia.org

A compassionate resource for people who have or may be at risk of having ataxia, and for their families. This book explains the nature and causes of ataxia, the basic genetics that underlie many kinds of ataxia, discusses medical management of ataxia, provides practical advice for everyday living, points the way to many useful resources and assures that living a good life is an entirely reasonable aspiration, even with ataxia.

112 pages

568 Ten Years to Live
National Ataxia Foundation
2600 Fernbrook Lane, Suite 119
Minneapolis, MN 55447
763-553-0020
Fax: 763-553-0167
e-mail: naf@ataxia.org
www.ataxia.org

Struggles of the Schut family with hereditary ataxia.
ISBN: 0-962716-63-1

Newsletters

569 A-TMRF Newsletter
A-T Medical Research Foundation
5241 Round Meadow Road
Hidden Hills, CA 91302
818-704-8146
Fax: 818-704-8310

Reports on the two major labs that are supported and funded by us.

570 Alert
Alliance of Genetic Support Groups
4301 Connecticut Ave NW, Suite 404
Washington, DC 20008
202-966-5557
Fax: 202-966-8553
e-mail: info@geneticalliance.org
www.geneticalliance.org

Functions as a vehicle of communication between the Alliance and its constituency. Provides timely and useful information on genetics research.
Monthly

Sharon Terry, MA, President/ CEO
Natasha Bonhomme, VP, Strategic Development
Ruth Evans, Director of Accounting

571 Generations
National Ataxia Foundation
2600 Fernbrook Lane, Suite 119
Minneapolis, MN 55447
763-553-0020
Fax: 763-553-0167
e-mail: naf@ataxia.org
www.ataxia.org

Contains reports on the organization and its chapters, offers research, advice and guides to other resources available.

Charlene Danielson, President
Camille Daglio, Vice-President
William P. Sweeney, Treasurer

572 MSRGSN Newsletter
Mountain States Regional Genetics Service Network
4300 Cherry Creek Drive S
Denver, CO 80222
303-692-2423
Fax: 303-782-5576

Joyce Hooker, Coordinator

573 NERG News
New England Regional Genetics Group
PO Box 670
Mount Desert, ME 4660
207-288-2701
Fax: 207-288-2705

574 SERGG Regional News
Southeast Regional Genetics Group
PO Box 1642
Decatur, GA 30031
404-775-8551
Fax: 404-775-8562
e-mail: mlane@sergginc.org
www.sergginc.org

Provides information on genetics services, public health departments, consumers, and related laboratory services.

Timothy C. Wood, PhD, President
Mary Rose Simpson, Administrator

Pamphlets

575 Alliance Brochure
Alliance of Genetic Support Groups
4301 Connecticut Ave NW, Suite 404
Washington, DC 20008
202-966-5557
Fax: 202-966-8553
e-mail: info@geneticalliance.org
www.geneticalliance.org

Explains the services and programs offered by the Alliance.

Sharon Terry, MA, President/ CEO
Natasha Bonhomme, VP, Strategic Development
Ruth Evans, Director of Accounting

576 Ataxia Fact Sheet
National Ataxia Foundation
2600 Fernbrook Lane, Suite 119
Minneapolis, MN 55447
763-553-0020
Fax: 763-553-0167
e-mail: naf@ataxia.org
www.ataxia.org

Describes ataxia as a symptom and its association with other medical problems as well as the hereditary types.

Charlene Danielson, President
Camille Daglio, Vice-President
William P. Sweeney, Treasurer

577 Consumer Indicators of Quality Genetic Services
Alliance of Genetic Support Groups
4301 Connecticut Avenue NW, #404
Washington, DC 20008
202-966-5557
800-336-4363
Fax: 202-966-8553
e-mail: info@geneticalliance.org
www.geneticalliance.org

Describes the Alliance of Genetic Support Groups Partnership Program, which strives to increase provider awareness of the unique needs and resources of genetic consumers, improve provider access to quality, consumer-oriented support group resources, and develop replacable educational materials for other programs.

Sharon Terry, MA, President/ CEO
Natasha Bonhomme, VP, Strategic Development
Ruth Evans, Director of Accounting

578 Facts About Friedreich's Ataxia
Muscular Dystrophy Association
222 S. Riverside Plaza, Suite 1500
Chicago, IL 60606   520-529-2000
                                           800-572-1717
                                     Fax: 520-529-5300
                                e-mail: mda@mdausa.org
                                               mda.org

Explains Friedreich's ataxia in layman's terms and answers commonly asked questions about the disease. Also in Spanish and on-line.
2006

Steven M. Derks, President/ CEO
Valerie A. Cwik, M.D., EVP/ CMO/ CSO
Julie Faber, EVP/ CFO

579 Friedrich's Ataxia
National Ataxia Foundation
2600 Fernbrook Lane, Suite 119
Minneapolis, MN 55447   763-553-0020
                                     Fax: 763-553-0167
                                 e-mail: naf@ataxia.org
                                           www.ataxia.org

Describes symptoms, diagnosis, genetics and hints on coping.

Charlene Danielson, President
Camille Daglio, Vice-President
William P. Sweeney, Treasurer

580 Gene Testing for Ataxia
National Ataxia Foundation
2600 Fernbrook Lane, Suite 119
Minneapolis, MN 55447   763-553-0020
                                     Fax: 763-553-0167
                                 e-mail: naf@ataxia.org
                                           www.ataxia.org

Describes the latest information about who should consider it and where to have it done.

Charlene Danielson, President
Camille Daglio, Vice-President
William P. Sweeney, Treasurer

581 Hereditary Ataxia: The Facts
National Ataxia Foundation
2600 Fernbrook Lane, Suite 119
Minneapolis, MN 55447   612-553-0020
                                     Fax: 612-553-0167
                                  e-mail: naf@mr.net
                                           www.ataxia.org

Describes recessive and dominant ataxias, information on how hereditary ataxia is transmitted and explanations of the NAF's role in education, service and prevention.

Charlene Danielson, President
Camille Daglio, Vice-President
William P. Sweeney, Treasurer

582 Incorporating Consumers into Regional Genetics Networks
Alliance of Genetic Support Groups
4301 Connecticut Avenue NW, Suite 404
Washington, DC 20008   301-652-5553
                                     Fax: 202-966-8553
                              e-mail: alliance@capaccess.org
                                    medhelp.org/www/agsg.htm

583 Informed Consent: Participation in Genetic Research Studies
Alliance of Genetic Support Groups
4301 Connecticut Avenue NW, Suite 404
Washington, DC 20008   202-966-5557
                                           800-336-4363
                                     Fax: 202-966-8553
                             e-mail: info@geneticalliance.org
                                    www.geneticalliance.org

This booklet explains the nature of genetic research with its benefits and risks.

Sharon Terry, MA, President/ CEO
Natasha Bonhomme, VP, Strategic Development
Ruth Evans, Director of Accounting

584 Pen-Pal Directory
National Ataxia Foundation
2600 Fernbrook Lane, Suite 119
Minneapolis, MN 55447   763-553-0020
                                     Fax: 763-553-0167
                                 e-mail: naf@ataxia.org
                                           www.ataxia.org

National, state and international directory of others who are affected by ataxia. Available to NAF Pen-Pal members only.

Charlene Danielson, President
Camille Daglio, Vice-President
William P. Sweeney, Treasurer

Description

585 ATRIAL SEPTAL DEFECTS

Synonyms: ASD, Atrioseptal defects

Involves the following Biologic System(s):

Cardiovascular Disorders

The term atrial septal defect, or ASD, refers to a group of congenital abnormalities characterized by the presence of a hole in the wall (septum) that separates the two upper chambers of the heart (atria). Atrial septal defects are classified according to their location and may occur as a single anomaly or in association with other heart (cardiac) defects. These types of abnormalities occur in approximately 2000 of every 100,000 births.

The upper left chamber of the heart (left atrium) receives blood that is rich with oxygen (oxygenated) from the lungs. The blood then passes into the lower left chamber (left ventricle) from which it is then pumped through the arteries of the body into the general circulation. The right atrium receives blood that has been depleted of oxygen (deoxygenated) that then passes into the right ventricle and is pumped to the lungs where it once again receives oxygen. Atrial septal defects may allow the passage of some oxygenated blood from the upper left side of the heart into the upper right side of the heart where it mixes with blood that is oxygen depleted. In some patients, this results in a reduced oxygen supply to the body and an increase in blood flow to the lungs. Physical findings associated with ASDs may include enlargement of the right atrium, the right ventricle, or both, and characteristic heart sounds. In some patients, symptoms may be completely absent, especially in early childhood. ASDs are often discovered during routine physical examination by the pressure of a systolic heart murmur. Some affected individuals may experience fatigue upon exertion or exercise. Other findings or symptoms may become apparent after the age of 30 years or when an affected woman becomes pregnant. In these patients, symptoms may include fatigue upon exercise (exercise intolerance), valve insufficiencies, and other, more serious problems such as heart failure and or arrhythmias.

The standard method for closure of atrial septal defects has been open-heart surgery. However, a new nonsurgical procedure has been developed and is done in the heart catheterization laboratory, thus avoiding the need for surgery. A patch, usually resembling a small umbrella, is inserted into the damaged area through a catheter. It is then put into place to close the hole.

Government Agencies

586 NIH/National Heart, Lung and Blood Institu te
National Institute of Health
31 Center Dr MSC 2486, Bldg 31, Rm 5A48
Bethesda, MD 10167
301-592-8573
Fax: 240-629-3246
TTY: 240-629-3255
e-mail: nhlbiinfo@nhlbi.nih.gov
www.nhlbi.nih.gov

The National Heart, Lung, and Blood Institute (NHLBI) provides global leadership for a research, training, and education program to promote the prevention and treatment of heart, lung, and blood diseases and enhance the health of all individuals so that they can live longer and more fulfilling lives.

Gary H Gibbons MD, Director
Susan Shurin, MD, Deputy Director
Nakela Cook MD, Chief of Staff

587 NIH/National Institute of Child Health and Human Development
31 Center Drive, Building 31 Room 2A32
Bethesda, MD 10168
800-370-2943
Fax: 301-496-1104
TTY: 888-320-6942
www.nichd.nih.gov

Established in 1962 by congress, today the institute conducts and supports laboratory research, clinical trials, and epidemiological studies that explore health processes; examines the impact of disabilities, diseases, and variations on the lives of individuals; and sponsors training programs for scientists, health care providers, and researchers to ensure that NICHD research can continue.

Alan E Guttmacher MD, Director
Lisa Kaeser, Program & Public Liaison

National Associations & Support Groups

588 American Academy of Pediatrics
141 Northwest Point Boulevard
Elk Grove Village, IL 60007
847-434-4000
800-433-9016
Fax: 847-434-8000
www.aap.org

The American Academy of Pediatrics and its member pediatricians are committed to the attainment of optimal physical, mental and social health and well-being for all infants, children, adolescents, and young adults.

Sandra Hassink, MD, FAAP, President

589 American Heart Association
7272 Greenville Avenue
Dallas, TX 10169
214-373-6300
800-242-8721
Fax: 214-706-1341
e-mail: inquire@amhrt.org
www.americanheart.org

Our mission is to build healthier lives, free of cardiovascular diseases and stroke.

Nancy Brown, CEO
Suzie Upton, Chief Development Officer
Sunder Joshi, CFO

590 Genetic Alliance
4301 Connecticut Avenue NW Suite 404
Washington, DC 10170
202-966-7955
800-336-4363
Fax: 202-966-8553
e-mail: info@geneticalliance.org
www.geneticalliance.org

World's leading nonprofit health advocacy organization committed to transforming health through genetics and promoting an environment of openness centered on the health of individuals, families, and communities.

Sharon Terry, President
Lisa Wise, Chief Operating Officer
Tetyana Murza MES, Programs and Policy Coordinator

591 March of Dimes Birth Defects Foundation
1275 Mamaroneck Avenue
White Plains, NY 10171
914-997-4488
888-663-4637
Fax: 914-997-4763
e-mail: answers@marchofdimes.com
www.marchofdimes.com

The March of Dimes helps moms have full-term pregnancies and research the problems that threaten the health of babies.

Kenneth A. May, Chair
Jennifer Howse, President & CEO
Alan Fleischman, Medical Director

Conferences

592 Genetic Alliance Annual Conference
Genetic Alliance
4301 Connecticut Avenue NW, Suite 404
Washington, DC 20008   202-966-5557
                                800-336-4363
                           Fax: 202-966-8553
              e-mail: info@geneticalliance.org
                    www.geneticalliance.org

Consistently inspirational and enables partnership among all
stakeholders: advocates and community leaders, health and industry professionals, policymakers, and academicians.

July

Sharon Terry, President/CEO
Tetyana Murza, Programs/Events Manager

Web Sites

593 Southern Illinois University School of Medicine
P O Box 19658
Springfield, IL 62794   217-545-8000
                  www.siumed.edu/peds/index.htm

Mission is to meet the health care needs of children and their families in Central and Southern Illinois through provision of high
quality, coordinated care of children with acute and chronic conditions with inpatient, ambulatory, and community-based
programs.

594 Yale University School of Medicine
333 Cedar Street
New Haven, CT 6510   203-432-4771
                            medicine.yale.edu

Offers information on congenital heart conditions such as Atrial
Septal Defects, including symptoms, causes and treatments.

Peter Salovey, President of the University
Richard Belitsky M.D., Deputy Dean for Education
Benjamin Polak B.A., M.A., Ph.D., Provost of the University

Book Publishers

595 Congenital Disorders Sourcebook 2nd Edition
Omnigraphics
PO Box 31-1640
Detroit, MI 48231   800-234-1340
                           Fax: 800-875-1340
              e-mail: info@omnigraphics.com
                    www.omnigraphics.com

Provides basic consumer health information about the most common types of nonhereditary birth defects and disorders related to
prematurity, gestational injuries, congenital infections, and birth
complications, including disorders of the heart, brain, gastrointestinal tract, musculoskeletal system, urinary tract, and reproductive system craniofacial disorders, cerebral palsy, spina bifida,
and fetal alcohol syndrome, and detailing the causes, diagnostic
tests, and treatments for each.

650 pages
ISBN: 0-780809-45-9

Description

596   ATTENTION DEFICIT HYPERACTIVITY DISORDER

Synonyms: ADHD, Hyperactive child syndrome, Hyperkinetic syndrome

Involves the following Biologic System(s):

Developmental/Behavioral/Psychiatric Disorders

Attention deficit hyperactivity disorder, or ADHD, is a syndrome of childhood and adolescence characterized by impulsive behavior, motor-related overactivity (hyperactivity), and inattention. The short attention span results in a decreased ability or inability to complete chores, assignments, or other tasks. ADHD is four to six times more prevalent among boys than it is in girls. In approximately 50 percent of cases, this disorder develops before the age of four years, while in others it appears before seven years of age. Over the last decade, it has been increasingly diagnosed in adults. Some behavioral symptoms associated with this disorder may be present at times in children with ADHD or in children with certain other disorders (e.g., conduct disorder, learning disabilities, hearing impairment, etc.). Therefore, specialists often base their diagnosis on the frequent presence of eight or more characteristic findings. Among these are restlessness, difficulty in remaining seated, difficulty in waiting for a turn in group activities, inclination to be easily distracted, impulsively answering questions before they are completed, difficulty following instructions, inability to sustain concentration while performing tasks or playing, shifting to other tasks before completing others, talking excessively, poor ability to play quietly, interrupting or butting in on others, not appearing to listen when others speak, losing things, and frequently taking part in dangerous physical activities.Evaluation of an individual with ADHD involves taking a detailed family and medical history, paying careful attention to such things as activity level, behavior, and temperament during the early years of the life of the affected child. Obtaining this information may be helpful in determining the extent of the disorder and the presence of additional difficulties (e.g., learning disabilities, anxiety disorders, conduct disorders, etc.).

ADHD is currently considered to be a persistent and chronic condition for which no medical cure is available. Although the cause of ADHD is not known, genetic influences may be a factor in the development of this disorder. In addition, children with neurological disorders and other abnormalities related to the central nervous system may be predisposed to the development of ADHD. Treatment of attention deficit hyperactivity disorder may include an ongoing behavioral and psychosocial therapeutic plan that includes the cooperation of school personnel, the child, and the child's parents or caregivers. In addition, psychostimulant drugs or other medications may be prescribed and carefully monitored. Affected children may also benefit from a structured environment at home and in school. Studies show that, in many phases children who receive multifaceted treatment are better able to cope with ADHD through their adolescent years and into adulthood. Other treatment is supportive.

Government Agencies

597   NIH/National Institute of Mental Health
6001 Executive Boulevard, Room 8184, MSC 9663
Bethesda, MD 10172

301-443-4513
866-615-6464
Fax: 301-443-4279
TTY: 301-443-8431
e-mail: nimhinfo@nih.gov
www.nimh.nih.gov

The mission of NIMH is to transform the understanding and treatment of mental illnesses through basic and clinical research, paving the way for prevention, recovery, and cure.

Dr Thomas R Insel, Director

598   NIH/National Institute of Neurological Dis orders and Stroke (NINDS)
PO Box 5801
Bethesda, MD 10173

301-496-5751
800-352-9424
Fax: 301-496-0296
TTY: 301-468-5981
www.ninds.nih.gov

The mission of NINDS is to reduce the burden of neurological disease - a burden borne by every age group, by every segment of society, by people all over the world.

Story C Landis Ph.D., Director
Walter J Koroshetz, Deputy Director
Caroline Lewis, Executive Officer

National Associations & Support Groups

599   AD-IN: Attention Deficit Information Network
475 Hillside Avenue
Needham, MA 10174

781-455-9895
Fax: 781-444-5466
e-mail: adin@gis.net
www.addinfonetwork.com

Provides information on training programs and speakers for those who work with individuals with ADD.

600   ADHD Challenge
PO Box 488
West Peabody, MA 01985

978-535-3276
800-233-2322
TDD: 508-535-3276
www.additudemag.com/adhd/article/8643.html

Provision of data and emotional assistance to both sufferers and medical professionals.

601   ARC of the United States
1010 Wayne Avenue, Suite 650
Silver Spring, MD 20910

301-565-3842
Fax: 301-565-5342
e-mail: info@thearc.org
www.thearc.org

The ARC of the United States advocates for the rights and full participation of all children and adults with intellectual and developmental disabilities. Together with our network of members and affiliated chapters, we improve systems of supports and services; connect families; inspire communities an influence public policy.

Peter V Barns, CEO
Nancy Webster, President
Ronald Brown, Vice President

602   American Academy of Pediatrics
141 Northwest Point Boulevard
Elk Grove Village, IL 60007

847-434-4000
800-433-9016
Fax: 847-434-8000
www.aap.org

The American Academy of Pediatrics and its member pediatricians are committed to the attainment of optimal physical, mental and social health and well-being for all infants, children, adolescents, and young adults.

Sandra Hassink, MD, FAAP, President

603 Attention Deficit Disorder Association
PO Box 7557
Wilmington, DE 10177

800-939-1019
Fax: 856-439-0525
e-mail: info@add.org
www.add.org

The Attention Deficit Disorder Association provides information, resources and networking opportunities to help adults with Attention Deficit Hyperactivity Disorder lead better lives.

Evelyn Polk Green, President
Linda Roggli, Vice President
Janet Kramer MD, Treasurer

604 CHADD: Children and Adults with Attention Deficit/Hyperactivity Disorders
8181 Professional Place, Suite 150
Landover, MD 10178

301-306-7070
800-233-4050
Fax: 301-306-7090
www.chadd.org

Children and Adults with Attention-Deficit/Hyperactivity Disorder (CHADD) was founded in 1987 in response to the frustration and sense of isolation experienced by parents and their children with ADHD.

1987

Barbara S Hawkins, President
Michael MacKay, Treasurer

605 Feingold Association of the US
11849 Suncatcher Drive
Fishers, IN 10179

631-369-9340
800-321-3287
Fax: 631-369-2988
e-mail: help@feingold.org
www.feingold.org

An organization of families and professionals founded in 1976 to provide a dietary management program for both children and adults

Annette Miller, President
Kathleen Bratby, Secretary
Larisa Scarbrough, Vice President

606 Genetic Alliance
4301 Connecticut Avenue NW Suite 404
Washington, DC 10180

202-966-7955
800-336-4363
Fax: 202-966-8553
e-mail: info@geneticalliance.org
www.geneticalliance.org

World's leading nonprofit health advocacy organization committed to transforming health through genetics and promoting an environment of openness centered on the health of individuals, families, and communities.

Sharon Terry, President
Lisa Wise, Chief Operating Officer
Tetyana Murza MES, Programs and Policy Coordinator

607 Learning Disabilities Association of Ameri ca
4156 Library Road
Pittsburgh, PA 15234

412-341-1515
888-300-6710
Fax: 412-344-0224
e-mail: info@LDAAmerica.org
www.ldaamerica.org

Helps families of the affected individual through information and referral to professionals in their area. A membership organization with affiliates across the country.

Sheila Buckley, Executive Director

608 March of Dimes Birth Defects Foundation
1275 Mamaroneck Avenue
White Plains, NY 10181

914-997-4488
888-663-4637
Fax: 914-997-4763
e-mail: answers@marchofdimes.com
www.marchofdimes.com

March of Dimes help moms have full-term pregnancies and research the problems that threaten the health of babies.The March of Dimes also acts globally: sharing best practices in perinatal health and helping improve birth outcomes where the needs are the most urgent.

Kenneth A. May, Chair
Jennifer Howse, President & CEO
Alan Fleischman, Medical Director

609 Mental Health America
2000 N Beauregard Street, 6th Floor
Alexandria, VA 10182

703-684-7722
800-969-6642
Fax: 703-684-5968
TTY: 800-433-5959
e-mail: info@mentalhealthamerica.net
www.mentalhealthamerica.net

MHA, the leading advocacy organization addressing the full spectrum of mental and substance use conditions and their effects nationwide, works to inform, advocate and enable access to quality behavioral health services for all Americans.

Ann Boughtin, Chair of the Board
Eric Ashton, Vice Chair
Elaine Crider, Secretary/Treasurer

610 National Alliance for the Mentally Ill
3803 N. Fairfax Dr., Suite 100
Arlington, VA 10183

703-525-7600
800-950-6264
Fax: 703-524-9094
TDD: 703-516-7227
e-mail: info@nami.org
www.nami.org

NAMI is a nonprofit, grassroots, self-help, support and advocacy organization of consumers, families and friends of people with severe mental illness, such as schizophrenia, bipolar disorder, major depressive disorder, obsessive compulsive disorder, anxiety disorders, autism and other severe and persistent mental illnesses that affect the brain.

Keris J,,n Myrick, President
Kevin B Sullivan, First Vice President
Jim Payne, Second Vice President

611 National Center for Learning Disabilities
381 Park Avenue S, Suite 1401
New York, NY 10184

212-545-7510
888-575-7373
Fax: 212-545-9665
e-mail: ncld@ncld.org
www.ncld.org

The National Center for Learning Disabilities improves the lives of all people with learning difficulties and disabilities by empowering parents, enabling young adults, transforming schools, and creating policy and advocacy impact.

Frederic M Poses, CEO
Anne Ford, Chairman Emeritus
Mary Kalikow, Vice Chair

612 National Mental Health Consumers' Self-Help Clearinghouse
1211 Chestnut Street, Suite 1207
Philadelphia, PA 10185

215-751-1810
800-553-4539
Fax: 215-636-6312
e-mail: info@mhselfhelp.org
www.mhselfhelp.org

The Clearinghouse works to foster peer empowerment through our website, up-to-date news and information announcements, a directory of peer-driven services, electronic and printed publications, training packages, and individual and onsite consultation

Joseph Rogers, Executive Director & Founder
Susan Rogers, Director of Special Projects
Britani Nestel, Program Specialist

613 Option Institute: Son Rise Program
Autism Treatment Center of America
2080 S Undermountain Road
Sheffield, MA 10186

413-229-2100
800-714-2779
Fax: 413-229-3202
e-mail: information@son-rise.org
www.son-rise.org

Describes an effective, loving and respectful method for treating children with autism. It teaches parents and healing professionals how to set up a home based program using the child's motivation to reach their special child.

Barry Neil Kaufman, Co-Founder/Co-Creator
Samahria Lyte Kaufman, Co-Founder/Co-Creator
Bryn Hogan, ATCA Senior Staff

614 The Council For Exceptional Children
2900 Crystal Drive, Suite 1000
Arlington, VA 10187

703-243-0446
888-232-7733
Fax: 703-264-9494
TTY: 866-915-5000
e-mail: service@cec.sped.org
www.cec.sped.org

wide mission of the Council for Exceptional Children is to improve educational outcomes for individuals with exceptionalities.

Bruce Ramirez, Executive Director
Veronica Browne-Barnes, Senior Executive Assistant for Gove
Sharon Rodriguez, Senior Executive Assistant for Admi

Conferences

615 Annual International Conference on ADHD
CHADD
8181 Professional Place, Suite 150
Landover, MD 20785

301-306-7070
800-233-4050
Fax: 301-306-7090
e-mail: webmaster@chadd.org
www.chadd.org

November

Marsha Bokman, Meetings/Events Director

616 Arc's National Convention
ARC
1825 K Street NW, Suite 1200
Washington, DC 20006

202-534-3700
800-433-5255
Fax: 202-534-3731
e-mail: info@thearc.org
www.thearc.org

Where members, staff, volunteers, professionals, experts, self advocates and their families gather for a dynamic convention to meet each other, learn from each other, and tackle the tough issues facing the intellectual and developmental disability (I/DD) community together.

Nanci Webster, President
Ronald Brown, Vice President
Elise McMillan, Secretary

617 CEC Convention & Expo
Council for Exceptional Children
2900 Crystal Drive Suite 1000
Arlington, VA 22202

703-243-0446
888-232-7733
Fax: 703-264-9494
TTY: 866-915-5000
e-mail: service@cec.sped.org
www.cec.sped.org

Offers an unparalleled experience with more than 800 sessions to help you learn the latest in evidence-based practices; explore innovative technologies, products, and services; and network with other professionals working with children with exceptionalities and their families.

April

Bruce Ramirez, Executive Director

618 Genetic Alliance Annual Conference
Genetic Alliance
4301 Connecticut Avenue NW, Suite 404
Washington, DC 20008

202-966-5557
800-336-4363
Fax: 202-966-8553
e-mail: info@geneticalliance.org
www.geneticalliance.org

Consistently inspirational and enables partnership among all stakeholders: advocates and community leaders, health and industry professionals, policymakers, and academicians.

July

Sharon Terry, President/CEO
Tetyana Murza, Programs/Events Manager

619 NAMI Convention
National Alliance on Mental Illness
3803 N Fairfax Drive, Suite 100
Arlington, VA 22203

703-524-7600
888-999-6264
Fax: 703-524-9094
TDD: 703-516-7227
e-mail: info@nami.org
www.nami.org

The NAMI Convention is packed with information, chances to network, leadership development opportunities, and lots more.

July

Keris Jan Myrick, President
Kevin B Sullivan, Vice President
Clarence Jordan, Secretary

Audio Video

620 ADD From A To Z-Understanding The Diagnosis & Treatment of ADD in Children & Adult
Connecticut Association for Children with LD
25 Van Zant Street, Suite 15-5
East Norwalk, CT 6855

203-838-5010
Fax: 203-866-6108
e-mail: cacld@optonline.net
www.cacld.org

Provides a comprehensive overview of this complicated and often misunderstood subject. Informative, authorative, and entertaining, this video will be useful to anyone who wants a clear understanding of what ADD is and what is not.

107 Minutes

621 ADHD: What Can We Do?
ADD WareHouse
300 NW 70th Avenue, Suite 102
Plantation, FL 33317

954-792-8100
800-233-9273
Fax: 954-792-8545
e-mail: websales@addwarehouse.com
www.addwarehouse.com

Can serve as a companion to ADHD: What Do We Know. This video focuses on the most effective ways to manage ADHD, both in the home and in the classroom. Scenes depict the use of behavior management at home and accommodations and interventions in the classroom which have proven to be effective in the treatment of ADHD. Thirty seven minutes.

1993
ISBN: 0-898629-82-1

622   ADHD: What Do We Know?

Russell A Barkley, author

Guilford Publications
370 Seventh Avenue, Suite 1200
New York, NY 10001

212-431-9800
800-365-7006
Fax: 212-966-6708
e-mail: info@guilford.com
www.guilford.com

An introduction for teachers and special education practitioners, school psychologists and parents of ADHD children. Topics outlined in this video include the causes and prevalence of ADHD, ways children with ADHD behave, other conditions that may accompany ADHD and long-term prospects for children with ADHD. DVD'36 minutes, Manual 31 pages.

Oct 2006 31 pages DVD & Manual

623   Concentration Video

Learning disAbilities Resources
PO Box 716
Bryn Mawr, PA 19010

610-525-8336
Fax: 610-525-8337

An instructional video which provides a perspective about attention problems, possible causes and solutions.

Video

624   Educating Inattentive Children

ADD WareHouse
300 NW 70th Avenue, Suite 102
Plantation, FL 33317

954-792-8100
800-233-9273
Fax: 954-792-8545
e-mail: websales@addwarehouse.com
www.addwarehouse.com

An excellent resources for teachers who encounter inattention and hyperactivity in the classroom. It helps teachers distinguish deliberate misbehavior from the incompetent, nonpurposeful behavior of the inattentive child.

1990 Video

625   How to Help Your Child Succeed in School

Peytral Publications
PO Box 1162
Minnetonka, MN 55345

952-949-8707
877-739-8725
Fax: 952-906-9777
e-mail: help@peytral.com
www.peytral.com

In this deeply powerful video, Sandra Reif presents the essential information needed by those who work with ADHD and/or Learning Disabilities to help children in school. The focus is on the key for success, a strong partnership in education between home and school.

56 Minutes

Donna Kaufman

626   Medication for ADHD

ADD WareHouse
300 NW 70th Avenue, Suite 102
Plantation, FL 33317

954-792-8100
800-233-9273
Fax: 954-792-8545
e-mail: websales@addwarehouse.com
www.addwarehouse.com

This comprehensive DVD program addresses the critical questions regarding the use of medicati in the treatment of ADD or ADHD. WGN-TV medical reporter Dina Bair interviews two long-time ADHD experts: psychiatrist Dr Jonathan Bloomberg and clinical psychologist Dr Thomas Phelan.

ISBN: 1-889140-18-X

627   Understanding Attention Deficit Disorder

Connecticut Association for Children with LD
25 Van Zant Street, Suite 15-5
East Norwalk, CT 6855

203-838-5010
Fax: 203-866-6108
e-mail: cacld@optonline.net
www.cacld.org

A video in an interview format for parents and professionals providing the history, symptoms, methods of diagnosis and three approaches used to ease the effects of attention deficit disorder.

45 minutes

628   Understanding Hyperactivity

Psychiatric Support Services
Houston, TX

281-580-0046

Designed for parents and teachers, a video explaining the symptoms and consequences of attention deficit hyperactivity disorder.

Video

629   Why Can't Michael Pay Attention?

Learning Seed
P.O. Box 617880
Chicago, IL 60661

800-634-4941
Fax: 800-998-0854
e-mail: info@learningseed.com
www.learningseed.com

After a multi-faceted assessment, six year old, Michael is diagnosed with Attention Deficit Hyperactivity Disorder. Michael's parents learn techniques such as consistent schedules, docking systems, star charts, and self-monitoring to help organize home life. ISBN: DVD 1-55740-973-0; VHS 1-55740-896-3

21 minutes

630   Why Won't My Child Pay Attention?

Wiley Publishing Inc
111 River Street
Hoboken, NJ 07030

317-572-3000
201-748-6000
Fax: 201-748-6088
e-mail: info@wiley.com
as.wiley.com/WileyCDA/Section/index.html

Practical and reassuring videotape. Noted child psychologist tells parents about two of the most common and complex problems of childhood: inattention and hyperactivity.

1993 Video
ISBN: 0-471303-19-4

Stephen M. Smith, President & CEO
John Kritzmacher, Executive Vice President
Edward J. May, Corporate Secretary

Web Sites

631   Attention Deficit Disorder Association
www.add.org

Provides children, adolescents and adults with ADD information, support groups, publications, videos, and referrals.

Evelyn Polk Green, President
Linda Roggli, Vice President
Celeste A. Jacque, Board of Director

632   Attention Deficit Disorder and Parenting Site
www.LD-ADD.com

Website has been created for parents to help them recognize and manage ADHD/LD in children.

633   Attention Deficit Information Network
www.addinfonetwork.com

Nonprofit volunteer organization. We offer support and information to families of children with ADD and adults with ADD, professionals through a network of AD-IN chapters.

634   CHADD: Children and Adults with Attention Deficit Disorders
4601 Presidents Drive, Suite 300
Lanham, MD 20706
301-306-7070
800-233-4050
Fax: 301-306-7090
e-mail: help@chadd.org
www.chadd.org

Many children and/or adults have a disorder characterized by deficits in attention span and impulse control, which is frequently accompanied by hyperactivity. C.H.A.D.D. (Children and Adults with Attention Deficit Disorders) provides parents, professionals and adults diagnosed with ADD information, support and educational material dealing with this disorder. C.H.A.D.D. has over 600 chapters across the country and over 28,000 active members.

Michael MacKay, President
April Gower, Chief Operations Officer
Khalilah Long, Director of Membership & Marketing

635   Feingold Association of the US
11849 Suncatcher Drive
Fishers, IN 46037
631-369-9340
e-mail: help@feingold.org
www.feingold.org

Helps families of children with learning and behavior problems, including attention deficit disorder. Also helps chemically-sensitive and salicylate-sensitive adults. Program is based upon a diet which primarily eliminates certain synthetic food additives.

636   Health Answers
410 Horsham Road
Horsham, PA 19044
215-442-9017
e-mail: Michael.tague@healthanswers.com
www.healthanswers.com

HealthAnswers offers a breadth of services in medical education, sales force training, patient support solutions, professional promotion and consumer solutions.

Michael Tague, Managing Director

637   Learning Disabilities Association of America
www.ldaamerica.org

Helps families of the affected individual through information and referral to professionals in their area. A membership organization with affiliates across the country.

638   National Center for Learning Disabilities
32 Laight Street, Second Floor
New York, NY 10013
212-545-7510
888-575-7373
Fax: 212-545-9665
e-mail: help@ncld.org
www.ld.org

The mission of the NCLD is to increase opportunities for all individuals with learning disabilities to achieve their potential. NCLD accomplishes this by increasing public awareness and understanding of learning disabilities, conducting educational programs and services that promote research-based knowledge and providing national leadership in shaping public policy.

Frederic M Poses, Chairman
Mary Kalikow, Vice Chairman
William Haney, Secretary

639   Option Institute: Son Rise Program
www.autismtreatmentcenter.org
877-766-7473
www.autismtreatmentcenter.org

Describes an effective, loving and respectful method for treating children with autism. It teaches parents and healing professionals how to set up a home based program using the child's motivation to reach their special child.

Barry Neil Kaufman, Co-Founder
Kate Wilde, Group Facilitator
Samahria Lyte Kaufman, Founder

Book Publishers

640   ADD & Learning Disabilities
Bantam Doubleday Dell Publishing
1745 Broadway, 10th Floor
New York, NY 10019
212-572-6066
Fax: 212-782-9700
e-mail: webmaster@randomhouse.com
www.randomhouse.com

For parents of children with learning disabilities and attention deficit disorder - and for educational and medical professionals who encounter these children - two experts in the field have devised a handbook to help identify the very best treatments.

256 pages
ISBN: 0-385469-31-4

641   ADD: Helping Your Child
Warner Books
1271 Avenue of the Americas
New York, NY 10020
212-484-2900
Fax: 617-263-2854

1994 224 pages Paperback
ISBN: 0-446670-13-8

642   ADHD Parenting Handbook: Practical Advice for Parents from Parents
Taylor Publishing
1550 W Mockingbird Lane
Dallas, TX 75235
214-637-2800
Fax: 214-819-8141

Provides guidelines, suggestions, and advice to help parents interact with their children who have ADHD.

1994 224 pages Paperback
ISBN: 0-878338-62-4

643   ADHD Survival Guide for Parents and Teachers
Hope Press
PO Box 188
Duarte, CA 91009
818-303-0644
800-321-4039
Fax: 626-358-3520
e-mail: dcomings@earthlink.net
hopepress.com

Guide for parents and teacher and other caretakers of ADHD children.
ISBN: 1-878267-43-4

644   ADHD in Schools: Assessment and Intervention Strategies
George DuPaul, Gary Stoner, author

Guilford Publications
72 Spring Street
New York, NY 10012
212-431-9800
800-365-7006
Fax: 212-966-6708
e-mail: info@guilford.com
www.guilford.com

Comprehensive and practical, the book includes several reproducible assessment tools and handouts, and emphasizes a team-based approach to intervetion. This is a popular reference providing essential guidance for school-based professionals meeting the challenges of ADHD at any grade level. Available in paperback or hardcover.

Oct 2004 330 pages Paperback
ISBN: 1-593850-89-0

645   ADHD in the Young Child
ADD WareHouse
300 NW 70th Avenue, Suite 102
Plantation, FL 33317
954-792-8100
800-233-9273
Fax: 954-792-8545
e-mail: websales@addwarehouse.com
www.addwarehouse.com

The authors sensitively and effectively describe what life is like living with a young child with ADHD. With the help of over 75 cartoon illustrations they provide practical solutions to common problems found at home, in school and elsewhere.

2006 202 pages
ISBN: 1-886941-32-7

646 ADHD: Handbook for Diagnosis & Treatment
Guilford Press
72 Spring Street
New York, NY 10012

800-365-7006
Fax: 212-966-6708
e-mail: info@guilford.com
www.guilford.com

This second edition helps clinicians diagnose and treat Attention Deficit Hyperactivity Disorder. Written by an internationally recognized authority in the field, it covers the history of ADHD, its primary symptoms, associated conditions, developmental course and outcome, and family context. A workbook companion manual is also available.

2005 770 pages
ISBN: 1-593852-10-8

647 All Kinds of Minds
ADD WareHouse
300 NW 70th Avenue, Suite 102
Plantation, FL 33317

954-792-8100
800-233-9273
Fax: 954-792-8545
e-mail: websales@addwarehouse.com
www.addwarehouse.com

Primary and elementary students with learning disorders can now gain insight into the difficulties they face in school. This book helps all children understand and respect all kinds of minds and can encourage children with learning disorders to maintain their motivation and keep from developing behavior problems stemming from their learning disorders.

1993 283 pages
ISBN: 0-838820-90-5

648 Alphabet Soup: A Recipe for Understanding & Treating ADD
Minerva Books
137 W 14th Street
New York, NY 10011

212-343-6100
Fax: 212-343-6934

1994 50 pages Paperback
ISBN: 0-934695-00-8

649 Attention Deficit Disorder and Learning Disabilities
Random House
1745 Broadway
New York, NY 10019

212-572-6066
e-mail: webmaster@randomhouse.com
www.randomhouse.com

Realities, myths, and controversial treatments. Section I tries to dispel the myths and discusses proven treatments for ADHD and LD. Section II explains how the scientific community evaluates new treatment methods, and Section III summarizes alternative treatments and discusses scientific evidence pertaining to its usefulness.

256 pages
ISBN: 0-385469-31-4

650 Attention Deficit Disorder: Concise Source of Information for Parents
Temeron Books
6531 111th Street NW
Edmonton, AB T6H 4
Canada

403-283-0900
855-283-0900
Fax: 403-283-6947
e-mail: contact@brusheducation.ca
www.brusheducation.ca

Help with a frustrating situation that many parents face.

2006 112 pages
ISBN: 1-550590-82-0

Glenn Rollans, Partner
Lauri Seidlitz, Managing Editor

651 Attention Deficit Hyperactivity Disorder: What Every Parent Wants to Know
Paul H Brookes & Company
PO Box 10624
Baltimore, MD 21285

301-337-9580
800-638-3775
Fax: 410-337-8539
e-mail: custserv@brookspublishing.com
www.brookespublishing.com

The new edition breaks down the complex issues surrounding ADHD today into easy-to-understand, non-technical terms. Now you can quickly get the information you need to help your child with ADHD, without taking the time to wade through heavy research or statistics.

2000 304 pages Paperback
ISBN: 1-557663-98-X

652 Beyond Ritalin: Facts About Medication and Other Strategies for Helping Children
ADD WareHouse
300 NW 70th Avenue, Suite 102
Plantation, FL 33317

954-792-8100
800-233-9273
Fax: 954-792-8545
e-mail: websales@addwarehouse.com
www.addwarehouse.com

The authors respond to concerns all parents and individuals have about using medication to treat disorders such as ADHD, explain the importance of a treatment program for those with this condition and discuss fads and fallacies in current treatments.

1996 272 pages
ISBN: 0-060977-25-6

653 Distant Drums, Different Drummers: A Guide for Young People with ADHD
ADD WareHouse
300 NW 70th Avenue, Suite 102
Plantation, FL 33317

954-792-8100
800-233-9273
Fax: 954-792-8545
e-mail: websales@addwarehouse.com
www.addwarehouse.com

This book presents a positive perspective of ADHD - one that stresses the value of individual differences. Written for children and adolescents struggling with ADHD, it offers young readers the opportunity to see themselves in a positive light and motivates them to face challenging problems. Ages 8-14.

1995 39 pages
ISBN: 0-964854-80-5

Barbara Ingersoll, PhD

654 Don't Give Up Kid
ADD WareHouse
300 NW 70th Avenue, Suite 102
Plantation, FL 33317

954-792-8100
800-233-9273
Fax: 954-792-8545
e-mail: websales@addwarehouse.com
www.addwarehouse.com

Alex, the hero of this book, is one of two million children in the US who have learning disabilities. This book gives children with reading problems and learning disabilities a clear understanding of their difficulties and the necessary courage to learn to live with them. Ages 5-12.

ISBN: 1-884281-10-9

655 Eagle Eyes A Child's View od Attention Deficit Disorder
Connecticut Association for Children with LD
25 Van Zant Street, Suite 15-5
East Norwalk, CT 06855

203-838-5010
Fax: 203-866-6108
e-mail: cacld@optonline.net
www.cacld.org

Story about a boy with ADHD. A valuable tool for parents and teachers to use with elementary school age children with ADHD, their siblings and classmates to help them understand the strengths as well as weaknesses of this population.

30 pages

656   Eagle Eyes: A Child's View of Attention Deficit Disorder
ADD WareHouse
300 NW 70th Avenue, Suite 102
Plantation, FL 33317   954-792-8100
                                                    800-233-9273
                                                Fax: 954-792-8545
                            e-mail: websales@addwarehouse.com
                                        www.addwarehouse.com

This book helps readers of all ages understand ADD and gives
practical suggestions for organization, social cues and self calm-
ing. Expressive illustrations enhance the book and encourage reluctant readers. Ages 5-12.

ISBN: 1-884281-11-7

Jeanne Gehret

657   Eukee the Jumpy, Jumpy Elephant
ADD WareHouse
300 NW 70th Avenue, Suite 102
Plantation, FL 33317   954-792-8100
                                                    800-233-9273
                                                Fax: 954-792-8545
                            e-mail: websales@addwarehouse.com
                                        www.addwarehouse.com

A story about a bright young elephant who is not like all the other
elephants. Eukee moves through the jungle like a tornado, unable
to pay attention to the other elephants. He begins to feel sad, but
gets help after a visit to the doctor who explains why Eukee is so
jumpy and hyperactive. With love, support and help, Eukee learns
ways to help himself and gain renewed self-esteem. Ideal for ages
3-8.

1995 22 pages
ISBN: 0-962162-98-1

Cliff Corman, MD
Esther Trevino

**658   Getting a Grip on ADD: A Kid's Guide to Understanding &
Coping with ADD**
Educational Media Corporation
6021 Wish Avenue
Encino, CA 91316   818-708-0962
1994 64 pages Paperback
ISBN: 0-932796-60-3

**659   Give Your ADD Teen a Chance: A Guide for Parents of
Teenagers with ADD**
ADD WareHouse
300 NW 70th Avenue, Suite 102
Plantation, FL 33317   954-792-8100
                                                    800-233-9273
                                                Fax: 954-792-8545
                            e-mail: websales@addwarehouse.com
                                        www.addwarehouse.com

Parenting teenagers is never easy, especially if your teen suffers
from ADD. This book provides parents with expert help by showing them how to determine which issues are caused by 'normal'
teenager development and which are caused by ADD.

1996 299 pages
ISBN: 0-891099-77-8

Lynn Weiss, PhD

**660   Hyperactive Child, Adolescent, and Adult: ADD Through the
Lifespan**
Connecticut Association for Children with LD
25 Van Zant Street, Suite 15-5
East Norwalk, CT 06855   203-838-5010
                                                Fax: 203-866-6108
                                   e-mail: cacld@optonline.net
                                               www.cacld.org

Comprehensive general review. Update on previous research by
the author, offering a basic text.

162 pages

661   Hyperactivity: Why Won't My Child Pay Attention?
John Wiley & Sons
1 Wiley Drive
Somerset, NJ 08875   732-469-4400
                                                Fax: 732-302-2300
                                     e-mail: custserv@wiley.com
                                               www.wiley.com

Deals with children who experience problems paying attention,
controlling their emotions and physical actions and acting without forethought. Helps parents and professionals to accept the hyperactive child's behavior and find ways to help the child
succeed. Provides and accurate understanding of the current state
of science concerning the cause, developmental course,
evaluation and outcome of this problem.

224 pages
ISBN: 0-471533-07-6

662   It's So Much Work to Be Your Friend
Active Parenting Publishers
1220 Kennestone Circle, Suite 130
Marietta, GA 30066   770-429-0565
                                                    800-825-0060
                                                Fax: 770-429-0334
                          e-mail: cservice@activeparenting.com
                                      www.activeparenting.com

Offers practical strategies to help learning disabled children ages
six through seventeen navigate the treacherous social waters of
their school, home, and community.

448 pages

**663   Jumpin' Johnny Get Back to Work! A Child's Guide to
ADHD/Hyperactivity**
Connecticut Association for Children with LD
25 Van Zant Street, Suite 15-5
East Norwalk, CT 06855   203-838-5010
                                                Fax: 203-866-6108
                                   e-mail: cacld@optonline.net
                                               www.cacld.org

Written primarily for elementary age youngsters with ADHD to
help them understand their disability. Also valuable as an educational tool for parents, siblings, friends, and classmates. Includes
two pages on medication.

24 pages

664   Kids With Incredible Potential Parent's Guide
Active Parenting Publishers
1220 Kennestone Circle, Suite 130
Marietta, GA 30066   770-429-0565
                                                    800-825-0060
                                                Fax: 770-429-0334
                          e-mail: cservice@activeparenting.com
                                      www.activeparenting.com

The guide for parents of ADHD children is designed as an add-on
to the Active Parenting Now video and discussion program. Adds
an ADHD emphasis that makes the parenting information more
immediate and practical for these parents' special needs.

665   Kids with Incredible Potential Leader's Guide
Active Parenting Publishers
1220 Kennestone Circle, Suite 130
Marietta, GA 30066   770-429-0565
                                                    800-825-0060
                                                Fax: 770-429-0334
                          e-mail: cservice@activeparenting.com
                                      www.activeparenting.com

Allows the facilitator to give parents specialized information that
is more immediate and practical to these parents' needs.

666   Learning To Slow Down and Pay Attention
Connecticut Association for Children with LD
25 Van Zant Street, Suite 15-5
East Norwalk, CT 06855   203-838-5010
                                                Fax: 203-866-6108
                                   e-mail: cacld@optonline.net
                                               www.cacld.org

Written for elementary school age children with ADHD to read with their parents. A checklist helps families decide if attention and concentration are problems. Interventions are given for parents, doctors and teachers. Includes practical strategies for paying better attention, getting more organized and problem solving.

62 pages

667 Managing Attention Deficit Hyperactivity Disorder in Children
John Wiley & Sons
1 Wiley Drive
Somerset, NJ 08875   732-469-4400
                                               Fax: 732-302-2300
                                       e-mail: custserv@wiley.com
                                                   www.wiley.com

This book explores symptoms of ADHD, the crossover into adulthood with such a disorder, and the latest and most controversial treatments.

1998 896 pages
ISBN: 0-471121-58-4

668 Maybe You Know My Kid: A Parent's Guide to Identifying ADHD
Birch Lane Press
120 Enterprise Avenue S
Secaucus, NJ 07094   212-407-1500
                                               Fax: 212-935-0699

The author writes about her family experiences with their son, David, who has attention deficit disorder. Contains a comprehensive review of important issues plus descriptions of some helpful management techniques.

222 pages

669 My Brother's a World Class Pain: A Sibling's Guide To ADHD/Hyperactivity
Connecticut Association for Children with LD
25 Van Zant Street, Suite 15-5
East Norwalk, CT 06855   203-838-5010
                                               Fax: 203-866-6108
                                     e-mail: cacld@optonline.net
                                                   www.cacld.org

A young girl tells what it's like to have a little brother with ADHD. She expresses the frustration, anger, embarrassment and resentment that often develop living with a sibling who has attention deficit. Her parents seek professional help to understand the disability and enlisted in trying to bring about positive changes in the family.

34 pages

670 Otto Learns About His Medicine A Story Abo ut Medication for Hyperative Children
Connecticut Association for Children with LD
25 Van Zant Street, Suite 15-5
East Norwalk, CT 06855   203-838-5010
                                               Fax: 203-866-6108
                                     e-mail: cacld@optonline.net
                                                   www.cacld.org

A book about Otto, a young, hyperactive car. Otto has difficulty paying attention in school, so his parents take him to a mechanic who prescribes medication that will help him control his behavior.

28 pages

671 Parenting Children with ADHD: Lessons That Medicine Cannot Teach
Active Parenting Publishers
1220 Kennestone Circle, Suite 130
Marietta, GA 30066   770-429-0565
                                                     800-825-0060
                                               Fax: 770-429-0334
                               e-mail: cservice@activeparenting.com
                                             www.activeparenting.com

Gives parents a framework for building a successful parenting program at home. Presents a series of ten lessons that are essential for promoting the success of kids with ADHD.

261 pages

672 Parents Helping Parents: A Directory of Support Groups for ADD
CibaGelgy, Pharmaceuticals Division
External Communications
Summit, NJ 07901   908-277-5000
                                               Fax: 973-781-2601
                                                   www.add.org

Evelyn Polk Green, President
Linda Roggli, Vice President
Janet Kramer, Treasurer

673 Parents' Hyperactivity Handbook: Helping the Fidgety Child
Plenum Press
233 Spring Street
New York, NY 10013   212-620-8000
                                               Fax: 212-463-0742
                                       e-mail: info@plenum.com

1993 306 pages
ISBN: 0-306444-65-8

674 Putting On The Brakes - Young People's Guide To Understanding ADHD
Connecticut Association for Children with LD
25 Van Zant Street, Suite 15-5
East Norwalk, CT 06855   203-838-5010
                                               Fax: 203-866-6108
                                     e-mail: cacld@optonline.net
                                                   www.cacld.org

Written from both a medical and educational perspective. Reviews what it is like to have ADHD. It explains what's going on in the brain, discusses feelings and tries to help children gain some control of their lives.

64 pages

675 Putting on the Brakes
Courage To Change
PO Box 486
Wilkes-Barres, PA 18703   800-440-4003
                                               Fax: 800-772-6499
                                          www.couragetochange.com

This book written for kids ages eight to thirteen tells all they need to know about ADHD. Also available is a companion activity book that teaches organizing, setting priorities, problem solving, maintaining control and other life management skills. The activity book is 88 pages and sells for $14.95.

676 Rethinking Attention Deficit Disorders
Brookline Books
8 Trumbell Rd, Suite B-001
Northampton, MA 01060   413-584-0184
                                                     800-666-2665
                                               Fax: 413-584-6184
                                    e-mail: brbooks@yahoo.com
                                          www.brooklinebooks.com

Gives the classroom teacher useful information that provides ideas and strategies for working with children suffering from ADD.

ISBN: 1-571290-37-0

677 Ritalin is Not the Answer
Jossey-Bass
111 River Street
Hoboken, NJ 07030   201-748-6000
                                                     800-956-7739
                                               Fax: 201-748-6088
                                              www.josseybass.com

A healthy, drug-free alternative to Ritalin and an absolute must read for every physician before prescribing it.

224 pages
ISBN: 0-787945-14-5

678 Self-Control Games & Workbook
Western Psychological Services
12031 Wilshire Boulevard
Los Angeles, CA 90025   310-478-2061
                                               Fax: 310-478-7838

This game is designed to teach self-control in academic and social situations. Addresses a total of 24 impulsive, inattentive and hyperactive behaviors. The companion workbook reinforces the use of positive self-statements, and problem-solving techniques, instead of expressing anger.

Game

679 Shelley The Hyperactive Turtle
Connecticut Association for Children with LD
25 Van Zant Street, Suite 15-5
East Norwalk, CT 06855
203-838-5010
Fax: 203-866-6108
e-mail: cacld@optonline.net
www.cacld.org

Delightful picture book for use with very young children. Sensitive text and wonderful colored illustrations help little ones understand ADHD.

20 pages

680 Taking Charge of ADHD: The Complete, Authoritative Guide for Parents
Guilford Press
72 Spring Street
New York, NY 10012
800-365-7006
Fax: 212-966-6708
e-mail: info@guilford.com
www.guilford.com

Provides a guide to understanding attention-deficit/hyperactivity disorder and relating to the children whose behavior can be frustrating and confusing. Hardcover, paperback, e-book.

2005 321 pages Paperback
ISBN: 1-572305-60-1

681 Teaching the Tiger
Hope Press
PO Box 188
Duarte, CA 91009
800-321-4039
Fax: 626-358-3520
e-mail: dcomings@earthlink.net
www.hopepress.com

A handbook for individuals involved in the education of students with Attention Deficit Disorder, Tourette Syndrome, or Obsessive Compulsive Disorder.

ISBN: 1-878267-34-5
David E Comings MD, Presenter

682 The 'Putting On The Brakes' Activity Book For Young People With ADHD
Connecticut Association for Children with LD
25 Van Zant Street, Suite 15-5
East Norwalk, CT 06855
203-838-5010
Fax: 203-866-6108
e-mail: cacld@optonline.net
www.cacld.org

A companion to the book 'Putting On The Brakes: Young People's Guide To Understanfing Attention Deficit Hyperactivity Disorder (ADHD)'. Offers various exercises to help children with ADHD learn to deal with their problems in a positive way. Some activities can be done independently, others need the collaboration of an adult.

88 pages

683 The ADHD Book of Lists
Courage To Change
PO Box 486
Wilkes-Barres, PA 18703
800-440-4003
Fax: 800-772-6499
www.couragetochange.com

Presented in list format and created for parents, school psychologists, and mental health professionals. A reliable source of answers, strategies, tools, interventions, support, and additional resources.

684 The LD Child and the ADHD Child: Ways Parents and Professionals Can Help
John F Blair Publishers
1406 Plaza Drive
Winston-Salem, NC 27103
336-768-1374
800-222-9796
Fax: 336-768-9194
e-mail: editorial@blairpub.com
www.blairpub.com

The author recommends other options that can be explored to treat LD and ADHD children without drugs.

261 pages Paperback
ISBN: 0-895871-42-4

Carolyn Sakowski, President
Steve Kirk, Editor In Chief

685 You and Your ADD Child
Nelson Publications
1 Gateway Plaza
Port Chester, NY 10573
914-937-8400
Fax: 914-937-8676

1995 252 pages Paperback
ISBN: 0-785278-95-8

Magazines

686 Attention
CHADD
4601 Presidents Drive, Suite 300
Lanham, MD 20706
301-306-7070
800-233-4050
Fax: 301-306-7090
e-mail: help@chadd.org
www.chadd.org

Available with membership.

Quarterly
Michael MacKay, President
April Gower, Chief Operations Officer
Khalilah Long, Director of Membership & Marketing

Newsletters

687 ADHD Report
Guilford Publications
370 Seventh Avenue, Suite 1200
New York, NY 10001
212-431-9800
800-365-7006
Fax: 212-966-6708
e-mail: info@guilford.com
www.guilford.com

Presents the most up-to-date information on the evaluation, diagnosis and management of ADHD in children, adolescents and adults. This important newsletter is an invaluable resource for all professionals interested in ADHD. 6 issues per year; content available online.

16 pages Subscription
ISBN: 1-065802-5 -
Russell A. Barkley, PhD, Editor

688 Chadder
CHADD
BOX.8181 Professional Place, Suite 201
Landover, MD 20785
301-306-7070
Fax: 301-306-7090
TTY: 301-429-0641
disabilityresourcejs.weebly.com/adhd.html

Quarterly

689 Pure Facts
Feingold Association of the US
11849 Suncatcher Drive
Fishers, IN 46037
631-369-9340
e-mail: help@feingold.org
www.feingold.org

Monthly newsletter with articles on nutrition and behavior and lists of approved brand-name foods.

monthly

Deborah Lehner, Executive Director

Pamphlets

690 ADHD
Learning Disabilities Association of America
4156 Library Road
Pittsburgh, PA 15234   412-341-1515
                                   Fax: 412-344-0224
                        e-mail: info@LDAAmerica.org
                                       ldaamerica.org

A booklet for parents offering information on Attention Deficit-Hyperactivity Disorders and learning disabilities.

Nancie Payne, President
Ed Schlitt, First Vice President
Beth McGaw, Secretary

691 Attention Deficit Disorders and Hyperactivity
ERIC Clearinghouse on Disabled and Gifted Children
1920 Association Drive
Reston, VA 20191   703-620-3660
                                   Fax: 703-620-2521

Dedicated to improving educational outcomes for individuals with exceptionalities, students with disabilities, and/or the gifted.

692 Attention Deficit-Hyperactivity Disorder: Is it a Learning Disability?
Georgetown University, School of Medicine
3800 Reservoir Road NW, Main Hospital Building, Fi
Washington, DC 20007   202-444-3960
                                   Fax: 202-687-2387
                               www.medstarhealth.org

Offers information on learning disabilities and related disorders.

Stephen Ray Mitchell, MD, MBA, Dean for Medical Education
Mikey Cassidy, Executive Assistant to the Dean
Diana Kassar, Sr. Associate Dean for Fin & Admin

693 COGREHAB
Life Science Associates
1 Fenimore Road
Bayport, NY 11705   631-472-2111
                                   Fax: 631-472-8146
                    e-mail: lifesciassoc@pipeline.com
                    www.lifesciassoc.home.pipeline.com

Divided into six groups for diagnosis and treatment of attention, memory and perceptual disorders to be used by and under the guidance of a professional.

$95 - $1,950

Frank Manoriota, Vice President

694 Children with ADD: A Shared Responsibility
Council for Exceptional Children
2900 Crystal Drive, Suite 1000
Arlington, VA 22202   703-264-9494
                                        888-232-7733
                                   TTY: 866-915-5000
                        e-mail: service@cec.sped.org
                                     www.cec.sped.org

This book represents a consensus of what professionals and parents believe ADD is all about and how children with ADD may best be served. Reviews the evaluation process under IDEA and 504 and presents effective classroom strategies.

35 pages
ISBN: 0-865862-33-8

James P. Heiden, President
Antonis Katsiyannis, President Elect
Sharon Raimondi, Treasurer

695 Coping with Your Inattentive Child
Connecticut Association for Children with LD
25 Van Zant Street, Suite 15-5
East Norwalk, CT 6855   203-838-5010
                                   Fax: 203-866-6108
                        e-mail: cacld@optonline.net
                                       www.cacld.org

Lists signs of ADHD and discusses managing the problems of children with ADHD from infancy through elementary school.

13 pages

696 Identification and Treatment of Attention Deficit Disorders
Therapro
225 Arlington Street
Framingham, MA 1701   508-872-9494
                                        800-257-5376
                                   Fax: 508-875-2062

This handbook contains information that is based on research and offers practical suggestions for parents, teachers and other professionals.

697 Out of Darkness
Connecticut Association for Children with LD
25 Van Zant Street, Suite 15-5
East Norwalk, CT 6855   203-838-5010
                                   Fax: 203-866-6108
                        e-mail: cacld@optonline.net
                                       www.cacld.org

Article by an adult who discovers at age 30 that he has ADD.

4 pages

698 Parenting Attention Deficit Disordered Teens
Connecticut Association for Children with LD
25 Van Zant Street, Suite 15-5
East Norwalk, CT 6855   203-838-5010
                                   Fax: 203-866-6108
                        e-mail: cacld@optonline.net
                                       www.cacld.org

Detailed outline of the various problems of adolescents with ADHD.

14 pages

699 School Based Assessment of Attention Deficit Disorders
National Clearinghouse of Rehabilitation Materials
5202 N Richmond Hill Drive
Stillwater, OK 74078   405-624-7650
                                        800-223-5219
                                   Fax: 405-624-0695
                                   TDD: 405-624-3156
                             www.nchrtm.okstate,edu

The 1992 OSEP ruling, placing more responsibility on schools for the assessment of students who may have attention deficit disorders, has raised questions concerning the assessment process. This guide was developed to help states formulate new policies. The paper seeks to: present an overview of current thoughts concerning ADD from an educational perspective, contrast traditional assessment strategies with an alternative model, and describe phases of evaluation.

David Brooks, Director
Carolyn Cain

Camps

700 Camp Buckskin
4124 Quebec Ave N, Ste 300
Minneapolis, MN 55427   763-208-4805
                                   Fax: 952-938-6996
                    e-mail: info@campbuckskin.com
                                 www.campbuckskin.com

LD and ADD/ADHD youth have often experienced frustration and a lack of success. Buckskin assists these individuals to realize and develop the potentials and abilities which they possess.

Thomas R Bauer, CCD, Camp Director

701   Camp Nuhop
404 Hillcrest Drive
Ashland, OH 44805   419-289-2227
                                    Fax: 419-289-2227
                              e-mail: info@campnuhop.org
                                    www.campnuhop.org

A summer residential program for any youngster from 6 to 18
with a learning disability, behavior disorder or Attention Deficit
Disorder. Sixty two campers and 35 staff members live on site in
groups of 7 campers to every 3 counselors. Activities focus on
positive self-concept and behaviors and teach children to learn
how to find their strengths, abilities and talents from a positive,
yet realistic viewpoint.

Jerry Dunlap, Director

702   Dallas Academy
950 Tiffany Way
Dallas, TX 75218   214-324-1481
                                    Fax: 214-327-8537
                              www.dallas-academy.com

7-week summer session for students who are having difficulty in
regular school classes.

Jim Richardson, Director

703   Developmental Center
6710 86th Avenue N
Pinellas Park, FL 33782   727-541-5716
                                    Fax: 727-544-8186
                            e-mail: infopp@centeracademy.com
                                    www.centeracademy.com

Specifically designed for the learning disabled child and other
children with difficulties in concentration, strategy, social skills,
impulsivity, distractibility and study strategies. Programs offered
include: attention training, visual-motor remediation, socialization skills training, relaxation training, horseback riding and
more. The day camp meets weekdays from 9-3 for 3,4 or 5 week
sessions.

Dr. Eric Larson

704   Eagle Hill School - Summer Program
242 Old Petersham Road, PO Box 116
Hardwick, MA 01037   413-477-6000
                                    Fax: 413-477-6837
                         e-mail: admission@eaglehillschool.com
                                    www.ehs1.org

For the child, age 9-19, with a specific learning disability or Attention Deficit Disorder, this summer program offers a structured
curriculum designed to build a basic foundation of academic competence. Extracurricular and outdoor activities complement the
educational program.

Erin E Wynne, Dean of Admission

705   Groves Academy
3200 Highway 100 South
Saint Louis Park, MN 55416   952-920-6377
                                    Fax: 952-920-2068
                                    www.grovesacademy.org

A nonprofit day school in Minnesota designed especially for children with learning differences. The Center has a full day academic program from September through June, as well as an 8
week summer program. Groves also offers community services
such as: psychoeducational testing for children and adults, consulting services, workshops on learning disabilities and other special learning needs, and afternoon/evening tutorial services for
children and adults.

John Alexander, Head of School

706   Hill School of Fort Worth
4817 Odessa Avenue
Fort Worth, TX 76133   817-923-9482
                                    Fax: 817-923-4894
                              e-mail: admission@hillschool.org
                                    www.hillschool.org

Provides an alternative learning environment for students having
average or above-average intelligence with learning differences.
Hill school is an established leader in North Texas with a 25 year
history of effectively serving LD children. Beginning in 1961 as
a tutorial service, Hill became a formal school in 1973. Our mission is to help those who learn differently develop skills and
strategies to succeed. We do this by developing academic/study
skills, and self-discipline.

Lucille H Helton, Principal
Cathy Allen, Admissions Director
Grey Owens, Principal

707   Lab School of Washington Summer Program
4759 Reservoir Road NW
Washington, DC 20007   202-965-6600
                                    Fax: 202-965-5106
                         e-mail: Alexandra.Freeman@labschool.org
                                    www.labschool.org

The Lab School 5-week summer session includes individualized
reading, spelling, writing, study skills, and math programs. A
multisensory approach addresses the needs of bright learning disabled children. Related services such as speech/language therapy
and occupational therapy are integrated into the curriculum. Ele-
mentary/Intermediate; Junior High/High School.

Sally Smith, Founder
Susan Feeley, Admissions Director

708   Maplebrook School
5142 Route 22
Amenia, NY 12501   845-373-8191
                                    Fax: 845-373-7029
                         e-mail: jscully@maplebrookschool.org
                                    www.maplebrookschool.org

A coeductional boarding school for students with learning differences and ADD. A New York State registered high school servicing ages 11-18. Post secondary options offered to 18-21.

Donna M Konkolios, Head of School
Jennifer Scully, Director Admissions

709   Round Lake Camp
21 Plymouth Street
Fairfield, NJ 7004   973-575-3333
                                          800-776-5657
                                    Fax: 973-575-4188
                              e-mail: rlc@njycamps.org
                                    www.njycamps.org

For ages 7-18, this camp provides individualized academics in
reading, language development and math for children with mild
learning disabilities, Round Lake also offers therapeutic recreation and Jewish cultural values to its participants.

Sheira Director, Asst. Director

710   Tourette Syndrome Camp Organization
6933 N Kedzie, Ste 816
Chicago, IL 60640   773-465-7536
                              e-mail: info@tourettecamp.com
                                    www.tourettecamp.com

Dedicated to promoting camping opportunities for children with
Tourette Syndrome and its assocaited disorders, Obsessive Com-
pulsive Disorder (OCD) and Attention Deficit/Hyperactivity
Disorder (ADD/ADHD).

Monica Newman, Camp Director

Description

711   AUTISTIC DISORDER

Synonyms: Infantile autism, Kanner's syndrome

Involves the following Biologic System(s):

Developmental/Behavioral/Psychiatric Disorders, Neurologic Disorders

Autistic disorder, also known as infantile autism, is classified as a developmental disability that results from a disorder of the human central nervous system. It usually becomes apparent by three years of age. It is thought to affect approximately four in 10,000 children and is about three to four times more common in males than females. Autistic disorder is characterized by deficient verbal and nonverbal communication, impaired social interactions, and a restricted range of interests and activities.

Children with autistic disorder may fail to acquire or have poorly developed verbal and nonverbal communication skills. If children do communicate verbally, abnormal speech patterns are typically present, such as repetition of another's words or phrases (echolalia); reversal of the proper use of pronouns, such as use of the term "you" rather than "I" when referring to themselves; and nonsensical rhyming. In addition, affected children may be withdrawn, make little or no eye contact, resist cuddling, lack awareness of others' thoughts or feelings, or fail to seek comfort when distressed. Children also typically engage in solitary play for hours, perform ritualistic behaviors and repeated body movements (e.g., rocking, flicking fingers) and have a strong need for a predictable, consistent environment. Certain behaviors (e.g., rubbing an object or surface) may demonstrate a heightened awareness of particular stimuli, whereas others, such as a lack of reaction to sudden, loud noises, may indicate a lowered sensitivity to other stimuli. In many children with autistic disorder, disruptions of rituals or routines may result in tantrum-like outbursts or rages. In addition, some children may exhibit self-injurious or outwardly aggressive behaviors. Because of impairment of language and socialization skills, it may be difficult to obtain accurate estimates of overall intelligence levels and potential. Although such testing often demonstrates functional retardation, some affected children perform adequately in nonverbal areas, such as spatial and motor skills, and those with speech skills may perform adequately in all test areas.

In most patients, the symptoms and findings associated with autistic disorder continue to affect them throughout life. The Food and Drug Administration (FDA) recently approved the use of an antipsychotic, risperidone, for the treatment of irritability associated with autistic disorder, including symptoms of aggression, deliberate self-injury, temper tantrums, and quickly changing moods. This is the first time the FDA has approved any medication for use in children and adolescents with autism. In addition, the management and treatment of affected children may include integrated, multidisciplinary techniques, such as language therapy, structured play and interpersonal exercises, and other behavioral therapies. Some patients, particularly those with speech development, may lead somewhat independent lives with proper support. However, other individuals with autistic disorder may require special, ongoing care.

The cause of autistic disorder is unknown. However, according to the medical literature, several underlying neurologic, infectious, and other disorders are known to produce or to increase a predisposition toward autistic-like behaviors in children. Genetic abnormalities are also thought to play some role in causing or resulting in susceptibility for the disorder. For example, some researchers theorize that autistic disorder may result from certain brain abnormalities during infancy (e.g., particular biochemical abnormalities, brain injury, etc.), potentially in combination with a genetic predisposition for the condition (multifactorial).

Government Agencies

712   NIH/National Institute of Neurological Disorders and Stroke (NINDS)
PO Box 5801
Bethesda, MD 10188
301-496-5751
800-352-9424
Fax: 301-496-0296
TTY: 301-468-5981
www.ninds.nih.gov

The mission of NINDS is to reduce the burden of neurological disease - a burden borne by every age group, by every segment of society, by people all over the world.

Story C Landis Ph.D., Director
Walter J Koroshetz, Deputy Director
Caroline Lewis, Executive Officer

713   NIH/National Institute on Deafness and Other Communication Disorders (NIDCD)
31 Center Drive, MSC 2320
Bethesda, MD 20892
800-241-1044
TTY: 800-241-1055
e-mail: nidcdinfo@nidcd.nih.gov
www.nidcd.nih.gov

Conducts and supports biomedical research and research training on normal mechanisms, as well as diseases and disorders of hearing, balance, smell, taste, voice, speech and language.

Dr James F Battey Jr, Director
Judith A Cooper, Deputy Director
W David Kerr, Executive Officer

National Associations & Support Groups

714   Achieve Beyond
7000 Austin Street, Suite 200
Forest Hills, NY 11375
718-762-7633
Fax: 212-679-7867
e-mail: info@achievebeyondusa.com
www.achievebeyondusa.com

Achieve Beyond was founded in 1995 to meet the needs of developmentally delayed and disabled children and their families, particularly children with bilingual needs.

Trudy Font Padron, Founder/ Programs Executive Dir
Robert Padron, Executive Director

715   Aging with Autism
704 Marten RD
Princeton, NJ 8540
908-904-9319
e-mail: contact@agingwithautism.org
www.agingwithautism.org

Aging with Autism is dedicated to enhancing programs and services for individuals with autism and other developmental disabilities as they transition to and through adulthood.

Dr. Cyndy Hayes, Founder/ President
Andria Prather, Administrator

716 American Academy of Pediatrics
141 Northwest Point Boulevard
Elk Grove Village, IL 60007   847-434-4000
                                                  800-433-9016
                                            Fax: 847-434-8000
                                                  www.aap.org

The American Academy of Pediatrics and its member pediatricians are committed to the attainment of optimal physical, mental
and social health and well-being for all infants, children, adolescents, and young adults.

Sandra Hassink, MD, FAAP, President

717 American Psychological Association
750 First St. NE
Washington, DC 20002   202-336-5500
                                                  800-374-2721
                                             TTY: 202-336-6123
                                                  www.apa.org

The mission is to advance the creation, communication and application of psychological knowledge to benefit society and improve
people's lives.

Norman B. Anderson, PhD, CEO/ EVP
L. Michael Honaker, PhD, Deputy Chief Executive Officer
Ellen G. Garrison, PhD, Senior Policy Advisor

718 American School Counselor Association
1101 King Street, Suite 310
Alexandria, VA 22314   703-683-2722
                                                  800-306-4722
                                            Fax: 703-997-7572
                             e-mail: asca@schoolcounselor.org
                                         www.schoolcounselor.org

The mission of ASCA is to represent professional school counselors and to promote professionalism and ethical practices.

Richard Wong, Executive Director
Jeff Broderson, Information Technology Admin.
Kathleen M Rakestraw, Director of Communications

719 Asperger/Autism Network
51 Water Street, Suite 206
Watertown, MA 2472   617-393-3824
                                                  866-597-AANE
                                            Fax: 617-393-3827
                                         e-mail: info@aane.org
                                                  www.aane.org

The Asperger/Autism Network (AANE) works with individuals,
families, and professionals to help people with Asperger Syndrome and similar autism spectrum profiles build meaningful,
connected lives.

Jayne Burke, President
Karen Boyd, Vice President
Stephen Burgay, B.A., J.D., Vice President

720 Association for Science in Autism Treatment
PO Box 188
Crosswicks, NJ 08515   781-397-8943
                                       e-mail: info@asatonline.org

To disseminate accurate information about autism and treatments,
and to improve access to effective, science-based treatments for
all people with autism.

David Celiberti PhD BCBA, President
Sharon A Reeve PhD BCBA, Vice President

721 Autism Action Network
550 East Chester Street
Long Beach, NY 11561   516-382-0081
                                            Fax: 888-995-6161
                      e-mail: jgilmore@autismactionnetwork.org
                                         autismactionnetwork.org

Autism Action Network is a national, non-partisan, grassroots,
political action organization formed by parents in support of children and adults with autism, vaccine injuries, and
neurodevelopmental and communication disorders.

722 Autism Consortium
10 Shattuck Street
Boston, MA 2115   866-518-0296
                                            Fax: 617-432-6960
                    e-mail: autismconsortium@hms.harvard.edu
                                         www.autismconsortium.org

The Autism Consortium catalyzes rapid advances in understanding of autism by fostering collaboration among families, researchers, clinicians, and donors. There mission is to improve the
care of children and families affected by autism and other
neurological disorders.

Deirdre B. Phillips, Executive Director
Laura K. Farfel, Digital Outreach Coordinator

723 Autism Inclusion Resources
www.autismir.com

                                       e-mail: info@autismir.com
                                                  www.autismir.com

AIR is the creative force behind services and solutions that will
enable today's generation of children with autism to participate
more fully in the world.

Wendy Ross, MD, FAAP, Founder
Roger Ideishi, JD, OT/L, Collaborator
Angela Jones, PhD, Collaborator

724 Autism National Committee
3 Bedford Green
South Burlington, VT 05403   800-378-0386
                    e-mail: sandra.mcclennen@emich.edu
                                                  www.autcom.org

Organization dedicated to social justice for all citizens with autism through a shared vision and a commitment to positive
approaches.

Anne Bakeman, Treasurer

725 Autism Network International
PO Box 35448
Syracuse, NY 10190   315-476-2462
                             e-mail: jisincla@mailbox.syr.edu
                                                  www.autreat.com

Supported by individuals who want to make a difference for the
sufferers, the foundation provides a variety of support and educational references to inform on the latest changes in the field.

Jim Sinclair, Coordinator
Jame Bordner, List-owners
Sola Shelly, Webmaster

726 Autism Network for Hearing and Visually Impaired Persons
7510 Ocean Front Avenue
Virginia Beach, VA 23451   757-428-9036
                                            Fax: 757-428-0019
                                                  www.autism.com

Provides communication, education, research and advocacy for
persons with autism combined with a hearing or visual disability,
their families, and professionals. Sharing of educational materials, phone help, support groups, referrals and conferences.

Dolores Bartel, Contact
Alan Bartel, Contact

727 Autism Research Foundation
C/O Moss-Rosene Lab, W701
72 East Concord Street, R-1014
Boston, MA 10192   617-414-7012
                                            Fax: 617-414-7207
                                         e-mail: tarf@ladders.org
                             www.theautismresearchfoundation.org/

he Autism Research Foundation is a 501(c)3 nonprofit organization dedicated to brain-based research and inclusion programs in
the community. Our goal is to fundraise for continuous
brain-based research, while providing tangible resources for families and providers managing autism right now.

Margaret Bauman MD, Fouding Director
Thomas Sabin MD, President
Thomas Kemper MD, Vice President

728 **Autism Research Institute**
4182 Adams Avenue
San Diego, CA 10193
619-281-7165
866-366-3361
Fax: 619-563-6840
e-mail: media@autismresearchinstitute.com
www.autism.com

ARI advocates for the rights of people with ASD, and operates without funding from special-interest groups. ARI is dedicated to developing a standard of care for individuals with autism spectrum disorders and their families. We rely on the generosity of donors to help us advance autism research and provide needed information and support for families and individuals with autism spectrum disorders.

Stephen Edelson, Executive Director
Jane Johnson, Managing Director
Rebecca McKenney, Office Manager

729 **Autism Research Institute Conference**
Autism Research Institute
4182 Adams Avenue
San Diego, CA 10194
619-281-7165
866-366-3361
Fax: 619-563-6840
www.autism.com/index.php/video

ARI advocates for the rights of people with ASD, and operates without funding from special-interest groups. ARI is dedicated to developing a standard of care for individuals with autism spectrum disorders and their families. We rely on the generosity of donors to help us advance autism research and provide needed information and support for families and individuals with autism spectrum disorders.

Stephen Edelson PhD, Executive Director
Jane Johnson, Managing Director
Rebecca McKenney, Office Manager

730 **Autism Science Foundation**
28 West 39th Street, Suite #502
New York, NY 10018
212-391-3913
Fax: 212-391-3954
e-mail: contactus@autismsciencefoundation.org
autismsciencefoundation.org

The Autism Science Foundation's mission is to support autism research by providing funding and other assistance to scientists and organizations conducting, facilitating, publicizing and disseminating autism research. The organization also provides information about autism to the general public and serves to increase awareness of autism spectrum disorders and the needs of individuals and families affected by autism.

Alison Singer, Co-Founder/ President
Karen Margulis London, Co-Founder
Gregg E. Ireland, SVP, Capital World Investors

731 **Autism Services Center**
929 4th Avenue, P.O. Box 507
Huntington, WV 10195
304-525-8014
Fax: 304-525-8026
www.autismservicescenter.org

Autism Services Center (ASC) is a nonprofit, licensed behavioral health center that was founded in 1979 by Ruth C. Sullivan, Ph.D. to provide services in Cabell, Wayne, Lincoln and Mason counties in the state of West Virginia. Though specializing in autism, ASC provides comprehensive, community-integrated services to all individuals with intellectual and developmental disabilities.

Mike Grady, CEO
Elaine Harvey, Vice President
Derek Hyman, President & Treasurer of the Greate

732 **Autism Society of America**
7910 Woodmont Avenue, Suite 300
Bethesda, MD 10196
301-657-0881
800-328-8476
e-mail: info@autism-society.org
www.autism-society.org

The Autism Society, the nation's leading grassroots autism organization, exists to improve the lives of all affected by autism. We do this by increasing public awareness about the day-to-day issues faced by people on the spectrum, advocating for appropriate services for individuals across the lifespan, and providing the latest information regarding treatment, education, research and advocacy

James Ball, Executive Chair
Ron E Simmons, Vice Chair
Scott Badesch, President & COO

733 **Autism Solution Center**
www.autismsolutioncenter.com
e-mail: dorrisphilpot@yahoo.com
www.autismsolutioncenter.com

The Autism Solution Center, Inc. (ASC) is a non-profit organization being developed to address an unmet, ongoing need within our communities for autism therapy, support services, research and other assistance.

734 **Autism Speaks**
1 East 33rd Street 4th Floor
New York, NY 10197
212-252-8584
Fax: 212-252-8676
e-mail: familyservices@autismspeaks.org
www.autismspeaks.org

At Autism Speaks, our goal is to change the future for all who struggle with autism spectrum disorder. We are dedicated to funding global biomedical research into the causes, prevention, treatments, and cure for autism; to raising public awareness about autism and its effects on individuals, families, and society; and to bringing hope to all who deal with the hardships of this disorder.

Liz Feld, President
Peter H Bell, Executive VP
Lisa Goring, Vice President

735 **Autism Treatment Center of America**
www.autismtreatmentcenter.org
413-229-2100
877-766-7473
www.autismtreatmentcenter.org

Welcome to the Autism Treatment Center of AmericaT, the worldwide teaching center for The Son-Rise Programr , a powerful and effective treatment for children and adults challenged by Autism, Autism Spectrum Disorders, Pervasive Developmental Disorder (PDD) , Asperger's Syndrome, and other developmental difficulties.

736 **Autistic Services**
4444 Bryant Stratton Way
Williamsville, NY 10198
716-631-5777
888-288-4764
Fax: 716-565-0671
e-mail: tpanzarella@autism-services-inc.org.
www.autisticservices.org

Agency exclusively dedicated to serving the unique lifelong needs of autistic individuals. Also a regional resource for parents, school districts, physicians and other professionals.

Veronica Federiconi, Executive Director

737 **Autreat**
Autism Network International
PO Box 35448
Syracuse, NY 13235
315-476-2462
e-mail: jisincla@mailbox.syr.edu
www.autreat.com

A retreat-style conference run by autistic people, for autistic people and friends. Focuses on positive living with autism, not on causes, cures, or ways to make individuals more normal.

August

Jim Sinclair, Coordinator
Jame Bordner, List-Owners
Sola Shelly, Webmaster

738   Center for Autism and Related Disorders
19019 Ventura Blvd., Suite 300
Tarzana, CA 91356   818-345-2345
                                     855-345-2273
                                Fax: 818-758-8015
                                www.centerforautism.com

The Center for Autism and Related Disorders (CARD) uses applied behavior analysis (ABA) in the treatment of autism spectrum disorder.

Doreen Granpeesheh, Founder/ Executive Director

739   Community Services for Autistic Adults & Children (CSAAC)
8615 East Village
Montgomery Village, MD 10201   204-912-2220
                                Fax: 301-926-9384
                                e-mail: csaac@csaac.org
                                www.csaac.org

To enable individuals with autism to achieve their highest potential and contribute as confident individuals to their community

Ian Paregol, Executive Director
Marcee Smith, Ph.D., Assistant Executive Director of Pro

740   Developmental Delay Resources (DDR)
5801 Beacon Street
Pittsburgh, PA 10202   412-422-3373
                                     800-497-0944
                                Fax: 412-422-1374
                                e-mail: devdelay@mindspring.com
                                www.devdelay.org

Dedicated to meeting the needs of those working with children who have developmental delays in sensory, motor, language, social, and emotional areas. Publicizes research into determining identifiable factors that would put a child at risk and maintains a registry, tracking possible trends.

Patricia Lemer, Owner

741   Facilitated Communication Institute at Syracuse University
307 Huntington Hall
Syracuse, NY 10203   315-443-9379
                                Fax: 315-443-2274
                                e-mail: ICIstaff@syr.edu
                                www.soe.syr.edu/centers_institutes/institute_communi

College offering facilitated learning research into communication with persons who have autism or severe disabilities. Offers books, videos and public awareness information on the research projects.

Timothy Eatman, Director
Kathleen Hinchman, Board of Directors
Nancy Cantor, Chancellor and President

742   Families for Early Autism Treatment
PO Box 255722
Sacramento, CA 10204   916-303-7405
                                Fax: 916-303-7405
                                e-mail: feat@feat.org
                                www.feat.org

A nonprofit organization of parents and professionals, designed to help families with children who are diagnosed with autism or pervasive developmental disorder. It offers a network of support for families. FEAT has a Lending Library, with information on autism and also offers Support Meetings on the third Wednesday of each month.

Nancy Fellmeth, President
Kathleen Berry, VP
Gordon Hall, Treasurer

743   Families of Adults Afflicted with Asperger's Syndrome
PO Box 514
Centerville, MA 2632   508-790-1930
                                e-mail: faaas@faaas.org
                                faaas.org

Offers support to the family members of adult individuals with Asperger's Syndrome.

Karen E. Rodman, President/ Founder
Jack Kelley, Events Coordinator
Thomas Rodman, Webmaster/ Docmaster

744   Federation of Families for Children's Mental Health
9605 Medical Center Drive, Suite 280
Rockville, MD 10205   240-403-1901
                                Fax: 240-403-1909
                                e-mail: ffcmh@ffcmh.org
                                www.ffcmh.org

The National family run organization is dedicated exclusively to helping children with mental health needs and their families achieve a better quality of life.

Teka Dempson, President
Sherri Luthe, Vice President
Sheila Pires, Treasurer

745   Generation Rescue
13636 Ventura Blvd. #259
Sherman Oaks, CA 91423   877-98 -UTIS
                                www.generationrescue.org

Provides hope, information and immediate treatment assistance to families affected by autism spectrum disorders.

JB Handley, Co-Founder
Lisa Handley, Co-Founder
Jenny McCarthy, President

746   Genetic Alliance Washington, DC 10206
                                     202-966-7955
                                     800-336-4363
                                Fax: 202-966-8553
                                e-mail: info@geneticalliance.org
                                www.geneticalliance.org

World's leading nonprofit health advocacy organization committed to transforming health through genetics and promoting an environment of openness centered on the health of individuals, families, and communities.

Sharon Terry, President
Lisa Wise, Chief Operating Officer
Tetyana Murza MES, Programs and Policy Coordinator

747   Global and Regional Asperger Syndrome Partnership
419 Lafayette Street
New York, NY 10003   888-474-7277
                                e-mail: info@grasp.org
                                grasp.org

GRASP works to improve the lives of teens and adults with autism spectrum disorder (ASD). It offers in-school programs to help students with autism learn advocacy skills and improve social skills. Through its website, it educates the public about autism, while also offering free online resources and networking opportunities for individuals with ASD and their families.

748   Groupworks West
11140 Washington Blvd.
Culver City, CA 90232   310-287-1640
                                Fax: 310-287-0851
                                www.groupworkswest.com

GroupWorks West utilizes innovative intervention programs designed to improve the quality of life of children, teens and young adults challenged by developmental, psychiatric, and behavior disorders.

Christopher Mulligan, L.C.S.W., Founder/ Clinical Director

749   Institute on Communication and Inclusion
307 Huntington Hall
Syracuse, NY 13244   315-443-9379
                                Fax: 315-443-2274
                                e-mail: icistaff@syr.edu
                                www.soe.syr.edu/about/

College offering facilitated learning research into communication with persons who have autism or severe disabilities. Offers books, videos and public awareness information on the research projects.

Douglas Biklen, Ph.D., Director
Christine Ashby, Ph.D., Research Director
Michele Paetow, Lead Trainer

750   Lovaas Institute
6167 Bristol Parkway, Suite 130
Culver City, CA 90230   310-410-4450
                                               Fax: 310-410-4455
                                          e-mail: info@lovaas.com
                                                   www.lovaas.com

Committed to providing the highest quality treatment available to children diagnosed with autism or a related disorder.

Scott Wright, President/ CEO:
Simone Stevens, Director of West Coast Ops/ COO
Matthew Sands, Director of East Coast Ops/ CFO

751   March of Dimes Birth Defects Foundation
1275 Mamaroneck Avenue
White Plains, NY 10208   914-997-4488
                                                     888-663-4637
                                               Fax: 914-997-4763
                                     e-mail: answers@marchofdimes.com
                                               www.marchofdimes.com

March of Dimes help moms have full-term pregnancies and research the problems that threaten the health of babies. The March of Dimes also acts globally: sharing best practices in perinatal health and helping improve birth outcomes where the needs are the most urgent.

Kenneth A. May, Chair
Jennifer Howse, President & CEO
Alan Fleischman, Medical Director

752   Mental Health America
2000 N Beauregard Street, 6th Floor
Alexandria, VA 10209   703-684-7722
                                                     800-969-6642
                                               Fax: 703-684-5968
                                  e-mail: info@mentalhealthamerica.net
                                            www.mentalhealthamerica.net

MHA, the leading advocacy organization addressing the full spectrum of mental and substance use conditions and their effects nationwide, works to inform, advocate and enable access to quality behavioral health services for all Americans.

Ann Boughtin, Chair of the Board
Eric Ashton, Vice Chair
Elaine Crider, Secretary/Treasurer

753   National Association of Residential Providers for Adults with Autism
www.narpaa.org

                                        e-mail: info@narpaa.org
                                                  www.narpaa.org

To assure the availability of residential services and other supports for adults with autism throughout their lives.

Gwen Lee, Treasurer
Mike Storz, Vice President
Barbara Boyett, President

754   National Association of Special Education Teachers
1250 Connecticut Avenue, N.W., Suite 200
Washington, DC 20036   800-754-4421
                                               Fax: 800-754-4421
                                       e-mail: contactus@naset.org
                                                   www.naset.org

A membership organization dedicated solely to meeting the needs of special education teachers and those preparing for the field of special education teaching.

Dr. Roger Pierangelo, Co-Executive Director
Dr. George Giuliani, Co-Executive Director

755   National Autism Association
One Park Avenue, Suite 1
Portsmouth, RI 2871   401-293-5551
                                                     877-622-2884
                                               Fax: 401-293-5342
                                  e-mail: naa@nationalautism.org
                                           nationalautismassociation.org

NAA is a parent-run advocacy organization and the leading voice on urgent issues related to severe autism, regressive autism, autism safety, autism abuse, and crisis prevention.

Wendy Fournier, President
Kelly Vanicek, Executive Director
Katie Wright-Hildebrand, Vice President

756   National Autism Hotline - Autism Services Center
605 Ninth Street Prichard Bldg PO Box 507
Huntington, WV 25710   304-525-8014
                                               Fax: 304-525-8026
                                       e-mail: info@autismlink.com
                            www.autismlink.com/listing/national_autism_hotline_a

Service agency for individuals with autism and developmental disabilities, and their families. Assists families and agencies attempting to meet the needs of individuals with autism and other developmental disabilities. Makes available technical assistance in designing treatment programs and more. The hotline provides informational packets to callers re: autism and assists via telephone when possible.

Cindy Walterman, Director
Rick Bryant, Board Member
Kathy Horvath, Board Member

757   National Dissemination Center for Children with Disabilities
1825 Connecticut Ave NW
Washington, DC 10211   202-884-8200
                                                     800-695-0285
                                               Fax: 202-884-8441
                                        e-mail: nichcy@fhi360.org
                                                   www.nichcy.org

A national information and referral center that provides information on disabilities and disability-related issues for families, educators and other professionals.

Suzanne Ripley, Executive Director

758   National Mental Health Consumers' Self-Help Clearinghouse
1211 Chestnut Street, Suite 1207
Philadelphia, PA 10212   215-751-1810
                                                     800-553-4539
                                               Fax: 215-636-6312
                                      e-mail: info@mhselfhelp.org
                                                  www.mhselfhelp.org

The Clearinghouse works to foster peer empowerment through our website, up-to-date news and information announcements, a directory of peer-driven services, electronic and printed publications, training packages, and individual and onsite consultation

Joseph Rogers, Executive Director & Founder
Susan Rogers, Director of Special Projects
Britani Nestel, Program Specialist

759   New England Center for Children
33 Turnpike Road
Southborough, MA 10213   508-481-1015
                                               Fax: 508-485-3421
                                           e-mail: info@necc.org
                                                   www.necc.org

Serving students between the ages of 3 and 22 diagnosed with autism, learning disabilities, language delays, mental retardation, behavior disorders and related disabilities; educational curriculum encompasses both the teaching of functional life skills and traditional academics; communication skills are taught throughout all activities in the school, residence, and community. Tuition and fees are set by the state. Consulting services also available.

Lisel Macenka, Chair of the Board
James C Burling, Vice Chair of Board
L Vincent Strully Jr, President

760   Oak-Leyden Developmental Services
411 Chicago Avenue
Oak Park, IL 10214   708-524-1050
                                               Fax: 708-524-2469
                                     e-mail: webmaster@oaklyden.org
                                                  www.oakleyden.org

The mission of Oak-Leyden Developmental Services is to serve people with developmental disabilities and their families in a manner which recognizes their dignity, is supportive of their personal choices and promotes their inclusion in the larger community.

Bob Atkinson, CEO
Nancy Thomas, Director of Human Resources
Mary Taylor, Vice President of Finance

761 Oasis at MAAP
PO Box 524
Crown Point, IN 10215   219-662-1311
                                          Fax: 219-662-0638
                              e-mail: info@aspergersyndrome.org
                                      www.aspergersyndrome.org

MAAP Services is a world wide 501-C-3 non profit organization providing information, networking, referrals and printed materials for families, challenged individuals and professionals concerned with the autism spectrum. Founded in 1984, MAAP Services, adheres to the basic principal that all individuals with autism spectrum challenges have the ability to learn, grow and enjoy a good quality of life.

Susan Moreno, Founder & President
Lara Blanchard, BCBA

762 Option Institute: Son Rise Program
Autism Treatment Center of America
2080 S Undermountain Road
Sheffield, MA 10216   413-229-2100
                                               800-714-2779
                                          Fax: 413-229-3202
                              e-mail: information@son-rise.org
                                            www.son-rise.org

Describes an effective, loving and respectful method for treating children with autism. It teaches parents and healing professionals how to set up a home based program using the child's motivation to reach their special child.

Barry Neil Kaufman, Co-Founder/Co-Creator
Samahria Lyte Kaufman, Co-Founder/Co-Creator
Bryn Hogan, ATCA Senior Staff

763 Organization for Autism Research
2000 North 14th Street, Suite 240
Arlington, VA 22201   703-243-9710
                                      www.researchautism.org

The Organization for Autism Research (OAR) was created in December 2001-the product of the shared vision and unique life experiences of OAR's seven founders. Led by these parents and grandparents of children and adults on the autism spectrum, OAR set out to use applied science to answer questions that parents, families, individuals with autism, teachers and caregivers confront daily. No other autism organization has this singular focus.

Peter F. Gerhardt, Ed.D., OAR Scientific Council
Lori Lapin Jones, Vice Chairperson
Michael V. Maloney, Executive Director/ Secretary

764 Raleigh TEACCH Center
University of North Carolina at Chapel Hill
100 Renee Lynne Court
Carrboro, NC 10217   919-966-2174
                                          Fax: 413-229-3202
                                   e-mail: TEACCH@unc.edu
                                            www.teacch.com

The University of North Carolina TEACCH Autism Program creates and cultivates the development of exemplary community-based services, training programs, and research to enhance the quality of life for individuals with Autism Spectrum Disorder and for their families across the lifespan.

Eric Schopler, Founder & Co-Director

765 Rethink autism
19 West 21st Street, Suite 403
New York, NY 10010   877-988-8871
                                          Fax: 646-257-2926
                              e-mail: info@rethinkfirst.com
                                        www.rethinkfirst.com

Offers parents and professionals immediate access to effective and affordable Applied Behavior Analysis-based treatment tools for the growing population affected by autism spectrum disorders.

Daniel A. Etra, Chief Executive Officer
Eran Rosenthal, President/ COO
Jamie Pagliaro, EVP/ Chief Learning Officer

766 Society for Autistic Children
NYS Society for Autistic Children
879 Madison Avenue
Albany, NY 10218   518-459-1418
                                 e-mail: info@autism-society.org
                                      www.autism-society.org/

The Autism Society, the nation's leading grassroots autism organization, exists to improve the lives of all affected by autism. We do this by increasing public awareness about the day-to-day issues faced by people on the spectrum, advocating for appropriate services for individuals across the lifespan, and providing the latest information regarding treatment, education, research and advocacy.

James Ball, Executive Chair
Ron E Simmons, Vice Chair
Scott Badesch, President & COO

767 Talk About Curing Autism
2222 Martin St., Suite 140
Irvine, CA 92612   949-640-4401
                                               855-726-7810
                                          Fax: 949-640-4424
                                             www.tacanow.org

Talk About Curing Autism (TACA) is a national non-profit 501(c)(3) organization dedicated to educating, empowering and supporting families affected by autism. For families who have just received the autism diagnosis, TACA aims to speed up the cycle time from the autism diagnosis to effective treatments.

Glen Ackerman, President
Lisa Ackerman, Founder/ Secretary
Dan Carney, CFO/ Board Member

768 The Daniel Jordan Fiddle Foundation
www.djfiddlefoundation.org

                              e-mail: info@djfiddlefoundation.org
                                      www.djfiddlefoundation.org

The Daniel Jordan Fiddle Foundation is a national organization focused on adults living with Autism Spectrum Disorders (ASD). The mission of the volunteer-run organization is to develop, advocate for and fund our Signature Programs that create innovative blueprints for grassroots organizations and service providers to develop their own programs for the diverse population of adults living with ASD.

Linda J. Walder, Esq., Founder and President
Frederick J. Fiddle, Founder/ Treasurer
James J. Scancarella, VP, Development Co-Chair

769 The Doug Flutie, Jr. Foundation for Autism
PO Box 767
Framingham, MA 1701   508-270-8855
                                          Fax: 508-270-6868
                                       www.flutiefoundation.org

The goal of the Flutie Foundation is to help families affected by autism live life to the fullest.

Douglas Flutie, President/ Co-Founder
Laurie Flutie, Vice President/ Co-Founder
Lisa Borges, Executive Director

770 The Golden Fund for Autism
P.O. BOX 424
Cold Spring Harbor, NY 11724 e-mail: admin@goldenfundautism.org
                                      www.goldenfundautism.org

The Golden Fund for Autism is a 501(c)(3) tax-exempt organization dedicated to raising funds for children diagnosed with Autism Spectrum Disorders and their families.

Joelle A. Perez, Executive Director

771 The Help Group
13130 Burbank Blvd.
Sherman Oaks, CA 91401   818-781-0360
                                               877-994-3588
                                          Fax: 818-779-5295
                                        www.thehelpgroup.org

Serves children with special needs related to autism spectrum disorder, learning disabilities, ADHD, developmental delays, abuse and emotional problems.

Barbara Firestone, PhD, President/ CEO
Susan Berman, PhD, Chief Operating Officer
Tom Komp, LCSW, Sr. Vice President

772 Train 4 Autism
904 Silver Spur Rd., #373
Rolling Hills Estates, CA 90274   e-mail: info@train4autism.org
www.train4autism.org

Train 4 Autism is a foundation dedicated to bringing together a community of athletes, physically active, and socially conscious people who are committed to raising awareness and funds for research and treatment for those living with Autism and their families.

Ben Fesagaiga, Founder
Sam Felsenfeld, Director of Technology
Shelly Overton, Director of Chapter Development

773 US Autism & Asperger Association
P.O. Box 532
Draper, UT 84020   888-9AU-ISM
www.usautism.org

US Autism & Asperger Association (USAAA) is a 501(c)(3) nonprofit organization for autism and Asperger education, support, and solutions.

Lawrence P. Kaplan, PhD, Chairman/ CEO
Richard Dunie, MPh, MBA, CPA, Secretary/ Treasurer
Phillip C. DeMio, MD, Chief Medical Officer

774 iCanShine
P.O. Box 541
Paoli, PA 19301   610-647-4176
icanshine.org

iCan Shine (formerly, Lose The Training Wheels) is a national charitable nonprofit organization. They collaborate with local organizations and individuals, and refer to as our program 'hosts', to conduct over 100 five-day iCan Bike programs in 32 States and 3 Provinces in Canada serving nearly 3,000 people with disabilities each year.

Lisa Ruby, Founder/ Executive Director
Jeff Sullivan, Co-Founder, Dir of Finance & Admin
Jillian Bonior, Floor Supervisor

New Jersey

775 New Jersey Center for Outreach & Services for the Autism Community (COSAC)
500 Horizon Drive Suite 530
Robbinsville, NJ 08691   609-588-8200
800-428-8476
Fax: 609-588-8858
e-mail: information@autismnj.org
www.njcosac.org

Autism New Jersey is a nonprofit agency committed to ensuring safe and fulfilling lives for individuals with autism, their families, and the professionals who support them. Through awareness, credible information, education, and public policy initiatives, Autism New Jersey leads the way to lifelong individualized services provided with skill and compassion.

James A. Paone, II, Esq, President
Genare Valiant, Vice President
Mary Jane Weiss, Ph.D., BCBA-D, Vice President

State Agencies & Support Groups

Alabama

776 Autism Society of Alabama
Autism Society of America
4217 Dolly Ridge Rd
Birmingham, AL 10219   205-951-1364
877-428-8476
Fax: 205-951-1366
e-mail: melanie@autism-alabama.org
www.autism-alabama.org

To improve services for persons with Autism Spectrum Disorders and their families through education and advocacy.

Melanie Jones, Executive Director
Debbie Bumbicka, Community and Program Coordinator
Angel Loewen, Community and program Coordinator

777 Autism Society of North Alabama
Autism Society of America
PO Box 2902
Huntsville, AL 10220   256-773-0549
e-mail: tntntwhite@msn.com
www.autism-alabama.org

To improve services for persons with Autism Spectrum Disorders and their families through education and advocacy.

Peggy Stevens, President
Jonathan Nelson, Vice President
Rod Harbin, Treasurer

Arizona

778 Autism Society of America Greater Phoenix Chapter
PO Box 10543
Phoenix, AZ 10221   480-940-1093
e-mail: cynthia.macluskie@phxautism.org
www.phxautism.org

The Autism Society of Greater Phoenix provides information, resources, and support to families affected by autism and helps families who have just received the autism diagnosis by providing information on effective treatments.

James B Adams, President
Jason Gellman, Co-Chair
Catina Hoffman, Co-Chair

779 Autism Society of America Northern Arizona Chapter
PO Box 2014
Flagstaff, AZ 86003   928-779-9948
e-mail: mary.lane-kelso@nau.edu
www.nazasa.org/board%20bios/mary.html

Supports the options policy adopted by the National Autism Society of America. Dedicated to increasing public awareness and providing support to family members and individuals with autism spectrum disorders within the Northern Arizona region.

Mary Lane Kelso, Coordinator
Lynn Morrison, Co-President

780 Autism Society of America Pima County Chapter
2600 N Wyatt DR
Tucson, AZ 10223   520-770-1541
Fax: 520-319-5979
e-mail: az-pimacounty@autismsocietyofamerica.org
www.autismsocietygreatertucson.org

Volunteer organization of parents, professionals, and friends of persons with autism, designed to promote the general welfare of persons with autism.

Wendy Swartz, President
Levon Lamy, Treasurer
Amanda Heyser, Secretary

Arkansas

781 Autism Society of America Arkansas Chapter
2001 Pershing Circle F-13
North Little Rock, AR 10224   501-626-9048
e-mail: ar-arkansas@autismsocietyofamerica.org
www.autism-society.org/

Offers information and support.

Cathy Pratt, Chairman
Joan Zaro, Executive Director
Lee Grossman, CEO

California

782   Autism Society of America Coachella Valley
Autism Society of America
77564 Country Club Dr.Building B Suite 363
Palm Desert, CA 10225   760-772-1000
e-mail: info@coachellavalleyautism.org
www.cvasa.org

The Coachella Valley Autism Society of America (CVASA) exists to provide support for families of individuals with autism in the Coachella Valley and surrounding desert areas.

Monica Bernaldo, Co-President
Dianne Tostado, Treasurer
Jannet Reyes, Secretary/Vice President

783   Autism Society of America Greater Long Beach/South Bay Chapter
Autism Society of America
P.O. Box 15247
Long Beach, CA 10226   562-943-3335
562-941-1931
Fax: 562-943-3335
e-mail: ca-longbeach@autismsocietyofamerica.org
www.greaterlongbeach-asa.org

We provide information and referrals about behavior problems, education and treatment programs, your child's right to a free appropriate public education (FAPE), inclusion, how and where to obtain an evaluation and diagnosis, specialized facilities such as camps or residential programs, federal and state legislation, how to be an advocate for your child and more.

Regina Moreno, President
Gloria McNeil, Co-President
Joe McNeil, Treasurer

784   Autism Society of America Inland Empire Chapter
Autism Society of America
2276 Griffin Way, Suite 105-194
Corona, CA 10227   909-220-6922
e-mail: ieautism@att.net
www.ieautism.org

The mission of the Autism Society Inland Empire is to improve the lives of all affected by an autism spectrum disorder. We do this by increasing public awareness about the day-to-day issues faced by people on the spectrum, advocating for appropriate services for individuals across the lifespan, and providing the latest information regarding treatment, education, research, support and advocacy.

Beth Burt, President
Lillian Vasquez, Vice President
Philip Hannawi, Treasurer

785   Autism Society of America Los Angeles Chapter
Autism Society of America
8939 S Sepulveda Blvd Suite 110-788
Los Angeles, CA 10228   562-804-5556
Fax: 562-425-4940
e-mail: execdirector@autismla.org
www.autismla.org/

To improve the lives of all affected by autism in Los Angeles County by empowering individuals with autism, their families, and professionals through advocacy, education, support, and community collaboration.

Caroline Wilson, President
Emily D Iland MA, President
Danny Delgadio, Vice President

786   Autism Society of America North California Chapter
Autism Society of America
976 Mangrove Avenue
Chico, CA 10229   530-897-0900
Fax: 530-897-0100
www.asaoc.org

Provides information and support.

787   Autism Society of America North San Diego County Chapter
Autism Society of America
4699 Murphy Canyon Road
San Diego, CA 10230   858-715-0678
Fax: 858-712-1510
e-mail: info@autismsocietysandiego.org
www.autismsocietysandiego.org/Home.php

Offers chapter meetings, local groups for support and information, family events, and a lending library.

Shirley Fett, President
Nichole Hope Moore, President Elect
Tina Huston, Treasurer

788   Autism Society of America Orange County Chapter
Autism Society of America
582 N. Waverly
Orange, CA 10231   714-282-9005
e-mail: paulap@mailcity.com
www.asaoc.tripod.com/Index.htm

The Autism Society of Orange County, in unison with the Autism Society of America, strives to promote lifelong access and opportunities for persons within the autistic spectrum and their families, to be fully included, participating members of their communities through advocacy, public awareness, education, and research related to autism.

Paula Peterson, President
Linda Molyneux, Vice President

789   Autism Society of America San Diego Chapter
Autism Society of America
PO Box 420908
San Diego, CA 10232   858-715-0678
Fax: 858-712-1510
e-mail: info@autismsocietysandiego.org
www.autismsocietysandiego.org/Home.php

Promotes lifelong access and opportunities for persons within the autism spectrum and their families, to be fully included, participating members of their communities through advocacy, public awareness, education, and research related to autism.

Shirley Fett, President
Nichole Hope Moore, President Elect
Tina Huston, Treasurer

790   Autism Society of America San Francisco Bay Chapter
Autism Society of America
PO Box 249
San Mateo, CA 94401   650-637-7772
e-mail: info@sfautismsociety.org
http://sfautismsociety.virtualave.net

Promotes lifelong access and opportunities for persons within the autism spectrum and their families, to be fully included, participating members of their communities through advocacy, public awareness, education, and research related to autism.

Connie Boyar, President
Sue Swezey, Secretary
Irma Velasquez, Treasurer

791   Autism Society of America San Gabriel Valley Chapter
Autism Society of America
PO Box 15247
Glendora, CA 10234   626-388-2134
www.greaterlongbeach-asa.org/

We provide information and referrals about behavior problems, education and treatment programs, your child's right to a free appropriate public education (FAPE), inclusion, how and where to obtain an evaluation and diagnosis, specialized facilities such as camps or residential programs, federal and state legislation, how to be an advocate for your child and more.

Regina Moreno, President
Bronwyn Estephan, Vice President
Joe McNiel, Treasurer

792   Autism Society of America Santa Barbara Chapter
Autism Society of America
PO Box 30364
Santa Barbara, CA 93130   805-560-3762
e-mail: sdshove@cox.net
www.asasb.org

Promote lifelong access and opportunity for all individuals within the autism spectrum, and their families, to be fully participating, included members of their community. Support, education, advocacy, and an active public awareness from the cornerstones of ASA Santa Barbara's efforts to carry forth its mission.

Marcia Eichelberger, Co-President
Patti Gaultney, Co-President

793   Autism Society of America Tulare County Chapter
Autism Society of America
3201 West Payson Avenue
Visalia, CA 93291   559-747-2126
e-mail: lori10677@aol.com
www.autism-society.org

Promote lifelong access and opportunity for all individuals within the autism spectrum, and their families, to be fully participating, included members of their community. Support, education, advocacy, and an active public awareness from the cornerstones of ASA Santa Barbara's efforts to carry forth its mission.

Lori Collins, President

794   Autism Society of California
Autism Society of America
PO Box 1355
Glendora, CA 10236   800-869-7069
e-mail: ca-california@autismsocietyofamerica.org
www.autismsocietyca.org

The mission of the Autism Society of California is to promote lifelong access and opportunities for persons within the autism spectrum and their families, and to be fully included, participating members of their communities through advocacy, public awareness, education and research related to autism.

Marcia Eichelberger, President
Beth Burt, First Vice President
Sandra Shove, 2nd Vice President

795   Kern Autism Network
Autism Society of America
8200 Stockdale Hwy, M-10#171
Bakersfield, CA 10237   661-588-4235
661-762-7528
Fax: 661-588-4235
e-mail: kernautism@gmail.com
www.kernautism.org

Autism Society Chapter-Kern Autism Network provides support, awareness, information and education to families, professionals and the public throughout Kern County.

Ramona Puget, parent and advocate
Carl Twisselman, Honorary Lifetime Board Member
Carol Baker-Willey, Parent

Colorado

796   Autism Society of America Larimer County Chapter
3331 Lochwood Dr
Fort Collins, CO 10238   970-377-9640
e-mail: aslc@autismlarimer.org
www.autismlarimer.org

The ASLC is a volunteer group of dedicated well-informed parents and professionals working together to increase public awareness about autism and the day-to-day issues faced by individuals with autism, their families and the professionals with whom they interact.

Phyllis Zimmerman, President
Tina Boyer, Vice President
Jennifer Cotton, Treasurer

797   Autism Society of America Pikes Peak Chapter
918 Crown Ridge Drive
Colorado Springs, CO 80904   719-630-7072
e-mail: co-pikespeak@autismsocietyofamerica.org
www.asappr.org

Sponsors training opportunities for educators and parents in Southern Colorado to learn best practice strategies that will help students with autism be successful in inclusive classrooms and communities.

Alison Seyler, President

798   Autism Society of America: Colorado Chapter
550 S. Wadsworth Boulevard, Suite 100
Lakewood, CO 10240   720-214-0794
Fax: 720-274-2744
www.autismcolorado.org

To improve the lives of all affected by Autism.

Kevin Custer, President
John Sheldon, Vice President
Jeffery Nickless, Treasurer

799   Autism Society of American Boulder County Chapter
P.O. Box 270300
Louisville, CO 10241   720-272-8231
Fax: 303-604-6656
e-mail: info@autismboulder.org
www.autismboulder.org

The Autism Society of Boulder County is an all-volunteer 501(c)(3) non-profit organization that offers all of its services for free to individuals and families affected by autism in Boulder and Broomfield Counties.

Emmy Conroy, President
Whitney Pinion, Secretary
Jill Sheldon, Treasurer

Connecticut

800   Autism Society of America Connecticut Chapter
PO Box 1404
Guilford, CT 10242   888-453-4975
e-mail: info@asconn.org
www.asconn.org

Worked with parents, educators, state government, and therapeutic and medical professionals to enhance the lives of those touched by Autism Spectrum Disorders. ASCONN serves the entire autism spectrum, across specific diagnosis, needs, challenges, and age ranges.

Kim R Newgass, President
Bruce Putterman, Vice President
Jonathan Stein, Treasurer

Delaware

801   Autism Society of Delaware
Autism Society of America
924 Old Harmony Road, Suite 201
Newark, DE 10243   302-224-6020
302-472-2639
Fax: 302-224-6014
e-mail: delautism@delautism.org
www.delautism.org

The Autism Delaware Mission: to create better lives for people with autism and their families in Delaware.

Marcy kempner, President
John Willey II, Vice President
Scott Young, Treasurer

District of Columbia

802 Autism Society of America District of Columbia Chapter
5167 7th Street NE
Washington, DC 10244   202-561-5300
                                    202-561-8634
e-mail: sondrakcunningham@verizon.net
www.autism-society.org/chapter130

Provides information and referrals for families affected by autism and related disabilities. Advocate for appropriate services in education, medical and other areas.

Ronald Hampton, President
Rhoda Mcleese Smith, Vice President
Franklin Davis SR, Treasurer

Florida

803 Autism Society of America Broward Chapter
10250 NW 53rd
Sunrise, FL 10245   954-577-4141
                                 954-474-5333
www.asabroward.org

ASB's full range of family support, children's programming, public outreach and autism awareness campaigns are available to all interested in the betterment of life for not only individuals and families with autism, but to the community of South Florida as a whole

Hugh J Keough Esq, President
Fabiola Anna Torrez, Vice President
Brent Boucaud, Treasurer

804 Autism Society of America Emerald Coast Chapter
8668 Navarre Parkway Suite # 216
Navarre, FL 10246   850-736-0879
e-mail: myra@ecautismsociety.com
www.ecautismsociety.com

Provides information and support.
Myra Fowler, President
Kristen Bowen, Vice-President
Greg Hasty, Treasurer

805 Autism Society of America Florida Chapter
PO Box 450476
Sunrise, FL 10247   954-577-4141
                                 855-529-6807
Fax: 954-571-2136
e-mail: ven@autismfl.com
www.autismfl.com

The Autism Society of Florida is a statewide organization that supports individuals with autism, their families, and caregivers. It includes individuals with autism and volunteers (including family members, professionals, and other interested persons). The Autism Society of Florida coordinates activities on behalf of people with autism on a statewide basis.

806 Autism Society of America Jacksonville Chapter
1526 University Blvd W #235
Jacksonville, FL 32217   904-399-4490
www.autism-society.org/chapter1003

Mission is to support, inform and empower the families of Jacksonville.

Jeenifer Nunes, President

807 Autism Society of America Manasota Chapter
2380 Wycliff Street, Suite 102
St Paul, MN 10249   651-647-1083
                                 941-780-5237
Fax: 651-642-1230
e-mail: info@ausm.org
www.ausm.org

Established in 1971, the Autism Society of Minnesota (AuSM) is a self-funded organization committed to education, support and advocacy designed to enhance the lives of those affected by autism from birth through retirement.

Todd Schwartzberg, President
Jean Bender, Vice President
Aaron R Deris, Treasurer

808 Autism Society of America Panhandle Chapter
P.O. Box 30213
Pensacola, FL 32503   850-450-0656
e-mail: info@autismpensacola.org
www.autismpensacola.org

A nonprofit, tax-exempt association of parents, professionals and other concerned community members dedicated to the education and welfare of children and adults with autism and related disorders of communication and behavior.

Fred Donovan, President
Julian Irby, Vice President
Bonnie Sferes, Treasurer

809 Autism Society of Greater Orlando
Autism Society of America
12720 S. Orange Blossom Trail Suite 8
Orlando, FL 10251   407-855-0235
Fax: 407-855-5129
e-mail: contact@asgo.org
www.asgo.org

ASGO was founded in 1996 by a group of volunteer parents to better assist families of children and adults with autism in the Central Florida area. The mission or goal of the ASGO is that all individuals within the autism spectrum will be provided a lifetime network of opportunities to become fully accepted, included, and actively participating members of our community, through family support, education, and advocacy, and public awareness.

Donna Lorman, President
Lorienda Crawford, Vice President
Angelica Taylor, Treasurer

Georgia

810 Autism Society of America Greater Georgia Chapter
P.O. Box 3707
Suwanee, GA 10252   770-904-4474
Fax: 678-935-1152
e-mail: office@asaga.com
www.asaga.com

Chapter of ASA, we offer resource info to individuals and their families and to professionals about autism, add, add and other developmental disabilities

Gailynn Gluth, President
Jason Cavin, 1st Vice President
Jon Basinger, 2nd Vice President

Hawaii

811 Autism Society of Hawaii
Autism Society of America
1600 Kapiolani Blvd. #620
Honolulu, HI 10253   808-282-3676
                                  808-228-0122
e-mail: autismhi@gmail.com
www.autismhi.org

The Autism Society of Hawaii is a 501(c)(3) organization serving families and individuals touched by autism and autism spectrum disorders.

Dr William Bolman, President
Jessica Wong, Executive Director
John P Dellera, Board Member

Idaho

812 Autism Society of America Treasure Valley Chapter
P.O. Box 44831
Boise, ID 10254   208-336-5676
e-mail: autism.asatvc@yahoo.com
www.asatvc.org

Top provide advocacy, support and information to individuals with autism, their families, professionals, and communities throughout Treasure Valley Chapter.

To provide advocacy, support and information to individuals with autism, their families, professionals, and communities throughout state Kansas.

Illinois

813 Autism Society of Illinois
Autism Society of America
2200 South Main Street, # 205
Lombard, IL 10255
630-691-1270
888-691-1270
Fax: 630-932-5620
e-mail: info@autismillinois.org
www.autismillinois.org

Partnering with families and communities living with autism in Illinois by generating awareness and providing education, training, support, and guidance as a compassionate and caring authority.

Mary K Betz, Executive Director
Jean C Thomas, Associate Executive Director
Dave Geslak, Treasurer

Indiana

814 Autism Society of Indiana
Autism Society of America
13295 Illinois Street Suite 213
Carmel, IN 10256
317-695-0252
800-609-8449
e-mail: info@inautism.org
www.autismsocietyofindiana.org

Since 1998, the Autism Society of America - Indiana (ASI) has worked to raise awareness about autism, to promote early diagnosis and early intervention thereby helping people on the autism spectrum have the fullest and most successful journey possible.

Joshua Carr, Executive Board President
Kylee Hope, Executive Board Vice President
Kelli McKinzie, Executive Board Treasurer

Iowa

815 Autism Society of Iowa
Autism Society of America
4340 East-West Hwy, Suite 350
Bethesda, ML 10257
301-657-0881
800-328-8476
e-mail: autism50ia@aol.com
www.autism-society.org

The Autism Society, the nation's leading grassroots autism organization, exists to improve the lives of all affected by autism.

Kris Steinmantz, Manager

816 The Link
Autism Society of Iowa
4549 Waterford Drive
West Des Moines, IA 50265
515-327-9075
888-457-7225
e-mail: autism50ia@aol.com
www.autismia.org

Provides information for parents, professionals and care givers on autism spectrum disorders.

Kris Steinmantz, Manager

Kansas

817 Autism Society of Kansas
Autism Society of America
2250 N Rock Road
Wichita, KS 67203
316-943-1191
e-mail: arkansas@att.net
www.ask.hostrack.net

Kentucky

818 Autism Society of America Bluegrass Chapter
Autism Society of America
243 Shady Lane
Lexington, KY 40503
859-299-9000
e-mail: ky-lexington@autismsocietyofamerica.org
www.asbg.org

A resource and support group for families and professionals in the Central Kentucky area who are involved with autism.

Sara Spragens, President

Louisiana

819 Autism Society of Louisiana
Autism Society of America
PO Box 80162
Baton Rouge, LA 70898
800-955-3760
e-mail: autismsociety_lastatechapter@yahoo.com
www.lastateautism.org

To provide information and referrals, advocacy and support for individuals with ASD and their families; to help families identify qualified professionals in their communities; to assist families in securing benefits and services provided by law; and, to promote lifelong opportunities for persons with autism spectrum disorder in order to be fully included members of their communities.

Pat Giamanco, President

Maine

820 Autism Society of Maine
Autism Society of America
72 Main Street, Suite B
Winthrop, ME 04364
207-377-9603
800-273-5200
Fax: 207-377-9434
e-mail: info@asmonline.org
www.asmonline.org

The Autism Society of Maine provides education and resources to support the valued lives of individuals on the autism spectrum and their families.

Janine Collins, President
Laurie Raymond', Vice President
Michael Lamoreau, Treasurer

Maryland

821 Autism Society of America Baltimore Chesapeake Chapter
PO Box 10822
Parkville, MD 21234
410-655-7933
e-mail: info@baltimoreautismsociety.org
www.bcc-asa.org

Serves families of children and adults with autism spectrum disorders in Baltimore County, Maryland, Baltimore City, and the State of Maryland by providing information, advocacy, and support for families and individuals with autism.

Debbie Page, Co- President
David Savick, Co- President
Kay Holman, Vice President

Massachusetts

822   **Autism Society of America Massachusetts Chapter**
Autism Society of America
47 Walnut Street
Wellesley Hills, MA 02481   781-237-0272
                                          Fax: 781-237-5020
                          e-mail: asamasschapter@hotmail.com
                                          www.massautism.org

Mission is to promote lifelong access and opportunity for all individuals within the autism spectrum and their families to be fully
participating, included members of their community.

Barry Neil Kaufman, Co-Founder/Co-Creator
Samahria Lyte Kaufman, Co-Founder/Co-Creator

823   **Option Institute: Son Rise Program**
Autism Treatment Center of America
2080 S Undermountain Road
Sheffield, MA 01257   413-229-2100
                                             800-714-2779
                                          Fax: 413-229-3202
                           e-mail: information@son-rise.org
                                          www.son-rise.org

Since 1983, the Autism Treatment Center of America has provided innovative training programs for parents and professionals
caring for children challenged by Autism, Autism Spectrum Disorders, Pervasive Developmental Disorder (PDD) and other developmental difficulties. The Son-Rise Program teaches a specific
yet comprehensive system of treatment and education designed to
help families and caregivers enable their children to dramatically
improve in all areas of learning.

Barry Neil Kaufman, Co-Founder/Co-Creator
Samahria Lyte Kaufman, Co-Founder/Co-Creator
Bryn Hogan, ACTA Senior Staff

Michigan

824   **Autism Society of Michigan**
Autism Society of America
2178 Commons Parkway
Okemos, MI 48864   517-882-2800
                                             800-223-6722
                                          Fax: 517-862-2816
                              e-mail: autism@autism-mi.org
                                          www.autism-mi.org

The Autism Society of Michigan is committed to empowering individuals with autism and their families by offering educational
resources and materials, workshops, seminars and other services.
ASM advocates that making human connections in a supportive,
integrated community is a right of all persons.

Bob Opsommer, President

Minnesota

825   **Autism Society of Minnesota**
Autism Society of America
2380 Wycliff Street, Suite 102
Saint Paul, MN 55114   651-647-1083
                                          Fax: 651-642-1230
                                     e-mail: info@ausm.org
                                          www.ausm.org

The Autism Society of Minnesota exists to enhance the lives of
individuals with autism spectrum disorders. AuSM seeks to realize its mission through education support, collaboration, and
advocacy.

Todd Schwartzberg, President
Jean Bender, Vice President
Aaron R Deris, Treasurer

Mississippi

826   **Autism Society of Mississippi**
Autism Society of America
5908 Tolar Road
Moss Point, MS 39562 e-mail: ms-mississippi@autismsocietyofamerica.or
                  www.autismnow.org/local/autism-society-of-mississipp

Offers information, referrals, and support to parents, professionals and caregivers.

Cathy Pratt, Chairman
Joan Zaro, Executive Director
Lee Grossman, CEO

Missouri

827   **Autism Society of America Gateway Chapter**
Autism Society of America
7777 Bonhomme Avenue, Suite 1600
St Louis, MO 63105   314-721-0042
                                          Fax: 314-863-7494
                                   e-mail: pegisues@aol.com

Provides information and support.

Pegi Price, President

Nebraska

828   **Autism Society of Nebraska**
Autism Society of America
PO Box 83559
Lincoln, NE 68501   402-637-5670
                                             800-580-9279
                      e-mail: autismsociety@autismnebraska.org
                                          www.autismnebraska.org

Supports and advocates for individuals with autism and their families through increasing education and awareness, fundraising,
and facilitating community involvement for persons with autism
spectrum disorders to achieve their potential by becoming a productive, accepted, and integral part of society.

Megan Misegadis, President
Wendy Hamilton, Vice President
Robyn Roberts, Treasurer

Nevada

829   **Autism Society of Northern Nevada Chapter**
Autism Society of America
3490 Southampton Drive
Reno, NV 89509   775-786-9315
                                          Fax: 775-786-0984
                                 e-mail: pd1989@yahoo.com
                                          www.nnasa.org

Promote and advocate for the general welfare of persons with autism. To further the education and training of parents and professional personnel for training, educating, and caring for persons
with autism.

Dinah Deane, President
Paul Deane, Vice President
Guy McKillip, Web Master

New Hampshire

830   **Autism Society of New Hampshire**
Autism Society of America
PO Box 68
Concord, NH 03302   603-679-2424
                                          Fax: 301-657-0869
                                 e-mail: info@nhautism.com
           www.autismnow.org/local/autism-society-of-new-hampsh

The Autism Society of New Hampshire is dedicated to individuals with Autism and Pervasive Developmental Disorders.

Stacey Shannon, President

New Jersey

831 New Jersey Center for Outreach & Services for the Autism Community (COSAC)
500 Horizon Drive Suite 530
Robbinsville, NJ 08691   609-588-8200
                               800-428-8476
                          Fax: 609-588-8858
           e-mail: information@autismnj.org
                              www.njcosac.org

Autism New Jersey is a nonprofit agency committed to ensuring safe and fulfilling lives for individuals with autism, their families, and the professionals who support them. Through awareness, credible information, education, and public policy initiatives, Autism New Jersey leads the way to lifelong individualized services provided with skill and compassion.

James A. Paone, II, Esq, President
Genare Valiant, Vice President
Mary Jane Weiss, Ph.D., BCBA-D, Vice President

New Mexico

832 New Mexico Autism Society
Autism Society of America
PO Box 30955
Albuquerque, NM 87190   505-332-0306
                       www.nmautismsociety.org

Our mission is to promote lifelong access and opportunities for persons within the autism spectrum, and their families, to be fully included participating members of their communities.

Roger Riley,, President
Sarah Baca, Executive Director
Pauline Riley, Treasurer

New York

833 Center for Family Support
333 7th Avenue, 9th Floor
New York, NY 10001   212-629-7939
                       Fax: 212-239-2211
           e-mail: svernikoff@cfsny.org
                       www.cfsny.org

The Center for Family Support is committed to providing support and assistance to individuals with developmental and related disabilities, and to the family members who care for them.

Steven Vernikoff, Executive Director
Eileen Berg, Director of Quality Assurance
Sharon Lax, Director of Human Resources

834 New York Autism Network
Autism Society of America
101 State Street
Schenectady, NY 12305   518-355-2191
                         Fax: 518-355-2191
           e-mail: info@albanyautism.org
                       www.albanyautism.org

Provide ongoing support to families and professionals, develop regional networks, provide technical assistance, and conduct conferences related to pervasive developmental disorders.

Gordon Zuckerman, President
Jenny DeBellis, Treasurer
Haley Knox, Secretary

North Carolina

835 Autism Society of North Carolina
Autism Society of America
505 Oberlin Road Suite 230
Raleigh, NC 27605   800-442-2762
                       Fax: 919-743-0204
           e-mail: info@autismsociety-nc.org
                       www.autismsociety-nc.org

For over 43 years, the Autism Society of North Carolina (ASNC) has worked to address areas of need and expand services for the autism community in North Carolina. ASNC is a statewide organization, supporting North Carolinians affected by autism

Beverly Moore, Chair
Sharon Jeffries-Jones, Vice Chair
Elizabeth Phillippi, Treasurer

Ohio

836 Autism Society of Greater Cincinatti
Autism Society of America
PO Box 58385
Cincinnati, OH 45258   513-561-2300
                         Fax: 513-561-4748
           e-mail: info@autismcincy.org
                       www.autismcincy.org

The mission of the Autism Society of Greater Cincinnati is to improve the quality of life for all people with autism spectrum disorders and their families.

Kay Brown, President
Sue Radabaugh, Vice President
James Keller, Treasurer

837 Autism Society of Ohio Tri-County Chapter
Autism Society of America
25 East Boardman Street, Suite 230
Youngstown, OH 44503   330-501-7553
                         Fax: 614-754-6332
   e-mail: mahoningvalley@autismohio.org
                       www.autismohio.org

To improve the quality of life for all people with autism spectrum disorders and their families.

Aundrea Cika, Director

Oklahoma

838 Autism Society of Oklahoma
Autism Society of America
PO Box 720103
Norman, OK 73070   405-370-3220
                       www.asofok.org

Dedicated to the education and welfare of all people with autism and other pervasive developmental disorders.

Oregon

839 Autism Society of Oregon
Autism Society of America
PO Box 396
Marylhurst, OR 97036   503-636-1676
                               888-288-4761
                          Fax: 503-636-1696
               www.autismsocietyoregon.org

Promote mutual communication, autism awareness and better service delivery across Oregon.

Tobi Burch, Executive Director
Leigh Ann Chapman, President
Brad Volchok, Treasurer

Pennsylvania

840 Autism Society of America Greater Harrisburg Area Chapter
PO Box 101
Enola, PA 17025   717-732-8400
                               800-244-2425
               www.autismharrisburg.org

To promote opportunities for individuals with autism spectrum disorders, to participate in the same value life experiences as do other citizens.

Esther Feirick, President
Kathleen Haigh, Vice President
Diana Fishlock, Treasurer

Rhode Island

841 Autism Society of Rhode Island
Autism Society of America
PO Box 16603
Rumford, RI 02916
401-595-3241
e-mail: lrego@asa-ri.org
www.asa-ri.org

Provides information and support.

Lisa Rego, President
Claudia Swiader, Vice President

South Carolina

842 Autism Society of South Carolina
Autism Society of America
806 12th Street
West Columbia, SC 29169
803-750-6988
800-438-4790
Fax: 803-750-8121
e-mail: scas@scautism.org
www.scautism.org

The purpose of the South Carolina Autism Society is to enable all individuals with autism spectrum disorders to reach their maximum potential.

Susan Kastner, Chair
Alex Holbert, Vice Chair
Mitchell Yell, Treasurer

South Dakota

843 Autism Society of South Dakota Black Hills Chapter
Autism Society of America
3650 Range Road
Rapid City, SD 57702
605-415-3739
e-mail: info@autismsd.org
www.autismsd.org

We have joined to enable all families and others associated with an autistic, Asperger's or Pervasive Development Disorder individual to have access to support groups, meetings, additional information and resources.

Tennessee

844 Autism Society of America East Tennessee Chapter
PO Box 30015
Knoxville, TN 37930
865-637-3914
e-mail: info@asaetc.org
www.asaetc.org

To promote lifelong access and opportunity of all individuals within the autism spectrum, and their families, to be fully participating, included members of their community.

Mike Manfredo, President
Roddey M. Coe, Vice President
Sara Hirtz, Treasurer

Texas

845 Autism Society of America Greater Austin Chapter
Autism Society of America
PO Box 160841
Austin, TX 78716
512-479-4199
e-mail: austinautismsociety@gmail.com
www.autism-society.org/chapter244

Mission is to promote lifelong access and opportunities for person within the autism spectrum, and their families, to be fully included, participating members of their communities through advocacy, public awareness, education, and research related to Autism.

Ann Hart, President
Sandra Batlouni, Vice President
Tom Ibis, Treasurer

Vermont

846 Autism Society of Vermont
Autism Society of America
PO Box 978
White River Junction, VT 05001
800-559-7398
e-mail: vt-vermont@autismsocietyofamerica.org
www.asvermont.org

The ASVT is a non-profit corporation serving the needs of Vermont's Autism community.

Cathy Pratt, Chairman
Joan Zaro, Executive Director
Lee Grossman, CEO

Virginia

847 Autism Society of America Northern Virginia Chapter
98 N. Washington Street
Falls Church, VA 22046
703-495-8444
Fax: 703-563-6099
e-mail: info@asanv.org
www.asanv.org

Provides information and support to individuals with autism and their families in Northern Virginia area.

Scott Campbell, President
Ray Nelson, Vice President
John J Wall, CPA, Treasurer

Washington

848 Autism Society of Washington
Autism Society of America
PO Box 503
Olympia, WA 98507
360-515-8910
888-279-4968
Fax: 253-503-1557
e-mail: info@autismsocietyofwa.org
www.autismsocietyofwa.org

The mission of the Autism Society of Washington is to promote lifelong access and opportunities for persons within the autism spectrum and their families, and to be fully included, participating members of their communities through advocacy, public awareness, education, and research related to autism.

Jeffrey Foster, President
Teresa McCann, Vice President
Stephen Peters, Treasurer

West Virginia

849 Autism Society of West Virginia
PO Box 7
Huntington, WV 25706
304-748-1331
e-mail: jfair3@comcast.net
http://autismwv.blogspot.com

ASA-WV is dedicated to increasing public awareness about autism and the day-to-day issues faced by individuals with autism, their families and the professionals with whom they interact. The Society's mission is to provide information and education, support research and advocate for programs and services for the autism population

Christina Lee Fair, President

Wisconsin

850 **Autism Society of Wisconsin**
Autism Society of America
1477 Kenwood Dr.
Menasha, WI 54952
920-558-4602
888-428-8476
Fax: 920-558-4611
e-mail: asw@asw4autism.org
www.asw4autism.org

To promote lifelong opportunities for persons within the autism spectrum and their families to be fully included, participating members of their communities through information and referral, advocacy, public awareness, and education and support for local Autism Society of America chapters, professionals and others who support individuals with autism in Wisconsin.

Kristen Cooper, Executive Director
Kelly Brodhagen, Office Manager
Melissa Vande Velden, Events Coordinator/WALN Project Coo

Libraries & Resource Centers

Georgia

851 **Emory Autism Resource Center**
Emory University
101 Woodruff Circle, Suite 4000
Atlanta, GA 30322
404-727-8382
Fax: 404-727-3969
e-mail: jsheikh@emory.edu
www.psychiatry.emory.edu/clinical_sites_autism_cente

Offers online bulletin boards which are relevant to autism.

Mark Hyman Rapaport, Chairman

Indiana

852 **Indiana Resource Center for Autism**
Inst. for the Study of Developmental Disabilities
2853 E 10th Street
Bloomington, IN 47408
812-855-6508
Fax: 812-855-9630
TTY: 812-855-9396
e-mail: iidc@indiana.edu
www.iidc.indiana.edu/irca

Conducts outreach training and consultation, engage in research, and develops and disseminate information on behalf of individuals across the autism spectrum, including autism, asperger's syndrome, and other pervasive developmental disorders.

Dr. Cathy Pratt, Director

Michigan

853 **Burger School for the Autistic**
30922 Beechwood Street
Garden City, MI 48135
734-762-8420
Fax: 734-762-8533
www.resa.net/gardencity/burger.htm

Committed to maximizing the potential of each student to gain independence and self-fulfillment.

Mary O'Neill, Manager

Missouri

854 **Judevine Center for Autism**
1101 Olivette Executive Parkway
Saint Louis, MO 63132
314-432-6200
800-780-6545
Fax: 314-849-2721
e-mail: contactus@judevine.org
www.judevine.org

Rooted in principles of applied behavior analysis within a social exchange framework, the Judevine Center has provided effective training and treatment to thousands of families locally, nationally and globally.

New Jersey

855 **New Jersey Center for Outreach and Service s for the Autism Community (COSAC)**
500 Horizon Drive, Suite 530
Robbinsville, NJ 8691
609-588-8200
800-428-8476
Fax: 609-588-8858
e-mail: information@autismnj.org
www.njcosac.org

Nonprofit agency providing information and advocacy, services, family and professional education and consultation. COSAC encourages responsible basic and applied research that would lead to a lessening of the effects and potential prevention of autism. COSAC is dedicated to ensuring that all people with autism receive appropriate, effective services to maximize their growth potential and to enhance the overall awareness of autism in the general public.

James A Paone, President
Genare Valiant, Vice President
Kathleen Moore, Secretary

New York

856 **Institute for Basic Research in Developmental Disabilities**
1050 Forest Hill Road
Staten Island, NY 10314
718-494-0600
Fax: 718-698-3803
www.omr.state.ny.us

To conduct basic and clinical research in order to further the prevention and early detection and treatment of mental retardation and developmental disabilities.

W Ted Brown, Manager

857 **State University of New York Health Sciences Center**
450 Clarkson Avenue, Box 32
Brooklyn, NY 11203
718-270-1000
Fax: 718-778-5397
www.downstate.edu

Child psychiatry research programs.

Richard Kream, Manager

North Carolina

858 **Autism Society of North Carolina**
505 Oberlin Road, Suite 230
Raleigh, NC 27605
919-743-0204
800-442-2762
Fax: 919-743-0208
e-mail: books@autismsociety-nc.org
www.autismbookstore.com

Offers a library that carries one of the largest selections of books about autism.

David Lax, Manager

West Virginia

859 **Autism Services Center**
929 4th Avenue, PO Box 507
Huntington, WV 25710
304-525-8014
Fax: 304-525-8026
www.autismservicescenter.org

Works to improve appropriate and professional training, advocacy, consulting and information for individuals responsible for the welfare and care of autistic individuals and others with developmental disabilities.

Mike Grady, CEO
Derek Hyman, President/Treasurer
Elaine Harvey, Vice President

860   Autism Training Center
Marshall University
1 John Marshall Drive, Suite 316
Huntington, WV 25755   304-696-2332
                                        800-344-5115
                                        Fax: 304-696-2846
                            e-mail: wvatc@marshall.edu.
                                    www.marshall.edu/atc/

To provide education, training and treatment programs for West Virginians who have autism, pervasive developmental disorders or Asperger's disorders and have been formally registered with the center.

Barbara Cottrill, Executive Director

Research Centers

861   Autism Research Foundation
BU School of Medicine
72 East Concord Street
Boston, MA 02118   617-414-7012
                                        Fax: 617-414-7207
            e-mail: hello@theautismresearchfoundation.org
                    www.theautismresearchfoundation.org

A nonprofit, tax-exempt organization dedicated to researching the neurological underpinnings of autism and other related developmental brain disorders. Seeking to rapidly expand and accelerate research into the pervasive developmental disorders. To do this, time and effort goes into investigating the neuropathology of autism in their laboratories, collecting and redistributing brain tissue to promising research groups for use by projects approved by the Tissue Resource Committee.

Margaret Bauman, MD, Founding Director
Thomas Sabin MD, President
Thomas Kemper MD, Vice President

862   Autism Research Institute
4182 Adams Avenue
San Diego, CA 92116   619-281-7165
                                        866-366-3361
                                        Fax: 619-563-6840
                e-mail: media@autismresearchinstitute.com
                                        www.autism.com

ARI advocates for the rights of people with ASD, and operates without funding from special-interest groups. ARI is dedicated to developing a standard of care for individuals with autism spectrum disorders and their families. We rely on the generosity of donors to help us advance autism research and provide needed information and support for families and individuals with autism spectrum disorders.

Stephen Edelson, Executive Director
Jane Johnson, Managing Director
Rebecca McKenney, Office Manager

863   Autism Speaks
1 East 33rd Street 4th Floor
New York, NY 10016   212-252-8584
                                        Fax: 212-252-8676
                e-mail: familyservices@autismspeaks.org
                                        www.autismspeaks.org

At Autism Speaks, our goal is to change the future for all who struggle with autism spectrum disorder. We are dedicated to funding global biomedical research into the causes, prevention, treatments, and cure for autism; to raising public awareness about autism and its effects on individuals, families, and society; and to bringing hope to all who deal with the hardships of this disorder.

Liz Feld, President
Peter H Bell, Executive VP
Lisa Goring, Vice President

864   Children's Center for Neurodevelopmental Studies
5430 West Glenn Drive
Glendale, AZ 85301   623-915-0345
                                        Fax: 623-937-5425
                            e-mail: admin@ccnsaz.org
                            www.thechildrenscenteraz.org

The Children's Center is a full service non-profit corporation (501-c3) offering comprehensive educational, therapeutic, and habilitative programs for children and adults

Kent Rideout, Director
Dawna Sterner, Preschool & Education Information
Catherine Orsak, Therapy Information

865   Facilitated Communication Institute at Syracuse University
230 Huntington Hall
Syracuse, NY 13244   315-443-4752
                                        Fax: 315-443-2258
                            e-mail: scstaff@sued.syr.edu
                                    www.soe.syr.edu/about/

Facilitated Communication Institute, the new name, the Institute on Communication and Inclusion, represents a broadened focus developed over the past 20 years, reflecting lines of research, training and public dissemination that focus on school and community inclusion, narratives of disability and ability, and disability rights. Its initiatives stress the important relationship of communication to inclusion.

Robert Bogdan, Distinguished Professor Emeritus
Joan Burstyn, Professor Emerita
John Centra, Professor Emeritus

866   Institute on Communication and Inclusion
203 Huntington Hall
Syracuse, NY 13244   315-443-4752
                                        Fax: 315-443-2258
                            e-mail: icistaff@syr.edu
                                    www.soe.syr.edu/about/

Facilitated Communication Institute, the new name, the Institute on Communication and Inclusion, represents a broadened focus developed over the past 20 years, reflecting lines of research, training and public dissemination that focus on school and community inclusion, narratives of disability and ability, and disability rights. Its initiatives stress the important relationship of communication to inclusion.

Robert Bogdan, Distinguished Professor Emeritus
Joan Burstyn, Professor Emerita
John Centra, Professor Emeritus

867   State University of New York Health Sciences Center
450 Clarkson Avenue
Brooklyn, NY 11203   718-270-1568
                                        Fax: 718-778-5397
                                        www.downstate.edu

Child psychiatry research programs.

Robert Furchgott, President

868   University of North Carolina at Chapel Hill, Brain Research Center
Matthew Gfeller Center 2207 Stallings-Evans Sports
Chapel Hill, NC 8700   919-962-0409
                                        Fax: 919-962-7060
                            e-mail: tbicenter@unc.edu
                www.tbicenter.unc.edu/MAG_Center/Home.html

The Matthew Gfeller Sport-Related Traumatic Brain Injury Research Center demonstrates its commitment to providing the highest level of care for athletes of all ages suffering from sport-related brain injuries, and to assist parents, coaches, and medical professionals in managing these student-athletes.

Kevin M. Guskiewicz, Faculty
Jason P. Mihalik, Faculty
Stephen W. Marshall, Faculty

Conferences

869 Annual TEACCH Conference
University of North Carolina at Chapel Hill
1418 Aversboro Road
Garner, NC 27529
919-662-4625
Fax: 919-662-4634
e-mail: raleighteacch@med.unc.edu
www.teacch.com

May

Eric Schopler, Founder & Co-Director

870 Autism National Committee Conference
Autism National Committee Conference
3 Bedford Green
South Burlington, VT 05403
800-378-0386
e-mail: sandra.mcclennen@emich.edu
www.autcom.org

October

871 Autism Society National Conference & Expo
Austim Society
4340 East-West Way, Suite 350
Bethesda, MD 20814
301-657-0881
800-328-8476
e-mail: info@autism-society.org
www.autism-society.org

Addresses the range of issues affecting people with autism including early intervention, education, employment, behavior,
communication, social skills, biomedical interventions and others,
across the entire lifespan. Bringing together the expertise and experiences of family members, professionals and individuals on the
spectrum, attendees are able to learn how to more effectively advocate and obtain supports for the individual with ASD.

July

James Ball, Executive Chair
Ron E Simmons, Vice Chair
Sergio Mariaca, Treasurer

872 FFCMH Annual Conference
Federation of Families for Childrens Mental Health
9605 Medical Center Drive, Suite 280
Rockville, MD 20850
240-403-1901
Fax: 240-403-1909
e-mail: ffcmh@ffcmh.org
www.ffcmh.org

Address the complex issue of trauma; the impact it has on children and families; the promotion of healing and prevention strategies; knowledge about how to address trauma through
resiliency-based interventions, utilizing a familydriven, youth
guided approach; and examples of how family organizations and
the partners they work with are raising awareness and improving
trauma-focused services and supports.

November

Teka Dempson, President
Sherri Luthe, Vice President
Sheila Pires, Treasurer

873 Genetic Alliance Annual Conference
Genetic Alliance
4301 Connecticut Avenue NW, Suite 404
Washington, DC 20008
202-966-5557
800-336-4363
Fax: 202-966-8553
e-mail: info@geneticalliance.org
www.geneticalliance.org

Consistently inspirational and enables partnership among all
stakeholders: advocates and community leaders, health and industry professionals, policymakers, and academicians.

July

Sharon Terry, President/CEO
Tetyana Murza, Programs/Events Manager

**874 International Conference On Young Children With Special
Needs & Their Famililies**
Division for Early Childhood
27 Fort Missoula Road, Suite 2
Missoula, MT 59804
406-543-0872
Fax: 406-543-0887
TTY: 703-264-9446
e-mail: dec@dec-sped.org
www.dec-sped.org

Attendees from around the world explore the evidence, present
practical strategies, and engage in discussions that will change
the way one thinks about early childhood special education. Topics include: policy, autism, recommended practices, tiered interventions, challenging behavior, personnel development, research,
assessment, cultural diversity and more.

Bonnie Keilty, President
Juliann Woods, Vice President
Misty Goosen, Secretary

Audio Video

**875 A Sense of Belonging: Including Students with Autism in their
School Community**
Indiana Resource Center for Autism
1905 North Range Rd.
Bloomington, IN 47408
812-855-6508
Fax: 812-855-9630
TTY: 812-855-9396
e-mail: iidc@indiana.edu
www.iidc.indiana.edu

Highlights the efforts of two elementary and one middle school in
Indiana in teaching students with autism in general education settings. Truly involoving students in their school community requires teamwork, the adoption of effective instructional practices,
and a school committed to supporting a diverse range of students.

David Mank, Director

876 Autism
Fanflight Productions
32 Court Street, 21st Floor
Brooklyn, NY 11201
718-488-8900
800-876-1710
Fax: 718-488-8642
e-mail: info@fanlight.com
www.fanlight.com

The stories of three families show us what the textbooks and
studies cannot — what it's really like to love and care for children with autism.

28 minutes

Kelli English, Publicity Coordinator

877 Autism Is a World
Syracuse University, Institute on Communication
370 Huntington Hall
Syracuse, NY 13244
315-443-9657
Fax: 315-443-2274
http://suedweb.syr.edu/thefci

Documentary that takes the viewer on a journey into the mind of
13 year old girl, into her world and her obsessions. Explores
Sue's world world, her writings, and the remarkable friendships
she has created while in college.

Videotape

878 Autism: A Strange, Silent World
Filmakers Library
3212 Duke Street
Alexandria, VA 22314
212-808-4980
703-212-8520
Fax: 212-808-4983
e-mail: sales@alexanderstreet.com
www.academicvideostore.com/filmakers

British educators and medical personnel offer insight into autism's characteristics and treatment approaches through the cam-
eos of three children.

52 Minute
Sue Oscar, Co-President

879 Autism: A World Apart
Fanlight Productions
32 Court Street, 21st Floor
Brooklyn, NY 11201

718-488-8900
800-876-1710
Fax: 718-488-8642
e-mail: info@fanlight.com
www.fanlight.com

In this documentary, three families show us what the textbooks and studies cannot, what it's like to live with autism day after day, raise and love children who may be withdrawn and violent and unable to make personal connections with their families.
ISBN: DVD: 1-57295-950-9; VHS: 1-57295-039-0

29 Minutes DVD or VHS

880 Autism: Being Friends
Indiana Resource Center for Autism
1905 North Range Rd.
Bloomington, IN 47408

812-855-6508
800-280-7010
Fax: 812-855-9630
TTY: 812-855-9396
e-mail: iidc@indiana.edu
www.iidc.indiana.edu

This autism awareness videotape was produced specifically for use with young children. The program portrays the abilities of the child with autism and describes ways in which peers can help the child to be a part of the everyday world.

David Mank, Director

881 Autism: The Child Who Couldn't Play
Films for the Humanities and Sciences
132 West 31st Street
New York, NY 10001

800-257-5126
Fax: 609-275-0266
e-mail: custserv@films.com
www.ffh.films.com

This program is a comprehensive overview of autism, the mysterious disorder that impedes normal child development. It was once believed that autism was caused by remote, cold parents; most often the mother was blamed. The program explores the frontiers of our understanding of autism, which today is recognized as a partly genetic biological disorder.

28 minutes
ISBN: 1-421373-28-7

882 Autism: The Unfolding Mystery
Aquarius Health Care Videos
Lot 2/12 Willmott Ave
Margaret River, WA 6285

508-650-1616
888-440-2963
Fax: 508-650-1665
e-mail: aquarius33@bigpond.com
www.aquariusproductions.com

Explores what it means to be autistic, how you can recognize the signs of autism in your child, and hear about new tretments and programs to help children learn to deal with the disorder.

26 Minutes

883 Children and Autism: Time is Brain
Aquarius Health Care Videos
Lot 2/12 Willmott Ave
Margaret River, WA 6285

508-650-1616
888-440-2963
Fax: 508-650-1665
e-mail: aquarius33@bigpond.com
www.aquariusproductions.com

A mother of an autistic child implores parents who suspect their child may be autisitc not to 'wait and see.' Don't wait, don't be afraid of that diagnosis, diagnosis is a tool, not a stigma. The term 'time is brain' is absolutely accurate for children with autism, because the sooner diagnosed, the sooner they can get excellent care.

27 Minutes
ISBN: 1-581404-44-1

884 Children of the Stars
Fanlight Productions
32 Court Street, 21st Floor
Brooklyn, NY 11201

718-488-8900
800-876-1710
Fax: 718-488-8642
e-mail: info@fanlight.com
www.fanlight.com

This film explores the harsh reality of raising children with autism in modern day China. It prodives moving insights into the hardships parents face and reminds us painfully of conditions that prevailed in the United States not so very many years ago.
49 Minutes DVD
ISBN: 1-572955-07-4

885 Developing Friendships: Wonderful People to Get to Know
Indiana Resource Center for Autism
1905 North Range Rd.
Bloomington, IN 47408

812-855-6508
Fax: 812-855-9630
TTY: 812-855-9396
e-mail: iidc@indiana.edu
www.iidc.indiana.edu

Individuals discuss the various social difficulties they experience, such as being bullied, missing subtle social cues, and following and maintaining conversations. Strategies for supporting social interactions are highlighted.

David Mank, Director

886 Developing and Writing IEPs Under the New IDEA
LRP Publications
P.O. Box 24668
West Palm Beach, FL 33416

215-784-0860
800-515-4577
Fax: 215-784-9639
TTY: 215-658-0938
e-mail: custserve@lrp.com
www.lrp.com

Addresses the new IEP content and IEP team requirements by explaining the new provisions, providing context and background to the changes, and predicting their potential impact on special education programs.

2005 90 minutes
Kenneth F. Kahn, President

887 Educating Students with Autism: Implementa tion of Applied Bahavior Analysis
LRP Publications
P.O. Box 24668
West Palm Beach, FL 33416

215-784-0860
800-515-4577
Fax: 215-784-9639
TTY: 215-658-0938
e-mail: custserve@lrp.com
www.lrp.com

During this taped audio conference, behavior and autism consultant Dr Susan Catlett discusses the practical aspects of using ABA in your public school programs for students with autism spectrum disorders.

2006 90 Minutes
Kenneth F. Kahn, President

888 Getting Started with Facilitated Communica tion
Syracuse University, Institute On Communication
230 Huntington Hall
Syracuse, NY 13244

315-443-4752
Fax: 315-443-2258
e-mail: ICIstaff@syr.edu
soe.syr.edu/centers_institutes/institute_communicati

Describes in detail how to help individuals with autism and/or severe communication difficulties to get started with facilitated communication.

Videotape
Christine Ashby, Director
Douglas Biklen, Senior Researcher
Dani Weinstein, Administrative Secretary

889 How I Am (Wie Ich Bin)
Fanlight Productions
32 Court Street, 21st Floor
Brooklyn, NY 11201   718-488-8900
                                      800-876-1710
                                      Fax: 718-488-8642
                                      e-mail: info@fanlight.com
                                      www.fanlight.com

With the dreams and fears of a teenager, but wisdom beyond his years, Patrick takes us into his emotional world through the words he painstakingly types into his computer.

49 Minutes DVD
ISBN: 1-572955-05-8

890 I Want My Little Boy Back
Autism Treatment Center of America
2080 S Undermountain Road
Sheffield, MA 1257   413-229-2100
                                      877-766-7473
                                      Fax: 413-229-8931
                                      e-mail: information@son-rise.org
                                      www.autismtreatmentcenter.org

This BBC documentary follows an English family with a child with autism before, during and after their time at the Son Rise Program. It uniquely captures the heart of the Son Rise Program and is extremely useful in understanding our techniques.

1981 379 pages Video
ISBN: 0-449201-08-2

Barry Neil Kaufman, Co-Founder
Kate Wilde, Group Facilitator
Samahria Lyte Kaufman, Founder

891 Sense of Belonging: Including Students with Autism in Their School Community
Indiana Resource Center for Autism
1905 North Range Rd.
Bloomington, IN 47408   812-855-9630
                                      Fax: 812-855-6508
                                      e-mail: iidc@indiana.edu
                                      www.iidc.indiana.edu

Highlights the efforts of two elementary and one middle school in Indiana in teaching students with autism in general education settings.

20 minutes

David Mank, Director

892 Two Worlds - One Planet
Fanlight Productions
32 Court Street, 21st Floor
Brooklyn, NY 11201   718-488-8900
                                      800-876-1710
                                      Fax: 718-488-8642
                                      e-mail: info@fanlight.com
                                      www.fanlight.com

This documentary brings Autism syndrome out of the shadows, stressing that young people with developmental disabilities can learn and grow, if their individual needs, styles, and abilities are respected. It takes an upbeat look at students attending a private day school.

62 minutes DVD
ISBN: 1-572954-99-X

893 Understanding Autism
Fanlight Productions
32 Court Street, 21st Floor
Brooklyn, NY 11201   718-488-8900
                                      800-876-1710
                                      Fax: 718-488-8642
                                      e-mail: info@fanlight.com
                                      www.fanlight.com

Parents of children with autism discuss the nature and symptoms of this lifelong disability, and outline a treatment program based on behavior modification principles. ISBN: DVD: 1-57295-951-7; VHS: 1-572951-11-1

19 minutes DVD or VHS

Kelli English, Publicity Coordinator

894 We've Climbed Mountains: Increasing Our Un derstanding of Autism Spectrum Disorders
Indiana Resource Center for Autism
1905 North Range Rd.
Bloomington, IN 47408   812-855-6508
                                      Fax: 812-855-9630
                                      TTY: 812-855-9396
                                      e-mail: iidc@indiana.edu
                                      www.iidc.indiana.edu

Provides general information about autism spectrum disorders with the hope of increasing overall awareness, especially about those with high-functioning autism/Asperger's syndrome. Specific topics addressed include sensory challenges, social understanding, and responses to the diagnosis.

David Mank, Director

Web Sites

895 Asperger Syndrome Education Network
9 Aspen Circle
Edison, NJ 8820   732-321-0880
                                      e-mail: aspenorg@aol.com
                                      www.aspennj.org

Regionally based nonprofit organization headquartered in NJ, with 12 local chapters, providing for families and those individuals affected with Asperger Syndrome, PDD-NOS, High Function Autism, and related disorders.

Lori Shery, President
Rich Meleo, Vice President
Elizabeth Yamashita, Vice President

896 Autism Network International
P.O. Box 35448
Syracuse, NY 13235   e-mail: webmaster@autreat.com.
                        www.autreat.com

An autistic-run self-help and advocacy organization for autistic people.

897 Autism Network for Dietary Intervention
www.autismndi.com

Providing help and support for families using a gluten and casein free diet in the treatment of autism and related developmental disabilities.

898 Autism Research Institute
4182 Adams Avenue
San Diego, CA 92116   www.autism.com

Provides information based on research to parents and professionals throughout the world.

Stephen Edelson, Executive Director
Jane Johnson, Managing Director
Rebecca McKenney, Office Manager

899 Autism Resources
www.autism-resources.com

Offers information and links regarding the developmental dsabilities of autism and aspergers syndrome.

900 Autism Society of America
4340 East-West Hwy, Suite 350
Bethesda, ML 20814   301-657-0881
                                      800-328-8476
                                      e-mail: info@autism-society.org
                                      www.autism-society.org

Information regarding autism.

James Ball, Executive Chair
Anne Holmes, Vice Chair
Lars Perner, Secretary

901 Autism Speaks
1 East 33rd Street, 4th Floor
New York, NY 10016
                                      212-252-8584
                                      888-288-4762
                                 Fax: 212-252-8676
              e-mail: familyservices@autismspeaks.org
                                 www.autismspeaks.org

Information about Autism Research.

Liz Field, President
Lisa Goring, Executive Vice President
Alec M Elbert, Chief Strategy Officer

902 Center for the Study of Autism
www.autism.org

Information about autism to parents and professionals.

903 Community Services for Autistic Adults & Children (CSAAC)
8615 East Village Avenue
Montgomery Village, MD 20886
                                      240-912-2220
                                 Fax: 301-926-9384
                                      www.csaac.org

Information about autism to parents and professionals.

Ian Paregol, Executive Director
Don Rodrick, Chief Financial Officer
Marcee Smith, Assistant Executive Director

904 Families for Early Autism Treatment
P. O. Box 255722
Sacramento, CA 95865   www.feat.org

Information about autism.

905 Institute on Communication and Inclusion
230 Huntington Hall
Syracuse, NY 13244
                                      315-443-4752
                                 Fax: 315-443-2258
                             e-mail: ICIstaff@syr.edu
          soe.syr.edu/centers_institutes/institute_communicati

College offering facilitated learning research into communication
with persons who have autism or severe disabilities. Offers
books, videos and public awareness information on the research
projects.

Christine Ashby, Director
Douglas Biklen, Senior Researcher
Dani Weinstein, Administrative Secretary

906 Online Mendelian Inheritance in Man
National Library of Medicine, Building 38A
Bethesda, MD 20894
                                      888-346-3656
                           e-mail: info@ncbi.nlm.nih.gov
                                      www.ncbi.nlm.nih.gov

This database is a catalog of human genes and genetic disorders.

Christine E. Seidman, M.D., Chair
David J. Lipman, M.D., Executive Secretary

**907 University Students with Autism and Asperger's Syndrome
Web Site**
www.users.dircon.co.uk/~cns

                                      207-704-7450
                                      77- 56- 774
                                 Fax: 207-359-9440
                          e-mail: judith.kerem@nas.org.uk
                                 www.users.dircon.co.uk/~cns

Helps to develop and understanding of the difficulties people
with Asperger Syndrome may face. We also work on a one to one
basis with the student and liase with staff and peers. help is also
given in setting up support networks such as mentors and providing effective strategies to aid independent learning.

Book Publishers

908 ABA Program Companion
Autism Society of North Carolina Bookstore
505 Oberlin Road, Suite 230
Raleigh, NC 27605
                                      919-743-0204
                                      800-442-2762
                                 Fax: 919-743-0208
                      e-mail: books@autismsociety-nc.org
                                 www.autismbookstore.com

A guide developed to help educational teams organize an implement Applied Behavior Analysis (ABA) programs, including
home, school, and center-based programs.

909 Activity Schedules for Children with Autism
Autism Society of North Carolina Bookstore
505 Oberlin Road, Suite 230
Raleigh, NC 27605
                                      919-743-0204
                                      800-442-2762
                                 Fax: 919-743-0208
                      e-mail: books@autismsociety-nc.org
                                 www.autismbookstore.com

Written to help parents and professionals utilize activity schedules to promote independence in children in a variety of settings.

910 Al Capone Does My Shirts: A Novel
Autism Society of North Carolina Bookstore
505 Oberlin Road, Suite 230
Raleigh, NC 27605
                                      919-743-0204
                                      800-442-2762
                                 Fax: 919-743-0208
                      e-mail: books@autismsociety-nc.org
                                 www.autismbookstore.com

Set in 1935, this colorful novels tells the story of Matthew
'Moose' Flanagan, a 12-year-old boy who moves with his family
(including sister with autism) to Alcatraz Island. For readers age
12 and up.

**911 Autism Acceptance Book: Being A Friend to Someone With
Autism**
Autism Society of North Carolina Bookstore
505 Oberlin Road, Suite 230
Raleigh, NC 27605
                                      919-743-0204
                                      800-442-2762
                                 Fax: 919-743-0208
                      e-mail: books@autismsociety-nc.org
                                 www.autismbookstore.com

Colorfully illustrated activity book was created to help
neurotypical children learn about autism spectrum disorder
(ASD) and the characteristics that make kids with ASD unique.
For readers age 6 and up.

912 Autism Spectrum Disorders: The Complete Guide
Autism Society of North Carolina Bookstore
505 Oberlin Road, Suite 230
Raleigh, NC 27605
                                      919-743-0204
                                      800-442-2762
                                 Fax: 919-743-0208
                      e-mail: books@autismsociety-nc.org
                                 www.autismbookstore.com

Written to help parents, professionals, and other members of the
community learn more about autism spectrum disorder (ASD),
and it presents a thorough overview of the disorder, from diagnosis through adulthood.

913 Autism and Learning
David Fulton Publishers
2 Park Square, Milton Park
Abingdon, 0X14 4RN,
United Kingdom
                                      207-017-7913
                                 Fax: 207-017-6707
                      e-mail: mail@fultonpublisher.co.uk
                      http://catalogue.fultonpublishers.co.uk

This book is about how a cognitive perception on the way in
which individuals with autism think and learn may be applied to
particular curriculum areas.

1997 180 pages Paperback
ISBN: 1-853464-21-X

914 Autism and the Family: Problems, Prospects and Coping with the Disorder
Charles C Thomas Publishing
2600 S 1st Street
Springfield, IL 62704
217-789-8980
800-258-8980
Fax: 217-789-9130
e-mail: books@ccthomas.com
www.ccthomas.com

Examination of certain issues such as stress, coping and stigma. Contains 33 interviews with parents whose children attended an autistic treatment center. An excellent resource text.

1998 210 pages Softcover
ISBN: 0-398068-43-7

915 Autism as an Executive Director
Oxford University Press
2001 Evans Road
Cary, NC 27513
919-677-0977
800-445-9714
Fax: 919-677-1303
e-mail: custserv.us@oup.com
www.us.oup.com

Provides a new and conroversial perspective from some of the leading researchers in this field.

1998 328 pages
ISBN: 0-198523-49-1

916 Autism: Effective Biomedical Treatments
Autism Society of North Carolina Bookstore
505 Oberlin Road, Suite 230
Raleigh, NC 27605
919-743-0204
Fax: 919-743-0208
e-mail: books@autismsociety-nc.org
www.autismbookstore.com

Written for clinicians, professionals, and parents who would like to understand more about specific biomedical treatments for autism spectrum disorder (ASD).

917 Autism: From Tragedy to Triumph
Branden Publishing Company
17 Station Street
Brookline Village, MA 02447
617-734-2045
Fax: 617-734-2046
e-mail: branden@branden.com
www.branden.com

A book that deals with the Lovaas method and includes a foreward by Dr. Ivar Lovaas. The book is broken down into two parts — the long road to diagnosis and then treatment.

ISBN: 0-828319-65-0

918 Autism: Mind and Brain
Oxford University Press
2001 Evans Road
Cary, NC 27513
919-677-0977
800-445-9714
Fax: 919-677-1303
e-mail: custserv.us@oup.com
www.us.oup.com

An important work describing the latest advances in autism research.

2004 320 pages
ISBN: 0-198529-24-4

919 Autism: The Facts
Oxford University Press
2001 Evans Road
Cary, NC 27513
919-677-0977
800-445-9714
Fax: 919-677-1303
e-mail: custserv.us@oup.com
www.us.oup.com

Contains valuable information for families and those afflicted with this condition.

1994 124 pages
ISBN: 0-192623-27-3

920 Beyond the Autism Diagnosis: A Professiona l's Guide to Helping Families
Autism Society of North Carolina Bookstore
505 Oberlin Road, Suite 230
Raleigh, NC 27605
919-743-0204
Fax: 919-743-0208
e-mail: books@autismsociety-nc.org
www.autismbookstore.com

Helps to change the way professionals communicate with parents of children with autism spectrum disorder (ASD), making the experience more effective and meaningful for all involved.

921 Children With Autism: A Parents Guide
Peytral Publications
P.O. Box 1162
Minnetonka, MN 55345
952-949-8707
877-739-8725
Fax: 952-906-9777
e-mail: help@peytral.com
www.peytral.com

Informative handbook for parents of children and teens; covers medical, educational, legal, family life, daily care, emotional issues and more.

456 pages

922 Children wIth Starving Brains
Autism Society of North Carolina Bookstore
505 Oberlin Road, Suite 230
Raleigh, NC 27605
919-743-0204
800-442-2762
Fax: 919-743-0208
e-mail: books@autismsociety-nc.org
www.autismbookstore.com

Written by an experienced physician who is the grandmother of a child with autism spectrum disorder (ASD), this book takes a biomedical approach toward the treatment of ASD.

Eric Schopler, Editor
Gary Mesibov, Co-Editor

923 Children with Autism and Asperger Syndrome A Guide for Practitioners and Carers
John Wiley & Sons
10475 Crosspoint Blvd
Indianapolis, IN 46256
877-762-2974
Fax: 800-597-3299
www.wiley.com

Covers the disorders of autism, understanding the causes and the different approaches of treatment for autistic children.

1999 342 pages
ISBN: 0-471983-28-4

924 Children with Autism: A Developmental Perspective
Harvard University Press
79 Garden Street
Cambridge, MA 02138
401-531-2800
800-405-1619
Fax: 401-531-2801
e-mail: hup@harvard.edu
www.hup.harvard.edu

Offers a rare close look at the mysterious condition that afflicts approximately 350,000 Americans and millions more.

1997
ISBN: 0-674053-13-3

925 Cowden Preautism Observation Inventory
Jo E. Cowden, author

Charles C Thomas Publisher
2600 S 1st Street
Springfield, IL 62704
217-789-8980
800-258-8980
Fax: 217-789-9130
e-mail: books@ccthomas.com
www.ccthomas.com

Contains effective intervention activities for sensory motor stimulation and joint attention.

226 pages
ISBN: 0-398086-43-5

Sue F V Rakow, Co-Author
Carol B Carpenter, Co-Author

926 Diagnosis Autism: Now What? 10 Steps to Improve Treatment Outcomes
Autism Society of North Carolina Bookstore
505 Oberlin Road, Suite 230
Raleigh, NC 27605
919-743-0204
800-442-2762
Fax: 919-743-0208
e-mail: books@autismsociety-nc.org
www.autismbookstore.com

Practical guide was written to help parents of children with autism spectrum disorder (ASD) form successful pediatric partnerships with physicians and other healthcare practitioners involved in their child's diagnosis and treatment.

927 Different Like Me: My Book of Autism Heroe s
Autism Society of North Carolina Bookstore
505 Oberlin Road, Suite 230
Raleigh, NC 27605
919-743-0204
800-442-2762
Fax: 919-743-0208
e-mail: books@autismsociety-nc.org
www.autismbookstore.com

This beautifully illustrated children's book tells the tales of many famous people throughout history who all had on thing in common: they didn't fit in. It's also possible they may have had autism spectrum disorder (ASD). For readers ages 7-12.

928 Does My Child Have Autism?
Autism Society of North Carolina Bookstore
505 Oberlin Road, Suite 230
Raleigh, NC 27605
919-743-0204
800-442-2762
Fax: 919-743-0208
e-mail: books@autismsociety-nc.org
www.autismbookstore.com

Written for parents of children age three and younger who have concerns about their child's development.

929 Education and Care for Adolescents and Adults with Autism
Kate Wall, author

Hamill Institute on Disabilities
2455 Teller Road
Thousand Oaks, CA 91320
800-818-7243
Fax: 800-583-2665
e-mail: info@sagepub.com
www.sagepub.com

Uses case studies and examples that show the reader how to put theory into practice in multi-disciplinary settings, this book clearly explains how changes in policy and provision have affected how young people and adults with autism are cared for and educated. With highlights of up-to-date and accessible information on the nature and affects of ASD, legislation information, family issues, positive intervention programs, and strategies. Hardcover or paperback.

2007 168 pages Paperback
ISBN: 1-412923-82-8

Sara Miller McCune, Founder/Chairman
Blaise R Simqu, President/CEO
Chris Hickok, Senior Vice President/CFO

930 Everybody is Different: A Book for Young P eople
Autism Society of North Carolina Bookstore
505 Oberlin Road, Suite 230
Raleigh, NC 27605
919-743-0204
800-442-2762
Fax: 919-743-0208
e-mail: books@autismsociety-nc.org
www.autismbookstore.com

Written for brothers and sisters of young persons with autism spectrum disorder (ASD). It not only explains the basic characterisitics of ASD, but also answers the questions often asked by a sibling of a child with ASD. For readers ages 8-16.
Hardbound

931 Everyday Solutions: A Practical Guide for Families of Children with Autism
Autism Society of North Carolina Bookstore
505 Oberlin Road, Suite 230
Raleigh, NC 27605
919-743-0204
800-442-2762
Fax: 919-743-0208
e-mail: books@autismsociety-nc.org
www.autismbookstore.com

Presents 37 everyday situations that may present difficulties for a child with autism spectrum disorder (ASD), along with recommendations and strategies.

932 Functional Behavior Assessment for People with Autism
Autism Society of North Carolina Bookstore
505 Oberlin Road, Suite 230
Raleigh, NC 27605
919-743-0204
800-442-2762
Fax: 919-743-0208
e-mail: books@autismsociety-nc.org
www.autismbookstore.com

provides and introduction to functional behavior assessment (FBA). FBA is a valuable tool that can be used by parents and professionals to understand and address the challenging behaviors of persons with autism spectrum disorder (ASD).

933 Handbook of Autism and Pervasive Developme ntal Disorders
Autism Society of North Carolina Bookstore
505 Oberlin Road, Suite 230
Raleigh, NC 27605
919-743-0204
800-442-2762
Fax: 919-743-0208
e-mail: books@autismsociety-nc.org
www.autismbookstore.com

Two-volume scholarly resource presents the latest scientific research on autism spectrum disorders (ASD).

934 Healthcare for Children on the Autism Spectrum
Autism Society of North Carolina Bookstore
505 Oberlin Road, Suite 230
Raleigh, NC 27605
919-743-0204
800-442-2762
Fax: 919-743-0208
e-mail: books@autismsociety-nc.org
www.autismbookstore.com

The first publication of its kind to focus on the health and medical care of children with autism spectrum disorder (ASD).

935 Helping Children with Autism Learn
Oxford University Press
2001 Evans Road
Cary, NC 27513
919-677-0977
800-445-9714
Fax: 919-677-1303
e-mail: custserv.us@oup.com
www.us.oup.com

A leading authority on autism offers practical, reliable advice on coping with learning disorders associated with autism.
2003 512 pages
ISBN: 0-195138-11-2

936 Ian's Walk: A Story About Autism
Autism Society of North Carolina Bookstore
505 Oberlin Road, Suite 230
Raleigh, NC 27605
919-743-0204
800-442-2762
Fax: 919-743-0208
e-mail: books@autismsociety-nc.org
www.autismbookstore.com

In this moving fictional story, a young girl named Julie realizes how much she cares for her brother, Ian, who has autism spectrum disorder (ASD). For readers ages 4-8.

937 Incredible 5-Point Scale
Autism Society of North Carolina Bookstore
505 Oberlin Road, Suite 230
Raleigh, NC 27605
919-743-0204
800-442-2762
Fax: 919-743-0208
e-mail: books@autismsociety-nc.org
www.autismbookstore.com

Shows parents and professionals how to implement a simple
5-point scale to help students with sutism spectrum disorder
(ASD) understand and control their emotional responses and
behavior.

**938 Just Take a Bite: Easy, Effective Answers to Food Aversions
and Eating Challenges**
Autism Society of North Carolina Bookstore
505 Oberlin Road, Suite 230
Raleigh, NC 27605
919-743-0204
800-442-2762
Fax: 919-743-0208
e-mail: books@autismsociety-nc.org
www.autismbookstore.com

A much-need resource that specifically addresses the eating challenges of children who may have autism spectrum disorder
(ASD), sensory processing disorder (SPD), or other developmental delays.

939 Kids In the Syndrome Mix
Autism Society of North Carolina Bookstore
505 Oberlin Road, Suite 230
Raleigh, NC 27605
919-743-0204
800-442-2762
Fax: 919-743-0208
e-mail: books@autismsociety-nc.org
www.autismbookstore.com

Children with autism spectrum disorder (ASD) often have coexisting neuropsychiatric diagnoses, and this handbook focuses on
the most common neuropsychiatric disorders and their symptoms.

940 Looking After Louis
Autism Society of North Carolina
505 Oberlin Road, Suite 230
Raleigh, NC 27605
919-743-0204
800-442-2762
Fax: 919-743-0208
e-mail: books@autismsociety-nc.org
www.autismbookstore.com

Colrfully illustrated fictional story introduces readers to Louis, a
new boy in school who has autism spectrum disorder (ASD). Told
from the perspective of a female classmate, the story describes
how Louis plays and interacts with students and teachers in a general education classroom. For readers ages 4-8.

941 Mindblindness: An Essay on Autism & Theory of Mind
MIT Press
55 Hayward Street
Cambridge, MA 02142
617-253-5646
800-405-1619
Fax: 617-258-6779
e-mail: mitpress-order-inq@mit.edu
http://mitpress.mit.edu

Interpretations and research into the theory of mindblindness in
children with autism.
1995 208 pages
ISBN: 0-262023-84-9

Ellen W Faran, Director
Rebecca Schrader, Associate Director

942 Miracle to Believe In
Fawcett

A group of people from all walks of life come together and are
transformed as they reach out, under the direction of the
Kaufmans, to help a little boy the medical world has given up as
hopeless. The heartwarming journey of loving a child back to life
will not only inspire you, the reader, but presents a compelling
new way to deal with life's traumas and difficulties.

1982 384 pages
ISBN: 0-449201-08-2

943 My Brother Sammy
Autism Society of North Carolina Bookstore
505 Oberlin Road, Suite 230
Raleigh, NC 27605
919-743-0204
800-442-2762
Fax: 919-743-0208
e-mail: books@autismsociety-nc.org
www.autismbookstore.com

Filled with beautiful watercolor illustrations, this book tells the
fictional story of Sammy, a young boy with autism spectrum disorder (ASD). The story is told from the perspective of Sammy's
older brother, who is sometimes frustrated by Sammy's behavior.
For readers ages 4-8.

944 My Friend With Autism
Autism Society of North Carolina Bookstore
505 Oberlin Road, Suite 230
Raleigh, NC 27605
919-743-0204
800-442-2762
Fax: 919-743-0208
e-mail: books@autismsociety-nc.org
www.autismbookstore.com

Created for teachers and students in her son's elementary school
class. The book is a valuable tool for helping typical children understand the traits and behaviors of their classmates with autism
spectrum disorder (ASD). For readers ages 4-10.

945 My Social Stories Book
Autism Society of North Carolina Bookstore
505 Oberlin Road, Suite 230
Raleigh, NC 27605
919-743-0204
800-442-2762
Fax: 919-743-0208
e-mail: books@autismsociety-nc.org
www.autismbookstore.com

The Social Stones in this book are written for children with autism spectrum disorder (ASD) ages 2 to 6, and they include over
150 everyday situations that are frequently encountered in early
childhood.

946 Neurobiology of Autism
Johns Hopkins University Press
2715 N Charles Street
Baltimore, MD 21218
410-516-6900
800-537-5487
Fax: 410-516-6998
e-mail: webmaster@press.jhu.edu
www.press.jhu.edu

This book discusses recent advances in scientific research that
point to a neurobiological basis for autism and examines the clinical implications of this research.

2006 424 pages
ISBN: 0-801880-47-5

Alfred R Berkeley, Chairman

947 Parenting Across the Autism Spectrum
Autism Society of North Carolina Bookstore
505 Oberlin Road, Suite 230
Raleigh, NC 27605
919-743-0204
800-442-2762
Fax: 919-743-0208
e-mail: books@autismsociety-nc.org
www.autismbookstore.com

Two mothers who have children on the opposite ends of the autism spectrum wrote this poignant and insightful book, and the
book also provides a look at what lies beyond the early intervention and elementary school years.

948 **Positive Behavioral Strategies to Support Children & Young People with Autism**

Martin Hanbury, author

Hamill Institute on Disabilities/Sage Publications
2455 Teller Road
Thousand Oaks, CA 91320
800-818-7243
Fax: 800-583-2665
e-mail: info@sagepub.com
www.sagepub.com

Offers advice on understanding and managing childrens' often challenging actions. Covering a range from birth to 19 years, this resource provides: practical advice on developing an appropriate learning environement; INSET materials for developing behavior management practices; self-audit tools for practioners; and reproducables and practical resources. Hardcover or paperback.

2007 120 pages Paperback
ISBN: 1-412929-11-0

Sara Miller McCune, Founder/Chairman
Blaise R Simqu, President/CEO
Chris Hickok, Senior Vice President/CFO

949 **Preschool Issues in Autism**

Plenum Publishing Corporation
233 Spring Street
New York, NY 10013
212-620-8000
Fax: 212-463-0742
www.springer.com

Combines some of the most important theory and data related to the early identifiction and intervention in autism and related disorders. Addresses clinical aspects, parental concerns and legal issues. Helps professionals understand and implement state-of-the-art services for young children and their families.

294 pages
ISBN: 0-306444-40-2

Derk Haank, CEO
Ulrich Vest, CFO
Martin Mos, COO

950 **Prescription for Success**

Autism Society of North Carolina Bookstore
505 Oberlin Road, Suite 230
Raleigh, NC 27605
919-743-0204
800-442-2762
Fax: 919-743-0208
e-mail: books@autismsociety-nc.org
www.autismbookstore.com

Written for medical professionals who work with patients who have autism spectrum disorder.

951 **Reaching the Autistic Child: A Parent Training Program**

Brookline Books/Lumen Editions
8 Trumbell Rd, Suite B-001
Northampton, MA 01060
413-584-0184
800-666-2665
Fax: 413-584-6184
e-mail: brbooks@yahoo.com
www.brooklinebooks.com

Detailed case studies of social and behavioral change in autistic children and their families show parents how to implement the principles for improved socialization and behavior.

1998 Softcover
ISBN: 1-571290-56-7

952 **Riddle of Autism: A Psychological Analysis**

Jason Aronson
4501 Forbes Blvd, Suite 200
Lanham, MD 20706
301-459-3366
800-462-6420
Fax: 301-429-5748
e-mail: custserv@rowman.com
www.aronson.com

Dr. Victor examines the myths that cloud an understanding of this disorder and describes the meanings of its specific behavioral symptoms.

356 pages Softcover
ISBN: 1-568215-73-8

953 **Social Skills Picture Book**

Autism Society of North Carolina Bookstore
505 Oberlin Road, Suite 230
Raleigh, NC 27605
919-743-0204
800-442-2762
Fax: 919-743-0208
e-mail: books@autismsociety-nc.org
www.autismbookstore.com

(Teaching Play, Emotions, and Communication to Children with Autism). Through photographs and conversation bubbles, the author demonstrates approximately 30 social skilld in the areas of communication, play, and emotion.

954 **Solving Behavior Problems in Autism**

Autism Society of North Carolina Bookstore
505 Oberlin Road, Suite 230
Raleigh, NC 27605
919-743-0204
800-442-2762
Fax: 919-743-0208
e-mail: books@autismsociety-nc.org
www.autismbookstore.com

In this guide, the author explains how to use effective communication techniques to reduce problem behaviors in persons with autism spectrum disorder (ASD).

955 **Son-Rise: The Miracle Continues**

Describes an effective, loving and respectful method for treating children with autism. It documents the development of the Son Rise Program throught the record of Raun Kaufman's astonishing development from a lifeless, autistic, retarded child into a highly verbal, loveable youngster with no traces of his former condition. It further details Raun's extraordinary progress from the age of four into young adulthood. It also shares moving accounts of five families who successfully used the program.

1995 384 pages
ISBN: 0-915811-61-8

956 **Stress and Coping in Autism**

Oxford University Press
2001 Evans Road
Cary, NC 27513
919-677-0977
800-445-9714
Fax: 919-677-1303
e-mail: custserv.us@oup.com
www.us.oup.com

Provides a theoretical framework for the usefukness of the stress construct in understanding and treating autism.

2006 472 pages
ISBN: 0-195182-26-X

957 **Taking Autism to School**

Autism Society of North Carolina Bookstore
505 Oberlin Road, Suite 230
Raleigh, NC 27605
919-743-0204
800-442-2762
Fax: 919-743-0208
e-mail: books@autismsociety-nc.org
www.autismbookstore.com

A fictional story about a girl named Angel and her friendship woth Sam, a classmate who has autism spectrum disorder (ASD). From her own point of view, Angel explains how Sam thinks and behaves in school and at home. For readers ages 5-10.

958 **Teaching Children with Autism to Mind-Read A Pratical Guide for Teachers & Parents**

John Wiley & Sons
10475 Crosspoint Blvd
Indianapolis, IN 46256
877-762-2974
Fax: 800-597-3299
www.wiley.com

This book explains the Theory of Mind, which is the ability to infer other's mental states and then interpret their speech and actions based on this information. The author applies this theory to autistic children to help their social and communicative abnormalities.

1999 302 pages
ISBN: 0-471976-23-7

959   Teaching Coversations to Children With Autism: Scripts and Script Fading
Autism Society of North Carolina Bookstore
505 Oberlin Road, Suite 230
Raleigh, NC 27605   919-743-0204
                                             800-442-2762
                                        Fax: 919-743-0208
                        e-mail: books@autismsociety-nc.org
                                  www.autismbookstore.com

Uses the principles of Apllied Behavior Analysis (ABA) to create strategies that facilitate communication in children who have autism spectrum disorder.

960   Ten Things Every Child With Autism Wishes You Know
Autism Society of North Carolina Bookstore
505 Oberlin Road, Suite 230
Raleigh, NC 27605   919-743-0204
                                             800-442-2762
                                        Fax: 919-743-0208
                        e-mail: books@autismsociety-nc.org
                                  www.autismbookstore.com

Describes how children with autism spectrum disorder (ASD) function and what they are trying to say to the world when they cannot always express it in a conventional way.

961   The Neurology of Autism
Oxford University Press
2001 Evans Road
Cary, NC 27513   919-677-0977
                                             800-445-9714
                                        Fax: 919-677-1303
                              e-mail: custserv.us@oup.com
                                            www.us.oup.com

A valuable resource for both the latest information from basic-science research and its application to the diagnosis and treatment of autism.

2005 272 pages
ISBN: 0-195182-22-7

962   Toilet Training for Individuals with Autism and Related Disorders
Autism Society of North Carolina Bookstore
505 Oberlin Road, Suite 230
Raleigh, NC 27605   919-743-0204
                                             800-442-2762
                                        Fax: 919-743-0208
                        e-mail: books@autismsociety-nc.org
                                  www.autismbookstore.com

Comprehensive guide for parents and professionals provides over 200 toilet training tips and more than 40 helpful case examples.

963   Treasure Chest of Behavioral Strategies for Individuals with Autism
Autism Society of North Carolina Bookstore
505 Oberlin Road, Suite 230
Raleigh, NC 27605   919-743-0204
                                             800-442-2762
                                        Fax: 919-743-0208
                        e-mail: books@autismsociety-nc.org
                                  www.autismbookstore.com

Comprehensive resource manual provides parents and teachers with numerous behavior management strategies for individuals with autism spectrum disorder (ASD).

964   Understanding and Treating Children with Autism
John Wiley & Sons
10475 Crosspoint Blvd
Indianapolis, IN 46256   877-762-2974
                                        Fax: 800-597-3299
                                            www.wiley.com

Aimed at those concerned with the education and welfare of the children with autism, particularly at teachers in Special education and the psychologists and care professionals who work with teachers and parents of children with autism.

1995 188 pages
ISBN: 0-471958-88-3

965   Visual Strategies for Improving Communicat ion
Autism Society of North Carolina Bookstore
505 Oberlin Road, Suite 230
Raleigh, NC 27605   919-743-0204
                                             800-442-2762
                                        Fax: 919-743-0208
                        e-mail: books@autismsociety-nc.org
                                  www.autismbookstore.com

This how-to manual describes a communication intervention strategy for teaching persons with autism spectrum disorder (ASD) that evolved from learning style research.

966   World of the Autistic Child
Oxford University Press
2001 Evans Road
Cary, NC 27513   919-677-0977
                                             800-445-9714
                                        Fax: 919-677-1303
                          e-mail: custserv.us@oup.com
                                            www.us.oup.com

Comprehensive guide for parents with children diagnosed or suspected of being autistic. Includes current thinking on causes, diagnosis, and treatment, using illustrative case studies.

1998 368 pages
ISBN: 0-195119-17-7

Magazines

967   Autism Advocate
Autism Society of America
4340 East-West Hwy, Suite 350
Bethesda, ML 20814   301-657-0881
                                             800-328-8476
                          e-mail: info@autism-society.org
                                      www.autism-society.org

Gathers a diverse collection of the latest autism news, chapter highlights, first-person accounts of families living with and growing with autism, and tips from paretns and professionals. Published 5 times a year.

James Ball, Executive Chair
Anne Holmes, Vice Chair
Lars Perner, Secretary

968   Newslink
Autism Society Ontario
4340 East-West Hwy, Suite 350
Bethesda, ML 20814
M6K 3C5   301-657-0881
                                             800-328-8476
                                        Fax: 416-246-9417
                          e-mail: info@autism-society.org
                                      www.autism-society.org

Covers society activities and contains information on autism. Recurring features include news of research, a calendar of events, reports of meetings, and book reviews.

10 pages
James Ball, Executive Chair
Anne Holmes, Vice Chair
Lars Perner, Secretary

Journals

969   Focus on Autism and Other Developmental Disabilities
Hammill Institute on Disabilities/Sage Publication
2455 Teller Road
Thousand Oaks, CA 91320   800-818-7243
                                        Fax: 800-583-2665
                          e-mail: journals@sagepub.com
                                            www.sagepub.com

Practical elements of management, treatment, planning and education for persons with autism or other pervasive developmental disabilities. FOCUS publishes articles representing diverse philosophical and theoretical positions and reflecting a wide range of disciplines, inclusing, education, psychology, psychiatry, medicine, physical therapy, occupational therapy, speech/language pathology and related areas. ISSN: Print: 0885-7288; Electronic: 1538-4837

Quarterly

970   The Journal of Positive Behavior Intervent ions
Hamill Institute on Disabilities/Sage Publications
2455 Teller Road
Thousand Oaks, CA 91320   800-818-7243
                                          Fax: 800-583-2665
                                    e-mail: journals@sagepub.com
                                             www.sagepub.com

The JPBI offers sound, research-based principles of positive behavior support for use in school, home, and community settings with people with challenges in bahvior adaptations. JPBI is an official journal of the Association of Positive Behavior Support. Subscriptions: Institutional - Print Only $146, Institutional - Print & E-access $149, Individual - Print & E-access $57.

Quarterly

V Mark Durand, PhD, Co-Editor
Robert L Koegel, PhD, Co-Editor

971   The Journal of Special Education
Hamill Institute on Disabilities/Sage Publications
2455 Teller Road
Thousand Oaks, CA 91320   800-818-7243
                                          Fax: 800-583-2665
                                    e-mail: journals@sagepub.com
                                             www.sagepub.com

For four decades professionals have relied on the JSE'for timely, sound research in the area of special education. JSE provides reseach articles and scholarly review by expert authors in all subspecialties of special education for individuals with disabilities ranging from mild to severe. JSE is an official journal of the Division for Research of the CEC. Subscriptions: Institutional - Print Only $172, Institutional - Print & E-access $176, Individual - Print & E-access $57.

Quarterly

Bob Algozzine, PhD, Co-Editor
Fred Spooner, PhD, Co-Editor

Newsletters

972   Autism Research Review International
Autism Research Institute
4182 Adams Avenue
San Diego, CA 92116   619-281-7165
                                          Fax: 619-563-6840
                                             www.autism.com

Discusses current research and provides information about the causes, diagnosis, and treatment of autism and related disorders.

8 pages Quarterly

Stephen Edelson, Executive Director
Jane Johnson, Managing Director
Rebecca McKenney, Office Manager

973   MAAP Newsletter
PO Box 524
Crown Point, IN 46308   219-662-1311
                                          Fax: 219-662-0638
                                    e-mail: chart@netnitco.net
                                          www.maapservices.org

Shares information that are not find in textbooks or read in other sources.

Pamphlets

974   Autism Fact Sheet
NINDS
PO Box 5801
Bethesda, MD 20824   301-496-5751
                                              800-352-9424
                                         TTY: 301-468-5981
                                            www.ninds.nih.gov

Also available in Spanish.

Walter J. Koroshetz, M.D., Acting Director
Alan L. Willard, Ph.D., Acting Deputy Director
Caroline Lewis, Executive Officer

975   Facts About Autism
Indiana Institute on Disability and Community
1905 North Range Rd.
Bloomington, IN 47408   812-855-6508
                                              800-280-7010
                                          Fax: 812-855-9630
                                         TTY: 812-855-9396
                                     e-mail: iidc@indiana.edu
                                            www.iidc.indiana.edu

Provides concise information describing autism, diagnosis, needs of the person with autism from diagnosis through adulthood. Information on the Autism Society of America chapters in Indiana is listed in the back, along with a description of the Indiana Resource Center for Autism and suggested books to look for in the local library. Also available in Spanish.

17 pages

David Mank, Director
Suzie Rimstidt
Susan Gray

976   Pervasive Developmental Disorders
National Inst. of Neurological Disorders/Stroke
31 Center Drive, MSC 2540, Building 31, Room 8A06
Bethesda, MD 20892   301-496-5751
                                              800-352-9424

Detailed booklet that describes symptoms, causes, and treatments, with information on getting help and coping.

Camps

977   Anchor Point Camp
RBM Ministries
PO Box 128
Plainwell, MI 49080   269-342-9879
                              e-mail: bobgoodenough@sbcglobal.net
                                          www.rbmministries.org

Accepts mentally and physically handicapped children ages 13 and up.

Bob Goodenough, Executive Director

978   Beech Brook
3737 Lander Road
Cleveland, OH 44124   216-831-2255
                                              877-546-1225
                                          Fax: 216-831-0436
                                             www.beechbrook.org

A year-round residential and day treatment center, accepts summer residents when there are openings in the regular enrollment. The program is designed for emotionally disturbed, learning disabled and autistic children, providing therapeutically oriented teaching and programming techniques in a camp setting.

Don Harris, Director

979   Big Crystal Camp
8533 Williams Road
DeWitt, MI 48820   517-669-9367

One week residential camp sponsored by Lansing Area Chapter of Michigan Association for Children with Learning Disabilities.

Florence Curtis

980   Camp Buckskin
4124 Quebec Ave N, Ste 300
Minneapolis, MN 55427   763-208-4805
                                    Fax: 952-938-6996
                            e-mail: info@campbuckskin.com
                                    www.campbuckskin.com

LD and ADD/ADHD youth have often experienced frustration
and a lack of success. Buckskin assists these individuals to realize and develop the potentials and abilities which they possess.

Thomas R Bauer, CCD, Camp Director

981   Camp Friendship
Friendship Ventures
10509 108th Street NW
Annandale, MN 55302   952-852-0101
                                         800-450-8376
                                    Fax: 952-852-0123
                        e-mail: info@friendshipventures.org
                                 www.friendshipventures.org

Camp Friendship offers kids, teens, and adults the chance to have
the time of their lives. The program focuses on building self-esteem and independence, and practicing social skills; and we nurture each person's strengths and abilities and encourage
participation in activies at their own pace. Specially designed for
persons with developmental, physical or multiple disabilities, special medical conditions, Down syndrome, autism or other conditions. Weekend camps and longer available.

Georgann Rumsey, Vice President, Programs
Laurie Tschetter, Program Director

982   Camp Krem
102 Brook Lane
Boulder Creek, CA 95006   510-222-6662
                            e-mail: campkrem@gmail.com
                                 www.campingunlimited.com

Camp with year-around recreational activities and summer camping for children and adults with developmental disabilities.

983   Camp Lotsafun
3660 Baker Lane, Suite 103
Reno, NV 89509   775-827-3866
                                    Fax: 775-827-0334
                         e-mail: camp@camplotsafun.com
                                    www.camplotsafun.com

Provides recreational, therapeutic, and educational opportunities
for individuals with developmental disabilities, while providing
respite care for their families.

Jill Gabel, Program Director

984   Camp Merrimack
3320 Triana Boulevard
Huntsville, AL 35805   256-534-6455
                        e-mail: ksimari@merrimackhall.com
                                    www.merrimackhall.com

A unique arts half-day camp for children ages 3 through 12; open
to children with special needs including Cerebral Palsy, Down
Syndrome, autism and others.

Ashley Dinges, Executive Director
Kim Simari, Managing Director

985   Camp New Hope
Friendship Ventures
53035 Lake Avenue
McGregor, MN 55760   952-852-0101
                                         800-450-8376
                                    Fax: 952-852-0123
                           e-mail: fv@friendshipventures.org
                                 www.friendshipventures.org

Camp New Hope is a great place for children, teens, and adults to
have the time of their lives. The program provides a unique opportunity for having fun, learning skills, boosting confidence, and
making friends. Services are specifically designed for persons
with developmental, phyisical or multiple disabilities, special
medical needs, Down syndrome, autism, or other conditions.
Weekend camps and longer available. Other services available
throughout the year.

Georgann Rumsey, Vice President, Programs
Laurie Tschetter, Program Director

986   Camp Nuhop
404 Hillcrest Drive
Ashland, OH 44805   419-289-2227
                                    Fax: 419-289-2227
                            e-mail: info@campnuhop.org
                                    www.campnuhop.org

A summer residential program for any youngster from 6 to 18
with a learning disability, behavior disorder or Attention Deficit
Disorder. Sixty two campers and 35 staff members live on site in
groups of 7 campers to every 3 counselors. Activities focus on
positive self-concept and behaviors and teach children to learn
how to find their strengths, abilities and talents from a positive,
yet realistic viewpoint.

Jerry Dunlap, Director

987   Camp Ramah in New England Tikvah Program
39 Bennett Street
Palmer, MA 01609   413-283-9771
                                    Fax: 413-283-6661
                           e-mail: info@campramahne.org
                                    www.campramahne.org

The Tikvah program is one of the first summer programs for Jewish children with special needs. It continues to grow and evolve
as it strives to serve campers with a wide range of special needs
including, but not limited to, congitive impairments, autism, cerebral palsy and seizure disorder.

Howard Blas, Tikvah Program Director
Talya Kalender, Director, Camper Care
Benjamin Greene, Director of Education

988   Crotched Mountain School & Rehabilitation Center
1 Verney Drive
Greenfield, NH 03047   603-547-3311
                                         800-800-966
                                    Fax: 603-547-3232
                      e-mail: info@crotchedmountain.org
                                    www.cmf.org

Currently serves children ages 6-22 with multiple-handicaps including: Cerebral Palsy, Spina Bifida, visual and hearing impairments and neurological disabilities, developmental disorders,
mental retardation, autism, behavioral and emotional disorders,
seizure disorders, spinal cord and head injuries. Member of the
National Association of Independent Schools and accredited with
the NE Association of Schools and Colleges, Independent
Schools of Northern NE.

Rita Phinney, Director Admissions
John Young, Registrar

989   Dallas Academy
950 Tiffany Way
Dallas, TX 75218   214-324-1481
                                    Fax: 214-327-8537
                                    www.dallas-academy.com

7-week summer session for students who are having difficulty in
regular school classes.

Jim Richardson, Director

990   Developmental Center
6710 86th Avenue N
Pinellas Park, FL 33782   727-541-5716
                                    Fax: 727-544-8186
                          e-mail: infopp@centeracademy.com
                                    www.centeracademy.com

Specifically designed for the learning disabled child and other
children with difficulties in concentration, strategy, social skills,
impulsivity, distractibility and study strategies. Programs offered
include: attention training, visual-motor remediation, socialization skills training, relaxation training, horseback riding and
more. The day camp meets weekdays from 9-3 for 3,4 or 5 week
sessions.

Dr. Eric Larson

991   Eagle Hill School - Summer Program
242 Old Petersham Road, PO Box 116
Hardwick, MA 01037   413-477-6000
                                        Fax: 413-477-6837
                        e-mail: admission@eaglehillschool.com
                                            www.ehs1.org

For the child, age 9-19, with a specific learning disability or Attention Deficit Disorder, this summer program offers a structured curriculum designed to build a basic foundation of academic competence. Extracurricular and outdoor activities complement the educational program.

Erin E Wynne, Dean of Admission

992   Groves Academy
3200 Highway 100 South
Saint Louis Park, MN 55416   952-920-6377
                                        Fax: 952-920-2068
                                        www.grovesacademy.org

A nonprofit day school in Minnesota designed especially for children with learning differences. The Center has a full day academic program from September through June, as well as an 8 week summer program. Groves also offers community services such as: psychoeducational testing for children and adults, consulting services, workshops on learning disabilities and other special learning needs, and afternoon/evening tutorial services for children and adults.

John Alexander, Head of School

993   Hill School of Fort Worth
4817 Odessa Avenue
Fort Worth, TX   817-923-9482
                                        Fax: 817-923-4894
                            e-mail: hillschool@hillschool.org
                                            www.hillschool.org

Provides an alternative learning environment for students having average or above-average intelligence with learning differences. Hill school is an established leader in North Texas with a 25 year history of effectively serving LD children. Beginning in 1961 as a tutorial service, Hill became a formal school in 1973. Our mission is to help those who learn differently develop skills and strategies to succeed. We do this by developing academic/study skills, and self-discipline.

John W. Wright, Chairman
Randall Canedy, Vice Chairman
Audrey Boda-Davis, Executive Director

994   Kris' Camp
1132 Green Hill Trace
Tallahassee, FL 32317   801-942-1750
                                        Fax: 877-267-9451
                                e-mail: info@kriscamp.org
                                            www.kriscamp.org

Therapy intensive/respite camp for children with special needs (thus far focusing on children with autism/autistic-like challenges) and their families.

Michelle Hardy, Program Director
Leidy Van Ispelen, Assistant Director

995   Lab School of Washington Summer Program
4759 Reservoir Road NW
Washington, DC 20007   202-965-6600
                                        Fax: 202-965-5106
                    e-mail: alexandra.freeman@labschool.org
                                            www.labschool.org

The Lab School 5-week summer session includes individualized reading, spelling, writing, study skills, and math programs. A multisensory approach addresses the needs of bright learning disabled children. Related services such as speech/language therapy and occupational therapy are integrated into the curriculum. Elementary/Intermediate; Junior High/High School.

Sally Smith, Founder
Susan Feeley, Admissions Director

996   Maplebrook School
5142 Route 22
Amenia, NY 12501   845-373-8191
                                        Fax: 845-373-7029
                        e-mail: jscully@maplebrookschool.org
                                        www.maplebrookschool.org

A coeductional boarding school for students with learning differences and ADD. A New York State registered high school servicing ages 11-18. Post secondary options offered to 18-21.

Donna M Konkolios, Head of School
Jennifer Scully, Director Admissions

997   Round Lake Camp
21 Plymouth Street
Fairfield, NJ   973-575-3333
                                            800-776-5657
                                        Fax: 973-575-4188
                                e-mail: rlc@njycamps.org
                                            www.njycamps.org

For ages 7-18, this camp provides individualized academics in reading, language development and math for children with mild learning disabilities, Round Lake also offers therapeutic recreation and Jewish cultural values to its participants.

Sheira Director, Asst. Director

998   Squirrel Hollow
5665 Milam Road
Fairburn, GA 30213   770-774-8001
                                        Fax: 770-774-8005
                        e-mail: bbox@thebedfordschool.org
                                        www.thebedfordschool.org

A remedial summer program of The Bedford School; serves children with academic needs due to learning difficulties. For students ages 6-16 and held on the campus of The Bedford School in Fairburn, GA. Campers participate in an individualized academic program as well as recreational activities. Students receive the proper academic remediation as well as specific remedial help with physical skills, peer interaction and self-esteem.

Betsy E Box, Director
Jeff James, Assistant Director
Bonnie Sides, Administrative Secretary

999   Summer Experience
Vanguard School
PO Box 730
Paoli, PA 19301   610-296-6700
                                        Fax: 610-640-0132
                        e-mail: info@vanguardshool-pa.org
                                        www.vanguardschool-pa.org

For students who are experiencing learning difficulties due to neurological impairment, social/emotional disturbance and/or autism/pervasive developmental disorder.

Susan Snyder, Admissions Director
John D Wilson, Education Director

1000   Wesley Woods
1001 Fiddlersgreen Rd
Grand Valley, PA 16420   814-430-7802
                                        Fax: 814-436-7669
                                            www.wesleywoods.com

Exceptional children's camp for children with emotional and intellectual handicaps.

Herb West

1001   Worthmore Academy
3535 Kessler Blvd East Drive
Indianapolis, IN 46220   877-700-6516
                                        Fax: 317-251-6516
                    e-mail: bjackson@worthmoreacademy.org
                                        www.worthmoreacademy.org

A K-12 non-profit school for children with learning differences providing educational assessments, alternative educational programs, academic guidance and public awareness services.

Brenda J Jackson, Director
Diana Buser, Assistant

Description

1002 BELL'S PALSY

Involves the following Biologic System(s):

Neurologic Disorders

Bell's palsy is the most common form of facial nerve paralysis and may affect children at any age from infancy through adolescence. The facial nerve, also known as the seventh cranial nerve, arises from a certain area of the brain (i.e., brainstem) and divides into several branches that supply (innervate) the forehead, scalp, eyelids, cheeks, jaws, and muscles of facial expression. The facial nerve also conveys taste sensations from the front two thirds of the tongue. Bell's palsy is a temporary form of facial paralysis that usually develops suddenly approximately two weeks after a widespread viral infection, such as Epstein-Barr virus, herpesvirus, or mumps virus. It is thought to represent a postinfectious demyelination of the facial nerve (neuritis) due to allergic or immune responses.

Bell's palsy typically affects one side of the face and may involve upper and lower areas on the affected side. Symptoms of Bell's palsy usually begin suddenly and reach their peak within 48 hours. Children with the condition may experience weakness or slight paralysis of the upper and lower face; drooping of the corner of the mouth; an inability to close the eye; loss of taste sensations from the front two thirds of the tongue; or abnormal sensitivity to loud sounds (hyperacusis). Because the affected eye may be overexposed to the air, some patients may develop inflammation (exposure keratitis) of the transparent, front region of the eye (cornea). In addition, saliva may dribble from the corner of the mouth and food may tend to collect between the teeth and lips.

There is no cure or standard course of treatment for Bell's palsy. Some cases are mild and do not require treatment since the symptoms usually subside on their own within 2 weeks. For others, treatment may include medications such as acyclovir, used to fight viral infections, combined with an anti-inflammatory drug such as the steroid prednisone, used to reduce inflammation and swelling. Pain medications, such as aspirin, acetaminophen, or ibuprofen may be helpful. Other treatment of children with Bell's palsy is supportive, including eye drops to lubricate the cornea, particularly at night. In over 85 percent of affected children, Bell's palsy spontaneously resolves with no remaining facial weakness. About 10 percent may have mild longstanding weakness, and approximately five percent may experience severe, permanent facial weakness.

Government Agencies

1003 NIH/National Institute of Neurological Dis orders and Stroke (NINDS)
PO Box 5801
Bethesda, MD 20824

301-496-5751
800-352-9424
Fax: 301-496-0296
TTY: 301-468-5981
www.ninds.nih.gov

The mission of NINDS is to reduce the burden of neurological disease - a burden borne by every age group, by every segment of society, by people all over the world.

Story C Landis Ph.D., Director
Walter J Koroshetz, Deputy Director
Caroline Lewis, Executive Officer

National Associations & Support Groups

1004 American Academy of Otolaryngology-Head and Neck Surgery
1650 Diagonal Road
Alexandria, VA 22314

703-836-4444
Fax: 703-683-5100
TTY: 703-519-1585
e-mail: webmaster@entnet.org
www.entnet.org

The missions of the AAO-HNS and its foundation are to advance the art and science of otolaryngology-head and neck surgery through state-of-the-art education, research and learning; and to unite, serve and represent the interests of its members and their patients to the public, government, other medical specialists and related organizations. Founded in 1896, the AAO-HNS is the world's largest organization of otolaryngologist-head and neck surgeons.

11,600 Members

James L Netterville, President
Richard W Waguespack MD, President Elect
J. Gavin Setzen MD, Treasurer/Secretary

1005 American Academy of Pediatrics
141 Northwest Point Boulevard
Elk Grove Village, IL 60007

847-434-4000
800-433-9016
Fax: 847-434-8000
www.aap.org

The American Academy of Pediatrics and its member pediatricians are committed to the attainment of optimal physical, mental and social health and well-being for all infants, children, adolescents, and young adults.

Sandra Hassink, MD, FAAP, President

1006 March of Dimes Birth Defects Foundation
1275 Mamaroneck Avenue
White Plains, NY 10605

914-997-4488
888-663-4637
Fax: 914-997-4763
e-mail: answers@marchofdimes.com
www.marchofdimes.com

March of Dimes help moms have full-term pregnancies and research the problems that threaten the health of babies.The March of Dimes also acts globally: sharing best practices in perinatal health and helping improve birth outcomes where the needs are the most urgent.

Jennifer L Howse, President

1007 National Centers for Facial Paralysis
18403 Woodfield Road, Suite D
Gaithersburg, MD 20879

301-330-3223
Fax: 301-330-9075
e-mail: lgamliel@targangroup.com
www.bellspalsy.com

Strives to evaluate, inform and assist patients with past and/or current history of Facial Palsy, Bell's Palsy, Ramsey-Hunt Syndrome, or Facial Paralysis from surgery, trauma, pregnancy, Lyme disease, or other causes.

Research Centers

1008 Bell's Palsy Research Foundation
19550 Club House Road
Montgomery Village, MD 20886

301-651-9605
Fax: 301-216-2477
e-mail: drtargan@erols.com
www.bellspalsy.com

An online support foundation for facial palsy patients, providing information and support to patients worldwide; also functions to educate the medical community about facial paralysis and to advance research and development in all aspects of facial palsy and facial pain.

Bob Targen, MD, Director

Conferences

1009 Annual Meeting & OTO Expo
American Academy of Otolaryngology
1650 Diagonal Road
Alexandria, VA 22314

703-836-4444
Fax: 703-683-5100
TTY: 703-519-1585
e-mail: webmaster@entnet.org
www.entnet.org

Held each fall, with thousands of Academy members, non-member physicians, allied health professionals, administrators, and exhibiting companies attending. It draws more than 6,000 medical experts and professionals from around the world. The conference will feature instruction courses, miniseminars, scientific oral presentations, honorary guest lectures, and numerous scientific posters.

September

James L Netterville, President
J Gavin Setzen, Secretary/Treasurer

Web Sites

1010 American Academy of Otolaryngology Head an d Neck Surgery
www.entnet.org

Mission is to advance the art and science of otolaryngology-head and neck surgery through state-of-the-art education, research and learning.

1011 Bell's Palsy Network
www.bellspalsy.net/

Provides information on facial paralysis, Bell's Palsy, Ramsey Hunt Syndrome and other forms of facial paralysis. We were the first dedicated web portal for Bell's palsy and facial paralysis informaton and host the largest and most popular forum about bell's palsy and facial palsy information.

1012 Bell's Palsy Research Foundation
www.bellspalsyresearch.com

Online support foundation for facial palsy patients, providing information and supprt to patients worldwide.

1013 NIH/National Institute of Neurological Dis orders and Stroke (NINDS)
PO Box 5801
Bethesda, MD 20824

301-496-5751
800-352-9424
www.ninds.nih.gov

Mission is to reduce the burden of neurological disease-a burden borne by every age group, by every segment of society, by people all over the world.

Walter J. Koroshetz, M.D., Acting Director
Alan L. Willard, Ph.D., Acting Deputy Director
Caroline Lewis, Executive Officer

Description

1014 BILIARY ATRESIA

Involves the following Biologic System(s):

Gastrointestinal Disorders

Biliary atresia is a rare condition that is present at birth (congenital) in approximately 1 in 12,500 births, and is characterized by the absence of or the abnormal or incomplete development (hypoplasia) of the bile ducts. These ducts carry bile from the liver and gallbladder into the small intestine. Bile, which is secreted by the liver, is a yellowish or greenish fluid that aids in the digestion of fats. Bile passes through the common bile duct and into the upper portion of the small intestine (duodenum). Absence or underdevelopment of the bile ducts interferes with or prevents the passage of bile into the intestine and, as a result, characteristic findings and symptoms may be noticed within the first few weeks of life.

Symptoms may include progressively darkening urine; pale stools (acholic); a persistent yellowing of the skin, eyes, and mucous membranes (jaundice); and enlargement of the liver (hepatomegaly). If untreated, additional symptoms and findings may become apparent within two or three months. These may include growth retardation, increased irritability, and itching (pruritus). A potential complication of biliary atresia involves an increase in pressure in the vein that conveys blood from the spleen, stomach, pancreas, and intestine to the liver (portal hypertension). In addition, untreated biliary atresia may result in a life-threatening condition known as biliary cirrhosis, in which the liver's function is impaired and, eventually, the liverbecomes irreversibly damaged.

Treatment for biliary atresia is often determined by the site of the obstruction and includes various surgical procedures. In some infants, surgery may be performed as a means to help postpone cirrhosis and growth retardation until liver transplantation is feasible.

National Associations & Support Groups

1015 American Academy of Pediatrics

141 Northwest Point Boulevard
Elk Grove Village, IL 60007

847-434-4000
800-433-9016
Fax: 847-434-8000
www.aap.org

The American Academy of Pediatrics and its member pediatricians are committed to the attainment of optimal physical, mental and social health and well-being for all infants, children, adolescents, and young adults.

Sandra Hassink, MD, FAAP, President

1016 American Association for the Study of Liver Diseases

1001 North Fairfax Street Suite 400
Alexandria, VA 22314

703-299-9766
Fax: 703-299-9622
e-mail: aasld@aasld.org
www.aasld.org

To Advance the Science and Practice of Hepatology, Liver Transplantation and Hepatobiliary Surgery, Thereby Promoting Liver Health and Optimal Care of Patients with Liver and Biliary Tract Diseases.

J Gregory Fitz MD, President
Adrian M. Di Bisceglie, MD, FACP, President Elect
Donald M. Jensen, MD, Treasurer

1017 CHARGE Syndrome Foundation

141 Middle Neck Rd.
Sands Point, NY 11050

516-684-4720
800-442-7604
Fax: 516-883-9060
e-mail: info@chargesyndrome.org
www.chargesyndrome.org

The mission of the CHARGE Syndrome Foundation is to provide support to individuals with CHARGE syndrome and their families; to gather, develop, maintain and distribute information about CHARGE syndrome; and to promote awareness and research regarding its identification, cause and management.

David Wolfe, President
Sheri Stanger, Director of Outreach
Lisa Weir, Vice President

1018 Children's Liver Association for Support Services

27023 McBean Parkway, #126
Valencia, CA 91355

661-263-9099
877-679-8256
Fax: 661-263-9099
e-mail: supportsru@aol.com
www.classkids.org

CLASS is an all volunteer, nonprofit organization dedicated to serving the emotional, educational and financial needs of families coping with childhood liver disease and transplantation. Our goal is to be both a service to families and a valuable resource for the medical community.

Diane Sumner, President
Ann Whitehead, VP

1019 Genetic Alliance

4301 Connecticut Avenue NW Suite 404
Washington, DC 20008

202-966-7955
800-336-4363
Fax: 202-966-8553
e-mail: info@geneticalliance.org
www.geneticalliance.org

World's leading nonprofit health advocacy organization committed to transforming health through genetics and promoting an environment of openness centered on the health of individuals, families, and communities.

Sharon Terry, President
Lisa Wise, Chief Operating Officer
Tetyana Murza MES, Programs and Policy Coordinator

Research Centers

1020 Clinical Research Center, Pediatrics

Children's Hospital Research Foundation
3333 Burnett Avenue
Cincinnati, OH 45229

513-636-4200
800-344-2462
Fax: 513-636-7151
TTY: 513-636-4900
www.cincinnatichildrens.org

Cincinnati Children's will improve child health and transform delivery of care through fully integrated, globally recognized research, education and innovation

Michael Fisher, President and CEO

1021 Univ. of Texas-Southwestern Med. Ctr. at D allas - Clinical Ctr. for Liver Disease

5323 Harry Hines Boulevard
Dallas, TX 75390

214-648-3111
Fax: 214-648-3715
e-mail: LIVER@UTSouthwestern.edu
www.utsouthwestern.edu/about-us/contact-us.html

To achieve optimal outcomes for patients with a variety of liver disorders, including but not limited to Hepatitis B, C, and acute liver failure.

Dr. William Lee, Director
Dr Marlyn Mayo, Specialist

Conferences

1022 CHARGE Syndrome Conference
141 Middle Neck Rd
Sands Point, NY 11050
516-684-4720
800-442-7604
Fax: 516-883-9060
e-mail: conference@chargesyndrome.org
www.chargesyndrome.org

Annual conference sponsored by CHARGE (Coloboma, Heart Malformations, Atresia Choanae, Retardation, Genital Abnormalities, Ear Abnormalities). Includes exhibitors, workshops, and networking for professionals, patients and parents.

July

Marilyn Ogan, Chairperson, Conference Committee

1023 Genetic Alliance Annual Conference
Genetic Alliance
4301 Connecticut Avenue NW, Suite 404
Washington, DC 20008
202-966-5557
800-336-4363
Fax: 202-966-8553
e-mail: info@geneticalliance.org
www.geneticalliance.org

Consistently inspirational and enables partnership among all stakeholders: advocates and community leaders, health and industry professionals, policymakers, and academicians.

July

Sharon Terry, President/CEO
Tetyana Murza, Programs/Events Manager

1024 International CHARGE Syndrome Conference
CHARGE Syndrome Foundation
141 Middle Neck Rd
Sands Point, NY 11050
516-684-4720
800-442-7604
Fax: 516-883-9060
e-mail: marion@chargesyndrome.org
www.chargesyndrome.org

July

Marion Norbury, Executive Director

Web Sites

1025 Children's Liver Association for Support Services
www.classkids.org

CLASS is an all volunteer, nonprofit organization dedicated to serving the emotional, educational and financial needs of families coping with childhood liver disease and transplantation. Our goal is to be both a service to families and a valuable resource for the medical community.

1026 Online Mendelian Inheritance in Man
National Library of Medicine, Building 38A
Bethesda, MD 20894
888-346-3656
e-mail: info@ncbi.nlm.nih.gov
www.ncbi.nlm.nih.gov

This database is a catalog of human genes and genetic disorders.

Christine E. Seidman, M.D., Chair
David J. Lipman, M.D., Executive Secretary

Book Publishers

1027 Liver Disease in Children
Lippincott Williams & Wilkins
530 Walnut Street
Philadelphia, PA 19106
215-521-8300
Fax: 215-521-8902
www.lww.com

This is a difinitive book on pediatric liver disease, providing extensive, well-edited information that is not easily accessible or available in other textbooks. A must-have for those interested in this rapidly growing subspecialty in pediatrics.

2000 1008 pages
ISBN: 0-781720-98-2

Pamphlets

1028 Biliary Atresia
American Liver Foundation
39 Broadway, Suite 2700
New York, NY 10006
212-668-1000
Fax: 212-483-8179
www.liverfoundation.org

Pamphlet with information and symptoms on biliary atresia

Tom Nealon, Chair
David Ticker, Chief Financial Officer
Lynn Seim, Chief Operating Officer

1029 Facts on Liver Transplantation
American Liver Foundation
39 Broadway, Suite 2700
New York, NY 10006
212-668-1000
800-223-0179
Fax: 212-483-8179
www.liverfoundation.org

Provides information on liver transplantation, and the effects.

Tom Nealon, Chair
David Ticker, Chief Financial Officer
Lynn Seim, Chief Operating Officer

Description

1030 BIPOLAR DISORDER

Synonyms: Manic-depressive disorder, Manic-depressive illness, Manic-depressive psychosis

Involves the following Biologic System(s):
Developmental/Behavioral/Psychiatric Disorders

Bipolar disorder, also known as manic-depressive disorder, is a condition characterized by alternating depression and mania or, in rare cases, mania alone. The disorder is thought to affect less than two percent of the general population. Although bipolar disorder usually becomes apparent during the third or fourth decade of life, a significant proportion of individuals are initially affected in childhood, adolescence, or early adulthood. Individuals with bipolar disorder may initially experience either a depressive or a manic episode. In some affected children and adolescents, manic episodes may be more frequent than depressive episodes during the first years of their illness. However, as the disease progresses, episodes of depression may become more frequent than manic episodes. Bipolar disorder is often further classified as unipolar in cases in which only depression is experienced and bipolar when mania occurs, with or without depression. In addition, mixed affected states are characterized by the occurrence of depressive and manic symptoms during a single episode.

In children and adolescents with bipolar disorder, associated symptoms resemble those seen in affected adults. Depressive states usually emerge gradually and may be characterized by feelings of sadness, despair, hopelessness, and discouragement; loss of self-esteem; physical and emotional exhaustion; and lack of interest of formerly enjoyed activities. In severe cases, affected individuals may have suicidal tendencies, and hospitalization in a pediatric, general, or psychiatric facility may be essential. In such cases, consultation with child psychiatrists is important for ongoing support and decision-making regarding treatment options.

In affected children and adolescents, manic states may be characterized by overactivity (hyperactivity); excessive talking; inability to sleep (insomnia); impulsive behavior and impaired judgment that may result in reckless spending; elation that may quickly change to irritability and anger; personal neglect that may result in poor hygiene; and, in some cases, delusions of grandeur and persecution (paranoid delusions). Initial episodes of depression or mania often last approximately six months without treatment. Although most manic or depressive episodes usually cease in months, some individuals may be affected for longer periods.

Adolescents with bipolar disorder may be misdiagnosed, e.g., with a psychotic disorder characterized by disturbances in behavior, cognition, and emotional reactions (schizophrenia) or a maladjusted reaction to a stressful life event (adjustment disorder). However, most affected individuals are correctly diagnosed with bipolar disorder during adulthood. According to reports in the literature, the earlier the onset of bipolar disorder, the more susceptible affected individuals may be to frequent episodes, rapid cycling between depressive and manic states, and severe episodes that may result in suicidal tendencies. In addition, earlier onset of the disorder is often associated with an increased incidence of depression and bipolar disorder in immediate (first-degree) relatives.

The treatment of children and adolescents with bipolar disorder may include therapy with certain medications (e.g., lithium carbonate, carbamazepine) and integrated, multidisciplinary management (e.g., behavioral therapy; individual, family, or group psychodynamic therapy; etc.). In children and adolescents with the disorder, thorough patient and family histories and specific medical evaluations are typically conducted before medications are prescribed. Pretreatment evaluation for lithium may include assessment of electrolyte levels, and kidney (renal) and thyroid function. Pretreatment evaluation for tricyclic antidepressants may include a cardiovascular examination including electrocardiography. If such medications are prescribed, regular blood levels should be taken until an adequate dose is determined.

Other treatment options include antipsychotics or tranquilizers if agitation or psychotic symptoms are present, especially at the initiation of treatment when acute manic episodes are likely. Recent studies have shown that about 80% of patients treated with electroconvulsive therapy (ECT) experienced improvement, and for some, it was the only treatment that worked. The exact cause of bipolar disorder is unknown. However, many researchers agree that genetic abnormalities may play some role in the etiology of the disorder.

Government Agencies

1031 Center for Mental Health Services Knowledge Exchange Network

US Department of Health and Human Services
PO Box 42557
Washington, DC 20015

800-789-2647
Fax: 240-747-5470
TDD: 866-889-2647
www.mentalhealth.samhsa.gov

Supplies the public with responses to their commonly asked questions about mental health issues and services.

1032 NIH/National Institute of Mental Health

6001 Executive Boulevard, Room 8184, MSC 9663
Bethesda, MD 20892

301-443-4513
866-615-6464
Fax: 301-443-4279
TTY: 301-443-8431
e-mail: nimhinfo@nih.gov
www.nimh.nih.gov

The mission of NIMH is to transform the understanding and treatment of mental illnesses through basic and clinical research, paving the way for prevention, recovery, and cure.

Dr Thomas R Insel, Director

National Associations & Support Groups

1033 American Academy of Pediatrics

141 Northwest Point Boulevard
Elk Grove Village, IL 60007

847-434-4000
800-433-9016
Fax: 847-434-8000
www.aap.org

The American Academy of Pediatrics and its member pediatricians are committed to the attainment of optimal physical, mental and social health and well-being for all infants, children, adolescents, and young adults.

Sandra Hassink, MD, FAAP, President

1034 American Counseling Association
6101 Stevenson Ave
Alexandria, VA 22304
703-823-9800
800-347-6647
Fax: 703-823-0252
e-mail: webmaster@counseling.org
www.counseling.org

Represents professional counselors in various practice settings, and stands ready to serve more than 55,000 members with the resources they need to make a difference. From webinars, publications, and journals to Conference education sessions and legislative action alerts, ACA is where counseling professionals turn for powerful, credible content and support.

Robert L. Smith, President

1035 American Group Psychotherapy Association
25 East 21st St, 6th Floor
New York, NY 10010
212-477-2677
Fax: 212-979-6627
e-mail: info@agpa.org
www.agpa.org

The American Group Psychotherapy Association is a dynamic, thriving community of mental health professionals of all disciplines dedicated to advancing knowledge and research, and providing quality training in group psychotherapy and other group interventions, consultation and direct services nationally and internationally.

Les R. Greene, Ph.D., President
Marsha S. Block, CAE, CFRE, Chief Executive Officer
Diane C. Feirman, CAE, Public Affairs Senior Director

1036 American Mental Health Counselors Association
801 N. Fairfax Street, Suite 304
Alexandria, VA 22314
703-548-6002
800-326-2642
Fax: 703-548-4775
e-mail: sgiunta@troy.edu
www.amhca.org

The American Mental Health Counselors Association (AMHCA) is a national organization for licensed clinical mental health counselors. AMHCA strives to be the go-to organization for LCMHCs for education, advocacy, leadership and collaboration.

Stephen A. Giunta, Ph.D., President
Keith Mobley, Ph.D., President-Elect
Joel Miller, Executive Director/ CEO

1037 American Psychiatric Association
1000 Wilson Boulevard, Suite 1825
Arlington, VA 22209
703-907-7300
888-35 -7924
e-mail: apa@psych.org
www.psychiatry.org

It is a medical specialty society representing growing membership of more than 36,000 psychiatrists.

1038 American Psychiatric Nurses Association
3141 Fairview Park Drive, Suite 625
Falls Church, VA 22042
571-533-1919
855-863-2762
Fax: 855-883-2762
e-mail: ncroce@apna.org
www.apna.org

The American Psychiatric Nurses Association (APNA) is a professional association organized to advance the science and education of psychiatric-mental health nursing. It is committed to the specialty practice of psychiatric-mental health nursing, health, wellness and recovery promotion through identification of mental health issues, prevention of mental health problems and the care and treatment of persons with psychiatric disorders.

Nicholas Croce, Jr., MS, Executive Director
Patricia L. Black, PhD, RN, Associate Executive Director
Lisa Deffenbaugh Nguyen, Director of Operations

1039 American Psychoanalytic Association
309 E 49th St
New York, NY 10017
212-752-0450
e-mail: deankstein@apsa.org
www.apsa.org

APsaA as a professional organization for psychoanalysts, focuses on education, research and membership development.

Mark Smaller, Ph.D., President
Dean K. Stein, Executive Director
Tina Faison, Admin Assis to Executive Director

1040 American Psychological Association
750 First St. NE
Washington, DC 20002
202-336-5500
800-374-2721
TTY: 202-336-6123
www.apa.org

The mission is to advance the creation, communication and application of psychological knowledge to benefit society and improve people's lives.

Norman B. Anderson, PhD, CEO/ EVP
L. Michael Honaker, PhD, Deputy Chief Executive Officer
Ellen G. Garrison, PhD, Senior Policy Advisor

1041 Anxiety and Depression Association of America
8701 Georgia Ave., Suite #412
Silver Spring, MD 20910
240-485-1001
Fax: 240-485-1035
www.adaa.org

ADAA is a national nonprofit organization dedicated to the prevention, treatment, and cure of anxiety, depression, OCD, PTSD, and related disorders and to improving the lives of all people who suffer from them through education, practice, and research.

Mark H. Pollack, MD, President
Alies Muskin, Executive Director
Jean Kaplan Teichroew, Communications Director

1042 Association for Psychological Science
1133 15th Street, NW, Suite 1000
Washington, DC 20005
202-293-9300
Fax: 202-293-9350
www.psychologicalscience.org

The Association for Psychological Science (previously the American Psychological Society) is a nonprofit organization dedicated to the advancement of scientific psychology and its representation at the national and international level.

Nancy Eisenberg, President
Alan Kraut, Executive Director
Sarah Brookhart, Deputy Director

1043 Brain & Behavior Research Foundation
90 Park Avenue, 16th Floor
New York, NY 10016
646-681-4888
800-829-8289
e-mail: info@bbrfoundation.org
bbrfoundation.org

The Brain & Behavior Research Foundation is committed to alleviating the suffering caused by mental illness by awarding grants that will lead to advances and breakthroughs in scientific research.

Steve Lieber, Chairman of the Board
Suzanne Golden, Vice President
Jeffrey Borenstein, M.D., President/ CEO

1044 Center for Psychiatric Rehabilitation
940 Commonwealth Ave. West
Boston, MA 2215
617-353-3549
Fax: 617-358-3066
e-mail: psyrehab@bu.edu
cpr.bu.edu

The Center is a research, training, and service organization dedicated to improving the lives of persons who have psychiatric disabilities.

Kim T. Mueser, Executive Director
Deborah Dolan, Director of Operations
Dori Hutchinson, Director of Services

1045 College of Psychiatric and Neurologic Pharmacists
8055 O Street, Suite S113
Lincoln, NE 68510
402-476-1677
Fax: 888-551-7617
e-mail: info@cpnp.org
cpnp.org

121

As the voice of the specialty, there mission is to advance the reach and practice of neuropsychiatric pharmacists.

Steven Burghart, DPh, MBA, BCPP, President
Ray Love, President-Elect
Julie Dopheide, PharmD, BCPP, Past President

1046 Depression and Bipolar Support Alliance
730 N Franklin Street, Suite 501
Chicago, IL 60654

800-826-3632
Fax: 312-642-7243
www.dbsalliance.org

Patient-directed organization focusing on the most prevalent mental illnesses- depression and bipolar disorder. Fosters an understanding about the impact and management of these life-threatening illnesses by providing up-to-date, scientifically-based tools and information written in language the general public can understand.

Lucinda Jewell ED. M, Chair
Rev. Cheryl T. Magrini, Ph.D., Vice Chair
Christy B. Beckmann,, Treasurer

1047 Families for Depression Awareness
395 Totten Pond Road, Suite 404
Waltham, MA 2451

781-890-0220
Fax: 781-890-2411
www.familyaware.org

Families for Depression Awareness is a national nonprofit organization helping families recognize and cope with depression and bipolar disorder to get people well and prevent suicides.

Julie Totten, Founder
Valerie Cordero, Interim Co-Executive Director
Susan Weinstein, Interim Co-Executive Director

1048 Federation of Families for Children's Mental Health
9605 Medical Center Drive, Suite 280
Rockville, MD 20850

240-403-1901
Fax: 240-403-1909
e-mail: ffcmh@ffcmh.org
www.ffcmh.org

The National family run organization is dedicated exclusively to helping children with mental health needs and their families achieve a better quality of life.

Teka Dempson, President
Sherri Luthe, Vice President
Sheila Pires, Treasurer

1049 Juvenile Bipolar Research Foundation
277 Martine Avenue, Suite 226
White Plains, NY 10601

e-mail: info@jbrf.org
www.jbrf.org

JBRF is a 501(c)(3) organization that actively promotes and supports scientific research focused on the cause of and treatments for bipolar disorder in children.

Charles Goldberg, Director of Development

1050 Kristin Brooks Hope Center
1250 24th Street NW, Suite 300
Washington, DC 20037

800-442-HOPE
Fax: 202-536-3206
e-mail: reese@hopeline.com
www.hopeline.com

Since the suicide of his wife Kristin in April 1998, KBHC Founder Reese Butler has been on a personal crusade. His mission the past 11 years has been to offer HOPE and the option to LIVE to those in the deepest emotional pain.

H. Reese Butler II, President/ CEO
Richard Rossell, Treasurer

1051 Mental Health America
2000 N Beauregard Street, 6th Floor
Alexandria, VA 22311

703-684-7722
800-969-6642
Fax: 703-684-5968
TTY: 800-433-5959
e-mail: info@mentalhealthamerica.net
www.mentalhealthamerica.net

Addresses all aspects of mental health and mental illness. NMHA with over 340 affiliates works to improve the mental health of all Americans.

Ann Boughtin, Chair
Eric Ashton, Vice-Chair
Elaine Crider, Secretary/Treasurer

1052 National Alliance for the Mentally Ill
3803 N. Fairfax Dr., Suite 100
Arlington, VA 22203

703-525-7600
800-950-6264
Fax: 703-524-9094
TDD: 703-516-7227
e-mail: info@nami.org
www.nami.org

NAMI is a nonprofit, grassroots, self-help, support and advocacy organization of consumers, families and friends of people with severe mental illness, such as schizophrenia, bipolar disorder, major depressive disorder, obsessive compulsive disorder, anxiety disorders, autism and other severe and persistent mental illnesses that affect the brain.

Keris J,,n Myrick, President
Kevin B Sullivan, First Vice President
Jim Payne, Second Vice President

1053 National Association of State Mental Health Program Directors
66 Canal Center Plaza, Suite 302
Alexandria, VA 22314

703-739-9333
Fax: 703-548-9517
e-mail: webmaster@nasmhpd.org
www.nasmhpd.org

National Association of State Mental Health Program Directors (NASMHPD) represents the $37.6 billion public mental health service delivery system serving 7.1 million people annually in all 50 states, 4 territories, and the District of Columbia.

Jay Meek, CPA, MBA, Chief Financial Officer
Robert W. Glover, PhD, Executive Director
David Miller, MPAff, Project Director

1054 National Council for Behavioral Health
1400 K Street NW, Suite 400
Washington, DC 20005

202-684-7457
e-mail: Communications@TheNationalCouncil.org
www.thenationalcouncil.org

The National Council for Behavioral Health (National Council) is the unifying voice of America's community mental health and addictions treatment organizations.

Linda Rosenberg, President/ CEO
Jeannie Campbell, EVP/ COO
Heather Cobb, Vice President, Communications

1055 The Jed Foundation
1140 Broadway, Ste. 803
New York, NY 10001

212-647-7544
Fax: 212-647-7542
www.jedfoundation.org

The Jed Foundation's mission is to promote emotional health and prevent suicide among college and university students.

John MacPhee, Executive Director/ CEO
Dr. Victor Dr. Schwartz, Medical Director
Dr. Nance Roy, Clinical Director

1056 The Ryan Licht Sang Bipolar Foundation
875 N. Michigan Avenue, Suite 3100
Chicago, IL 60611

888-944-4408
www.ryanlichtsangbipolarfoundation.org

The Ryan Licht Sang Bipolar Foundation is dedicated to fostering awareness, understanding and research for early-onset Bipolar Disorder.

Joyce Licht Sang, Founder Director
Jaynee Licht Luntz, Founder Director
Joyce Licht Sang, President

State Agencies & Support Groups

1057 Center for Family Support
333 7th Avenue, 9th Floor
New York, NY 10001
212-629-7939
Fax: 212-239-2211
e-mail: svernikoff@cfsny.org
www.cfsny.org

The Center for Family (CFS) is a not-for-profit human service agency providing support and assistance to individuals with developmental disabilities and traumatic brain injuries throughout New York City, Long Island, the lower Hudson Valley region and New Jersey.

Eileen Berg, Corporate Compliance Officer

1058 Depressive and Manic-Depressive Assocation of Mount Sinai
100 LaSalle Street, Suite 5A
New York, NY 10027
917-445-2399
e-mail: jgg17@columbia.edu
www.columbia.edu/~jgg17/DMDA/PAGE_1.html

The NYC Depressive and Manic-Depressive Group is a support group for persons with mood disorders, depression and bipolar disorder, as well as their family members and friends.

Research Centers

1059 National Alliance for Research on Schizophrenia and Depression
60 Cutter Mill Road, Suite 404
Great Neck, NY 11021
516-829-0091
800-829-8289
Fax: 516-487-6930
e-mail: info@bbrfoundation.org.
www.bbrfoundation.org/

NARSAD raises and distributes funds for scientific research into the causes, cures, treatments, and prevention of severe mental illnesses, primarily schizophrenia.

Steve Lieber, Chairman of the Board
Suzanne Golden, Vice President
Arthur Radin, Treasurer

Conferences

1060 DBSA National Conference
Depression and Bipolar Support Alliance
730 N Franklin Street, Suite 501
Chicago, IL 60654
800-826-3632
Fax: 312-642-7243
www.dbsalliance.org

Offers a unique peer-centered conference for individuals living with depression or bipolar disorder, as well as for family members or health care providers looking for ways to best help their loved ones, patients, or clients by partnering with them on their path to recovery. The conference consists of compelling keynote presentations, educational workshops, and pre-conference institutes.

Lucinda Jewel, Chair
Rev. Cheryl T Magrini, Vice Chair
Mike Kuhl, Secretary

1061 FFCMH Annual Conference
Federation of Families for Childrens Mental Health
9605 Medical Center Drive, Suite 280
Rockville, MD 20850
240-403-1901
Fax: 240-403-1909
e-mail: ffcmh@ffcmh.org
www.ffcmh.org

Address the complex issue of trauma; the impact it has on children and families; the promotion of healing and prevention strategies; knowledge about how to address trauma through resiliency-based interventions, utilizing a familydriven, youth guided approach; and examples of how family organizations and the partners they work with are raising awareness and improving trauma-focused services and supports.

November

Teka Dempson, President
Sherri Luthe, Vice President
Sheila Pires, Treasurer

1062 NAMI Convention
National Alliance on Mental Illness
3803 N Fairfax Drive, Suite 100
Arlington, VA 22203
703-524-7600
888-999-6264
Fax: 703-524-9094
TDD: 703-516-7227
e-mail: info@nami.org
www.nami.org

The NAMI Convention is packed with information, chances to network, leadership development opportunities, and lots more.

July

Keris Jan Myrik, President
Kevin B Sullivan, Vice President
Clarence Jordan, Secretary

Audio Video

1063 Families Coping with Mental Illness
Mental Illness Education Project
25 West Street
Westborough, MA 1581
USA
617-562-1111
800-343-5540
Fax: 617-779-0061
e-mail: info@miepvideos.org
miepvideos.org

Ten family members share their experiences of having a family member with schizophrenia or bipolar disorder. Designed to provide insights and support to other families, the tape also profoundly conveys to professionals the needs of families when mental illness strikes. In two versions: a 22-minute version ideal for short classes and workshops, and a richer 43-minute version with more examples and details. Discounted price for families/consumers.

Video

Michael M Faenza, Executive Director

Web Sites

1064 Bipolar World
www.bipolarworld.net

A support and educational web site for individuals diagnosed with Bipolar Affective Disorder and for the families and friends who care for them.

1065 CyberPsych
www.cyberpsych.org

CyberPsych presents information about psychoanalysis, psychotherapy, and special topics such as anxiety disorder, the problematic use of alcohol, homophobia, and the traumatic effects of racism. CyberPsych is a nonprofit network which offers free web hosting and technical support for internet communication to nonprofit groups and individuals.

Carol Lindemann, Ph.D., Contact

1066 Internet Mental Health
www.mentalhealth.com

Our goal is to improve understanding, diagnosis, and treatment of mental illness throughout the world.

Phillip W. Long, M.D., Psychiatrist

1067 Mental Health Net
P.O. Box 20709
Columbus, OH 43220
614-448-4055
e-mail: info@centersite.net
www.mentalhelp.net

We wish to provide the following: to discuss, develop and debate in an open forum the future of the mental health field in America and throughout the world. To help coordinate various components of the mental health field so as to bring about greater communication between them.

1068 Planetpsych
www.planetpsych.com

e-mail: webmaster@planetpsych.com
www.planetpsych.com

Online resource for mental health information.

Book Publishers

1069 Bipolar Disorders: A Guide to Helping Children & Adolescents
O'Reilly and Associates
1005 Gravenstein Highway N
Sebastopol, CA 95472
707-827-7019
800-998-8969
Fax: 707-824-8268
e-mail: patientguides@oreilly.com
www.patientcenters.com

A million children and adolescents in the US may have childhood-onset bipolar disorder, including an estimated 23 percent of those currently diagnosed with ADHD. Bipolar Disorders helps parents and professionals recognize, treat, and cope with bipolar disorders in children and adolescents. It covers diagnosis, family life, medications, talk therapies, other interventions (improving sleep patterns, diet, preventing seasonal mood swings), insurance and school.

1999 460 pages
ISBN: 1-565926-56-0

1070 Bipolar Puzzle Solutions
Taylor & Francis
7625 Empire Drive
Florence, KT 41042
800-634-7064
Fax: 800-248-4724
e-mail: orders@taylorandfrancis.com
www.taylorandfrancis.com

187 answers to questions asked by support group members about living with manic depressive illness.

ISBN: 1-560324-93-7

1071 Covert Modeling and Reinforcement
New Harbinger Publications
5674 Shattuck Avenue
Oakland, CA 94609
510-652-0215
800-748-6273
Fax: 800-652-1613
e-mail: customreservice@newharbinger.com
www.newharbinger.com

Audio programs based on our essential book of cognitive behavioral techniques for effecting change in your life, Thoughts & Feelings. Listeners learn step-by-step protocols for controlling destructive behaviors such anxiety, obessional thinking, uncontrolled anger, and depression.

ISBN: 0-934986-29-0

1072 Touched with Fire-Manic Depressive Illness & the Artistic Temperament
Free Press
866 3rd Avenue
New York, NY 10022
USA
212-832-2101
800-323-7445
Fax: 800-943-9831
www.simonsays.com

Describing and discussing the markedly increased rates of severe mood disorders and suicides among the artistically creative and the reasons why.

384 pages
ISBN: 0-684831-83-X

Newsletters

1073 Outreach
Depression and Bipolar Support Alliance
55 E. Jackson Blvd, Suite 490
Chicago, IL 60604
800-826-3632
Fax: 312-642-7243
www.dbsalliance.org

Quarterly publication serving members and constituents of the organization. National DMDA educates patients, families, professionals, and the public concerning the nature of depressive and manic-depressive illnesses as treatable medical diseases; fosters self-help for patients and families; eliminates discrimination and stigma; improves access to care; advocates for research toward the elimination of these illnesses.

Cheryl T. Magrini, Chair
Allen Doederlein, President
Cindy Specht, Executive Vice President

Pamphlets

1074 Bipolar Disorder
National Institutes of Health
9000 Rockville Pike
Bethesda, MD 20892
301-443-3706
Fax: 301-443-6349
www.nih.gov

A short booklet offering a concise description of this disorder, which is also called manic-depressive illness.

Francis S. Collins, Director

1075 Child and Adolescent Bipolar Disorder
Child and Adolescent Bipolar Foundation
730 N. Franklin Street,Suite 501
Chicago, IL 60654
312-642-0049
Fax: 847-920-9498
e-mail: info@thebalancedmind.org
www.thebalancedmind.org

To educate families, professsionals and the public about early onset bipolar disorder.

Julia Small, Staff Leader
Karen Cruise, Volunteer Leaders
Kathy Karle, Support Network Coordinator

1076 Mood Disorders
Center for Mental Health Services
PO Box 42557
Washington, DC 20015
800-789-2647
Fax: 240-747-5470
TDD: 866-889-2647
e-mail: nmhic-info@samhsa.HHS.gov
http://mentalhealth.samhsa.gov

This fact sheet provides basic information on the symptoms, formal diagnosis, and treatment for bipolar disorder.

3 pages

Description

1077 BRAIN TUMORS

Involves the following Biologic System(s):

Neurologic Disorders

Brain tumors are abnormal growths in or on the brain. They may be cancerous (malignant) or noncancerous (benign), and may be classified as primary tumors that arise directly from brain tissue or as secondary tumors, which are almost always malignant and have spread or metastasized to the brain from cancers in other parts of the body. By contrast, tumors that begin in the brain or spinal cord rarely spread to other parts of the body.

All types of brain tumors, whether they are primary tumors that begin within the brain or secondary tumors that spread to the brain, originate from aberrations or mutations in the genes of a cell, causing the cell to divide and replicate itself into the large numbers of identical cells that constitute a tumor.

Space-occupying benign tumors may also present complications resulting from increasing intracranial pressure. Symptoms and characteristic findings associated with brain tumors depend upon their location as well as their size and rate of growth. However, many symptoms are common to most types of brain tumors and may include recurrent or constant headache, irregularities of vision, difficulties in balance and the coordination of voluntary movements, muscle weakness, speech difficulties, and sometimes seizures. Nausea, vomiting, fever, and fluctuations in pulse rate, breathing rate, and blood pressure may be later and more foreboding manifestations. Although there are many different types of brain tumors, children are most commonly affected by primary tumors, especially those that develop toward the back of the brain (posterior fossa tumor).

The most common of the posterior fossa tumors in children is the cerebellar astrocytoma. This type of tumor may be fluid-filled (cystic) or relatively solid and may often have a low grade of malignancy. However, cerebellar astrocytomas may sometimes invade the fibers on each side of the cerebellum that connect with other areas of the brain as well as the spinal cord (cerebellar peduncles). Symptoms and findings may include an abnormal accumulation of cerebrospinal fluid, often under increased pressure, within the skull (hydrocephalus) that is characterized by an increase in head size in infants as well as irritability, vomiting, lethargy, irregular reflex action, and leg rigidity followed by drowsiness and seizures. Older children may have a headache and may vomit, lose coordination, and exhibit deteriorating mental capabilities. Effective treatment for low-grade cerebellar astrocytoma includes surgical removal. Radiation treatment may be indicated for children with cerebellar astrocytoma of high-grade malignancy or in children who exhibit evidence of tumor growth after surgery.

Medulloblastoma is the second most common of the posterior fossa tumors in children and, in children younger than seven years of age, is the most common brain tumor. This type of malignant tumor usually grows relatively fast and spreads to other parts of the brain, the spinal cord, and sometimes other areas of the body. Symptoms associated with medulloblastoma may include headache, recurrent vomiting,

and frequent falling. Diagnosis is achieved through imaging studies such as magnetic resonance imaging (MRI) or computer tomography (CT scan) which give a detailed picture of the size and extent of the tumor. Treatment may include surgical excision. In addition, children older than four years of age may receive radiation therapy, especially if the tumor is small and has not yet spread. Children who have evidence of some remaining tumor growth after surgery and those whose tumor has spread may benefit from chemotherapy in addition to further surgery and radiation therapy. Due to the possibility of adverse effects on the brain, radiation is delayed in very young children with medulloblastoma.

Craniopharyngioma is a tumor that appears most often in children and adolescents, and arises from the pituitary, an endocrine gland that is located at the base of the skull. This type of tumor may sometimes interfere with pituitary gland and other endocrine functions as well as cause compression resulting in hydrocephalus and its associated symptoms. Other findings may include headache, vomiting, irregularities in vision, and short stature resulting from hormonal irregularities. Treatment for craniopharyngioma includes surgical excision. Additional treatment with radiation may be indicated for those children whose tumor is not able to be completely removed through surgery or who experience a recurrence. Subsequent to surgery, some children may develop such hormonal abnormalities as an underactive thyroid (hypothyroidism), growth hormone deficiency, diabetes insipidus, and other problems. Evaluation for these hormonal disorders is indicated and treatment is dependent upon the particular abnormality.

Government Agencies

1078 NIH/National Cancer Institute
BG 9609 MSC 9760 9609 Medical Center Drive
Bethesda, MD 20892   800-422-6237
                                       www.cancer.gov

The National Cancer Institute coordinates the National Cancer Program, which conducts and supports research, training, health information dissemination, and other programs with respect to the cause, diagnosis, prevention, and treatment of cancer, rehabilitation from cancer, and the continuing care of cancer patients and the families of cancer patients.

Harold Varmus MD, Director

1079 NIH/National Institute of Neurological Disorders and Stroke (NINDS)
PO Box 5801
Bethesda, MD 20824   301-496-5751
                                       800-352-9424
                                       Fax: 301-496-0296
                                       TTY: 301-468-5981
                                       www.ninds.nih.gov

The mission of NINDS is to reduce the burden of neurological disease - a burden borne by every age group, by every segment of society, by people all over the world.

Story C Landis Ph.D., Director
Walter J Koroshetz, Deputy Director
Caroline Lewis, Executive Officer

National Associations & Support Groups

1080 A Kids' Brain Tumor Cure Foundation
98 Random Farms Drive
Chappaqua, NY 10514   e-mail: contact@akidsbraintumorcure.org.
                        akidsbraintumorcure.org

A Kids' Brain Tumor Cure Foundation (aka The Pediatric Low Grade Astrocytoma (PLGA) Foundation) was founded in August 2007, as a 501(c)(3) organization by families and friends dedicated to giving hope to children battling the most common forms of pediatric brain tumors, by raising funds for targeted scientific and medical research.

Andrew Janower, President
John Ragnoni, Secretary
Amy Weinstein, Treasurer

1081 Accelerate Brain Cancer Cure
1717 Rhode Island Avenue, NW Suite 700
Washington, DC 20036
202-419-3140
e-mail: info@abc2.org
www.abc2.org

Provides researchers with the pivotal support they need to make critical breakthroughs.

Stacey Case, Co-Founder
Steve Case, Co-Founder
Jean Case, Co-Founder

1082 American Academy of Pediatrics
141 Northwest Point Boulevard
Elk Grove Village, IL 60007
847-434-4000
800-433-9016
Fax: 847-434-8000
www.aap.org

The American Academy of Pediatrics and its member pediatricians are committed to the attainment of optimal physical, mental and social health and well-being for all infants, children, adolescents, and young adults.

Sandra Hassink, MD, FAAP, President

1083 American Association for Cancer Research
615 Chestnut St., 17th Floor
Philadelphia, PA 19106
215-440-9300
866-423-3965
Fax: 215-440-9313
e-mail: aacr@aacr.org
www.aacr.org

Helps prevent and cure cancer through research, education, communication, and collaboration.

Carlos L Arteaga, President
Jose Baselga, President Elect
Maragaret Foti, Chief Executive Officer

1084 American Association of Neurological Surgeons
5550 Meadowbrook Drive
Rolling Meadows, IL 60008
847-378-0500
888-566-2267
Fax: 847-378-0600
e-mail: info@aans.org
www.aans.org

The AANS is dedicated to advancing the specialty of neurological surgery in order to promote the highest quality of patient care.

Robert E Harbaugh, President
H. Hunt Batjer, President Elect
Frederick A Boop, Secretary

1085 American Brain Tumor Association
8550 W. Bryn Mawr Ave. Ste 550
Chicago, IL 60631
773-577-8750
800-886-2282
Fax: 773-577-8738
e-mail: info@abta.org
www.abta.org

Services include over 20 publications which address brain tumors, their treatment, and coping with the disease. Materials address brain tumors in all age groups. Provides free social service consultations; a mentorship program for new brain tumor support group leaders; a nationwide database of established support groups; the Connections pen-pal program; networking with organizations that provide services to patients and families; a resource listing of physicians offering investigative treatments

Ronald Petrocelli, M.D., Chair
Michael Cathey, Vice Chair
Brian Olson, Treasurer

1086 American Brain Tumor Association Patient Line
8550 W. Bryn Mawr Ave. Ste 550
Chicago, IL 60631
773-577-8750
800-886-2282
Fax: 773-577-8738
e-mail: info@abta.org
www.abta.org

Offers emergency support, information and referrals for patients and their families.

Ronald Petrocelli, M.D., Chair
Michael Cathey, Vice Chair
Brian Olson, Treasurer

1087 American Cancer Society
Brain Tumor Support Group
8900 John W Carpenter Freeway
Dallas, TX 75247
214-819-1200
800-227-2345
Fax: 214-631-3869
www.cancer.org

Your American Cancer Society is in your corner around the clock to help you stay well and get well, to find cures, and to fight back.

Gary M Reedy, Chair of the Board
Vincent T DeVita Jr., MD, President
Pamela K Meyerhoffer, FAHP, Chair Elect

1088 American Childhood Cancer Organization
10920 Connecticut Ave Suite A
Kensington, MD 20895
301-962-3520
855-858-2226
Fax: 301-962-3521
e-mail: rhoffman@acco.org
www.acco.org

One of the nation's largest grassroots organizations at the forefront of the crucial battle against childhood cancer.

Naomi Bartley, President
Janine Lynne, Vice President
Ruth I. Hoffman MPH, Executive Director

1089 Association for Neurologically Impaired Brain Injured Children
61-35 220th Street
Oakland Gardens, NY 11364
718-423-9550
Fax: 718-423-9838
e-mail: mail@anibic.org
www.anibic.org

ANIBIc is a voluntary, multi-service organization that is dedicated to serving individuals with severe learning disabilities, neurological impairments and other developmental disabilities. Services include: residential, vocational, family support services, recreation (children and adults), respite (adult), summer day camp, counseling, and tramatic brain injury services (adults).

Michael Steward, President
Phyllis Kaye, Vice President
Helene Nieman, Vice President

1090 Beez Foundation (The)
26H World's Fair Drive
Somerset, NJ 08873
732-563-1144
www.beezfoundation.org

To raise money to support pediatric brain cancer research projects, related support activities for pediatric patients in cancer hospitals and education regarding the prevalence of pediatric brain cancer.

Joseph J. Giardina, President/Co-Founder
Gail Kurtzhals, VP/Marketing Director
Susan Giardina, Sec/Treas./Co-Founder

1091 Ben and Catherine Ivy Foundation
6710 North Scottsdale Road Suite 235
Scottsdale, AZ 85253
480-659-9621
Fax: 480-659-9651
e-mail: beth@mcraeagency.com
www.ivyfoundation.org

At the Ivy Foundation, the long-term, ultimate goal is to cure brain cancer.

Catherine E. Ivy, Founder and Board President
Stephanie A. McRae, Secretary
Megan Edwards, Treasurer

1092 Brain Tumor Foundation - National
National Brain Tumor Foundation
22 Battery Street, Suite 612
San Francisco, CA 94111   617-924-9997
                                           800-934-2873
                                    Fax: 415-834-9980
                           e-mail: nbtf@braintumor.org
                                      www.braintumor.org

National Brain Tumor Society is fiercely committed to finding better treatments, and ultimately a cure, for people living with a brain tumor today and anyone who will be diagnosed tomorrow. This means effecting change in the system at all levels.

Jeffrey Kolodin, Chair
Michael Nathanson, Vice Chair
Michael Corkin, Treasurer

1093 Brain Tumor Foundation for Children
6065 Roswell Road NE, Suite 505
Atlanta, GA 30328   404-252-4107
                                    Fax: 404-252-4108
                      e-mail: info@braintumorkids.org
                                   www.braintumorkids.org

The mission of the Brain Tumor Foundation for Children is to provide financial assistance, social support, and information for families of children with brain and spinal cord tumors; fund research projects that improve treatment options and search for a cure; and raise public awareness of the disease and advocate on behalf of children who are affected.

Pamela B Ellis, President
Robert Flamini MD, Vice President
William A Guzak, Treasurer

1094 Brain Tumor Trials Collaborative
www.bttconline.org

The mission of the BTTC is to develop and perform hypothesis-based, state-of-the-art clinical trials in a collaborative and collegial environment emphasizing innovation and meticulous attention to data quality.

1095 CERN Foundation
6450 Poe Avenue, Suite 201
Dayton, OH 45414   937-264-2574
                                    Fax: 937-264-7877
                                      cern-foundation.org

To develop new treatments for ependymoma, improve the outcomes and care of patients, ultimately leading to a cure.

Glenn Lesser, Advisory Board
Mary Lovely, Advisory Board
Robert Jenkins, Advisory Board

1096 CancerCare
275 7th Avenue (between 25th and 26th Streets)
New York, NY 10001   212-712-6120
                                           800-813-4673
                                    Fax: 212-712-8495
                          e-mail: info@cancercare.org
                                      www.cancercare.org

CancerCare provides free, professional support services to individuals, families, caregivers and the bereaved to help them cope with and manage the emotional and practical challenges of cancer.

Helen H Miller, Chief Executive Officer
John Rutigliano, Chief Operating Officer
Jan McDavitt, Chief Development Officer

1097 Candlelighters Childhood Cancer Foundation
10920 Connecticut Ave. Suite A
Kensington, MD 20895   301-962-3520
                                           855-858-2226
                                    Fax: 310-962-3521
                             e-mail: staff@acco.org
                                      www.acco.org

The American Childhood Cancer Organization (ACCO) was founded in 1970 by a group of parents whose children had been diagnosed with cancer. Today, ACCO is one of the largest grassroots, national organizations dedicated to improving the lives of children and adolescents with cancer and their families.

Naomi Bartley, President
Janine Lynne, Vice President
Ken Phillips, Treasurer

1098 Central Brain Tumor Registry of the United States
244 East Ogden Ave Suite 116
Hinsdale, IL 60521   630-655-4786
                                    Fax: 630-655-1756
                             e-mail: cbtrus@aol.com
                                      www.cbtrus.org

It is a not-for-profit corporation established to provide a resource for descriptive statistical data on all primary brain tumors irrespective of behavior.

Carol Kruchko, President
Steven Brem, Vice President
Donald Segal, Treasurer

1099 Childhood Brain Tumor Foundation
20312 Watkins Meadow Drive
Germantown, MD 20876   301-515-2900
                                           877-217-4166
                                    Fax: 301-540-8367
                  e-mail: cbtf@childhoodbraintumor.org
                                   www.childhoodbraintumor.org

A major service this organization provides is the Childhood Cancer Ombudsman Program, a free service consisting of volunteers trained in the disciplines of medicine, law, and education who provide assistance in : 1) seeking second opinions, 2) access to healthcare, and 3) combating discrimination. The foundation also funds research, has a hotline and publishes a newsletter three times a year.

Jeanne P Young, President
Carol Cornman, Vice President
Kiren Day, Vice President/Secretary

1100 Childhood Brain Tumor Foundation (The)
20312 Watkins Meadow Drive
Germantown, ML 20876   301-515-2900
                                           877-217-4166
                  e-mail: cbtf@childhoodbraintumor.org
                                   www.childhoodbraintumor.org

It is an all-volunteer organization founded by families, friends and physicians of children with brain tumors.

Jeanne P Young, President
Carol Comman, Vice President
Kiren Day, Secretary

1101 Children's Brain Tumor Foundation
274 Madison Avenue Suite 1004
New York, NY 10016   866-228-4673
                               e-mail: info@cbtf.org
                                      www.cbtf.org

To improve the treatment, quality of life and the long term outlook for children with brain and spinal cord tumors through research.

Robert Budlow, President
Eric Snyder, Vice President
Miriam Barry, Secretary

1102 Cushing's Support and Research Foundation
60 Robbins Rd, #12
Plymouth, MA 02360   csrf.net

To be a resource for information and support to health care professionals.

Louise Pace, Founding President
Karen Campbell, Director
John P. Gulielmetti, Treasurer

1103 Epidermoid Brain Tumor Society
epidermoidbraintumorsociety.org

To inform, educate, and to provide a support and research organization for those affected by the epidermoid brain tumor.

1104 Glenn Garcelon Foundation
PO Box 2104
Lake Oswego, OR 97035   503-969-7651
                    e-mail: glenngarcelonfoundation@msn.com
                    glenngarcelonfoundation.org

Exists to improve the quality of life of brain tumor survivors,
caregivers and their families by providing emotional and financial
support.

Gail Garcelon, President
Danielle Hess, Vice President
Nicole Smith, Secretary

1105 Heads Up Brain Tumor Support Group
Dominican Hospital
18300 Roscoe Boulevard
Northridge, CA 91325   818-885-5432
                    e-mail: robert.salazar@chw.edu
                    www.braintumor.org/

Robert Salazar, Contact
Michael Nathanson, Vice Chair
Michael Corkin, Treasurer

1106 Healing Exchange Brain Trust
459 Broadway, Suite 302
Everett, MA 02149   877-252-8480
                    Fax: 617-623-0086
                    e-mail: info@braintrust.org
                    www.braintrust.org

The mission of The Healing Exchange BRAIN TRUST is to improve quality of life for people living with brain tumors and related conditions TODAY.

Samantha J Scolamiero, President & Founding Director

1107 Hope for Hypothalamic Hamartomas
P. O. Box 721
Waddell, AZ 85355   e-mail: admin@hopeforhh.org.
                    hopeforhh.org

A volunteer-based nonprofit organization founded by parents of
children with hypothalamic hamartomas.

Lisa Dunn Soeby, President
Ilene Penn Miller, Vice President
Erica Webster, Secretary

1108 James S. McDonnell Foundation
1034 S. Brentwood Blvd. Suite 1850
St. Louis, MO 63117   314-721-1532
                    e-mail: info@jsmf.org
                    www.jsmf.org

The Foundation has pursued his goals by supporting scientific,
educational, and charitable causes locally, nationally, and internationally.

John T Bruer, President
John F. McDonnell, Board of Director
Marcella M. Stevens, Board of Director

**1109 Musella Foundation for Brain Tumor Research and
       Information**
1100 Peninsula Blvd
Hewlett, NY 11557   888-295-4740
                    www.virtualtrials.com

Nonprofit public charity dedicated to helping brain tumor patients
through emotional and financial support, education, advocacy and
raising money for brain tumor research.

Al Musella, President
Mitchell Siegel, Vice President
Neal Houslanger, Secretary

1110 National Association for Proton Therapy
1301 Highland Drive
Silver Spring, ML 20910   301-587-6100
                    e-mail: lenarzt@proton-therapy.org
                    www.proton-therapy.org

The National Association for Proton Therapy (NAPT) is registered as an independent, non-profit, public benefit corporation
providing education and awareness for the public, professional
and governmental communities.

Leonard Arzt, Executive Director

1111 National Brain Research Association
1439 Rhode Island Avenue NW
Washington, DC 20005   202-483-6272

Also provides support groups for parents.

1112 National Brain Tumor Foundation
22 Battery Street, Suite 612
San Francisco, CA 94111   617-924-9997
                    800-934-2873
                    Fax: 510-834-9980
                    e-mail: nbtf@braintumor.org
                    www.braintumor.org

NBTF is a national nonprofit health organization dedicated to
providing information and support for brain tumor patients, family members, and healthcare professionals, while supporting innovative research into better treatment options and a cure for brain
tumors.

Jeffrey Kolodin, Chair
Michael Nathanson, Vice Chair
Michael Corkin, Treasurer

1113 National Brain Tumor Society
124 Watertown Street, Suite 2D
Watertown, MA 02472   617-924-9997
                    800-770-8287
                    Fax: 617-924-9998
                    e-mail: info@braintumor.org
                    www.braintumor.org

The Brain Tumor Society exists to find a cure for brain tumors. It
strives to improve the quality of life of brain tumor patients and
their families. It disseminates educational information and provides access to psychosocial support. It raises funds to advance
carefully selected scientific research projects, improve clinical
care and find a cure.

N Paul TonThat, Executive Director
Jeffrey Kolodin, Chair
Michael Nathanson, Vice Chair

1114 National Childhood Cancer Foundation
4600 East West Highway, Suite 600
Bethesda, MD 20814   301-718-0042
                    800-458-6223
                    Fax: 301-718-0047
                    e-mail: info@curesearch.org
                    www.curesearch.org

CureSearch for Children's Cancer is a national non-profit foundation that accelerates the cure for children's cancer by driving innovation, eliminating research barriers and solving the field's
most challenging problems.

Stuart Siegal MD, Chair of the Board
Timothy Harmon, Vice Chair
Mary Payne, Treasurer

1115 National Children's Cancer Society
500 North Broadway, Suite 800 St.
Louis, MO 63102   314-241-1600
                    Fax: 314-241-1996
                    www.thenccs.org

The National Children's Cancer Society (NCCS) provides emotional, financial and educational support to children with cancer,
their families and survivors.

Mark Slocomb, Chairman
Maria Taxman, Vice Chairman
Mark Stolze, President

1116 National Comprehensive Cancer Network
275 Commerce Dr, Suite 300
Fort Washington, PA 19034   215-690-0300
                    Fax: 215-690-0280
                    www.nccn.org

Devoted to patient care, research, and education, is dedicated to
improving the quality, effectiveness, and efficiency of cancer
care so that patients can live better lives.

Samuel M. Silver, Chair
Timothy J. Eberlein, Vice Chair
Mara G. Bloom, Secretary

1117 Nevus Outreach
600 SE Delaware Ave., Suite 200
Bartlesville, OK 74003
918-331-0595
877-426-3887
e-mail: ahouseal@nevus.org
www.nevus.org

Nevus Outreach is dedicated to improving awareness and providing support for people affected by congenital melanocytic nevi and finding a cure.

Anne Houseal, Chairman
Mark Beckwith, Executive Director
Michael Kushner, Secretary

1118 Pituitary Network Association
P.O. Box 1958
Thousand Oaks, CA 91358
805-499-9973
Fax: 805-480-0633
e-mail: info@pituitary.org
www.pituitary.org

The PNA is an international non-profit organization for patients with pituitary tumors and disorders, their families, loved ones, and the physicians and health care providers who treat them.

Robert Knutzen, CEO / Chairman
Paula Gallegos-Maxfield, Treasurer
Christina Bourne, Board of Director

1119 Preuss Foundation
2223 Avenida de la Playa, Suite 220
La Jolla, CA 92037
858-454-0200
Fax: 858-454-4449
e-mail: fari@preuss.org
www.ninds.nih.gov/find_people/voluntary_orgs/volorg2

Foundation that provides information on support groups, brochures and pamphlets.

Story C Landis, Director
Walter J Koroshetz, Deputy Director
Caroline Lewis, Executive Officer

1120 Society for NeuroOncology
PO Box 273296
Houston, TX 77277
281-554-6589
Fax: 713-583-1345
e-mail: linda@soc-neuro-onc.org
www.soc-neuro-onc.org

Multi-disciplinary organization dedicated to promoting advances in neuro-oncology through research and education.

David A. Reardon, President
E. Antonio Chiocca, Vice President
Eva Galanis, Secretary/Treasurer

1121 Sontag Foundation
sontagfoundation.org
e-mail: info@sontagfoundation.org
sontagfoundation.org

Our primary focus is on brain cancer, with additional support for rheumatoid arthritis.

Frederick B Sontag, President
Frederick T Sontag, Vice President
Kay W Verble, Executive Director

1122 Students Supporting Brain Tumor Research
8390 E. Via de Ventura, F-110
Scottsdale, AZ 85258
888-772-8729
e-mail: admin@ssbtr.org
www.ssbtr.org

Mission is to provide education and leadership development to our youth.

1123 Tug McGraw Foundation
100 California Drive
Yountville, CA 94599
707-947-7124
707-676-4398
e-mail: info@tugmcgraw.org
www.tugmcgraw.org

To provide resources and hands-on support, foster understanding, promote awareness, and stimulate research.

Tom Higgins, Chairman
Jennifer Brusstar, President & CEO
Tom McGraw, Chief Executive Officer

State Agencies & Support Groups

Alabama

1124 Pediatric Brain Tumor Support Group
Children's Hospital
1600 7th Avenue S
Birmingham, AL 35233
205-939-9090
Fax: 205-939-9010
e-mail: info@braintumorkids.org
www.braintumorkids.org

Groups for parents and siblings of brain tumor patients. Related to Children's Hospital of Alabama. Babysitting available.

Pamela B Ellis, President
Robert Flamini MD, Vice President
William A Guzak, Treasurer

Arizona

1125 Brain Tumor Support Group at NovaCare Rehabilitation Institute of Tucson
2650 N Wyatt Drive
Tucson, AZ 85712
520-293-8040
www.tmcaz.com

Scott Gulbrandsen

1126 Brain Tumor Support Group at Phoenix
350 W Thomas Road
Phoenix, AZ 85013
602-873-2757
www.braintumorsupportgroup.com/hospital/children/pho

The Jaydie Lynn King Neuro-oncology Program at Phoenix Children's Hospital is the only comprehensive pediatric program of its kind in Arizona, combining the expertise of subspecialists in the Children's Neuroscience Institute and the Center for Cancer and Blood Disorders (CCBD).

Steve Westerhoff

California

1127 Brain Tumor Patient & Family Support Group
Saint Jude Medical Center
2151 N Harbor Blvd, St Jude Medical Plaza, Rm 2266
Fullerton, CA 92635
714-446-7182
www.stjudemedicalcenter.org

Periodic guest presentations.

Robert Merlino

1128 Brain Tumor Support Group at Newport Beach
301 Newport Blvd.
Newport Beach, CA 92658
949-760-2350
www.bettyclooneyfoundation.org

Speakers once a month, education materials available.

Kris O'Neal

1129 Brain Tumor Support Group at San Diego
8555 Aero Drive #340
San Diego, CA 92103
858-467-1065
www.bettyclooneyfoundation.org

Speakers once a month, education materials available.

Donna Gilpatrick RN, MS, FNP

1130 Brain Tumor Support Group at San Luis Obispo
1911 Johnson Avenue
San Luis Obispo, CA 93401
805-461-3989
www.bettyclooneyfoundation.org

Speakers once a month, education materials available.

Becky Nunez

1131 Brain Tumor Support Group at Santa Monica
2200 Colorado Boulevard
Santa Monica, CA 90404 310-453-2200
www.bettyclooneyfoundation.org

Speakers once a month, education materials available.

Michael Slater, Program Director

1132 Brain Tumor Support Program Cedars-Sinai Neurosurgical Inst. & Wellness Communit
8631 W 3rd Street, Suite 800 E
Los Angeles, CA 90048 310-855-7900
Fax: 310-423-0777
www.bettyclooneyfoundation.org

Last Wednesday of month 6-7:30 pm with an RSVP.

Jennice Vilhauer, Contact

1133 Fresno Brain Tumor Support Group
7130 North Millbrook Avenue
Fresno, CA 93720 559-450-5528
Fax: 559-449-3990
e-mail: karen.kennedy@samc.com
www.braintumor.org

Speakers once a month, education materials available.

Karen Kennedy, Contact
Jeffrey Kolodin, Chair
Michael Nathanson, Vice Chair

1134 Inland Empire Brain Tumor Support Group
Medical Annex Building
Riverside Community Hospital, 4445 Magnolia Avenue
Riverside, CA 92502 951-222-8090
http://events.pe.com/riverside-ca

Meets third Saturday, once a month.

Sue Melton, Contact

1135 Neuroscience Institute Brain Tumor Support Group
637 S Lucas Avenue, Suite 501
Los Angeles, CA 90017 213-977-2234
800-762-1692
www.mhmni.com/support/

The group meets the second Wednesday of every month at 6 p.m. in the Heart & Vascular Institute, 3rd floor, conference room A.

Cherrie Valacruz, Manager

1136 Northridge Hospital: Leavey Cancer Center
18300 Roscoe Boulevard
Northridge, CA 91328 818-885-5431
www.northridgehospital.org

We are fully-accredited by the American College of Surgeons Commission on Cancer as a Comprehensive Cancer Center since 1980.

Marylou Perelmutter, Manager

1137 Palo Alto Brain Tumor Support Group
920 Bryant Street, 2nd Floor Room B
Palo Alto, CA 94301 415-284-0208
www.pamf.org

Joanie Taylor, RN

1138 Peninsula Support & Education Group for Parents of Children with Brain Tumors
3041 Olcott
Santa Clara, CA 95054 650-325-4523
www.supportforfamilies.org

Sheri Sobrato, MA, MFC

1139 Sacramento Area Brain Tumor Support Group Lawrence J Ellison Ambulatory Care Ctr
UC Davis Medical Center, Camellia Cottage
4860 Y Street Suite 3740
Sacramento, CA 95817 916-734-3658
Fax: 916-703-5368
e-mail: kksmith@ucdavis.edu
www.ucdmc.ucdavis.edu/neurosurg/contactus/contact_in

First Thursday of month 6:30-8:30 pm.

J. Paul . Muizelaar, M.D., Ph.D, Program Director
James E Boggan MD, Professor and Acting Chair
Kee D Kim MD, Associate Professor

1140 San Francisco Brain Tumor Support Group
UC San Francisco, Clinical Sciences Building
521 Parnassus Avenue, Room C130
San Francisco, CA 94188 415-990-4461
e-mail: mary.lovely@sbcglobal.net
www.ucsfhealth.org/support_groups/neurology/

First Wednesday of each month, 7:00 - 8:30 pm

Sharon Lamb, Contact
Mary Lovely, Contact

1141 Santa Barbara Brain Tumor Support Group
Cancer Foundation of Santa Barbara
540 West Pueblo Street
Santa Barbara, CA 93105 805-682-7300
www.braintumor.org

Third Thursday of each month, 5:15-6:30 pm.

Rosario Campuzano, Contact
Jeffrey Kolodin, Chair
Michael Nathanson, Vice Chair

1142 Santa Cruz County Brain Tumor Support Group
3031 Main Street
Soquel, CA 95073 831-438-8344
www.braintumor.org

Gregory Valki-Tarsy
Jeffrey Kolodin, Chair
Michael Nathanson, Vice Chair

1143 Santa Rosa Brain Tumor Support Group
North Coast Rehab Hospital Fulton Campus Conf Room
1287 Fulton
Santa Rosa, CA 95401 415-353-2966
www.braintumor.org

Last Wednesday of each month, 6:30-8:00 pm.

Jane Rabbitt RN, Contact
Jeffrey Kolodin, Chair
Michael Nathanson, Vice Chair

1144 South Bay Brain Tumor Support Group
667 Chapman Street
San Jose, CA 95126 650-725-8630
www.braintumor.org

Genny See-Tho RN
Jeffrey Kolodin, Chair
Michael Nathanson, Vice Chair

1145 Southern California Pediatric Brain Tumor Network
UCLA Medical Center
10833 LeConte Avenue, Suite 501
Los Angeles, CA 310-825-7354
www.braintumor.org

For parents of children with brain tumors, and for teenagers with brain tumors.

Patricia Park
Jeffrey Kolodin, Chair
Michael Nathanson, Vice Chair

1146 Support Group for Caregivers of Brain Tumor Patients
UCLA Medical Center
UCLA Medical Plaza Building
Los Angeles, CA 90052 310-206-6731
www.braintumor.org

Guest speakers on occasion.

Pamela Hoff, LCSW
Jeffrey Kolodin, Chair
Michael Nathanson, Vice Chair

1147 Support Group for Parents of Children with Brain Tumors
Oakland Children's Hospital
747 52nd Street, Auditorium Sd II
Oakland, CA 94609   510-428-3885
                                            www.braintumor.org

Contact can be reached at extension 2161.

Trish Murphy
Jeffrey Kolodin, Chair
Michael Nathanson, Vice Chair

1148 Vital Options
4419 Coldwater Canyon Ave., Suite I
Studio City, CA 91604   818-508-5657
                                         Fax: 818-788-5260
                                 e-mail: info@vitaloptions.org
                                        www.vitaloptions.org

Vital Options International is a 501(c)(3) not-for-profit cancer
communications organization with a mission, to facilitate a global
cancer dialogue

Selma R Schimmel, CEO and Founder
Derek Alpert, President
Terry Merrill Wilcox, Creative Director and Supervising P

1149 Wellness Community San Francisco/East Bay
3276 McNutt Avenue
Walnut Creek, CA 94597   925-933-0107
                                         Fax: 925-933-0249
                                        www.twc-bayarea.org

To help people affected by cancer enhance their health and
well-being through participation in a professional program of
emotional support, education, and hope.

James R Bouquin, Executive Director
Margaret Stauffer MFT, Program Director
Amy Alanes, Development Manager

1150 West Los Angeles Brain Tumor Support Group
2716 Ocean Park Boulvard, Suite 1040
Santa Monica, CA 90405   310-314-2555
                                            www.braintumor.org

Michael States, Program Director
Jeffrey Kolodin, Chair
Michael Nathanson, Vice Chair

Colorado

1151 Brain Tumor Patient & Family Support Group
Swedish Medical Center Conference Center
701 E Hampden Avenue #330
Englewood, CO 80113   303-806-7420
                                 e-mail: lgibson@thecni.org
                                            www.braintumor.org

Sponsored by Colorado Neurological Institute Center for Brain
and Spinal Tumors. First Wednesday of month, 6:30-8:00 pm.

Lorre Gibson, Contact

1152 Brain Tumor Patient/Family Group
Anchutz Cancer Pavillion, University of Colorado
Fitzsimons Campus, 1635 Ursula Street
Aurora, CO 80045   303-315-6635
                                e-mail: amy.ebert@uchsc.edu
                                            www.braintumor.org

First Wednesday of each month, 5:00-7:00 pm. call to confirm location.

Amy Ebert, Contact
Jeffrey Kolodin, Chair
Michael Nathanson, Vice Chair

1153 Brain Tumor Support Group
Poudre Valley Hospital
1024 S Lemay, Neuroscience Floor
Ft. Collins, CO 80521   970-495-8320
                                        e-mail: ryjj@aol.com
                                            www.braintumor.org

Second Thursday of each month at 5:00 pm. Call to confirm location.

Georgie Knaub, Contact
Jeffrey Kolodin, Chair
Michael Nathanson, Vice Chair

Connecticut

1154 Brain Tumor Support Group
Cancer Program
80 Seymour Street
Hartford, CT 06102   860-545-5000
                                               860-545-2318
                                         Fax: 860-545-5066
                                            www.braintumor.org

First Thursday of each month, 5:30-7:00 pm. Call in advance to
RSVP.

Hillary Keller, Contact
Jeffrey Kolodin, Chair
Michael Nathanson, Vice Chair

1155 Connecticut Brain Tumor Support Group (Adult)
Yale New Haven Hospital, Children's Hospital
20 York Street, Room 201
New Haven, CT 06510   203-688-7528
                                            www.braintumor.org

Second Tuesday of each month, 2:00-3:30 pm (please call to confirm date and time).

Betsy D'Andrea, Contact
Angela Thomas MSW, Contact
Michael Nathanson, Vice Chair

Delaware

1156 Pediatric Brain Tumor Support Group
1901 Rockland Road
Wilmington, DE 19803   302-995-0938
                                            www.braintumor.org

Cathy Francisco
Jeffrey Kolodin, Chair
Michael Nathanson, Vice Chair

District of Columbia

1157 Washington DC Metropolitan Area Support Group
2121 Eye Street, NW
Washington, DC 20052   202-994-1000
                                            www.braintumor.org

Jeffrey Kolodin, Chair
Michael Nathanson, Vice Chair

Florida

1158 Angels in the Sun Brain Tumor Support Group
3251 Proctor Road
Sarasota, FL 34231   941-364-9105
                                        www.braintumorkids.org

Anna Browder
Jeffrey Kolodin, Chair
Michael Nathanson, Vice Chair

1159 Brain Tumor Support Group
1703 W Colonial Drive
Orlando, FL 32804   407-740-0007
                                            www.braintumor.org

David Cox, MD
Jeffrey Kolodin, Chair
Michael Nathanson, Vice Chair

1160 Brain Tumor Support Group at Miami
Miami Children's Hospital Foundation
3000 SW 62nd Avenue, Founders Lounge
Miami, FL 33155   305-662-8386
                                    www.braintumor.org

Call to confirm time and date.

Maria Penate RN, Contact
Jeffrey Kolodin, Chair
Michael Nathanson, Vice Chair

1161 Brain Tumor Support Group at St. Petersburg
Saint Anthony's Hospital
Saint Petersburg, FL 33730   813-825-1100
                                    www.braintumor.org

Contact can be reached at extension 4231.

Karen McGough
Jeffrey Kolodin, Chair
Michael Nathanson, Vice Chair

1162 Brain Tumor Support Group at Tampa
12902 Magnolia Drive
Tampa, FL 33612   813-979-7258
                                    800-456-3434
                                    www.braintumor.org

Inez Rodriquez
Jeffrey Kolodin, Chair
Michael Nathanson, Vice Chair

1163 Cancer Support Group for Children
3501 Johnson Street, 4th Floor
Hollywood, FL 33021   954-987-2000
            www.ped-onc.org/resources/supportorg.html

Sub-groups for children with brain tumors and their parents. Contact at ext. 4193.

Suzanne Baxter RN

1164 South Florida Brain Tumor Association Lynn Regional Cancer Center
Boca Raton Community Hospital
800 Meadows Road, Education Center
Boca Raton, FL 33486   561-955-7100
                                    561-955-5897
            www.brrh.com/Cancer_Institute.aspx

Neuropsychologist Dr. Laurence Miller and therapist Marjorie O'Sullivan are present to facilitate the meetings. Second and Fourth Thursdays of each month, 7:30-8:30 pm.

Jerry Fedele, President and Chief Executive Offic
Karen Poole, FACHE, Vice President, Chief Operating Off
Dawn P Javersack, Vice President and Chief Financial

1165 Tampa Bay Area Brain Tumor Support Group
St Joseph's Hospital, Medical Arts Building
3000 West Martin Luther King Boulevard
Tampa Bay, FL 33630   813-870-4101
                                    www.braintumor.org

Third Tuesday of each month, 6:30-7:30 pm.

Jeffrey Kolodin, Chair
Michael Nathanson, Vice Chair
Michael Corkin, Treasurer

Georgia

1166 All Ages Support Group
1835 Savoy Drive, Suite 316
Atlanta, GA 30341   770-458-5554
                        e-mail: btfc@bellsouth.net
                        www.braintumorkids.org

Contact for details.
Mary Campbell, Contact

1167 Brain Tumor Foundation for Children
6065 Roswell Road NE, Suite 505
Atlanta, GA 30328   404-252-4107
                                    Fax: 404-252-4108
                        e-mail: info@braintumorkids.org
                        www.braintumorkids.org

The mission of the Brain Tumor Foundation for Children is to provide financial assistance, social support, and information for families of children with brain and spinal cord tumors; fund research projects that improve treatment options and search for a cure; and raise public awareness of the disease and advocate on behalf of children who are affected.

Pamela B Ellis, President
Robert Flamini MD, Vice President
William A Guzak, Treasurer

1168 Brain Tumor Support Group
Emory Clinic, Neurosurgery Conference Room
1365 Clifton Road, Building B, 2nd Floor
Atlanta, GA 30341   404-778-4153
                                    404-778-3091
                                    www.braintumor.org

First Thursday of each month, 12:30-2:30 pm. Please RSVP to attend.

Karen Shires, Contact
Linda Phillips, Contact
Jeffrey Kolodin, Chair

1169 Southeastern Brain Tumor Foundation Brain Tumor Support Group
Wellness Community, Peachtree Dunwoody Pavillion
PO Box 422471
Atlanta, GA 30342   404-843-3700
                        e-mail: info@sbtf.org
                        www.sbtf.org/home.html

Second Monday of each month, 7:00-8:30 pm.

Costas G. Hadjipanayis, MD, PhD, President
Jennifer Keenan Giliberto, Vice President
Suzanne Boeren, Treasurer

Hawaii

1170 Brain Tumor Support Group
93 N Kainalu, Kailu
Oahu, HI   808-254-1989
                                    www.braintumor.org

Chuck Rogers
Kari Rogers
Jeffrey Kolodin, Chair

Idaho

1171 Treasure Valley Brain Injury Support Group
Idaho Elks Rehabilitation Hospital
600 North Robbins Road
Boise, ID 83702   208-489-4558
                        e-mail: bjaundalderis@elksrehab.org
                        www.idahoelksrehab.org

Through our expertise in rehab and uncompromising commitment to care, education and research, we help you live life to its fullest. Fourth Tuesday of each month 7:00-9:00 pm.

Bob Jaundalderis, Marketing Director
Katie McCurdy, Brain Injury Program Director

Illinois

1172 Brain Tumor Resource & Support Group
Central DuPage Hospital, Neuro-Spine Unit
25 North Winfield Road
Winfield, IL 60190   630-933-6955
                        e-mail: debbie_brunelle@cdh.org
                        www.braintumor.org

Second and Fourth Wednesday of each month, 7:30-9:00 pm.

Deborah Brunelle RN, Contact
Jeffrey Kolodin, Chair
Michael Nathanson, Vice Chair

1173 Brain Tumor Support Group
303 E Superior
Chicago, IL 60611
312-908-8177
www.braintumor.org

Mary Ellen Maher Deleon
Jeffrey Kolodin, Chair
Michael Nathanson, Vice Chair

1174 Brain Tumor Support Group at Northwestern Memorial Hospital
251 East Huron, Suite 3-520
Chicago, IL 60611
312-695-8143
www.braintumor.org

Educational program offered at each meeting by members of the professional committee. Third Monday of each month, 5:00-6:00 pm.

Mary Ellen Maher Deleon, Contact
Jeffrey Kolodin, Chair
Michael Nathanson, Vice Chair

1175 Brain Tumor Support Group at Park Ridge
Lutheran General Hospital, Cancer Care Center
1775 Dempster St.
Park Ridge, IL 60302
847-696-5475
www.braintumor.org

Third Wednesday of each month, 7:30-9:00 pm.

Syril Gilbert LCSW, Contact
Jeffrey Kolodin, Chair
Michael Nathanson, Vice Chair

1176 Parents of Children with Brain Tumors (PCBT)
Children's Memorial Hospital
2300 Children's Plaza
Chicago, IL 60614
773-880-4553
www.cbtrf.org/

Monthly newsletter. Library available at meetings (at CMH). Educational speakers and family functions. Call to confirm meetings.

Teresa Berry, Contact

Indiana

1177 Benign Brain Tumor Support Group
Howard Regional Health Systems
322 North Main Street
Kokomo, IN 46901
765-455-2613
www.braintumor.org

Third Wednesday of each month, 5:00-6:30 pm. Meet in southeast corner of the building, enter at set of double doors on corner of North Main and Taylor Street.

Marsha Mahoney, Contact
Jeffrey Kolodin, Chair
Michael Nathanson, Vice Chair

1178 Brain Tumor Support Group
205 E Kirkwood Avenue
Bloomington, IN 47408
812-332-4459
Fax: 812-332-4479
www.braintumor.org

Jean Bauer
Jeffrey Kolodin, Chair
Michael Nathanson, Vice Chair

1179 Brain Tumor Support Group at Indianapolis
Community Hospital North
Regional Cancer Center
Indianapolis, IN 46256
317-485-6616
317-842-1229
e-mail: m.w.kempf@sbcglobal.net
www.braintumor.org

Third Wednesday of each month, 6:3-7:30 pm. The Regional Cancer Center is in a building just to the south of the main hospital, across Clearvista Drive.

Lisa Peters RN, Contact
Michael Kempf, Contact
Marcia Cline, Contact

1180 Primary Brain Cancer Support Group
Women's Cancer Center at Lutheran Hospital
7910 W Jefferson Boulevard, Suite 112
Fort Wayne, IN 46804
260-435-7959
www.cancercenter.com/

First Tuesday of every month, 6:00 pm.

Linda Jordan RN, Contact

Iowa

1181 Brain Tumor Support Group
University Of Iowa Hospitals
200 Hawkins Drive
Iowa City, IA 52242
319-356-4125
319-356-2301
e-mail: suzanne-witte@uiowa.edu
www.braintumor.org

First Tuesday of each month with exception of July, August, January. Meeting held at the Cancer Center Waiting Room from 7-8:30 pm.

Sue Witte, Contact
Sue May, Contact
Jeffrey Kolodin, Chair

1182 Quad Cities Brain Tumor Support Group
Genesis Medical Center
1401 W Central Park
Davenport, IA 52804
563-421-1905
e-mail: christyp@genesishealth.com
www.braintumor.org

Fourth Monday of each month, 6:30-8:00 pm.

Pat Christy RN, Contact
Jeffrey Kolodin, Chair
Michael Nathanson, Vice Chair

Kansas

1183 Headstrong Brain Tumor Support Group
Victory in the Valley
Victory House, 3755 East Douglas,
Witchita, KS 67214
316-634-2801
e-mail: phyllis.jacobs@wichita.edu
www.braintumor.org

Second Wednesday of each month at 7pm. Call for information.

Phyllis Jacob, Contact
Jeffrey Kolodin, Chair
Michael Nathanson, Vice Chair

Kentucky

1184 Brain Injury Support Group
2050 Versailles Road
Lexington, KY 40504
859-254-5701
www.braininjuryguide.org/braininjurysupportgroups.ht

First Thursday of each month at 6:00 pm. Meeting will be held in Conference Room A or B in the Center of Learning.

Tonia Wells, Contact

Louisiana

1185 Brain Injury Support And Education Group
Touro Infirmary
1401 Foucher Street
New Orleans, LA 70115
504-897-7011
e-mail: babies@touro.com
www.touro.com

1331 National Fire Protection Association
1 Batterymarch Park
Quincy, MA 02169

617-770-3000
800-844-6058
Fax: 617-770-0700
www.nfpa.org

Providing and advocating scientifically-based consensus codes and standards, research, training and education.

Ernest J. Grant, Chair
Randolph W. Tucker, 1st Vice Chair
Keith E. Williams, 2nd Vice Chair

1332 Society for Pediatric Dermatology
8365 Keystone Crossing, Suite 107
Indianapolis, IN 46240

317-202-0224
Fax: 317-205-9481
e-mail: info@pedsderm.net
www.pedsderm.net

Promotes, develop and advance education, research and care of skin disease in all pediatric age groups.

Beth Drolet, President
Howard Pride, VP Finance and Administration
Karen Wiss, VP Education

Book Publishers

1333 Burns Sourcebook
Omnigraphics
PO Box 31-1640
Detroit, MI 48231

800-234-1340
Fax: 800-875-1340
e-mail: info@omnigraphics.com
www.omnigraphics.com

Basic consumer health information on various types of burns and scalds.

604 pages
ISBN: 0-780802-04-7

Camps

1334 Firefighters Kids Camp Camp Concord
1000 Mount Tallac Road
South Lake Tahoe, CA 96150

916-739-8525
e-mail: catharine@ffburn.org
www.ffburn.org

One-week program to benefit young burn survivors who are age six to age seventeen. Our mission is to provide young burn survivors with a fun and safe camp environment that encourages healing, personal growth and character development within a natural setting.

Catharine Shaw, Director

Description

1335 CELIAC DISEASE

Synonyms: CD, Celiac sprue, Gluten-sensitive enteropathy, GSE, Nontropical sprue

Involves the following Biologic System(s):

Gastrointestinal Disorders

Celiac disease (CD) is a digestive disorder in which the lining of the small intestine is damaged by gluten, a protein found in wheat, barley, rye, and oats. People with CD are thought to have an abnormal immune response to dietary gluten, resulting in the body's own immune system attacks and causes degeneration (atrophy) and flattening of the tiny projections (villi) that line the small intestine. These villi play a vital role in absorbing fats and other nutrients from food products (malabsorption). This damage to the intestinal villi seriously impairs their ability to absorb these nutrients. Although the specific cause of CD is unknown, it is thought to be multifactorial, resulting from interactions between multiple genes (polygenic) and certain environmental factors. CD may affect both children and adults. The frequency with which it occurs varies greatly among countries and among different populations, and more cases occur in Europe than in the United States. Approximately one in 10,000 infants is thought to be affected by CD in the U.S. Celiac disease is genetic, meaning it runs in families. Diagnosis is usually made by a gastroenterologist, through special blood tests and the testing of tissue from the small intestine.

The symptoms associated with celiac disease do not become apparent until gluten is introduced into the diet, and its symptoms may occur in the digestive system or elsewhere in the body. In most children with CD, symptoms begin between the ages of one to five years. Although the symptoms and findings in CD may vary, many children initially have diarrhea, and their stools become abnormally bulky, pale, frothy, and offensive smelling, the result of an abnormally increased fat content (steatorrhea). Other abnormalities in CD may include excessive gas (flatulence); a failure to grow and gain weight at the expected rate (failure to thrive), the result of a decreased intake of nutrients; lack of appetite (anorexia); hair loss; weight loss; vomiting; and swelling (distension) of the abdomen. Many children also experience muscle wasting, are unusually clingy and irritable, and have abnormally pale skin (pallor). As a result of the malabsorption of fats and other nutrients, children with this condition typically have deficiencies of certain vitamins, and some may have abnormally reduced levels of the oxygen-carrying protein hemoglobin in the blood, because of deficient intestinal absorption of iron (iron-deficiency anemia), which is an important component of hemoglobin.

The key step in treating celiac disease is eliminating gluten from the diet. Wheat and rye products must be completely eliminated, although some children with CD may be able to tolerate barley and oat products. Because gluten is widely used in various food products, parents and children may initially require assistance and guidance from an experienced dietitian in avoiding foods that contain it. Specially manufactured, gluten-free food products are available commercially, including gluten-free pasta, bread, and flour. Treatment may also include iron and vitamin supplementation as required.

National Associations & Support Groups

1336 American Academy of Pediatrics
141 Northwest Point Boulevard
Elk Grove Village, IL 60007
847-434-4000
800-433-9016
Fax: 847-434-8000
www.aap.org

The American Academy of Pediatrics and its member pediatricians are committed to the attainment of optimal physical, mental and social health and well-being for all infants, children, adolescents, and young adults.

Sandra Hassink, MD, FAAP, President

1337 American Autoimmune Related Diseases Association, Inc.
22100 Gratiot Avenue
East Detroit, MI 48021
586-776-3900
Fax: 586-776-3903
e-mail: aarda@aarda.org
www.aarda.org

The American Autoimmune Related Diseases Association is dedicated to the eradication of autoimmune diseases and the alleviation of suffering and the socioeconomic impact of autoimmunity through fostering and facilitating collaboration in the areas of education, public awareness, research, and patient services in an effective, ethical and efficient manner.

Stanley M Finger, PhD, Chairman of the Board
Noel R Rose, MD, PhD, Chairman Emeritus
Virginia T Ladd RT, President and Executive Director

1338 American Celiac Disease Alliance
americanceliac.org
e-mail: feedback@americanceliac.org
americanceliac.org

In early 2003, an ad hoc group of 15 leaders in the celiac community came together to help persuade Congress to require food labels to include information about allergens.

1339 American Celiac Society
PO Box 23455
New Orleans, LA 70183
504-737-3293
Fax: 504-737-3283
e-mail: americanceliacsociety@yahoo.com
www.americanceliacsociety.org

Nonprofit, tax exempt organization that supports efforts in education, research and natural support. Helps to set up support groups, sponsors conferences, seeks funding for education and research, identifies ingredients in foods and educates the public about problems facing its members.

Annette C Bentley, President
James R Bentley, VP

1340 American Celiac Society Dietary Support
www.americanceliacsociety.org
504-305-2968
www.americanceliacsociety.org

The American Celiac Society Dietary Support Coalition, a non-profit tax exempt organization, serves individuals suffering with dietary disorders.

Annette C. Bentley, President
James R. Bentley, Vice President

1341 American Dietetic Association
120 South Riverside Plaza, Suite 2000
Chicago, IL 60606
312-899-0040
800-877-1600
e-mail: foundation@eatright.org
www.eatright.org

Nation's largest organization of food and nutrition professionals.

Ethan A Bergman PhD, RD, FADA, C, President
Glenna R McCollum DMOL, MPH, RD, President Elect
Patricia M Babjak, Chief Executive Officer

1342 American Society for Gastrointestinal Endoscopy
3300 Woodcreek Dr.
Downers Grove, IL 60515
630-573-0600
866-353-2743
Fax: 630-963-8332
e-mail: info@asge.com
www.asge.org

ASGE has been dedicated to advancing patient care and digestive health by promoting excellence and innovation in gastrointestinal endoscopy.

Colleen M. Schmitt, President
Douglas O. Faigel, President Elect
Kenneth R. McQuaid, Secretary

1343 Association of Gastrointestinal Motility Disorders
12 Roberts Drive
Bedford, MA 01730
781-275-1300
Fax: 781-275-1304
e-mail: digestive.motility@gmail.com
www.agmd-gimotility.org

AGMD is a non-profit organizations in existence with a focus on digestive motility diseases and disorders.

Thomas Abell, Advisor
Carlo Di Lorenzo, Advisor
Alex Flores, Advisor

1344 Asthma & Allergy Foundation of America
8201 Corporate Drive Suite 1000
Landover, MD 20785
800-727-8462
www.aafa.org

AAFA is a patient organization for people with asthma and allergies, and the oldest asthma and allergy patient group in the world.

Kelli Wilson, Chair
Lynn Hanessian, Immediate Past Chair
David Stukus, Secretary

1345 Catholic Celiac Society
www.catholicceliacs.org

Catholic Celiac Society's three-fold mission will be to educate Catholic celiacs about their options for Holy Communion as provided for by Canon Law and the U.S. Conference of Catholic Bishops; to inform Catholic clergy and lay ministers about the special needs of Catholic celiacs in their dioceses and parishes; and to reconcile those Catholic celiacs who have left the Church through lack of understanding, exclusion from the Eucharist, and isolation from their church community.

1346 Celiac Disease Foundation
20350 Ventura Blvd Ste 240
Woodland Hills, CA 91364
818-716-1513
Fax: 818-267-5577
e-mail: cdf@celiac.org
www.celiac.org

Provides services and support to persons with celiac disease and dermatitus herpetiformis, through programs of awareness, education, advocacy and research; telephone information and referral services; medical advisory board; and special educational seminars and quarterly meetings.

Marc Riches, President
Richard Tasoff, Vice President
Christopher J. Holland, Treasurer

1347 Celiac Sprue Association/USA
PO Box 31700
Omaha, NE 68131
402-558-0600
877-272-4272
Fax: 402-643-4108
e-mail: celiacs@csaceliacs.org
www.csaceliacs.org

National support organization that provides information and referral services for persons with celiac sprue and dermatitis herpetiformis and parents of celiac children. Made up of six regions in the United States, with 84 chapters and 36 resource units.

Bill Locke, President
Mary Schuluckebier, Executive Director
Clark Kolterman, Treasurer

1348 Celiac Support Association
P.O. Box 31700
Omaha, NE 68131
402-643-4101
877-272-4272
Fax: 402-643-4108
e-mail: celiacs@csaceliacs.org
www.csaceliacs.org

Works to increase awareness, improve diagnosis and treatment, and help celiacs and gluten sensitive individuals to love living gluten-free.

1349 Children's National Health System
111 Michigan Avenue, NW
Washington, DC 20010
202-476-5000
888-884-2327
childrensnational.org

At Children's National, we are champions for children, with our entire team focused on pediatric care.

Kurt Newman, President & CEO
Anthony Sandler, Senior Vice President
Brian Jacobs, Vice President

1350 Food Allergy Research & Education
7925 Jones Branch Dr., Suite 1100
McLean, VA 22102
703-691-3179
800-929-4040
Fax: 703-691-2713
www.foodallergy.org

FARE works on behalf of the 15 million Americans with food allergies, including all those at risk for life-threatening anaphylaxis.

Janet Atwater, Chair
Robert Nichols, Vice Chair
Sharyn T. Mann, Secretary

1351 GLC Annual Education Conference
Gluten Intolerance Group
31214 124th Ave SE
Auburn, WA 98092
253-833-6655
Fax: 206-833-6675
e-mail: CustomerService@gluten.net
www.gluten.net

For individuals that are following a gluten-free diet, or want to know all you need about it.

July

David Kline, President
Joe Spancic, Vice President of Business Administ
Kim Kelly, Vice President of Programs

1352 Gluten Intolerance Group of North America (GIG)
31214 124th Ave SE
Auburn, WA 98092
253-833-6655
Fax: 206-833-6675
e-mail: CustomerService@gluten.net
www.gluten.net

The mission of the Gluten Intolerance Group of North America™ is to provide support to persons with gluten intolerances, including celiac disease, dermatitis herpetiformis, and other gluten sensitivities, in order to live healthy lives.

David Kline, President
Joe Spancic, Vice President of Business Administ
Kim Kelly, Vice President of Programs

1353 Kids with Food Allergies
5049 Swamp Rd, Ste 303, PO Box 554
Fountainville, PA 18923
215-230-5394
215-340-7674
www.kidswithfoodallergies.org

Helps to mprove the day-to-day lives of families raising children with food allergies and empower them to create a safe and healthy future for their children.

Heidi Bayer, Chair
Colette Martin, Vice Chair
Amy Recob, Board of Director

1354 National Celiac Disease Society
34 Audrey Avenue, 3rd Floor
Oyster Bay, NY 11771
516-680-8873
e-mail: info@celiacnation.org
www.celiacnation.org

It is an IRS recognized 501(c)(3) non-profit organization with a mission to raise celiac disease education and awareness.

Craig Pinto, Founder
Gary Leuis, Legal Advisor
Lawrence Baronciani, Creative Director

1355 National Foundation for Celiac Awareness
PO Box 544
Ambler, PA 19002
215-325-1306
Fax: 215-643-1707
www.celiaccentral.org

The National Foundation for Celiac Awareness advances widespread understanding of celiac disease as a serious genetic autoimmune condition and works to secure early diagnosis and effective management.

Wendi L. Wasik, Chair
David H. Cohen, Vice Chair
Alice Bast, President & CEO

1356 North American Society for the Study of Ce
P.O. Box 812180
Wellesley, MA 02482
781-431-8138
www.nasscd.org

The NASSCD is the U.S. national society of medical, scientific and allied health professionals in the field of celiac disease.

Joseph A. Murray, President
Peter H.R. Green, President Elect
Alessio Fasano, Secretary

Conferences

1357 Annual Education Conference & Food Faire
Celiac Disease Foundation
20350 Ventura Boulevard, #240
Woodland Hills, CA 91364
818-716-1513
Fax: 818-267-5577
e-mail: cdf@celiac.org
www.celiac.org

Provides people with a greater understanding of Celiac disease, gluten sensitivity, dietary compliance, future therapies, associated conditions and the effect on family members. They networked with other people following the gluten-free lifestyle. Everyone met with exhibitors, sampled and discovered the latest gluten-free foods and services.

May

Mark Riches, President
Richard Tasoff, Vice President
Judy Thomas, Secretary

1358 CSA Annual Conference
Celiac Sprue Association
PO Box 31700
Omaha, NE 68131
402-643-4101
877-272-4272
Fax: 402-643-4108
e-mail: celiacs@csaceliacs.org
www.csaceliacs.org

Invites experts from a broad spectrum of disciplines relating to celiac disease and the required gluten-free diet to share current information. Researchers, healthcare professionals, dietitians, authors, chefs, restaurant owners, and gluten-free food vendors from across the United States participate in this annual educational event.

September

Mary Schluckebier, Executive Director

Audio Video

1359 Unmarking Celiac Disease
American Celiac Society
PO Box 23455
New Orleans, LA 70183
504-737-3293
Fax: 504-737-3283
e-mail: amerceliacsoc@onebox.com

Annette Bentley, President
James Bentley, Vice President

Web Sites

1360 Celiac Disease Foundation
20350 Ventura Boulevard, Suite 240
Woodland Hills, CA 91364
818-716-1513
www.celiac.org

Provides support, information and assistance to people affected by Celiac Disease/Dermatitis Herpetiformis.

Elaine Monarch, Founder
Marc Riches, Chair
Chad Hines, Vice Chair

1361 Celiac Support Page
20350 Ventura Boulevard, Suite 240
Woodland Hills, CA 91364
818-716-1513
www.celiac.com

To help as many people as possibe with celiac disease get diagnosed and live happy, healthy gluten-free lives.

Elaine Monarch, Founder
Marc Riches, Chair
Chad Hines, Vice Chair

1362 Gluten-Free Page
donwiss.com

Offers links about Gluten Free Pages about the Celiac Disease/Gluten Intolerance, gluten free food vendors, and other types of gluten free food sites.

1363 Health Answers
410 Horsham Road
Horsham, PA 19044
215-442-9017
e-mail: Michael.tague@healthanswers.com
www.healthanswers.com

The vision was to provide a breadth of services to clients through the formation of a network of companies. Each company plays a key role in meeting out clients' needs.

Michael Tague, Managing Director

Book Publishers

1364 Digestive Diseases & Disorders Sourcebook
Omnigraphics
PO Box 625
Holmes, PA 19043
610-461-3548
800-234-1340
Fax: 610-532-9001
e-mail: info@omnigraphics.com
www.omnigraphics.com

Basic consumer health information including celiac disease, Crohn's disease, diarrhea, hernias, irritable bowel syndrome and ulcers.

2000 335 pages
ISBN: 0-780803-27-2

Newsletters

1365 GIG Quarterly
Gluten Intolerance Group of North America
31214 124th Avenue SE
Auburn, WA 98092
253-833-6655
Fax: 253-833-6675
e-mail: info@gluten.net
www.gluten.net

The mission of the Gluten Intolerance Group of North America™ is to provide support to persons with gluten intolerances, including celiac disease, dermatitis herpetiformis, and other gluten sensitivities, in order to live healthy lives.

Quarterly

David Kline, President
Kim Kelly, Vice President
Mark Evans, Vice President

1366 Lifeline
Celiac Sprue Association/USA
PO Box 31700
Omaha, NE 68131
402-558-0600
877-272-4272
Fax: 402-643-4108
e-mail: celiacs@csaceliacs.org
www.csaceliacs.org

Quarterly newsletter for celiacs with membership forms, chapter information, resource unit information and promotion brochure.

Bruce Homstead, President
Mary A. Schluckebier, Executive Director
Jeanine Morgan, Recording Secretary

1367 Whoo's Report
PO Box 23455
New Orleans, LA 70183
504-737-3293
Fax: 504-737-3283

Provides practical assistance to members and individuals with celiac disease and information about the disease to the public.

Annette Bentley, President
James Bentley, Vice President

Pamphlets

1368 A Diet Management
Celiac Sprue Association/USA
PO Box 31700
Omaha, NE 68131
402-558-0600
877-272-4272
Fax: 402-643-4108
e-mail: celiacs@csaceliacs.org
www.csaceliacs.org

A personalized chart that shows how to make your diet work.

Bruce Homstead, President
Mary A. Schluckebier, Executive Director
Jeanine Morgan, Recording Secretary

1369 A Success Story
Celiac Sprue Association/USA
PO Box 31700
Omaha, NE 68131
402-558-0600, 877-272-4272
Fax: 402-643-4108
e-mail: celiacs@csaceliacs.org
www.csaceliacs.org

Tells about the history of CSA. Also provides the information of how the CSA Gluten-Free Product Listing Book came about.

Bruce Homstead, President
Mary A. Schluckebier, Executive Director
Jeanine Morgan, Recording Secretary

1370 American Celiac Society
PO Box 23455
New Orleans, LA 71083
504-305-2968
Fax: 504-737-3283
e-mail: info@americanceliacsociety.org
www.americanceliacsociety.org

Information package on American Celiac Society, a national support organization that provides information on celiac disease and related disorders. Provides information on local support groups throughout the US and the world.

Annette Bentley, President
James Bentley, Vice President

1371 Basics for the Gluten-free Diet
Celiac Sprue Association/USA
PO Box 31700
Omaha, NE 68131
402-558-0600
877-272-4272
Fax: 402-643-4108
e-mail: celiacs@csaceliacs.org
www.csaceliacs.org

Information sheets by the Celiac Sprue Association/USA Inc, a national support organization that provides information and referral services for persons with celiac sprue and dermatitis herpetiformis and parents of celiac children. Made up of 6 regions in the United States, with 84 chapters and 36 resource units.

Bruce Homstead, President
Mary A. Schluckebier, Executive Director
Jeanine Morgan, Recording Secretary

1372 Diet Instruction
Gluten Intolerance Group of North America
31214 124th Avenue SE
Auburn, WA 98092
253-833-6655
Fax: 253-833-6675

1373 Gluten-free Commercial Products
Celiac Sprue Association/USA
PO Box 31700
Omaha, NE 68131
402-558-0600, 877-272-4272
Fax: 402-643-4108
e-mail: celiacs@csaceliacs.org
www.csaceliacs.org

Information sheets by the Celiac Sprue Association/USA.

Bruce Homstead, President
Mary A. Schluckebier, Executive Director
Jeanine Morgan, Recording Secretary

1374 Introductory Packet Brochure
Gluten Intolerance Group of North America
31214 124th Avenue SE
Auburn, WA 98092
253-833-6655; Fax: 253-833-6675

Offers facts and statistics on celiac sprue and dermatitis herpetiformis.

1375 Living a Full Life with Celiac Sprue
Celiac Sprue Association/USA
PO Box 31700
Omaha, NE 68131
402-558-0600, 877-272-4272
Fax: 402-643-4108
e-mail: celiacs@csaceliacs.org
www.csaceliacs.org

Provides information on celiac-symptoms, treatments and where it was derived from.

Bruce Homstead, President
Mary A. Schluckebier, Executive Director
Jeanine Morgan, Recording Secretary

1376 Patient Packets For Celiac Disease
Gluten Intolerance Group of North America
31214 124th Avenue SE
Auburn, WA 98092
253-833-6655
Fax: 253-833-6675

Includes various brochures and research reports on celiac sprue, recipes, diet instruction and more.

Description

1377 CEREBRAL PALSY

Synonym: CP

Covers these related disorders: Ataxic cerebral palsy,
Choreoathetoid cerebral palsy, Mixed cerebral palsy, Spastic
cerebral palsy

Involves the following Biologic System(s):

Neurologic Disorders, Orthopedic and Muscle Disorders

Cerebral palsy (CP) is a nonprogressive condition characterized by stiff, rigid, and awkward movements (spasticity); involuntary, slow writhing movements (athetosis); and poor
balance and coordination of voluntary movement (ataxia).
Approximately two of every 1,000 infants are affected with
cerebral palsy. Both premature and low birth weight infants
are particularly at risk for this condition. Cerebral palsy may
occur as the result of an injury to the brain during pregnancy,
birth, or the early childhood years. Such brain injuries may be
caused by a decrease in the supply of oxygen to the brain during the birthing period; an infection passed from the mother
to the fetus during pregnancy; or an excess of bile pigment
(bilirubin) in the developing fetus, usually arising from a
blood incompatibility between mother and child. After birth,
cerebral palsy may result from head trauma, an infection of
the brain (e.g., encephalitis), an infection of the membranes
surrounding the brain (meningitis), or other insult to the brain
or surrounding tissue.

This condition is divided into four main types, based on the
movement disorder. These include spastic, choreoathetoid,
ataxic, and mixed cerebral palsy. Spastic cerebral palsy is the
most common type of this condition and is characterized by
stiff and weak muscles in the arms and legs on one or both
sides of the body. Choreoathetoid cerebral palsy is characterized by poorly controlled, spontaneous slow movements of
the muscles and accounts for approximately 20 percent of affected children. Ataxic cerebral palsy affects approximately
10 percent of all those with cerebral palsy and is characterized by poor coordination and shaky movements. Mixed cerebral palsy is a combination of two or more types of this
abnormality and is characterized by the physical characteristics of the types. Although some children with cerebral palsy
have below-average intelligence or are mentally retarded, others are of average or above-average intelligence.

There is no cure for cerebral palsy, but the disabilities associated with CP can be reduced. The type and extent of
treatment depends upon the degree and type of disability experienced by the individual child. Medications are prescribed
to reduce spasticity and abnormal movements and to prevent
seizures. Surgery can also be used to reduce spasticity. Occupational and physical therapy may aid affected children with
walking and muscle coordination and control. Some children
may benefit from the use of braces or other orthopedic intervention. Speech therapy may be useful for improvement of
speech and eating difficulties. Physical and emotional
stimulation and support are very important aspects of
treatment and will aid in helping children with cerebral palsy
to realize their full potential.

Government Agencies

**1378 NIH/National Institute of Child Health and Human
Development**
31 Center Drive, Building 31
Bethesda, MD 20892
800-370-2943
Fax: 301-496-1104
TTY: 888-320-6942
e-mail: NICHDInformationResourceCenter@mail.nih.
www.nichd.nih.gov

Established in 1962 by congress, today the institute conducts and
supports laboratory research, clinical trials, and epidemiological
studies that explore health processes; examines the impact of disabilities, diseases, and variations on the lives of individuals; and
sponsors training programs for scientists, health care providers,
and researchers to ensure that NICHD research can continue

Alan E Guttmacher MD, Director
Lisa Kaeser, Program & Public Liaison

**1379 NIH/National Institute of Neurological Dis orders and Stroke
(NINDS)**
PO Box 5801
Bethesda, MD 20824
301-496-5751
800-352-9424
Fax: 301-496-0296
TTY: 301-468-5981
www.ninds.nih.gov

The mission of NINDS is to reduce the burden of neurological
disease - a burden borne by every age group, by every segment of
society, by people all over the world.

Story C Landis Ph.D., Director
Walter J Koroshetz, Deputy Director
Caroline Lewis, Executive Officer

National Associations & Support Groups

1380 ADA Technical Assistance Program
401 North Washington Street, Suite 450
Rockville, MD 20805
703-448-6155
800-949-4232
Fax: 301-251-3762
TTY: 301-217-0124
e-mail: adata@adata.org
www.adainfo.org/

A federally funded network of grantees which provides information, training and technical assistance to businesses and agencies
with duties and responsibilities under the ADA (American with
Disabilities Act) and to people with disabilities with rights under
the ADA. Materials-the ADA and newsletters are available.

Marian Vessels, Director
Karen Goss, Assistant Director
Del Rae Conley, Office Manager

**1381 American Academy for Cerebral Palsy and Developmental
Medicine**
555 E Wells Street, Suite 1100
Milwaukee, WI 53202
414-918-3014
Fax: 414-276-2146
e-mail: info@aacpdm.org
www.aacpdm.org

The American Academy for Cerebral Palsy and Developmental
Medicine is a multidisciplinary scientific society devoted to the
study of cerebral palsy and other childhood onset disabilities, to
promoting professional education for the treatment and management of these conditions, and to improving the quality of life for
people with these disabilities.

Maureen O'Donnell, President
Richard Stevenson, MD, First Vice President
Darcy Fehlings, Second Vice President

1382 American Academy of Pediatrics
141 Northwest Point Boulevard
Elk Grove Village, IL 60007
847-434-4000
800-433-9016
Fax: 847-434-8000
www.aap.org

The American Academy of Pediatrics and its member pediatricians are committed to the attainment of optimal physical, mental and social health and well-being for all infants, children, adolescents, and young adults.

Sandra Hassink, MD, FAAP, President

1383 American School Counselor Association
1101 King Street, Suite 310
Alexandria, VA 22314
703-683-2722
800-306-4722
Fax: 703-997-7572
e-mail: asca@schoolcounselor.org
www.schoolcounselor.org

The mission of ASCA is to represent professional school counselors and to promote professionalism and ethical practices.

Richard Wong, Executive Director
Jeff Broderson, Information Technology Admin.
Kathleen M Rakestraw, Director of Communications

1384 Center for Disabilities and Development
University of Iowa Hospitals and Clinics
100 Hawkins Drive
Iowa City, IA 52242
319-353-6900
877-686-0031
Fax: 319-356-8284
e-mail: cdd-webmaster@uiowa.edu
www.uichildrens.org/cdd/

A trusted resource for healthcare, training, research and information for people with disabilities that include: behavior disorders, brain injury, cerebral palsy, diabetes, down syndrome, learning disabilities, mental retardation, sleep disorders and spina bifida.

Raphael Hirsch, MD, Physician-in-Chief, UI Children's H
Scott Turner, Executive Director, University of I
Joel Shilyansky, MD,, Associate Professor and Director, D

1385 Children's Neurobiological Solutions Foundation
1223 Wilshire Blvd., #937
Santa Barbara, CA 90403
310-889-8611
866-267-5580
Fax: 805-965-8838
e-mail: info@cnsfoundation.org
www.cnsfoundation.org

Children's Neurobiological Solutions Foundation (CNS), is a national, nonprofit, 501(c)(3) organization, whose mission is to orchestrate cutting-edge, collaborative research with the goal of expediting the creation of effective treatments and therapies for children with neurodevelopmental abnormalities, birth injuries to the nervous system, and related neurological problems.

Carol Abrams JD, President
Fia Richmond, Founder & President, CNS
Phillip H Richmond, Co-Founder, CNS

1386 Easter Seals
233 South Wacker Drive, Suite 2400
Chicago, IL 60606
312-575-0243
800-221-6827
Fax: 312-726-1494
TTY: 312-726-4258
www.easterseals.com

Easter Seals offers a variety of services to help people with disabilities address life's challenges and achieve personal goals.

Stephen F. Rossman, Chairman
Richard W. Davidson, 1st Vice Chairman
Sandra L Bouwman, 2nd Vice Chairman

1387 Easter Seals Disability Services
233 South Wacker Drive, Suite 2400
Chicago, IL 60606
800-221-6827
Fax: 312-726-1494
TTY: 312-726-4258
e-mail: extranetinfo@easterseals.com
www.extraneteasterseals.com

Easter Seals has been helping individuals with disabilities and special needs, and their families, live better lives for more then 80 years. From child development centers to physical rehabilitation and jobs training for peoplewith disabilities, Easter Seals offers a variety of services to help people with disabilities address life's challenges and achieve personal goals.

1388 Epilepsy Foundation
8301 Professional Place
Landover, MD 20785
866-330-2718
800-332-1000
Fax: 301-459-1569
e-mail: ContactUs@efa.org
www.epilepsyfoundation.org

A toll free information and referral service staffed by specially trained people who will answer questions and discuss concerns about seizure disorders and their treatment. Staff will direct callers to local affiliates of the foundation and provide information about a broad range of services that respond to the needs of people with seizure disorders.

18,000 members

Phil Gattone, President and CEO
Gloria Uchegbu, Program Manager
Michele Dawson, Manager of Executive Operations

1389 Family Support Network
Tuberous Sclerosis Alliance
801 Roeder Road, Suite 750
Silver Spring, MD 20910
301-562-9890
800-225-6872
Fax: 301-562-9870
e-mail: info@tsalliance.org
www.tsalliance.org

The Support Network is an organized partnership of individuals whose lives have been affected by tuberous sclerosis. Across the nation, the Support Network is providing the latest medical information, education and support to those individuals who are seeking understanding about the genetic disease and offering them words of encouragement and empowerment.

Matt Bolger, Chair
Keith Hall, Vice Chair
David Michaels, Treasurer

1390 March of Dimes Birth Defects Foundation
1275 Mamaroneck Avenue
White Plains, NY 10605
914-997-4488
888-663-4637
Fax: 914-997-4763
e-mail: answers@marchofdimes.com
www.marchofdimes.com

March of Dimes help moms have full-term pregnancies and research the problems that threaten the health of babies.The March of Dimes also acts globally: sharing best practices in perinatal health and helping improve birth outcomes where the needs are the most urgent.

Kenneth A. May, Chair
Jennifer Howse, President & CEO
Alan Fleischman, Medical Director

1391 National Disability Sports Alliance
25 W Independence Way
Kingston, RI 02881
401-792-7130
Fax: 401-792-7132
e-mail: info@ndsaonline.org
www.nationaldisabilitysportsalliance.webs.com/

Nonprofit organization. Coordinates sports, recreation and fitness activities for individuals with physical disabilities. Main focus is on cerebral palsy, traumatic brain injury and stroke.

Jerry McCole, Executive Director

1392 National Dissemination Center for Children with Disabilities
1825 Connecticut Ave NW
Washington, DC 20009
202-884-8200
800-695-0285
Fax: 202-884-8441
e-mail: nichcy@fhi360.org
www.nichcy.org

A national information and referral center that provides information on disabilities and disability-related issues for families, educators and other professionals.

Suzanne Ripley, Executive Director

1393 United Cerebral Palsy Associations
1825 K Street NW Suite 600
Washington, DC 20036

202-776-0406
800-872-5827
Fax: 202-776-0414
TTY: 202-973-7197
e-mail: info@ucp.org
www.ucp.org

A network of approximately 119 state and local voluntary agencies which provide services, conduct public and professional education programs and support research in cerebral palsy.

Stephen Bennett, Ceo
Woody Connette, Chair
Ian Ridlon, Vice Chair

1394 WE MOVE (Worldwide Education and Advocacy for Movement Disorders)
Mt. Sinai Medical Center
5731 Mosholu Avenue
Bronx, NY 10471

212-875-8312
800-437-6682
Fax: 212-875-8389
e-mail: wemove@wemove.org
www.wemove.org

WE MOVE provides movement disorder information and educational materials to physicians, patients and families, the media, and the public via its comprehensive Web sites, training courses, and more. Its goal is to make early diagnosis, up-to-date treatment and patient support a reality for all people living with movement disorders.

Susan Bressman MD, President
Mo Moadeli, Vice President
Arlene Ploshnick, Treasurer

State Agencies & Support Groups

Alabama

1395 United Cerebral Palsy of Alabama
C/O UCP of East Central Alabama
301 EA Darden Drive, Box 694
Anniston, AL 36202

256-237-8203
Fax: 256-235-2388
e-mail: inda@ecaucp.org
www.ecaucp.org

United Cerebral Palsy provides information, advocacy, referral services for persons with disabilities and/or their families. UCP also operates an equipment loan program, conducts parent workshops, disseminates written literature on topics of interest to people with disabilities.

Donald Turner, Chairman of the Board
Kathy Wood, First Vice-Chairman
John Rogers, Treasurer

1396 United Cerebral Palsy of Greater Birmingham
120 Oslo Circle
Birmingham, AL 35211

205-944-3944
Fax: 205-226-9112
e-mail: dlittlepage@ucpbham.com
www.ucpbham.com

United Cerebral Palsy provides information, advocacy, referral services for persons with disabilities and/or their families. UCP also operates an equipment loan program, conducts parent workshops, disseminates written literature on topics of interest to people with disabilities.

Tom Hinton, Chair
Melva Tate, Executive Vice Chair
Eddie Denaburg, Treasurer

1397 United Cerebral Palsy of Huntsville & Tennessee Valley
2075 Max Luther Drive NW
Huntsville, AL 35810

256-852-5600
256-852-5673
Fax: 256-852-6722
e-mail: therapy@ucphuntsville.org
www.ucphuntsville.org

United Cerebral Palsy provides information, advocacy, referral services for persons with disabilities and/or their families. UCP also operates an equipment loan program, conducts parent workshops, disseminates written literature on topics of interest to people with disabilities.

John Jeffery, President
Cathy Scholl, President-Elect
Gretchen Jensen, Treasurer

1398 United Cerebral Palsy of Mobile
3058 Dauphin Square Connector
Mobile, AL 36607

251-479-4900
Fax: 251-479-4998
e-mail: info@ucpmobile.org
www.ucpmobile.org

United Cerebral Palsy provides information, advocacy and referral services for persons with disabilities and/or their families. UCP also operates an equipment loan program, conducts parent workshops, disseminates written literature on topics of interest to people with disabilities and provides early intervention, supported employment, pre-school, therapy, and inclusive camp and adolescent services.

Allen Ladd, Chairman
Brooke Grehan, Vice Chairman
Keith Graham, Treasurer

1399 United Cerebral Palsy of Northwest Alabama
507 N. Hook Street
Tuscumbia, AL 35674

256-381-4310
Fax: 256-381-4378
e-mail: alison@ucpshoals.org
www.ucpshoals.org

United Cerebral Palsy provides information, advocacy, referral services for persons with disabilities and/or their families. UCP also operates an equipment loan program, conducts parent workshops, disseminates written literature on topics of interest to people with disabilities.

Alison Isbell, Executive Director
Martha Martha, Office Manager
Gena Williams, Respite Coordinator/Billing

1400 United Cerebral Palsy of West Alabama
1100 UCP Parkway
Northport, AL 35476

205-345-3031
Fax: 205-345-3035
e-mail: tfrankucp@comcast.net
www.ucpwa.org

Provides early intervention for birth through age 3, preschool services, afternoon and summer CARE services, (child and adult respite/education), Start on Success Alabama (high school transition to work program), Adult Day Habilitation Program (adults with mental retardation), UCP Miracle Riders (equestrian physical therapy program).

Nancy Rhodes, President
Brandon Stough, Vice President
Bruce Boner, Treasurer

Alaska

1401 United Cerebral Palsy of Alaska/PARENTS
4743 E Northern Lights Boulevard
Anchorage, AK 99508

907-337-7678
Fax: 907-337-7671
e-mail: sanja@parentsinc.org
www.parentsinc.org

United Cerebral Palsy provides information, advocacy, referral services for persons with disabilities and/or their families. UCP also operates an equipment loan program, conducts parent workshops, disseminates written literature on topics of interest to people with disabilities.

Sanja Bolling, Executive Director

Arizona

1402 United Cerebral Palsy of Central Arizona
1802 W Parkside Lane
Phoenix, AZ 85027
602-943-5472
888-943-5472
Fax: 602-943-4936
e-mail: info@ucpofcentralaz.org
www.ucpofaz.org

United Cerebral Palsy provides information, advocacy, referral services for persons with disabilities and/or their families. UCP also operates an equipment loan program, conducts parent workshops, disseminates written literature on topics of interest to people with disabilities.

Veronica De La O, Board Chairwoman. President,
Dr. Cristina Carballo Perelman, Vice Chairman
Nathan Anspach, Treasurer

1403 United Cerebral Palsy of Southern Arizona
635 N. Craycroft Road
Tucson, AZ 85711
520-795-3108
Fax: 520-795-3196
e-mail: staff@ucpsa.org
www.ucpsa.org/?contact

United Cerebral Palsy provides information, advocacy, referral services for persons with disabilities and/or their families. UCP also operates an equipment loan program, conducts parent workshops, disseminates written literature on topics of interest to people with disabilities.

Alexis Cruz, Program Manager
Sean Hammond, Program Manager
Rita Lopez, Program Manager

Arkansas

1404 United Cerebral Palsy of Central Arkansas
9720 N Rodney Parham Road
Little Rock, AR 72227
501-224-6067
800-228-6174
Fax: 501-227-5591
e-mail: info@ucpcark.org
www.ucpcark.org

United Cerebral Palsy provides information, advocacy, referral services for persons with disabilities and/or their families. UCP also operates an equipment loan program, conducts parent workshops, disseminates written literature on topics of interest to people with disabilities.

Stephen Jones, Chair
Gary Wells, Vice Chair
Bill Yee, Treasurer

California

1405 United Cerebral Palsy of Central California
4224 N Cedar Avenue
Fresno, CA 93726
559-221-8272
Fax: 559-221-9347
e-mail: jeffreys@ccucp.org
www.ccucp.org

United Cerebral Palsy provides information, advocacy, referral services for persons with disabilities and/or their families. UCP also operates an adult day program - the Center for Arts and Technology in Fresno, CA, and services to children and their parents in Kings County, CA.

Jeffrey Snyder, Executive Director

1406 United Cerebral Palsy of Greater Sacramento
4350 Auburn Blvd.
Sacramento, CA 95841
916-565-7700
Fax: 916-565-7773
e-mail: ucp@ucpsacto.org
www.ucpsacto.org

UCP provides programs and services for people with all types of developmental disabilities. These services include: day programs for adults, an in-home respite service, transportation, independent living services, information and referral services, a toy lending library, a recreational program for children, and advocacy at the State and National levels. UCP will, upon request, furnish written literature regarding their programs and services or information regarding a variety of disabilities.

Dennis Hart md, Chair
Annie Granucci, Treasurer
Kristoffer Kalmbach, Secretary

1407 United Cerebral Palsy of Los Angeles, Ventura and Santa Barbara Counties
6430 Independence Avenue
Woodland Hills, CA 91367
818-782-2211
Fax: 818-909-9106
e-mail: mail@ucpla.org
www.ucpla.org

Serving Los Angeles, Ventura and Santa Barbara counties. Serves hundreds of adults and children with disabilities every day with housing, education programs and professional and personal support for people with disabilities and their families. In addition to the high volume of people assisted, UCP is known for a caring, personal approach to each family's individual situation and choices.

Ronald Cohen, Executive Director
Ellen Kessler, President

1408 United Cerebral Palsy of Orange County
980 Roosevelt, Suite 100
Irvine, CA 92620
949-333-6400
Fax: 949-333-6440
e-mail: info@ucp-oc.org
www.ucp-oc.org

United Cerebral Palsy of Orange County operaptes an infant stimulation program with physical, occupational and speech therapy consultation. Aditionally, UCP provides information and referral services for the families of children having developmental disabilities as well as an equiptment loan program, Respitality program, parent support groups and individulized support, respite/babysitter programs, and consultation/training to childcare providers.

James Corbett, President
Michele Maryott, Vice President
Thomas Quinn, Treasurer

1409 United Cerebral Palsy of San Diego County
8525 Gibbs Drive, #209
San Diego, CA 92123
858-571-7803
Fax: 858-571-0919
e-mail: info@ucpsd.org
www.ucpsd.org

United Cerebral Palsy provides information, advocacy, referral services for persons with disabilities and/or their families. UCP also operates an equipment loan program, conducts parent workshops, disseminates written literature on topics of interest to people with disabilities.

Stephen Holland, President
Mike Crossley, Vice President
Greg Wells, Treasurer

1410 United Cerebral Palsy of San Joaquin, Calaveras & Amador Counties
333 W Benjamin Holt Drive, Suite 1
Stockton, CA 95207
209-956-0290
800-479-0311
Fax: 209-956-6707
e-mail: rcall@ucpsj.org
www.ucpsj.org

United Cerebral Palsy provides early intervention, information, advocacy, assistive technology and referral services for persons with disabilities and/or their families. UCP also operates an equipment loan program, conducts parent workshops, disseminates written literature on topics of interest to people with disabilities.

Daniel Platt, President
Martin J. Herzog, Vice-President
Eddie Lira, Treasurer

1411 United Cerebral Palsy of San Luis Obispo
3620 Sacramento Drive, Suite 201C
San Luis Obispo, CA 93401   805-543-2039
                                        Fax: 805-543-2045
                                   e-mail: shaftmt@aol.com
                                        www.ucp-slo.org

United Cerebral Palsy provides information, advocacy, referral services for persons with disabilities and/or their families. UCP also operates an equipment loan program, conducts parent workshops, disseminates written literature on topics of interest to people with disabilities.

Mark Shaffer, Executive Director
Jason Portugal, Technology Coordinator
Many Aslanzadeh, Youth Services

1412 United Cerebral Palsy of Santa Clara & San Mateo Counties
512 E Maude Avenue
Sunnyvale, CA 94085   408-737-7112
                                   650-917-6900
                                   Fax: 408-737-7225
                                   e-mail: ucp@ucpscsm.org
                                        www.ucpscsm.org

United Cerebral Palsy provides information, advocacy, referral services for persons with disabilities and/or their families. UCP also operates an equipment loan program, conducts parent workshops, disseminates written literature on topics of interest to people with disabilities.

Jane Lefferdink, Executive Director

1413 United Cerebral Palsy of Stanislaus County Stanislaus
4265 Spyres Way #2
Modesto, CA 95356   209-577-2122
                                   Fax: 209-577-2392
                                   e-mail: rlonczak@ucpstan.org
                                        www.ucpstan.org

United Cerebral Palsy provides information, advocacy, referral services for persons with disabilities and/or their families. Conducts parent workshops, disseminates written literature on topics of interest to people with disabilities.

Chris Peterson, Chair
Russ Hayward, Interim Executive Director
Michelle Gallegher, Treasurer

1414 United Cerebral Palsy of the Golden State
1970 Broadway, Suite 115
Oakland, CA 94612   510-832-7430
                                   Fax: 510-839-1329
                                   e-mail: info@ucpgg.org
                                        www.ucpgg.org

United Cerebral Palsy provides information, advocacy, referral services for persons with disabilities and/or their families. UCP also operates an equipment loan program, conducts parent workshops, disseminates written literature on topics of interest to people with disabilities.

Barry N Gardin, President
Patricia Peck, Vice President
Henry Gusman, Treasurer

1415 United Cerebral Palsy of the Inland Empire
35-325 Date Palm Drive, Suite 139
Cathedral City, CA 92234   760-321-8184
                                   877-512-2224
                                   Fax: 760-321-8284
                                   e-mail: info@ucpie.org
                                        www.ucpie.org

United Cerebral Palsy provides information, advocacy, referral services for persons with disabilities and/or their families. UCP conducts parent workshops, disseminates written literature on topics of interest to people with disabilities.

Greg Wetmore, President/CEO
Sofia Campos, Director of Program Services
Amber Fleming, Support Services Administrator

1416 United Cerebral Palsy of the North Bay
3835 Cypress Drive, #103
Petaluma, CA 94954   707-766-9990
                                   e-mail: mchughe@sonoma.edu
                                        www.ucpa.org

United Cerebral Palsy provides information, advocacy, referral services for persons with disabilities and/or their families. UCP also operates an equipment loan program, conducts parent workshops, disseminates written literature on topics of interest to people with disabilities.

Steve Lohrer, Board President
Elaine McHugh, Board Vice-President
Janet Hart, Treasurer

Connecticut

1417 United Cerebral Palsy of Eastern Connecticut
42 Norwich Road
Quaker Hill, CT 06375   860-443-3800
                                   Fax: 860-443-8272
                                   e-mail: mmorisson@ucpect.org
                                        www.ucpect.org

United Cerebral Palsy provides information, advocacy, referral services for persons with disabilities and/or their families. UCP also operates an equipment loan program, conducts parent workshops, disseminates written literature on topics of interest to people with disabilities.

Margaret (Peg) Morrison, Executive Director
Jennifer Keatley, Associate Executive Director of Adm
Steven Smigiel, Financial Manager

1418 United Cerebral Palsy of Greater Hartford
80 Whitney Street
Hartford, CT 06105   860-236-6201
                                   Fax: 860-218-2454
                                   e-mail: preid@sunrisegroup.org
                                        www.ucphartford.org/

United Cerebral Palsy provides information, advocacy, referral services for persons with disabilities and/or their families. UCP also operates an equipment loan program, conducts parent workshops, disseminates written literature on topics of interest to people with disabilities.

Pam Reid, Regional Administrator
Sarah Winiarski, Director of Development & Communica
Peter Cavanagh, Camp Coordinator

1419 United Cerebral Palsy of Southern Connecticut
94-96 South Turnpike Road (Halycon Office Park)
Wallingford, CT 06492   203-269-3511
                                   Fax: 203-269-7411
                                   e-mail: ucpasouthernct@yahoo.com
                                        www.ucpasouthernct.com

United Cerebral Palsy provides information, advocacy, referral services for persons with disabilities and/or their families. UCP also operates an equipment loan program, conducts parent workshops, disseminates written literature on topics of interest to people with disabilities.

Arcangelo DiStefano, M.D., President
Peter DiDomizio, Vice President
Strick Woods MD, Treasurer

Delaware

1420 United Cerebral Palsy of Delaware
700A River Road
Wilmington, DE 19809   302-764-2400
                                   Fax: 302-764-8713
                                   e-mail: wmccool@ucpde.org
                                        www.ucpde.org

United Cerebral Palsy provides information, advocacy, referral services for persons with disabilities and/or their families. UCP also operates an equipment loan program, conducts parent workshops, disseminates written literature on topics of interest to people with disabilities.

Donna M Hopkins, President
D. Bruce McClenathan, Vice President
Daniel Edgar, Treasurer

1421 United Cerebral Palsy of Washington DC & Northern Virginia
3135 8th Street NE
Washington, DC 20017   202-269-1500
Fax: 202-526-0519
e-mail: webmaster@ucpdc.org
www.ucpdc.org

United Cerebral Palsy provides information, advocacy, referral services for persons with disabilities and/or their families. UCP also operates an equipment loan program, conducts parent workshops, disseminates written literature on topics of interest to people with disabilities.

Mark A Simione, Board President
George Connors, 1st Vice President
Roderick Johnson, 2nd Vice President

Florida

1422 New Heights (formerly Cerebral Palsy of No rtheast Florida)
3311 Beach Boulevard
Jacksonville, FL 32207   904-396-1462
Fax: 904-396-1199
e-mail: agency@cpnef.org
www.newheightsnefl.org

United Cerebral Palsy provides information, advocacy, referral services for persons with disabilities and/or their families. UCP also operates an equipment loan program, conducts parent workshops, disseminates written literature on topics of interest to people with disabilities, and provides individual and family counseling. Locations also in Kissimme, Winter Garden, Sanford and East Orange.

Sue Driscoll, President & CEO
Michelle Abner, Chief Development Officer
Joel Weaver, Secretary-Treasurer

1423 United Cerebral Palsy of Central Florida
1221 W. Colonial Dr., Ste. 300
Orlando, FL 32804   407-852-3300
Fax: 407-852-3301
e-mail: iwilkins@ucpcfl.org
www.ucpcfl.org

United Cerebral Palsy provides information, advocacy, referral services for persons with disabilities and/or their families. UCP also operates an equipment loan program, conducts parent workshops, disseminates written literature on topics of interest to people with disabilities, and provides individual and family counseling. Locations also in Kissimme, Winter Garden, Sanford and East Orange.

Dr. Ilene Wilkins, CEO
Paul Brown, Chair
Lynn Fleeger, Vice-Chair

1424 United Cerebral Palsy of East Central Florida
1100 Jimmy Ann Drive
Daytona Beach, FL 32117   386-274-6474
Fax: 386-274-6532
e-mail: info@ucpworc.org
www.ucpecf.org

United Cerebral Palsy provides information, advocacy, referral services for persons with disabilities and/or their families. UCP also operates an equipment loan program, conducts parent workshops, disseminates written literature on topics of interest to people with disabilities, and provides individual and family counseling. Locations also in Kissimme, Winter Garden, Sanford and East Orange.

Brooks Casey, Chair
Ed Best, Treasurer
Parker Mynchenberg, Treasurer

1425 United Cerebral Palsy of Florida
2700 W. 81 Street
Hialeah, FL 33016   305-325-9018
Fax: 850-922-1258
e-mail: ucpinfo@ucpsouthflorida.org
www.ucpsouthflorida.org

United Cerebral Palsy provides information, advocacy, referral services for persons with disabilities and/or their families. UCP also operates an equipment loan program, conducts parent workshops, disseminates written literature on topics of interest to people with disabilities.

Joseph A. Aniello, Ed.D., President and CEO
Debbie Terenzio, Ed.D., Vice President & COO
Linda Gluck, CPA, Vice President & CFO

1426 United Cerebral Palsy of North Florida/ Tender Loving Care
1241 N East Avenue
Panama City, FL 32401   850-769-7960
Fax: 850-769-1060
e-mail: ucpstlc@aol.com
www.ucpa.org

United Cerebral Palsy provides information, advocacy, referral services for persons with disabilities and/or their families. UCP also operates an equipment loan program, conducts parent workshops, disseminates written literature on topics of interest to people with disabilities.

1427 United Cerebral Palsy of Northwest Florida
2912 North E Street
Pensacola, FL 32501   850-432-1596
Fax: 850-432-1930
e-mail: info@ucpnwfl.org
www.ucpnwfl.org

The number one service provider in Northwest Florida for individuals with cerebral palsy and other developmental disabilities, UCP provides information, advocacy and referral services for persons with disabilities and/or their families. Additionally, UCP offers individuals assistance with daily living skills training, computer training, basic education, speech, physical and occupational therapy, residential, supported living and finding long-term employment.

Brian P Bell SR, Chair
Michele W Fielder, Vice Chair
Norman Smith, Treasurer

1428 United Cerebral Palsy of Sarasota-Manatee
1090 S Tamiami Trail
Sarasota, FL 34236   941-957-3599
Fax: 941-957-3499
e-mail: dwalker@sunrisegroup.org
www.ucpsarasota.org

United Cerebral Palsy provides information, advocacy, referral services for persons with disabilities and/or their families. UCP also operates an equipment loan program, conducts parent workshops, disseminates written literature on topics of interest to people with disabilities.

Barnett A Greenberg, Chairperson
Norma Israel, Executive Director

1429 United Cerebral Palsy of South Florida
2700 West 81 Street
Hialeah, FL 33016   305-325-9018
Fax: 305-325-1313
e-mail: ucpinfo@ucpsouthflorida.org
www.ucpsouthflorida.org

United Cerebral Palsy provides information, advocacy, referral services for persons with disabilities and/or their families. UCP also operates an equipment loan program, conducts parent workshops, disseminates written literature on topics of interest to people with disabilities.

Joseph Aniello Ed.D, President & CEO
Linda Gluck, Vice President & CFO
Debbie Terenzio, Ed.D., Vice President & COO

1430 United Cerebral Palsy of Tampa Bay
2215 E Henry Avenue
Tampa, FL 33610   813-239-1179
800-749-5155
Fax: 813-237-3091
e-mail: lwhite@ucptampa.org.
www.ucptampa.org

United Cerebral Palsy provides information, advocacy, referral services for persons with disabilities and/or their families. UCP also operates an equipment loan program, conducts parent workshops, disseminates written literature on topics of interest to people with disabilities.

Jim King, Executive Director
Dawn Gosselin, Executive Development Assistant / E
Laura White, Director of Program Development

Georgia

1431 United Cerebral Palsy of Georgia
3300 Northeast Expressway, Building 9
Atlanta, GA 30341

770-676-2000
888-827-9455
Fax: 770-455-8040
e-mail: info@ucpga.org
www.ucpga.org

United Cerebral Palsy provides information, advocacy, referral services for persons with disabilities and/or their families. UCP also operates an equipment loan program, conducts parent workshops, disseminates written literature on topics of interest to people with disabilities.

Diane Wilush, Executive Director
Angela Easter, Associate Executive Director, Opera
R. Curt Harrison, Associate Executive Director, Strat

Hawaii

1432 United Cerebral Palsy of Hawaii
414 Kuwili Street, Suite 105
Honolulu, HI 96817

808-532-6744
800-606-5654
Fax: 808-532-6747
e-mail: ucpa@ucpahi.org
www.ucpahi.org

United Cerebral Palsy provides information, advocacy, referral services for persons with disabilities and/or their families. UCP also operates an equipment loan program, conducts parent workshops, disseminates written literature on topics of interest to people with disabilities.

Ted Jung Jr, President
Derek Lau, Vice President
Jan Choy, Treasurer

Idaho

1433 United Cerebral Palsy of Idaho
5420 W Franklin, Suite A
Boise, ID 83705

208-377-8070
Fax: 208-322-7133
e-mail: info@ucpidaho.org
www.ucpidaho.org

United Cerebral Palsy provides information, advocacy, referral services for persons with disabilities and/or their families.

Lynn Cundick, Executive Director
Kathy Griffen, Program Director

Illinois

1434 United Cerebral Palsy Land of Lincoln
101 North 16th Street
Springfield, IL 62703

217-525-6522
Fax: 217-525-9017
e-mail: ucpll@ucpll.org
www.ucpll.org

United Cerebral Palsy provides information, advocacy, referral services for persons with disabilities and/or their families. UCP also operates an equipment loan program, conducts parent workshops, disseminates written literature on topics of interest to people with disabilities.

Brenda Yarnell, President
Kathy Leuelling, Chief Operating Officer
Char Fanning, Chief Financial Officer

1435 United Cerebral Palsy of Greater Chicago
7550 West 183rd Street
Tinley Park, IL 60477

708-444-8460
800-476-2836
Fax: 708-429-3981
e-mail: pdulle@ucpnet.org
www.ucpnet.org

United Cerebral Palsy provides information and referral services for persons with disabilities and/or their families. UCP also operates an equipment loan program, conducts parent workshops, disseminates written literature on topics of interest to people with disabilities.

Paul Dulle, President and CEO
Peggy Childs, Executive Vice President
Mei Hong Zhang, Chief Financial Officer

1436 United Cerebral Palsy of Illinois
310 East Adams
Springfield, IL 62701

217-528-9681
Fax: 217-528-9739
e-mail: ucpillinois.org
www.ucpillinois.org

United Cerebral Palsy provides information, advocacy, referral services for persons with disabilities and/or their families. UCP also operates an equipment loan program, conducts parent workshops, disseminates written literature on topics of interest to people with disabilities.

Don Moss, Executive Director

1437 United Cerebral Palsy of Southern Illinois
9 Cusumano Professional Pplaza Drive
Mt Vernon, IL 62864

618-244-2505
800-332-9745
Fax: 618-244-3568
e-mail: ucpsi@onemain.com
http://home.onemain.com/~ucpsi

United Cerebral Palsy provides information, advocacy, referral services for persons with disabilities and/or their families. UCP also operates an equipment loan program, conducts parent workshops, disseminates written literature on topics of interest to people with disabilities.

Sharon Hale, Executive Director

1438 United Cerebral Palsy of Will County
311 South Reed Street
Joliet, IL 60436

815-744-3500
Fax: 815-744-3504
e-mail: ucpilprairieland@ucpilprairieland.org
www.ucpilprairieland.org

United Cerebral Palsy provides information, advocacy, referral services for persons with disabilities and/or their families. UCP also operates an equipment loan program, conducts parent workshops, disseminates written literature on topics of interest to people with disabilities.

Bret Mitchell, Chair
Larry Johnson, Vice Chair - Administrative Service
Jim Keck, Vice Chair - Program Services

Indiana

1439 United Cerebral Palsy of Greater Indiana
107 N Pennsylvania St Suite 804
Indianapolis, IN 46220

317-632-3561
800-732-7620
Fax: 317-632-3338
e-mail: donnar@ucpaindy.org
www.ucpaindy.org

United Cerebral Palsy provides information, advocacy, referral services for persons with Cerebal Palsy and/or their families. UCP also provides funding for equipment and operates an equipment loan program, disseminates written literature on topics of interest to people with disabilities.

Lee White, Board and Development Committee Mem
Craig Burns, Board President and Development Com
Gavin MCNAMARA, Board Treasurer and Finance Committ

1440   United Cerebral Palsy of the Wabash Valley
621 Poplar Street
Terre Haute, IN 47807   812-232-6305
                                          Fax: 812-234-3683
                                       e-mail: info@ucpwv.org
                                                www.ucpwv.org

United Cerebral Palsy provides information, advocacy, referral
services for persons with disabilities and/or their families. UCP
also operates an equipment loan program, conducts parent workshops, disseminates written literature on topics of interest to
people with disabilities.

Brian Garcia, President
Anna Wetnight, First Vice-President
Pam Deady, Treasurer

Kansas

1441   United Cerebral Palsy of Greater Kansas City
3100 Broadway, Suite 330
Kansas City, MO 64111   816-531-4454
                                          Fax: 816-531-3383
                                       e-mail: info@ucpkc.org
                                                www.ucpkc.org

United Cerebral Palsy provides information, advocacy, referral
services for persons with disabilities and/or their families. UCP
also operates an equipment loan program, conducts parent workshops, disseminates written literature on topics of interest to
people with disabilities.

Bruce Scott, President and CEO
Sam Switzer, Senior Vice President & Chief Finan
Bill Koch, Chairperson

1442   United Cerebral Palsy of Kansas
5111 E 21st Street N
Wichita, KS 67208   316-688-1888
                                          Fax: 316-688-5687
                                       e-mail: davej@cprf.org
                                                www.cprf.org

United Cerebral Palsy provides information, advocacy, referral
services for persons with disabilities and/or their families. UCP
also operates an equipment loan program, conducts parent workshops, disseminates written literature on topics of interest to
people with disabilities.

Daniel M Carney, Chairman of the Board
Deryl K. Schuster, Vice Chairman
Daniel J Taylor, Treasurer

Louisiana

**1443   United Cerebral Palsy of Baton Rouge McMains Children's
Developmental Center**
1805 College Drive
Baton Rouge, LA 70808   225-923-3420
                                          Fax: 225-922-9316
                                  e-mail: cdcjanet@gmail.com
                                             www.mcmainscdc.org

United Cerebral Palsy provides information, advocacy, referral
services for persons with disabilities and/or their families. UCP
also operates an equipment loan program, conducts parent workshops, disseminates written literature on topics of interest to
people with disabilities.

Michael McNulty, President
Gina Dugas, Vice President
Mike Krumholt, Secretary-Treasurer

1444   United Cerebral Palsy of Greater New Orleans
2200 Veterans Memorial Boulevard, Suite 103
New Orleans, LA 70062   504-461-4266
                                          Fax: 504-461-9976
                                    e-mail: info@ucpgno.com
                                                www.ucpgno.org

United Cerebral Palsy provides information, advocacy, referral
services for persons with disabilities and/or their families. UCP
also operates an equipment loan program, conducts parent workshops, disseminates written literature on topics of interest to
people with disabilities.

Tommy Freel, Chair
p.Alden kellog, Vice Chair
Jeffery Smith, Executive Vice chair

Maine

1445   United Cerebral Palsy of Northeastern Maine
700 Mount Hope Avenue, Suite 320
Bangor, ME 04401   207-941-2952
                                          Fax: 207-941-2955
                          e-mail: bobbijo.yeager@ucpofmaine.org
                                             www.ucpofmaine.org

United Cerebral Palsy provides information, advocacy, referral
services for persons with disabilities and/or their families. UCP
also operates an equipment loan program, conducts parent workshops, disseminates written literature on topics of interest to
people with disabilities.

Micheal S. Haenn, Director
Ron Cote, Vice President
Valerie Roy, Treasurer

Maryland

1446   United Cerebral Palsy of Central Maryland
1700 Reistertown Road, Suite 226
Baltimore, MD 21208   410-484-4540
                                          Fax: 410-486-3825
                                          TTY: 800-451-2452
                                     e-mail: info@ucp-cm.org
                                                www.ucp-cm.org

United Cerebral Palsy provides information, advocacy, referral
services for persons with disabilities and/or their families. UCP
also operates an equipment loan program, conducts parent workshops, disseminates written literature on topics of interest to
people with disabilities.

Diane Coughlin, President

**1447   United Cerebral Palsy of Prince Georges & Montgomery
Counties**
4409 Forbes Boulevard
Lanham, MD 20706   301-459-0566
                                          Fax: 301-459-7691
                                          TTY: 301-262-4982
                                    e-mail: ucppgmc@aol.com
                                                www.ucppgmc.com

United Cerebral Palsy provides information, advocacy, referral
services for persons with disabilities and/or their families. UCP
also operates an equipment loan program, conducts parent workshops, disseminates written literature on topics of interest to
people with disabilities.

Charles Mc Nelly, Manager

1448   United Cerebral Palsy of Southern Maryland
211 Chinquapin Round Road
Annapolis, MD 21401   410-280-2003
                                          Fax: 410-269-5757
                                    e-mail: ucpinfo@ucpsm.org
                                                www.ucpsm.org

United Cerebral Palsy provides information, advocacy, referral
services for persons with disabilities and/or their families. UCP
also operates an equipment loan program, conducts parent workshops, disseminates written literature on topics of interest to
people with disabilities.

Massachusetts

1449   United Cerebral Palsy of Berkshire County
208 West Street
Pittsfield, MA 01201   413-442-1562
                                          Fax: 413-499-4077
                                  e-mail: info@ucpberkshire.org
                                             www.upcberkshire.org

United Cerebral Palsy provides information, advocacy,assistive technology, referral services for persons with disabilities and/or their families. UCP also operates an equipment loan program, conducts parent workshops, disseminates written literature on topics of interest to people with disabilities.

Anthony Hyte, President
Sarah Gaffey, 1st Vice President
Warren Buhl, 2nd Vice president

1450 United Cerebral Palsy of MetroBoston
71 Arsenal Street
Watertown, MA 02472
617-926-5480
Fax: 617-926-3059
e-mail: ucpboston@ucpboston.org
www.ucpboston.org

United Cerebral Palsy provides information, advocacy, referral services for persons with disabilities and/or their families. UCP also operates an equipment loan program, conducts parent workshops, disseminates written literature on topics of interest to people with disabilities.

Richard Merson, President
Linda Cox Maguire, Vice President
Desmond Brown, Board of Director

Michigan

1451 United Cerebral Palsy Michigan
3498 Lake Lansing road Suite. 170
East Lansing, MI 48823
517-203-1200
800-828-2714
Fax: 517-203-1203
e-mail: ucp@ucpmichigan.org
www.ucpmichigan.org

United Cerebral Palsy provides information, advocacy, referral services for persons with disabilities and/or their families. UCP also operates an equipment loan program, conducts parent workshops, disseminates written literature on topics of interest to people with disabilities.

Dan Vivian, President
Judy Cerano, Vice President
Jackie Doig, Chairperson

1452 United Cerebral Palsy of Metropolitan Detroit
23077 Greenfield, Suite 205
Southfield, MI 48075
248-557-5070
800-827-4843
Fax: 248-557-0224
e-mail: main@ucpdetroit.org
www.ucpdetroit.org

United Cerebral Palsy provides information, advocacy, referral services for persons with disabilities and/or their families. UCP also operates an equipment loan program, conducts parent workshops, disseminates written literature on topics of interest to people with disabilities.

Leslynn R Angel, President
Thomas H. Landry, Chairman
Diann G. Dudash, 1st Vice Chair

Minnesota

1453 United Cerebral Palsy of Central Minnesota
510 25th Avenue N, Suite 8A
Saint Cloud, MN 56303
320-253-0765
Fax: 320-253-6753
e-mail: info@ucpcentralmn.org
www.ucpcentralmn.org

United Cerebral Palsy provides information, advocacy, referral services for persons with disabilities and/or their families. UCP also operates an equipment loan program, conducts parent workshops, disseminates free newsletter. Computers Go Round recycles quality used computers to persons with disabilities.

Shelley Gaetz, President/Treasurer
Sue Schlosser, Vice President/Secretary
Kristin Schmidt, Treasurer

1454 United Cerebral Palsy of Minnesota
1821 University Avenue W Suite 219 South
Saint Paul, MN 55104
651-646-7588
800-328-4827
Fax: 651-646-3045
e-mail: ucpmn@cpinternet.com
www.ucpmn.org

United Cerebral Palsy provides information, advocacy, referral services for persons with disabilities and/or their families. UCP also operates an equipment loan program, conducts parent workshops, disseminates written literature on topics of interest to people with disabilities.

Stacey Vogele, Executive Director

Missouri

1455 United Cerebral Palsy of Greater Kansas City
Suite 400
Kansas City, MO 64111
816-531-4454
Fax: 816-531-3383
e-mail: info@ucpkc.org
www.ucpkc.org

United Cerebral Palsy provides information, advocacy, referral services for persons with disabilities and/or their families. UCP also operates an equipment loan program, conducts parent workshops, disseminates written literature on topics of interest to people with disabilities.

Bruce Scott, President/CEO
Sam Switzer, Senior Vice President
Vincent Bustamante, Vice President, community living

1456 United Cerebral Palsy of Greater St. Louis
8645 Old Bonhomme Road
Saint Louis, MO 63132
314-994-1600
Fax: 314-994-0179
e-mail: forkoshr@ucpstl.org
www.ucpstl.org

Offers skill development and training programs in the areas of independent living, human relations, social and leisure activities, assistive technology, sensory and tactile stimulation, community integration, career exploration, job placement, and functional academics to individuals eighteen years of age and older with developmental disabilities.

Richard Forkosh, Executive Director

1457 United Cerebral Palsy of Northwest Missouri
3303 Frederick Avenue
Saint Joseph, MO 64506
816-364-3836
Fax: 816-390-8546
e-mail: ucp@ucpnwmo.org
www.ucpnwmo.org

United Cerebral Palsy provides information, advocacy, referral services for persons with disabilities and/or their families. UCP also operates an equipment loan program, conducts parent workshops, disseminates written literature on topics of interest to people with disabilities.

Teresa Gagliano, Executive Director
Jared Brooner, President
Shawn Drew, Vice president

Nebraska

1458 United Cerebral Palsy of Nebraska
920 S. 107th Avenue, Suite 302
Omaha, NE 68114
402-502-3572
800-729-2556
Fax: 402-502-6791
e-mail: ucp@ucpnebraska.org
www.ucpnebraska.org

United Cerebral Palsy provides information, advocacy, referral services for persons with disabilities and/or their families. UCP also operates an equipment loan program, conducts parent workshops, disseminates written literature on topics of interest to people with disabilities.

Carol Hahn, Executive Director
Christopher Scott, President
Dave Prough, Treasurer

New Jersey

1459 United Cerebral Palsy of Hudson County
721 Broadway
Bayonne, NJ 07002   201-436-2200
                                      Fax: 201-436-6642
                   e-mail: info@ucpofhudsoncounty.org
                            www.ucpofhudsoncounty.org

United Cerebral Palsy provides information, advocacy, referral services for persons with disabilities and/or their families. UCP also operates an equipment loan program, conducts parent workshops, disseminates written literature on topics of interest to people with disabilities.

Paul E. Venino, President
Paul Maffei, President
James Dooley, Treasurer

1460 United Cerebral Palsy of Northern, Central & Southern New Jersey
245 Main Street Suite 113
Chester, NJ 07930   908-879-2243
                                      Fax: 908-879-8363
                          e-mail: info@ucpncsnj.org
                                      www.ucp.org

United Cerebral Palsy provides information, advocacy, referral services for persons with disabilities and/or their families. UCP also operates an equipment loan program, conducts parent workshops, disseminates written literature on topics of interest to people with disabilities.

Deborah Miller, Executive Director

New York

1461 Aspire of WNY
2356 N Forest Road
Getzville, NY 14068   716-505-5610
                                      Fax: 716-894-8257
                     e-mail: AJHoldna@aspirewny.org
                                  www.aspirewny.org

Aspire of WNY is a provider of comprehensive programs and services for developmentally disabled children and adults in Western New York. Services areas include residential, bocational, therapeutic, clinical, habilitative and educational services amoung others. Aspire also offers advocacy, case management, work shops and referral services for the disabled and their families.

Nixon Peabody LLP, Chairperson
Eileen Nosek, Vice Chairperson
Leslie Wangelin, CTP, Treasurer

1462 Center for the Disabled
314 S Manning Boulevard
Albany, NY 12208   518-437-5700
                                      Fax: 518-437-5931
                   www.cfdsny.org/htmlweb/CFDShome2.html

Center Health Care offers a wide variety of medical dental and therapy services provided in an outpatient practice setting, serving individuals with developmental disabilities and chronic disabling conditions. In addition, educational diagnostic and evaluation services are offered to children of different ages. parent workshops and support groups are conducted throughout the year.

Allan Krafchin, President
Donna Lamkin, Chief Program Officer
Gregory Sorrentino, Chief Financial Officer

1463 Cerebral Palsy Associations of New York State
330 West 34th Street, 15th floor
New York, NY 10001   212-947-5770
                                      Fax: 212-594-4538
                   e-mail: information@cpofnys.org
                                  www.cpofnys.org

Cerebral Palsy provides information, advocacy, and services for persons with disabilities and/or their families. CP also operates an equipment loan program, conducts parent workshops, disseminates written literature on topics of interest to people with disabilities.

Susan Constantino, President & CEO
Joseph M Pancari, COO
Thomas N Mandelkow, CFO,CAO

1464 Inspire - Cerebral Palsy Center
2 Fletcher Street
Goshen, NY 10924   845-294-8806
                                      Fax: 845-294-8650
                          e-mail: info@inspirecp.org.
                                      www.inspirecp.org

An affiliate of Cerebral Palsy Associations of New York, provides information, advocacy, referral services for persons with disabilities and/or their families. Inspire runs a rehabilitative clinic and special needs preschool, conducts parent workshops, disseminates written literature on topics of interest to people with disabilities.

Katharine Fitzgerald, Chairman
Suzanne Schindler, Vice-Chairman
Allen Zick, Treasurer

1465 UCP of Greater Suffolk
250 Marcus Boulevard, PO Box 18045
Hauppauge, NY 11788   631-232-0011
                                      Fax: 631-232-4422
                          e-mail: info@ucp-suffolk.org
                                      www.ucp-suffolk.org

UCP Suffolk provides information, advocacy, referral services for persons with disabilities and/or their families. UCP also operates an equipment loan program, conducts parent workshops, disseminates written literature on topics of interest to people with disabilities.

Stephen H Friedman, President/CEO
Janine Klein, CFO
Colleen West-Levy, Chairperson

1466 United Cerebral Palsy of Nassau County
380 Washington Avenue
Roosevelt, NY 11575   516-378-2000
                                      Fax: 516-378-0357
                              e-mail: info@ucpn.org
                                      www.ucpn.org

United Cerebral Palsy provides information, advocacy, referral services for persons with disabilities and/or their families. UCP also operates an equipment loan program, conducts parent workshops, disseminates written literature on topics of interest to people with disabilities.

Robert Masterson, President
Thomas Connolly, Executive Vice President
Anthony Galano, Vice president

1467 United Cerebral Palsy of New York City
80 Maiden Lane, 8th Floor
New York, NY 10038   212-683-6700
                                      Fax: 212-685-8394
                              e-mail: info@ucpnyc.org
                                      www.ucpnyc.org

United Cerebral Palsy provides information, advocacy, referral services for persons with disabilities and/or their families. UCP also operates an equipment loan program, conducts parent workshops, disseminates written literature on topics of interest to people with disabilities.

Edward R Matthews, Ceo
Gary Geresi, President
Jerome Belsome, Chairman

North Carolina

1468 United Cerebral Palsy of North Carolina
2315 Myron Drive
Raleigh, NC 27607
919-863-3859
800-662-7119
Fax: 919-782-5486
e-mail: info@nc.eastersealsucp.com
www.nc.eastersealsucp.com

United Cerebral Palsy provides information, advocacy, referral services for persons with disabilities and/or their families. UCP also operates an equipment loan program, conducts parent workshops, disseminates written literature on topics of interest to people with disabilities.

Connie Cochran, President

Ohio

1469 United Cerebral Palsy of Central Ohio
440 Industrial Mile Road
Columbus, OH 43228
614-279-0109
Fax: 614-279-2527
e-mail: gthorpe@ucpofcentralohio.org
www.ucpofcentralohio.org

United Cerebral Palsy provides information, advocacy, referral services for persons with disabilities and/or their families. UCP also operates an equipment loan program, conducts parent workshops, disseminates written literature on topics of interest to people with disabilities.

Kathy Streblo, Executive Director

1470 United Cerebral Palsy of Cincinnati
3601 Victory Parkway
Cincinnati, OH 45229
513-221-4606
Fax: 513-872-5262
e-mail: info@ucp-cincinnati.org
www.ucp-cincinnati.org

United Cerebral Palsy provides information, advocacy, referral services for persons with disabilities and/or their families. UCP also operates an equipment loan program, conducts parent workshops, disseminates written literature on topics of interest to people with disabilities.

Michael P. Folley, Chairperson
Thomas R Williams, President
Peter J. Cardullias, ll, Vice president

1471 United Cerebral Palsy of Greater Cleveland
1011 Euclid Avenue
Cleveland, OH 44115
216-791-8363
Fax: 216-721-3372
e-mail: wmorgan@ucpcleveland.org
www.ucpcleveland.org

United Cerebral Palsy provides information, advocacy, referral services for persons with disabilities and/or their families. UCP also operates an equipment loan program, conducts parent workshops, disseminates written literature on topics of interest to people with disabilities.

Matthew R Cox, President
Sean D. Wenger, Vice Chairperson
Jeffrey D. Minnick, Treasurer

Oklahoma

1472 United Cerebral Palsy of Oklahoma
10400 Greenbriar Place, Suite 101
Oklahoma City, OK 73159
405-759-3562
800-827-2289
Fax: 405-917-7082
e-mail: info@ucpok.org
www.ucpok.org

United Cerebral Palsy provides information, advocacy, referral services for persons with disabilities and/or their families. UCP also operates an equipment loan program, disseminates written literature on topics of interest to people with disabilities.

Jim Rankin, Executive Director

Oregon

1473 United Cerebral Palsy of Oregon & SW Washington
305 NE 102nd Ave, Suite 100
Portland, OR 97220
503-777-4166
800-473-4581
Fax: 503-771-8048
e-mail: ucpa@ucpaorwa.org
www.ucpaorwa.org

United Cerebral Palsy provides information, advocacy, referral services for persons with disabilities and/or their families. UCP also operates an equipment loan program, conducts parent workshops, disseminates written literature on topics of interest to people with disabilities.

Nancy Cicirello, President
Jerrold Pattee, Vice president
John R. Hancock, Board of Director

Pennsylvania

1474 Alleghenies United Cerebral Palsy
119 Jari Drive
Johnstown, PA 15904
814-262-9600
877-371-1110
Fax: 814-262-9650
e-mail: contact-us@alucp.org
www.alucp.org

United Cerebral Palsy provides information, advocacy, referral services for persons with disabilities and/or their families. UCP also operates an equipment loan program, conducts parent workshops, disseminates written literature on topics of interest to people with disabilities.

Marie Polinsky, Ceo
Mark Malzi, Chief Financial Officer
Stacey Zometsky, Executive Assistant

1475 United Cerebral Palsy Central PA
925 Linda Lane
Camp Hill, PA 17011
717-737-3477
800-998-4827
Fax: 717-975-3333
e-mail: mainoffice@ucpcentralpa.org
www.ucpcentralpa.org

United Cerebral Palsy provides information, advocacy, referral services for persons with disabilities and/or their families. UCP also operates an equipment loan program, conducts parent workshops, disseminates written literature on topics of interest to people with disabilities.

Jeffrey W. Cooper, President/CEO
John M. Coles, Chairperson
William K. Wilkison, Vice Chairperson

1476 United Cerebral Palsy of Northeastern Pennsylvania
425 Wyoming Avenue
Scranton, PA 18503
570-347-3357
877-827-8324
Fax: 570-341-5308
TTY: 570-347-3117
e-mail: ucpnepa@epix.net
www.ucpnepa.com

United Cerebral Palsy provides information, advocacy, referral services for persons with disabilities and/or their families. UCP also operates an equipment loan program, conducts parent workshops, disseminates written literature on topics of interest to people with disabilities.

Daniel Ginsberg, President
Sarah A. Drob, Executive Director
Edward Karpovich, Treasurer

1477 United Cerebral Palsy of Northwestern Pennsylvania
3745 W 12th Street
Erie, PA 16505
814-836-9113
Fax: 814-833-3919
e-mail: leaton@mecaucp.com
www.mecaucp.com

United Cerebral Palsy provides information, advocacy, referral services for persons with disabilities and/or their families. UCP also operates an equipment loan program, conducts parent workshops, disseminates written literature on topics of interest to people with disabilities.

1478   United Cerebral Palsy of Pennsylvania
908 North Second Street
Harrisburg, PA 17102

717-441-6049
866-761-6129
Fax: 717-236-2046
e-mail: info@ucpofpa.org
www.ucpofpa.org

United Cerebral Palsy provides information, advocacy, referral services for persons with disabilities and/or their families. UCP also operates an equipment loan program, conducts parent workshops, disseminates written literature on topics of interest to people with disabilities.

Joan Martin, Executive Director

1479   United Cerebral Palsy of Philadelphia & Vicinity
102 E Mermaid Lane
Philadelphia, PA 19118

215-242-4200
Fax: 215-247-4229
e-mail: ucpkravitz@aol.com
www.ucpphila.org

United Cerebral Palsy provides information, advocacy, referral services for persons with disabilities and/or their families. UCP also operates an equipment loan program, conducts parent workshops, disseminates written literature on topics of interest to people with disabilities.

Stephen A Sheridan, Ceo

1480   United Cerebral Palsy of Pittsburgh
4638 Centre Avenue
Pittsburgh, PA 15213

412-683-7100
1 8-8 9-4 24
Fax: 412-683-4160
e-mail: info@ucpclass.org
www.ucpclass.org

United Cerebral Palsy provides information, advocacy, referral services for persons with disabilities and/or their families. UCP also operates an equipment loan program, conducts parent workshops, disseminates written literature on topics of interest to people with disabilities.

Al Condelusci, Executive Director
Sally Balogh, Board Member
Shirley Biancheria, Board Member

1481   United Cerebral Palsy of South Central Pennsylvania
788 Cherry Tree Court
Hanover, PA 17331

717-632-5552
1 8-0 3-3 38
Fax: 717-632-2315
e-mail: phoughton@ucpsouthcentral.org
www.ucpsouthcentral.org

United Cerebral Palsy provides information, advocacy, referral services for persons with disabilities and/or their families. UCP also operates an equipment loan program, conducts parent workshops, disseminates written literature on topics of interest to people with disabilities.

Donald C McVay, President
K Scott Burns, Board Member
Scott Ganley, Board Member

1482   United Cerebral Palsy of Southwestern Pennsylvania
Washington Federal Square
190 North Main Street, Suite 306
Washington, PA 15301

724-229-0851
Fax: 724-229-9252
e-mail: info@ucpswpa.org
www.ucpswpa.org

United Cerebral Palsy provides information, advocacy, referral services for persons with disabilities and/or their families. UCP also operates an equipment loan program, conducts parent workshops, disseminates written literature on topics of interest to people with disabilities.

1483   United Cerebral Palsy of Western Pennsylvania
2904 Seminary Drive
Greensburg, PA 15601

724-832-8272
Fax: 724-837-8278
e-mail: ucp@ucpofwesternpa.org
www.ucpofwesternpa.org

United Cerebral Palsy provides information, advocacy, referral services for persons with disabilities and/or their families. UCP also operates an equipment loan program, conducts parent workshops, disseminates written literature on topics of interest to people with disabilities.

Debra Forsha, Children's Services Director

Rhode Island

1484   United Cerebral Palsy of Rhode Island
200 Main Street, Suite 210, PO Box 36
Pawtucket, RI 02862

401-728-1800
Fax: 401-728-0182
e-mail: info@ucpri.org
www.ucpri.org

United Cerebral Palsy provides information, advocacy, referral services for persons with disabilities and/or their families. UCP also operates an equipment loan program, conducts parent workshops, disseminates written literature on topics of interest to people with disabilities.

Stacey Johnson, President
Kenneth MacDonald, Vice president
Jennifer Spagnole, Treasurer

South Carolina

1485   United Cerebral Palsy of South Carolina
1101 Harbor Drive
West Columbia, SC 29169

803-926-8878
888-827-7277
Fax: 803-926-1272
e-mail: info@ucpsc.org
www.ucpsc.org

United Cerebral Palsy provides information, advocacy, referral services for persons with disabilities and/or their families. UCP also operates an equipment loan program, conducts parent workshops, disseminates written literature on topics of interest to people with disabilities.

Ray E. Gentry, Chairperson
Ouida Spencer, Vice Chairperson
Diane Wilush, Executive Director

Tennessee

1486   United Cerebral Palsy of Middle Tennessee
1200 9th Avenue North Suite 110
Nashville, TN 37208

615-242-4091
Fax: 615-242-3582
e-mail: request@ucpnashville.org
www.ucpmidtn.org

United Cerebral Palsy provides information, advocacy, referral services for persons with disabilities and/or their families. UCP also operates an equipment loan program, conducts parent workshops, disseminates written literature on topics of interest to people with disabilities.

Deana Claiborne, Executive Director
Diane Dietrich,, Director of Development
Margaret Eighmy, Equipment Exchange Program Director

1487   United Cerebral Palsy of the Mid-South
3239 Players Club Parkway
Memphis, TN 38125

901-761-4277
Fax: 901-761-7876
e-mail: ucp@ucpmemphis.org
www.ucpmemphis.org

United Cerebral Palsy provides information, advocacy, referral services for persons with disabilities and/or their families. UCP also operates an equipment loan program, conducts parent workshops, disseminates written literature on topics of interest to people with disabilities.

Michael Nolen, Ceo
Clint Sidle, Chairperson
Brunetta Garner, Chair ,personal committee

Texas

1488   United Cerebral Palsy of Greater Houston
4500 Bissonet, Suite 340
Bellaire, TX 77401   713-838-9050
Fax: 713-838-9098
e-mail: info@eastersealshouston.org
www.eastersealshouston.org

United Cerebral Palsy provides information, advocacy, referral services for persons with disabilities and/or their families. UCP also operates an equipment loan program, conducts parent workshops, disseminates written literature on topics of interest to people with disabilities.

Elise Hough, CEO
Wendy Dawson, President
Clark Varner, Vice President

1489   United Cerebral Palsy of Metropolitan Dallas
8802 Harry Hines Boulevard
Dallas, TX 75235   214-351-2500
800-999-1898
Fax: 214-351-2610
e-mail: billknudsen@ucpdallas.org
www.ucpdallas.org

United Cerebral Palsy provides information, advocacy, referral services for persons with disabilities and/or their families. UCP also operates an equipment loan program, conducts parent workshops, disseminates written literature on topics of interest to people with disabilities.

Bill Knudsen, President
Rebecca Adams

1490   United Cerebral Palsy of Texas
1016 La Posada Drive, Suite 145
Austin, TX 78752   512-472-8696
800-798-1492
Fax: 512-472-8026
e-mail: info@ucptexas.org
www.ucptexas.org

United Cerebral Palsy provides information, advocacy, referral services for persons with disabilities and/or their families. UCP also operates an equipment loan program, conducts parent workshops, disseminates written literature on topics of interest to people with disabilities.

Jean Langendorf, Executive Director

Utah

1491   United Cerebral Palsy of Utah
3550 S. 700 W
Salt Lake, UT 84119   801-266-1805
Fax: 801-266-2404
e-mail: Petes@ucputah.org
www.ucputah.org

United Cerebral Palsy information, advocacy, referral services for persons with disabilities and/or their families. UCP also operates an equipment loan program, conducts parent workshops, and disseminates written literature on topics of interest to people with disabilities.

Peter M. Shingledecker, Contact

Virginia

1492   United Cerebral Palsy of Washington DC & Northern Virginia
1818 New York Avenue NE, Suite 101
Washington, DC 20002   202-526-0146
Fax: 202-526-0238
e-mail: webmaster@ucpdc.org
www.ucpdc.org

United Cerebral Palsy provides information, advocacy, referral services for persons with disabilities and/or their families. UCP also operates an equipment loan program, conducts parent workshops, disseminates written literature on topics of interest to people with disabilities.

Dawn Carter, Executive Director

Washington

1493   United Cerebral Palsy of South Puget Sound
633 North Mildred Street, Suite C
Tacoma, WA 98406   253-565-1463
Fax: 253-565-0153
e-mail: info@ucp-sps.org
www.ucp-sps.org

United Cerebral Palsy provides information, advocacy, referral services for persons with disabilities and/or their families. UCP also operates an equipment loan program, conducts parent workshops, disseminates written literature on topics of interest to people with disabilities.

Joan Lornez, Manager

Wisconsin

1494   United Cerebral Palsy of Greater Dane County
2801 Coho Street, Suite 300
Madison, WI 53713   608-273-4434
Fax: 608-273-3426
e-mail: ucpgdc@ucpdane.org
www.ucpdane.org

United Cerebral Palsy provides information, advocacy, referral services for persons with disabilities and/or their families. UCP also conducts parent workshops and disseminates written literature on topics of interest to people with disabilities.

Wade Harrison, President
Rich Cooper, Vice President
Melanie Patterson, Treasurer

1495   United Cerebral Palsy of Southeastern Wisconsin
6102 W. Layton Avenue
Greenfield, WI 53220   414-329-4500
888-482-7739
Fax: 414-329-4510
e-mail: info@ucpsew.org
www.ucpsew.org

United Cerebral Palsy provides information, advocacy, referral services for persons with disabilities and/or their families. UCP also operates an equipment loan program, conducts parent workshops, disseminates written literature on topics of interest to people with disabilities.

Scott D. Anderson, President
Sally M. Lyne, Vice President
Ryan Engelhardt, Treasurer

1496   United Cerebral Palsy of West Central Wisconsin
206 Water Street
Eau Claire, WI 54703   715-832-1782
Fax: 715-832-8203
e-mail: ucp1dave@sbcglobal.net
www.ucpwcw.org

United Cerebral Palsy provides information, advocacy, referral services for persons with disabilities and/or their families. UCP also operates an equipment loan program, conducts parent workshops, disseminates written literature on topics of interest to people with disabilities.

Connie Werlein, President
Randi Johnson, Vice President
Jennifer Napolitano, Secretary

Libraries & Resource Centers

1497 National Rehabilitation Information Center
8400 Corporate Drive, Suite 500
Landover, MD 20785
301-459-5900
800-346-2742
Fax: 301-459-4263
TTY: 301-459-5984
e-mail: naricinfo@heitechservices.com
www.naric.com

Committed to providing direct, personal and high quality information services to anyone interested in disability rehabilitation issues; Committed to serving consumers, researchers, family members, health professionals, educators, counselors, students, librarians and the administrators throughout the country.

Mark Odum, Director

Research Centers

1498 Orthopaedic Biomechanics Laboratory
Shriners Hospital for Crippled Children
1701 19th Avenue
San Francisco, CA 94122
415-665-1100
Fax: 415-661-3615

Offers research and studies into cerebral palsy.

Stephen R Skinner, Clinical Director

1499 United Cerebral Palsy Research and Educational Foundation
186 Princeton Hightstown Road Building 4 2nd Floor
Princeton Junction, NJ 08550
609-452-1200
800-872-5827
Fax: 609-452-1201
e-mail: cpirf@cpirf.org
www.cpirf.org

Provides research grants to prevent cerebral palsy and to improve treatment, management and functioning of persons with cerebral palsy.

Glenn R Tringali, Chief Executive Officer/President
James A Blackman, M.D., M.P.H, Medical Director
Jacqueline M Carmosino, Manager of Administration

Conferences

1500 American Academy for Cerebral Palsy and Developmental Medicine Annual Meeting
555 E Wells Street, Suite 1100
Milwaukee, WI 53202
414-918-3014
Fax: 414-276-2146
e-mail: info@aacpdm.org
www.aacpdm.org

October

Maureen O'Donnell, President
Richard Stevenson, Vice President
Annette Majnemer, Secretary

Audio Video

1501 Accidents of Nature
Random House
1745 Broadway
New York, NY 10019
212-782-9000
e-mail: rhkidspublicity@randomhouse.com
www.randomhouse.com

About a girl who goes to a camp and has experiences that will change her life forever. Audio book feature.

2006
ISBN: 0-739335-30-8

1502 Cerebral Palsy: What Every Parent Should Know
Films for the Humanities and Sciences
132 West 31st Street
New York, NY 10001
800-257-5126
Fax: 609-275-0266
e-mail: custserv@films.com
www.ffh.films.com

This program covers the causes, symptoms, and range of possible treatments of cerebral palsy, including the relationship between physical and mental handicaps, and the role of medications and physical therapy treatment.

28 minutes
ISBN: 1-421336-41-1

Web Sites

1503 American Academy for Cerebral Palsy and Developmental Medicine
555 East Wells, Suite 1100
Milwaukee, WI 53202
414-918-3014
Fax: 414-276-2146
e-mail: info@aacpdm.org
www.aacpdm.org

Organization of professionals involved in the care of people with Cerebral Palsy, developmental disorders, and related diseases.

Darcy Fehlings, President
Eileen Fowler, 1st Vice President
Unni Narayanan, 2nd Vice President

1504 Children's Neurobiological Solutions Foundation
1223 Wilshire Blvd., #937
Santa Monica, CA 90403
310-889-8611
e-mail: info@cnsfoundation.org
www.cnsfoundation.org

Children's Neurobiological Solutions Foundation (CNS), is a national, nonprofit, 501(c)(3) organization, whose mission is to orchestrate cutting-edge, collaborative research with the goal of expediting the creation of effective treatments and therapies for children with neurodevelopmental abnormalities, birth injuries to the nervous system, and related neurological problems.

Fia Richmond, Founder
Phill Richmond, Founder
Jeffrey D. Macklis, Board Member

1505 Easter Seals Disability Services
233 South Wacker Drive, Suite 2400
Chicago, IL 60606
800-221-6827
www.easterseals.com

For more than 80 years, Easter Seals has helped people with disabilities in communities nationwide. From creating the first national voluntary act on behalf of children with disabilities in the 1920's to leading the creation and implementation of the Americans with Disabilities Act in the 1990's. Easter Seals child development services build strong foundations for children of all abilities.

Brad Halverson, Chair
Don Young, 1st Vice Chair
Wes Blumenshine, 2nd Vice Chair

1506 Family Support Network
www.tsalliance.org

The Support Network is an organized partnership of individuals whose lives have been affected by tuberous sclerosis. Across the nation, the Support Network is providing the latest medical information, education and support to those individuals who are seeking understanding about the genetic disease and offering them words of encouragement and empowerment.

1507 Health Answers
410 Horsham Road
Horsham, PA 19044
215-442-9017
e-mail: Michael.tague@healthanswers.com
www.healthanswers.com

The vision was to provide a breadth of services to clients through the formation of a network of companies. Each company plays a key role in meeting out clients' needs.

Michael Tague, Managing Director

1508 Infinitec
547 W. Jackson Street, Suite 225
Chicago, IL 60661
312-765-0419
Fax: 312-765-0503
e-mail: mbettlach@ucpnet.org
www.infinitec.org

The mission of Infinitec is to advance independence and promote inclusive opportunities for children and adults with disabilities throught technology.

Mary Bettlach, Managing Director

1509 My Child Without Limits
www.mychildwithoutlimits.org

An authoritative early intervention resource for families of young children ages 0-5 with developmental delays or disabilities, and professionals looking for a single, trusted, aggregate source of information that relates to their needs and interests. All medical information is reviewed by the My Child Without Limits medical advisory board, a panel composed of doctors in the fields of developmental disability and delay.

1510 National Dissemination Center for Children with Disabilities
35 Halsey St., Fourth Floor
Newark, NJ 7102
e-mail: malizo@spannj.org
www.nichcy.org

A national information and referral center that provides information on disabilities and disability-related issues for families, educators and other professionals.

Debra Jennings, Project Director
Indira Medina, Coordinator of Communication
Lisa Kupper, Product Coordinator

1511 Scope (UK)
www.scope.org.uk/

Our aim is that disabled people achieve equality: a society in which they are as valued and have the same human and civil rights as everyone else.

Andrew McDonald, Chair
John Gilbert, Treasurer
Richard Hawkes, Chief Executive

1512 United Cerebral Palsy Associations
1825 K Street NW Suite 600
Washington, DC 20006
202-776-0406
800-872-5827
www.ucp.org

The UCP is the leading source of information on cerebral palsy and is a pivitol advocate for the rights of persons with any disability. As one of the largest health charities in America, UCP's mission is to advance the independence, productivity and full citizenship of people with Cerebral Palsy and other diabilities.

Stephen Bennett, President/ CEO
Connie Garner, EVP, Public Policy
Anita Porco, VP, Affiliate Network

1513 WE MOVE (Worldwide Education and Advocacy for Movement Disorders)
www.wemove.org

WE MOVE provides movement disorder information and educational materials to physicians, patients and families, the media, and the public via its comprehensive Web sites, training courses, and more. Its goal is to make early diagnosis, up-to-date treatment and patient support a reality for all people living with movement disorders.

Book Publishers

1514 A Mother's Touch: The Tiffany Callo Story
United Cerebral Palsy Associations
1825 K Street NW, Suite 600
Washington, DC 20006
202-776-0406
800-872-5827
Fax: 202-776-0414
e-mail: info@ucp.org
www.ucp.org

A vivid portrayal of a woman with cerebral palsy who faced discrimination because of her disability.

Woody Connette, Chair
Ian Ridlon, Vice Chair
Pamela Talkin, Secretary

1515 After the Tears: Parents Talk About Raising a Child with a Disability
United Cerebral Palsy Associations
1825 K Street NW, Suite 600
Washington, DC 20006
202-776-0406
800-872-5827
Fax: 202-776-0414
e-mail: info@ucp.org
www.ucp.org

Book draws on stories of parents who have struggled, learned and grown in the years since their child was born with a disability.

89 pages Softcover

Woody Connette, Chair
Ian Ridlon, Vice Chair
Pamela Talkin, Secretary

1516 An Introduction to Your Child Who Has Cerebral Palsy
Medic Publishing Company
PO Box 89
Redmond, WA 98073
425-881-2883

Information and answers to questions for parents of children with cerebral palsy.

1517 Breaking Ground: Ten Families Building Opportunities Through Integration
United Cerebral Palsy Associations
1825 K Street NW, Suite 600
Washington, DC 20006
202-776-0406
800-872-5827
Fax: 202-776-0414
e-mail: info@ucp.org
www.ucp.org

Gives examples of strategies families have used to integrate the children fully into their schools and communities.

75 pages Softcover

Woody Connette, Chair
Ian Ridlon, Vice Chair
Pamela Talkin, Secretary

1518 Can't You be Still?
Gemma B Publishing
101-478 River Avenue, #779
Winnipeg, Manitoba, R3L 0
Canada
204-452-7566
Fax: 204-475-9903
e-mail: gempub@shaw.ca
www.gemmab.ca

This wonderfully written children's book features a heroine, Ann, with cerebral palsy who goes to school for the first time. First in a trilogy, the book is written in the first person since Ann cannot speak out loud intelligibly but has lots of words inside her head.

28 pages Softcover

Sarah Yates
Anne Allan

1519 Children With Cerebral Palsy: A Parents Guide
Peytral Publications
PO Box 1162
Minnetonka, MN 55345

952-949-8707
877-739-8725
Fax: 952-906-9777
e-mail: help@peytral.com
www.peytral.com

Informative handbook for parents of children and teens; covers medical, educational, legal, family life, daily care, emotional issues and more.

470 pages

1520 Congenital Disorders Sourcebook 2nd Edition
Omnigraphics
PO Box 31-1640
Detroit, MI 48231

800-234-1340
Fax: 800-875-1340
e-mail: info@omnigraphics.com
www.omnigraphics.com

Provides basic consumer health information about the most common types of nonhereditary birth defects and disorders related to prematurity, gestational injuries, congenital infections, and birth complications, including disorders of the heart, brain, gastrointestinal tract, musculoskeletal system, urinary tract, and reproductive system, craniofacial disorders, cerebral palsy, spina bifida, and fetal alcohol syndrome, and detailing the causes, diagnostic tests, and treatments for each.

650 pages
ISBN: 0-780809-45-9

1521 Connecting Students: A Guide to Thoughtful Friendship Facilitation
United Cerebral Palsy Associations
1660 L Street NW, Suite 700
Washington, DC 20036

202-776-0406
800-872-5823
Fax: 202-776-0414
e-mail: info@ucp.org
www.ucp.org

Contains helpful strategies on real-life experiences on building friendships.

48 pages Softcover

Woody Connette, Chair
Ian Ridlon, Vice Chair
Pamela Talkin, Secretary

1522 Discovery Book
United Cerebral Palsy Association
1825 K Street NW, Suite 600
Washington, DC 20006

202-776-0406
800-872-5827
Fax: 202-776-0414
e-mail: info@ucp.org
www.ucp.org

Created within a United Cerebral Palsy group for children with physical disabilities, The Discovery Book is an exploration of social and psychological aspects of childhood disability. Accompanied by their artwork, children speak in their own words about important areas of life such as: What about friends?; Doctors and hospitals; Problems and challenges; and Goals, wishes & dreams.

96 pages

Woody Connette, Chair
Ian Ridlon, Vice Chair
Pamela Talkin, Secretary

1523 Each of Us Remembers: Parents of Children With Cerebral Palsy
United Cerebral Palsy Associations
1825 K Street NW, Suite 600
Washington, DC 20006

202-776-0406
800-872-5827
Fax: 202-776-0414
e-mail: info@ucp.org
www.ucp.org

Parents of children with cerebral palsy answer questions that people really need to know.

Woody Connette, Chair
Ian Ridlon, Vice Chair
Pamela Talkin, Secretary

1524 Gemma B Publishing
101-478 River Avenue, Suite 779
Winnipeg, MB R3L 0
Canada

204-452-7566
Fax: 204-475-9903
e-mail: gempub@shaw.ca
www.gemmab.ca

Gemma B Publishing was formed to develop literary heroines for the disabled, emphasizing their active participation in life.

Sarah Yates, Founder

1525 Handling the Young Cerebral Palsied Child at Home
United Cerebral Palsy Associations
1825 K Street NW, Suite 600
Washington, DC 20006

202-776-0406
800-872-5827
Fax: 202-776-0414
e-mail: info@ucp.org
www.ucp.org

Offers chapters on bathing, feeding, dressing and play for parents of children with cerebral palsy.

337 pages Softcover

Woody Connette, Chair
Ian Ridlon, Vice Chair
Pamela Talkin, Secretary

1526 Here's What I Mean to Say
Gemma B Publishing
101-478 River Avenue, #779
Winnipeg, Manitoba, R3L 0
Canada

204-452-7566
Fax: 204-475-9903
e-mail: gempub@shaw.ca
www.gemmab.ca

Third in the Ann trilogy, Ann learns to read and uncovers the magic of literacy. She uses a speech program in her computer and wonders, when she succeeds in reading, 'Is it me or is it my angel?'

24 pages
ISBN: 0-969647-72-7

Sarah Yates
Anne Allan

1527 Lucky Lou Gets Game
Gemma B Publishing
101-478 River Avenue, #779
Winnipeg, Manitoba, R3L 0
Canada

204-452-7566
Fax: 204-475-9903
e-mail: gempub@shaw.ca
www.gemmab.ca

A coming of age young adult novel about 17-year old Lucky Lou who takes on a neighborhood, learns how to play baseball, and meets the boy who was never in her dreams. In this funny and insightful book, Lou gets game and the results are unexpected.

24 pages
ISBN: 0-969647-71-9

Sarah Yates, Autor
Anne Allan

1528 Natural Supports in School/Work/Community for the Severely Disabled
United Cerebral Palsy Associations
1825 K Street NW, Suite 600
Washington, DC 20006

202-776-0406
800-872-5827
Fax: 202-776-0414
e-mail: info@ucp.org
www.ucp.org

Promotes the position that assistance must be defined by the needs of individuals rather than the requirements of the service systems.

361 pages Softcover
Woody Connette, Chair
Ian Ridlon, Vice Chair
Pamela Talkin, Secretary

1529 No Time for Jello: One Family's Experience
Brookline Books
8 Trumbell Rd, Suite B-001
Northampton, MA 01060
                             413-584-0184
                        Fax: 413-584-6184
                e-mail: brbooks@yahoo.com
                http://brooklinebooks.com

One family's story of their attempts to remediate and cure the effects of cerebral palsied condition the oldest son was born with. The Bratts traveled traditional routes, through distinguished medical centers in Boston, and nontraditional routes in a search for treatments that would help their son.

Softcover
ISBN: 0-253363-65-9

1530 Nobody Knows
Gemma B Publishing
101-478 River Avenue, #779
Winnipeg, Manitoba, R3L 0
Canada
                             204-452-7566
                        Fax: 204-475-9903
                e-mail: gempub@shaw.ca
                www.gemmab.ca

Sequel to 'Can't You Be Still,' Ann gets frustrated that nobody knows what she wants and is trying to say; they find it hard to understand her. She goes out to find someone who can understand and in the process, learns that there are many ways to communicate.

24 pages
ISBN: 0-969647-71-9
Sarah Yates
Anne Allan

1531 Opening Doors: Strategies for Including All Students in Regular Education
United Cerebral Palsy Associations
1825 K Street NW, Suite 600
Washington, DC 20006
                             202-776-0406
                             800-872-5827
                        Fax: 202-776-0414
                e-mail: info@ucp.org
                www.ucp.org

Contains practical information for including and supporting all students in regular classes.

55 pages Softcover
Woody Connette, Chair
Ian Ridlon, Vice Chair
Pamela Talkin, Secretary

1532 Teaching Motor Skills to Children with Cerebral Palsy & Similar Movement Disorders
Woodbine House
6510 Bells Mill Road
Bethesda, MD 20817
                             301-897-3570
                             800-843-7323
                        Fax: 301-897-5838
                e-mail: info@woodbinehouse.com
                www.woodbinehouse.com

The resource that parents, therapists, and other caregivers can consult to help children with gross motor delays learn and practice motor skills outside of therapy sessions.

2006 275 pages
ISBN: 1-890627-72-0

1533 Walk with Me
United Cerebral Palsy Associations
1825 K Sreet NW, Suite 600
Washington, DC 20006
                             202-776-0406
                             800-872-5827
                        Fax: 202-776-0414
                e-mail: info@ucp.org
                www.ucp.org

A story written by eight-year-old Eric Grimm covering his thoughts on living with cerebral palsy.
Woody Connette, Chair
Ian Ridlon, Vice Chair
Pamela Talkin, Secretary

Newsletters

1534 Family Support Bulletin
United Cerebral Palsy Associations
1825 K Street NW Suite 600
Washington, DC 20006
                             202-776-0406
                             800-872-5827
                        Fax: 202-776-0414
                e-mail: info@ucp.org
                www.ucp.org

A detailed quarterly journal that takes a comprehensive look at the latest policies, resources and legislative information enacted in Washington and state capitals.

Quarterly
Stephen Bennett, President/ CEO
Connie Garner, EVP, Public Policy
Anita Porco, VP, Affiliate Network

1535 My Child Without Limits Newsletter
United Cerebral Palsy
1825 K Street NW Suite 600
Washington, DC 20006
                             202-776-0406
                             800-872-5827
                        Fax: 202-776-0414
                e-mail: info@ucp.org
                www.ucp.org

A monthly publication that highlights new and relevant content from the 'My Child Without Limits' web site and online community, which provides an early intervention resource for families of young children ages 0-5 with developmental delays or disabilities, and the professionals who serve them.

Stephen Bennett, President & CEO
Connie Garner, EVP, Public Policy
Anita Porco, VP, Affiliate Network

1536 Networker
United Cerebral Palsy Associations
1825 K Street NW Suite 600
Washington, DC 20006
                             202-776-0406
                             800-872-5827
                        Fax: 202-776-0414
                e-mail: info@ucp.org
                www.ucp.org

Offers the latest information on the newest technology available for persons with cerebral palsy.

Quarterly
Stephen Bennett, President/ CEO
Connie Garner, EVP, Public Policy
Anita Porco, VP, Affiliate Network

1537 UCP Newsletter
United Cerebral Palsy
1825 K Street NW Suite 600
Washington, DC 20006
                             202-776-0406
                             800-872-5827
                        Fax: 202-776-0414
                e-mail: info@ucp.org
                www.ucp.org

A monthly e-publication formerly known as Life Without Limits. The newsletteris not only for UCP affiliates, but also volunteers, activists and information seekers. Each issue highlights stories centered around advocacy efforts, affiliate news, information and referral sources, upcoming events, inspiring events and more.

Stephen Bennett, President & CEO
Connie Garner, EVP, Public Policy
Anita Porco, VP, Affiliate Network

1538 UCP Washington Wire
United Cerebral Palsy
1825 K Street NW Suite 600
Washington, DC 20006
202-776-0406
800-872-5827
Fax: 202-776-0414
e-mail: info@ucp.org
www.ucp.org

A weekly publication that provides a comprehensive source of information on federal legislation, agency regulations, court decisions and other issues of interest to the disability community.

Stephen Bennett, President & CEO
Connie Garner, EVP, Public Policy
Anita Porco, VP, Affiliate Network

Pamphlets

1539 Cerebral Palsy-Facts & Figures
United Cerebral Palsy Associations
1825 K Street NW Suite 600
Washington, DC 20006
202-776-0406
800-872-5827
Fax: 202-776-0414
www.ucp.org

Offers information on what cerebral palsy is, the effects, causes, types, and prevention.

Stephen Bennett, President/ CEO
Connie Garner, EVP, Public Policy
Anita Porco, VP, Affiliate Network

Camps

1540 Camp Merrimack
3320 Triana Boulevard
Huntsville, AL 35805
256-534-6455
e-mail: ksimari@merrimackhall.com
www.merrimackhall.com

A unique arts half-day camp for children ages 3 through 12; open to children with special needs including Cerebral Palsy, Down Syndrome, autism and others.

Ashley Dinges, Executive Director
Kim Simari, Managing Director

1541 Camp Merry Heart/Easter Seals Easter Seal Society
21 O'Brian Road
Hackettstown, NJ 07840
908-852-3896
Fax: 908-852-9263
e-mail: camp@nj.easterseals.com
www.nj.easterseals.com

An organized program of swimming, arts and crafts, boating, nature study and travel offered to the physically disabled, developmentally disabled, cerebral palsied, brain damaged and head injured children, ages 5-18, adults 19-75+. Fall and spring travel programs for adults.

Mary Ellen Ross, Camping Director

1542 Camp Ramah in New England Tikvah Program
39 Bennett Street
Palmer, MA 01609
413-283-9771
Fax: 413-283-6661
e-mail: info@campramahne.org
www.campramahne.org

The Tikvah program is one of the first summer programs for Jewish children with special needs. It continues to grow and evolve as it strives to serve campers with a wide range of special needs including, but not limited to, congitive impairments, autism, cerebral palsy and seizure disorder.

Howard Blas, Tikvah Program Director
Talya Kalender, Director, Camper Care
Benjamin Greene, Director of Education

1543 Cerebral Palsy Center Summer Program
7 Sanford Avenue
Belleville, NJ
201-751-0200
e-mail: info@kidscamps.com
www.kidscamps.com

1544 Charles Campbell Children's Camp
PO Box 23342
Billings, MT 59104
e-mail: campbellcamp@msn.com
www.billingslions.org

Camp for children with physical disabilities including but not limited to: sight or hearing impairment, cerebral palsy, spina bifida, amputee, gross motor skill impairments, and other disabilities.

Doug Hanson, Director

1545 Crotched Mountain School & Rehabilitation Center
1 Verney Drive
Greenfield, NH 03047
603-547-3311
800-800-966
Fax: 603-547-3232
e-mail: info@crotchedmountain.org
www.cmf.org

Currently serves children ages 6-22 with multiple-handicaps including: Cerebral Palsy, Spina Bifida, visual and hearing impairments and neurological disabilities, developmental disorders, mental retardation, autism, behavioral and emotional disorders, seizure disorders, spinal cord and head injuries. Member of the National Association of Independent Schools and accredited with the NE Association of Schools and Colleges, Independent Schools of Northern NE.

Rita Phinney, Director Admissions
John Young, Registrar

1546 Easter Seals Wisconsin Camp Respite
1550 Waubeek Road
Wisconsin Dells, WI 53965
608-254-2502
Fax: 608-253-0327
e-mail: dfourness@easterselaswisconsin.com
www.easterselaswisconsin.com

Camp for individuals age 3 to adult with moderate to severe disabilities. The campers have a variety of different diagnosis such as: autism, cerebral palsy, traumatic brain injury, developmental disabilities, and behavioral issues.

Dan Fournes, Camp Director

1547 Eric RicStar Winter Music Therapy Summer Camp
4930 S Hagadorn Rd
East Lansing, MI 48823
517-353-7661
Fax: 517-355-3292
e-mail: commusic@msu.edu
www.cms.msu.edu

The purpose of this camp is to provide opportunities for musical expression, enjoyment and interaction for all people with special needs and their siblings.

Cindy Edgerton, Director
Judy Winter, Co-Chair

Description

1548 CHARCOT-MARIE-TOOTH DISEASE

Charcot-Marie-Tooth (CMT) disease belongs to a group of disorders known as hereditary motor-sensory neuropathies or HMSNs. The HMSNs are progressive disorders of nerves outside of the central nervous system that extend from the brain and spinal cord to particular areas of the body (peripheral nervous system). Symptoms and findings associated with these disorders are primarily the result of involvement of motor nerve fibers (those that affect motion). These nerves transmit various nerve impulses away from the brain and spinal cord to their termination (e.g., muscle tissue). As these disorders progress, affected individuals may experience some symptoms due to sensory and autonomic involvement. Sensory nerve fibers carry impulses to the brain and spinal cord. The autonomic nervous system is the portion of the peripheral nervous system that regulates involuntary functioning of particular tissues and organs.

There are different types of Charcot-Marie-Tooth disease that have varying modes of inheritance. Charcot-Marie-Tooth disease (in all its forms) is the most prevalent hereditary peripheral neuropathy, affecting approximately one in 2,500 individuals. The most common form of the disease, known as Charcot-Marie-Tooth disease type 1A or CMT1A, is inherited as an autosomal dominant trait. A disease gene for CMT1A is located on the short arm of chromosome 17.

Children with CMT type 1A usually do not have associated symptoms until late childhood or early adolescence. However, some may experience abnormalities in their manner of walking (gait disturbances) as early as the second year of life. In other, rare instances, associated symptoms may not become apparent until middle adulthood. CMT1A initially affects muscles supplied by nerves of the lower legs (peroneal and tibial nerves), causing muscle degeneration (atrophy) in the lower legs and feet. This is accompanied by muscle weakness and a distinctive stork-like contour of the legs. Bending movements of the ankles become progressively weaker, eventually resulting in footdrop, a condition in which the foot does not flex or bend upward. In addition, the arch of the foot becomes unusually increased in height (pescavus deformities). An unstable gait may develop, and children may appear clumsy, easily tripping or falling. Although muscles of both legs are affected, disease progression and associated findings usually differ slightly from one side of the body to the other.

As the disorder progresses, individuals with CMT1A also usually develop a loss of muscle tissue mass and weakness in the forearms and hands. These areas seem to be less severely affected than the lower legs. However, patients may eventually develop permanent fixation of certain joints in a bend position. This typically occurs in the fingers and wrists. Some patients also experience gradual sensory involvement, such as abnormal burning or tingling sensations (paresthesias) in the feet. Associated autonomic abnormalities may include unusual paleness (pallor) or blotching of the skin, especially of the feet. In individuals with CMT1A, specialized testing typically reveals a marked reduction in the transmission of motor and sensory nerve signals to affected muscles (reduced conduction velocities).

Although CMT1A is progressive, most affected individuals maintain the ability to walk. However, the use of special orthopedic appliances, such as stiff boots that reach to the midcalf, plastic splints, or light leg braces, are typically necessary to help stabilize the ankles. Surgical measures may be considered, such as surgical fusion of the ankles. In addition, certain medications may help to alleviate burning sensations in the feet (e.g., carbamazepine or phenytoin). Other treatment is symptomatic and supportive.

In addition to Charcot-Marie-Tooth disease type 1A, additional autosomal dominant, autosomal recessive, and X-linked forms of the disease have been identified. Specific symptoms and findings and the nature of the disorder progression may vary, depending upon the specific form of the disease.

National Associations & Support Groups

1549 American Academy of Pediatrics
141 Northwest Point Boulevard
Elk Grove Village, IL 60007
847-434-4000
800-433-9016
Fax: 847-434-8000
www.aap.org

The American Academy of Pediatrics and its member pediatricians are committed to the attainment of optimal physical, mental and social health and well-being for all infants, children, adolescents, and young adults.

Sandra Hassink, MD, FAAP, President

State Agencies & Support Groups

New York

1550 CMTA Chapter - New York (Greater)
CMT Association
333 East 34th StreetSuite 1J
Manhattan, NY 10016
212-535-4314
Fax: 212-535-6392
e-mail: david.younger@nyumc.org
www.cmtnyc.org

Every other month (Third Saturday from 1:00 - 3:00 p.m.) - check website
Dr David Younger, Contact

Ohio

1551 CMTA Chapter - Ohio
CMT Association
405 Wagner Avenue
Greenville, OH 45331
937-548-3963
e-mail: Greenville-Ohio-CMT@who.rr.com
www.charcot-marie-tooth.org

Fourth Thursday, April - October
Dot Cain, Contact

Pennsylvania

1552 CMTA Chapter - Pennsylvania
CMT Association
PO Box 105
Glenolden, PA 19036
610-499-9264
800-606-2682
Fax: 610-499-9267
e-mail: info@cmtausa.org.
www.cmtausa.org

Bi-monthly (3rd Saturday, 10:00 a.m. - 12:00 p.m.)

Herbert Beron, Chairman
Gary J Gasper, Treasurer
Elizabeth Ouellette, Secretary

Web Sites

1553 CMT Net
275 Madison Ave (corner of 40th St)
New York, NY 10016   www.rcn.com

CMTNet is intended to provide information for both the medical and non-medical communities.

1554 Charcot-Marie-Tooth Association
PO Box 105
Glenolden, PA 19036   610-499-9264
                                    800-606-2682
                                Fax: 610-499-9267
                            e-mail: info@cmtausa.org
                                    www.cmtausa.org

Information regarding patient support, public education, promotion of research and ultimately the treatment and cure of CMT.

Patrick A. Livney, Chief Executive Officer
Kim Magee, Director of Finance
Susan Ruediger, Director of Development

1555 Health Answers
410 Horsham Road
Horsham, PA 19044   215-442-9017
              e-mail: Michael.tague@healthanswers.com
                           www.healthanswers.com

The vision was to provide a breadth of services to clients through the formation of a network of companies. Each company plays a key role in meeting our clients' needs.

Michael Tague, Managing Director

1556 Muscular Dystrophy Association
222 S. Riverside Plaza, Suite 1500
Chicago, IL 60606   800-572-1717
                          e-mail: mda@mdausa.org
                                    mda.org

Information regarding neuromuscular diseases through programs of worldwide research, comprehensive medical and community services, and far-reaching professional and public health education; including publications.

Steven M. Derks, President/ CEO
Valerie A. Cwik, M.D., EVP/ CMO/ CSO
Julie Faber, EVP/ CFO

Book Publishers

1557 Charcot-Marie-Tooth Disorders: A Handbook for Primary Care Physicians
Charcot-Marie-Tooth Association
PO Box 105
Glenolden, PA 19036   610-499-9264
                                    800-606-2682
                                Fax: 610-499-9267
                            e-mail: info@cmtausa.org
                                    www.cmtausa.org

Excellent source of information about the causes, symptoms, and treatment/management of CMT.

1995 130 pages

Patrick A Livney, CEO
Patricia Dreibelbis, Director Of Program Services
Kim Magee, Director Of Finance

1558 Let's Talk About Going to the Hospital
Rosen Publishing Group's PowerKids Press
29 E 21st Street
New York, NY 10010   212-777-3017
                                    800-237-9932
                                Fax: 888-436-4643
                      e-mail: rosenpub@tribeca.ios.com
                                    www.rosenpublishing.com

If a child has to check into the hospital, chances are he or she is already upset about being ill. Knowing how a hospital functions and what the procedures are, such as when family members can visit, will help in what is already a stressful situation. Grades K-5.

24 pages
ISBN: 0-823950-36-0

Magazines

1559 Quest Magazine
MDA Publications
222 S. Riverside Plaza, Suite 1500
Chicago, IL 60606   520-529-2000
                                    800-572-1717
                                Fax: 520-529-5300
                            e-mail: mda@mdausa.org
                                    mda.org

A national magazine that goes out to everyone registered with MDA, MDA clinics, researchers and subscribers. It presents news related to muscular dystrophy and other neuromuscular diseases including research, personal profiles, fund raising activities, patient services, and lifestyle information including products and trends.

Bimonthly

Steven M. Derks, President/ CEO
Valerie A. Cwik, M.D., EVP/ CMO/ CSO
Julie Faber, EVP/ CFO

Newsletters

1560 CMTA Report
CMT Association
PO Box 105
Glenolden, PA 19036   610-499-9264
                                    800-606-2682
                                Fax: 610-499-9267
                    e-mail: info@charcot-marie-tooth.org
                                    www.cmtausa.org

Contains articles on CMT topics, research news and patient profiles. Free with membership.

Bi-Monthly

Patrick A. Livney, Chief Executive Officer
Kim Magee, Director of Finance
Susan Ruediger, Director of Development

Pamphlets

1561 CMT Brochure
Charcot-Marie-Tooth Association
PO Box 105
Glenolden, PA 19036   610-499-9264
                                    800-606-2682
                                Fax: 610-499-9267
                    e-mail: info@charcot-marie-tooth.org
                                    www.cmtausa.org

Provides a quick overview of CMT.

2005 8 pages

Patrick A. Livney, Chief Executive Officer
Kim Magee, Director of Finance
Susan Ruediger, Director of Development

1562 CMT Facts I
Charcot-Marie-Tooth Association
PO Box 105
Glenolden, PA 19036   610-499-9264
                                    800-606-2682
                                Fax: 610-499-9267
                    e-mail: info@charcot-marie-tooth.org
                                    www.cmtausa.org

Offers information on the neurotrophic drugs, genetics and therapies for CMT, surgical options and an overview of the disorder.

1993 16 pages

Patrick A. Livney, Chief Executive Officer
Kim Magee, Director of Finance
Susan Ruediger, Director of Development

1563 CMT Facts II
Charcot-Marie-Tooth Association
PO Box 105
Glenolden, PA 19036   610-499-9264
                                       800-606-2682
                                  Fax: 610-499-9267
              e-mail: info@charcot-marie-tooth.org
                                   www.cmtausa.org

Offers information on adaptive devices, feature specialists and
the Americans with disabilities act.

1993 24 pages

Patrick A. Livney, Chief Executive Officer
Kim Magee, Director of Finance
Susan Ruediger, Director of Development

1564 CMT Facts III
Charcot-Marie-Tooth Association
PO Box 105
Glenolden, PA 19036   610-499-9264
                                       800-606-2682
                                  Fax: 610-499-9267
              e-mail: info@charcot-marie-tooth.org
                                   www.cmtausa.org

Offers information on neurotrophic drugs, neuromuscular disorders, genetic news and doctor's questions and answers.

1995 24 pages

Patrick A. Livney, Chief Executive Officer
Kim Magee, Director of Finance
Susan Ruediger, Director of Development

1565 CMT Facts IV
Charcot-Marie-Tooth Association
PO Box 105
Glenolden, PA 19036   610-499-9264
                                       800-606-2682
                                  Fax: 610-499-9267
              e-mail: info@charcot-marie-tooth.org
                                   www.cmtausa.org

Provides information for Charcot-Marie-Tooth patients.

1998 32 pages

Patrick A. Livney, Chief Executive Officer
Kim Magee, Director of Finance
Susan Ruediger, Director of Development

1566 CMT Facts V
Charcot-Marie-Tooth Association
PO Box 105
Glenolden, PA 19036   610-499-9264
                                       800-606-2682
                                  Fax: 610-499-9267
              e-mail: info@charcot-marie-tooth.org
                                   www.cmtausa.org

Source for information on orthotics, pain, emotional, HNPP,
physical and occupational therapy, Social Security Disability and
more.

2002 56 pages

Patrick A. Livney, Chief Executive Officer
Kim Magee, Director of Finance
Susan Ruediger, Director of Development

**1567 Charcot-Marie-Tooth Disorders: A Guide abo ut Genetics for
Patients**
Charcot-Marie-Tooth Association
PO Box 105
Glenolden, PA 19036   610-499-9264
                                       800-606-2682
                                  Fax: 610-499-9267
              e-mail: info@charcot-marie-tooth.org
                                   www.cmtausa.org

Illustrated with easy-to-understand diagrams, this booklet outlines the basics of genetics inheritance and CMT.

2000 21 pages

Patrick A. Livney, Chief Executive Officer
Kim Magee, Director of Finance
Susan Ruediger, Director of Development

**1568 Facts About Charcot-Marie-Tooth Disease an d
Dejerine-Sottas**
Muscular Dystrophy Association
222 S. Riverside Plaza, Suite 1500
Chicago, IL 60606   520-529-2000
                                       800-572-1717
                                  Fax: 520-529-5300
                         e-mail: mda@mdausa.org
                                           mda.org

This booklet has been prepared to give you the basic knowledge
about CMT and Dejerine-Sottas disease that you'll need in order
to help you prepare for changed that may offur in your future. It
cover research, explaining the causes, treatments, and cures. Also
available in Spanish and online.

2009 15 pages Paperback

Steven M. Derks, President/ CEO
Valerie A. Cwik, M.D., EVP/ CMO/ CSO
Julie Faber, EVP/ CFO

1569 MDA Fact Sheet
Muscular Dystrophy Association
222 S. Riverside Plaza, Suite 1500
Chicago, IL 60606   520-529-2000
                                       800-572-1717
                                  Fax: 520-529-5300
                         e-mail: mda@mdausa.org
                                           mda.org

Provides information about the association, how it got started,
and what muscular dystrophy can affect the body. Also in Spanish and online.

2008

Steven M. Derks, President/ CEO
Valerie A. Cwik, M.D., EVP/ CMO/ CSO
Julie Faber, EVP/ CFO

Description

1570 CHILDHOOD DERMATOMYOSITIS

Synonym: Juvenile dermatomyositis (JDMS)

Involves the following Biologic System(s):

Connective Tissue Disorders, Dermatologic Disorders, Orthopedic and Muscle Disorders

Dermatomyositis is a connective tissue disorder characterized by inflammatory and degenerative changes of the muscles and distinctive lesions of the skin. Although the disorder may become apparent at any time, it most commonly occurs in children between five to 15 years of age or adults between the ages of 40 to 60 years. In children, the average age at onset is eight or nine years. More females than males are affected by dermatomyositis.

The cause of dermatomyositis is unknown. However, immune, genetic, and environmental factors are thought to play some role. Many researchers suggest that dermatomyositis is an autoimmune disorder resulting from abnormal immune responses directed against the body's own tissues.

The symptoms and findings associated with childhood dermatomyositis are similar to those seen in the adult form of the disease. However, involvement of the gastrointestinal (GI) tract and the development of abnormal calcium deposits (calcifications) within skin and muscle tissues are more frequent and widespread in childhood dermatomyositis. Affected children usually have widespread inflammation of small blood vessels (vasculitis) within connective tissues of the skin, muscles, tissues beneath the skin (subcutaneous tissues), and tissues underlying the nails (nail beds). In addition, cancerous growths (malignancies) occur in approximately 20 percent of affected adults; malignancies are rarely seen in those with childhood dermatomyositis.

In most patients with childhood dermatomyositis, the onset of symptoms is relatively gradual and subtle. Children initially experience slowly progressive muscle weakness affecting the upper arms, shoulders, hips, and thighs (proximal muscles) as well as the trunk. Involved muscles tend to be sore, stiff, tender, or abnormally hard. Affected children may develop an awkward manner of walking and gradually lose the ability to perform certain tasks, such as lifting the arms above the shoulders, combing their hair, dressing, climbing stairs, or rising from the floor unassisted. Involved muscles may eventually show varying degrees of degeneration (atrophy) and, in severe cases, permanent bending or extension in various fixed postures (joint contractures). Although muscles of the upper arms or legs are typically most severely affected, any muscle may become involved. In severe cases, affected muscles may include those of the roof of the mouth and those involved in respiration, resulting in a nasal quality to the voice; breathing difficulties; hyperventilation; inadvertent breathing of foreign materials into the respiratory passages (bronchial aspiration); and potentially life-threatening complications. In addition, involvement of muscles of the gastrointestinal tract may cause difficulties swallowing; abdominal pain; passage of dark, tarry stools containing digested blood (melena); and infrequent bowel movements or difficulty passing stools (constipation). In severe cases, gastrointestinal bleeding (hemorrhage) or other associated abnormalities (e.g., intestinal perforations) may cause potentially life-threatening conditions.

Patients with childhood dermatomyositis also develop characteristic skin changes, such as a reddish-purple rash of the upper eyelids (heliotrope rash); an abnormal accumulation of fluid in body tissues surrounding the eyes and in other facial areas (periorbital and facial edema); a reddish rash across the skin of the nose and cheeks (butterfly rash); and reddish-purple, raised, scaling skin lesions (papules) on the surfaces of certain joints, particularly the knuckles (Gottron's sign), elbows, and knees. These scaling lesions develop a central area of tissue loss (atrophy) that lacks color (vitiligo) or has increased pigmentation (hyperpigmentation). Patients may also have a dusky reddish rash covering the upper arms and legs and the upper trunk.

Approximately 20 to 50 percent of affected children also develop abnormal calcium deposits (calcifications) within muscle, skin, and subcutaneous tissues. These deposits may contribute to localized areas of muscle loss or the freezing of joints in permanently bent positions. Some patients may also experience additional symptoms and findings, such as a low-grade fever, joint inflammation (arthritis), enlargement of the liver and spleen (hepatosplenomegaly), or other abnormalities. In most patients, childhood dermatomyositis gradually becomes inactive over several years.

The treatment of patients with childhood dermatomyositis requires early, aggressive measures to help prevent potentially life-threatening complications. Such measures include evaluation to detect possible involvement of the respiratory or gastrointestinal systems and provision of ongoing nursing care for those with such involvement. Such care may include mechanical suctioning of the throat by way of the nose (nasopharyngeal suction), the creation of a temporary opening in the throat to ease breathing difficulties (tracheostomy), or mechanical breathing support (e.g., endotracheal intubation or respirator). In addition, the treatment of patients typically includes the use of corticosteroids (e.g., prednisone) to help suppress the inflammatory process of the disease. Blood levels of certain muscle enzymes are regularly measured to help gauge the effectiveness of such therapy. Once such enzyme levels are reduced to normal ranges, the steroid dosage may gradually be decreased to as low as possible while still being effective, owing to the numerous problems associated with prolonged administration or high-dose steroids. After about two years, such treatment may be discontinued without the reemergence of symptoms. In patients who do not respond to steroid therapy, certain immunosuppressant drugs such as methotrexate, azathioprine, or cyclosporine or, in some patients, intravenous immunoglobulin therapy may be beneficial. In addition, treatment may include surgical removal of calcium deposits. Physical therapy (e.g., passive exercises, eventual progression to active exercises) is important in helping to rebuild muscle strength and prevent permanent, disabling contractures. Splints may be required to help ensure proper positioning of certain limbs. Proper skin hygiene is also important in patients with childhood dermatomyositis.

National Associations & Support Groups

1571 American Academy of Pediatrics
141 Northwest Point Boulevard
Elk Grove Village, IL 60007
847-434-4000
800-433-9016
Fax: 847-434-8000
www.aap.org

The American Academy of Pediatrics and its member pediatricians are committed to the attainment of optimal physical, mental and social health and well-being for all infants, children, adolescents, and young adults.

Sandra Hassink, MD, FAAP, President

1572 American Autoimmune Related Diseases Association
22100 Gratiot Avenue
East Detroit, MI 48021
586-776-3900
800-598-4668
Fax: 586-776-3903
e-mail: aarda@aarda.org
www.aarda.org

Dedicated to the eradication of autoimmune diseases and the alleviation of suffering and the socio-economic impact of autoimmunity through fostering and facilitating collaboration in the areas of education, public awareness, research and patient services in an effective, ethical and efficient manner.

Betty Diamond, Chair of Advisory Board
Stanley M Finger Phd, Chairman of Board of Directors
Noel R Rose, Chairman Emeritus

1573 American Osteopathic College of Dermatology
1501 E Illinois Street, PO Box 7525
Kirksville, MO 63501
660-665-2184
800-449-2623
Fax: 660-627-2623
e-mail: ExecDirector@AOCD.org
www.aocd.org

Strives to improve the standards of the practice of dermatology, to stimulate the study and extend knowledge in the field of dermatology, and to promote a more general understanding of the nature and scope of services rendered by osteopathic dermatologists to other divisions of practice, hospitals, clinics and the public.

David Grice, President
Suzanne Rozenberg, President-Elect
Rick Lin, First Vice-President

1574 Arthritis Foundation
1330 W. Peachtree Street.,Suite 100
Atlanta, GA 30309
404-872-7100
800-568-4045
Fax: 404-872-0457
www.arthritis.org

The only nonprofit organization that supports the more than 100 types of arthritis and related conditions with advocacy, programs, services and research.

Daniel T McGowan, Chair
Rowland W. Chang, Vice Chairs
Patricia Novak Nelson, Vice Chairs

1575 Juvenile Dermatomyositis
Arthritis Foundation
PO Box 7669
Atlanta, GA 30357
404-872-7100
800-283-7800
Fax: 404-872-0457
e-mail: info@jdfcure.com
www.atrhritis.org

1576 Myositis Association of America
1737 King Street, Suite 600
Alexandria, VA 22314
703-299-4850
800-821-7356
Fax: 703-535-6752
e-mail: tma@myositis.org
www.myositis.org

The mission of The Myositis Association is to find a cure for inflammatory and other related myopathies, while serving those affected by these diseases.

Kanneboyina Nagaraju DVM, PhD, Chair
David Fiorentino M.D., PhD, Vice Chair
Alan Pestronk M.D., Research Chair

1577 Society for Pediatric Dermatology
8365 Keystone Crossing, Suite 107
Indianapolis, IN 46240
317-202-0224
Fax: 317-205-9841
e-mail: spd@hp-assoc.com
www.pedsderm.net

National organization dedicated to promote, develop and advance education, research and care of skin disease in all pediatric age groups.

Sheila Friedlander, MD, President
Richard Antaya, MD, President Elect
Anthony Mancini, MD, Secretary/Treasurer

Libraries & Resource Centers

California

1578 University of California, San Francisco Dermatology Drug Research
515 Spruce
San Francisco, CA 94143
415-476-2001
Fax: 415-476-6014
cc.ucsf.edu/people

Conducts clinical testing of new or existing pharmalogic agents used in the treatment of skin disorders.

John Koo, MD, Director

Delaware

1579 Delaware Division of Libraries for the Blind and Physically Handicapped
43 S Dupont Highway
Dover, DE 19901
302-736-4748
800-282-8676
Fax: 302-736-6787
TDD: 302-739-4748
e-mail: bedpg@lib.de.us

Braille readers receive service from Philadelphia and Pennsylvania, summer reading program, braille writer and cassettes.

Beth Landon, Librarian

Illinois

1580 Dermatology Information Network (DERMINFONET)
American Academy of Dermatology
PO Box 4014
Schaumburg, IL 60168
847-330-0230
Fax: 847-330-0050

Consists of a collection of dermatologic databases that are available to members on a subscription and/or purchase basis. These databases are designed to run on a wide variety of personal computers.

1581 National Library of Dermatologic Teaching Slides
American Academy of Dermatology
930 E Woodfield Road
Schaumburg, IL 60173
847-240-1280
866-503-7546
Fax: 847-240-1859
www.aad.org

A collection of dermatologic teaching slides offering the most comprehensive series ever assembled. Each set offers a realistic presentation of classic clinical skin conditions encountered by the dermatologist.

Dirk M Elston, President
Lisa A Garner, Vice President
Suzanne M Olbricht, Secretary/Treasurer

ISBN: 7-032994-85-0

Bob Goldberg, Executive Director

New York

1582 Laboratory of Dermatology Research
Memorial Sloan-Kettering Cancer Center
1275 York Avenue
New York, NY 10065   212-639-2000
                                  Fax: 212-639-3576
                                      www.mskcc.org

Specific studies on the identification of skin disorders and dermatology.

Craig B Thompson, President/CEO

1583 Rockefeller University Laboratory for Investigative Dermatology
1230 York Avenue
New York, NY 10065   212-327-7490
                                  Fax: 212-327-7459

Research into skin disorders and the whole specialty of dermatology in general.

Barry Coller, Head

Research Centers

1584 University of California, San Francisco Dermatology Drug Research
515 Spruce Street
San Francisco, CA 94115   41-76-701
                                  Fax: 415-502-4126
        www.dermatology.ucsf.edu/research/areasofresearch.as

Conducts clinical testing of new or existing pharmacologic agents used in the treatment of skin disorders.

Mounira Kenaani, MBA, Department Manager
Darrell Young, Associate Director of Development
Leslie Chau, Assistant to Chair

Conferences

1585 AOCD Annual Meeting
American Osteopathic College of Dermatology
1501 E Illinois Street, PO Box 7525
Kirksville, MO 63501   660-665-2184
                                       800-449-2623
                                  Fax: 660-627-2623
                                  e-mail: info@aocd.org
                                       www.aocd.org

November

Marsha Wise, Executive Director

1586 Society for Pediatric Dermatology Annual Meeting
8365 Keystone Crossing, Suite 107
Indianapolis, IN 46240   317-202-0224
                                  Fax: 317-205-9841
                              e-mail: spd@hp-assoc.com
                                     www.pedsderm.net

Kent Lindeman, Executive Director

1587 TMA Annual Patient Conference
Myositis Association
1737 King Street, Suite 600
Alexandria, VA 22314   800-821-7356
                                  Fax: 703-535-6752
                              e-mail: tma@myositis.org
                                     www.myositis.org

To meet other myosentis patients, hear from TMA's medical advisors about myositis research, and benefit from the support and practical ideas of others with your disease. The Conference regularly includes sessions on research, exercise, advocacy and coping skills, and disease-specific question and answer sessions as well as new and interesting sessions each year.

Web Sites

1588 American Autoimmune Related Diseases Association
22100 Gratiot Ave.
Eastpointe, MI 48021   586-776-3900
                                       800-598-4668
                                  Fax: 586-776-3903
                                      www.aarda.org

Dedicated to the eradication of autoimmune diseases and the alleviation of suffering and the socio-economic impact of autoimmunity through fostering and facilitating collaboration in the areas of education, public awareness, research and patient services in an effective, ethical and efficient manner.

Virginia T. Ladd, President/ Executive Director
Patricia Barber, Asst. Director
Eula Hoover, Exec. Assistant/ Newsletter Editor

1589 American Osteopathic College of Dermatology
2902 North Baltimore Street
Kirksville, MI 63501   660-665-2184
                                       800-449-2623
                                  Fax: 660-627-2623
                                      www.aocd.org

Improving the standards of the practice of dermatology, to stimulate the study and extend knowledge in the field of dermatology, and to promote a more general understanding of the nature and scope of services rendered by osteopathic dermatologists to other divisions of practice, hospitals, clinics and the public.

Rick Lin, President
Karthik Krishnamurthy, 1st Vice President
Daniel Ladd, 2nd Vice President

1590 Arthritis Foundation
1330 W. Peachtree Street, Suite 100
Atlanta, GA 30309   404-872-7100
                                      www.arthritis.org

Supports more than 100 types of arthritis and related conditions with advocacy, programs, services and research.

Ann M. Palmer, President/ CEO
Meagan Fulmer, Chief Development Officer
Wayne Guthrie, SPHR, SVP, Staff Operations

1591 Myosentis Association of America
1737 King Street, Suite 600
Alexandria, VA 22314   703-299-4850
                                       800-821-7356
                                  Fax: 703-535-6752
                              e-mail: TMA@myositis.org
                                     www.myositis.org

Mission is to find a cure for inflammatory and other related myopathies, while serving those affected by these diseases.

Augie DeAugustinis, Chair
Patrick Zenner, Vice Chairman
Bob Goldberg, Executive Director

1592 Society for Pediatric Dermatology
8365 Keystone Crossing, Suite 107
Indianapolis, IN 46240   317-202-0224
                                  Fax: 317-205-9481
                              e-mail: info@pedsderm.net
                                     www.pedsderm.net

Objective is to promote, develop and advance education, research and care of skin disease in all pediatric age groups.

Beth Drolet, President
Howard Pride, VP Finance and Administration
Karen Wiss, VP Education

Book Publishers

1593 Let's Talk About Going to the Hospital
Rosen Publishing Group's PowerKids Press
29 E 21st Street
New York, NY 10010
212-777-3017
800-237-9932
Fax: 888-436-4643
e-mail: rosenpub@tribeca.ios.com
www.rosenpublishing.com

If a child has to check into the hospital, chances are he or she is already upset about being ill. Knowing how a hospital functions and what the procedures are, such as when family members can visit, will help in what is already a stressful situation. Grades K-5.

24 pages
ISBN: 0-823950-36-0

Magazines

1594 International Journal of Dermatology
International Society of Dermatology
2323 North State Street #30
Bunnell, FL 32110
386-437-4405
Fax: 386-437-4427
e-mail: info@intsocdermatol.org
www.intsocderm.org

Focuses on information for dermatologists and the whole specialty of dermatology research and education.

10 times a year

Evangeline Handog, President
Nellie Konnikov, Secretary-General
Marcia Ramos-e-Silva, Assistant Secretary-General

1595 JM Companion
The Myositis Association
1737 King Street, Suite 600
Alexandria, VA 22314
703-299-4850
800-821-7356
Fax: 703-535-6752
e-mail: TMA@myositis.org
www.myositis.org

Focuses on special concerns and also has an 'Ask the doctor' column with answers from leading JM physicians, a special insert for children, and clinical trial listings for JM patients.

Quarterly

Augie DeAugustinis, Chair
Patrick Zenner, Vice Chairman
Bob Goldberg, Executive Director

1596 Journal of Dermatologic Surgery and Oncology
International Society for Dermatologic Surgery
350 Main Street
Malden, MA 2148
781-388-8598
800-835-6770
Fax: 847-330-1135
e-mail: cs-journals@wiley.com
onlinelibrary.wiley.com

Focuses on medical updates and information on dermatology.

Monthly

Newsletters

1597 Awareness
NAPVI
PO Box 317
Watertown, MA 2471
617-972-7441
800-562-6265
Fax: 617-972-7444
www.spedex.com/napvi

Newsletter offering regional news, sports and activities, conferences, camps, legislative updates, book reviews, audio reviews, professional question and answer column and more for the visually impaired and their families.

Quarterly

1598 DVH Quarterly
University of Arkansas at Little Rock
2801 S University Avenue
Little Rock, AR 72204
Fax: 501-663-3536

Offers information on upcoming events, conferences and workshops on and for visual disabilities. Book reviews, information on the newest resources and technology, educational programs, want ads and more.

Quarterly

Bob Brasher, Editor

1599 Dermatology Focus
Dermatology Foundation
1560 Sherman Avenue, Suite 870
Evanston, IL 60201
847-328-2256
Fax: 847-328-0509
e-mail: dfgen@dermatologyfoundation.org
dermatologyfoundation.org

Includes membership activities, research articles and lists recipients of foundation awards.

Quarterly

Bruce U. Wintroub, Chairman
Michael D. Tharp, President
Stuart R. Lessin, Vice President

1600 Dermatology World
American Academy of Dermatology
P.O. Box 4014
Schaumburg, IL 60168
847-240-1280
866-503-7546
Fax: 847-240-1859
www.aad.org

Offers Academy members information outside the clinical realm. It carries news of government actions, reports of socioeconomic issues, societal trends and other events which impinge on the practice of dermatology.

Monthly

Brett M. Coldiron, MD, President
Elise A. Olsen, MD, Vice President
Mark Lebwohl, MD, President-Elect

1601 Keep In Touch (KIT) Forum
The Myositis Association
1737 King Street, Suite 600
Alexandria, VA 22314
703-299-4850
800-821-7356
Fax: 703-535-6752
e-mail: TMA@myositis.org
www.myositis.org

Allows KIT leaders to share information and raise awareness. Provide a forum for members to exchange information and ideas for day-to-day living.

Augie DeAugustinis, Chair
Patrick Zenner, Vice Chairman
Bob Goldberg, Executive Director

1602 Progress in Dermatology
Dermatology Foundation
1560 Sherman Avenue, Suite 870
Evanston, IL 60201
847-328-2256
Fax: 847-328-0509
e-mail: dfgen@dermatologyfoundation.org
dermatologyfoundation.org

Bulletin offering information on research reports and clinical trials.

Quarterly

Bruce U. Wintroub, Chairman
Michael D. Tharp, President
Stuart R. Lessin, Vice President

1603 The OutLook
The Myositis Association
1737 King Street, Suite 600
Alexandria, VA 22314   703-299-4850
                                              800-821-7356
                                         Fax: 703-535-6752
                                   e-mail: TMA@myositis.org
                                          www.myositis.org

Newsletter featuring articles for patients with polymyositis,
dermatomyositis, inclusion-body myositis, and juvenile forms of
myositis.

Quarterly

Augie DeAugustinis, Chair
Patrick Zenner, Vice Chairman
Bob Goldberg, Executive Director

Pamphlets

1604 Arthritis in Children
Arthritis Foundation
1330 W. Peachtree Street, Suite 100
Atlanta, GA 30309   404-872-7100
                                              800-568-4045
                                           www.arthritis.org

Includes definitions of nine types of juvenile arthritis and related
conditions, diagnosis, treatment options, emotional coping,
school issues, federal laws and financial assistance.

28 pages

Ann M. Palmer, President/ CEO
Meagan Fulmer, Chief Development Officer
Wayne Guthrie, SPHR, SVP, Staff Operations

1605 Juvenile Dermatomyositis
Arthritis Foundation
PO Box 7669
Atlanta, GA 30357   404-872-7100
                                         Fax: 404-872-0457
                                   e-mail: info@jdfcure.com
                                          www.jdfcure.com

Camps

1606 Camp Discovery
American Academy of Dermatology
930 E Woodfield Road
Schaumburg, IL 60173   847-240-1280
                                              866-503-7546
                                         Fax: 847-240-1859
                                 e-mail: jmueller@aad.org
                                       www.campdiscovery.org

For children with chronic skin conditions; no fee and transportation is provided. Call for locations.

David M Pariser, MD, President
Janine Mueller, Program Coordinator

Description

1607 CHILDHOOD SCHIZOPHRENIA

Involves the following Biologic System(s):

Developmental/Behavioral/Psychiatric Disorders

Childhood schizophrenia is characterized by disturbances in behavior, thought, and emotional reactions. These changes initially become apparent between approximately seven years of age and the onset of adolescence. Affected children may become increasingly withdrawn, have flat or blunted emotions that do not appear to change in response to environmental or external stimuli, experience episodes of unexplained silliness (hebephrenic silliness), exhibit aggressive behaviors, and have distortions in thinking. For example, some children may regularly repeat the same responses to different questions; experience sudden blockages in thought; perceive sights, sounds, or other sensations in the absence of external stimuli (hallucinations); and hold false beliefs in spite of evidence to the contrary (psychotic delusions), such as delusions of persecution (paranoid delusions). Affected children often appear to be chaotic in their emotions, thought, and behavioral patterns.

The relationship of childhood schizophrenia and adult schizophrenia remains unclear. Because schizophrenia typically becomes apparent during late adolescence or early adulthood and affects approximately one percent of the general population, only a small percentage of children exhibit symptoms that meet the criteria for a diagnosis of schizophrenia. In addition, many children who are diagnosed with schizophrenia before puberty are later diagnosed with mood disorders, such as bipolar disorder, or other conditions, such as mental retardation or a metabolic disorder. Although there is no clear relationship between childhood and adult schizophrenia, childhood symptoms that most likely predict adult psychotic disorders appear to include social withdrawal, disturbed interpersonal relationships, and blunted emotions. Though the specific underlying abnormalities that may contribute to childhood schizoid behaviors are unknown, genetic factors and certain biochemical abnormalities of the brain play some role in their development.

The treatment of children with schizoid behaviors may include therapy with certain medications known as neuroleptics to manage psychotic delusions, hallucinations, and severe agitation. In addition, an integrated, multidisciplinary approach may include individual therapy or parental training to help modify the child's behavior. In severe cases, hospitalization may be required to ensure appropriate medication adjustments, to prevent children from harming themselves, or to prevent them from hurting others if they exhibit aggressive or violent behavior.

Although certain medications can help treat children with schizoid behaviors, these drugs should be prescribed with great caution due to the potential for side effects. For example, such therapy may result in tardive dyskinesia (TD), a usually nonreversible condition characterized by tics or spasms of facial muscles and involuntary, rapid or writhing movements of the limbs (choreoathetoid movements). In other cases, therapy may cause abnormally slow movement (bradykinesis); involuntary hand movements; abnormal twisting of the neck (torticollis); drooling; and other findings.

If TD develops, treatment with other medications may be indicated and the neuroleptic medication may be decreased or discontinued.

Government Agencies

1608 Center for Mental Health Services Knowledge Exchange Network
US Department of Health and Human Services
PO Box 42557
Washington, DC 20015

800-662-4357
800-789-2647
Fax: 240-747-5470
TTY: 800-487-4889
TDD: 866-889-2647
e-mail: samhsa.media@ees.hhs.gov
www.store.samhsa.gov/home

Develops national mental health policies that promote Federal/State coordination and benefit from input from consumers, family members and providers. Ensures that high quality mental health services programs are implemented to benefit seriously mentally ill populations, disasters or those involved in the criminal justice system.

Mirtha R. Beadle M.P.A., Deputy for Operations
Kana . Enomoto, M.A, Principal Deputy Administrator
Pamela S. Hyde, J.D., Administrator

1609 NIH/National Institute of Mental Health
6001 Executive Boulevard, Room 8184, MSC 9663
Bethesda, MD 20892

301-443-4513
866-615-6464
Fax: 301-443-4279
TTY: 301-443-8431
e-mail: nimhinfo@nih.gov
www.nimh.nih.gov

The mission of NIMH is to transform the understanding and treatment of mental illnesses through basic and clinical research, paving the way for prevention, recovery, and cure.

Dr Thomas R Insel, Director

National Associations & Support Groups

1610 American Academy of Pediatrics
141 Northwest Point Boulevard
Elk Grove Village, IL 60007

847-434-4000
800-433-9016
Fax: 847-434-8000
www.aap.org

The American Academy of Pediatrics and its member pediatricians are committed to the attainment of optimal physical, mental and social health and well-being for all infants, children, adolescents, and young adults.

Sandra Hassink, MD, FAAP, President

1611 American Mental Health Foundation (AMHF)
PO Box 3
Riverdale, NY 10471

212-737-9027
e-mail: elomke@americanmentalhealthfoundation.or
americanmentalhealthfoundation.org

Dedicated to the extensive and intensive research in the theories and techniques of treatment of emotional illness and to the implementation of reforms in the mental health system. Efforts have resulted in development of better and less expensive treatment methods. Findings are disseminated in English and other major languages.

Sister Joan Curtin. CND, Director
Evander Lomke, President & Executive Director
Eugene Gollogly, Vice President

1612 Federation of Families for Children's Mental Health
9605 Medical Center Drive, Suite 280
Rockville, MD 20850

240-403-1901
Fax: 240-403-1909
e-mail: ffcmh@ffcmh.org
www.ffcmh.org

The National family run organization is dedicated exclusively to helping children with mental health needs and their families achieve a better quality of life.

Teka Dempson, President
Sherri Luthe, Vice President
Sheila Pires, Treasurer

1613 NADD: National Association for the Dually Diagnosed
132 Fair Street
Kingston, NY 12401

845-331-4336
800-331-5362
Fax: 845-331-4569
e-mail: info@thenadd.org
www.thenadd.org

Nonprofit organization designed to promote the interests of professional and care providers for individuals who have the coexistence of mental illness and mental retardation. NADD provides conferences, educational services and training materials to professionals, parents, concerned citizens and service organizations.

Dr Robert Fletcher, CEO
Michelle Jordan, Office Manager
Judie Johnston, Administrative Assistant

1614 National Alliance for Research on Schizophrenia and Depression
60 Cutter Mill Road, Suite 404
Great Neck, NY 11021

516-829-0091
800-829-8289
Fax: 516-487-6930
e-mail: info@bbrfoundation.org.
www.bbrfoundation.org

Largest private 501 (c) (3) not for profit corporation and registered public charity. Raises and distributes funds for scientific research into the causes, cures, treatments and prevention of brain disorders.

Steve Lieber, Chairman of the Board
Suzanne Golden, Vice President
Anne Abramson, Director

1615 National Alliance for the Mentally Ill
3803 N. Fairfax Dr., Suite 100
Arlington, VA 22203

703-525-7600
800-950-6264
Fax: 703-524-9094
TDD: 703-516-7227
e-mail: info@nami.org
www.nami.org

NAMI is a nonprofit, grassroots, self-help, support and advocacy organization of consumers, families and friends of people with severe mental illness, such as schizophrenia, bipolar disorder, major despressive disorder, obsessive compulsive disorder, anxiety disorders, autism and other severe and persistent mental illnesses that affect the brain.

Keris J,,n Myrick, President
Kevin B Sullivan, First Vice President
Jim Payne, Second Vice President

1616 National Mental Health Association
2000 N Beauregard Street, 6th Floor
Alexandria, VA 10182

703-684-7722
800-969-6642
Fax: 703-684-5968
TTY: 800-433-5959
e-mail: info@mentalhealthamerica.net
www.mentalhealthamerica.net

MHA, the leading advocacy organization addressing the full spectrum of mental and substance use conditions and their effects nationwide, works to inform, advocate and enable access to quality behavioral health services for all Americans.

Ann Boughtin, Chair of the Board
Eric Ashton, Vice Chair
Elaine Crider, Secretary/Treasurer

1617 National Mental Health Consumers' Self-Help Clearinghouse
1211 Chestnut Street, Suite 1207
Philadelphia, PA 19107

215-751-1810
800-553-4539
Fax: 215-636-6312
e-mail: info@mhselfhelp.org
www.mhselfhelp.org

The Clearinghouse works to foster peer empowerment through our website, up-to-date news and information announcements, a directory of peer-driven services, electronic and printed publications, training packages, and individual and onsite consultation

Joseph Rogers, Executive Director & Founder
Susan Rogers, Director of Special Projects
Britani Nestel, Program Specialist

1618 National Schizophrenia Foundation
403 Seymour Avenue, Suite 202
Lansing, MI 48933

517-485-7168
Fax: 517-485-7180
e-mail: inquiries@nsfoundation.org
www.nsfoundation.org

Mission is to develop and maintain support groups for individuals, and their friends and family members, affected by schizophrenia and related disorders; and to be broad resource for all persons regarding schizophrenia and related disorders through education, information, and public awareness services.

Eric Hufnagel, President
Sharon Pederson, Director of Programs

1619 North American Society for Childhood Onset Schizophrenia - NACOS
88 Briarwood Drive East
Berkeley Heights, NJ 07922

e-mail: info@nascos.org
www.nascos.org

Non-profit, internet based group formed to provide a Web site devoted solely to childhood onset schizophrenia (COS). Families, caregivers and medical professionals will be able to locate and contact each other in order to access and share information related to this rare, devastating disease.

Karen Sniezek, Director
Meredith Morgan, Director
Edward Orton, Director

1620 Schizophrenics Anonymous Forum
Mental Health Association in Michigan
30233 Southfield Road, Suite 220
Southfield, MI 48076

248-647-1711
Fax: 248-647-1732
e-mail: schizanon@aol.com
schizophrenia.org

Self-help organization sponsored by American Schizophrenia Association. Groups are comprised of dignosed schizophrenics who meet to share experiences, strengths and hopes in an effort to help each other cope with common problems and recover from the disease. Rehabilitation program follows the 12 principles of Alcoholics Anonymous. Publications: Newsletter, semi-annual. Monthly support group meeting.

State Agencies & Support Groups

1621 Center for Family Support
333 7th Avenue, 9th Floor
New York, NY 10001

212-629-7939
Fax: 212-239-2211
e-mail: svernikoff@cfsny.org
www.cfsny.org

The Center for Family Support is committed to providing support and assistance to individuals with developmental and related disabilities, and to the family members who care for them.

Steven Vernikoff, Executive Director
Eileen Berg, Director of Quality Assurance
Sharon Lax, Director of Human Resources

Libraries & Resource Centers

1622 National Alliance for Research on Schizophrenia and Depression
50 West Hawthorne Avenue
Valley Stream, NY 11580

516-569-6600
800-829-8289
Fax: 516-374-2261
e-mail: info@narsad.org
www.pccli.org

Largest private 501 (c) (3) not for profit corporation and registered public charity. Raises and distributes funds for scientific research into the causes, cures, treatments and prevention of brain disorders.

David Schimel, President

Research Centers

1623 National Alliance for Research on Schizophrenia and Depression
60 Cutter Mill Road, Suite 404
Great Neck, NY 11021

516-829-0091
800-829-8289
Fax: 516-487-6930
e-mail: info@bbrfoundation.org
www.bbrfoundation.org

Largest private 501 (c) (3) not for profit corporation and registered public charity. Raises and distributes funds for scientific research into the causes, cures, treatments and prevention of brain disorders.

Steve Lieber, Chairman of the Board
Suzanne Golden, Vice President
Anne Abramson, Director

1624 Suncoast Residential Training Center/Developmental Services Program
Goodwill Industries-Suncoast
10596 Gandy Boulevard
Saint Petersburg, FL 33702

727-523-1512
888-279-1988
Fax: 727-563-9300
TTY: 727-579-1068
www.goodwill-suncoast.org

A large group home which serves individuals diagnosed as mentally retarded with a secondary diagnosis of psychiatric difficulties as evidenced by problem behavior. Providing residential, behavioral and instructional support and services that will promote the development of adaptive, socially appropriate behavior. Each individual is assessed to determine, socialization, basic academics and recreation. The primary intervention strategy is applied behavior analysis.

Oscar J. Horton, Chair
Martin W. Gladysz, Sr. Vice Chair
Steven M Erickson, Vice Chair

Conferences

1625 FFCMH Annual Conference
Federation of Families for Childrens Mental Health
9605 Medical Center Drive, Suite 280
Rockville, MD 20850

240-403-1901
Fax: 240-403-1909
e-mail: ffcmh@ffcmh.org
www.ffcmh.org

Address the complex issue of trauma; the impact it has on children and families; the promotion of healing and prevention strategies; knowledge about how to address trauma through resiliency-based interventions, utilizing a familydriven, youth guided approach; and examples of how family organizations and the partners they work with are raising awareness and improving trauma-focused services and supports.

November

Teka Dempson, President
Sherri Luthe, Vice President
Sheila Pires, Treasurer

1626 NAMI Convention
National Alliance on Mental Illness
3803 N Fairfax Drive, Suite 100
Arlington, VA 22203

703-524-7600
888-999-6264
Fax: 703-524-9094
TDD: 703-516-7227
e-mail: info@nami.org
www.nami.org

The NAMI Convention is packed with information, chances to network, leadership development opportunities, and lots more

July

Keris Jan Myrick, President
Kevin B Sullivan, Vice President
Clarence Jordan, Secretary

Audio Video

1627 Bonnie Tapes
Mental Illness Education Project
25 West Street
Westborough, MA 1581

617-562-1111
800-343-5540
Fax: 617-779-0061
e-mail: info@miepvideos.org
www.miepvideos.org

Bonnie's account of coping with schizophrenia will be a relevation to people whose view of mental illness has been shaped by the popular media. She and her family provide an intimate view of the frequently feared, often misrepresented and much stigmatized illness and the human side of learning to live with a psychiatric disability. Tape 1: Mental Illness in the Family (26 minutes); Tape 2: Recovering from Mental Illness (27 minutes); Tape 3: My Sister Is Mentally Ill (22 minutes) $99.95 each

1997 $143.88 for 3

1628 Families Coping with Mental Illness
Mental Illness Education Project
25 West Street
Westborough, MA 1581

617-562-1111
800-343-5540
Fax: 617-779-0061
e-mail: info@miepvideos.org
miepvideos.org

10 family members share their experiences of having a family member with schizophrenia or bipolar disorder. Designed to provide insights and support to other families, the tape also profoundly conveys to professionals the needs of families when mental illness strikes. In two versions: a twenty two minute version ideal for short classes and workshops, and a richer forty three minute version with more examples and details. Discounted price for families/consumers.

Michael M Faenza, Executive Director

1629 Living with Schizophrenia
Guilford Press
370 Seventh Avenue, Suite 1200
New York, NY 10001

800-365-7006
Fax: 212-966-6708
e-mail: info@guilford.com
www.guilford.com

Offers essential information and huidance for individuals and families coping with schizophrenia diagnosis. Features illuminating first-hand accounts from three people with schizophrenia and one person with schizoaffective disorder, along with commentary from treatment expert Dr Andy Campbell. Learn clear steps to take to lead fuller, more successful lives.

2006 DVD, 39 minutes
ISBN: 1-593853-86-6

1630 Pharmacotherapy of Schizophrenia
American Psychiatric Publishing
1000 Wilson Boulevard, Suite 1825
Arlington, VA 22209

703-907-7322
800-368-5777
Fax: 703-907-1091
e-mail: appi@psych.org
www.appi.org

Presented by John M Kane MD, Chairman of Psychiatry at LI Jewish Medical Center, and Professor of Psychiatry at Albert Einstein College of Medicine. Illustrates the major issues and treatment considerations, and the latest findings on the effectiveness as well as on the side effects of the many and varied psychopharmacological agents are carefully illustrated and discussed. 75 minutes. ISBN # 9780880483803

1995

Robert E. Hales, Editor-in-Chief
Rebecca D. Rinehart, Publisher
John McDuffie, Associate Publisher

Web Sites

1631 CyberPsych
www.cyberpsych.org

CyberPsych presents information about psychoanalysis, psychotherapy, and special topics such as anxiety disorder, the problematic use of alcohol, homophobia, and the traumatic effects of racism. CyberPsych is a nonprofit network which offers free web hosting and technical support for internet communication to nonprofit groups and individuals.

Carol Lindemann, Ph.D., Contact

1632 Internet Mental Health
www.mentalhealth.com

Our goal is to improve understanding, diagnosis, and treatment of mental illness throughout the world.

Phillip W. Long, M.D., Psychiatrist

1633 Mental Health Net
P.O. Box 20709
Columbus, OH 43220

614-448-4055
e-mail: info@centersite.net
www.mentalhelp.net

We wish to provide the following: to discuss, develope and debate in an open forum the future of the mental health field in America and throughout the world. To help coordinate various components of the mental health field so as to bring about greater communication between them. To educate the public about mental health issues, to promote active collaboration between professionals in all segments of mental health development, implementation and policy.

1634 Mental Wellness
www.choicesinrecovery.com

800-526-7736
www.choicesinrecovery.com

Mental Wellness is an online resource for bipolar disorder, schizophrenia and general mental health information.

1635 NADD: National Association for the Dually Diagnosed
www.thenadd.org

Nonprofit organization designed to promote the interests of professional and care providers for individuals who have the coexistence of mental illness and mental retardation. NADD provides conferences, educational services and training materials to professionals, parents, concerned citizens and service organizations.

Donna McNelis, President
Dan Baker, Vice President
Robert J. Fletcher, Chief Executive Officer

1636 Online Mendelian Inheritance in Man
National Library of Medicine, Building 38A
Bethesda, MD 20894

888-346-3656
e-mail: info@ncbi.nlm.nih.gov
www.ncbi.nlm.nih.gov

This database is a catalog of human genes and genetic disorders.

Christine E. Seidman, M.D., Chair
David J. Lipman, M.D., Executive Secretary

1637 Planetpsych
www.planetpsych.com

e-mail: webmaster@planetpsych.com
www.planetpsych.com

Planetpsych is an online resource for mental health information.

1638 Psych Central
55 Pleasant St., Suite 207
Newburyport, MA 1950

e-mail: talkback@psychcentral.com
www.psychcentral.com

Offers free informational and educational articles and resources on psychology, support and mental health online.

John M. Grohol, CEO & Founder

1639 Schizophrenia Support Organizations
www.members.aol.com/leonardjk/USA.htm

Contains a listing of support organizations for people with schizophrenia and their families.

1640 Schizophrenia.com
www.schizophrenia.com

Is a leading web commuity dedicated to providing high quality information, support and education to the family members, caregivers and individuals who's lives have been impacted by schizophrenia.

Brain Chiko, Executive Director
J. Megginson Hollister, Editor

1641 Schizophrenia.com Home Page
www.schizophrenia.com/discuss/Disc3.html

On-line support for patients and families.

Brain Chiko, Executive Director
J. Megginson Hollister, Editor

1642 Schizophrenia: Handbook for Families
www.mentalhealth.com/book/p40-sc01.html

This handbook is dedicated to the families and to their loved ones who carry the burden of schizophrenia, a major psychiatric disorder.

Phillip W. Long, M.D., Psychiatrist

Book Publishers

1643 Biology of Schizophrenia and Affective Disease
American Psychiatric Publishing
1000 Wilson Boulevard, Suite 1825
Arlington, VA 22209

703-907-7322
800-368-5777
Fax: 703-907-1091
e-mail: appi@psych.org
www.appi.org

Provides a state-of-the-art look at the biological bases of severe mental illness from the perspective of the researchers making these exceptional discoveries. ISBN # 9780880487467

1995 560 pages

Stanley J Watson PhD MD, Author

1644 Contemporary Issues in the Treatment of Schizophrenia
American Psychiatric Press
1000 Wilson Boulevard, Suite 1825
Arlington, VA 22209

703-907-7322
800-368-5777
Fax: 703-907-1091
e-mail: appi@psych.org
www.appi.org

Covers approaches to the patient by investigating biological, pharmacological, and psychological treatments. ISBN #: 9780880486811

1995 889 pages

Christian L Shriqui, MD, Editor
Henry A Nasrallah, MD, Editor

1645 Diagnosis Schizophrenia: A Comprehensive Resource
Columbia University Press
116th and Broadway
New York, NY 10027

212-854-1754
Fax: 212-459-3678
www.columbia.edu/cu/cup

Has alot of consumers' stories in the first person and sketches of their faces sprinkled throughout.

2002

Rachel Miller, Author
Susan E Mason, Author

1646 Encyclopedia of Schizophrenia and the Psychotic Disorders
Facts on File
11 Penn Plaza
New York, NY 10001

212-290-8090
800-322-8755
Fax: 212-678-3633

This volume details recent theories and research findings on schizophrenia and psychotic disorders, together with a complete overview of the field's history.

368 pages

1647 Getting Your Life Back Together When You Have Schizophrenia
New Harbinger Publications
5674 Shattuck Ave
Oakland, CA 94609

800-748-6273
Fax: 800-652-1613
e-mail: customerservice@newharbinger.com
www.newharbinger.com

Provides good information for someone who has just been diagnosed with schiophrenia.

2002

Roberta Temes PhD, Author

1648 Medical Illness and Schizophrenia
American Psychiatric Publishing
1000 Wilson Boulevard, Suite 1825
Arlington, VA 22209

703-907-7322
800-368-5777
Fax: 703-907-1091
e-mail: appi@psych.org
www.appi.org

Examines the links between medical conditions and severe chronic mental illness, with a focus on the need for better medical assessment and treatment to improve outcomes in patients; links between schizophrenia and conditions such as obesity, cardiovascular disease, diabetes, HIV and hepatitis C, endocrine-related diorders, and others; the association between therapy with certain antipsychotics and adverse health outcomes; the importance of improving community health. ISBN # 9781585621064

2003 256 pages

Jonathan M Meyer MD, Author
Henry A Nasrallah MD, Author

1649 Negative Symptom and Cognitive Deficit Tre atment Response in Schizophrenia
American Psychiatric Publishing
1000 Wilson Boulevard, Suite 1825
Arlington, VA 22209

703-907-7322
800-368-5777
Fax: 703-907-1091
e-mail: appi@psych.org
www.appi.org

Addresses the complex issues-issues rarely confronted in empirical studies of patients with schizophrenia-and controversial research surrounding the assessment of negative symptoms and cognitive deficits in patients with schizophrenia. ISBN # 9780880487856

2001 216 pages

Richard S E Keefe PhD, Author
Joseph P McEvoy MD, Author

1650 New Pharmacotherapy of Schizophrenia
American Psychiatric Press
1000 Wilson Boulevard, Suite 1825
Arlington, VA 22209

703-907-7322
800-368-5777
Fax: 703-907-1091
e-mail: appi@psych.org
www.appi.org

Discusses the new class of antipsychotic agents that promises superior efficiency and more favorable side-effects; offers an improved understanding of how to employ exsisting pharmachotherapeutic agents. ISBN # 9780880484916

1996 264 pages

1651 Plasma Homovanillic Asid in Schhizophrenia
American Psychiatric Publishing
1000 Wilson Boulevard, Suite 1825
Arlington, VA 22209

703-907-7322
800-368-5777
Fax: 703-907-1091
e-mail: appi@psych.org
www.appi.org

Provides the most comprehensive and current collection of information on plasma HVA levels to be found anywhere. Provides a consice synthesis and critique of current data as well as interesting proposals for future research. ISBN # 9780880484893

1997 216 pages

Arnold J Friedhoff MD, Author
Farooq Amin MD, Author

1652 Prenatal Exposures in Schizophrenia
American Psychiatric Press
1000 Wilson Boulevard, Suite 1825
Arlington, VA 22209

703-907-7322
800-368-5777
Fax: 703-907-1091
e-mail: appi@psych.org
www.appi.org

Considers a range of epigenetic elements thought to interact with abnormal genes to produce the onset of illness. Attention to the evidence implicating obstetric complications, prenatal infection, autoimmunity and prenatal malnutrition in brain disorders. ISBN # 9780880484992

1999 296 pages Hardcover

Ezra S Susser MD, Author
Alan S Brown MD, Author
Jack M Gorman MD, Author

1653 Schizophrenia
American Psychiatric Publishing
1000 Wilson Boulevard, Suite 1825
Arlington, VA 22209

703-907-7322
800-368-5777
Fax: 703-907-1091
e-mail: appi@psych.org
www.appi.org

Ideas in treating the disease, and how many patients can lead productive lives without relapse. ISBN # 9780880489508

1994 294 pages

Nancy C Andleasen MD, Author

1654 Schizophrenia Into Later Life: Treatment, Research, and Policy

American Psychiatric Publishing
1000 Wilson Boulevard, Suite 1825
Arlington, VA 22209

703-907-7322
800-368-5777
Fax: 703-907-1091
e-mail: appi@psych.org
www.appi.org

Multidisciplinary reference on this important topic-a landmark work for researchers, service providers, and policy makers. ISBN # 9781585620371

2003 344 pages

Carl I Cohen MD, Author

1655 Schizophrenia Revealed: From Neurons to Social Interactions

W.W. Norton
500 Fifth Avenue
New York, NY 10110

212-354-5500
800-233-4830
Fax: 212-869-0856
www.wwnorton.com

Educational, informational, scientific and yet readable.

2003

1656 Schizophrenia and Comorbid Conditions Diagnosis and Treatment

American Psychiatric Publishing
1000 Wilson Boulevard, Suite 1825
Arlington, VA 22209

703-907-7322
800-368-5777
Fax: 703-907-1091
e-mail: appi@psych.org
www.appi.org

Lays diagnostic oversimplification of schizophrenia to rest once and for all. Editors are criticizing the reductionist view of schizophrenia as a single unitary disorder- a view that has led many psychiatrists and mental health care professionals to overlook potentially important syndromes. ISBN # 9780880487719

2001 256 pages

1657 Scizophrenia in a Molecular Age

American Psychiatric Publishing
1000 Wilson Boulevard, Suite 1825
Arlington, VA 22209

703-907-7322
800-368-5777
Fax: 703-907-1091
e-mail: appi@psych.org
www.appi.org

Reviews neuroscience mechanisms and analyzes genetic determinants. ISBN # 9780880489614

1999 204 pages

Carol A Tamminga MD, Author

1658 Surviving Schizophrenia: A Manual for Families, Consumers and Providers

Harper Collins
10 E 53rd Street
New York, NY 10022

212-207-7528
800-242-7737
Fax: 212-207-2586
e-mail: orders@harpercollins.com
harpercollins.com

The third edition of this indispensable manual throughly details everything patients, families and mental health professionals need to know about one of the most widespread and misunderstood illnesses. Paperback.

464 pages
ISBN: 0-060950-76-5

1659 The American Psychiatric Publishing Text book of Schizophrenia

American Psychiatric Publishing
1000 Wilson Boulevard, Suite 1825
Arlington, VA 22209

703-907-7322
800-368-5777
Fax: 703-907-1091
e-mail: appi@psych.org
www.appi.org

Offers broad coverage that encompasses the current state of knowledge the cause, nature, and treatment of schizophrenia. ISBN # 9781585621910

2006 453 pages

Jeffrey A Lieberman MD, Author
T Scott Stroup MD MPH, Author
Diana O Perkins MD MPH, Author

1660 The Complete Family Guide to Schizophrenia

Kim Mueser, Susan Gingerich, author

Guilford Press
72 Spring Street
New York, NY 10012

800-365-7006
Fax: 212-966-6708
e-mail: info@guilford.com
www.guilford.com

The authors, noted therapists, deepen the reader's understanding of the illness and discuss a wide range of effective treatments. This volume walks the reader through a range of treatment and support options that can lead to a better life for the entire family.Topics include prioritizing needs, solving everyday problems, life-goals, symptoms, and the life-long journey of recovery. Hardcover, paperback, e-book.

2006 480 pages Paperback
ISBN: 1-593851-80-4

Kim T Mueser, Author
Susan Gingerich, Author

1661 The Early Stages of Schizophrenia

American Psychiatric Publishing
1000 Wilson Boulevard, Suite 1825
Arlington, VA 22209

703-907-7322
800-368-5777
Fax: 703-907-1091
e-mail: appi@psych.org
www.appi.org

Divided into three major parts: Early Intervention, Epidemiology, and Natural History of Schizophrenia; Management of the Early Stages of Schizophrenia; and Neurobiological Investigations of the Early Stages of Schizophrenia. ISBN # 9780880488402

2002 280 pages

Robert B Zipursky MD, Author
S Charles Schulz MD, Author

1662 The Natural History of Mania, Depression, and Schizophrenia

American Psychiatric Publishing
1000 Wilson Boulevard, Suite 1825
Arlington, VA 22209

703-907-7322
800-368-5777
Fax: 703-907-1091
e-mail: appi@psych.org
www.appi.org

Takes an unusual look at the course of mental illness, based on data from the Iowa 500 Research Project. This project involved the long-term (30-40 yrs) follow-up of patients diagnosed with schizophrenia, depression, and bipolar illness. ISBN # 9780880487269

1996 384 pages

George Winokur MD, Author
Ming T Tsuang MD PhD, Author

1663 Water Balance in Schizophrenia
American Psychiatric Publishing
1000 Wilson Boulevard, Suite 1825
Arlington, VA 22209

703-907-7322
800-368-5777
Fax: 703-907-1091
e-mail: appi@psych.org
www.appi.org

Represents the first attempt to provide clinicians with a consolidated guide to polydipsia-hyponatremia, associated with schizophrenia. ISBN # 9780880484855

1996 360 pages

David B Schnur MD, Author
Darrell G Kirch MD, Author

Newsletters

1664 NADD Bulletin
NADD Press
132 Fair Street
Kingston, NY 12401

845-331-4336
800-331-5362
Fax: 845-331-4569
e-mail: info@thenadd.org
www.thenadd.org

Official publication of the National Association for the Dually Diagnosed. It features articles that address clinical, programmatic, research or family oriented issues concerning mental health aspects in persons with disabilities.

20 pages Bimonthly

Donna McNelis, President
Dan Baker, Vice President
Robert J. Fletcher, Chief Executive Officer

Pamphlets

1665 Schizophrenia
National Institute of Mental Health
PO Box 5801
Bethesda, MD 20824

301-496-5751
800-352-9424
Fax: 301-443-4279
TTY: 866-415-8051
e-mail: nimhinfo@nih.gov
www.nimh.nih.gov

This booklet answers many common questions about schizophrenia, one of the most chronic, severe and disabling mental disorders. Current research-based information is provided for people with schizophrenia, their family members, friends and the general public about the symptoms and diagnosis of schizophrenia, possible causes, treatments and treatment resources.

2006 28 pages

Walter J. Koroshetz, M.D., Acting Director
Alan L. Willard, Ph.D., Acting Deputy Director
Caroline Lewis, Executive Officer

1666 Schizophrenia Fact Sheet
Center for Mental Health Services
PO Box 42557
Washington, DC 20015

800-789-2647
Fax: 240-747-5470
TDD: 866-889-2647
mentalhealth.samhsa.gov

This fact sheet provides information on the symptoms, diagnosis, and treatment for schizophrenia.

2 pages

Phillip W. Long, M.D., Psychiatrist

1667 Understanding Schizophrenia
National Alliance on Mental Illness
3803 N. Fairfax Drive, Suite 100
Arlington, VA 22203

703-524-7600
800-950-6264
Fax: 703-524-9094
TDD: 703-516-7227
www.nami.org

An excellent introduction to schizophrenia. Appropriate for supprt groups, physicians offices, coventions, health fairs, and the workplace.

Jim Payne, President
Ralph E. Nelson, 1st Vice President
Marilyn Ricci, 2nd Vice President

Description

1668 CHOREA

Covers these related disorders: Benign familial chorea, Drug-induced chorea, Sydenham's chorea

Involves the following Biologic System(s):

Neurologic Disorders

Chorea is a neuromuscular condition characterized by irregular, rapid, jerky movements that may appear to be well coordinated but actually occur involuntarily. These movements may be simple or highly complex. In addition, the arms and legs may have abnormally diminished muscle tone (hypotonia) and therefore may be abnormally loose or slack. Choreic movements are often subtle. However, if several of these movements are present, they may essentially flow into one another, causing them to appear relatively slow, sinuous, and writhing in nature (athetosis).

The specific underlying cause of chorea is unknown. However, some researchers suspect that it may result due to overactivity of certain neurotransmitters (dopamine) in the brain. Neurotransmitters are naturally produced chemicals that regulate the transmission of messages between certain nerve cells (neurons). In some children, chorea may result from the use of particular drugs, such as certain antiseizure medications, particularly phenytoin, or antipsychotic (neuroleptic) drugs, such as haloperidol or phenothiazines. Chorea may also occur in association with certain underlying disorders, such as systemic lupus erythematosus (lupus) or Wilson's disease, a disorder of copper metabolism. In addition, chorea is a primary feature of a rare genetic disorder known as benign familial chorea in which nonprogressive chorea begins in infancy or early childhood in the absence of other neurologic abnormalities. Associated symptoms and findings include delays in attaining certain motor milestones during childhood and poorly coordinated movements of the arms and legs. Benign familial chorea is likely inherited as an autosomal dominant trait.

In addition, chorea is the dominant feature of a disorder known as Sydenham's chorea. This disorder is the most common cause of acquired chorea during childhood. Sydenham's chorea occurs in association with rheumatic fever, which is an inflammatory disease following throat infection with certain strains of streptococcal bacteria. Patients with rheumatic fever may experience fever, inflammation and swelling of one or more large joints, or inflammation of the heart (carditis), potentially causing thickening, scarring, and associated disease of heart valves. If rheumatic fever affects the nervous system, Sydenham's chorea may result. Although Sydenham's chorea previously occurred in as many as half of those with rheumatic fever, recent studies suggest that it more likely affects approximately 10 percent of rheumatic patients in the United States.

Sydenham's chorea most commonly occurs in children between ages five and 15. The condition may begin subtly and gradually, sometimes as long as several months after other symptoms associated with rheumatic fever have resolved. Patients may initially experience increasing clumsiness. As symptoms progress, involuntary movements may become prominent in the face, trunk, and arms and legs; move from one muscle group to another; and eventually affect all motor movements, including walking and speech. In some patients, chorea may be restricted to one side of the body (hemichorea). If children have severe chorea and abnormally diminished muscle tone (hypotonia), they may become unable to dress, feed themselves, or walk. Many children with the condition also experience rapid mood swings and episodes of uncontrollable crying (emotional lability).

Sydenham's chorea is usually a self-limited disorder that subsides in weeks or months. However, in some patients, the condition may persist for up to one to two years. In approximately 20 percent of children, the condition may recur within two years of the initial episode. If patients experience mild symptoms, treatment may include symptomatic and supportive measures, including minimizing stress as much as possible. In children with more severe symptoms, treatment may be attempted with the drug diazepam.

Government Agencies

1669 NIH/National Institute of Neurological Dis orders and Stroke (NINDS)
PO Box 5801
Bethesda, MD 20824

301-496-5751
800-352-9424
Fax: 301-496-0296
TTY: 301-468-5981
www.ninds.nih.gov

The mission of NINDS is to reduce the burden of neurological disease - a burden borne by every age group, by every segment of society, by people all over the world.

Story C Landis Ph.D., Director
Walter J Koroshetz, Deputy Director
Caroline Lewis, Executive Officer

National Associations & Support Groups

1670 American Academy of Child and Adolescent Psychiatry
3615 Wisconsin Avenue NW
Washington, DC 20016

202-966-7300
Fax: 202-966-2891
e-mail: communications@aacap.org
www.aacap.org

The AACAP (American Academy of Child and Adolescent Psychiatry) is the leading national professional medical association dedicated to treating and improving the quality of life for children, adolescents, and families affected by these disorders.

Martin J. Drell M.D, President
Paramjit T Joshi, M.D, President-Elect
Steven P Cuffe, M.D., Treasurer

1671 American Academy of Pediatrics
141 Northwest Point Boulevard
Elk Grove Village, IL 60007

847-434-4000
800-433-9016
Fax: 847-434-8000
www.aap.org

The American Academy of Pediatrics and its member pediatricians are committed to the attainment of optimal physical, mental and social health and well-being for all infants, children, adolescents, and young adults.

Sandra Hassink, MD, FAAP, President

1672 Genetic Alliance
4301 Connecticut Avenue NW Suite 404
Washington, DC 20008

202-966-7955
800-336-4363
Fax: 202-966-8553
e-mail: info@geneticalliance.org
www.geneticalliance.org

World's leading nonprofit health advocacy organization committed to transforming health through genetics and promoting an environment of openness centered on the health of individuals, families, and communities.

Sharon Terry, President
Lisa Wise, Chief Operating Officer
Tetyana Murza MES, Programs and Policy Coordinator

1673 March of Dimes Birth Defects Foundation
1275 Mamaroneck Avenue
White Plains, NY 10605

914-997-4488
888-663-4637
Fax: 914-997-4763
e-mail: answers@marchofdimes.com
www.marchofdimes.com

March of Dimes help moms have full-term pregnancies and research the problems that threaten the health of babies.The March of Dimes also acts globally: sharing best practices in perinatal health and helping improve birth outcomes where the needs are the most urgent.

Kenneth A. May, Chair
Jennifer Howse, President/CEO
Alan Fleischman, Medical Director

1674 Muscular Dystrophy Association
3300 E Sunrise Drive
Tucson, AZ 85718

520-529-2000
800-572-1717
Fax: 520-529-5300
e-mail: mda@mdausa.org
www.mda.org

Voluntary health agency aimed at conquering nueromuscular diseases that affect more than 1,000,000 Americans. The diseases in MDA's program include nine forms of muscular dystrophy, amyotrophic lateral sclerosis (Lou Gehrig's disease), spinal muscular atrophy, Charcot-Marie-Tooth disease, and other neuromuscular conditions. With over 200 offices across the country, MDA conducts research, medical and community services, clinics, support groups, summer camps for youngsters and much more.

Jennifer Lopez, Associate Director-Health Care Svcs

1675 WE MOVE (Worldwide Education and Advocacy for Movement Disorders)
5731 Mosholu Avenue
Bronx, NY 10471

212-875-8312
800-437-6682
Fax: 212-875-8389
e-mail: wemove@wemove.org
www.wemove.org

Gives the general public the knowledge that they desire regarding any disorder involving movement difficulties.

Susan Bressman MD, President
Mo Moadeli, Vice President
Arlene Ploshnick, Treasurer

Conferences

1676 AACAP & CACAP Joint Annual Meeting
American Academy of Child & Adolescent Psychiatry
3615 Wisconsin Avenue NW
Washington, DC 20016

202-966-7300
Fax: 202-966-2891
e-mail: meetings@aacap.org
www.aacap.org

The world's largest gathering place for leaders in the field of child and adolescent psychiatry, children's mental health, and other allied disciplines.

Laurence Lee Greenhill MD, President

Web Sites

1677 Online Mendelian Inheritance in Man
National Library of Medicine, Building 38A
Bethesda, MD 20894

888-346-3656
e-mail: info@ncbi.nlm.nih.gov
www.ncbi.nlm.nih.gov

This database is a catalog of human genes and genetic disorders.

Christine E. Seidman, M.D., Chair
David J. Lipman, M.D., Executive Secretary

Book Publishers

1678 Diagnostic and Statistical Manual of Mental Disorders
American Psychiatric Association
1000 Wilson Boulevard, Suite 1825
Arlington, VA 22209

703-907-7300
888-357-7924
e-mail: apa@psych.org
www.psych.org

Includes updated information on diagnoses, etiology, and research on mental illness.

1679 Merck Manual of Diagnosis and Therapy 18th Edition
Wiley Publishers
10475 Crosspoint Boulevard
Indianapolis, IN 46256

317-572-3000
877-762-2974
Fax: 800-597-3299
e-mail: consumer@wiley.com
www.wiley.com

Packed with essential information on diagnosing and treating medical disorders to help health care professionals and medical students deliver the best care.

2006
ISBN: 0-911910-18-2

1680 Neuroanatomy: Text and Atlas 3rd Edition
McGraw-Hill Medical
860 Taylor Station Road
Blacklick, OH 43004

877-833-5524
Fax: 614-759-3823
e-mail: pbg.ecommerce_custserv@mcgraw-hill.com
http://books.mcgraw-hill.com

Comprehensive appraoch to neuroanatomy from both functional and regional perspective! Examines how parts of the nervous system work together to regulate body systems and produce behavior.

2003 532 pages
ISBN: 0-071381-83-X

Pamphlets

1681 Sydenham Chorea Information Page
National Inst. of Neurological Disorders/Stroke
PO Box 5801
Bethesda, MD 20824

301-496-5751
800-352-9424
TTY: 301-468-5981
www.ninds.nih.gov/disorders/sydenham/sydenham.htm

Provides information on the disease, treatment options, and the prognosis, as well as provides some research centers regarding the disease.

Walter J. Koroshetz, M.D., Acting Director
Alan L. Willard, Ph.D., Acting Deputy Director
Caroline Lewis, Executive Officer

Description

1682 CLEFT LIP AND CLEFT PALATE
Involves the following Biologic System(s):
Dermatologic Disorders, Orthopedic and Muscle Disorders

Cleft lip and cleft palate are birth defects that may occur together or as isolated conditions. Newborns with cleft lip have a groove in the upper lip that may be a small notch or, in more severe cases, may be deep and extend up to the nose. Cleft palate is characterized by incomplete closure of the roof of the mouth (palate). In affected newborns, an abnormal gap runs along the midline of the soft, fleshy area of the palate (soft palate) and, in some patients, extends into one or both sides of the bony, front region of the palate (hard palate). As a result, the nasal cavity may open into the palate. Cleft lip with or without cleft palate affects approximately one in 600 newborns, whereas cleft palate alone occurs in about one in 1,000 births.

In newborns with cleft lip, the defect may occur on one or both sides of the upper lip and typically affects the bony ridge of the upper jaw (upper alveolar ridge). This ridge contains the sockets in which the roots of the teeth are held (dental alveoli). As a result, affected children often experience improper development of certain teeth, potentially resulting in absent, malformed, improperly positioned, or extra teeth and increased risk of dental decay (dental caries). In addition, infants with cleft lip and cleft palate typically have feeding difficulties associated with poor suckling capability and excessive swallowing of air. Affected children with cleft palate are also prone to repeated infections of the middle ear (otitis media) that, in some cases, may contribute to associated hearing loss. Many children also experience speech defects that may be due to inadequate functioning of certain muscles of the throat and palate (pharyngeal and palatal muscles).

In affected newborns, treatment initially consists of measures to ensure improved feeding and proper intake of nutrients. In many patients, a plastic device (a prosthetic known as an obturator) may be fitted that covers the gap in the palate, thereby improving suction and intake of fluids, milk, and or formula. The obturator is typically replaced every few weeks due to rapid growth during infancy. In addition, in those with cleft palate, modified artificial nipples may help to improve feeding. In many cases, cleft lip may be surgically closed by approximately two months of age and additional corrective surgery may be performed later during childhood. If affected children do not have associated physical abnormalities, surgical correction of cleft palate may be performed before the age of one year to help improve normal speech development. However, if surgery is delayed until the age of three years or later, a device (such as a contoured speech bulb) may be used to help close off the uppermost portion of the throat (nasopharynx) during the production of certain sounds. This helps children to develop understandable speech. Treatment may also include dental procedures to correct improperly positioned teeth or to replace absent teeth (e.g., with prosthetic devices). Speech therapy may be beneficial for some affected children. Additional treatment for infants and children with cleft lip and cleft palate is symptomatic and supportive.

Cleft lip and cleft palate may occur as isolated conditions or in association with several underlying chromosomal disorders or malformation syndromes. Isolated cleft lip and/or cleft palate may potentially result due to certain environmental factors, occur randomly for unknown reasons (sporadically), or be familial. Many cases have been reported in which several individuals in multigenerational families (kindreds) have been affected by isolated cleft lip and cleft palate. In such cases, the specific modes of inheritance are not understood. The frequent association of cleft lip and cleft palate is thought to result from certain developmental abnormalities during embryonic growth.

National Associations & Support Groups

1683 AmeriFace
PO Box 751112
Las Vegas, NV 89136
702-769-9264
888-486-1209
Fax: 702-341-5351
e-mail: info@ameriface.org
www.ameriface.org

Provides information, services, emotional support and educational programs for and on behalf of individuals with facial differences and their families. Working to increase understanding through public awareness and education.

3M members

Debbie Oliver, Executive Director
Robin Remele, Program Driector
Joyce Bentz, National Action Team Coordinator

1684 American Academy of Pediatrics
141 Northwest Point Boulevard
Elk Grove Village, IL 60007
847-434-4000
800-433-9016
Fax: 847-434-8000
www.aap.org

The American Academy of Pediatrics and its member pediatricians are committed to the attainment of optimal physical, mental and social health and well-being for all infants, children, adolescents, and young adults.

Sandra Hassink, MD, FAAP, President

1685 Cleft Palate Foundation
1504 East Franklin Street, Suite 102
Chapel Hill, NC 27514
919-933-9044
800-242-5338
Fax: 919-933-9604
e-mail: info@cleftline.org
www.cleftline.org

Provides comprehensive information to educate patients, families, and professionals; Makes referrals to cleft/craniofacial treatment teams; Funds research to learn all we can about prevention and care; Offers telephone and online counseling and support service through the Cleftline, 1-800-24-CLEFT

Nancy Smythe, Executive Director
Samantha Jennings, MSW, Director of Family Services
Emily Kiser, Foundation Administrator

1686 Craniofacial Foundation of America
975 E 3rd Street
Chattanooga, TN 37403
423-778-7000
800-418-3223
Fax: 423-778-8172
e-mail: Mickey.Milita@erlanger.org
www.erlanger.org

Organization assists families with both the physical and emotional aspects, trying to make the everyday events a little easier.

Kevin Spiegel,, President/CEO
J. Britton Tabor, Senior Vice President and Chief Fin
Alana B Sullivan, Senior Vice President and Chief Com

1687 FACES: National Association for the Craniofacially Handicapped
PO Box 11082
Chattanooga, TN 37401

423-266-1632
800-332-2373
Fax: 423-267-3124
e-mail: faces@faces-cranio.org
www.faces-cranio.org

Assists individuals with facial disfigurations and their families They maintain a registry of centers offering corrective surgery for craniofacial deformities and financial assistance to qualified applicants.

Lynne Mayfield, President

1688 Genetic Alliance
4301 Connecticut Avenue NW Suite 404
Washington, DC 20008

202-966-7955
800-336-4363
Fax: 202-966-8553
e-mail: info@geneticalliance.org
www.geneticalliance.org

World's leading nonprofit health advocacy organization committed to transforming health through genetics and promoting an environment of openness centered on the health of individuals, families, and communities.

Sharon Terry, President
Lisa Wise, Chief Operating Officer
Tetyana Murza MES, Programs and Policy Coordinator

1689 March of Dimes Birth Defects Foundation
1275 Mamaroneck Avenue
White Plains, NY 10605

914-997-4488
888-663-4637
Fax: 914-997-4763
e-mail: answers@marchofdimes.com
www.marchofdimes.com

March of Dimes help moms have full-term pregnancies and research the problems that threaten the health of babies.The March of Dimes also acts globally: sharing best practices in perinatal health and helping improve birth outcomes where the needs are the most urgent.

Kenneth A. May, Chair
Jennifer Howse, President/CEO
Alan Fleischman, Medical Director

1690 Prescription Parents
45 Brentwood Circle
Needham, MA 02492

617-499-1936
www.samizdat.com/pp1.html

Organization that gives information and support to children with cleft lip and cleft palate through its educational and support materials, including its directory, newsletter and brochures.

1691 Wide Smiles
PO Box 5153
Stockton, CA 95205

209-942-2812
Fax: 209-464-1497
e-mail: josmiles@yahoo.com
www.widesmiles2.org/index.html

Wide Smiles was formed to ensure that parents of cleft-affected children do not have to feel alone. We offer support, inspiration, information and networking for families everywhere who may be dealing with the challenges associated with clefting.

Joanne Green, Founding Director

Conferences

1692 Connections Conference
Cleft Palate Foundation
1504 East Franklin Street, Suite 102
Chapel Hill, NC 27514

919-933-9044
800-242-5338
Fax: 919-933-9604
e-mail: info@cleftline.org
www.cleftline.org

Nancy Smythe, Executive Director
Samantha Jennings, MSW, Director of Family Services
Emily Kiser, Foundation Administrator

1693 Genetic Alliance Annual Conference
Genetic Alliance
4301 Connecticut Avenue NW, Suite 404
Washington, DC 20008

202-966-5557
800-336-4363
Fax: 202-966-8553
e-mail: info@geneticalliance.org
www.geneticalliance.org

Consistently inspirational and enables partnership among all stakeholders: advocates and community leaders, health and industry professionals, policymakers, and academicians.

July

Sharon Terry, President/CEO
Tetyana Murza, Programs/Events Manager

Web Sites

1694 AboutFace USA
1057 Steeles Ave. West
North York, ON M2R 3

416-597-2229
800-597-3223
Fax: 416-597-8494
e-mail: info@aboutface.ca
www.aboutface.ca

Provides information, services, emotional support and educational programs for and on behalf of individuals with facial differences and their families. Working to increase understanding through public awareness and education.

Anna Pileggi, Executive Director
Colleen Wheatley, Manager, Programs & Services
Emily Rivers, Manager, Communications

1695 Cleft Palate/Craniofacial Birth Defects: Cleft Palate Foundation
1504 East Franklin Street, Suite 102
Chapel Hill, NC 27514

919-933-9044
800-242-5338
Fax: 919-933-9604
www.cleftline.org

The Cleft Palate Foundation operates a toll-free CLEFTLINE for parents with children born with cleft lip, palate and other craniofacial birth defects. Referrals are made to cleft palate/craniofacial healthcare teams and to parent-support groups. Free information is available to parents.

Marilyn A. Cohen, LSLP, President
Nichelle Berry Weintraub, Secretary
Emily Kiser, Administrator

1696 Craniofacial Foundation of America
www.erlanger.org/cranio

Organization assists families with both the physical and emotional aspects, trying to make the everyday events a little easier.

1697 FACES: National Association for the Craniofacially Handicapped
P.O. Box 11082
Chattanooga, TN 37401

423-266-1632
800-332-2373
e-mail: faces@faces-cranio.org
www.faces-cranio.org

Assists individuals with facial disfigurations and their families They maintain a registry of centers offering corrective surgery for craniofacial deformities and financial assistance to qualified applicants.

Lynne Mayfield, President
Kim Teems, Communications & Program Director

1698 March of Dimes Birth Defects Foundation
1275 Mamaroneck Avenue
White Plains, NY 10605

914-997-4488
888-663-4637
Fax: 914-997-4763
www.marchofdimes.com

The March of Dimes Resource Center answers questions about preparing for pregnancy, pregnancy, genetic diseases, birth defects and related topics.

1699 Online Mendelian Inheritance in Man
National Library of Medicine, Building 38A
Bethesda, MD 20894   888-346-3656
e-mail: info@ncbi.nlm.nih.gov
www.ncbi.nlm.nih.gov

This database is a catalog of human genes and genetic disorders.

Christine E. Seidman, M.D., Chair
David J. Lipman, M.D., Executive Secretary

1700 Prescription Parents
www.samizdat.com/pp1.html

Organization that gives information and support to children with cleft lip and cleft palate through its educational and support materials, including its directory, newsletter and brochures.

1701 Wide Smiles
P.O. Box 5153
Stockton, CA 95205   209-942-2812
Fax: 209-464-1497
e-mail: josmiles@yahoo.com
www.widesmiles2.org

Wide Smiles was formed to ensure that parents of cleft-affected children do not have to feel alone. We offer support, inspiration, information and networking for families everywhere who may be dealing with the challenges associated with clefting.

Newsletters

1702 AmeriFace Newsletter
AmeriFace
PO Box 75112
Las Vegas, NV 89136   702-769-9264
888-486-1209
Fax: 702-341-5351
e-mail: info@ameriface.org
www.ameriface.org

A free newsletter.

8 pages

David Reisberg, DDS, President
Christina Corsiglia, Vice President
Debbie Oliver, Executive Director

Pamphlets

1703 As You Get Older
Cleft Palate Foundation
1504 East Franklin Street, Suite 102
Chapel Hill, NC 27514   919-933-9044
800-242-5338
Fax: 919-933-9604
e-mail: info@cleftline.org
www.cleftline.org

Describes medical treatment and social skills that may be necessary for teens born with clefts. There are sections on surgery, braces, speech and ear/nose/throat concerns, as well as social relationships and planning for the future.

2002 17 pages

Marilyn A. Cohen, LSLP, President
Nichelle Berry Weintraub, Secretary
Emily Kiser, Administrator

1704 CPF Teddy Bears
Cleft Palate Foundation
1504 East Franklin Street, Suite 102
Chapel Hill, NC 27514   919-933-9044
800-242-5338
Fax: 919-933-9604
e-mail: info@cleftline.org
www.cleftline.org

Marilyn A. Cohen, LSLP, President
Nichelle Berry Weintraub, Secretary
Emily Kiser, Administrator

1705 Cleft Lip & Palate
March of Dimes Pregnancy & Newborn Health Edu Ctr
1275 Mamaroneck Avenue
White Plains, NY 10605   914-977-4488
888-663-4637
Fax: 914-997-4763
e-mail: answers@marchofdimes.com
www.marchofdimes.com/phnec/pnhec.asp

Discusses how oral-palate clefts affect a baby's face, when and why they develop, special challenges that arise due to clefts, and repair oprtions.

1706 Cleft Surgery
Cleft Palate Foundation
1504 East Franklin Street, Suite 102
Chapel Hill, NC 27514   919-933-9044
800-242-5338
Fax: 919-933-9604
e-mail: info@cleftline.org
www.cleftline.org

Provides general information about primary cleft lip and cleft palate surgeries. Complete with drawing explaining the surgical procedures and before and after photos, this brochure addresses general considerations about surgery, post-operative care, and a list of questions to ask your surgeon. Available for newborns, toddlers, preschoolers and school-aged children, teens, and adults. Available in Spanish (Preparando para la Cirug a).

2001 8 pages

Marilyn A. Cohen, LSLP, President
Nichelle Berry Weintraub, Secretary
Emily Kiser, Administrator

1707 Developing Good Speech
Cleft Palate Foundation
1504 East Franklin Street, Suite 102
Chapel Hill, NC 27514   919-933-9044
800-242-5338
Fax: 919-933-9604
e-mail: info@cleftline.org
www.cleftline.org

Describes additional procedures that may be needed to improve speech in people with repaired cleft palate. Explains surgical procedures including palate lengthening, pharyngeal flap, spincter pharyngoplasty, and pharyngeal wall augmentation. Non-surgical prosthetic treatments are also described. (This information is most relevant to patients ages 4 to adult). Also available in Spanish (Desarrollando Bien el Habla).

2004 10 pages

Marilyn A. Cohen, LSLP, President
Nichelle Berry Weintraub, Secretary
Emily Kiser, Administrator

1708 Feeding Your Baby
Cleft Palate Foundation
1504 East Franklin Street, Suite 102
Chapel Hill, NC 27514   919-933-9044
800-242-5338
Fax: 919-933-9604
e-mail: info@cleftline.org
www.cleftline.org

Provides information on how best to feed your baby. Intended for use by parents, caregivers, and nurses caring for infants with cleft lip and/or cleft palate, not for infants with more complicated craniofacial conditions. Also avaible in Spanish (Alimentando a su BebS).

1999 15 pages

Marilyn A. Cohen, LSLP, President
Nichelle Berry Weintraub, Secretary
Emily Kiser, Administrator

1709 Genetics and You
Cleft Palate Foundation
1504 East Franklin Street, Suite 102
Chapel Hill, NC 27514

919-933-9044
800-242-5338
Fax: 919-933-9604
e-mail: info@cleftline.org
www.cleftline.org

Contains a brief overview of genetic biology and a summary of what is known about the causes of clefting. Features a graph for affected individuals, parents, and siblings, showing each group's approximate chances of having a child with a cleft. Details the steps involved i a genetic evaluation, which can help a family to determine its own particular recurrence risks. (The information presented is only applicable to patients with isolated cleft lip and/or palate).

2001 11 pages

Marilyn A. Cohen, LSLP, President
Nichelle Berry Weintraub, Secretary
Emily Kiser, Administrator

1710 Helping with Hearing
Cleft Palate Foundation
1504 East Franklin Street, Suite 102
Chapel Hill, NC 27514

919-933-9044
800-242-5338
Fax: 919-933-9604
e-mail: info@cleftline.org
www.cleftline.org

Provides information on types of hearing loss, middle ear disease and its treament, and speech concerns resulting from hearing problems. Also available in Spanish (Ayuda con el Oido).

2002 9 pages

Marilyn A. Cohen, LSLP, President
Nichelle Berry Weintraub, Secretary
Emily Kiser, Administrator

1711 Information for Adults
Cleft Palate Foundation
1504 East Franklin Street, Suite 102
Chapel Hill, NC 27514

919-933-9044
800-242-5338
Fax: 919-933-9604
e-mail: info@cleftline.org
www.cleftline.org

Designed to empower adults to make informed decisions about what additional treatment, if any, they want to seek out in relation to their clefts.

2000 25 pages

Marilyn A. Cohen, LSLP, President
Nichelle Berry Weintraub, Secretary
Emily Kiser, Administrator

1712 The First Year
Cleft Palate Foundation
1504 East Franklin Street, Suite 102
Chapel Hill, NC 27514

919-933-9044
800-242-5338
Fax: 919-933-9604
e-mail: info@cleftline.org
www.cleftline.org

Also available in Spanish (Los Cuatro Primeros Aos).

Marilyn A. Cohen, LSLP, President
Nichelle Berry Weintraub, Secretary
Emily Kiser, Administrator

1713 The School-Aged Child
Cleft Palate Foundation
1504 East Franklin Street, Suite 102
Chapel Hill, NC 27514

919-933-9044
800-242-5338
Fax: 919-933-9604
e-mail: info@cleftline.org
www.cleftline.org

Divided into two sections, one addressing the medical concerns of a school-aged child born with a cleft and other providing information about the school experience for these children. The medical section contains information about surgery, dental care, and speech providing simple diagrams of how the speech mechanism may be affected by cleft palate. Also available in Spanish (Los nios de Edad Escolar).

1995 29 pages

Marilyn A. Cohen, LSLP, President
Nichelle Berry Weintraub, Secretary
Emily Kiser, Administrator

1714 Toddlers and Preschoolers
Cleft Palate Foundation
1504 East Franklin Street, Suite 102
Chapel Hill, NC 27514

919-933-9044
800-242-5338
Fax: 919-933-9604
e-mail: info@cleftline.org
www.cleftline.org

Marilyn A. Cohen, LSLP, President
Nichelle Berry Weintraub, Secretary
Emily Kiser, Administrator

Description

1715 CLUBFOOT

Synonym: Talipes

Covers these related disorders: Talipes equinovarus

Involves the following Biologic System(s):

Orthopedic and Muscle Disorders

The term clubfoot describes a deformity in which the foot is rotated inward and downward, rather than being in its normal position. The deformity in clubfoot is congenital or inborn, and is present at birth. It has several variants, all of which are referred to collectively under the Latin name "talipes" because they stem from structural aberrations in the anklebone, or talus, and dislocation of the ankle (i.e., talonavicular joint). In the most common type of clubfoot, known as congenital talipes equinovarus, the foot is abnormally twisted inward and the toes point downward (plantar flexion). Other deformities classified as types of clubfoot include defects in which the inner portion of the foot is raised with the sole turned inward (metatarsus varus), or the front area of the foot is raised and the heel is turned outward (talipes calcaneovalgus).

In about half of all cases of clubfoot, both feet are affected. A clubfoot tends to be smaller than an unaffected foot, and muscles of the foot and calf are typically underdeveloped, which may become more apparent with advancing age, and depending upon the severity of the deformity, the affected foot may have varying levels of stiffness and inflexibility.

Talipes equinovarus occurs in about 1 of every 1000 births, and is approximately twice as common in males as in females, and may be familiar or idiopathic, occurring as an isolated condition of unknown cause. In infants in whom the condition affects only one foot, the right side is most often involved. Familial talipes equjinovarus is thought to result from the interaction of an abnormal (mutated) gene with other genes or certain environmental factors (multifactorial inheritance). Although deformity of the ankle bone was once considered the primary abnormality in talipes, researchers speculate that a neuromuscular abnormality may be the underlying cause of the talus deformities and associated findings.

In some cases, talipes may occur in association with a neuromuscular disorder (e.g., arthrogryposis multiplex congenita) or with other underlying disorders or syndromes.

The treatment of talipes usually begins soon after birth, since failure to correct this deformity can result in walking on the edge of the foot rather than with the sole of the foot flat on the floor, and in reduced size and strength of muscles in the affected leg. Treatment typically involves the use of taping, casting, or splinting (e.g., malleable splints, serial plaster casts) to move the foot and ankle toward their normal positions. This is often done gradually and over a period of months, through successive, repeated taping, splinting, or casting procedures that each provide a small degree of correction until the proper position of the foot and ankle is achieved. The treatment may involve the use of other orthopedic appliances and corrective shoes to assist with walking. If the use of taping, splints, or casts does not result inappropriate correction, or if a clubfoot is rigid, with shortness or tightness of the Achilles tendon or other structural deformi-

ties in the connective tissues or bones of the foot and ankle, corrective surgery may be needed. This is typically delayed until at least the age of 4 months in order to allow natural growth and strengthening of these structures. Regular monitoring of children with a clubfoot is needed to ensure their continued improvement.

Although clubfoot is not always completely correctible, treatment can improve both the appearance and function of the foot, and in most cases the prognosis for children with a clubfoot is good.

Government Agencies

1716 National Center for Environmental Health

Division of Birth Defects & Developmental Disabled
1600 Clifton Road
Atlanta, GA 30333

404-639-3311
800-232-4636
TTY: 888-232-6348
www.cdc.gov

Strives to promote health and quality of life by preventing or controlling those diseases or deaths that result from interactions between people and their enviroment.

Thomas R. Frieden, MD, MPH,, Director
Ileana Arias, PhD, Principal Deputy Director of DC/ATS
Ursula E. Bauer, PhD, MPH, Director, National Center for Chron

National Associations & Support Groups

1717 American Academy of Pediatrics

141 Northwest Point Boulevard
Elk Grove Village, IL 60007

847-434-4000
800-433-9016
Fax: 847-434-8000
www.aap.org

The American Academy of Pediatrics and its member pediatricians are committed to the attainment of optimal physical, mental and social health and well-being for all infants, children, adolescents, and young adults.

Sandra Hassink, MD, FAAP, President

1718 Center for Pediatric Orthopaedic Surgery

NYU Hospital for Joint Diseases
301 E 17th Street, Suite 413
New York, NY 10003

212-598-6606
Fax: 212-598-6084

A specialized sector of the Center for Children at the Hospital for Joint Diseases, offering information, consultation, and comprehensive treatment of clubfoot deformities.

Paul Gusmorino, Physician

1719 Genetic Alliance

4301 Connecticut Avenue NW, Suite 404
Washington, DC 20008

202-966-7955
800-336-4363
Fax: 202-966-8553
e-mail: info@geneticalliance.org
www.geneticalliance.org

World's leading nonprofit health advocacy organization committed to transforming health through genetics and promoting an environment of openness centered on the health of individuals, families, and communities.

Sharon Terry, President
Lisa Wise, Chief Operating Officer
Tetyana Murza MES, Programs and Policy Coordinator

1720 March of Dimes Birth Defects Foundation
1275 Mamaroneck Avenue
White Plains, NY 10605   914-997-4488
888-663-4637
Fax: 914-997-4763
e-mail: answers@marchofdimes.com
www.marchofdimes.com

March of Dimes help moms have full-term pregnancies and research the problems that threaten the health of babies.The March of Dimes also acts globally: sharing best practices in perinatal health and helping improve birth outcomes where the needs are the most urgent.

Kenneth A. May, Chair
Jennifer Howse, President/CEO
Alan Fleischman, Medical Director

Conferences

1721 Genetic Alliance Annual Conference
Genetic Alliance
4301 Connecticut Avenue NW, Suite 404
Washington, DC 20008   202-966-5557
800-336-4363
Fax: 202-966-8553
e-mail: info@geneticalliance.org
www.geneticalliance.org

Consistently inspirational and enables partnership among all stakeholders: advocates and community leaders, health and industry professionals, policymakers, and academicians.

July

Sharon Terry, President/CEO
Tetyana Murza, Programs/Events Manager

Web Sites

1722 CLIPS: Clubfoot Information and Parental Support
ixprss.com/clubfoot

A web site dedicated to providing clubfoot information and parental support, created by a parent as a resource for information, support and understanding.

1723 Children with Talipes (Clubfoot)
www.clubfoot.co.uk

Created by a parent of a child with talipes, the web site offers a first-hand account of treatment and description of clubfoot, as well as links to other sites.

1724 Johns Hopkins Department of Orthopaedic Surgery
601 North Caroline Street , JHOC #5215
Baltimore, MD 21287   443-997-2663
e-mail: hopkinsortho@jhmi.edu
www.hopkinsmedicine.org/orthopedicsurgery

A web site serving as a learning resource for patients and physicians alike, offering insight into the services provided by the university's professional staff members.

John V. Ingari, MD, Associate Professor
Adam S. Levin, Othopaedic Oncology
Carrol D. Morris, MD, MS, Division Chief,Othopaedic Oncology

1725 Orthoseek
www.orthoseek.com/articles/clubfoot.html

e-mail: admin@orthoseek.com
www.orthoseek.com/articles/clubfoot.html

A source of authoritative information on pediatric orthopedics and pediatric sports medicine.

Andrew Chong, MD, Founder

1726 TIPS: Talipes Information and Parental Support
www.clubfootaustralia.com/about-us

A support group run by parents whose children have, or had, talipes, offering comprehensive information and many web links, as well as a bi-monthly newletter, stories from parents, email correspondence, and emotional support.

1727 Virtual Children's Hospital: Treatment of Congenital Clubfoot
200 Hawkins Drive
Iowa City, IA 52242   800-777-8442
www.vh.org/pediatric/provider/orthopaedics/clubfoot

A digital library of pediatric information committed to educating patients, healthcare providers and students for the purpose of improving patients' care, outcome and lives; uses current, authoritative, trustworthy health information created by the University of Iowa, while serving as a platform for research into the challenges facing world-wide information distribution.

Jean E. Robillard, MD, UI VP for Medical Affairs
Theresa Brennan, MD, Chief Medical Officer
Sabi Singh, MS, MA, Co-Chief Operating Officer

1728 Wheeless' Textbook of Orthopaedics
www.wheelessonline.com

Derives from a variety of sources, including journals, articles, national meetings, lectures and other textbooks.

Clifford R. Wheeless, III, M.D., Author

Pamphlets

1729 Club Foot & Other Physical Deformities
March of Dimes Pregnancy & Newborn Health Edu Ctr
1275 Mamaroneck Avenue
White Plains, NY 10605   914-977-4488
888-663-4637
Fax: 914-997-4763
e-mail: answers@marchofdimes.com
www.marchofdimes.com/phnec/pnhec.asp

Provides information on Club Foot and other deformities, discussing the affects on the child, diagnoses, causes, prevention, and treatment. Online.

1730 Club Foot and Other Foot Deformities
March of Dimes Resource Center
1275 Mamaroneck Avenue
White Plains, NY 10605   914-977-4488
888-663-4637
Fax: 914-997-4763
TTY: 914-997-4764
e-mail: resourcecenter@modimes.org
www.modimes.org

Fact Sheets: one to two page review written for the general public. Also available electronically from our website www.modimes.org. Brochures: 3 panel color brochures written for the general public.

Camps

1731 Hemlocks Easter Seals Recreation
85 Jones Street
Amston, CT 06231   860-228-9496
800-832-4409
Fax: 860-228-2091
e-mail: cmerkent@eastersealsct.org
www.ct_easterseals.com

Accepts campers, ages 6 and under, whose major disability is orthopedic. First preference is given to Connecticut residents. A computer camp is also available.

Carl Larson

Description

1732 COARCTATION OF THE AORTA

Involves the following Biologic System(s):

Cardiovascular Disorders

Coarctation of the aorta is a congenital heart defect character-ized by a narrowing or constriction of the body's main artery. This artery, known as the aorta, carries blood away from the heart to nourish the tissues of the body. Most of these defects are located just below the origin of the artery that supplies blood to the left arm, (left subclavian artery). Because this constriction reduces blood flow to the lower portion of the body, affected individuals may have unusually low blood pressure and weak or absent pulses in their legs. In addition, there may be higher blood pressure and strong pulses in the arms.

The severity of associated symptoms relates to the degree of pressure changes resulting from aortic narrowing. Although some children have no symptoms, others may experience diz-ziness, headache, weakness, fainting, nosebleeds, cold legs, and leg pain or cramps. Some affected infants may develop heart failure within the first few days or weeks of life. In some newborns, heart failure may result in decreased blood flow and abnormally high levels of acid in the blood (meta-bolic acidosis), sometimes accompanied by severe diarrhea and kidney (renal) failure. This life-threatening situation re-quires immediate treatment. Treatment of coarctation in a newborn requires surgery. (As these infants age, the narrow-ing may recur [restenosis] necessitating dilation or opening of the vessel through a procedure called balloon angioplasty, during which a balloon-tipped tube [catheter] is inflated in-side the aorta, thus helping to expand the narrowed area of the vessel.) Correction of coarctation of the aorta through sur-gery or balloon catheterization may be recommended in older children with significant impairment. Because coarctation of the aorta is very often accompanied by other heart defects, early intervention is crucial. Other cardiac anomalies often associated with this defect include bicuspid aortic valve (i.e., the heart valve between the left ventricle and the aorta is composed of only two leaflets, or cusps, instead of the normal three); abnormalities of the mitral valve (located between the left atrium and the left ventricle); and an abnormal opening in the wall between the left and right ventricles (ventricular septal defect).

The cause of coarctation of the aorta is unknown. Some re-searchers think that it develops in the fetus in association with certain types of cardiac abnormalities. Coarctation of the aorta is more prevalent in males than in females by a ratio of about two to one.

Government Agencies

1733 NIH/National Heart, Lung and Blood Institu te
National Institute of Health
31 Center Dr MSC 2486, Bldg 31, Room 5A48
Bethesda, MD 20892   301-592-8573
                                        Fax: 240-629-3246
                                        TTY: 240-629-3255
                    e-mail: nhlbiinfo@nhlbi.nih.gov
                                        www.nhlbi.nih.gov

The National Heart, Lung, and Blood Institute (NHLBI) provides global leadership for a research, training, and education program to promote the prevention and treatment of heart, lung, and blood diseases and enhance the health of all individuals so that they can live longer and more fulfilling lives

Gary H Gibbons MD, Director
Susan Shurin, MD, Deputy Director
Nakela Cook MD, Chief of Staff

1734 NIH/National Institute of Child Health and Human Development
31 Center Drive, Building 31
Bethesda, MD 20892   800-370-2943
                                        Fax: 301-496-1104
                                        TTY: 888-320-6942
            e-mail: NICHDInformationResourceCenter@mail.nih.
                                        www.nichd.nih.gov

Established in 1962 by congress, today the institute conducts and supports laboratory research, clinical trials, and epidemiological studies that explore health processes; examines the impact of dis-abilities, diseases, and variations on the lives of individuals; and sponsors training programs for scientists, health care providers, and researchers to ensure that NICHD research can continue

Alan E Guttmacher MD, Director
Lisa Kaeser, Program & Public Liaison

National Associations & Support Groups

1735 American Academy of Pediatrics
141 Northwest Point Boulevard
Elk Grove Village, IL 60007   847-434-4000
                                              800-433-9016
                                        Fax: 847-434-8000
                                        www.aap.org

The American Academy of Pediatrics and its member pediatri-cians are committed to the attainment of optimal physical, mental and social health and well-being for all infants, children, adoles-cents, and young adults.

Sandra Hassink, MD, FAAP, President

1736 American Heart Association
7272 Greenville Avenue
Dallas, TX 10169   214-373-6300
                                              800-242-8721
                                        Fax: 214-706-1341
                    e-mail: inquire@amhrt.org
                                        www.americanheart.org

Our mission is to build healthier lives, free of cardiovascular dis-eases and stroke.

Nancy Brown, CEO
Suzie Upton, Chief Development Officer
Sunder Joshi, CFO

1737 Genetic Alliance
4301 Connecticut Avenue NW Suite 404
Washington, DC 20008   202-966-7955
                                              800-336-4363
                                        Fax: 202-966-8553
                    e-mail: info@geneticalliance.org
                                        www.geneticalliance.org

World's leading nonprofit health advocacy organization commit-ted to transforming health through genetics and promoting an en-vironment of openness centered on the health of individuals, families, and communities.

Sharon Terry, President
Lisa Wise, Chief Operating Officer
Tetyana Murza MES, Programs and Policy Coordinator

1738 March of Dimes Birth Defects Foundation
1275 Mamaroneck Avenue
White Plains, NY 10605   914-997-4488
                                              888-663-4637
                                        Fax: 914-997-4763
                    e-mail: answers@marchofdimes.com
                                        www.marchofdimes.com

March of Dimes help moms have full-term pregnancies and research the problems that threaten the health of babies.The March of Dimes also acts globally: sharing best practices in perinatal health and helping improve birth outcomes where the needs are the most urgent.

Kenneth A. May, Chair
Jennifer Howse, President/CEO
Alan Fleischman, Medical Director

Research Centers

1739 Children's Hospital: Academic Pediatric Surgery Department
1056 E 19th Avenue
Denver, CO 80218
303-493-8333
800-624-6553
Fax: 303-764-5997
www.chipteam.org

Strives to improve the health of children through the provision of high quality, coordinated programs of patient care, education, research and advocacy.

Emily L Dobyns

Conferences

1740 Genetic Alliance Annual Conference
Genetic Alliance
4301 Connecticut Avenue NW, Suite 404
Washington, DC 20008
202-966-5557
800-336-4363
Fax: 202-966-8553
e-mail: info@geneticalliance.org
www.geneticalliance.org

Consistently inspirational and enables partnership among all stakeholders: advocates and community leaders, health and industry professionals, policymakers, and academicians.

July

Sharon Terry, President/CEO
Tetyana Murza, Programs/Events Manager

Web Sites

1741 Congenital Heart Information Network
www.tchin.org

An international organization that provides reliable information, support services and resources to families of children with congenital heart defects and acquired heart disease, adults with congenital heart defects, and the professionals who work with them.

1742 Southern Illinois University School of Medicine
PO Box 19658
Springfield, IL 62794
217-545-8000
www.siumed.edu/peds/index.htm

Mission is to meet the health care needs of children and their families in central and Southern Illinois through provision of high quality, coordinated care of children with acute and chronic conditions with inpatient, ambulatory, and community-based programs.

1743 Yale University School of Medicine
333 Cedar St.
New Haven, CT 6510
203-737-1770
medicine.yale.edu

A site that offers information on congential heart conditions including Coarctation of the Aorta.

Peter Salovey, AB, MA, PhD, President
Richard Belitsky, MD, Deputy Dean of Education
Benjamin Polak, MA, MA, PhD, Provost

Book Publishers

1744 Congenital Disorders Sourcebook
Omnigraphics
PO Box 31-1640
Detroit, PA 48231
800-234-1340
Fax: 800-875-1340
e-mail: info@omnigraphics.com
www.omnigraphics.com

Basic consumer health information on disorders aquired during gestation, including spina bifida, hydrocephalus, cerebral palsy, heart defects, craniofacial abnormalities and fetal alcohol syndrome.

650 pages
ISBN: 0-780809-45-9

Description

1745 COLIC

Synonyms: Infantile colic, Three-month colic

Involves the following Biologic System(s):

Gastrointestinal Disorders, Neonatal and Infant Disorders

Colic refers to a condition in which infants experience frequent episodes of abdominal pain, accompanied by irritability and intense crying. These episodes usually begin suddenly and continue for several hours. Symptoms and physical findings of colic may also include flushing of the face, swelling of the abdomen, repeated extending or flexing of the legs, and unusually cold feet.

It is suspected that colic is intestinal in origin; however, its exact cause is not known. Contributing factors may include the excessive swallowing of air during episodes of unceasing crying, overfeeding, hunger, certain foods, intestinal allergy, and environmental stress. Attacks of colic usually commence within the first few weeks of life and occur most often in the afternoon or evening. Colic often resolves spontaneously within three or four months, without residual effects.

Infants with symptoms associated with colic should be evaluated to determine if another, perhaps more serious disorder, is causing the pain and discomfort. The treatment of colic may include soothing, comforting gestures such as holding, patting, stroking, rocking, and other repetitive movements. Some affected infants may benefit from white noise or other comforting background sounds; the application of a warm wash cloth, hot water bottle, or warm heating pad under the stomach when the child is lying prone; or a ride in the car. Some episodes of colic may resolve with the passing of gas or stool. In addition, parents and caregivers may be advised to refrain from overstimulating, overfeeding, or underfeeding babies with colic. The toll colic takes on parents can be considerable. Physicians often advise that parents or caregivers try to get enough sleep as fatigue, may sometimes add to the already stressful situation.

National Associations & Support Groups

1746 American Academy of Pediatrics
141 Northwest Point Boulevard
Elk Grove Village, IL 60007
847-434-4000
800-433-9016
Fax: 847-434-8000
www.aap.org

The American Academy of Pediatrics and its member pediatricians are committed to the attainment of optimal physical, mental and social health and well-being for all infants, children, adolescents, and young adults.

Sandra Hassink, MD, FAAP, President

1747 American College of Gastroenterology
6400 Goldsboro Road Suite 200
Bethesda, MD 20827
301-263-9000
www.gi.org

To advance the scientific study and medical practice of diseases of the gastrointestinal tract.

1932

Ronald J Vender, President
Stephen B. Hanauer MD, Vice President
Harry E Sarles Jr. MD, President-Elect

1748 American Medical Association
AMA Plaza, 330 North Wabash Ave., Suite 39300
Chicago, IL 60611
800-262-3211
www.ama-assn.org/ama

AMA is dedicated to ensuring sustainable physician practices that result in better health outcomes for patients.

James L. Madara, MD, CEO/ EVP
Bernard L. Hengesbaugh, Chief Operating Officer
Kenneth J. Sharigian, SVP/ Chief Strategy Officer

1749 American Pregnancy Association
1425 Greenway Drive, Suite 440
Irving, TX 75038
e-mail: info@americanpregnancy.org
americanpregnancy.org

The American Pregnancy Association is a 501(c)(3) nonprofit organization committed to promoting pregnancy wellness through education, advocacy and community awareness.

1750 American Urological Association
1000 Corporate Boulevard
Linthicum, MD 21090
410-689-3700
Fax: 410-689-3800
e-mail: aua@AUAnet.org
www.auanet.org

Urology is a surgical specialty which deals with diseases of the male and female urinary tract and the male reproductive organs.

1751 Digestive Disease National Coalition
507 Capitol Court NE, Suite 200
Washington, DC 10039
202-544-7497
Fax: 202-546-7105
e-mail: ddnc@hmcw.org
www.ddnc.org

Advocacy organization comprised of 22 voluntary and professional societies concerned with the many diseases of the digestive tract and liver.

Diane Paley, Chairperson
James DeGerome, President
Andrew Spiegel, Vice-Chairperson

1752 International Chiropractic Pediatric Assoc
icpa4kids.org
610-565-2360
icpa4kids.org

ICPA is a non-profit organization of chiropractic family practitioners dedicated to advancing public awareness and attainment of the chiropractic family wellness lifestyle.

Jeanne Ohm, Executive Director
Gabe Small, Webmaster

1753 North American Society for Pediatric Gastroenterology/Hepatology/Nutrition
PO Box 6
Flourtown, PA 19031
215-233-0808
Fax: 215-233-3918
e-mail: naspghan@naspghan.org
www.naspghan.org

Strives to improve the care of infants, children and adolescents with digestive disorders by promoting advances in clinical care of children with chronic abdominal pain, diarrhea, constipation, vomiting, bleeding from the GI tract, inflammatory bowel disease, liver diseases, diseases of the pancreas, poor weight gain and nutritional problems.

Philip Sherman, President
Margaret K Stallings, Executive Director

Libraries & Resource Centers

1754 Family Resource Center at Lucile Packard Children's Hospital
725 Welch Road
Palo Alto, CA 94304
650-497-8102
www.lpch.org/healthLibrary

Provides hospital patients, their families and staff with access to a wide variety of information about child and maternal health and well-being. The FRC collection includes books, periodicals and pamphlets on a variety of topics from coping with chronic illness such as colic to parenting skills and child development. The Family Resource Center also maintains a large collection of recreational reading materials and video tapes.

1755 National Digestive Diseases Information Clearinghouse
31 Center Drive, MSC 2560
Bethesda, MD 20892
301-496-3583
800-891-5389
Fax: 301-907-8906
e-mail: nddic@info.niddk.nih.gov
www.niddk.nih.gov

The National Institute of Diabetes and Digestive and Kidney Diseases conducts and supports research on many of the most serious diseases affecting public health. The Institute supports much of the clinical research on the diseases of internal medicine and related subspecialty fields as well as many basic science disciplines.

Dr. Griffin P Rodgers, President

Research Centers

1756 CRI Worldwide Pediatric Center for Excellence
CRI Worldwide
130 White Horse Pike
Clementon, NJ 08021
856-566-9000
Fax: 856-566-4302
e-mail: dkrefetz@cnsresearchinstitute.com
www.cnsresearchinstitute.com

Formerly called CNS Research Institute; Psychiatrists and Child Psychologists maintains a major emphasis in the area of pediatric research. Working hard with parents and their children to educate and treat the entire family.

Dr David Krefetz, Director

1757 Central DuPage Hospital Center for Digestive Disorders
25 N Winfield Road
Winfield, IL 60190
630-933-1600
Fax: 630-933-1300
TTY: 630-933-4833
www.cdh.org

Bringing together the best research about colic and weighed up the evidence about how to treat it.

Michael Vivoda, President/CEO
Brian Lemon, President of Delnor Hospital, Execu
Brian Lemon, President of Central DuPage Hospita

1758 Cincinnati Digestive Diseases Research Development Center
Cincinnati Children's Hospital Medical Center
3333 Burnet Avenue
Cincinnati, OH 45229
513-636-4200
800-344-2462
TTY: 513-636-4900
www.cincinnatichildrens.org

Promote research that will yield insights into the fundamental processes of growth and development in the digestive tract and lead to novel or improved therapies.

Michael Fisher, President/CEO
Jorge Bezerra, MD, Associate Director

1759 Infant Behavior, Cry and Sleep Clinic
Women & Infants Hospital of Rhode Island
50 Holden Street, 1st Floor
Providence, RI 02908
401-453-7690
Fax: 401-453-7697
e-mail: Barry_Lester@brown.edu
www.womenandinfants.org/Services/Infant-Behavior-Cry

A clinical service developed to diagnose and treat infants with crying, sleeping, feeding and associated early behavior problems by helping parents understand and manage their infant and to adjust to the disruption caused by having an infant who has behavioral problems in the first few months of life.

Constance A. Howes, FACHE, President/CEO of Women & Infants Ho

Conferences

1760 NASPGHAN Annual Meeting and Postgraduate Course
NASPGHAN
PO Box 6
Flourtown, PA 19031
215-233-0808
Fax: 215-233-3918
e-mail: naspghan@naspghan.org
www.naspghan.org

October
Margaret K Stallings, Executive Director

Journals

1761 Journal of Pediatric Gastroenterology and Nutrition
NASPGHAN, author

Lippincott Williams & Wilkins
Two Commerce Square, 2001 Market Street
Philadelphia, PA 19103
215-521-8300
Fax: 215-521-8902
www.wolterskluwerhealth.com

Publication of the North American Society for Pediatric Gastroenterolgy, Hepatology and Nutrition, which strives to improve the care of infants, children and adolescents with digestive disorders by promoting advances in clinical care of children with chronic abdominal pain, diarrhea, constipation, vomiting, bleeding from the GI tract, inflammatory bowel disease, liver diseases, diseases of the pancreas, poor weight gain and nutritional problems.

Bob Becker, President/ CEO
Susan Yules, Chief Financial Officer
Cathy Wolfe, President/ CEO, Medical Research

Newsletters

1762 NASPGHAN News
PO Box 6
Flourtown, PA 19031
215-233-0808
Fax: 215-233-3939
e-mail: naspghan@naspghan.org
www.naspgn.org

Publication of the North American Society for Pediatric Gastroenterolgy, Hepatology and Nutrition, which strives to improve the care of infants, children and adolescents with digestive disorders by promoting advances in clinical care of children with chronic abdominal pain, diarrhea, constipation, vomiting, bleeding from the GI tract, inflammatory bowel disease, liver diseases, diseases of the pancreas, poor weight gain and nutritional problems.

Description

1763 CONDUCT DISORDER

Covers these related disorders: Group conduct disorder, Solitary aggressive conduct disorder, Undifferentiated conduct disorder

Involves the following Biologic System(s):
Developmental/Behavioral/Psychiatric Disorders

Conduct disorder refers to a group of distinct behavioral abnormalities characterized by the repetition of certain types of disruptive or antisocial behaviors. Children or adolescents with conduct disorder may often lie, steal, skip school, run away from home, use drugs or alcohol, hurt animals, commit arson or vandalism, engage in physical violence, use weapons, and commit other criminal acts. Those affected with solitary aggressive conduct disorder are usually selfish, rarely get along with or relate well to others, and often lack remorse for their behavior. Children and adolescents with group conduct disorder, however, may be attached and faithful to a particular clique, gang, or other group of friends while at the same time violating the rights of or displaying antisocial behavior toward those outside of the group. In some cases, affected individuals may display behavior characteristic of both solitary aggressive and group conduct disorders and, subsequently, may be diagnosed with undifferentiated conduct disorder.

Conduct disorder may be caused by a variety of factors including genetic as well as environmental influences (e.g., childrearing, etc.). In many cases, children with this type of behavioral irregularity have parents or caregivers who display similar patterns of conduct. In addition, parents or caregivers often have inconsistent parenting skills or may be overly aggressive in punishing or disciplining. Some parents or caregivers may be unsupportive of the child, or may lack other basic skills that help the child to develop a sense of self-worth, respect for others, etc. Several factors may influence whether affected children carry these characteristic patterns of behavior into adulthood. Some factors include parental or caregiver influences, the age of onset, the severity and type of behavior, the number of different types of antisocial behaviors exhibited, and whether the episodes of disruptive behavior continue to increase.

Treatment of conduct disorder may include individual, group, and family therapy, as well as parental or caregiver management training. In some cases, children with severe conduct disorder may benefit from hospitalization for psychiatric evaluation and treatment. Medication is, in most cases, not indicated for the treatment of conduct disorder; however, it is sometimes prescribed to treat other underlying disorders (e.g, depression, attention deficit hyperactivity disorder, etc.). Other treatment is supportive.

Government Agencies

1764 NIH/National Institute of Mental Health
6001 Executive Boulevard, Room 8184, MSC 9663
Bethesda, MD 20892   301-443-4513
                            866-615-6464
                            Fax: 301-443-4279
                            TTY: 301-443-8431
                            e-mail: nimhinfo@nih.gov
                            www.nimh.nih.gov

The mission of NIMH is to transform the understanding and treatment of mental illnesses through basic and clinical research, paving the way for prevention, recovery, and cure.

Dr Thomas R Insel, Director

National Associations & Support Groups

1765 American Academy of Pediatrics
141 Northwest Point Boulevard
Elk Grove Village, IL 60007   847-434-4000
                                     800-433-9016
                                     Fax: 847-434-8000
                                     www.aap.org

The American Academy of Pediatrics and its member pediatricians are committed to the attainment of optimal physical, mental and social health and well-being for all infants, children, adolescents, and young adults.

Sandra Hassink, MD, FAAP, President

1766 American Mental Health Foundation (AMHF)
PO Box 3
Riverdale,, NY 10471
USA   212-737-9027
     e-mail: elomke@americanmentalhealthfoundation.or
                  americanmentalhealthfoundation.org

Dedicated to the extensive and intensive research in the theories and techniques of treatment of emotional illness and to the implementation of reforms in the mental health system. Efforts have resulted in development of better and less expensive treatment methods. Findings are disseminated in English and other major languages.

Sister Joan Curtin. CND, Director
Evander Lomke, President/Executive Director
Eugene Gollogly, Vice President

1767 Association for Behavioral and Cognitive Therapies
305 7th Avenue, 16th Floor
New York, NY 10001   212-647-1890
                                     Fax: 212-647-1865
                                     e-mail: membership@abct.org
                                     www.abct.org/Home/

Formerly known as the Association for Advancement of Behavior Therapy; this organization is concerned with the application of behavioral and cognitive sciences to understanding human behavior, developing interventions to enhance the human condition, and promoting the appropriate utilization of these interventions.

Stefan G. Hofmann, Ph.D., President
Dean McKay, Ph.D, President- Elect
Denise D. Davis, Ph.D., Secretary/Treasurer

1768 Center for Disabilities and Development
University of Iowa Hospitals and Clinics
100 Hawkins Drive
Iowa City, IA 52242   319-353-6900
                                     877-686-0031
                                     Fax: 319-356-8284
                                     e-mail: cdd-webmaster@uiowa.edu
                                     www.uichildrens.org/cdd/

A trusted resource for healthcare, training, research and information for people with disabilities that include: behavior disorders, brain injury, cerebral palsy, diabetes, down syndrome, learning disabilities, mental retardation, sleep disorders and spina bifida.

Raphael Hirsch, MD, Physician-in-Chief, UI Children's H
Scott Turner, Executive Director, University of I
Joel Shilyansky, MD,, Associate Professor and Director, D

1769 Center for Mental Health Services Knowledge Exchange Network
US Department of Health and Human Services
PO Box 42557
Washington, DC 20015   800-662-4357
                                     800-789-2647
                                     Fax: 240-747-5470
                                     TTY: 800-487-4889
                                     TDD: 866-889-2647
                                     e-mail: samhsa.media@ees.hhs.gov
                                     www.store.samhsa.gov/home

197

Develops national mental health policies that promote Federal/State coordination and benefit from input from consumers, family members and providers. Ensures that high quality mental health services programs are implemented to benefit seriously mentally ill populations, disasters or those involved in the criminal justice system.

Mirtha R. Beadle M.P.A., Deputy for Operations
Kana . Enomoto, M.A, Principal Deputy Administrator
Pamela S. Hyde, J.D., Administrator

1770 Federation of Families for Children's Mental Health
9605 Medical Center Drive, Suite 280
Rockville, MD 10205
240-403-1901
Fax: 240-403-1909
e-mail: ffcmh@ffcmh.org
www.ffcmh.org

The National family run organization is dedicated exclusively to helping children with mental health needs and their families achieve a better quality of life.

Teka Dempson, President
Sherri Luthe, Vice President
Sheila Pires, Treasurer

1771 NADD: National Association for the Dually Diagnosed
132 Fair Street
Kingston, NY 12401
845-331-4336
800-331-5362
Fax: 845-331-4569
e-mail: info@thenadd.org
www.thenadd.org

Nonprofit organization designed to promote the interests of professional and care providers for individuals who have the coexistence of mental illness and mental retardation. NADD provides conferences, educational services and training materials to professionals, parents, concerned citizens and service organizations.

Dr Robert Fletcher, CEO
Michelle Jordan, Office Manager
Judie Johnston, Administrative Assistant

1772 National Alliance for the Mentally Ill
3803 N. Fairfax Dr., Suite 100
Arlington, VA 22203
703-525-7600
800-950-6264
Fax: 703-524-9094
TDD: 703-516-7227
e-mail: info@nami.org
www.nami.org

NAMI is a nonprofit, grassroots, self-help, support and advocacy organization of consumers, families and friends of people with severe mental illness, such as schizophrenia, bipolar disorder, major despressive disorder, obsessive compulsive disorder, anxiety disorders, autism and other severe and persistent mental illnesses that affect the brain.

Keris J,,n Myrick, President
Kevin B Sullivan, First Vice President
Jim Payne, Second Vice President

1773 National Mental Health Association
2000 N Beauregard Street, 6th Floor
Alexandria, VA 10182
703-684-7722
800-969-6642
Fax: 703-684-5968
TTY: 800-433-5959
e-mail: info@mentalhealthamerica.net
www.mentalhealthamerica.net

MHA, the leading advocacy organization addressing the full spectrum of mental and substance use conditions and their effects nationwide, works to inform, advocate and enable access to quality behavioral health services for all Americans.

Ann Boughtin, Chair of the Board
Eric Ashton, Vice Chair
Elaine Crider, Secretary/Treasurer

1774 National Mental Health Consumers' Self-Help Clearinghouse
1211 Chestnut Street, Suite 1207
Philadelphia, PA 19107
215-751-1810
800-553-4539
Fax: 215-636-6312
e-mail: info@mhselfhelp.org
www.mhselfhelp.org

The Clearinghouse works to foster peer empowerment through our website, up-to-date news and information announcements, a directory of peer-driven services, electronic and printed publications, training packages, and individual and onsite consultation

Joseph Rogers, Executive Director & Founder
Susan Rogers, Director of Special Projects
Britani Nestel, Program Specialist

Research Centers

1775 Menninger Child & Family Program
Menninger Clinic
2801 Gessner Drive, PO Box 809045
Houston, TX 77280
713-275-5000
800-351-9058
Fax: 713-275-5117
www.menninger.edu

Menninger's research strategies are developed through the Menninger Child & Family Program. Projects are designed to develop a better understanding of the mind in order to more effectively treat mental disorders.

Ian Aitken, Ceo

1776 National Technical Assistance Center for Children's Mental Health
Georgetown University
Center for Child and Human Development Georgetown
Washington, DC 20057
202-687-5000
Fax: 202-687-8899
TDD: 202-687-5503
e-mail: gucdc@georgetown.edu
www.gucchd.georgetown.edu/67211.html

Devoted to helping states, tribes, territories, and communities discover, apply, and sustain innovative and collaborative solutions that improve the social, emotional, and behavioral well being of children and families.

James Wotring MSW, Director

1777 Research & Training Center for Children's Mental Health at University of South FL
Louis de la Parte Florida Mental Health Institute
13301 Bruce B. Downs Boulevard
Tampa, FL 33612
813-974-3154
Fax: 813-974-3078
e-mail: friedman@fmhi.usf.edu
www.rtckids.fmhi.usf.edu/default.cfm

Working towards increasing the effectiveness of service systems by strengthening the empirical base for such systems through research and dissemination to key audiences. With its new, five-year research program, the Center expands its mission with an integrated research, training, and dissemination program targeted specifically at implementation issues for developing effective systems of care.

Robert M. Friedman, Ph.D, Center Director
Albert Duchnowski, Ph.D, Deputy Director
Krista Kutash, Ph.D, Deputy Director

1778 Research and Training Center on Family Support and Children's Mental Health
1600 SW 4th Avenue, Suite 900
Portland, OR 97201
503-725-4040
Fax: 503-725-4180
e-mail: flemingd@pdx.edu
www.rtc.pdx.edu

Funded to pursue an integrated set of research, training, technical assistance, and dissemination activities. The center's work will focus on two related themes; community integration for children and adolescents with emotional and behavioral disorders and their families; and strengthening family and youth participation in child and adolescent mental health services.

Donna Flemming, Information Director

1779 Technical Assistance Partnership for Child and Family Mental Health
1000 Thomas Jefferson Street NW, Suite 400
Washington, DC 20007 202-403-6827
Fax: 202-342-5007
e-mail: tapartnership@air.org
www.tapartnership.org

A staff of family members and professionals with extensive practice experience, grounded in an organization with vast research experience in children with serious emotional disturbance and their families.

Sharon Hunt, Deputy Director of Operations
Jeffrey Poirier, Continuous Quality Improvement
Regenia Hicks, Project Director Continuous Quality

Conferences

1780 FFCMH Annual Conference
Federation of Families for Childrens Mental Health
9605 Medical Center Drive, Suite 280
Rockville, MD 20850 240-403-1901
Fax: 240-403-1909
e-mail: ffcmh@ffcmh.org
www.ffcmh.org

Address the complex issue of trauma; the impact it has on children and families; the promotion of healing and prevention strategies; knowledge about how to address trauma through resiliency-based interventions, utilizing a familydriven, youth guided approach; and examples of how family organizations and the partners they work with are raising awareness and improving trauma-focused services and supports.

November

Teka Dempson, President
Sherri Luthe, Vice President
Sheila Pires, Treausrer

1781 NADD Conference & Exhibit Show
National Association for the Dually Diagnosed
132 Fair Street
Kingston, NY 12401 845-331-4336
800-331-5362
Fax: 845-331-4569
e-mail: info@thenadd.org
www.thenadd.org

Educating professionals, families and clients of services on standard and state-of-the-art information across many specialties; Enhancing specific skills required to provide maximum benefit to individuals with special or specific cognitive and/or developmental needs; Providing a forum for an exchange of ideas and information among professionals, families and those who may receive services.

November

Dr Robert Fletcher, CEO

1782 NAMI Convention
National Alliance on Mental Illness
3803 N Fairfax Drive, Suite 100
Arlington, VA 22203 703-524-7600
888-999-6264
Fax: 703-524-9094
TDD: 703-516-7227
e-mail: info@nami.org
www.nami.org

The NAMI Convention is packed with information, chances to network, leadership development opportunities, and lots more

July

Keris Jan Myrick, President
Kevin B Sullivan, Vice President
Clarence Jordan, Secretary

Audio Video

1783 Managing the Defiant Child
Courage To Change Publishing
PO Box 486
Wilkes-Barres, PA 18703 800-440-4003
Fax: 800-772-6499
www.couragetochange.com

An information-packed video brings to life a proven approach to behavior management. Shows clinicians, school practitioners, teachers, parents and students how enhanced parenting skills can dramatically improve the parent-child relationship.

Russell A Barkley, Editor

1784 Understanding and Treating the Hereditary Psychiatric Spectrum Disorders
Hope Press
PO Box 188
Duarte, CA 91009 818-303-0644
800-321-4039
Fax: 818-358-3520
hopepress.com

Learn with ten hours of audio tapes from a two day seminar given in May 1997 by David E Comings MD. Tapes cover: ADHD, Tourette syndrome, Obsessive-Compulsive Disorder, Conduct Disorder, Oppositional Defiant Disorder, Autism and other Hereditary Psychiatric Spectrum Disorders. Eight audio tapes.

David E Comings, MD, Presenter

1785 Understanding the Defiant Child
Courage To Change
PO Box 486
Wilkes-Barres, PA 18703 800-440-4003
Fax: 800-772-6499
www.couragetochange.com

Provides a vivid picture of what we know about Oppositional Defiant Disorder and presents real-life scenes of family interactions and commentary from parents. Illuminates the nature and causes of ODD, why it should be dealt with early, and what can be done. Ideal viewing for school practitioners, clinical child psychologists, counselors and parents coping with a defiant child.

Russell A Barkley, Editor

Web Sites

1786 Conductdisorders.com
www.conductdisorders.com

Site for parents, teachers, and family members who deal with a child with one of the defined behavioral disorders.

1787 Internet Mental Health
www.mentalhealth.com

e-mail: internetmentalhealth@shaw.ca
www.mentalhealth.com

Our goal is to improve understanding, diagnosis, and treatment of mental illness throughout the world.

Phillip W. Long, M.D., Psychiatrist

1788 NADD: National Association for the Dually Diagnosed
132 Fair Street
Kingston, NY 12401 845-331-4336
800-331-5362
Fax: 845-331-4569
e-mail: info@thenadd.org
www.thenadd.org

Nonprofit organization designed to promote the interests of professional and care providers for individuals who have the coexistence of mental illness and mental retardation. NADD provides conferences, educational services and training materials to professionals, parents, concerned citizens and service organizations.

Robert J. Fletcher, DSW, CEO
Michelle Jordan, Office Manager
Lisa Christie, Conference Planner

1789 Online Mendelian Inheritance in Man
National Library of Medicine, Building 38A
Bethesda, MD 20894
888-346-3656
e-mail: info@ncbi.nlm.nih.gov
www.ncbi.nlm.nih.gov

This database is a catalog of human genes and genetic disorders.

Christine E. Seidman, M.D., Chair
David J. Lipman, M.D., Executive Secretary

1790 Planetpsych
www.planetpsych.com

e-mail: webmaster@PlanetPsych.com
www.planetpsych.com

Planetpsych is an online resource for mental health information.

Book Publishers

1791 Aggression and Violence Throughout the Life Span
Sage Publications
2455 Teller Road
Thousand Oaks, CA 91320
800-818-7243
Fax: 800-583-2665
e-mail: info@sagepub.com
www.sagepub.com

A unique life span developmental perspective on some of society's most perplexing and pernicious problems, aggressive and violent behaviors. Examines issues in the development of aggressive behaviors in young children, the progression of these behaviors to older children and adolescents and cause, effect and treatment of aggressive and violent behaviors in adults. Integrates empirical research with clinical applications.

360 pages Softcover
ISBN: 0-803945-51-5

Sara Miller McCune, Founder/Chairman
Blaise R Simqu, President/CEO
Chris Hickok, Senior Vice President/CFO

1792 Antisocial Behavior by Young People
Cambridge University Press
32 Avenue of the Americas
New York, NY 10013
617-264-2300
Fax: 617-264-2323
e-mail: info@cambridge.org
www.cambridge.org

Written by a child psychiatrist, a criminologist and a social psychologist, this book is a major international review of research evidence on anti-social behavior. Covers all aspects of the field, including descriptions of different types of delinquency and time trends, the state of knowledge on the individuals, social-psychological and cultural factors involved and recent advances in prevention and intervention.

490 pages Paperback
ISBN: 0-521646-08-1

Michael Rutter, Editor
Ann Hagell, Editor
Henri Giller, Editor

1793 Conduct Disorders in Childhood and Adolescence (Developmental Clinical)
Sage Publications
2455 Teller Road
Thousand Oaks, CA 91320
800-818-7243
800-818-7243
Fax: 800-583-2665
e-mail: info@sagepub.com
www.sagepub.com

Conduct disorder is a clinical problem among children and adolescents that includes aggressive acts, theft, vandalism, firesetting, running away, truancy, defying authority and other antisocial behaviors. This book describes the nature of conduct disorder and what is currently known from research and clinical work. Topics include psychiatric diagnosis, parent psychopathology and child-rearing processes.

192 pages Hardcover
ISBN: 0-803971-81-8

Sara Miller McCune, Founder/Chairman
Blaise R Simqu, President/CEO
Chris Hickok, Senior Vice President/CFO

1794 Conduct Disorders in Children and Adolescents
American Psychiatric Publishing
1000 Wilson Boulevard, Suite 1825
Arlington, VA 22009
703-907-7322
800-368-5777
Fax: 703-907-1091
e-mail: appi@psych.org
www.appi.org

Examines the phenomenology, etiology, and diagnosis of conduct disorders, and describes therapeutic and preventive interventions. Includes the range of treatments now available, including individual, family, group, and behavior therapy; hospitalization; and residential treatment.

1995 414 pages Hardcover
ISBN: 0-880485-17-5

G Pirooz Sholevar, MD, Editor

1795 Conduct Problem/Emotional Problem Interventions: A Holistic Perspective
Slosson Educational Publications
PO Box 544
East Aurora, NY 14052
716-625-0930
888-756-7766
Fax: 800-655-3840
e-mail: slosson@slosson.com
www.slosson.com

This innovative book is broad in scope and addresses the now what sensation that many professionals get when charged with the education or treatment of individuals with conduct disorders or emotional disturbance. Distinct intervention and screening strategies and patient involvement strategies are offered in clear and practical terms.

Edward J Kelly, Editor

1796 Difficult Child
Random House
1745 Broadway
New York, NY 10019
212-782-9000
Fax: 212-572-6066
www.randomhouse.com

One of the nation's most respected experts on children and discipline; Dr. Stanley Turecki a father of a once difficult child offers compassionate and practical advice to parents of hard-to-raise children.

320 pages Paperback

Stanley Turecki, Writer

1797 Disruptive Behavior Disorders in Children and Adolescents
Robert L Hendren, DO, author

American Psychiatric Publishing
1000 Wilson Boulevard, Suite 1825
Arlington, VA 22209
703-907-7322
800-368-5777
Fax: 703-907-1091
e-mail: appi@psych.org
www.appi.org

Discusses attention deficit hyperactivity disorder, conduct disorder, substance abuse and disruptive behavior disorders. Examines the relationship between violence and mental illness in adolescence.

1999 216 pages Paperback
ISBN: 0-880489-60-7

1798 Preventing Antisocial Behavior: Interventions
Guilford Press
72 Spring Street
New York, NY 10012
212-431-9800
800-365-7006
Fax: 212-966-6708
e-mail: info@guilford.com
www.guilford.com

Establishes the crucial link between theory, measurement and intervention. Brings together a collection of studies that utilize experimental approaches for evaluating intervention programs, both the feasibility, and necessity of independent evaluation. Also shows how the information obtained in such studies can be used to test and refine prevailing theories about human behavior in general, and behavior changes in particular.

1992 391 pages
ISBN: 0-898628-82-1

Joan McCord, Editor
Richard Tremblay, Editor

1799 Skills Training for Children with Behavior Disorders
Courage To Change
PO Box 486
Wilkes-Barres, PA 18703
800-440-4003
Fax: 800-772-6499
www.couragetochange.com

Designed for use by both parents and therapists, provides background information, step-by-step instructions and many useful, reproducible worksheets. Techniques offered help children with anger management, compliance and following rules, academic success, emotional well-being and self-esteem and much more.

272 pages

Michael L Bloomquist, Editor

Pamphlets

1800 Conduct Disorder in Children and Adolescents
National Mental Health Information Center
PO Box 42557
Washington, DC 20015
800-789-2647
Fax: 240-747-5470
TDD: 866-889-2647
e-mail: ken@mentalhealth.org
www.mentalhealth.samhsa.gov

This fact sheet defines conduct disorder, identifies risk factors, discusses types of help available, and suggests what parents or other caregivers can do.

1997 2 pages

1801 Mental, Emotional, and Behavior Disorders in Children and Adolescents
National Mental Health Information
PO Box 42557
Washington, DC 20015
240-747-5484
800-789-2647
Fax: 240-747-5470
mentalhealth.samhsa.gov

This fact sheet describes mental, emotional, and behavioral problems that can occur during childhood and adolescence and discusses related treatment, support services, and research.

4 pages

1802 Treatment of Children with Mental Disorder
National Institute of Mental Health
PO Box 5801
Bethesda, MD 20824
301-496-5751
800-352-9424
Fax: 301-443-4279
TTY: 301-443-8431
e-mail: nimhinfo@nih.gov
www.nimh.nih.gov

A short booklet that contains questions and answers about therapy for children with mental disorders. Includes a chart of mental disorders and medications used.

Walter J. Koroshetz, M.D., Acting Director
Alan L. Willard, Ph.D., Acting Deputy Director
Caroline Lewis, Executive Officer

Camps

1803 Adventure Learning Center Camp Programs
Eagle Village
4507 170th Avenue
Hersey, MI 49639
231-832-2234
800-748-0061
Fax: 231-832-1468
e-mail: summercamp@eaglevillage.org
www.eaglevillage.org

Offers a variety of fun camp experiences for children, including those with emotional and/or behavioral impairments. A low staff-to-camper ratio and exciting, challenging activities make the camps rewarding experiences. As funding is available, we will offer camp scholarships to eligible participants.

Sara Kofal, Camp Director

1804 Life Adventure Center
Life Adventure Center of the Bluegrass
PO Box 447
Versailles, KY 40383
859-873-3271
Fax: 859-873-2410
www.lifeadventurecamp.org

A unique experience of discovery and development where lifelong lessons are learned. Through purposeful play, using a combination of physical and mental problem-solving exercises, participants engage in opportunities to make positive choices, gain self-confidence, improve decision making, build on group strengths and much more.

1805 Talisman Summer Camps
Talisman Schools
64 Gap Creek Road
Zirconia, NC 28790
855-588-8254
Fax: 828-669-2521
e-mail: summer@talismancamps.com
www.talismansummercamp.com/

Camps for children ages 6 to 17 and young adults 18-21 with LD, ADD and ADHD, Asperger's Syndrome, and high functioning autism. Talisman has been offering such experiences since 1980 and is ACA accredited. The unique summer camps specialize in creating camps that offer not only adventure, but learning experiences, for children and teenagers with learning disabilities, attention deficit hyperactivity disorder, Asperger's syndrome and high-functioning autism.

Linda Tatsapaugh, Director
Aaron McGinley, Base Camp Program Manager

Description

1806 CONGENITAL ADRENAL HYPERPLASIA

Synonyms: CAH, Androgenital syndrome, Congenital virilizing adrenal hyper, 21-hydroxylase deficiency, 11-beta-hydroxylase deficiency

Involves the following Biologic System(s):

Endocrinologic Disorders

Congenital adrenal hyperplasia (CAH) refers to a group of genetic diseases that leads to the inability of the adrenal glands to make cortisol. Cortisol is a steroid hormone needed to maintain metabolism, energy, blood pressure, and a normal responses to stress or injury. There are many different steps in the production of cortisol; each step requires an enzyme for completion and as a result, a deficiency in any enzyme along the path leads to one of the forms of CAH. The inability to make cortisol leads to symptoms from both the lack of cortisol as well as from the build-up of the cortisol precursors. In CAH, male hormones (androgens) are made in excess and this will lead to exaggerated male characteristics in these patients. Some people with CAH also have deficiency in another hormone, aldosterone. Aldosterone regulates salt (sodium)levels in the body.

Symptoms of CAH can vary in girls and boys, and also may vary according to the specific type of CAH. In girls, the excess of androgens leads to masculinization of the female external genitalia (ambiguous genitalia). Symptoms in girls with milder forms of CAH include irregular menstrual periods, excessive or male pattern hair growth, or infertility. In boys, symptoms of salt-wasting CAH include adrenal crisis which typically consists of low blood pressure and sodium abnormalities. Girls can also have salt abnormalities, but are often diagnosed before an adrenal crisis because of their ambiguous external genitalia can be seen. In boys with non-salt wasting CAH, the effect of excess androgens leads to pubertal changes earlier than expected (precocious puberty).

The treatment of CAH is replacement of cortisol with glucocorticoid medications, and if needed, replacement of aldosterone with mineralocorticoid medications. It is important to remember to give extra medication (stress dose steroids during times of stress, illness, or injury because of the body's greater demand for steroids during those times.)

National Associations & Support Groups

1807 American Academy of Pediatrics
141 Northwest Point Boulevard
Elk Grove Village, IL 60007

847-434-4000
800-433-9016
Fax: 847-434-8000
www.aap.org

The American Academy of Pediatrics and its member pediatricians are committed to the attainment of optimal physical, mental and social health and well-being for all infants, children, adolescents, and young adults.

Sandra Hassink, MD, FAAP, President

1808 CARES Foundation
2414 Morris Avenue, Suite 110
Union, NJ 07083

973-912-3895
866-227-3737
Fax: 973-912-8990
e-mail: karenf@caresfoundation.org
www.caresfoundation.org

CARES Foundation is a nonprofit, educational organization. Its purpose is to educate the public and physicians about all forms of Congenital Adrenal Hyerplasia, its symptoms, diagnostic protocols, treatment, genetic frequency, the necessity for early intervention and benefits of newborn screening. It is also dedicated to providing support and information to affected individuals and their families.

Dina Matos, Executive Director
Cindy Rogers, Director of Finance and Operations
Karen Fountain, Program Manager

1809 MAGIC Foundation: Major Aspects of Growth in Children
6645 W North Avenue
Oak Park, IL 60302

708-383-0808
800-362-4423
Fax: 708-383-0899
e-mail: ContactUs@magicfoundation.org
www.magicfoundation.org

A national nonprofit organization providing support and education regarding growth disorders in children and related adult disorders. Provides educational information, networking, a national conference, a kids' program and an extensive medical library.

10,000 members

Rich Buckley, Chairman
Ken Dickard, Vice Chairman
Teresa Tucker, Director at Large

1810 National Adrenal Diseases Foundation
505 Northern Boulevard
Great Neck, NY 11021

516-487-4992
e-mail: nadfmail@aol.com
www.nadf.us/nadf/index.htm

NADF is committed to bringing information regarding adrenal diseases into the public's awareness to facilitate early diagnosis and treatment.NADF sponsors support groups across the countrty allowing for an exchange of ideas and feelings by individuals who share a common illness. NADF members receive quaterly newsletters, educational materials, and access to a library of related information.

Kalina Warren, President
Timothy Skodon, Treasurer
Paul Margulies, M.D, FACP, FACE-Medical Director

Libraries & Resource Centers

1811 University of Iowa Birth Defects and Genetic Disorders Unit
2614 JCP
Iowa City, IA 52242
James M Smith, Director

319-335-9901

Conferences

1812 Adult GHD Educational Convention
Magic Foundation
6645 W North Avenue
Oak Park, IL 60302

708-383-0808
800-362-4423
Fax: 708-383-0899
e-mail: contactus@magicfoundation.org
www.magicfoundation.org

An educational program for adults who are affected with Growth Hormone Deficiency and/or other endocrine disorders.

June

Rich Buckley, Chairman
Ken Dickard, Vice Chairman
Courtney Lance, Secretary

Web Sites

1813 CARES Foundation
2414 Morris Ave., Suite 110
Union, NJ 7083
                                  908-364-0272
                                  866-227-3737
                              Fax: 908-686-2019
              e-mail: contact@caresfoundation.org
                          www.caresfoundation.org

Provides education to the public and physicians about all forms of
Congenital Adrenal Hyperplasia — symptoms, diagnostic protocols, treatment, genetic frequency, the necessity for early intervention and benefits of newborn screening. The web site also
provides support and information to affected individuals and their
families.

Katherine L. Fowler, President
Chad Lapp, Vice President
Alexandra Dubois, Secretary

1814 MAGIC Foundation: Major Aspects of Growth in Children
6645 W. North Avenue
Oak Park, IL 60302
                                  708-383-0808
                                  800-362-4423
          e-mail: ContactUs@magicfoundation.org
                          www.magicfoundation.org

Created to provide support services for the families of children
afflicted with a wide variety of chronic and/or critical disorders,
syndromes, and diseases that affect a child's growth.

Rich Buckley, Chair
Ken Dickard, Vice Chair
Mary Andrews, CEO

1815 National Adrenal Diseases Foundation
505 Northern Boulevard
Great Neck, NY 11021
                                  516-487-4992
                  e-mail: nadfsupport@nadf.us
                                  www.nadf.us

Committed to bringing information regarding rare diseases to the
publics awareness to facilitate early diagnosis and treatment.

Kalina Warren, President
Melanie G. Wong, Executive Director
Paul Margulies, MD, FACP, Medical Director

Newsletters

1816 CARES Foundation Newsletter
2414 Morris Avenue, Suite 110
Union, NJ 7083
                                  973-912-3895
                                  866-227-3737
              e-mail: kelly@caresfoundation.org
                          www.caresfoundation.org

Provides support and information to affected individuals and their
families.

3x year

Kelly R Leight, Executive Director

1817 NADF News
505 Northern Boulevard
Great Neck, NY 11021
                                  516-487-4992
                  e-mail: nadfsupport@nadf.us
                                  www.nadf.us

Features important information on adrenal disorders, support
groups and the latest research.

quaterly

Kalina Warren, President
Melanie G Wong, Executive Director
Paul Margulies, MD, FACP, Medical Director

Description

1818 CONGENITAL CATARACTS
Involves the following Biologic System(s):
Genetic/Chromosomal/Syndrome/Metabolic Disorders,
Ophthalmologic Disorders

Congenital cataracts refers to a condition in which cloudiness or opacities in the lens of the eye or eyes are present at birth. These opacities may vary in severity, with some resolving spontaneously as in cataracts of prematurity. Other congenital cataracts, if left untreated, may result in loss of transparency of the lens and subsequent visual impairment. In addition, in some newborns, remnants of other eye tissues may contribute to the formation of a stationary opacity of the cornea. In most instances , this type of stationary cloudiness does not contribute to visual impairment.

Congenital cataracts may occur as the result of many different factors (multifactorial), including genetic influences, associated metabolic and chromosomal disorders, congenital infections, and toxic exposure. If inherited as an isolated event, congenital cataracts are usually transmitted as an autosomal dominant or autosomal recessive trait. Several metabolic disorders are characterized by congenital cataracts, including galactosemia, in which an enzyme deficiency results in the inability to process the simple sugar galactose; oculocerebrorenal syndrome (Lowe's syndrome), an X-linked metabolic disorder that affects many systems of the body; certain metabolic diseases known as lyosomal storage disorders; and several other diseases related to inborn errors of metabolism. Other contributing metabolic factors may include low blood levels of calcium (hypocalcemia) or glucose (hypoglycemia). In addition, cataracts are sometimes diagnosed in newborns whose mothers have diabetes mellitus. Several chromosomal disorders are also characterized by congenital opacities including Down's syndrome (trisomy 21), trisomy 13 syndrome, Turner's syndrome (45XO), and others. Congenital cataracts are sometimes the result of maternal infections that occur during pregnancy. Such infections may include German measles (rubella), syphilis, measles, influenza, certain herpes infections, and others. Additional contributing factors may include toxic influences from drug substances taken by the mother during pregnancy.

Treatment for congenital cataracts depends upon the extent of the defect and its influence on vision. To restore lost transparency of the lens resulting from cataracts, surgery may be performed in which the cataract and lens are removed. To reestablish the ability of the eye to deflect light that was lost with lens removal, special contact lenses or implants are then fitted to the eye. In some cases, additional surgery may be indicated. Because congenital opacities of the lens are so often associated with other eye irregularities (e.g., amblyopia, glaucoma, strabismus, etc.) and in order to obtain the best outcome, treatment may also be directed toward any associated abnormalities. In addition, patients are followed carefully after surgery in order to prevent, correct, or treat any possible complications.

Government Agencies

1819 NIH/National Eye Institute
31 Center Drive MSC 2510
Bethesda, MD 10027
301-496-5248
e-mail: 2020@nei.nih.gov
www.nei.nih.gov

Conducts and supports research that helps prevent and treat eye diseases and other disorders of vision. This research leads to sight-saving treatments, reduces visual impairment and blindness, and improves the quality of life for people of all ages. NEI-supported research has advanced our knowledge of how the eye functions in health and disease.

Paul A Sieving M.D., Ph.D., Director

National Associations & Support Groups

1820 American Academy of Pediatrics
141 Northwest Point Boulevard
Elk Grove Village, IL 60007
847-434-4000
800-433-9016
Fax: 847-434-8000
www.aap.org

The American Academy of Pediatrics and its member pediatricians are committed to the attainment of optimal physical, mental and social health and well-being for all infants, children, adolescents, and young adults.

Sandra Hassink, MD, FAAP, President

1821 American Council of the Blind
2200 Wilson Boulevard Suite 650
Arlington, VA 22201
202-467-5081
800-424-8666
Fax: 202-467-5085
e-mail: info@acb.org
www.acb.org

The American Council of the Blind strives to increase the independence, security, equality of opportunity, and quality of life, for all blind and visually-impaired people.

Melanie Brunson, Executive Director
Mitch Pomerantz, President
Kim Charlson, First Vice President

1822 Association for Education & Rehabilitation of the Blind & Visually Impaired
1703 N Beauregard Street, Suite 440
Alexandria, VA 22311
703-671-4500
877-492-2708
Fax: 703-671-6391
e-mail: markr@aerbvi.org
www.aerbvi.org

The Association for Education and Rehabilitation of the Blind and Visually Impaired (AER) is the only international membership organization dedicated to rendering all possible support and assistance to the professionals who work in all phases of education and rehabilitation of blind and visually impaired children and adults. Our membership is comprised of more than 4,200 professionalswho provide services to people with visual impairment.

Lou Tutt, Executive Director
Ginger Croce, Senior Director, Marketing and Offi
Barbara James, Director, Membership and Office Ope

1823 Genetic Alliance
4301 Connecticut Avenue NW Suite 404
Washington, DC 20008
202-966-7955
800-336-4363
Fax: 202-966-8553
e-mail: info@geneticalliance.org
www.geneticalliance.org

World's leading nonprofit health advocacy organization committed to transforming health through genetics and promoting an environment of openness centered on the health of individuals, families, and communities.

Sharon Terry, President
Lisa Wise, Chief Operating Officer
Tetyana Murza MES, Programs and Policy Coordinator

1824 National Association for Parents of Children with Visual Impairments
175 N Beacon Street
Watertown, MA 00247
617-972-7441
800-562-6265
Fax: 617-972-7444
e-mail: napvi@guildhealth.org
www.spedex.com/napvi/

NAPVI is a national organization that enables parents to find information and resources for their children who are blind or visually impaired, including those with additional disabilities. NAPVI provides leadership, support, and training to assist parents in helping children reach their potential.

Susan LaVenture, Executive Director
Julie Urban, President
Venetia Hayden, Vice President

1825 National Association for Visually Handicapped
111 East 59th Street The Sol and Lillian Goldman B
New York, NY 10022
212-821-9200
800-829-0500
Fax: 212-821-9707
TTY: 212-821-9713
e-mail: info@lighthouse.org
www.lighthouse.org/navh

The only nonprofit health organization in the world solely dedicated to providing assistance to the partially sighted. Serves as a clearinghouse for information about all services available to the partially-sighted from public and private sources. Conducts self-help groups. Provides information on large print books, textbooks and educational tools.

Mark G. Ackermann, President and Chief Executive Offic
Maura J. Sweeney, Senior Vice President, Chief Operat
John Vlachos, Senior Vice President, Chief Financ

State Agencies & Support Groups

Alabama

1826 Alabama Institute for the Deaf & Blind
PO Box 698 (35161) 205 East South Street
Talladega, AL 35160
256-761-3331
Fax: 256-761-3344
www.aidb.org

Services include central directory, representatives of agencies, service providers, families, and coordinators of infant, toddler, and preschool special education programs.

Charlotte Lowry, Principal
Martha Waites, Director, Academic Department
Teresa Lacy, Director, Library and Resource Cent

Arizona

1827 National Association for Parents of the Visually Impaired
175 N Beacon Street
Watertown, MA 02472
617-972-7441
800-562-6265
Fax: 617-972-7444
e-mail: napvi@guildhealth.org
www.spedex.com/napvi/

NAPVI is a national organization that enables parents to find information and resources for their children who are blind or visually impaired, including those with additional disabilities. NAPVI provides leadership, support, and training to assist parents in helping children reach their potential.

Susan LaVenture, Executive Director
Julie Urban, President
Venetia Hayden, Vice President

Ohio

1828 Region 2 of the National Association for Parents of the Visually Impaired
3910 Pocahontas Avenue
Cincinnati, OH 45227
513-561-8542
e-mail: napvi@guildhealth.org
www.spedex.com/napvi

Susan LaVenture, Executive Director
Julie Urban, President
Venetia Hayden, Vice President

Pennsylvania

1829 East Central Region-Helen Keller National Center
4351 Garden City Drive
New Carrollton, MD 20785
301-459-5474
Fax: 301-459-5070
e-mail: hkncreg3cl@aol.com
www.helenkeller.org

Christopher D Maher, Chairman
Richard T. Arkwright, Vice-Chairman
John R Caughey, Treasurer

South Carolina

1830 Region 4 of the National Association for Parents of the Visually Impaired
1032 Trail Road
Belton, SC 29627
864-338-9593

Washington

1831 Northwestern Region-Helen Keller National Center
1620 18th Ave Suite 201
Seattle, WA 98122
206-324-9120
Fax: 206-324-9159
TTY: 206-324-1133
e-mail: nwhknc@juno.com
www.hknc.org/FieldServicesREGREPADD.htm

The Regional Representatives of HKNC are located in ten offices across the country. They are responsible for assessing the needs of individuals, communities and states within their regions; developing strategies of collaboration, coordination and cooperation to help meet those needs; advocating for those who are deaf-blind in local, state, national and international forums.

Libraries & Resource Centers

Arizona

1832 Educational Services for the Visually Impaired
PO Box 668
Little Rock, AR 72203
501-371-5710

Offers textbooks, braille books and more to the visually impaired grades K-12 in the Arkansas area.

David Beavers, Director

Arkansas

1833 Arkansas Regional Library for the Blind and Physically Handicapped
900 W Capitol, Suite 100
Little Rock, AR 72201
501-682-2053
Fax: 501-682-1533
TDD: 501-682-1002
e-mail: nlsbooks@asl.lib.ar.us
www.asl.lib.ar.us/ASL_LBPH.htm

Public library books in recorded or braille format. Popular fiction and nonfiction books for all ages, books and players are on free loan, sent to patrons by mail and may be returned postage free. Anyone who cannot see well enough to read regular print with glasses on or who has a disability that makes it difficult to hold a book or turn the pages is eligible.

John D Hall, Director

California

1834 American Action Fund for Blind Children and Adults
1800 Johnson Street
Baltimore, MD 21230   410-659-9315
                                   Fax: 818-343-3219
                            e-mail: lucyabba@aol.com
                                   www.actionfund.org

A lending library for the visually impaired. We send out a weekly Braille newspaper for the deaf-blind (worldwide), we also send out pocket-sized Braille calendars. Our lending library is for pre-school thru high school. All of our services are free.

Barbara Loos, President
Ramona Walhof, Vice President
Gary Mackenstadt, Secretary

1835 Blind Children's Center
4120 Marathon Street
Los Angeles, CA 90029   323-664-2153
                                   Fax: 323-665-3828
                            www.blindchildrenscenter.org

Offers support and informational groups.

Midge Horton, Executive Director

1836 Braille Institute Desert Center
741 N Vermont Avenue
Los Angeles, CA 90029   323-663-1111
                                   Fax: 323-663-0867
                            e-mail: la@brailleinstitute.org
                                   www.brailleinstitute.org

Dedicated to providing blind and visually impaired men, women and children with the training, programs and services they need to enjoy productive lives. Services offered include child development, youth programs, library services and adult education.

Lars Hansen, Manager

1837 Braille Institute Sight Center
741 N Vermont Avenue
Los Angeles, CA 90029   323-663-1111
                                   Fax: 323-663-0867
                            e-mail: la@brailleinstitute.org
                                   www.brailleinstitute.org

Offers help, programs, services and information to the blind and visually impaired children and adults.

Les Stocker, President

1838 Braille Institute Youth Center
3450 Cahuenga Boulevard W
Los Angeles, CA 90068   213-851-5695

Offers various youth programs and services for the blind and visually impaired youngster.

1839 New Beginnings - Blind Children's Center
4120 Marathon, Street
Los Angeles, CA 90029   323-664-2153
                                        800-222-3566
                                   Fax: 323-665-3828

Helps children and their families become independent by creating a climate of safety and trust. Services include an infant stimulation program, educational preschool, interdisciplinary assessment services, family services, correspondence program, toll-free national hotline and a publication and research service.

1840 San Francisco Public Library for the Blind and Print Disabled
PO Box 9428327
Sacramento, CA 94237   916-654-0261
                                   Fax: 415-557-4252
                            e-mail: lbphmgr@sfpl.lib.ca.us
                                   www.library.ca.us

Foreign-language books on cassette, children's books on cassettes and more.

Luis Herrera, Manager

1841 Variety Audio
PO Box 5731
San Jose, CA 95150   408-277-4839

Summer reading programs, braille writer, magnifiers, closed-circuit TV, large-print photocopier, cassette books and magazines, children's books on cassette, home visits and other reference materials on blindness and other handicaps.

Louisa Griehshammer

District of Columbia

1842 Council of Families with Visual Impairment
1155 15th Street NW
Washington, DC 20005   202-467-5081

Members are sighted parents of blind or visually impaired children. Offers a forum for support and outreach, sharing of experiences in parent-child relationships, and educational and cultural information about child development. Monitors developments in technical and legislative arenas.

Nola Webb, President

Florida

1843 Florida Bureau of Braille and Talking Book Library Services
420 Platt Street
Daytona Beach, FL 32114   386-239-6000
                                   Fax: 386-239-6069
                                   TDD: 800-226-6079
                            e-mail: mike_gunde@dbs.doe.state.fl.us
                                   www.state.fl.us/dbs/lswel.html

Discs, cassettes, closed-circuit TV, large-print photocopier, films, children's books on cassettes and more.

Michael Gunde, Librarian

1844 Talking Book Library, Jacksonville Public Library
2233 Park Avenue, Suite 402
Orange Park, FL 32073   904-278-5620
                                   Fax: 904-278-5625
                                   TDD: 904-768-7822
                            e-mail: jerryr@coj.net
                                   www.neflin.org

Discs, cassettes and reference materials on blindness and other disabilities.

Jerry Reynolds, Librarian Senior

1845 Talking Book Service - Manatee County Central Library
1112 Manatee Avenue West
Bradenton, FL 34205   941-748-4501
                                   Fax: 941-751-7089
                                   TDD: 941-742-5951
                            e-mail: webmaster@mymanatee.org
                                   www.mymanatee.org

Offers children's books on disc and cassette and more reference materials for the blind and physically handicapped.

Patricia Schubert, Librarian

Georgia

1846 Albany Library for the Blind and Physical Handicapped
300 Pine Avenue
Albany, GA 31701   229-420-3220
                              Fax: 229-420-3215
e-mail: sinquefk@mail.dougherty.public.lib.ga.us
www.docolib.org/LBPH/index.html

Offers discs, cassettes, reference materials on blindness and other handicaps, large-print photocopiers, summer reading programs, cassette books and more.

Katy Sinquefield, Manager

1847 Bainbridge Subregional Library for the Blind and Physically Handicapped
215 Sycamore Street
Decatur, GA 30030   404-370-8450
                                    800-795-2680
                              Fax: 404-370-8469
                              TDD: 912-248-2665
e-mail: lbph@mail.deccatur.public.lib.ga.us
www.dekalblibrary.org

Discs, cassettes, summer reading programs, closed-circuit TV, magnifiers and more.

Jon Abercrombie, Chairman
Julia H Jones, Vice Chairman
Elizabeth Joyner, Treasurer

1848 CEL Subregional Library for the Blind and Physically Handicapped
2708 Mechanics
Savannah, GA 31404   912-354-5864
                              Fax: 912-354-5534
                              TDD: 912-652-3635
e-mail: stokesl@cel.co.chatman.ga.us

Summer reading programs, braille writer, magnifiers, closed-circuit TV, large-print photocopier, cassette books and magazines, children's books on cassette, home visits and other reference materials on blindness and other handicaps.

Linda Stokes, Librarian

Idaho

1849 Idaho State Talking Book Library
325 W State Street
Boise, ID 83702   208-334-2150
                                    800-458-3271
                              Fax: 208-334-4016
                              TDD: 800-377-1363
e-mail: tblbooks@isl.state.id.us
www.lili.org/isl/tblinfo.htm

Summer reading programs, braille writer, magnifiers, closed-circuit TV, large-print photocopier, cassette books and magazines, children's books on cassette, home visits and other reference materials on blindness and other handicaps.

Sue Walker, Manager

Illinois

1850 Chicago Library Service for the Blind
1055 W Roosevelt Road
Chicago, IL 60608   312-746-9210

Summer reading programs, braille writer, magnifiers, closed-circuit TV, large-print photocopier, cassette books and magazines, children's books on cassette, home visits and other reference materials on blindness and other handicaps.

Carol Pellish, Librarian

1851 Illinois State Library, Talkng Book and Braille Service
213 State Capitol
Springfield, IL 62756   217-785-5600
                              Fax: 217-785-4326
                              TDD: 800-665-5576
e-mail: sruda@ilsos.net
www.cyberdriveillinois.com

Summer reading programs, braille writer, magnifiers, closed-circuit TV, large-print photocopier, cassette books and magazines, descriptive videos, children's books on cassette, home visits and other reference materials on blindness and other handicaps.

Anne Craig, Executive Director

1852 Mid Illinois Talking Book System
515 York Street
Quincy, IL 62301   217-224-6619
                              Fax: 217-224-9818

Summer reading programs, braille writer, magnifiers, closed-circuit TV, large-print photocopier, cassette books and magazines, children's books on cassette, home visits and other reference materials on blindness and other handicaps.

1853 Mid-Illinois Talking Book Center
600 High Point Lane
East Peoria, IL 61611   309-353-4110
                                    800-426-0709
                              Fax: 309-353-8281
e-mail: hitbc@darkstar.rsa.lib.il.us
www.mitbc.org

Summer reading programs, braille writer, magnifiers, closed-circuit TV, large-print photocopier, cassette books and magazines, children's books on cassette, home visits and other reference materials on blindness and other handicaps.

Eileen Sheppard, Librarian

1854 Talking Book Center of Northwest Illinois
Ste 2
East Peoria, IL 61611   309-694-9200
                              Fax: 309-799-7916
e-mail: kodean@libby.rbls.lib.il.us
www.rbls.lib.il.us

Subregional library provides Talking Book and Braille Book programs to eligible persons unable to use standard print materials due to visual or physical disabilities. Includes cassette books and magazines; summer reading program.

Indiana

1855 Northwest Indiana Subregional Library for Blind and Physically Handicapped
1919 W Lincoln Highway
Merrillville, IN 46410   219-769-3541
                              Fax: 219-769-0690

Summer reading programs, braille writer, magnifiers, closed-circuit TV, large-print photocopier, cassette books and magazines, children's books on cassette, home visits and other reference materials on blindness and other handicaps.

Renee Lewis

Iowa

1856 Iowa Library for the Blind and Physically Handicapped
Iowa Department for the Blind
524 4th Street
Des Moines, IA 50309   515-281-1333
                              Fax: 515-281-1378
                              TDD: 515-281-1355
e-mail: keninger.karen@blind.state.ia.us
www.blind.state.ia.us

Summer reading programs, magnifiers, closed-circuit TV, large-print photocopier, children's books on cassette, children's books in Braille and Print Braille, cassette magazines, home visits and reference materials on blindness and other handicaps.

Karen Keninger, Program Manager/Librarian

1857 University of Iowa Birth Defects and Genetic Disorders Unit
2614 JCP
Iowa City, IA 52242   319-335-9901
James M Smith, Director

Kansas

1858 CKLS Headquarters
PO Box 515
Northampton, MA 01061   413-268-7660
                                          888-622-8527
                                     Fax: 316-792-5495
                              e-mail: amdf@mascular.org
                                       www.macular.org

Summer reading programs, braille writer, magnifiers, closed-circuit TV, large-print photocopier, cassette books and magazines, children's books on cassette, home visits and other reference materials on blindness and other handicaps.

Chip Goehring, President/Treasurer
Mark E Torrey, Vice President
Paul F Gariepy, Secretary

1859 Services for the Visually Disabled
629 Poyntz Avenue
Manhattan, KS 66502   785-776-4741
                                     Fax: 785-776-1545
                       e-mail: marionr@manhattan.lib.ks.us

Summer reading programs, braille writer, magnifiers, closed-circuit TV, large-print photocopier, cassette books and magazines, children's books on cassette, home visits and other reference materials on blindness and other handicaps.

Marion Rice, Librarian

Kentucky

1860 Kentucky Library for the Blind and Physically Handicapped
PO Box 818
Frankfort, KY 40602   502-564-8300
                                          800-372-2968
                                     Fax: 502-564-5773
                        e-mail: richard.feindel@kdla.net
                              www.kdla.net/libserv/ktbl.htm

Large-print photocopier, cassette books and magazines, children's books on cassette, and other reference materials on blindness and other handicaps.

5,200 members

Richard Feindel, Librarian

Maryland

1861 Maryland State Library for the Blind and Physically Handicapped
415 Park Avenue
Baltimore, MD 21201   410-230-2424
                                     Fax: 410-333-2095
                                     TTY: 800-934-2541
                                     TDD: 410-333-8679
                          e-mail: recept@lbta.lib.md.us
                                     www.lbph.lib.md.us

Summer reading programs, braille writer, magnifiers, large-print photocopier, cassette books and magazines, children's books on cassette, and other reference materials on blindness and other handicaps.

Jill Lewis, Manager

1862 Prince George's County Memorial Library Talking Book Center
6530 Adelphi Road
Hyattsville, MD 20782   301-779-9330

Summer reading programs, braille writer, magnifiers, closed-circuit TV, large-print photocopier, cassette books and magazines, children's books on cassette, home visits and other reference materials on blindness and other handicaps.

Shirley Tuthill, Librarian

Massachusetts

1863 Braille and Talking Book Library Perkins School for the Blind
175 N Beacon Street
Watertown, MA 02472   617-924-3434
                                     Fax: 617-972-7315
                              e-mail: info@perkins.org
                                       www.perkins.org

Steven M Rothstein, President
Micheal Schnitman, Secretary
Charles C J Platt, Treasurer

Michigan

1864 Downtown Detroit Subregional Library for the Blind and Handicapped
5201 Woodward Avenue
Detroit, MI 48202   313-224-0580
                                     Fax: 313-965-1977
                                     TDD: 313-224-0584
                     e-mail: dir@detroitpubliclibrary.org
                                   www.detroit.lib.mi.us

Summer reading programs, braille writer, magnifiers, closed-circuit TV, large-print photocopier, cassette books and magazines, children's books on cassette, home visits and other reference materials on blindness and other handicaps.

Russell Bellant, President
Gregory Hicks, Vice President
Jonathan C Kinloch, Secretary

1865 Kent County Library for the Blind
775 Ball Avenue NE
Grand Rapids, MI 49503   616-336-3250
                                     Fax: 616-336-3201
                          e-mail: kdlem@lakeland.lib.mi.us

Summer reading programs, braille writer, magnifiers, closed-circuit TV, large-print photocopier, cassette books and magazines, children's books on cassette, home visits and other reference materials on blindness and other handicaps.

Claudya Muller, Librarian

1866 Library of Michigan Service for the Blind
PO Box 30007
Lansing, MI 48909   517-373-1300
                                     Fax: 517-373-5700
                       e-mail: info@sbph.libomich.lib.mi.us

Summer reading programs, braille writer, magnifiers, closed-circuit TV, large-print photocopier, cassette books and magazines, children's books on cassette, home visits and other reference materials on blindness and other handicaps.

Nancy Robertson, Manager

1867 Macomb Library for the Blind and Physically Handicapped
16480 Hall Road
Clinton Township, MI 48038   586-286-1580
                                     Fax: 586-286-0634
                                     TDD: 810-869-40
                           e-mail: macbld@libcoop.net
                              www.macomb.lib.mi.us/macspe/

Summer reading programs, braille writer, closed-circuit TV, cassette books and magazines, children's books on cassette, reference materials on blindness and other handicaps.

Beverlee Babcock, Executive Director

1868 Mideastern Michigan Library Co-op
G-4195 W Pasadena Avenue
Flint, MI 48504   810-732-1120
                                     Fax: 810-732-1715
                       e-mail: cnash@genesse.freeret.org
                              www.fakon.edu/gdl/talking.htm

Summer reading programs, braille writer, magnifiers, large-print photocopier, cassette books and magazines, children's books on cassette, home visits and other reference materials on blindness and other handicaps.

Carolyn Nash, Librarian

1869 Muskegon County Library for the Blind
635 Ottawa Street
Muskegon, MI 49442

231-724-6361
Fax: 231-724-6675
TDD: 231-722-4103
www.muskcolib.org

Summer reading programs, braille typewriter, magnifiers, closed-circuit TV, large-print photocopier, cassette books and magazines, children's books on cassette, home visits and other reference materials on blindness and other handicaps, The Reading Edge, Perkins Brailler and large print books.

Linda Clapp, Librarian

1870 Upper Peninsula Library for the Blind Physically Handicapped
1615 Presque Isle Avenue
Marquette, MI 49855

906-228-7697
Fax: 906-228-5627
e-mail: uproc.lib.mi.us
www.upesc.lib.mi.us/uplbph

Summer reading programs, braille writer, magnifiers, closed-circuit TV, large-print photocopier, cassette books and magazines, children's books on cassette, home visits and other reference materials on blindness and other handicaps.

Suzanne Dees, Executive Director

1871 Washtenaw County Library
PO Box 8645
Ann Arbor, MI 48107

734-994-4912
Fax: 734-663-2430
e-mail: contact us@ewashtenaw.org
www.ewashtenaw.org

Summer reading programs, braille writer, magnifiers, closed-circuit TV, large-print photocopier, cassette books and magazines, children's books on cassette, home visits and other reference materials on blindness and other handicaps.

Kyeena Slater, Executive Director

1872 Washtenaw County Library for the Blind and Physically Disabled
PO Box 8645
Ann Arbor, MI 48107

734-222-4357
Fax: 734-222-6850
e-mail: lbpd@co.washtennaw.mi.us
www.ewashtenaw.org

Book lovers club.adaptive technology,cassette equipment, cassette books and magazines, described videos, low vision aids reference and referral services.

Kyeena Slater, Executive Director

1873 Wayne County Regional Library for the Blind
30555 Michigan Avenue
Westland, MI 48186

734-727-7300
888-968-2737
Fax: 734-727-7333
TTY: 734-727-7330
e-mail: wcrlbph@wayneregional.lib.mi.us
www.wayneregional.lib.mi.us

Summer reading programs, braille writer, magnifiers, closed-circuit TV, large-print photocopier, cassette books and magazines, children's books on cassette, home visits and other reference materials on blindness and other handicaps.

Reginald Williams, Wayne County Librarian

Minnesota

1874 Minnesota Library for the Blind & Physically Handicapped
Highway 298, PO Box 68
Fairbault, MN 55021

507-333-4828
800-722-0550
Fax: 507-333-4832
e-mail: libblnd@state.mn.us
www.nfb.org/libraries for the blind

Summer reading programs, braille writer, magnifiers, closed-circuit TV, large-print photocopier, cassette, large print, braille books and magazines, children's books on cassette, and other reference materials on blindness and other handicaps.

Catherine A Durivage, Program Director

Missouri

1875 Adriene Resource Center for Blind Children
1445 N. Boonville Avenue
Springfield, MO 65802

417-862-2781
800-641-4310
Fax: 417-862-7566
e-mail: blind@ag.org
www.gospelpublishing.com

Offers braille and cassette lending library, braille and cassette Sunday school materials for all ages, braille and cassette periodicals and resource assistance, and resources for blind children and children of blind parents.

Paul Weingariner, Director

1876 Assemblies of God National Center for the Blind
1445 N. Boonville Avenue
Springfield, MO 65802

417-862-2781
877-840-4800
Fax: 417-863-6614
e-mail: info@aq.org
www.ag.org

Offers braille and cassette lending library, braille and cassette Sunday school materials for all ages, braille and cassette periodicals and resource assistance, and resources for blind children and children of blind parents.

Thomas Trask, Manager
Greg Mundis, Executive Director

1877 Wolfner Memorial Library for the Blind
PO Box 387
Jefferson City, MO 65102

573-751-8720
Fax: 573-526-2985
TDD: 800-347-1379
e-mail: beckles@mail.sos.state.mo.us
www.nfb.org/libraries for the blind

Summer reading programs, braille writer, magnifiers, closed-circuit TV, large-print photocopier, cassette books and magazines, children's books on cassette, home visits and other reference materials on blindness and other handicaps.

Richard J Smith, Executive Director

Nebraska

1878 Nebraska Library Commission Talking Book & Braille Services
1200 N Street
Lincoln, NE 68508

402-471-2045
800-742-7691
Fax: 402-471-2083
TDD: 402-471-4038
e-mail: david.oertli@nebraska.gov
www.nlc.nebraska.gov

Free loan of books and magazines on cartridge, cassette, and in Braille, including children's materials, along with specially designed playback equipment. Summer reading program for children, Braille embossing, closed circuit TV, large-print copier. Reference materials on blindness and other disabilities.

David Oerti, Librarian

New Jersey

1879 New Jersey State Library Talking Book and Braille Center
185 West State Street
Trenton, NJ 08625

609-278-2640
800-792-8322
Fax: 609-278-2647
TDD: 877-882-5593
e-mail: njlbh@njstatelib.org
www.njstatelib.org

Free home delivery of large-print, audio, and braille books and magazines, children's books on cassettes in braille and other reference materials on blindness and other handicaps. Services are for New Jersey residents with print disabilities.

Adan Szczepaniak, Director
Anne McArthur, Head of Outreach and Audiovision

New Mexico

1880 New Mexico State Library for the Blind and Physically Handicapped
1209 Camino Carlos Ray
Santa Fe, NM 87507

505-476-9700
Fax: 505-476-9761
e-mail: jbrewstr@stlib.state.nm.us
www.stlib.state.nm.us

Summer reading programs, braille writer, magnifiers, closed-circuit TV, large-print photocopier, cassette books and magazines, children's books on cassette, home visits and other reference materials on blindness and other handicaps.

Susan Overland, Manager

New York

1881 New York State Talking Book & Braille Library
National Library Service/NYS Library
Empire State Plaza, CEC
Albany, NY 12230

518-474-5935
800-342-3688
Fax: 518-486-1957
e-mail: tbbl@mail.nysed.gov
www.nysl.nysed.gov/tbbl

Recorded books and players, recorded magazines, braille books, braille writers, magnifiers, closed-circuit TV, children's books on cassette, reference materials on blindness and other disabilities. Service is completely free to eligible borrowers, including loan of equipment to listen to books. Over 60,000 titles available.

Sharon B Phillips, Library Program Director

North Carolina

1882 North Carolina Library for the Blind
1811 Capital Boulevard
Raleigh, NC 27635

919-733-4376
Fax: 919-733-6910
TDD: 919-733-1462
e-mail: nclbph@ncsl.der.state.nc
www.nfb.org/libraries for the blind

Summer reading programs, braille writer, magnifiers, closed-circuit TV, large-print photocopier, cassette books and magazines, children's books on cassette, home visits and other reference materials on blindness and other handicaps.

Francine Martin, Manager

Ohio

1883 American Council of Blind Parents
34400 Cedar Road, Apartment 108
University Heights, OH 44121

800-424-8666

Members are sighted parents of blind or visually impaired children. Offers a forum for support and outreach, sharing of experiences in parent-child relationships, and educational and cultural information about child development. Monitors developments in technical and legislative arenas.

Nola Webb, President

Oregon

1884 Oregon State Library, Talking Book and Braille Services
250 Winter Street NE
Salem, OR 97301

503-378-5389
800-452-0292
Fax: 503-585-8059
TDD: 503-378-4276
e-mail: tbabs@sparkie.osl.state.or.us
www.tbabs.org

Cassette books and magazines, children's books on cassette, home visits and other reference materials on blindness and other handicaps.

Susan Westin, Manager

Virginia

1885 Alexandria Library Talking Book Service
5005 Duke Street
Alexandria, VA 22304

703-746-1702
Fax: 703-519-5916
TDD: 703-838-4568
e-mail: emccaffr@lea.eda
www.alexandria.lib.va.us

Summer reading programs, braille writer, magnifiers, closed-circuit TV, large-print photocopier, cassette books and magazines, children's books on cassette, home visits and other reference materials on blindness and other handicaps.

Karen Russell, Manager

1886 Division for the Visually Handicapped
1920 Association Drive
Reston, VA 20191

703-620-3660

Members are teachers, college faculty members, administrators, supervisors and others concerned with the education and welfare of visually handicapped and blind children and youth. This is a division of the Council For Exceptional Children.

Dr. Kay Ferrell, President

1887 Division on Visual Impairments
Council for Exceptional Children
1110 North Glebe Road, Suite 300
Arlington, VA 22201

800-224-6830
Fax: 703-264-9494
TTY: 866-915-5000
www.ed.arizona.edu/dvi/welcome.htm; www.cec.sped.org

A division within the CEC, it handles concerns for Federal, state and local issues and policies related to education of youths, children and infants with visual impairments.

Ellyn Ross, President
Shirley J Wilson, Secretary
Phyllis T Simmons, President Elect

1888 Virginia State Library for the Visually and Physically Handicapped
1901 Roane Street
Richmond, VA 23222

804-367-0014

Summer reading programs, braille writer, magnifiers, closed-circuit TV, large-print photocopier, cassette books and magazines, children's books on cassette, home visits and other reference materials on blindness and other handicaps.

Mary Ruth Halapatz, Librarian

The purpose of the Center is to turn initial fears into hope. Helps children and their families become independent by creating a climate of safety and trust. Children learn to develop self confidence and to master a wide range of skills. Services include an infant stimulation program, educational preschool, interdisciplinary assessment services, family services, correspondence program, toll free national hotline and a publication and research service.

1895 Pediatric Ophathalmology and Adult Strabis mus Service Research
Indiana University
702 Rotary Circle
Indianapolis, IN 46202
317-274-2128
Fax: 317-274-2277
e-mail: dplager@iupui.edu
www.iupui.edu/~ophthal/

Improve techniques and treatment modalities for children with eye and vision problems, such as cataracts, glaucoma, retinopathy of prematurity, and for both children and adults with eye muscle abnormalities.

David A Plager, MD, Director

1896 Research to Prevent Blindness
645 Madison Avenue Floor 21
New York, NY 10022
212-752-4333
800-621-0026
Fax: 212-688-6231
e-mail: inforequest@rpbusa.org
www.rpbusa.org/rpb/about/overview/

Provides research grants to scientists interested in eye disease and vision disorders.

David F Weeks, Chairman Emeritus
Brian F. Hofland, PhD, President/Secretary
John I Bloomberg, Vice President

Conferences

1897 AADB National Symposium
American Association of the Deaf-Blind
PO Box 2831
Kensington, MD 20891
301-495-4403
Fax: 301-495-4404
TTY: 301-495-4402
e-mail: aadb-info@aadb.org
www.aadb.org

The symposium offers a training workshop, keynote speakers, full day exhibit hall, demonstration room, awards lunch and ceremony, talent show, Walk-A-Thon, and a banquet and dance.

Jill Gaus, President
Lynn Jansen, Vice President
Debby Lieberman, Secretary

1898 AER Regional Conference
1703 N Beauregard Street, Suite 440
Alexandria, VA 22311
703-671-4500
877-492-2708
Fax: 703-671-6391
e-mail: markr@aerbvi.org
www.aerbvi.org

August

Lou Tutt EdD, Executive Director
Ginger Croce, Senior Director

1899 Genetic Alliance Annual Conference
Genetic Alliance
4301 Connecticut Avenue NW, Suite 404
Washington, DC 20008
202-966-5557
800-336-4363
Fax: 202-966-8553
e-mail: info@geneticalliance.org
www.geneticalliance.org

Consistently inspirational and enables partnership among all stakeholders: advocates and community leaders, health and industry professionals, policymakers, and academicians.

1889 Washington Library for the Blind and Physically Handicapped
1000 Fourth Avenue
Seattle, WA 98104
206-386-4636
Fax: 206-386-4685
e-mail: wtbbl@spl.lib.wa.us
www.spl.lib.wa.us

Summer reading programs, braille writer, magnifiers, closed-circuit TV, large-print photocopier, cassette books and magazines, children's books on cassette, home visits and other reference materials on blindness and other handicaps.

Jan Ames, Librarian

West Virginia

1890 West Virginia School for the Blind
301 E Main Street
Romney, WV 26757
304-822-4801
Fax: 304-822-3370
e-mail: cjohn@access.mountain.net

Summer reading programs, braille writer, magnifiers, closed-circuit TV, large-print photocopier, cassette books and magazines, children's books on cassette, home visits and other reference materials on blindness and other handicaps.

Patsy Shank, Administrator

Research Centers

1891 American Association for Pediatric Ophthalmology and Strabismus
PO Box 193832
San Francisco, CA 94119
415-561-8505
Fax: 415-561-8531
e-mail: aapos@aao.org
www.aapos.org

Provides support and resources for Pediatric Ophthalmologists, Strabismologists, related personnel and their patients by way of its Internet Website.

David K. Epley MD, President
Christie L Morse, MD, Executive Vice President
Sharon F. Freedman, M.D, Vice President

1892 Center for the Partially Sighted
7462 North Figueroa Boulevard Suite 103
Los Angeles, CA 90041
310-988-1970
Fax: 310-988-1980
e-mail: info@low-vision.org
www.low-vision.org

Our mission is to provide the tools and techniques that maximize the ability of partially sighted children and adults to live successful and independent lives

James Adler, Esq., Board
Steve Edwards, Board
Brenda Premo, Board

1893 Mobile Association for the Blind
2440 Gordon Smith Drive
Mobile, AL 36617
251-473-3585
877-292-5463
Fax: 251-470-8622
e-mail: sales@mobile.blind.com
www.mobileblind.org

The American Foundation for the Blind removes barriers, creates solutions, and expands possibilities so people with vision loss can achieve their full potential

Jim Bullock, Executive Director

1894 New Beginnings - The Blind Children's Center
4120 Marathon Street
Los Angeles, CA 90029
213-664-2153
Fax: 323-665-3828
www.blindchildrenscenter.org/about.html

July
Sharon Terry, President/CEO
Tetyana Murza, Programs/Events Manager

Audio Video

1900 Heart to Heart
Blind Children's Center
4120 Marathon Street
Los Angeles, CA 90029   323-644-2153
                                     Fax: 323-665-3828
                                     www.blindcntr.org

Parents of blind and partially sighted children talk about their
feelings.
Videotape

1901 Let's Eat
Blind Children's Center
4120 Marathon Street
Los Angeles, CA 90029   323-664-2153
                                     Fax: 323-665-3828
                               www.blindchildrenscenter.org

Teaches competent feeding skills to children with visual impairments.
Videotape

1902 See What I Feel
Britannica Film Co.
345 4th Street
San Francisco, CA 94107   415-597-5555

A blind child tells her friends about her trip to the zoo. Each experience was explained as a blind child would experience it. A
teacher's guide comes with this video.
Films

Web Sites

**1903 American Association for Pediatric Ophthalmology and
Strabismus**
P.O. Box 193832
San Francisco, CA 94119   415-561-8505
                                     Fax: 415-561-8531
                                     www.aapos.org

Provides support and resources for Pediatric Ophthalmologists,
Strabismologists, related personnel and their patients by way of
its Internet Website.

Sherwin J. Isenberg, MD, President
M. Edward Wilson, MD, Vice President
Christie L. Morse, MD, Executive Vice President

1904 Lighthouse International
111 E 59th St
New York, NY 10022   800-284-4422
                              e-mail: info@lighthouseguild.org
                                     www.lighthouseguild.org

The mission is to overcome vision impairment for people of all
ages through worldwide leadership in rehabilitation services, education, research, prevention and advocacy.

1905 National Alliance of Blind Students
Los Angeles, CA   608-332-4147
                            e-mail: smwhalenpsp@gmail.com
                                     nabslink.org

The leading national advocacy and consumer organization for students in high school or college who are blind or visually
impaired.

Sean Whalen, President
Karen Anderson, 1st Vice President
Gabe Cazares, 2nd Vice President

1906 National Association for Visually Handicapped
111 E 59th St
New York, NY 10022   800-284-4422
                              e-mail: info@lighthouseguild.org
                                     www.lighthouseguild.org

Helps to cope with the difficulties of vision impairment.

1907 Online Mendelian Inheritance in Man
National Library of Medicine, Building 38A
Bethesda, MD 20894   888-346-3656
                              e-mail: info@ncbi.nlm.nih.gov
                                     www.ncbi.nlm.nih.gov

This database is a catalog of human genes and genetic disorders.

Christine E. Seidman, M.D., Chair
David J. Lipman, M.D., Executive Secretary

1908 Royal National Institute of the Blind
www.rnib.org.uk

                                          303-123-9999
                              e-mail: helpline@rnib.org.uk
                                     www.rnib.org.uk

Offering information, support and advice to people with sight
problems.

Lesley-Anne Alexander CBE, Chief Executive
Wanda Hamilton, Group Director (Fundraising)
Sally Harvey, Managing Director (RNIB Places)

Book Publishers

1909 Children with Visual Impairments: A Parents' Guide
Peytral Publications
PO Box 1162
Minnetonka, MN 55345   952-949-8707
                                          877-739-8725
                                     Fax: 952-906-9777
                                     www.peytral.com

Covers visual impairments ranging from low vision to total blindness. Offers authoritative information and empathy, parental insight on diagnosis and treatment, orientation and mobility,
literacy, legal issues and more. Valuable to parents, educators and
support staff.
395 pages
M Cay Holbrook PhD, Editor

1910 Ophthalmic Disorders Sourcebook
Omnigraphics Editorial Office
615 Griswold
Detroit, MI 48226   313-961-1340
                                          800-234-1340
                                     Fax: 313-961-1383
                              e-mail: editorial@omnigraphics.com
                                     www.omnigraphics.com

Basic consumer information about glaucoma, cataracts, macular
degeneration, strabismus, refractive disorders and more.
1996 631 pages Hardcover
ISBN: 0-780800-81-8
Linda M Ross, Editor

Magazines

1911 Journal of Visual Impairment and Blindness
American Foundation for the Blind
2 Penn Plaza, Suite 1102
New York, NY 10121   212-502-7600
                                     Fax: 888-545-8331
                              e-mail: contributions@afb.net
                                     www.afb.org

Published in braille, regular print and on cassette this journal
contains a wide variety of subjects including rehabilitation, psychology, education, legislation, medicine, technology, employment, sensory aids and childhood development as they relate to
visual impairments.

10x Year
Larry Kimbler, Chair
James H. McLaughlin, Vice Chair
Carl S. Augusto, President & CEO

1912 Reaching, Crawling, Walking - Let's Get Moving
Blind Children's Center
4120 Marathon Street
Los Angeles, CA 90029
323-664-2153
Fax: 323-665-3828
e-mail: info@blindchildrenscenter.org
www.blindchildrenscenter.org

Orientation and mobility for visually impaired preschool children.
24 pages

1913 Tactic
Clovernook Home and School for the Blind
7000 Hamilton Avenue
Cincinnati, OH 45231
513-522-3860
Fax: 513-728-3950
e-mail: clovernook@aol.com

Quarterly

Newsletters

1914 Gleams
Glaucoma Research Foundation
251 Post Street, Suite 600
San Francisco, CA 94108
415-986-3162
800-826-6693
Fax: 415-986-3763
e-mail: question@glaucoma.org
www.glaucoma.org

Includes information about glaucoma, new treatments, updates on research findings, and more.
3x/year

Thomas M. Brunner, President/ CEO
Nancy Graydon, Executive Director of Development
Andrew L. Jackson, Director of Communications

1915 NAVH Update
National Association for Visually Handicapped
111 E 59th St
New York, NY 10022
212-889-3141
800-284-4422
Fax: 212-727-2931
e-mail: info@lighthouseguild.org
lighthouse.org

Quarterly

Alan R. Morse, JD, PhD, President/ CEO
Mark G. Ackermann, EVP/ COO
Elliot J. Hagler, CPA, EVP/ CFO

1916 National Library Service for the Blind & Physically Handicapped
Library of Congress Reference Section
1291 Taylor Street NW
Washington, DC 20542
202-707-5100
800-424-8567
Fax: 202-707-0712
TTY: 202-707-0744
TDD: 202-707-0744
e-mail: nis@loc.gov
www.loc.gov/nls

Provides information and advocacy resources for families and professionals, including listings of organizations focusing on more specific areas of concern to families and young adults who have disabilities. Administers a natural library service that provides recorded and braille reading materials to eligible children and adults who cannot read standard print.

12 pages Quarterly
ISSN: 1046-1663

Vicki Fitzpatrick, Editor

1917 Talking Book Topics
National Library Services for the Blind
1291 Taylor Street NW
Washington, DC 20542
202-707-5100
Fax: 202-707-0712
TDD: 202-707-0744
e-mail: nls@loc.gov
www.loc.gov/nls

Offers hundreds of listings of books, fiction and nonfiction, for adults and children on cassette. Also offers listings on foreign language books on cassette, talking magazines and reviews.
Bimonthly

Pamphlets

1918 Dancing Cheek to Cheek
Blind Children's Center
4120 Marathon Street
Los Angeles, CA 90029
323-664-2153
Fax: 323-665-3828
www.blindchildrenscenter.org

Discusses beginning social, play and language interactions.
33 pages

1919 Family Guide - Growth and Development of the Partially Seeing Child
National Association for Visually Handicapped
111 E 59th St
New York, NY 10022
212-889-3141
800-284-4422
Fax: 212-727-2931
e-mail: info@lighthouseguild.org
www.lighthouseguild.org

Offers information for parents and guidelines in raising a partially seeing child.

1920 Family Guide to Vision Care
American Optometric Association
243 N Lindbergh Boulevard
Saint Louis, MO 63141
314-991-4100
Fax: 314-991-4101
www.aoanet.org

Offers information on the early developmental years of your vision, finding a family optometrist and how to take care of your eyesight through the learning years, the working years and the mature years.

1921 Heart to Heart
Blind Children's Center
4120 Marathon Street
Los Angeles, CA 90029
323-664-2153
Fax: 323-665-3828
www.blindchildrenscenter.org

Parents of blind and partially sighted children talk about their feelings.
12 pages

1922 Learning to Play
Blind Children's Center
4120 Marathon Street
Los Angeles, CA 90029
323-664-2153
Fax: 323-665-3828
www.blindchildrenscenter.org

Discusses how to present play activities to the visually impaired preschool child.
12 pages

1923 Let's Eat
Blind Children's Center
4120 Marathon Street
Los Angeles, CA 90029
323-664-2153
Fax: 323-665-3828
www.blindchildrenscenter.org

Teaches competent feeding skills to children with visual impairments.

28 pages

1924 Move with Me
Blind Children's Center
4120 Marathon Street
Los Angeles, CA 90029
323-664-2153
Fax: 323-665-3828
www.blindchildrenscenter.org

A parent's guide to movement development for visually impaired babies.

12 pages

1925 Selecting a Program
Blind Children's Center
4120 Marathon Street
Los Angeles, CA 90029
323-664-2153
Fax: 323-665-3828
www.blindchildrenscenter.org

A guide for parents of infants and preschoolers with visual impairments.

28 pages

1926 Standing on My Own Two Feet
Blind Children's Center
4120 Marathon Street
Los Angeles, CA 90029
323-664-2153
Fax: 323-665-3828
e-mail: info@blindchildrenscenter.org
www.blindchildrenscenter.org

A step-by-step guide to designing and constructing simple, individually tailored adaptive mobility devices for preschool-age children who are visually impaired.

36 pages

1927 Talk to Me
Blind Children's Center
4120 Marathon Street
Los Angeles, CA 90029
323-664-2153
Fax: 323-665-3828
www.blindchildrenscenter.org

A language guide for parents of deaf children.

11 pages

1928 Talk to Me II
Blind Children's Center
4120 Marathon Street
Los Angeles, CA 90029
323-664-2153
Fax: 323-665-3828
www.blindchildrenscenter.org

A sequel to Talk To Me, available in English and Spanish.

15 pages

Camps

1929 Bloomfield
5300 Angeles Vista Boulevard
Los Angeles, CA 90043
323-295-4555
800-352-2290
Fax: 323-296-0424
e-mail: info@juniorblind.org
www.juniorblind.org

This camp is dedicated to serving blind and developmentally disabled children and adults.

Miki Jordan, President

1930 Breckenridge Outdoor Education Center
PO Box 697
Breckenridge, CO 80424
970-453-6422
800-383-2632
Fax: 970-453-4676
e-mail: boec@boec.org
www.boec.org

Camp with a mission to expand the potential of people with disabilities and special needs through meaningful, educational and inspiring outdoor experiences.

Tim Casey, Chair

1931 Camp Civitan
3519 East Shea Blvd # 133
Phoenix, AZ 85028
602-953-2944
Fax: 602-953-2946
e-mail: info@campcivitan.org
www.campcivitan.org

A 501c3 non-profit organization, that has been providing multiple ever-changing programs to meet the needs of children and adults who are developmentally disabled.

Shannon Valenzuela, Director
Jane Armstrong, Director

1932 Camp Tushmehata
10500 Lincoln Lake Rd, PO Box 46
Greenville, MI 48838
616-754-5410
e-mail: gwen@campt.org
www.campt.org

Mission is to create and foster unlimited opportunities for blind and partially sighted people throughout Michigan and the world. The camp is comprised mainly of blind adults who have a passion for blind youth. The camp gained the opportunity to implement longer camping sessions, hire a large number of blind role models and steer the camp program into a bright, determined and promising future.

Gwen Botting, Director

1933 Enchanted Hills Camp
Lighthouse
214 Van Ness Avenue
San Francisco, CA 94102
415-694-7319
Fax: 415-863-7568
TTY: 415-431-4572
e-mail: afletcher@lighthouse-sf.org
www.lighthouse-sf.org

For blind, deaf/blind children and adults, ages 5 and up. This program offers a basic camping experience. Activities include music, art, dance, hiking and riding. Camperships are available to California residents.

Tony Fletcher, Camp Director

1934 Florida School-Deaf and Blind Summer Camp
207 N San Marco Avenue
Saint Augustine, FL 32084
904-827-2200
800-344-3732
e-mail: info@fsdb.k12.fl.us
www.fsdb.k12.fl.us

The Florida School for the Deaf and the Blind hosts summer campers from all over teh state of Florida for a week of fun and adventure. FSDB's 80 acre campus is where campers participate in a variety of activities including rock climbing, archery, swimming, kayaking, team games, arts and crafts, dance music, and much more.

L Daniel Hutto, President
Cindy Day, Executive Director of Parent Svcs
Terri Wiseman, Administrator of Business Services

1935 Highbrook Lodge Camp
12944 Aquilla Road
Chardon, OH 44024
216-791-8118
Fax: 216-791-1101
e-mail: camp@clevelandsightcenter.org
www.clevelandsightcenter.org

A summer residential camp for blind and disabled children, adults and families.

Mike Mullin, Director

1936 National Camps for Blind Children
Christian Record
4444 S 52nd Street
Lincoln, NE 68516
402-488-0981
Fax: 402-488-7582
e-mail: info@christianrecord.org
www.christianrecord.org

Camps throughout the US and Canada are offered at no cost to the legally blind, ages 9-65. Activities include archery, beeper basketball, water sports, hiking and rock climbing and horseback riding.

Peggy Hansen, Director

1937 Texas Lions Camp
Lions Clubs of Texas
PO Box 290247
Kerrville, TX 78029

830-896-8500
830-896-8500
Fax: 830-896-3666
e-mail: tlc@ktc.com
www.lionscamp.com

The primary purpose of Texas Lions camp is to provide, without charge, a camp for physically disabled, hearing/vision impaired and diabetic children from the State of Texas, regardless of race, religion, or national origin. Our goal is to create an atmosphere wherein campers will learn the can do philosophy and be allowed to achieve maximum personal growth and self esteem. The camp welcomes boys and girls ages 7-16.

Stephen Mabry, Executive Director
Doug Parker, Business Manager
Steven King, Program/Client Service Director

1938 VISIONS/Vacation Camp for the Blind
500 Greenwich Street, 3rd Floor
New York, NY 10013

212-625-1616
888-245-8333
Fax: 212-219-4078
e-mail: info@visions.org
www.visions.org

Family programs at Vacation Camp for the Blind in Rockland County, NY for children who are blind, severely visually impaired or multi-handicapped. Parent or guardian must attend winter weekends and summer session.

Thomas M Decker, Camp Director
Nancy D Miller, Executive Director

1939 Wisconsin Lions Camp
3834 County Road A
Rosholt, WI 54473

715-677-4969
Fax: 715-677-3297
TTY: 715-677-6999
e-mail: info@wisconsinlionscamp.org
www.wisconsinlionscamp.com

Serves children who have either a visual, hearing or mild cognitive disability. Many of the children also have multiple disabilities or medical conditions. Program activities include sailing, ropes course, bike and canoe trips, environmental education, swimming, camping, canoeing, outdoor living skills and handicrafts. ACA accredited, located in central Wisconsin, near Stevens Point.

Russell Link, Camp Director

Description

1940 CONGENITAL DIAPHRAGMATIC HERNIA

Synonym: CDH

Involves the following Biologic System(s):

Gastrointestinal Disorders, Respiratory Disorders

Congenital diaphragmatic hernia (CDH) is a birth defect characterized by projection or bulging of organs of the abdomen into the chest cavity. This occurs as a result of an abnormal opening in the diaphragm, the dome-shaped muscle that separates the abdomen from the chest and plays an essential role in breathing. Approximately one in 5,000 newborns are affected by the condition. CDH is thought to result due to failed closure of a certain area of the embryonic diaphragm (i.e., the foramen of Bochdalek) during fetal development. In some cases, disrupted development in other areas of the growing fetus may also cause CDH. This birth defect may occur as an isolated condition or, in about 20 to 30 percent of patients, in association with other abnormalities or underlying malformation syndromes, such as Down syndrome (trisomy 21), trisomy 18 syndrome, or trisomy 13 syndrome. There are reports of several infants with isolated CDH in certain families (kindreds). In such cases, the condition is thought to result from abnormal changes (mutations) of different genes, possibly in association with certain environmental factors (multifactorial inheritance).

In newborns with CDH, the diaphragmatic defect may be small or can affect up to half of the diaphragm. The left side of the diaphragm is most commonly involved. The lungs may also be unusually small and underdeveloped (pulmonary hypoplasia), and abnormalities of the blood vessels supplying the lungs may also be present. In addition, the intestines may not be positioned properly (intestinal malformation). Most newborns with CDH experience increasing difficulties breathing (respiratory distress) within the first 24 hours after birth. Associated symptoms include labored breathing (dyspnea), grunting upon exhalation, drawing in of the chest wall during inhalation, and a bluish discoloration of the skin and mucous membranes (cyanosis). These findings may potentially result in life-threatening complications. In addition, in some affected newborns, air may collect in the chest cavity, causing the lung(s) to collapse (pneumothorax). Symptoms associated with CDH may not become apparent until after the first few weeks of life. These infants may experience mild respiratory symptoms or intestinal obstruction and associated vomiting (emesis).

In newborns with CDH, immediate measures may be necessary to prevent or treat potentially life-threatening complications. Surgery to repair the diaphragmatic defect is deferred until the newborn's respiratory status has been stabilized. Ongoing supportive measures may be employed before surgery, such as use of a device known as an extracorporeal membrane oxygenator (ECMO). This device supplies oxygen to the infant's blood and returns this oxygenated blood to the body. In addition, certain medications may also be used (e.g., surfactant therapy to help improve oxygenation, etc.).

Government Agencies

1941 NIH/National Institute of Child Health and Human Development
31 Center Drive, Building 31
Bethesda, MD 20892

800-370-2943
Fax: 301-496-1104
TTY: 888-320-6942
e-mail: NICHDInformationResourceCenter@mail.nih.
www.nichd.nih.gov

Established in 1962 by congress, today the institute conducts and supports laboratory research, clinical trials, and epidemiological studies that explore health processes; examines the impact of disabilities, diseases, and variations on the lives of individuals; and sponsors training programs for scientists, health care providers, and researchers to ensure that NICHD research can continue.

Alan E Guttmacher MD, Director
Lisa Kaeser, Program & Public Liaison

National Associations & Support Groups

1942 American Academy of Pediatrics
141 Northwest Point Boulevard
Elk Grove Village, IL 60007

847-434-4000
800-433-9016
Fax: 847-434-8000
www.aap.org

The American Academy of Pediatrics and its member pediatricians are committed to the attainment of optimal physical, mental and social health and well-being for all infants, children, adolescents, and young adults.

Sandra Hassink, MD, FAAP, President

1943 CHERUBS: Association of Congenital Diaphragmatic Hernia Research & Advocacy
3650 Rogers Rd Suite 290
Wake Forest, NC 27587

919-610-0129
866-603-1944
Fax: 815-425-9155
e-mail: info@cherubs-cdh.org
www.cherubs-cdh.org

Goal is to not only help parents of children born with CDH but to lead the medical community into finding the cause and prevention of this devastating birth defect

Dawn Williamson, President/Founder

1944 Digestive Disease National Coalition
507 Capitol Court NE, Suite 200
Washington, DC 10039

202-544-7497
Fax: 202-546-7105
e-mail: ddnc@hmcw.org
www.ddnc.org

Advocacy organization comprised of 22 voluntary and professional societies concerned with the many diseases of the digestive tract and liver.

Diane Paley, Chairperson
James DeGerome, President
Andrew Spiegel, Vice-Chairperson

1945 Genetic Alliance
4301 Connecticut Avenue NW Suite 404
Washington, DC 20008

202-966-7955
800-336-4363
Fax: 202-966-8553
e-mail: info@geneticalliance.org
www.geneticalliance.org

World's leading nonprofit health advocacy organization committed to transforming health through genetics and promoting an environment of openness centered on the health of individuals, families, and communities.

Sharon Terry, President
Lisa Wise, Chief Operating Officer
Tetyana Murza MES, Programs and Policy Coordinator

1946 International CDH Conference
CHERUBS
3650 Rogers Rd Suite 290
Wake Forest, NC 27587
919-610-0129
866-603-1944
Fax: 815-425-9155
e-mail: info@cherubs-cdh.org
www.cherubs-cdh.org

Designed for families of CDH survivors, grieving CDH families, adult survivors and CDH researchers.

June

Dawn Williamson, President/Founder

Libraries & Resource Centers

1947 National Digestive Diseases Information Clearinghouse
2 Information Way
Bethesda, MD 20892
301-654-3810
800-891-5389
Fax: 301-907-8906
e-mail: nddic@info.niddk.nih.gov
www.niddk.nih.gov

The National Institute of Diabetes and Digestive and Kidney Diseases conducts and supports research on many of the most serious diseases affecting public health. The Institute supports much of the clinical research on the diseases of internal medicine and related subspecialty fields as well as many basic science disciplines.

Kathy Kranzfelder, Project Officer

1948 University of Iowa Birth Defects and Genetic Disorders Unit
2614 JCP
Iowa City, IA 52242
319-335-9901
James M Smith, Director

Conferences

1949 Genetic Alliance Annual Conference
Genetic Alliance
4301 Connecticut Avenue NW, Suite 404
Washington, DC 20008
202-966-5557
800-336-4363
Fax: 202-966-8553
e-mail: info@geneticalliance.org
www.geneticalliance.org

Consistently inspirational and enables partnership among all stakeholders: advocates and community leaders, health and industry professionals, policymakers, and academicians.

July

Sharon Terry, President/CEO
Tetyana Murza, Programs/Events Manager

Web Sites

1950 Family Village
www.familyvillage.wisc.edu

A global community that integrates information, resources and communication opportunities on the Internet for persons with cognitive and other disabilities, for their families and for those that provide them services and support.

Book Publishers

1951 Digestive Diseases & Disorders Sourcebook
Omnigraphics Editorial Office
615 Griswold
Detroit, MI 48226
313-961-1340
800-234-1340
Fax: 313-961-1383
e-mail: editorial@omnigraphics.com
www.omnigraphics.com

Provides basic information for the layperson about common disorders of the upper and lower digestive tract. It also includes information about medications and recommendations for maintaining a healthy digestive tract. A glossary of important terms and a directory of digestive diseases organizations are also provided.

2000 335 pages Hardcover
ISBN: 0-780803-27-2

Karen Bellenir, Editor

Description

1952 CONGENITAL DYSPLASIA OF THE HIP

Synonyms: CDH, Congenital dislocation of the hip, DDH, Developmental dysplasia of the hip

Covers these related disorders: Teratologic congenital dysplasia of the hip, Typical congenital dysplasia of the hip (Developmental dysplasia)

Involves the following Biologic System(s):

Neonatal and Infant Disorders, Orthopedic and Muscle Disorders

Congenital dysplasia of the hip (CDH) refers to a condition present at birth or soon thereafter in which one or both hips are dislocated. This occurs when the ball-shaped head of the upper thigh bone (femur) does not fit appropriately into the hip socket of the pelvis (acetabulum). Congenital hip dysplasia may be classified as typical, which occurs shortly after birth in infants with no underlying neurologic irregularities, or teratologic, which develops before birth. The typical form of this condition is commonly referred to as developmental dysplasia of the hip.

The cause of CDH is unknown, although it is more prevalent in newborns who were surrounded by an unusually small amount of amniotic fluid during the gestational period (oligohydramnios). Those infants who present in a breech position; those with other close family members with this condition may also be at increased risk for CDH. In addition, it is more predominant in girls than it is in boys by a ratio of nine to one. Teratologic dysplasia of the hip in the developing fetus may occur as part of a pattern of abnormalities associated with certain underlying disorders affecting the neuromuscular system such as arthrogryposis multiplex congenita and myelodysplasia.

Assessment of the hips is part of the newborn physical exam. The Ortalani and Barlow maneuvers help to detect both anterior and posterior dislocations for the femoral head. Children with certain risk factors (i.e. breech delivery) should have a hip ultrasound at 3 months.

Treatment during infancy may include manipulation of the hip joint into its proper position followed by immobilization and splinting of the thigh for a period of several months. Some infants may benefit from wearing two or three diapers at a time. In some patients, delayed detection of this birth defect may necessitate the use of traction to restore the femoral head to its correct position. However, if the dislocation is not discovered until late childhood, surgery followed by fitting with a plaster cast may be necessary to correct this condition. Delayed treatment may result in chronic difficulties with walking. Untreated dysplasia of the hip may result in degenerative changes in the joint (osteoarthritis). Approximately 4 of every 1,000 infants are affected by congenital dysplasia of the hip; however, in approximately 70 percent of these children, the dislocation corrects itself.

Government Agencies

1953 NIH/National Institute of Arthritis & Musculoskeletal & Skin Diseases
National Institutes of Health
1 AMS Circle
Bethesda, MD 20892
301-495-4484
877-226-4267
Fax: 301-718-6366
TTY: 301-565-2966
TDD: 301-565-2966
e-mail: niamsinfo@mail.nih.gov
www.niams.nih.gov

The mission of the National Institute of Arthritis and Musculoskeletal and Skin Diseases is to support research into the causes, treatment, and prevention of arthritis and musculoskeletal and skin diseases; the training of basic and clinical scientists to carry out this research; and the dissemination of information on research progress in these diseases

Stephen I Katz, MD/Ph.D, Director
Robert H Carter MD, Deputy Director
Gahan Breithaupt, Assoc Dir. Management & Operations

1954 NIH/National Institute of Child Health and Human Development
31 Center Drive, Building 31
Bethesda, MD 20892
800-370-2943
Fax: 301-496-1104
TTY: 888-320-6942
e-mail: NICHDInformationResourceCenter@mail.nih.
www.nichd.nih.gov

Established in 1962 by congress, today the institute conducts and supports laboratory research, clinical trials, and epidemiological studies that explore health processes; examines the impact of disabilities, diseases, and variations on the lives of individuals; and sponsors training programs for scientists, health care providers, and researchers to ensure that NICHD research can continue.

Alan E Guttmacher MD, Director
Lisa Kaeser, Program & Public Liaison

National Associations & Support Groups

1955 American Academy of Pediatrics
141 Northwest Point Boulevard
Elk Grove Village, IL 60007
847-434-4000
800-433-9016
Fax: 847-434-8000
www.aap.org

The American Academy of Pediatrics and its member pediatricians are committed to the attainment of optimal physical, mental and social health and well-being for all infants, children, adolescents, and young adults.

Sandra Hassink, MD, FAAP, President

1956 Genetic Alliance
4301 Connecticut Avenue NW
Washington, DC 20008
202-966-7955
800-336-4363
Fax: 202-966-8553
e-mail: info@geneticalliance.org
www.geneticalliance.org

World's leading nonprofit health advocacy organization committed to transforming health through genetics and promoting an environment of openness centered on the health of individuals, families, and communities.

Sharon Terry, President

1957 March of Dimes Birth Defects Foundation
1275 Mamaroneck Avenue
White Plains, NY 10605
914-997-4488
888-663-4637
Fax: 914-997-4763
e-mail: answers@marchofdimes.com
www.marchofdimes.com

Partnership of volunteers and professionals dedicated to improving the health of babies by preventing birth defects and infant mortality. Over 100 chapters are located across the country and can be located through the National Office.

Jennifer L Howse, President
Thomas A Russo, Board-Directors Vice Chairman
Jane Massey, EVP/Chief Operating Officer

1958 National Dissemination Center for Children with Disabilities
1825 Connecticut Ave NW, PO Box 1492
Washington, DC 20009   202-884-8200
                                                        800-695-0285
                                                   Fax: 202-884-8441
                                           e-mail: nichcy@fhi360@org
                                                       www.nichcy.org

A national information and referral center that provides information on disabilities and disability-related issues for families, educators and other professionals.

Suzanne Ripley, Executive Director

Libraries & Resource Centers

1959 University of Iowa Birth Defects and Genetic Disorders Unit
2614 JCP
Iowa City, IA 52242   319-335-9901
James M Smith, Director

Conferences

1960 Genetic Alliance Annual Conference
Genetic Alliance
4301 Connecticut Avenue NW, Suite 404
Washington, DC 20008   202-966-5557
                                                        800-336-4363
                                                   Fax: 202-966-8553
                                      e-mail: info@geneticalliance.org
                                                 www.geneticalliance.org

Consistently inspirational and enables partnership among all stakeholders: advocates and community leaders, health and industry professionals, policymakers, and academicians.

July

Sharon Terry, President/CEO
Tetyana Murza, Programs/Events Manager

Web Sites

1961 Dr. Koop
www.drkoop.com/

Information on the condition, causes, symptoms, tests and treatment.

Book Publishers

1962 Let's Talk About Going to the Hospital
Rosen Publishing Group's PowerKids Press
29 E 21st Street
New York, NY 10010   212-777-3017
                                                       800-237-9932
                                                  Fax: 888-436-4643
                                     e-mail: rosenpub@tribeca.ios.com
                                                  www.powerkidspress.com

If a child has to check into the hospital, chances are he or she is already upset about being ill. Knowing how a hospital functions and what the procedures are, such as when family members can visit, will help in what is already a stressful situation. Grades K-5.

24 pages
ISBN: 0-823950-36-0

Description

1963 CONGENITAL GLAUCOMA

Synonym: Infantile glaucoma

Covers these related disorders: Primary glaucoma, Secondary glaucoma

Involves the following Biologic System(s):

Ophthalmologic Disorders

Glaucoma refers to a condition in which the fluid pressure within the eyes (intraocular pressure) is abnormally elevated. This may occur as a result of the buildup of fluid (aqueous humor) due to obstruction or other problems with the eyes. Glaucoma that develops by the third year of life is referred to as congenital or infantile glaucoma, which is a very rare occurrence. Primary glaucoma refers to the condition as it relates to an irregularity in the mechanism that drains the eye. Secondary glaucoma refers to increased intraocular pressure that results from other types of irregularities that may or may not be accompanied by a drainage deficit.

Symptoms associated with congenital glaucoma may include an abnormal sensitivity to light (photophobia), involuntary, repeated squeezing and closing of the eyelids (blepharospasm), abnormal tearing, swelling and enlargement of the cornea, difficulty in seeing, and other ocular irregularities. Affected infants under three months of age are at additional risk of incurring tissue damage due to heightened sensitivity of the cornea to elevated fluid pressure within the eye. Eye irregularities may be observed by a physician upon ophthalmic examination.

Congenital glaucoma may develop subsequent to certain congenital problems such as trauma, bleeding (hemorrhage) within the eye, or tumors and inflammation. Other associated abnormalities may include the lack of transparency (opacity) of the lenses of the eye (cataracts), displacement of the lenses (ectopia lentis), partial absence of the iris (aniridia), and other abnormalities. Disorders often associated with congenital glaucoma include certain chromosomal disorders that may affect various systems of the body such as Sturge-Weber syndrome, oculocerebrorenal syndrome, neurofibromatosis, and Marfan syndrome.

Treatment for congenital glaucoma includes surgery to relieve the pressure within the eye to prevent optic nerve damage and preserve vision. In some cases, more than one surgery may be necessary and follow-up therapy may be required. Additional treatment is directed toward associated irregularities and complications.

Government Agencies

1964 NIH/National Eye Institute
31 Center Drive MSC 2510
Bethesda, MD 20892
301-496-5248
e-mail: 2020@nei.nih.gov
www.nei.nih.gov

Conducts and supports research that helps prevent and treat eye diseases and other disorders of vision. This research leads to sight-saving treatments, reduces visual impairment and blindness, and improves the quality of life for people of all ages. NEI-supported research has advanced our knowledge of how the eye functions in health and disease.

Paul A Sieving M.D., Ph.D., Director

National Associations & Support Groups

1965 American Academy of Pediatrics
141 Northwest Point Boulevard
Elk Grove Village, IL 60007
847-434-4000
800-433-9016
Fax: 847-434-8000
www.aap.org

The American Academy of Pediatrics and its member pediatricians are committed to the attainment of optimal physical, mental and social health and well-being for all infants, children, adolescents, and young adults.

Sandra Hassink, MD, FAAP, President

1966 Children's Glaucoma Foundation
2 Longfellow Place, Suite 201
Boston, MA 02114
617-227-3011
Fax: 617-227-9538
e-mail: walton.blackey@gmail.com
www.childrensglaucoma.com

A nonprofit organization dedicated to supporting programs for children with glaucoma. Serves to increase awareness of the symptoms and encourage parents and doctors to screen infants and children for glaucoma, and supports research programs.

David S Walton, MD, President

1967 Genetic Alliance
4301 Connecticut Avenue NW, Suite 404
Washington, DC 20008
202-966-5557
800-336-4363
Fax: 202-966-8553
e-mail: info@geneticalliance.org
www.geneticalliance.org

A coalition of voluntary genetic support groups, consumers and professionals addressing the needs of individuals and families affected by genetic disorders from a national perspective.

Sharon Terry, President
Natasha Bonhomme, Vice President of Strategic Develop
Vaughn Edelson, Assistant Director of Health Commun

1968 Glaucoma Research Foundation
251 Post Street, Suite 600
San Francisco, CA 94108
415-986-3162
800-826-6693
Fax: 415-986-3763
e-mail: questions@glaucoma.org
www.glaucoma.org

Mission is to preserve the sight and independence of individuals with glaucoma through research and education with the ultimate goal of finding a cure.

Tom Brunner, CEO
Andrew Iwach, Executive Director
H.Allen Bouch, Vice Chair

1969 National Association for Visually Handicapped
22 W 21st Street, 6th Floor
New York, NY 10010
212-889-3141
888-205-5951
Fax: 212-727-2931
e-mail: navh@navh.org
www.navh.org

The only nonprofit health organization in the world solely dedicated to providing assistance to the partially sighted. Serves as a clearinghouse for information about all services available to the partially-sighted from public and private sources. Conducts self-help groups. Provides information on large print books, textbooks and educational tools.

Lorianie Marchi, CEO

1970 Prevent Blindness America
211 West Wacker Drive, Ste 1700
Chicago, IL 60606
847-843-2020
800-331-2020
Fax: 847-843-8458
e-mail: info@preventblindness.org
www.preventblindness.org

A volunteer eye health and safety organization dedicated to fighting blindness and saving sight. Focused on promoting a continuum of vision care, Prevent Blindness America touches the lives of millions of people each year through public and professional education, advocacy, certified vision screening training, community and patient service programs and research.

Pary Hugh, President
Corbett Sue, Manager
Bilazer Arzu, Creative Director

State Agencies & Support Groups

Alabama

1971 Alabama Institute for the Deaf & Blind
205 East South Street, PO Box 698
Talladega, AL 35160
256-761-3331
Fax: 256-761-3344
www.aidb.org

Services include central directory, representatives of agencies, service providers, families, and coordinators of infant, toddler, and preschool special education programs.

Dr. John Mascia, President

Arizona

1972 National Association for Parents of the Visually Impaired
PO Box 317
Watertown, MA 02471
617-972-7441
800-562-6265
Fax: 617-972-7444
e-mail: napvi@guildhealth.org
www.spedex.com/napvi

Mary Ellen Simmons

Ohio

1973 Region 2 of the National Association for Parents of the Visually Impaired
3910 Pocahontas Avenue
Cincinnati, OH 45227
513-561-8542
Victoria Gorman Miller

Pennsylvania

1974 East Central Region-Helen Keller National Center
141 Middle Neck Road
Sands Point, NY 11050
516-944-8900
Fax: 516-944-7302
e-mail: HKNCinfo@hknc.org
www.helenkeller.org

Christopher D Maher, Chairman
Richard T Arkwright, Vice Chairman
John R. Caughey, Treasurer

South Carolina

1975 Region 4 of the National Association for Parents of the Visually Impaired
1032 Trail Road
Belton, SC 29627
864-338-9593

Washington

1976 Northwestern Region-Helen Keller National Center
141 Middle Neck Road
Sands Point, NY 11050
516-944-8900
Fax: 516-944-7302
e-mail: HKNCinfo@hknc.org
www.helenkeller.org

Christopher D Maher, Chairman
Richard T Arkwright, Vice Chairman
John R. Caughey, Treasurer

Libraries & Resource Centers

Alabama

1977 Mobile Association for the Blind
2440 Gordon Smith Drive
Mobile, AL 36617
251-473-3585
Fax: 251-470-8622
www.mobileblind.org

Offers work adjustment training, activities of daily living, mobility, communication skills and sheltered employment for adults and children who are visually impaired.

Jim Bullock, Executive Director

Arizona

1978 Educational Services for the Visually Impaired
PO Box 668
Little Rock, AR 72203
501-371-5710

Offers textbooks, braille books and more to the visually impaired grades K-12 in the Arkansas area.

David Beavers, Director

Arkansas

1979 Arkansas Regional Library for the Blind and Physically Handicapped
900 W. Capitol, Suite 100
Little Rock, AR 72201
501-682-2053
Fax: 501-682-1533
TDD: 501-682-1002
e-mail: nlsbooks@asl.lib.ar.us
www.asl.lib.ar.us/ASL_LBPH.htm

Public library books in recorded or braille format. Popular fiction and nonfiction books for all ages, books and players are on free loan, sent to patrons by mail and may be returned postage free. Anyone who cannot see well enough to read regular print with glasses on or who has a disability that makes it difficult to hold a book or turn the pages is eligible.

John D Hall, Director

California

1980 American Action Fund for Blind Children and Adults
18440 Oxnard Street
Tarzana, CA 91356
818-343-2022
Fax: 818-343-3219
e-mail: lucyabba@aol.com
www.actinfund.org

A lending library for the visually impaired. We send out a weekly Braille newspaper for the deaf-blind (worldwide), we also send out pocket-sized Braille calendars. Our lending library is for pre-school thru high school. All of our services are free.

Lucille Abbazia, Manager

1981 Blind Children's Center
4120 Marathon Street
Los Angeles, CA 90029
323-664-2153
Fax: 323-665-3828
www.blindchildrenscenter.org

Offers support and informational groups.

Midge Horton, Executive Director

1982 Braille Institute Desert Center
741 N Vermont Avenue
Los Angeles, CA 90029

323-663-1111
Fax: 323-663-0867
e-mail: la@brailleinstitute.org
www.brailleinstitute.org

Dedicated to providing blind and visually impaired men, women and children with the training, programs and services they need to enjoy productive lives. Services offered include child development, youth programs, library services and adult education.

Lars Hansen, Manager

1983 Braille Institute Sight Center
741 N Vermont Avenue
Los Angeles, CA 90029

323-663-1111
Fax: 323-663-0867
e-mail: la@brailleinstitute.org
www.brailleinstitute.org

Offers help, programs, services and information to the blind and visually impaired children and adults.

Les Stocker, President

1984 Braille Institute Youth Center
3450 Cahuenga Boulevard W
Los Angeles, CA 90068

213-851-5695

Offers various youth programs and services for the blind and visually impaired youngster.

1985 New Beginnings - Blind Children's Center
4120 Marathon, Street
Los Angeles, CA 90029

323-664-2153
800-222-3566
Fax: 323-665-3828

Helps children and their families become independent by creating a climate of safety and trust. Services include an infant stimulation program, educational preschool, interdisciplinary assessment services, family services, correspondence program, toll-free national hotline and a publication and research service.

1986 San Francisco Public Library for the Blind and Print Disabled
P.O Box 942837
Sacramento, CA 94237

415-557-4400
800-952-5666
Fax: 415-557-4252
e-mail: lbphmgr@sfpl.lib.ca.us
www.library.ca.gov

Foreign-language books on cassette, children's books on cassettes and more.

Luis Herrera, Manager

1987 Variety Audio
PO Box 5731
San Jose, CA 95150

408-277-4839

Summer reading programs, braille writer, magnifiers, closed-circuit TV, large-print photocopier, cassette books and magazines, children's books on cassette, home visits and other reference materials on blindness and other handicaps.

Louisa Griehshammer

District of Columbia

1988 Council of Families with Visual Impairment
1155 15th Street NW
Washington, DC 20005

202-467-5081

Members are sighted parents of blind or visually impaired children. Offers a forum for support and outreach, sharing of experiences in parent-child relationships, and educational and cultural information about child development. Monitors developments in technical and legislative arenas.

Nola Webb, President

Florida

1989 Florida Bureau of Braille and Talking Book Library Services
421 Platt Street
Daytona Beach, FL 32114

386-239-6000
800-226-6075
Fax: 386-239-6069
TDD: 800-226-6079
e-mail: mike_gunde@dbs.doe.state.fl.us
www.state.fl.us/dbs/lswel.html

Discs, cassettes, closed-circuit TV, large-print photocopier, films, children's books on cassettes and more.

Michael Gunde, Librarian

1990 Talking Book Library, Jacksonville Public Library
1755 Edgewood Avenue W, Suite 1
Jacksonville, FL 32208

904-765-5588
Fax: 904-768-7404
TDD: 904-768-7822
e-mail: jerryr@coj.net
www.neflin.org/neflin/members/jackspub.html

Discs, cassettes and reference materials on blindness and other disabilities.

Jerry Reynolds, Librarian Senior

1991 Talking Book Service - Manatee County Central Library
6081 26th Street W
Bradenton, FL 34207

941-742-5914
Fax: 941-751-7089
TDD: 941-742-5951
e-mail: patricia.schubert@co.manatee.fl.us
www.co.manatee.fl.us

Offers children's books on disc and cassette and more reference materials for the blind and physically handicapped.

Patricia Schubert, Librarian

Georgia

1992 Albany Library for the Blind and Physical Handicapped
300 Pine Avenue
Albany, GA 31701

229-420-3220
Fax: 229-420-3215
e-mail: sinquefk@mail.dougherty.public.lib.ga.us
www.docolib.org/LBPH/index.html

Offers discs, cassettes, reference materials on blindness and other handicaps, large-print photocopiers, summer reading programs, cassette books and more.

Katy Sinquefield, Manager

1993 Bainbridge Subregional Library for the Blind and Physically Handicapped
301 S Monroe Street
Bainbridge, GA 39819

912-248-2680
800-795-2680
Fax: 912-248-2670
TDD: 912-248-2665
e-mail: lbph@mail.deccatur.public.lib.ga.us
www.decatur.public.lib.ga.us/local/lbph/lbph1.htm

Discs, cassettes, summer reading programs, closed-circuit TV, magnifiers and more.

Kathy Hutchins, Librarian

1994 CEL Subregional Library for the Blind and Physically Handicapped
2708 Mechanics
Savannah, GA 31404

912-354-5864
Fax: 912-354-5534
TDD: 912-652-3635
e-mail: stokesl@cel.co.chatman.ga.us

Summer reading programs, braille writer, magnifiers, closed-circuit TV, large-print photocopier, cassette books and magazines, children's books on cassette, home visits and other reference materials on blindness and other handicaps.

Linda Stokes, Librarian

Idaho

1995 Idaho State Talking Book Library
325 W State Street
Boise, ID 83702
Fax: 208-334-2117
Fax: 208-334-4016
TDD: 800-377-1363
e-mail: tblbooks@isl.state.id.us
www.lili.org/isl/tblinfo.htm

Summer reading programs, braille writer, magnifiers, closed-circuit TV, large-print photocopier, cassette books and magazines, children's books on cassette, home visits and other reference materials on blindness and other handicaps.

Sue Walker, Manager

Illinois

1996 Chicago Library Service for the Blind
1055 W Roosevelt Road
Chicago, IL 60608
312-746-9210

Summer reading programs, braille writer, magnifiers, closed-circuit TV, large-print photocopier, cassette books and magazines, children's books on cassette, home visits and other reference materials on blindness and other handicaps.

Carol Pellish, Librarian

1997 Illinois State Library, Talkng Book and Braille Service
213 State Capitol
Springfield, IL 62756
217-785-5600
800-252-980
Fax: 217-785-4326
TDD: 800-665-5576
e-mail: sruda@ilsos.net
www.cyberdriveillinois.com

Summer reading programs, braille writer, magnifiers, closed-circuit TV, large-print photocopier, cassette books and magazines, descriptive videos, children's books on cassette, home visits and other reference materials on blindness and other handicaps.

Anne Craig, Executive Director

1998 Mid Illinois Talking Book System
515 York Street
Quincy, IL 62301
217-224-6619
Fax: 217-224-9818

Summer reading programs, braille writer, magnifiers, closed-circuit TV, large-print photocopier, cassette books and magazines, children's books on cassette, home visits and other reference materials on blindness and other handicaps.

1999 Mid-Illinois Talking Book Center
600 High Point Lane
East Peoria, IL 61611
309-353-4110
800-426-0709
Fax: 309-353-8281
e-mail: hitbc@darkstar.rsa.lib.il.us
www.mitbc.org

Summer reading programs, braille writer, magnifiers, closed-circuit TV, large-print photocopier, cassette books and magazines, children's books on cassette, home visits and other reference materials on blindness and other handicaps.

Eileen Sheppard, Librarian
Chenoweth Rose, Director
Boucher Nancy, Reader Advisor

2000 Talking Book Center of Northwest Illinois
PO Box 125
Coal Valley, IL 61240
309-799-3137
800-747-3137
Fax: 309-799-7916
e-mail: kodean@libby.rbls.lib.il.us
www.rbls.lib.il.us

Subregional library provides Talking Book and Braille Book programs to eligible persons unable to use standard print materials due to visual or physical disabilities. Includes cassette books and magazines; summer reading program.

Indiana

2001 Northwest Indiana Subregional Library for Blind and Physically Handicapped
1919 W Lincoln Highway
Merrillville, IN 46410
219-769-3541
Fax: 219-769-0690

Summer reading programs, braille writer, magnifiers, closed-circuit TV, large-print photocopier, cassette books and magazines, children's books on cassette, home visits and other reference materials on blindness and other handicaps.

Renee Lewis

Iowa

2002 Iowa Library for the Blind and Physically Handicapped
Iowa Department for the Blind
524 4th Street
Des Moines, IA 50309
515-281-1333
800-362-2587
Fax: 515-281-1263
TTY: 515-281-1355
TDD: 515-281-1355
e-mail: information@blind.state.ia.us
www.blind.state.ia.us

Summer reading programs, magnifiers, closed-circuit TV, large-print photocopier, children's books on cassette, children's books in Braille and Print Braille, cassette magazines, home visits and reference materials on blindness and other handicaps.

Eis Karen, Program Manager/Librarian
Richard Sorey, Director
Aldini Jodi, Library Support Staff

2003 University of Iowa Birth Defects and Genetic Disorders Unit
2614 JCP
Iowa City, IA 52242
319-335-9901
James M Smith, Director

Kansas

2004 CKLS Headquarters
1409 Williams Street
Great Bend, KS 67530
620-792-4865
800-362-2642
Fax: 620-792-5495
e-mail: cenks@ink.org
www.ckls.org

Summer reading programs, braille writer, magnifiers, closed-circuit TV, large-print photocopier, cassette books and magazines, children's books on cassette, home visits and other reference materials on blindness and other handicaps.

Jerri Robinson, Librarian

2005 Services for the Visually Disabled
629 Poyntz Avenue
Manhattan, KS 66502
785-776-4741
Fax: 785-776-1545
e-mail: marionr@manhattan.lib.ks.us

Summer reading programs, braille writer, magnifiers, closed-circuit TV, large-print photocopier, cassette books and magazines, children's books on cassette, home visits and other reference materials on blindness and other handicaps.

Marion Rice, Librarian

Kentucky

2006 Kentucky Library for the Blind and Physically Handicapped
PO Box 818
Frankfort, KY 40602
502-564-8300
800-372-2968
Fax: 502-564-5773
e-mail: richard.feindel@kdla.net
www.kdla.net/libserv/ktbl.htm

Large-print photocopier, cassette books and magazines, children's books on cassette, and other reference materials on blindness and other handicaps.

5,200 members

Richard Feindel, Librarian

Maryland

2007 Maryland State Library for the Blind and Physically Handicapped
415 Park Avenue
Baltimore, MD 21201   410-230-2424
                                                        Fax: 410-333-2095
                                                        TTY: 800-934-2541
                                                        TDD: 410-333-8679
                                              e-mail: recept@lbta.lib.md.us
                                                        www.lbph.lib.md.us

Summer reading programs, braille writer, magnifiers, large-print photocopier, cassette books and magazines, children's books on cassette, and other reference materials on blindness and other handicaps.

Jill Lewis, Manager

2008 Prince George's County Memorial Library Talking Book Center
6530 Adelphi Road
Hyattsville, MD 20782   301-779-9330

Summer reading programs, braille writer, magnifiers, closed-circuit TV, large-print photocopier, cassette books and magazines, children's books on cassette, home visits and other reference materials on blindness and other handicaps.

Shirley Tuthill, Librarian

Massachusetts

2009 Braille and Talking Book Library Perkins School for the Blind
175 N Beacon Street
Watertown, MA 02472   617-924-3434
                                                        Fax: 617-926-2027
                                                 e-mail: perkins@bpl.org
                                                        www.perkins.org

Patricia Kirk

2010 Carroll Center for the Blind
770 Centre Street
Newton, MA 02458   617-969-6200
                                                             800-852-3131
                                                        Fax: 617-969-6204
                                                        www.carroll.org

Assists blind and visually impaired adults and adolescents to adjust to loss of vision. The goal of this dynamic program is to help the person become more independent, to restore self-confidence, prepare for employment and improve the quality of life. Programs of individual counseling are offered as part of the program.

Rachel Rosenbaum, President

Michigan

2011 Downtown Detroit Subregional Library for the Blind and Handicapped
5201 Woodward Avenue
Detroit, MI 48202   313-224-0580
                                                        Fax: 313-965-1977
                                                        TDD: 313-224-0584
                                          e-mail: deveans@cms.xx.wayne.edu
                                                        www.detroit.lib.mi.us

Summer reading programs, braille writer, magnifiers, closed-circuit TV, large-print photocopier, cassette books and magazines, children's books on cassette, home visits and other reference materials on blindness and other handicaps.

Deborah Evans, Librarian
Jo Anne Mondowney, Library Director

2012 Kent County Library for the Blind
775 Ball Avenue NE
Grand Rapids, MI 49503   616-336-3250
                                                        Fax: 616-336-3201
                                         e-mail: kdlem@lakeland.lib.mi.us

Summer reading programs, braille writer, magnifiers, closed-circuit TV, large-print photocopier, cassette books and magazines, children's books on cassette, home visits and other reference materials on blindness and other handicaps.

Claudya Muller, Librarian

2013 Library of Michigan Service for the Blind
PO Box 30007
Lansing, MI 48909   517-373-1300
                                                        Fax: 517-373-5700
                                        e-mail: info@sbph.libomich.lib.mi.us
                                           www.nfb.org/libraries for the blind

Summer reading programs, braille writer, magnifiers, closed-circuit TV, large-print photocopier, cassette books and magazines, children's books on cassette, home visits and other reference materials on blindness and other handicaps.

Nancy Robertson, Manager

2014 Macomb Library for the Blind and Physically Handicapped
16480 Hall Road
Clinton Township, MI 48038   586-286-1580
                                                        Fax: 586-286-0634
                                                        TDD: 810-869-40
                                            e-mail: macbld@libcoop.net
                                          www.macomb.lib.mi.us/macspe/

Summer reading programs, braille writer, closed-circuit TV, cassette books and magazines, children's books on cassette, reference materials on blindness and other handicaps.

Beverlee Babcock, Executive Director

2015 Mideastern Michigan Library Co-op
G-4195 W Pasadena Avenue
Flint, MI 48504   810-732-1120
                                                        Fax: 810-732-1715
                                        e-mail: cnash@genesse.freeret.org
                                           www.fakon.edu/gdl/talking.htm

Summer reading programs, braille writer, magnifiers, closed-circuit TV, large-print photocopier, cassette books and magazines, children's books on cassette, home visits and other reference materials on blindness and other handicaps.

Carolyn Nash, Librarian

2016 Muskegon County Library for the Blind
635 Ottawa Street
Muskegon, MI 49442   231-724-6361
                                                        Fax: 231-724-6675
                                                        TDD: 231-722-4103
                                                        www.muskcolib.org

Summer reading programs, braille typewriter, magnifiers, closed-circuit TV, large-print photocopier, cassette books and magazines, children's books on cassette, home visits and other reference materials on blindness and other handicaps, The Reading Edge, Perkins Brailler and large print books.

Linda Clapp, Librarian

2017 Upper Peninsula Library for the Blind Physically Handicapped
1615 Presque Isle Avenue
Marquette, MI 49855   906-228-7697
                                                        Fax: 906-228-5627
                                               e-mail: uproc.lib.mi.us
                                           www.upesc.lib.mi.us/uplbph

Summer reading programs, braille writer, magnifiers, closed-circuit TV, large-print photocopier, cassette books and magazines, children's books on cassette, home visits and other reference materials on blindness and other handicaps.

Suzanne Dees, Executive Director

2018 Washtenaw County Library
PO Box 8645
Ann Arbor, MI 48107
734-994-4912
Fax: 734-663-2430
e-mail: contact us@ewashtenaw.org
www.ewashtenaw.org

Summer reading programs, braille writer, magnifiers, closed-circuit TV, large-print photocopier, cassette books and magazines, children's books on cassette, home visits and other reference materials on blindness and other handicaps.

Kyeena Slater, Executive Director

2019 Washtenaw County Library for the Blind and Physically Disabled
PO Box 8645
Ann Arbor, MI 48107
734-994-4912
Fax: 734-663-2430
e-mail: lbpd@co.washtennaw.mi.us
www.ewashtenaw.org

Book lovers club.adaptive technology,cassette equipment, cassette books and magazines, described videos, low vision aids reference and referral services.

Kyeena Slater, Executive Director

2020 Wayne County Regional Library for the Blind
30555 Michigan Avenue
Westland, MI 48186
734-727-7300
Fax: 734-727-7333
TTY: 734-727-7330
e-mail: werlbph@tln.lib.mi.us
www.wayneregional.lib.mi.us

Summer reading programs, braille writer, magnifiers, closed-circuit TV, large-print photocopier, cassette books and magazines, children's books on cassette, home visits and other reference materials on blindness and other handicaps.

Reginald Williams, Wayne County Librarian

Minnesota

2021 Minnesota Library for the Blind & Physically Handicapped
Highway 298, PO Box 68
Fairbault, MN 55021
507-333-4828
800-722-0550
Fax: 507-333-4832
e-mail: libblnd@state.mn.us
www.nfb.org/libraries for the blind

Summer reading programs, braille writer, magnifiers, closed-circuit TV, large-print photocopier, cassette, large print, braille books and magazines, children's books on cassette, and other reference materials on blindness and other handicaps.

Catherine A Durivage, Program Director

Missouri

2022 Adriene Resource Center for Blind Children
1445 N. Boonville Avenue
Springfield, MO 65802
417-862-2781
Fax: 417-862-7566
e-mail: blind@ag.org
www.gospelpublishing.com

Offers braille and cassette lending library, braille and cassette Sunday school materials for all ages, braille and cassette periodicals and resource assistance, and resources for blind children and children of blind parents.

Paul Weingariner, Director

2023 Assemblies of God National Center for the Blind
1445 Boonville Avenue
Springfield, MO 65802
417-862-2781
Fax: 417-863-6614
e-mail: blind@ag.org
www.ag.org

Offers braille and cassette lending library, braille and cassette Sunday school materials for all ages, braille and cassette periodicals and resource assistance, and resources for blind children and children of blind parents.

Thomas Trask, Manager
George O Wood, General Superintendent

2024 Wolfner Memorial Library for the Blind
PO Box 387
Jefferson City, MO 65102
573-751-8720
Fax: 573-526-2985
TDD: 800-347-1379
e-mail: beckles@mail.sos.state.mo.us
www.nfb.org/libraries for the blind

Summer reading programs, braille writer, magnifiers, closed-circuit TV, large-print photocopier, cassette books and magazines, children's books on cassette, home visits and other reference materials on blindness and other handicaps.

Richard J Smith, Executive Director

Nebraska

2025 Nebraska Library Commission Talking Book & Braille Services
1200 N Street
Lincoln, NE 68508
402-471-2045
800-742-7691
Fax: 402-471-2083
TDD: 402-471-4038
e-mail: david.oertli@nebraska.gov
www.nlc.nebraska.gov

Free loan of books and magazines on cartridge, cassette, and in Braille, including children's materials, along with specially designed playback equipment. Summer reading program for children, Braille embossing, closed circuit TV, large-print copier. Reference materials on blindness and other disabilities.

David Oerti, Librarian

New Jersey

2026 New Jersey State Library Talking Book and Braille Center
185 West State Street
Trenton, NJ 08625
609-278-2640
800-792-8322
Fax: 609-278-2647
TDD: 877-882-5593
e-mail: njlbh@njstatelib.org
www.njstatelib.org

Free home delivery of large-print, audio, and braille books and magazines, children's books on cassettes in braille and other reference materials on blindness and other handicaps. Services are for New Jersey residents with print disabilities.

Adanrah Szczepaniak, Director
Anne McArthur, Head of Outreach and Audiovision

New Mexico

2027 New Mexico State Library for the Blind and Physically Handicapped
1209 Camino Carlos Ray
Santa Fe, NM 87507
505-476-9700
Fax: 505-476-9761
e-mail: jbrewstr@stlib.state.nm.us
www.stlib.state.nm.us

Summer reading programs, braille writer, magnifiers, closed-circuit TV, large-print photocopier, cassette books and magazines, children's books on cassette, home visits and other reference materials on blindness and other handicaps.

Susan Overland, Manager

New York

2028 New York State Talking Book & Braille Library
CEC, 222 Madison Avenue
Albany, NY 12230
518-474-5935
800-342-3688
Fax: 518-474-5786
TDD: 518-474-7121
e-mail: tbbl@mail.nysed.gov
www.nysl.nysed.gov/contact.htm

Books on audio cassette, cassette players, Braille books, summer reading programs, Braille writer, magnifiers, closed-circuit TV, large-print photocopier, cassette books and magazines, children's books on cassette, reference materials on blindness and other handicaps.

loretta ebert, Director
Bernard A Margolis, State Librarian

North Carolina

2029 North Carolina Library for the Blind
1841 Capital Boulevard
Raleigh, NC 27635
919-733-4376
888-388-2460
Fax: 919-733-6910
TDD: 919-733-1462
e-mail: nclbph@ncdcr.gov
http://statelibrary.ncdcr.gov/lbph/

Summer reading programs, Braille writer, magnifiers, closed-circuit TV, large-print photocopier, cassette books and magazines, children's books on cassette, home visits and other reference materials on blindness and other handicaps.

Mary Boone, State Librarian

Ohio

2030 American Council of Blind Parents
14400 Cedar Road, Apartment 108
University Heights, OH 44121
216-791-8118
800-424-8666

Members are sighted parents of blind or visually impaired children. Offers a forum for support and outreach, sharing of experiences in parent-child relationships, and educational and cultural information about child development. Monitors developments in technical and legislative arenas.

Nola Webb, President

Oregon

2031 Oregon State Library, Talking Book and Braille Services
250 Winter Street NE
Salem, OR 97301
503-378-5389
800-452-0292
Fax: 503-585-8059
TDD: 503-838-4276
e-mail: tbabs@sparkie.osl.state.or.us
www.tbabs.org

Cassette books and magazines, children's books on cassette, home visits and other reference materials on blindness and other handicaps.

Susan Westin, Manager

Virginia

2032 Alexandria Library Talking Book Service
5005 Duke Street
Alexandria, VA 22304
703-746-1702
Fax: 703-746-1747
TDD: 703-838-4568
e-mail: rdawson@alexandria.lib.va.us
www.alexandria.lib.va.us

Summer reading programs, Braille writer, magnifiers, closed-circuit TV, large-print photocopier, cassette books and magazines, children's books on cassette, home visits and other reference materials on blindness and other handicaps.

Rose Dawson, Director
Linden Renner, Deputy Director

2033 Division for the Visually Handicapped
1920 Association Drive
Reston, VA 20191
703-620-3660
Fax: 703-264-9494
e-mail: cec@cec.sped.org
www.cecp.air.org/teams/stratpart/cec.asp

Members are teachers, college faculty members, administrators, supervisors and others concerned with the education and welfare of visually handicapped and blind children and youth. This is a division of the Council For Exceptional Children.

Dr. Kay Ferrell, President

2034 Division on Visual Impairments
Council for Exceptional Children
2900 Crystal Drive Suite 1000
Arlington, VA 22202
888-233-7733
Fax: 703-264-9494
TTY: 866-915-5000
www.cec.sped.org/AM/

A division within the CEC, it handles concerns for Federal, state and local issues and policies related to education of youths, children and infants with visual impairments.

Ellyn Ross, President
Shirley J Wilson, Secretary
Phyllis T Simmons, President Elect

2035 Virginia State Library for the Visually and Physically Handicapped
395 Azalea Ave
Richmond, VA 23227
804-371-3661
800-552-7015
Fax: 804-371-3328
e-mail: barbara.mccarthy@dbvi.virginia.gov
www.vdbvi.org/lrcservices.htm

Summer reading programs, Braille writer, magnifiers, closed-circuit TV, large-print photocopier, cassette books and magazines, children's books on cassette, home visits and other reference materials on blindness and other handicaps.

Barbara McCarthy, Librarian

Washington

2036 Washington Library for the Blind and Physically Handicapped
2021 9th Ave
Seattle, WA 98121
206-615-0400
800-542-0866
Fax: 206-615-0437
TTY: 206-615-0418
e-mail: wtbbl@sos.wa.gov
www.wtbbl.org/

Summer reading programs, Braille writer, magnifiers, closed-circuit TV, large-print photocopier, cassette books and magazines, children's books on cassette, home visits and other reference materials on blindness and other handicaps.

Danielle Miller, Librarian

West Virginia

2037 West Virginia School for the Blind
301 E Main Street
Romney, WV 26757
304-822-4800
Fax: 304-822-3370
e-mail: pshank@access.k12.wv.us
www.sdb2.state.k12.wv.us/About%20WVSDB.htm

Summer reading programs, Braille writer, magnifiers, closed-circuit TV, large-print photocopier, cassette books and magazines, children's books on cassette, home visits and other reference materials on blindness and other handicaps.

Patsy Shank, Administrator

Research Centers

2038 Center for the Partially Sighted
6101 W. Centinela Ave, Suite 150
Culver City, CA 90230
310-988-1970
Fax: 310-988-1980
e-mail: info@low-vision.org
www.low-vision.org

Provides professional, comprehensive vision rehabilitation services to visually impaired people of all ages. For those whose sight is severely limited due to macular degeneration, diabetic retinopathy, glaucoma, retinal detachment, stroke or other conditions not correctable medically or surgically.

La Donna Ringering, President
Phillis Amaral, Director
Marc Gerberick, IT Manager

2039 Florida Ophthalmic Institute
7106 NW 11th Place Suite B
Gainesville, FL 32605
352-377-8364

Nonprofit organization that understands and treats ocular diseases including glaucoma.

Norman S Levy, Director

2040 Foundation for Glaucoma Research
251 Post Street, Suite 600
San Francisco, CA 94108
415-986-3162
Fax: 415-986-3763
e-mail: questions@glaucoma.org
www.glaucoma.org

Clinical and laboratory studies of glaucoma.

Tom Brunner, CEO
Andrew Iwach, Executive Director
H.Allen Bouch, Vice Chair

2041 Glaucoma Laser Trabeculoplasty Study
29275 Northwestern Highway
Southfield, MI 48034
248-493-5157

Examines the effectiveness and safety of the treatments of glaucoma.

Hugh Beckman, Chairman

2042 Glaucoma Research Foundation
251 Post Street, Suite 600
San Francisco, CA 94108
415-986-3162
800-826-6693
Fax: 415-986-3763
e-mail: questions@glaucoma.org
www.glaucoma.org

Conducts patient education activities, maintains eye donor network, provides multi-disciplinary seminars and conducts collaborative studies.

Tom Brunner, CEO
Andrew Iwach, Executive Director
H.Allen Bouch, Vice Chair

2043 Mobile Association for the Blind
2440 Gordon Smith Drive
Mobile, AL 36617
251-473-3585
877-292-5463
Fax: 251-470-8622
e-mail: sales@MobileBlind.org
www.mobileblind.org

Offers work adjustment training, activities of daily living, mobility, communication skills and sheltered employment for adults and children who are visually impaired.

Jim Bullock, Executive Director

2044 National Eye Research Foundation
910 Skokie Boulevard, Suite 207A
Northbrook, IL 60662
847-564-4652
800-621-2258
Fax: 847-564-0807
e-mail: info@nerf.org
www.nerf.com

Devoted to the enhancement of care and study of eye related diseases.

Andrew Kim

2045 National Ophthalmic Research Institute
Retina Consultants of Southwest, Florida
6901 International Center Boulevard
Ft. Myers, FL 33912
239-938-1284
800-282-8281
Fax: 239-938-1270
e-mail: NORI@eye.md
www.nori.md/index.htm

A physician-owned clinical research center specializing in innovative investigational treatments for ophthalmic, retinal and vitreous diseases.

Glen Wing MD, Research Director
Eileen Knips, RN, Clinical Research Coordinator
Glenn L Wing, MD, Medical Director

2046 New Beginnings - The Blind Children's Center
4120 Marathon Street
Los Angeles, CA 90029
323-664-2153
Fax: 323-665-3828
www.blindchildrenscenter.org/

The purpose of the Center is to turn initial fears into hope. Helps children and their families become independent by creating a climate of safety and trust. Children learn to develop self confidence and to master a wide range of skills. Services include an infant stimulation program, educational preschool, interdisciplinary assessment services, family services, correspondence program, toll free national hotline and a publication and research service.

2047 Research to Prevent Blindness
645 Madison Avenue, Floor 21
New York, NY 10022
212-752-4333
800-621-0026
Fax: 212-688-6231
e-mail: inforequest@rpbusa.org
www.rpbusa.org

Provides research grants to scientists interested in eye disease and vision disorders.

Diane Swift, President
David Weeks, Chairman

Conferences

2048 AADB National Symposium
American Association of the Deaf-Blind
8630 Fenton Street, Suite 121
Silver Spring, MD 20910
301-495-4403
Fax: 301-495-4404
TTY: 301-495-4402
e-mail: aadb-info@aadb.org
www.aadb.org

The symposium offers a training workshop, keynote speakers, full day exhibit hall, demonstration room, awards lunch and ceremony, talent show, Walk-A-Thon, and a banquet and dance.

Jill Gaus, President
Lynn Jansen, Vice President
Debby Lieberman, Secretary

2049 Genetic Alliance Annual Conference
Genetic Alliance
4301 Connecticut Avenue NW, Suite 404
Washington, DC 20008   202-966-5557
                                        800-336-4363
                                   Fax: 202-966-8553
               e-mail: info@geneticalliance.org
                         www.geneticalliance.org

Consistently inspirational and enables partnership among all
stakeholders: advocates and community leaders, health and industry professionals, policymakers, and academicians.

July

Sharon Terry, President/CEO
Tetyana Murza, Programs/Events Manager

Audio Video

2050 Heart to Heart
Blind Children's Center
4120 Marathon Street
Los Angeles, CA 90029   323-644-2153
                                   Fax: 323-665-3828
                                        www.blindcntr.org

Parents of blind and partially sighted children talk about their
feelings.
Videotape

2051 Let's Eat
Blind Children's Center
4120 Marathon Street
Los Angeles, CA 90029   323-664-2153
                                   Fax: 323-665-3828
                            www.blindchildrenscenter.org

Teaches competent feeding skills to children with visual impairments.
Videotape

2052 See What I Feel
Britannica Film Co.
345 4th Street
San Francisco, CA 94107   415-597-5555

A blind child tells her friends about her trip to the zoo. Each experience was explained as a blind child would experience it. A
teacher's guide comes with this video.
Films

Web Sites

2053 Glaucoma Associates
310 East 14th Street
New York, NY 10003   212-477-7540
                                   Fax: 212-420-8743
                                        www.glaucoma.net

Developed to promote research into the basic causes of Glaucoma, develop new treatments for Glaucoma, and to develop public education into the treatment of Glaucoma.

2054 Glaucoma Research Foundation
251 Post Street, Suite 600
San Francisco, CA 94108   e-mail: question@glaucoma.org
                                        www.glaucoma.org

Mission is to preserve the sight and independence of individuals
with glaucoma through research and education with the ultimate
goal of finding a cure.

Thomas M. Brunner, President/ CEO
Nancy Graydon, Executive Director of Development
Andrew L. Jackson, Director of Communications

2055 Lighthouse International
111 E 59th St
New York, NY 10022   800-284-4422
               e-mail: info@lighthouseguild.org
                         www.lighthouseguild.org

The mission is to overcome vision impairment for people of all
ages through worldwide leadership in rehabilitation services, education, research, prevention and advocacy.

2056 National Alliance of Blind Students
Los Angeles, CA   608-332-4147
               e-mail: smwhalenpsp@gmail.com
                         nabslink.org

The leading national advocacy and consumer organization for students in high school or college who are blind or visually
impaired.

Sean Whalen, President
Karen Anderson, 1st Vice President
Gabe Cazares, 2nd Vice President

2057 National Association for Visually Handicapped
111 E 59th St
New York, NY 10022   800-284-4422
               e-mail: info@lighthouseguild.org
                         www.lighthouseguild.org

Helps to cope with the difficulties of vision impairment.

2058 Online Mendelian Inheritance in Man
National Library of Medicine, Building 38A
Bethesda, MD 20894   888-346-3656
               e-mail: info@ncbi.nlm.nih.gov
                         www.ncbi.nlm.nih.gov

This database is a catalog of human genes and genetic disorders.

Christine E. Seidman, M.D., Chair
David J. Lipman, M.D., Executive Secretary

2059 Royal National Institute of the Blind
www.rnib.org.uk
                                        303-123-9999
               e-mail: helpline@rnib.org.uk
                         www.rnib.org.uk

Offering information, support and advice to over two million
people with sight problems.

Lesley-Anne Alexander CBE, Chief Executive
Wanda Hamilton, Group Director (Fundraising)
Sally Harvey, Managing Director (RNIB Places)

Book Publishers

2060 Childhood Glaucoma: A Reference Guide for Families
Nat'l Assn for Parents of Children with Visual
PO Box 317
Watertown, MA 02272   617-972-7441
                                        800-562-6265
                                   Fax: 617-972-7444
                                        www.spedex.com/napvi

Provides nontechnical information about childhood glaucoma and
its treatment. The book also discusses educational issues and
family concerns, gives a resource list, and includes a glossary.
1997 36 pages

Susan LaVenture, Editor/Executive Director

2061 Children with Visual Impairments: A Parents' Guide
Peytral Publications
PO Box 1162
Minnetonka, MN 55345   952-949-8707
                                        877-739-8725
                                   Fax: 952-906-9777
                                        www.peytral.com

Covers visual impairments ranging from low vision to total blindness. Offers authoritative information and empathy, parental insight on diagnosis and treatment, orientation and mobility, literacy, legal issues and more. Valuable to parents, educators and support staff.

395 pages

M Cay Holbrook PhD, Editor

2062 Ophthalmic Disorders Sourcebook
Omnigraphics Editorial Office
615 Griswold
Detroit, MI 48226

610-461-3548
800-234-1340
Fax: 610-532-9001
e-mail: editorial@omnigraphics.com
omnigraphics.com

Basic Information about glaucoma, cataracts, macular degeneration, strabismus, refractive disorders, and more.

1996 631 pages
ISBN: 0-780800-81-8

Linda M Ross, Editor

Magazines

2063 Journal of Visual Impairment and Blindness
American Foundation for the Blind
2 Penn Plaza, Suite 1102
New York, NY 10121

212-502-7600
Fax: 888-545-8331
e-mail: contributions@afb.net
www.afb.org

Published in braille, regular print and on cassette this journal contains a wide variety of subjects including rehabilitation, psychology, education, legislation, medicine, technology, employment, sensory aids and childhood development as they relate to visual impairments.

10x Year

Larry Kimbler, Chair
James H. McLaughlin, Vice Chair
Carl S. Augusto, President & CEO

2064 Reaching, Crawling, Walking - Let's Get Moving
Blind Children's Center
4120 Marathon Street
Los Angeles, CA 90029

323-664-2153
Fax: 323-665-3828
e-mail: info@blindchildrenscenter.org
www.blindchildrenscenter.org

Orientation and mobility for visually impaired preschool children.

24 pages

2065 Tactic
Clovernook Home and School for the Blind
7000 Hamilton Avenue
Cincinnati, OH 45231

513-522-3860
Fax: 513-728-3950
e-mail: clovernook@aol.com

Quarterly

Newsletters

2066 NAVH Update
National Association for Visually Handicapped
111 E 59th St
New York, NY 10022

212-889-3141
800-284-4422
Fax: 212-727-2931
e-mail: info@lighthouseguild.org
www.lighthouseguild.org

NAVH is committed to distributing its printed newsletters free in order to make certain every low-vision person has access to it's important infomation. The newsletter provides vision specific and general information in large print.

Quarterly

2067 National Library Service for the Blind & Physically Handicapped
Library of Congress Reference Section
1291 Taylor Street NW
Washington, DC 20542

202-707-5100
800-424-8567
Fax: 202-707-0712
TTY: 202-707-0744
TDD: 202-707-0744
e-mail: nis@loc.gov
www.loc.gov/nls

Provides information and advocacy resources for families and professionals, including listings of organizations focusing on more specific areas of concern to families and young adults who have disabilities. Administers a natural library service that provides recorded and braille reading materials to eligible children and adults who cannot read standard print.

12 pages Quarterly
ISSN: 1046-1663

Vicki Fitzpatrick, Editor

2068 Talking Book Topics
National Library Services for the Blind
1291 Taylor Street NW
Washington, DC 20542

202-707-5100
Fax: 202-707-0712
TDD: 202-707-0744
e-mail: nls@loc.gov
www.loc.gov/nls

Offers hundreds of listings of books, fiction and nonfiction, for adults and children on cassette. Also offers listings on foreign language books on cassette, talking magazines and reviews.

Bimonthly

Pamphlets

2069 Dancing Cheek to Cheek
Blind Children's Center
4120 Marathon Street
Los Angeles, CA 90029

323-664-2153
Fax: 323-665-3828
www.blindchildrenscenter.org

Discusses beginning social, play and language interactions.

33 pages

2070 Family Guide - Growth and Development of the Partially Seeing Child
National Association for Visually Handicapped
111 E 59th St
New York, NY 10022

212-889-3141
800-284-4422
Fax: 212-727-2931
e-mail: info@lighthouseguild.org
www.lighthouseguild.org

Offers information for parents and guidelines in raising a partially seeing child.

2071 Family Guide to Vision Care
American Optometric Association
243 N Lindbergh Boulevard
Saint Louis, MO 63141

314-991-4100
Fax: 314-991-4101
www.aoanet.org

Offers information on the early developmental years of your vision, finding a family optometrist and how to take care of your eyesight through the learning years, the working years and the mature years.

2072 Glaucoma
Foundation for Glaucoma Research
251 Post Street, Suite 600
San Francisco, CA 94108
415-986-3162
800-826-6693
Fax: 415-986-3763
e-mail: question@glaucoma.org
www.glaucoma.org

Offers information on what glaucoma is, the causes, treatments, types of glaucoma, eye exams and prevention.

Thomas M. Brunner, President/ CEO
Nancy Graydon, Executive Director of Development
Andrew L. Jackson, Director of Communications

2073 Glaucoma: The Sneak Thief of Sight
National Association for Visually Handicapped
111 E 59th St
New York, NY 10022
212-889-3141
800-284-4422
Fax: 212-727-2931
e-mail: info@lighthouseguild.org
www.lighthouseguild.org

A pamphlet describing the disease, treatment and medications.

Donna A Esposito, MD, Editor

2074 Heart to Heart
Blind Children's Center
4120 Marathon Street
Los Angeles, CA 90029
323-664-2153
Fax: 323-665-3828
www.blindchildrenscenter.org

Parents of blind and partially sighted children talk about their feelings.
12 pages

2075 Learning to Play
Blind Children's Center
4120 Marathon Street
Los Angeles, CA 90029
323-664-2153
Fax: 323-665-3828
www.blindchildrenscenter.org

Discusses how to present play activities to the visually impaired preschool child.
12 pages

2076 Let's Eat
Blind Children's Center
4120 Marathon Street
Los Angeles, CA 90029
323-664-2153
Fax: 323-665-3828
www.blindchildrenscenter.org

Teaches competent feeding skills to children with visual impairments.
28 pages

2077 Move with Me
Blind Children's Center
4120 Marathon Street
Los Angeles, CA 90029
323-664-2153
Fax: 323-665-3828
www.blindchildrenscenter.org

A parent's guide to movement development for visually impaired babies.
12 pages

2078 Selecting a Program
Blind Children's Center
4120 Marathon Street
Los Angeles, CA 90029
323-664-2153
Fax: 323-665-3828
www.blindchildrenscenter.org

A guide for parents of infants and preschoolers with visual impairments.

28 pages

2079 Standing on My Own Two Feet
Blind Children's Center
4120 Marathon Street
Los Angeles, CA 90029
323-664-2153
Fax: 323-665-3828
e-mail: info@blindchildrenscenter.org
www.blindchildrenscenter.org

A step-by-step guide to designing and constructing simple, individually tailored adaptive mobility devices for preschool-age children who are visually impaired.
36 pages

2080 Talk to Me
Blind Children's Center
4120 Marathon Street
Los Angeles, CA 90029
323-664-2153
Fax: 323-665-3828
www.blindchildrenscenter.org

A language guide for parents of deaf children.
11 pages

2081 Talk to Me II
Blind Children's Center
4120 Marathon Street
Los Angeles, CA 90029
323-664-2153
Fax: 323-665-3828
www.blindchildrenscenter.org

A sequel to Talk To Me, available in English and Spanish.
15 pages

Camps

2082 Bloomfield
5300 Angeles Vista Boulevard
Los Angeles, CA 90043
323-295-4555
800-352-2290
Fax: 323-296-0424
e-mail: info@juniorblind.org
www.juniorblind.org

This camp is dedicated to serving blind and developmentally disabled children and adults.

Miki Jordan, President

2083 Camp Civitan
3519 East Shea Blvd # 133
Phoenix, AZ 85028
602-953-2944
Fax: 602-953-2946
e-mail: info@campcivitan.org
www.campcivitan.org

A 501c3 non-profit organization, that has been providing multiple ever-changing programs to meet the needs of children and adults who are developmentally disabled.

Shannon Valenzuela, Director
Jane Armstrong, Director

2084 Enchanted Hills Camp
Lighthouse
214 Van Ness Avenue
San Francisco, CA 94102
415-694-7319
Fax: 415-863-7568
TTY: 415-431-4572
e-mail: afletcher@lighthouse-sf.org
www.lighthouse-sf.org

For blind, deaf/blind children and adults, ages 5 and up. This program offers a basic camping experience. Activities include music, art, dance, hiking and riding. Camperships are available to California residents.

Tony Fletcher, Camp Director

2085 Florida School-Deaf and Blind Summer Camp

207 San Marco Avenue
Saint Augustine, FL 32084

904-827-2200
800-800-344
e-mail: info@fsdb.k12.fl.us
www.fsdb.k12.fl.us

The Florida School for the Deaf and the Blind hosts summer campers from all over teh state of Florida for a week of fun and adventure. FSDB's 80 acre campus is where campers participate in a variety of activities including rock climbing, archery, swimming, kayaking, team games, arts and crafts, dance music, and much more.

L Daniel Hutto, President
Cindy Day, Executive Director of Parent Svcs
Terri Wiseman, Administrator of Business Services

2086 Highbrook Lodge Camp

12944 Aquilla Road
Chardon, OH 44024

216-791-8118
Fax: 216-791-1101
e-mail: camp@clevelandsightcenter.org
www.clevelandsightcenter.org

A summer residential camp for blind and disabled children, adults and families.

Mike Mullin, Director

2087 National Camps for Blind Children

Christian Record
4444 S 52nd Street
Lincoln, NE 68516

402-488-0981
Fax: 402-488-7582
e-mail: info@christianrecord.org
www.christianrecord.org

Camps throughout the US and Canada are offered at no cost to the legally blind, ages 9-65. Activities include archery, beeper basketball, water sports, hiking and rock climbing and horseback riding.

Peggy Hansen, Director

2088 Texas Lions Camp

Lions Clubs of Texas
PO Box 290247
Kerrville, TX 78029

830-896-8500
Fax: 830-896-3666
e-mail: tlc@ktc.com
www.lionscamp.com

The primary purpose of Texas Lions camp is to provide, without charge, a camp for physically disabled, hearing/vision impaired and diabetic children from the State of Texas, regardless of race, religion, or national origin. Our goal is to create an atmosphere wherein campers will learn the can do philosophy and be allowed to achieve maximum personal growth and self esteem. The camp welcomes boys and girls ages 7-16.

Stephen Mabry, Executive Director
Doug Parker, Business Manager
Steven King, Program/Client Service Director

2089 VISIONS/Vacation Camp for the Blind

500 Greenwich Street, 3rd Floor
New York, NY 10013

212-625-1616
888-245-8333
Fax: 212-219-4078
e-mail: info@visions.org
www.visions.org

Family programs at Vacation Camp for the Blind in Rockland County, NY for children who are blind, severely visually impaired or multi-handicapped. Parent or guardian must attend winter weekends and summer session.

Thomas M Decker, Camp Director
Nancy D Miller, Executive Director

2090 Wisconsin Lions Camp

3834 County Road A
Rosholt, WI 54473

715-677-4969
Fax: 715-677-3297
TTY: 715-677-6999
e-mail: info@wisconsinlionscamp.org
www.wisconsinlionscamp.com

Serves children who have either a visual, hearing or mild cognitive disability. Many of the children also have multiple disabilities or medical conditions. Program activities include sailing, ropes course, bike and canoe trips, environmental education, swimming, camping, canoeing, outdoor living skills and handicrafts. ACA accredited, located in central Wisconsin, near Stevens Point.

Russell Link, Camp Director

Description

2091 CONJUNCTIVITIS

Synonym: Pinkeye

Covers these related disorders: Infectious conjunctivitis, Noninfectious conjunctivitis

Involves the following Biologic System(s):

Infectious Disorders, Ophthalmologic Disorders

Conjunctivitis refers to a condition characterized by acute inflammation of the delicate mucous membranes (conjunctiva) that line the inside of the eyelids and the whites of the eyes (sclerae). This condition may be caused by a virus or bacterium. Allergic reactions or exposure to certain chemicals and other environmental factors may also play a role in certain types of conjunctivitis. Neonatal conjunctivitis (also known as neonatal ophthalmia or ophthalmia neonatorum) becomes apparent during the first four weeks of life and is considered an infectious disease resulting from bacterial or viral infections carried by the mother and passed to the child during the birthing process. Bacteria responsible for neonatal conjunctivitis infections may be common disease-causing organisms (pathogens) or may include Chlamydia trachomatis, the bacteria that causes the sexually transmitted disease (STD) chlamydia or Neisseria gonorrhoeae, responsible for the STD gonorrhea. In addition, viral transmission may be caused by herpes simplex type 2 virus, which is responsible for genital herpes. In addition, bacterial contamination may occur in a hospital nursery (Pseudomonas aeruginosa) and may, in some cases, cause severe infection.

The characteristic symptoms associated with infectious neonatal conjunctivitis include redness and severe swelling of the conjunctiva, including the eyelids and whites of the eyes, and a discharge from the eyes that may or may not contain pus (purulent). Symptoms of neonatal infection resulting from transmission during the birthing process may be present at birth or may appear during the second week of life, depending on the bacterium or virus responsible. Any early conjunctival infection should be evaluated as soon as possible to determine its cause and, subsequently, the appropriate course of treatment in order to prevent complications that could potentially lead to impaired vision or blindness.

Soon after delivery, erythromycin, or tetracycline drops or ointment are routinely administered to the eyes of the newborn to prevent gonococcal (gonorrheal) conjunctivitis. The use of 1% silver nitrate drops as prophylaxis (prevention) against gonococcal ophthalmia soon after birth has reduced its incidence in the United States to less than 0.03% of infants. Although silver nitrate is effective, it also may cause a chemical conjunctival inflammation that typically resolves on its own within 48 hours. Other preventive measures are directed toward identification and treatment of pregnant women with gonococcal infection.

Treatment for bacteria-caused neonatal conjunctivitis includes the use of particular antibiotics. In addition, washing (irrigating) the eye with a solution containing salt (saline) or direct application of antibiotic ointment to the eyes is often effective in relieving itching and discomfort and clearing up the discharge. Conjunctivitis caused by viral transmission may be treated with antiviral eye drops or ointment. Sometimes the antiviral drug acyclovir may be administered to prevent viral spread.

Additional causes of conjunctivitis in children may include other viruses associated with systemic diseases such as measles, some viruses of the adenovirus family, and intestinal viruses of the enterovirus family. This type of conjunctivitis is usually characterized by a watery discharge from the eyes, is usually self-limited, and treatment is symptomatic. However, one such adenovirus may cause severe itching and burning of the eyes, sensitivity to light (photophobia), and involvement of the cornea. This type of conjunctivitis is known as keratoconjunctivitis and affects the membranes lining the eyelids as well as the corneas. This virus is transmitted by direct contact. Conjunctivitis caused by allergies is usually seasonal and is characterized by swelling, tearing, and itching. Treatment is symptomatic and may include the application of antihistamine eye drops. Certain chemicals or environmental factors may also cause noninfectious, allergic-type conjunctivitis. In addition to silver nitrate used in preventive treatment in newborns, other irritating substances may include cleaning products, different types of sprays, smoke, pollen, and other materials. Treatment is directed toward prevention and relief of symptoms.

In the United States, as mentioned, the occurrence of neonatal conjunctivitis caused by Neisseria gonorrhoeae is extremely rare, while that caused by Chlamydia trachomatis is slightly more than eight out of every 1,000 births.

Government Agencies

2092 NIH/National Eye Institute
31 Center Drive MSC 2510
Bethesda, MD 20892

301-496-5248
e-mail: 2020@nei.nih.gov
www.nei.nih.gov

Conducts and supports research that helps prevent and treat eye diseases and other disorders of vision. This research leads to sight-saving treatments, reduces visual impairment and blindness, and improves the quality of life for people of all ages. NEI-supported research has advanced our knowledge of how the eye functions in health and disease.

Paul A Sieving M.D., Ph.D., Director

2093 NIH/National Institute of Allergy and Infectious Diseases
6610 Rockledge Drive, MSC 6612
Bethesda, MD 20892

301-496-5717
866-284-4101
Fax: 301-402-3573
TDD: 800-877-8339
e-mail: niaidnews@niaid.nih.gov
www.niaid.nih.gov

Conducts and supports basic and applied research to better understand, treat, and ultimately prevent infectious, immunologic, and allergic diseases.

Anthony S Fauci MD, Director

National Associations & Support Groups

2094 American Academy of Pediatrics
141 Northwest Point Boulevard
Elk Grove Village, IL 60007

847-434-4000
800-433-9016
Fax: 847-434-8000
www.aap.org

The American Academy of Pediatrics and its member pediatricians are committed to the attainment of optimal physical, mental and social health and well-being for all infants, children, adolescents, and young adults.

Sandra Hassink, MD, FAAP, President

2095 American Institute for Preventive Medicine
30445 Northwestern Highway, Suite 350
Farmington Hills, MI 48334
248-539-1800
800-345-2476
Fax: 248-539-1808
e-mail: aipm@healthylife.com
www.healthylife.com

An internationally recognized authority on the development and implementation of health promotion, wellness, medical self-care, and disease management programs and publications.

Larry Chapman, President
Dee Edington, Director
Bill Hettler, Cofounder

2096 World Health Organization
Avenue Appia 20
Geneva, SW
Switzerland
122-791-2111
Fax: 122-791-3111
e-mail: ÿerecruit@who.int
www.who.int

WHO is the directing and coordinating authority for health within the United Nations system.

Dr Margaret Chan, Director General

Web Sites

2097 American Academy of Family Physicians
11400 Tomahawk Creek Parkway
Leawood, KS 66211
913-906-6000
800-274-2237
Fax: 913-906-6075
e-mail: contactcenter@aafp.org
www.aafp.org

Represents more than 94,300 family physicians, family practice residents and medical students nationwide. Its mission is to preserve and promote the science and art of family medicine and to ensure high-quality, cost effective health care for patients of all ages.

Reid B. Blackwelder, MD, FAAFP, Board Chair
Robert L. Wergin, MD, FAAFP, President
Carl R. Olden, MD, FAAFP, Director

2098 Dr. Koop
www.drkoop.com

Information on the condition, causes, symptoms, tests and treatment.

2099 LSU Health Sciences Center
433 Bolivar Street
New Orleans, LA 70112
504-568-4808
e-mail: webmaster@lsuhsc.edu
www.lsuhsc.edu

An online library of resources.

Larry H. Hollier, MD, FACS, FACC, Chancellor
Evana Morales, Staff Accountant
Martha Hotard, Collections Manager

2100 MedicineNet.com
www.medicinenet.com

An online, healthcare media publishing company providing easy-to-read, in-depth, authoritative medical information for consumers via its user-friendly, interactive web site. MedicineNet.com has had a highly accomplished, uniquely experienced team of qualified executives in the fields of medicine, healthcare, internet tehnology, and business to bring you the most comprehensive, sought after healthcare information anywhere.

2101 Virtual Children's Hospital
200 Hawkins Drive
Iowa City, IA 52242
800-777-8442
www.vh.org

Mission is to educate patients, healthcare providers, and students in a free and anonymous manner, for the purpose of improving patients' care, outcome and lives.

Jean E. Robillard, MD, UI VP for Medical Affairs
Theresa Brennan, MD, Chief Medical Officer
Sabi Singh, MS, MA, Co-Chief Operating Officer

Description

2102 CORNELIA DE LANGE SYNDROME

Synonyms: BDLS, Brachmann-de Lange syndrome, CdLS, De
Lange syndrome

Involves the following Biologic System(s):
Genetic/Chromosomal/Syndrome/Metabolic Disorders

Cornelia de Lange syndrome is a genetic disorder characterized by growth delays before and after birth (prenatal growth
retardation); delays in the acquisition of skills that require the
coordination of physical and mental activities (psychomotor
retardation), and mild to severe mental retardation. Characteristic physical abnormalities include delays in the maturation
of bone; malformations of the head and facial (craniofacial)
area that result in a distinctive facial appearance; abnormalities of the arms, legs, hands, and feet (limbs); or other abnormalities. Associated symptoms and findings may vary in
range and severity from case to case.

Infants with Cornelia de Lange syndrome often have feeding
difficulties (e.g., projectile vomiting, regurgitation, swallowing difficulties); fail to grow and gain weight at the expected
rate (failure to thrive); and have a weak, growling cry. Affected infants usually experience breathing problems, such as
episodes in which there is temporary cessation of breathing
(apnea), inhalation (aspiration) of food into the air passages
of the lungs, and increased susceptibility to repeated respiratory infections. Affected infants and children also typically
have arched, bushy eyebrows that grow together (synophrys);
unusually long, curly eyelashes; a low hair line; and generalized excessive hair growth (hirsutism). Characteristic
craniofacial abnormalities may include an abnormally prominent vertical groove in the center of the upper lip (philtrum);
thin, downturned lips; and a small jaw (micrognathia). In addition, in many affected children, the teeth may erupt later
than expected and are widely spaced.

Many infants and children with Cornelia de Lange syndrome
also have malformations of the upper limbs, such as small
hands or abnormal positioning of the fifth fingers
(clinodactyly) or thumbs. In rare cases, the forearms, hands,
and fingers may be absent (phocomelia and oligodactyly).
Many affected infants and children also may have abnormally
small, short feet with webbing of the second and third toes
(syndactyly).

In many cases, additional symptoms and findings are present.
For example, in most affected males, the testes may fail to descend into the scrotum (cryptorchidism). Some affected infants may also have digestive abnormalities (e.g.,
gastroesophageal reflux, pyloric stenosis, bowel obstruction);
heart defects (e.g., ventricular septal defects); episodes of uncontrolled electrical activity in the brain (seizures); or other
physical abnormalities. In addition, many affected children
experience hearing loss and speech delays and may demonstrate behavioral problems, such as self-destructive tendencies.

Treatment of infants and children with Cornelia de Lange
syndrome includes symptomatic and supportive measures,
such as the prescription of certain medications to help prevent or control seizures (i.e., anticonvulsants); supportive
therapies to ensure the proper intake of nutrients and to
helpprevent or treat respiratory problems; and surgical or
other appropriate methods to treat heart or digestive defects.

In most cases, Cornelia de Lange syndrome appears to occur
randomly for unknown reasons. However, in a few reported
cases, autosomal dominant inheritance has been suggested.
The disorder is thought to affect approximately one in 10,000
newborns.

National Associations & Support Groups

2103 American Academy of Pediatrics
141 Northwest Point Boulevard
Elk Grove Village, IL 60007
847-434-4000
800-433-9016
Fax: 847-434-8000
www.aap.org

The American Academy of Pediatrics and its member pediatricians are committed to the attainment of optimal physical, mental
and social health and well-being for all infants, children, adolescents, and young adults.
Sandra Hassink, MD, FAAP, President

2104 Children's Craniofacial Association
13140 Colt Road, Suite 517
Dallas, TX 75240
214-570-9099
800-535-3643
Fax: 214-570-8811
e-mail: contactCCA@ccakids.com
www.ccakids.com

A national, nonprofit organization dedicated to improving the
quality of life for people with facial differences and their families. CCA's mission is to empower and give hope to facially dis-
figured children and their families.
Charlene Smith, Executive Director
Annie Reeves, Program Director
Jill Patterson, Development Director

2105 Cornelia de Lange Syndrome Foundation
302 W Main Street, Suite 100
Avon, CT 06001
860-676-8166
800-223-8355
Fax: 860-676-8337
e-mail: info@cdlsusa.org
www.cdlsusa.org

Provides a host of services that attract, educate, and unite fami-
lies touched by this rare birth disorder which causes individuals
to develop at a slower rate, both physically and mentally.
Liana Fresher, Executive Director
Antonie Kline MD, Medical Director
Kelley Brown, Assistant Executive Director

2106 FACES: The National Craniofacial Association
PO Box 11082
Chattanooga, TN 37401
423-266-1632
800-332-2373
e-mail: faces@faces-cranio.org
www.faces-cranio.org

Serving children and adults throughout the United States with severe craniofacial deformities resulting from birth defects, injuries
or disease. There is never a charge for any service provided by
the association.

2107 Genetic Alliance
4301 Connecticut Avenue NW Suite 404
Washington, DC 20008
202-966-5557
800-336-4363
Fax: 202-966-8553
e-mail: info@geneticalliance.org
www.geneticalliance.org

A coalition of voluntary genetic support groups, consumers and
professionals addressing the needs of individuals and families affected by genetic disorders from a national perspective.

Sharon Terry, President
Natasha Bonhomme, Vice President
Vaughn Edelson, Assistant Director of Health Commun

2108 March of Dimes Birth Defects Foundation
1275 Mamaroneck Avenue
White Plains, NY 10605   914-997-4488
                                          888-663-4637
                                      Fax: 914-997-4763
                        e-mail: askus@marchofdimes.com
                                 www.marchofdimes.com

Partnership of volunteers and professionals dedicated to improving the health of babies by preventing birth defects and infant mortality. Over 100 chapters are located across the country and can be located through the National Office.

Jennifer L Howse, President

Conferences

2109 CdLS Biennial Conference
302 W Main Street, Suite 100
Avon, CT 06001   860-676-8166
                                          800-223-8355
                                      Fax: 860-676-8337
                            e-mail: info@cdlsusa.org
                                     www.cdlsusa.org

Provides education and support to families of individuals with CdLS. Attendees receive free head-to-toe consultations with experts from a range of medical and educational fields; attend workshops on legal concerns, educational issues and medical/behaviors challenges; and have opportunities to meet other families facing similar challenges.

June

Liana Fresher, Executive Director
Gail Speers, Development/Events Coordinator
Marc Needlman, President

2110 Genetic Alliance Annual Conference
Genetic Alliance
4301 Connecticut Avenue NW, Suite 404
Washington, DC 20008   202-966-5557
                                          800-336-4363
                                      Fax: 202-966-8553
                       e-mail: info@geneticalliance.org
                                 www.geneticalliance.org

Consistently inspirational and enables partnership among all stakeholders: advocates and community leaders, health and industry professionals, policymakers, and academicians.

July

Sharon Terry, President/CEO
Tetyana Murza, Programs/Events Manager

Web Sites

2111 Online Mendelian Inheritance in Man
National Library of Medicine, Building 38A
Bethesda, MD 20894   888-346-3656
                            e-mail: info@ncbi.nlm.nih.gov
                                    www.ncbi.nlm.nih.gov

This database is a catalog of human genes and genetic disorders.

Christine E. Seidman, M.D., Chair
David J. Lipman, M.D., Executive Secretary

Journals

2112 Facing the Challenges
Cornelia de Lange Syndrome Foundation
302 W Main Street, Suite 100
Avon, CT 6001   860-676-8166
                                          800-223-8355
                                      Fax: 860-676-8337
                            e-mail: info@cdlusa.org
                                 www.cdlsusa.org/publications

The purpose of this book is to provide emotional support and factual information to those facing the challenges of caring for a person with Cornelia de Lange Syndrome.

Robert Boneberg, Esq., President
Richard Haaland, Ph.D., Vice President
David Barnes, Esq., Treasurer

Newsletters

2113 Reaching Out
Cornelia de Lange Syndrome Foundation
302 W Main Street, Suite 100
Avon, CT 6001   860-676-8166
                                          800-223-8355
                                      Fax: 860-676-8337
                            e-mail: info@cdlusa.org
                                 www.cdlsusa.org/publications

Up-to-date on issues relevant to the syndrome and connected to a community of families who share in the joys and sorrows of CdLS.

1977 Bi-Monthly

Robert Boneberg, Esq., President
Richard Haaland, Ph.D., Vice President
David Barnes, Esq., Treasurer

Description

2114 CRANIOSYNOSTOSIS

Synonyms: Craniostenosis, Craniostosis

Covers these related disorders: Frontal plagiocephaly, Kleeblattschadel deformity, Scaphocephaly, Trigonocephaly, Turricephaly (oxycephaly or acrocephaly)

Involves the following Biologic System(s):
Orthopedic and Muscle Disorders

Craniosynostosis is a developmental abnormality in which early closure of one or more of the fibrous joints (sutures) between bones of the skull results in deformity of the skull and an abnormally shaped head. The severity of the deformity depends upon which fibrous joint or joints close prematurely as well as the ability of other joints in the skull to expand and compensate for the other closed joint or joints. Craniosynostosis may occur as an isolated condition or in association with certain chromosomal or malformation syndromes. In most instances of isolated craniosynostosis, the condition appears to occur randomly for unknown reasons. However, there have been reports of isolated craniosynostosis in members of several multigenerational families (kindreds), indicating autosomal dominant or autosomal recessive inheritance. Many genetic malformation syndromes have been identified in the medical literature that are associated with craniosynostosis. The specific underlying cause of craniosynostosis is not fully understood. Craniosynostosis occurs in approximately one in every 1,000 to 2,000 births and is more prevalent in males than females.

In infants with craniosynostosis, because the skull is unable to enlarge in certain directions relative to the affected fibrous joint in the skull, there is compensatory growth and enlargement in other directions at the sites of open joints. This causes deformity of the skull and an abnormally shaped head. For example, in the most common form of craniosynostosis, there is premature closure of the joint between the upper sides of the skull (sagittal suture), causing the head to appear abnormally long and narrow (scaphocephaly). Affected infants also tend to have a broad forehead and a prominent back portion of the head (occiput). This condition appears to be more common in males than females.

In the form of craniosynostosis known as frontal plagiocephaly, there is early closure of a suture between the upper sides of the head and one of the bones of the forehead (e.g., coronal suture). This results in flattening of one side of the forehead, prominence of the ear, and elevation of the eyebrow and eye on the affected side. Frontal plagiocephaly appears to affect females more commonly than males.

Trigonocephaly, another form of craniosynstosis, is characterized by premature fusion of the suture between the bones forming the forehead (metopic suture). Affected infants have a keel-shaped forehead and closely spaced eyes (hypotelorism). In infants with the form of craniosynostosis known as turricephaly (also called oxycephaly or acrocephaly), premature fusion of coronal and sagittal sutures causes the head to have an abnormally long, narrow, cone-like appearance. In addition, a rare form of craniosynostosis, known as Kleeblattschadel deformity, is characterized by premature closure of multiple cranial su-

tures, causing the skull to appear cloverleaf-like in shape. Affected infants have a high forehead, marked protrusion of the eyes (proptosis), abnormal prominence of the lower sides of the skull (temporal bones), and other associated abnormalities. Many affected infants also experience hydrocephalus, a condition in which obstruction or impaired absorption of the fluid surrounding the brain and spinal cord (cerebrospinal fluid) causes fluid accumulation under increasing pressure within the brain, resulting in abnormal enlargement of the brain.

In infants with craniosynostosis, premature closure of one suture is rarely associated with increased pressure within the skull or associated neurologic abnormalities, such as mental retardation. In such patients, surgery may be considered for cosmetic purposes. Premature closure of two or more sutures is more likely to cause increased pressure within the skull, potentially resulting in brain damage and associated mental retardation. Additional findings associated with increased pressure may include vomiting, headaches, and swelling of the area where the optic nerve enters the eye and joins with the nerve-rich membrane at the back of the eye (papilledema). In these infants, surgery is necessary to increase the capacity of the skull in order to prevent excessive pressure within the skull. If craniosynostosis is diagnosed before three months of age, surgery may be conducted to create artificial cranial joints in the skull, allowing skull growth and preventing abnormal shaping of the head.

National Associations & Support Groups

2115 AmeriFace
PO Box 751112
Las Vegas, NV 89136

702-769-9264
888-486-1209
Fax: 702-341-5351
e-mail: info@ameriface.org
www.ameriface.org

Provides information, services, emotional support and educational programs for and on behalf of individuals with facial differences and their families. Working to increase understanding through public awareness and education.

3M members

Debbie Oliver, Executive Director

2116 American Academy of Pediatrics
141 Northwest Point Boulevard
Elk Grove Village, IL 60007

847-434-4000
800-433-9016
Fax: 847-434-8000
www.aap.org

The American Academy of Pediatrics and its member pediatricians are committed to the attainment of optimal physical, mental and social health and well-being for all infants, children, adolescents, and young adults.

Sandra Hassink, MD, FAAP, President

2117 Children's Craniofacial Association
13140 Coit Road, Suite 307
Dallas, TX 75240

214-570-9099
800-535-3643
Fax: 214-570-8811
e-mail: contactCCA@ccakids.com
www.ccakids.com

Devoted to the dispersion of medical knowledge of this and similar disorders, along with providing emotional support for the sufferers and their families.

Charlene Smith, Executive Director
Annie Reeves, Program Director
Jill Patterson, Development Director

2118 Craniosynostosis and Positional Plagiocephaly Support
massapequa, NY 11758

515-232-7015
888-572-5526
Fax: 516-977-3164
e-mail: info@cappskids.org
www.cappskids.org/

Established by a mother whose child had Craniosynostosis to offer support and information to other families who had a child
with Craniosynostosis.

Amy Galm, Director

2119 FACES: National Association for the Craniofacially Handicapped
PO Box 11082
Chattanooga, TN 37401

423-266-1632
800-332-2373
Fax: 423-267-3124
e-mail: faces@faces-cranio.org
www.faces-cranio.org

Assists individuals with facial disfigurations and their families
They maintain a registry of centers offering corrective surgery for
craniofacial deformities and financial assistance to qualified
applicants.

2120 FACES: National Craniofacial Foundation
PO Box 11082
Chattanooga, TN 37401

423-266-1632
800-332-2373
Fax: 423-267-3124
e-mail: faces@faces-cranio.org
www.faces-cranio.org

A nonprofit organization serving children and adults throughout
the United States with severe craniofacial deformities resulting
from birth defects, injuries, or disease. There is never a charge for
any service provided by the foundation.

2121 Forward Face
317 E 34th Street, Suite 901A
New York, NY 10016

212-684-5860
Fax: 212-684-5864
e-mail: info@forwardface.org
www.forwardface.org

Mission is to help children and their families find immediate support to manage the medical and social effects of facial differences. Working to educate, advocate and raise public awareness.

Camille Walsh, Manager
Camille Walsh, Assistant to Executive Director

2122 Genetic Alliance
4301 Connecticut Avenue NW
Washington, DC 20008

202-966-5557
800-336-4363
Fax: 202-966-8553
e-mail: info@geneticalliance.org
www.geneticalliance.org

A coalition of voluntary genetic support groups, consumers and
professionals addressing the needs of individuals and families affected by genetic disorders from a national perspective.

Sharon Terry, President
Natasha Bonhomme, Vice President
Vaughn Edelson, Assistant Director of Health Commun

2123 Guardians of Hydrocephalus Research Foundation
2618 Avenue Z
Brooklyn, NY 11235

718-743-4473
800-458-8655
Fax: 718-743-1171
e-mail: ghrf2618@aol.com
www.ghrforg.org

Non-profit organization made up of concerned parents and dedicated volunteers. The goal of this foundation is to wipe out this
top ranking birth defect.

Kathy Soriano

2124 Hydrocephalus Parent Support Group
Exceptional Family Resource Center
9245 Sky Park Court, Suite 130
San Diego, CA 92123

619-594-7416
800-281-8252
Fax: 858-268-4275
e-mail: efrcproject@sdsu.edu
www.efrconline.org

Determined to provide support to the parents and relatives of the
children stricken with the disorder.

Sherry Torok, Executive Director

2125 Let's Face It
University of Michigan
1011 N University
Ann Arbor, MI 48109

360-676-7325

A nonprofit network for people with facial difference, their families, friends and professionals. The mission is to advance knowledge about, by, and for people with facial differences and to
promote their full and equal participation in society.

Betsy Wilson, Founder/Director

2126 March of Dimes Birth Defects Foundation
1275 Mamaroneck Avenue
White Plains, NY 10605

914-997-4488
888-663-4637
Fax: 914-997-4763
e-mail: askus@marchofdimes.com
www.marchofdimes.com

Partnership of volunteers and professionals dedicated to improving the health of babies by preventing birth defects and infant
mortality. Over 100 chapters are located across the country and
can be located through the National Office.

Jennifer L Howse, President

2127 National Foundation for Facial Reconstruction
333 East 30th Street, Lobby Unit
New York, NY 10016

212-263-6656
Fax: 212-263-7534
e-mail: info@nffr.org
www.nffr.org

Created to address the plight of children with a facial disfigure-
ment by supporting state-of-the-art treatment, innovative research, psychosocial support and medical training that inspires a
new generation of pediatric doctors.

Whitney Burnett, Executive Director
Adam Conrad, Associate Executive Director
Kelly Strantz, Director of Development and Event

2128 National Hydrocephalus Foundation
12413 Centralia Road
Lakewood, CA 90715

562-924-6666
888-857-3434
e-mail: nhf@earthlink.net
www.nhfonline.org

Nonprofit public service organization that assembles and disseminates information about Hydrocephalus. Promotes communication
networks among those affected and their families, helps others
gain a deeper understanding of those areas affected by Hydrocephalus, such as education, tax and estate planning, employment
and family. Also promotes and supports research on the causes,
treatment and prevention of Hydrocephalus.

Debie Fields, President/Treasurer
Debbie Fields, Executive Director

Libraries & Resource Centers

2129 University of Illinois at Chicago, Craniofacial Center
College of Medicine
808 S Wood Street
Chicago, IL 60612

312-996-7870
Fax: 312-413-1526
www.medicine.uic.edu

Richard M Novak, Director

Research Centers

2130 Craniofacial Center at University of Illinois, Chicago
811 S Paulina
Chicago, IL 60612   312-996-7546
                                            Fax: 312-413-1157
                                    e-mail: tkaislin@uic.edu
                uic.edu/com/surgery/plastic/craniofacial_cntr.htm
Maya Shahani, Director
Mimis Cohen, Professor of Surgery

Conferences

2131 Genetic Alliance Annual Conference
Genetic Alliance
4301 Connecticut Avenue NW, Suite 404
Washington, DC 20008   202-966-5557
                                                 800-336-4363
                                            Fax: 202-966-8553
                                    e-mail: info@geneticalliance.org
                                            www.geneticalliance.org

Consistently inspirational and enables partnership among all
stakeholders: advocates and community leaders, health and industry professionals, policymakers, and academicians.

July

Sharon Terry, President/CEO
Tetyana Murza, Programs/Events Manager

Audio Video

2132 Face First
Fanlight Productions
32 Court Street, 21st Floor
Brooklyn, NY 11201   718-488-8900
                                                 800-876-1710
                                            Fax: 718-488-8642
                                    e-mail: info@fanlight.com
                                            www.fanlight.com

Profiles of several people born with facial deformities; they
chronicle both physical pain and the pain of rejection, as well as
the strengths that have enabled them to achieve successful adult
lives. ISBN: DVD: 1-57295-886-3; VHS: 1-572952-59-8

29 minutes DVD or VHS

Nicole Johnson, Publicity Coordinator

Web Sites

2133 National Hydrocephalus Foundation
www.nhfonline.org

Promotes information and educational assistance. Establishes and
facilitates a communication network and works to increase public
awareness. Promote and support research. Also has brochures,
help sheets and more. Quarterly newsletter included with annual
membership fee of $35.00.

Book Publishers

2134 Congenital Disorders Sourcebook
Omnigraphics
PO Box 8002
Aston, PA 19014   800-234-1340
                                            Fax: 800-875-1340
                                    e-mail: info@omnigraphics.com
                                            www.omnigraphics.com

Basic consumer health information on disorders aquired during
gestation, including spina bifida, hydrocephalus, cerebral palsy,
heart defects, craniofacial abnormalities and fetal alcohol
syndrome.

650 pages
ISBN: 0-780809-45-9

Newsletters

2135 National Hydrocephalus Foundation Newsletter
12413 Centralia Road
Lakewood, CA 90715   562-924-6666
                                                 888-598-3434
                                            Fax: 415-732-7044
                                    e-mail: debbifields@nhfonline.org
                                            www.nhfonline.org

The Foundation is a national organization whose purpose is to
provide information and education, along with peer support
newsletter quarterly.

12-15 pages Quarterly

Michael Fields, President/ Treasurer
Debbie Fields, Executive Director
Jaynie Dunn, Secretary

Camps

2136 Camp About Face
Riley Hospital # 2514, 702 Barnhill Drive
Indianapolis, IN 46202   317-274-2489
                www.headsupfoundation.org/camp_about_face.htm

Camp designed to benefit youth ages 8-18 with craniofacial
anomalies.

Description

2137 CROHN'S DISEASE

Synonym: Regional enteritis

Involves the following Biologic System(s):

Gastrointestinal Disorders

Crohn's disease is an inflammatory bowel disease (IBD) characterized by chronic inflammation of any region of the digestive (gastrointestinal) tract from the mouth to the anus. The disease most commonly involves the lower region of the small intestine (ileum) and the major part of the large intestine (colon). Chronic inflammation of these areas causes thickening and scarring of the intestinal wall. The range and severity of Crohn's disease is extremely variable and depends on the intestinal region affected, the severity of symptoms and findings of inflammation, and associated complications. In children, Crohn's disease usually becomes apparent during the late teens; however, symptoms may begin during early childhood. In developed countries, inflammatory bowel disease, including Crohn's disease, is the most common cause of chronic intestinal inflammation during mid-childhood. Crohn's disease affects males and females in equal numbers. In the U.S., the disease affects approximately 30 to 100 per 100,000 individuals in the general population and occurs more frequently among Caucasians and African-Americans, (and is more common in Jewish individuals than in Hispanic-Americans and Asian-Americans. Although the exact cause of Crohn's disease is unknown, genetic, immune, and environmental factors are thought to play a role. Some researchers suspect that the disorder may result from an exaggerated immune response to an invading microorganism, such as a particular virus or bacterium.

In most children, Crohn's disease initially involves both the lower region of the small intestine and the major part of the large intestine (ileocolitis). However, initial inflammation may be restricted to the small intestine or the colon. The inflammatory process tends to be segmental in nature, and diseased regions of the intestine are often separated by apparently normal segments (skip lesions). Chronic inflammation causes thickening, ulceration, and scarring of affected areas of the intestinal walls and may lead to the development of abnormal channels (fistulas) between regions of the colon, the intestine and the urinary bladder, or the intestine and the surface of the skin. Additional complications may include the development of pus-filled pockets of infection (abscesses) or intestinal obstruction due to abnormal narrowing of certain intestinal regions.

Many children with Crohn's disease experience episodes of cramping; abdominal discomfort and pain; diarrhea that may contain blood; persistent spasms of the rectum (tenesmus); and a compelling urge to defecate. Additional symptoms and findings typically include fever, chills, easy fatigability, a general feeling of ill health (malaise), lack of appetite (anorexia), weight loss, and malnutrition due to impaired intestinal absorption of fats and nutrients (malabsorption). Many patients also develop deep grooves or cracks (fissures) in the mucous membranes of the anus. Some children have delayed bone maturation, retarded physical growth, or delayed sexual development as much as one to two years before the onset of other symptoms.

Many patients with Crohn's disease may also develop more generalized, systemic symptoms. These may include joint swelling and inflammation (arthritis); inflammation of the outermost layers of the eye's tough, white, outer coat (episcleritis); eruption of multiple, inflamed, reddish-purplish swellings on the legs and possibly the arms (erythema nodosum); and abnormal concentrations of mineral salts (calculi or stones) in the kidneys or the muscular sac (gall bladder) that stores and concentrates bile from the liver. Patients may also be prone to developing ankylosing spondylitis, a chronic, progressive, inflammatory disease that affects joints of the spine and results in pain, stiffness, and possible loss of spinal mobility. In addition, it is suspected that patients who have Crohn's disease for many years may have an increased risk of colon cancer as compared with the general population.

Symptoms typically flare up at irregular intervals throughout life. These episodes may be mild or severe and last for relatively short or prolonged periods. The treatment of Crohn's disease is directed at minimizing symptoms. Therapy may include the use of certain medication, such as sulfasalazine, azathioprine, or metronidazole. For example, azathioprine or metronidazole may be helpful in treating anal fistulas, and metronidazole has been beneficial in treating some patients who have not responded to other medications. Oral steroids may be added if needed. They are highly effective in reducing symptoms but should be used for short-term treatment only. Steroids should be tapered as soon as possible to reduce the risk of long-term side effects. In many children, treatment may include the administration of nutrients in liquid form (total parenteral nutrition) via a tube through the nose to the stomach (nasogastric tube). Some patients who experience severe, sudden episodes may require hospitalization to ensure proper intake of nutrients and fluids and to receive appropriate medical therapy. In addition, some patients may eventually require surgery to remove diseased portions of the intestine. However, such surgery is reserved for very specific indications, because the recurrence rate is high and the risk of needing additional surgery increases after such a procedure. Additional treatment is symptomatic and supportive.

National Associations & Support Groups

2138 American Academy of Pediatrics
141 Northwest Point Boulevard
Elk Grove Village, IL 60007
847-434-4000
800-433-9016
Fax: 847-434-8000
www.aap.org

The American Academy of Pediatrics and its member pediatricians are committed to the attainment of optimal physical, mental and social health and well-being for all infants, children, adolescents, and young adults.

Sandra Hassink, MD, FAAP, President

2139 American Autoimmune Related Diseases Association, Inc.
22100 Gratiot Avenue
East Detroit, MI 48021
586-776-3900
800-598-4668
Fax: 586-776-3903
www.aarda.org

The American Autoimmune Related Diseases Association is dedicated to the eradication of autoimmune diseases and the alleviation of suffering and the socioeconomic impact of autoimmunity through fostering and facilitating collaboration in the areas of education, public awareness, research, and patient services in an effective, ethical and efficient manner.

Stanley M Finger, PhD, Chairman of the Board
Noel R Rose, MD, PhD, Chairman Emeritus

2140 Crohn's & Colitis Foundation of America Hotline
Crohn's & Colitis Foundation of America
386 Park Avenue S, 17th Floor
New York, NY 10016   212-685-8707
                                                800-932-2423
                                           Fax: 212-779-4098
                                       e-mail: info@ccfa.org
                                                www.ccfa.org

The mission of the Crohn's & Colitis Foundation of America
(CCFA), is to cure and prevent Crohn's disease and ulcerative colitis through research and to improve the quality of life of children and adults affected by these digestive diseases through
education and support. Known collectively as inflammatory
bowel disease (IBD), these painful chronic illnesses affect up to
one million Americans, including approximately 100,000 children
under the age of 18. CCFA was founded in 1967.

2141 Digestive Disease National Coalition
507 Capitol Court NE, Suite 200
Washington, DC 20002   202-544-7497
                                           Fax: 202-546-7105
                                      e-mail: ddnc@hmcw.org
                                                www.ddnc.org

Advocacy organization comprised of 22 voluntary and professional societies concerned with the many diseases of the digestive
tract and liver.

Linda Aukett, Chairperson
James Degerome, President
Dr. Peter Banks, VP

2142 Genetic Alliance
4301 Connecticut Avenue NW
Washington, DC 20008   202-966-5557
                                                800-336-4363
                                           Fax: 202-966-8553
                               e-mail: info@geneticalliance.org
                                         www.geneticalliance.org

A coalition of voluntary genetic support groups, consumers and
professionals addressing the needs of individuals and families affected by genetic disorders from a national perspective.

Sharon Terry, President
Natasha Bonhomme, Vice President
Vaughn Edelson, Assistant Director of Health Commun

2143 International Foundation for Bowel Dysfunction
700 W. Virginia St.201
Milwaukee, WI 53204   414-964-1799
                                                888-964-2001
                                           Fax: 414-964-7176
                                       e-mail: iffgd@iffgd.org
                                                www.iffgd.org

A nonprofit education and research organization. Our mission is
to inform, assist, and support people affected by gastrointestinal
disorders.

Nancy J Norton, Founder
William Norton, VP

**2144 International Foundation for Functional Gastrointestinal
Disorders**
PO Box 170864
Milwaukee, WI 53217   414-964-1799
                                                888-964-2001
                                           Fax: 414-964-7176
                                       e-mail: iffgd@iffgd.org
                                                www.iffgd.org

Nonprofit education and research organization founded in 1991.
IFFGD addresses the issues surrounding life with gastrointestinal
(GI) functional and mobility disorders and increases the awareness about these disorders among the general public, researchers
and the clinical care community.

Nancy J Norton, Founder
William Norton, VP

2145 March of Dimes Birth Defects Foundation
1275 Mamaroneck Avenue
White Plains, NY 10605   914-997-4488
                                                888-663-4637
                                           Fax: 914-997-4763
                                  e-mail: askus@marchofdimes.com
                                           www.marchofdimes.com

Partnership of volunteers and professionals dedicated to improving the health of babies by preventing birth defects and infant
mortality. Over 100 chapters are located across the country and
can be located through the National Office.

Jennifer L Howse, President

State Agencies & Support Groups

Alabama

**2146 Alabama/Northwest Florida Chapter of Crohn s Colitis
Foundation of America**
244 Goodwin Crest Drive, Suite 120
Birmingham, AL 35259   646-387-2149
                                                800-249-1993
                                           Fax: 205-941-1411
                                    e-mail: jshugart@ccfa.org
                                                www.ccfa.org

Crohn's and Colitis Foundation of America is a nonprofit, voluntary health organization dedicated to improving the quality of life
for persons with Crohn's disease or ulcerative colitis.

Pat Talty, Executive Director
Maura Breen, Chairman

Arizona

2147 Arizona Chapter of Crohn's & Colitis Foundation of America
8098 Via de Negocio, Suite 201
Scottsdale, AZ 85258   480-246-3676
                                                877-259-2104
                                           Fax: 480-246-3679
                                   e-mail: southwest@ccfa.org
                                                www.ccfa.org

Crohn's and Colitis Foundation of America is a nonprofit, voluntary health organization dedicated to improving the quality of life
for persons with Crohn's disease or ulcerative colitis.

Bridgette Haley, Executive Director
Maura Breen, Chairman

California

**2148 Greater Los Angeles/Orange County Chapter of Chron's &
Colitis Foundation**
1640 S Sepulveda Boulevard, Suite 214
Los Angeles, CA 90025   310-478-4500
                                                866-831-9157
                                           Fax: 310-478-4546
                                   e-mail: losangeles@ccfa.org
                                                www.ccfa.org

Crohn's and Colitis Foundation of America is a nonprofit, voluntary health organization dedicated to improving the quality of life
for persons with Crohn's disease or ulcerative colitis.

Ronni Epstein, Executive Director
Lindsay Brown, Support Manager

**2149 Greater San Diego/Desert Chapter of Crohn' s & Colitis
Foundation of America**
7850 Mission Center Ct. Suite 100
San Diego, CA 92108   619-497-1300
                                           Fax: 619-497-1304
                                     e-mail: sandiego@ccfa.org
                                                www.ccfa.org

Crohn's and Colitis Foundation of America is a nonprofit, voluntary health organization dedicated to improving the quality of life
for persons with Crohn's disease or ulcerative colitis.

Pamela Meistrell, Executive Director

2150 Northern California Chapter of Crohn's and Colitis Foundation
5 Third Street, Suite 625
San Francisco, CA 94103
415-356-2232
800-241-0758
Fax: 415-356-0880
e-mail: ncal@ccfa.org
www.ccfa.org

Supports basic and clinical scientific research to find the cause of, and cure for, Crohn's disease and ulcerative colitis; provides educational programs for patients, medical professionals and the general public; offers supportive services for patients, their families and friends including support groups, information packets, education seminars, physician referral hotline and a quarterly newsletter called Rumblings.

Tamara Block, Executive Director

Colorado

2151 Rocky Mountain Chapter of Crohn's & Colitis Foundation of America
1777 S Bellaire Street, Suite 230
Denver, CO 80222
303-639-9163
800-768-2232
Fax: 303-639-9166
e-mail: rockymountain@ccfa.org
www.ccfa.org

Crohn's and Colitis Foundation of America is a nonprofit, voluntary health organization dedicated to improving the quality of life for persons with Crohn's disease or ulcerative colitis.

Michele L Basche, Executive Director
Maura Breen, Chairman

Connecticut

2152 Central Connecticut Chapter of Crohn's & Colitis Foundation of America
PO Box 34
New London, CT 06320
646-499-0159
e-mail: mbfecteau@ccfa.org
www.ccfa.org

Crohn's and Colitis Foundation of America is a nonprofit, voluntary health organization dedicated to improving the quality of life for persons with Crohn's disease or ulcerative colitis.

Maura Breen, Chairman

2153 Fairfield/Westchester Chapter of Crohn's & Colitis Foundation of America
200 Bloomingdale Road
White Plains, NY 10603
914-328-2874
Fax: 914-468-2133
e-mail: westfield@ccfa.org
www.ccfa.org

Crohn's and Colitis Foundation of America is a nonprofit, voluntary health organization dedicated to improving the quality of life for persons with Crohn's disease or ulcerative colitis.

Russell P Girolamo, Board President
Maura Breen, Chairman

2154 Northern Connecticut Affiliate Chapter of Crohn's & Colitis Foundation of America
PO Box 370614
West Hartford, CT 06137
www.ccfa.org

Crohn's and Colitis Foundation of America is a nonprofit, voluntary health organization dedicated to improving the quality of life for persons with Crohn's disease or uilcerative colitis.

Maura Breen, Chairman

Florida

2155 Florida Chapter of Crohn's & Colitis Found ation of America
21301 Powerline Road #301
21301 Powerline Rd., Suite 301
Boca Raton, FL 33433
561-218-2929
877-664-2929
Fax: 561-218-2240
e-mail: florida@ccfa.org
www.ccfa.org

Crohn's and Colitis Foundation of America is a nonprofit, voluntary health organization dedicated to improving the quality of life for persons with Crohn's disease or ulcerative colitis.

Amy Gray, Executive Director
Maura Breen, Chairman

Georgia

2156 Georgia Chapter of Crohn's & Colitis Foundation of America
2250 N Druid Hills Road, Suite 250
Atlanta, GA 30329
404-982-0616
800-472-6795
Fax: 404-982-0656
e-mail: sprimm@ccfa.org
www.ccfa.org

Crohn's and Colitis Foundation of America is a nonprofit, voluntary health organization dedicated to improving the quality of life for persons with Crohn's disease or ulcerative colitis.

Marcia Greenburg, Regional Executive Director
Karen Rittenbaum, Deputy Director

Illinois

2157 Crohn's & Colitis Foundation of America Carol Fisher Chapter
2200 E Devon Avenue, Suite 351
Des Plaines, IL 60018
847-827-0404
800-886-6664
Fax: 847-827-6563
e-mail: illinois@ccfa.org
www.ccfa.org

Crohn's and Colitis Foundation of America is a nonprofit, voluntary health organizaiton dedicated to finding the cause of, and cure for Crohn's disease and ulcerative colitis. The foundation is committed to conquering these devastating diseases.

$25.00 Dues

Marianne Floriano, Executive Director
Maura Breen, Chairman

Indiana

2158 Indiana Chapter of Crohn's & Colitis Found ation of America
931 e. 86th St Suite 210
Indianapolis, IN 46240
317-259-8071
800-332-6029
Fax: 317-259-8091
e-mail: jbender@ccfa.org
www.ccfa.org

Provides support and education to adults, children, and families dealing with Crohn's disease and ulcerative colitis. Raises funds for research and programs. Quarterly newsletter, national magazine, award winning website. 55 chapters nationwide.

Jo Bender, Community Development Director
Maura Breen, Chairman

Iowa

2159 Iowa Chapter of Crohn's Colitis Foundation of America
8031 West Center Rd Suite 322
Omaha, NE 68124
402-505-9901
e-mail: iowa@ccfa.org
www.ccfa.org

Crohn's and Colitis Foundation of America is a nonprofit, voluntary health organization dedicated to improving the quality of life for persons with Crohn's disease or ulcerative colitis.

Melissa Cupich, Development Manager
Maura Breen, Chairman

Kansas

2160 Mid-America Chapter of Crohn's & Colitis Foundation of America
1034 S. Brentwood Suite 1510
St. Louis, MO 63117
314-863-4747
800-783-8006
Fax: 314-863-4749
e-mail: awillet@ccfa.org
www.ccfa.org

Crohn's and Colitis Foundation of America is a nonprofit, voluntary health organization dedicated to improving the quality of life for persons with Crohn's disease or ulcerative colitis.

Steve Skodak, Development Director
Maura Breen, Chairman

Kentucky

2161 Kentucky Chapter of Crohn's & Colitis Foundation of America
PO Box 573
Prospect, KY 40059
646-623-2620
e-mail: kentucky@ccfa.org
www.ccfa.org

Crohn's and Colitis Foundation of America is a nonprofit, voluntary health organization dedicated to improving the quality of life for persons with Crohn's disease or ulcerative colitis.

Jenny Silberisen, Community Development Manager
Maura Breen, Chairman

Louisiana

2162 Louisiana/Mississippi Chapter of Crohn's & Colitis Foundation of America
8019 Maple Street
New Orleans, LA 70175
504-861-3433
866-382-2232
Fax: 504-861-3466
e-mail: lams@ccfa.org
www.ccfa.org

Crohn's and Colitis Foundation of America is a nonprofit, voluntary health organization dedicated to improving the quality of life for persons with Crohn's disease or ulcerative colitis.

David Lee Thomas, Executive Director
Maura Breen, Chairman

Maryland

2163 Maryland/South Delaware Chapter of Crohn's & Colitis Foundation of America
10400 Little Patuxent Parkway, Suite 270
Columbia, MD 21044
443-276-0861
800-618-5583
Fax: 443-276-0865
e-mail: maryland@ccfa.org
www.ccfa.org

Our mission is to fund research to find a cure for Crohn's disease and ulcerative colitis and to educate and provide support to patients and families with these diseases.

Allison Coffey, Community Development Director
Maura Breen, Chairman

Massachusetts

2164 New England Chapter of Crohn's & Colitis Foundation of America
280 Hillside Avenue
Needham, MA 02494
781-449-0324
800-314-3459
Fax: 781-449-0325
e-mail: ne@ccfa.org
www.ccfa.org

Crohn's and Colitis Foundation of America is a nonprofit, voluntary health organization dedicated to improving the quality of life for persons with Crohn's disease or ulcerative colitis.

Craig Comins, Regional Executive Director
Maura Breen, Chairman

Michigan

2165 Michigan Chapter of Crohn's & Colitis Foundation of America
31313 Northwestern Highway, Suite 204
Farmington Hills, MI 48334
248-737-0900
Fax: 248-737-0904
e-mail: michigan@ccfa.org
www.ccfa.org

Crohn's and Colitis Foundation of America is a nonprofit, voluntary health organization dedicated to improving the quality of life for persons with Crohn's disease or ulcerative colitis.

Anthonie Burke, Community Development Director
Maura Breen, Chairman

Minnesota

2166 Minnesota/Dakotas Chapter of Crohn's & Colitis Foundation of America
1885 University Avenue W, Suite 355
Saint Paul, MN 55104
651-917-2424
888-422-3266
Fax: 651-917-2425
e-mail: minnesota@ccfa.org
www.ccfa.org

Voluntary health organization providing education service and support to Crohn's disease and ulcerative colitis patients and the professional community.

Danielle L Baxter, Executive Director
Ruby Lanoux, Development Coordinator

Mississippi

2167 Louisiana/Mississippi Chapter of Crohn's & Colitis Foundation of America
8019 Maple Street
New Orleans, LA 70175
504-861-3433
866-382-2232
Fax: 504-861-3466
e-mail: lams@ccfa.org
www.ccfa.org

Crohn's and Colitis Foundation of America is a nonprofit, voluntary health organization dedicated to improving the quality of life for persons with Crohn's disease or ulcerative colitis. Your local chapter can supply you with a list of CCFA physician members in your area.

David Lee Thomas, Executive Director
Maura Breen, Chairman

Missouri

2168 Saint Louis Chapter of Crohn's & Colitis Foundation of America
8420 Delmar Boulevard, Suite 303
Saint Louis, MO 63124
314-997-4466
Fax: 314-991-8756
e-mail: missouri@ccfa.org
www.ccfa.org

Crohn's and Colitis Foundation of America is a nonprofit, voluntary health organization dedicated to improving the quality of life for persons with Crohn's disease or ulcerative colitis.

Charise Cross, Owner
Maura Breen, Chairman

New Jersey

2169 New Jersey Chapter of Crohn's & Colitis Foundation of America
45 Wilson Avenue
Manalapan, NJ 07726
732-786-9960
Fax: 732-786-9964
e-mail: newjersey@ccfa.org
www.ccfa.org

Crohn's and Colitis Foundation of America is a nonprofit, voluntary health organization dedicated to improving the quality of life for persons with Crohn's disease or ulcerative colitis.

Rosemarie Golombos, Executive Director
Maura Breen, Chairman

New Mexico

2170 Southwest Chapter of Crohn's & Colitis Foundation of America
8098 Via de Negocio, Suite 201
Scottsdale, AZ 85254
480-246-3676
877-259-2104
Fax: 480-246-3679
e-mail: southwest@ccfa.org
www.ccfa.org

Crohn's and Colitis Foundation of America is a nonprofit, voluntary health organization dedicated to improving the quality of life for persons with Crohn's disease or ulcerative colitis.

Cindy Sorensen, Regional Edu. & Support Manager
Maura Breen, Chairman

New York

2171 Central New York Chapter of Crohn's & Colitis Foundation of America
2117 Buffalo Rd Suite 299
Rochester, NY 14624
585-617-4771
e-mail: smassaro@ccfa.org
www.ccfa.org

Crohn's and Colitis Foundation of America is a nonprofit, voluntary health organization dedicated to improving the quality of life for persons with Crohn's disease or ulcerative colitis. Your local chapter can supply you with a list of CCFA physician members in your area.

Maura Breen, Chairman

2172 Fairfield/Westchester Chapter of Crohn's & Colitis Foundation of America
200 Bloomingdale Road
White Plains, NY 10605
914-328-2874
Fax: 914-328-2946
e-mail: westfield@ccfa.org
www.ccfa.org

Crohn's and Colitis Foundation of America is a nonprofit, voluntary health organization dedicated to improving the quality of life for persons with Crohn's disease or ulcerative colitis. Your local chapter can supply you with a list of CCFA physician members in your area.

Russell P Girolamo, Board President
Maura Breen, Chairman

2173 Greater New York Chapter of Crohn's & Colitis Foundation of America
386 Park Avenue S, 14th Floor
New York, NY 10016
212-679-1570
Fax: 212-679-3567
e-mail: newyork@ccfa.org
www.ccfa.org

Crohn's and Colitis Foundation of America is a nonprofit, voluntary health organization dedicated to improving the quality of life for persons with Crohn's disease or ulcerative colitis.

Stacy Clark, Manager
Maura Breen, Chairman

2174 Long Island Chapter of Crohn's & Colitis Foundation of America
585 Stewart Avenue, Suite 580
Garden City, NY 11530
516-222-5530
Fax: 516-222-5535
e-mail: longisland@ccfa.org
www.ccfa.org

Crohn's and Colitis Foundation of America is a nonprofit, voluntary health organization dedicated to improving the quality of life for persons with Crohn's disease or ulcerative colitis.

Edda Ramsdell, Executive Director
Maura Breen, Chairman

2175 Rochester Chapter of Crohn's & Colitis Foundation of America
2117 Buffalo Rd Suite 299
Rochester, NY 14624
585-617-4771
e-mail: smassaro@ccfa.org
www.ccfa.org

Crohn's and Colitis Foundation of America is a nonprofit, voluntary health organization dedicated to improving the quality of life for persons with Crohn's disease or ulcerative colitis.

Adam Urbanski, President
Maura Breen, Chairman

2176 Upstate/Northeast New York Chapter of Crohn's & Colitis Foundation of America
103 Patroon Dr 10
Guilderland, NY 12084
518-608-5069
e-mail: upstateny@ccfa.org
www.ccfa.org

The chapter encompasses the following: Albany, Schenectady, Rensselaer, Northern Dutchess, Jefferson, Sullivan, Greene, Columbia, Schoharie, Fulton, Montgomery, Oneida, Saratoga, Ulster, Washington, Warren, Essex, Clinton, Franklin, and Herkimer counties.

Linda Winston, Community Development Director
Maura Breen, Chairman

2177 Western New York Chapter of Crohn's & Colitis Foundation of America
651 Deleware Ave Suite 214
Buffalo, NY 14202
716-362-1232
e-mail: jpetri@ccfa.org
www.ccfa.org

Crohn's and Colitis Foundation of America is a nonprofit, voluntary health organization dedicated to improving the quality of life for persons with Crohn's disease or ulcerative colitis. Your local chapter can supply you with a list of CCFA physician members in your area.

Jeanenne Petri, Development Manager
Maura Breen, Chairman

North Carolina

2178 Carolinas Chapter of Crohn's & Colitis Foundation of America
2424 N. Davidson St, Suite 110
Charlotte, NC 28205
704-332-1611
Fax: 704-332-1612
e-mail: jgolombos@ccfa.org
www.ccfa.org

Crohn's and Colitis Foundation of America is a nonprofit, voluntary health organization dedicated to improving the quality of life for persons with Crohn's disease or ulcerative colitis.

Joanne Colombos, National Walk Specialist
Maura Breen, Chairman

Ohio

2179 Central Ohio Chapter of Crohn's & Colitis Foundation of America
5500 Frantz Rd , Suite 155
Dublin, OH 43017
614-889-6060
Fax: 614-889-6655
e-mail: centralohio@ccfa.org
www.ccfa.org

Crohn's and Colitis Foundation of America is a nonprofit, voluntary health organization dedicated to improving the quality of life for persons with Crohn's disease or ulcerative colitis.

Deborah Shub, Community Development Director
Maura Breen, Chairman

2180 Northeast Ohio Chapter of Crohn's & Colitis Foundation of America
4700 Rockside Rd. #425
Independence, OH 44131
216-524-7700
866-345-2232
Fax: 216-524-7701
e-mail: neohio@aol.com
www.ccfa.org

Crohn's and Colitis Foundation of America is a nonprofit, voluntary health organization dedicated to improving the quality of life for persons with Crohn's disease or ulcerative colitis.

Lesley Hoover, Chapter Director
Maura Breen, Chairman

2181 Southwest Ohio Chapter of Crohn's & Colitis Foundation of America
8 Triangle Park Drive, Suite 800
Cincinnati, OH 45246
513-772-3550
877-283-7513
Fax: 513-772-7599
e-mail: swohio@ccfa.org
www.ccfa.org

CCFA is the only national nonprofit organization dedicated to finding the cause of and cure for Crohn's disease and ulcerative colitis. We offer monthly connection and education groups, education symposium, one-on-one support through our Ambassador Program and for our children, a four day regional camp. CCFA offers free Teacher's Guides, Parent's Guide and Children's Guides to Crohn's Disease and Ulcerative Colitis. This chapter also serves Greater Dayton, Northern Kentucky and SW Indiana.

Jenny Southers, Development Director
Rachel Miller, Take Steps Walk Mgr

Oklahoma

2182 Oklahoma Chapter of Crohn's & Colitis Foundation of America
4504 E 67th Street, Suite 125
Tulsa, OK 74136
918-523-8540
Fax: 918-523-8560
e-mail: oklahoma@ccfa.org
www.ccfa.org

Crohn's and Colitis Foundation of America is a nonprofit, voluntary health organization dedicated to improving the quality of life for persons with Crohn's disease or ulcerative colitis.

Mike Gramm, Board of Trustees
Maura Breen, Chairman

Pennsylvania

2183 Pennsylvania/Delaware Valley Chapter of Crohn's & Colitis Foundation of America
367 E Street Road
Trevose, PA 19053
215-396-9100
888-340-4744
Fax: 215-396-1170
e-mail: philaelphia@ccfa.org
www.ccfa.org

Crohn's and Colitis Foundation of America is a nonprofit, voluntary health organization dedicated to improving the quality of life for persons with Crohn's disease and ulcerative colitis.

Barbara Berman, Executive Director
Maura Breen, Chairman

2184 Western Pennsylvania Chapter of Crohn's & Colitis Foundation of America
300 Penn Center Suite 401
Pittsburgh, PA 15235
412-823-8272
877-823-8272
Fax: 412-823-8276
e-mail: wpawv@ccfa.org
www.ccfa.org

National nonprofit research-oriented voluntary health organization dedicated to improving the quality of life for people with Crohn's disease and ulcerative colitis. Our mission: support basic and clinical scientific research to find a cause and cure for Crohn's disease and ulcerative colitis, provide educational programs for patients, medical professioinals, and general public, and offer supportive services for patients, their families and friends.

600 Members

Susan Kukic, Executive Director

South Carolina

2185 South Carolina Chapter of Crohn's & Colitis Foundation of America
2424 N. Davidson St, Suite 110
Charlotte, NC 28205
704-332-1611
877-632-1611
Fax: 704-332-1612
e-mail: carolinas@ccfa.org
www.ccfa.org

Crohn's and Colitis Foundation of America is a nonprofit, voluntary health organization dedicated to improving the quality of life for persons with Crohn's disease.

Kelli King, Development Director
Maura Breen, Chairman

Tennessee

2186 Tennessee Chapter of Crohn's & Colitis Foundation of America
95 White Bridge Rd Suite 209
Nashville, TN 37205
615-356-0444
866-814-2232
Fax: 615-356-0445
e-mail: tennessee@ccfa.org
www.ccfa.org

Crohn's and Colitis Foundation of America is a nonprofit, voluntary health organization dedicated to improving the quality of life for persons with Crohn's disease or ulcerative colitis.

Steve Wallace, Executive Director
Maura Breen, Chairman

Texas

2187 Houston-Gulf Coast/South Texas Chapter of Crohn's & Colitis Foundation of America
5120 Woodway, Suite 8008
Houston, TX 77056   713-752-2232
800-785-2232
Fax: 713-572-2433
e-mail: infohouston@ccfa.org
www.ccfa.org

Crohn's and Colitis Foundation of America is a nonprofit, voluntary health organization dedicated to cure and prevent Crohn's disease and ulcerative colitis through research and to improve the quality of life of children and adults affected by those digestive diseases through education and support.

Charles Weiss, IOM, Executive Director
Maura Breen, Chairman

2188 North Texas Chapter of Crohn's & Colitis Foundation of America
12801 N Central Expressway Suite 270
Dallas, TX 75243   972-386-0607
Fax: 972-386-0509
e-mail: ntexas@ccfa.org
www.ccfa.org

Crohn's and Colitis Foundation of America is a nonprofit, voluntary health organization dedicated to improving the quality of life for persons with Crohn's disease or ulcerative colitis.

Teresa Sheffield, Executive Director
Maura Breen, Chairman

Washington

2189 Washington State Chapter of Crohn's & Colitis Foundation of America
9 Lake Bellevue Drive, Suite 203
Bellevue, WA 98005   425-451-8455
Fax: 425-451-1708
e-mail: northwest@ccfa.org
www.ccfa.org

Crohn's and Colitis Foundation of America is a nonprofit, voluntary health organization dedicated to improving the quality of life for persons with Crohn's disease or ulcerative colitis.

Linda Huse, Regional Director
Maura Breen, Chairman

Wisconsin

2190 Wisconsin Chapter of Crohn's & Colitis Foundation of America
1126 S 70th Street, Suite S210A
West Allis, WI 53214   414-475-5520
877-586-5588
Fax: 414-475-5502
e-mail: wisconsin@ccfa.org
www.ccfa.org

Crohn's and Colitis Foundation of America is a nonprofit, voluntary health organization dedicated to improving the quality of life for persons with Crohn's disease or ulcerative colitis.

Tyler Hillstrom, Executive Director
Maura Breen, Chairman

Libraries & Resource Centers

2191 National Digestive Diseases Information Clearinghouse
2 Information Way
Bethesda, MD 20892   800-891-5389
Fax: 703-738-4929
e-mail: nddic@info.niddk.nih.gov
www.niddk.nih.gov

The National Institute of Diabetes and Digestive and Kidney Diseases conducts and supports research on many of the most serious diseases affecting public health. The Institute supports much of the clinical research on the diseases of internal medicine and related subspecialty fields as well as many basic science disciplines.

Research Centers

2192 Crohn's & Colitis Foundation of America
386 Park Avenue S, 17th Floor
New York, NY 10016   800-932-2423
e-mail: info@ccfa.org
www.ccfa.org

Since 1967, CCFA has been the only national voluntary health agency dedicated to funding research to find a cure for Crohn's disease and ulcerative colitis. The Foundation provides educational and patient support services to both the lay and medical communities and plans to provide grants dedicated to pediatric research.

Maura Breen, Chairman

2193 Krancer Center for Inflammatory Bowel Disease Research
Hahnemann University
Broad & Vine Streets
Philadelphia, PA 19102   215-762-8618
Fax: 215-762-1998

Research into the causes and treatments of ulcerative colitis and Crohn's disease.

Harris Clearfield, Director

Conferences

2194 Genetic Alliance Annual Conference
Genetic Alliance
4301 Connecticut Avenue NW, Suite 404
Washington, DC 20008   202-966-5557
800-336-4363
Fax: 202-966-8553
e-mail: info@geneticalliance.org
www.geneticalliance.org

Consistently inspirational and enables partnership among all stakeholders: advocates and community leaders, health and industry professionals, policymakers, and academicians.

July

Sharon Terry, President/CEO
Tetyana Murza, Programs/Events Manager

2195 IFFGD Professional Symposia
Int'l Foundation for Functional Gastrointestinal
700 W. Virginia St, Suite 201
Milwaukee, WI 53204   414-964-1799
888-964-2001
Fax: 414-964-7176
e-mail: iffgd@iffgd.org
www.iffgd.org

Aimed at promoting education and awareness among professionals from multiple disciplines who treat gastrointestinal disorders and incontinence.

April

Nancy J Norton, President
William Norton, Co-founder of IFFGD

Web Sites

2196 Crohn's & Colitis Foundation of America
733 Third Avenue, Suite 510
New York, NY 10017   800-932-2423
800-932-2423
Fax: 212-779-4098
e-mail: info@ccfa.org
www.ccfa.org

Information regardin Crohn's disease and ulcerative colitis.

Maura Breen, Chairman
Richard Geswell, President & CEO
Judi Brown, Chief Development Officer

2197 Health Answers
410 Horsham Road
Horsham, PA 19044
215-442-9017
e-mail: Michael.tague@healthanswers.com
www.healthanswers.com

HealthAnswers offers a breadth of services in medical education, sales force training, patient support, solutions, professional promotion and consumer solutions.

Michael Tague, Managing Director

Book Publishers

2198 Crohn's Disease and Ulcerative Colitis Fact Book
Crohn's & Colitis Foundation of America
386 Park Avenue S, 17th Floor
New York, NY 10016
212-685-3440
800-932-2423
Fax: 212-779-4098
e-mail: info@ccfa.org
www.ccfa.org

Written in layman's language, this first, complete guide is helpful in understanding and coping with inflammatory bowel diseases.

2199 Digestive Diseases & Disorders Sourcebook
Omnigraphics
PO Box 625
Holmes, PA 19043
800-234-1340
Fax: 800-875-1340
e-mail: info@omnigraphics.com
omnigraphics.com

Basic consumer health information including celiac disease, Crohn's disease, diarrhea, hernias, irritable bowel syndrome and ulcers.

335 pages
ISBN: 0-780803-27-2

2200 Let's Talk About Going to the Hospital
Rosen Publishing Group's PowerKids Press
29 E 21st Street
New York, NY 10010
212-777-3017
800-237-9932
Fax: 888-436-4643
e-mail: rosenpub@tribeca.ios.com
www.powerkidspress.com

If a child has to check into the hospital, chances are he or she is already upset about being ill. Knowing how a hospital functions and what the procedures are, such as when family members can visit, will help in what is already a stressful situation. Grades K-5.

24 pages
ISBN: 0-823950-36-0

2201 Managing Your Child's Crohn's Disease or Ulcerative Colitis
Crohn's & Colitis Foundation of America
386 Park Avenue S, 17th Floor
New York, NY 10016
212-685-3440
800-932-2423
Fax: 212-779-4098
e-mail: info@ccfa.org
www.ccfa.org

This first full-length book on Crohn's disease and ulcerative colitis, specifically targeted for parents of children and teenagers, includes topics on cause and diagnosis, treatment, surgery, hospitalization, diet and nutrition, school and social issues, and resources for the patient.

$16.95 Members

2202 New People...Not Patients: a Source Book for Living with Bowel Disease
Crohn's & Colitis Foundation of America
386 Park Avenue S, 17th Floor
New York, NY 10016
212-685-3440
800-932-2423
Fax: 212-779-4098
e-mail: info@ccfa.org
www.ccfa.org

This book contains the essential information you need to help you cope with Crohn's disease and ulcerative colitis after you leave the doctor's office.

2203 Treating IBD
Crohn's & Colitis Foundation of America
386 Park Avenue S, 17th Floor
New York, NY 10016
212-685-3440
800-932-2423
e-mail: info@ccfa.org
www.ccfa.org

A patient's guide to the medical and surgical management of Inflammatory Bowel Disease, this book gives information on treating Crohn's disease and ulcerative colitis, including drug therapies, advances in nutritional care, and recently developed surgical alternatives.

2204 Understanding Crohn Disease and Ulcerative Colitis
University Press of Mississippi
3825 Ridgewood Road, Unit 9
Jackson, MS 39211
601-432-6205
800-737-7788
Fax: 601-432-6246
e-mail: press@ihl.state.ms.us
www.upress.state.ms.us

For patients and caregivers, an overview of the nature and treatments of inflammatory bowel disease.

128 pages Paperback
ISBN: 1-578062-03-9

Leila W Salisbury Director

Magazines

2205 Take Charge
Crohn's & Colitis Foundation of America
733 Third Avenue, Suite 510
New York, NY 10017
800-932-2423
e-mail: info@ccfa.org
www.ccfa.org

Offers the most up-to-date information on IBD research, treatment, and legislative initiatives for patients, families, and friends.

Maura Breen, Chairman
Richard Geswell, President & CEO
Judi Brown, Chief Development Officer

Newsletters

2206 Under the Microscope
Crohn's & Colitis Foundation of America
733 Third Avenue, Suite 510
New York, NY 10017
800-932-2423
800-932-2423
Fax: 212-779-4098
e-mail: info@ccfa.org
www.ccfa.org

Includes a variety of relevant information such as information on new research projects, clinical trials, conference notes, and breaking news about partnerships and grants.

Maura Breen, Chairman
Richard Geswell, President & CEO
Judi Brown, Chief Development Officer

Pamphlets

2207 CCFA: A Case for Support
Crohn's & Colitis Foundation of America
733 Third Avenue, Suite 510
New York, NY 10017
800-932-2423
800-932-2423
Fax: 212-779-4098
e-mail: info@ccfa.org
www.ccfa.org

Reviews the work of the Crohn's and Colitis Foundation of America, sponsors a nationally recognized research program, which seeks to improve treatment, and ultimately find the cure for inflammatory bowel disease.

Maura Breen, Chairman
Richard Geswell, President & CEO
Judi Brown, Chief Development Officer

2208 Coping with Crohn's and Colitis is Tough
Crohn's & Colitis Foundation of America
733 Third Avenue, Suite 510
New York, NY 10017
800-932-2423
800-932-2423
Fax: 212-779-4098
e-mail: info@ccfa.org
www.ccfa.org

Offers information on the Crohn's and Colitis Association. Also offers factual information and statistics on the diseases.

Maura Breen, Chairman
Richard Geswell, President & CEO
Judi Brown, Chief Development Officer

2209 Crohn's Disease, Ulcerative Colitis, and Your Child
Crohn's & Colitis Foundation of America
733 Third Avenue, Suite 510
New York, NY 10017
800-932-2423
800-932-2423
Fax: 212-779-4098
e-mail: info@ccfa.org
www.ccfa.org

Answers questions about IBD in children, providing information on early signs, growth and developments, treatments and special problems in school.

Maura Breen, Chairman
Richard Geswell, President & CEO
Judi Brown, Chief Development Officer

2210 Guide for Children and Teenagers to Crohn's Disease/Ulcerative Colitis
Crohn's & Colitis Foundation of America
733 Third Avenue, Suite 510
New York, NY 10017
800-932-2423
800-932-2423
Fax: 212-779-4098
e-mail: info@ccfa.org
www.ccfa.org

Offers important information on these illnesses to children and teens.

Maura Breen, Chairman
Richard Geswell, President & CEO
Judi Brown, Chief Development Officer

2211 Questions & Answers About Diet and Nutrition
Crohn's & Colitis Foundation of America
733 Third Avenue, Suite 510
New York, NY 10017
800-932-2423
800-932-2423
Fax: 212-779-4098
e-mail: info@ccfa.org
www.ccfa.org

Raises important facts about how diet and nutrition affect persons with Crohn's Disease.

Maura Breen, Chairman
Richard Geswell, President & CEO
Judi Brown, Chief Development Officer

2212 Questions and Answers About Complications
Crohn's & Colitis Foundation of America
733 Third Avenue, Suite 510
New York, NY 10017
800-932-2423
800-932-2423
Fax: 212-779-4098
e-mail: info@ccfa.org
www.ccfa.org

Medical facts and complications from surgery.

Maura Breen, Chairman
Richard Geswell, President & CEO
Judi Brown, Chief Development Officer

2213 Questions and Answers About Crohn's Disease & Ulcerative Colitis
Crohn's & Colitis Foundation of America
733 Third Avenue, Suite 510
New York, NY 10017
800-932-2423
800-932-2423
Fax: 212-779-4098
e-mail: info@ccfa.org
www.ccfa.org

Offers information on the illness and answers the most frequently asked questions about Crohn's Disease. Also includes a glossary of IBD terms.

Maura Breen, Chairman
Richard Geswell, President & CEO
Judi Brown, Chief Development Officer

2214 Questions and Answers About Emotional Factors In Ileitis and Colitis
Crohn's & Colitis Foundation of America
733 Third Avenue, Suite 510
New York, NY 10017
800-932-2423
800-932-2423
Fax: 212-779-4098
e-mail: info@ccfa.org
www.ccfa.org

Answers some of the most commonly asked questions about ileitis and colitis and the role of emotional factors in their cause and course.

Maura Breen, Chairman
Richard Geswell, President & CEO
Judi Brown, Chief Development Officer

2215 Teacher's Guide to Crohn's Disease & Ulcerative Colitis
Crohn's & Colitis Foundation of America
733 Third Avenue, Suite 510
New York, NY 10017
800-932-2423
800-932-2423
Fax: 212-779-4098
e-mail: info@ccfa.org
www.ccfa.org

Maura Breen, Chairman
Richard Geswell, President & CEO
Judi Brown, Chief Development Officer

Description

2216 CRYPTORCHIDISM

Synonyms: Cryptorchidy, Cryptorchism

Covers these related disorders: Ectopic (maldescended) testes, True undescended testes

Involves the following Biologic System(s):

Renal and Urologic Disorders

Cryptorchidism is characterized by failure of one or both testes to descend into the pouch-like structure known as the scrotum. The testes are the paired, oval-shaped glands that produce the male reproductive cells (sperm). Early during male fetal growth, the testes develop within the abdomen near the kidneys. The testes then descend into the scrotum through a tubular canal that passes through lower muscular layers of the abdominal wall (inguinal canal). In males with cryptorchidism, one or both testes fail to complete their descent into the scrotum. Undescended testes that are located along the proper path of descent are known as true undescended testes, whereas those that have completed their descent through the inguinal canal yet have become located in areas other than the scrotum are referred to as ectopic or maldescended testes.

In most cases, one testis is affected (unilateral cryptorchidism); however, both testes may fail to descend (bilateral cryptorchidism) in up to 30 percent of affected male infants. In many cases, undescended testes may move down into the scrotum before one year of age. However, testes that fail to spontaneously descend during the first year of life typically fail to develop properly, may decrease in size, and have decreased numbers of reproductive cells. Without treatment, affected males are at an increased risk of infertility; malignant tumor development in affected testes during the third or fourth decade of life; or pain, swelling, and, in some cases, localized areas of tissue loss (necrosis).

Treatment of cryptorchidism often includes early surgery to relocate undescended testes into the scrotum (i.e., orchiopexy) and to correct inguinal hernias, which typically occur in association with true undescended testes and ectopic testes. Inguinal hernias are characterized by bulging of portions of the intestine into the inguinal canal. Surgical correction of cryptorchidism is typically recommended in the first years of life to help improve proper testicular development and fertility in adulthood.

Cryptorchidism affects about three and a half percent of full-term male newborns and increases in incidence in newborns who are born before 37 weeks of pregnancy (preterm). The condition may occur as an isolated abnormality or, in some cases, due to or in association with a number of different underlying syndromes or conditions.

Government Agencies

2217 NIH/National Institute of Child Health and Human Development

31 Center Drive, Building 31
Bethesda, MD 20892

301-496-1333
800-370-2943
Fax: 866-760-5947
TTY: 888-320-6942
www.nichd.nih.gov

Established in 1962 by congress, today the institute conducts and supports research on topics related to the health of children, adults, families and populations. Some of these topics include: developmental disabilities, growth and development, infant death, reproductive health and birth defects.

Jay H Hoofnagle, Director
Lisa Kaeser, Program & Public Liaison

National Associations & Support Groups

2218 American Academy of Pediatrics

141 Northwest Point Boulevard
Elk Grove Village, IL 60007

847-434-4000
800-433-9016
Fax: 847-434-8000
www.aap.org

The American Academy of Pediatrics and its member pediatricians are committed to the attainment of optimal physical, mental and social health and well-being for all infants, children, adolescents, and young adults.

Sandra Hassink, MD, FAAP, President

2219 Genetic Alliance

4301 Connecticut Avenue NW, Suite 404
Washington, DC 20008

202-966-5557
Fax: 202-966-8553
e-mail: info@geneticalliance.org
www.geneticalliance.org

A coalition of voluntary genetic support groups, consumers and professionals addressing the needs of individuals and families affected by genetic disorders from a national perspective.

Sharon Terry, President
Natasha Bonhomme, Vice President
Vaughn Edelson, Assistant Director of Health Commun

2220 March of Dimes Birth Defects Foundation

1275 Mamaroneck Avenue
White Plains, NY 10605

914-997-4488
888-663-4637
Fax: 914-997-4763
e-mail: info@marchofdimes.com
www.marchofdimes.com

Partnership of volunteers and professionals dedicated to improving the health of babies by preventing birth defects and infant mortality. Over 100 chapters are located across the country and can be located through the National Office.

Jennifer L Howse, President

2221 NIH/National Institute of Mental Health

6001 Executive Boulevard, Room 8184, MSC 9663
Bethesda, MD 20892

301-443-4513
866-615-6464
Fax: 301-443-4279
TTY: 301-443-8431
e-mail: nimhinfo@nih.gov
www.nimh.nih.gov

Conducts strategic planning for specific research areas as well as for the Institute as a whole.

Dr Thomas R Insel, NIMH Director

Conferences

2222 Genetic Alliance Annual Conference
Genetic Alliance
4301 Connecticut Avenue NW, Suite 404
Washington, DC 20008   202-966-5557
                                        800-336-4363
                                  Fax: 202-966-8553
                     e-mail: info@geneticalliance.org
                           www.geneticalliance.org

Consistently inspirational and enables partnership among all
stakeholders: advocates and community leaders, health and industry professionals, policymakers, and academicians.

July

Sharon Terry, President/CEO
Tetyana Murza, Programs/Events Manager

Web Sites

2223 European Society for Pediatric Urology
www.espu.org

                                        025-503-8690
                                  Fax: 025-503-2546
                        e-mail: president@espu.org
                                  www.espu.org

A nonprofit society whose main purpose is to promote pediatric
urology, appropriate practice, education as well as exchanges between practitioners involved in the treatment of genito urinary
disorders in children.

Ramnath Subramaniam, Chairman, Educational Committee
Gianantonio Manzoni, President
Dr. Emilio Merlini, Treasurer

2224 National Center for Biotechnology Information
National Library of Medicine, Building 38A
Bethesda, MD 20894   888-346-3656
                      e-mail: info@ncbi.nlm.nih.gov
                              www.ncbi.nlm.nih.gov

NCBI's mission is to develop new information technologies to aid
in the understanding of fundamental molecular and genetic processes that control health and disease.

Christine E. Seidman, M.D., Chair
David J. Lipman, M.D., Executive Secretary
Michael Boehnke, Ph.D., Board Member

2225 Online Mendelian Inheritance in Man
National Library of Medicine, Building 38A
Bethesda, MD 20894   888-346-3656
                      e-mail: info@ncbi.nlm.nih.gov
                              www.ncbi.nlm.nih.gov

This database is a catalog of human genes and genetic disorders.

Christine E. Seidman, M.D., Chair
David J. Lipman, M.D., Executive Secretary
Michael Boehnke, Ph.D., Board Member

Description

2226 CUSHING'S SYNDROME

Synonyms: Cushing's basophilism, Hyperadrenocorticism, Pituitary basophilism

Involves the following Biologic System(s):

Endocrinologic Disorders

Cushing's syndrome refers to a condition characterized by excessive levels of the corticosteroid hormone, cortisol, in the blood. Cortisol is produced in the outer portion (cortex) of the adrenal glands in response to the secretion of adrenocorticotropic hormone (ACTH; corticotropin). ACTH stimulates the growth of the adrenal cortex and thus the production of cortisol. Cushing's syndrome may be caused by a variety of factors including tumors of the adrenal glands or the pituitary gland, tumors of certain other organs, and excessive intake of corticosteroid drugs. In the very young, Cushing's syndrome occurs in more girls than boys by a ratio of approximately three to one.

Because cortisol assists in the metabolism of fat, protein, and glucose, many characteristic symptoms and findings associated with this disorder are related to the levels and distribution of body fat. For example, children with Cushing's syndrome may be somewhat obese with very full cheeks, a reddish moonface appearance, double chin, and excessive fat deposits on the back of the neck. In addition, the adrenal glands may be stimulated to secrete excessive amounts of other hormones that are converted in the liver to testosterone and estrogen. Overproduction of these androgenic hormones may result in symptoms such as increased amounts of hair on the face and trunk (hypertrichosis), the development of acne, and deepening of the voice as well as other masculine traits. Other findings that may appear over a period of time include elevated blood pressure (hypertension), kidney (renal) stones, and increased vulnerability to infection. Children with Cushing's syndrome may also experience growth delays or may not achieve height (short stature). However, those children who develop masculinization symptoms may reach average or above average height. Older children may experience a delay in onset of puberty and develop purplish stretch marks (striae) on the abdomen, breasts, hips, and thighs. In addition, their skin may become thin and fragile, leading to easy tissue injury. Affected children may develop headaches and weakness, experience increasing difficulty with school work, or become depressed or experience other emotional disturbances.

Treatment of Cushing's syndrome is dependent upon the underlying cause. If the disease results from a benign or malignant tumor or enlargement of the adrenal gland, surgical removal of the tumor or the adrenal gland (adrenalectomy) may be advised. A tumor in the pituitary gland may either be surgically removed or treated with radiation. Subsequent management of surgical or other procedures often includes appropriate hormone replacement therapy. Cushing's syndrome associated with prolonged or excessive intake of corticosteroids may be re|versed by a monitored and gradual (tapered) withdrawal of the medication. Other treatment is symptomatic and supportive.

National Associations & Support Groups

2227 American Academy of Pediatrics
141 Northwest Point Boulevard
Elk Grove Village, IL 60007
847-434-4000
800-433-9016
Fax: 847-434-8000
www.aap.org

The American Academy of Pediatrics and its member pediatricians are committed to the attainment of optimal physical, mental and social health and well-being for all infants, children, adolescents, and young adults.

Sandra Hassink, MD, FAAP, President

2228 American Association of Clinical Endocrinologists
245 Riverside Avenue, Suite 200
Jacksonville, FL 32202
904-353-7878
Fax: 904-353-8185
e-mail: info@aace.com
www.aace.com

A professional medical organization aimed at promoting the quality of clinical epidemiologic research and improving the knowledge base for the diagnosis, prognosis, prevention and treatment of health conditions through the advancement and application of innovative methods.

Jeffrey I Mechanick, President
George Grunberger, Vice President
Jonathan D Leffert, Secretary

2229 Cushing's Support & Research Foundation
65 E India Row, Suite 22B
Boston, MA 02110
617-723-3674
Fax: 617-723-3674
e-mail: cushinfo@csrf.net
www.csrf.net

To provide information and support for Cushing's Disease and Cushing's Syndrome to patients and their families to increase awareness and to educate the public about Cushing's Disease and Cushing's Syndrome. To be a resource for information and support to healthcare professionals, to raise and distribute funds for Cushing's Disease and Cushing's Syndrome research.

Louise Pace, Founding President

2230 Human Growth Foundation
997 Glen Cove Avenue, Suite 5
Glen Head, NY 11545
516-671-4041
800-451-6434
Fax: 516-671-4055
e-mail: hgfl@hgfound.org
www.hgfound.org

A voluntary, nonprofit organization whose mission is to help children and adults with disorders of growth and growth hormones through research, education, support and advocacy. The foundation is dedicated to helping medical science to better understand the process of growth. It is composed of concerned parents and friends of children and adults with growth problems and interested health professionals.

Patricia D Costa, Executive Director

2231 Lawson Wilkins Pediatric Endocrine Society
6728 Old McLean Village Drive
McLean, VA 22101
703-556-9222
Fax: 703-556-8729
e-mail: secretary@lwpes.org
www.lwpes.org

To promote the acquisition and dissemination of knowledge of endocrine and metabolic disorders from conception through adolescence.

Morey W Haymond, President
Karen Rubin, Treasurer
Peter A Lee, Secretary

2232 National Adrenal Diseases Foundation
505 Northern Boulevard
Great Neck, NY 11021
516-487-4992
e-mail: nadfmail@aol.com
www.nadf.us

A nonprofit organization dedicated to providing support, information and education to individuals having Addison's disease as well as related diseases such as Cushing's Syndrome and Congenital Adrenal Hyperplasia. Promotes early diagnosis and treatment, and sponsors support groups and offers a quarterly newsletter, educational materials and access to a library of related information.

Kalina Warren, President
Timothy Skodon, Treasurer
Phyllis Speiser, Medical Advisor

Conferences

2233 AACE Annual Meeting and Clinical Congress
American Association of Clinical Endocrinologists
245 Riverside Avenue, Suite 200
Jacksonville, FL 32202
904-353-7878
Fax: 904-353-8185
e-mail: info@aace.com
www.aace.com

April

Yehuda Handelsman, President
Donald C Jones, Chief Executive Officer

Web Sites

2234 Cushing's Support and Research Foundation
60 Robbins Road, #12
Plymouth, MA 2360
617-723-3674
Fax: 617-723-3674
e-mail: cushinfo@csrf.net
csrf.net

The mission is to provide information and support for Cushing's Disease and Cushing's Syndrome patients and their families, to increase awareness and to educate the public about Cushing's Disease and Cushing's Syndrome, to be a resource for information and support to health care professionals, to raise and distribute funds for Cushing's Disease and Cushing's Syndrome research.

Louise Pace, Founding President
John P. Gulielmetti, Treasurer
Karen Campbell, Director

Book Publishers

2235 Endocrine & Metabolic Disorders Sourcebook
Omnigraphics
PO Box 8002
Aston, PA 19014
800-234-1340
Fax: 800-875-1340
e-mail: info@omnigraphics.com
www.omnigraphics.com

Basic information for the lay person about pancreatic and insulin-related disorders such as pancreatitis, diabetes and hypoglycemia; adrenal gland disorders such as Cushing's syndrome, Addison's disease and congenital adrenal hyperplasia; pituitary gland disorders such as growth hormone deficiency, acromegaly and pituitary tumors; and thyroid disorders such as hypothyroidism, Grave's disease, Hashimoto's disease and goiter.

574 pages hardcover
ISBN: 0-780802-07-1

2236 Let's Talk About Going to the Hospital
Rosen Publishing Group's PowerKids Press
29 E 21st Street
New York, NY 10010
212-777-3017
800-237-9932
Fax: 888-436-4643
e-mail: rosenpub@tribeca.ios.com
www.powerkidspress.com

If a child has to check into the hospital, chances are he or she is already upset about being ill. Knowing how a hospital functions and what the procedures are, such as when family members can visit, will help in what is already a stressful situation. Grades K-5.

24 pages
ISBN: 0-823950-36-0

Journals

2237 Endocrine Practice
245 Riverside Avenue, Suite 200
Jacksonville, FL 32202
904-353-7878
Fax: 904-353-8185
e-mail: info@aace.com
www.aace.com

Peer-reviewed journal published six-times a year and is the official journal of the American College of Endocrinology (ACE) and the American Association of Clinical Endocrinologists (AACE).

R. Mack Harrell, MdD, FACP, FACE, President
Paulin M. Camacho, MD, FACE, Vice President
Donald C. Jones, CEO

Newsletters

2238 NADF News
National Adrenal Diseases Foundation
505 Northern Boulevard
Great Neck, NY 11021
516-487-4992
e-mail: nadfsupport@nadf.us
www.nadf.us

Provides support and information to those living with adrenal diseases.

Kalina Warren, President
Melanie G. Wong, Executive Director
Edward A. Wong, Executive Director's Assistant

Description

2239 CYSTIC FIBROSIS

Synonyms: CF, Mucoviscidosis

Involves the following Biologic System(s):

Respiratory Disorders

Cystic fibrosis (CF) is an inherited multisystem disorder that results in the abnormal production of mucus by almost all exocrine glands, causing obstruction of those glands and ducts. Glands of the respiratory and reproductive systems as well as pancreatic glands and sweat glands are affected. CF is considered one of the most common autosomal recessive disorders affecting Caucasians. Cystic fibrosis occurs in approximately one in 2,500 to 3,000 Caucasian infants and about one in 17,000 African-American infants. It is considered extremely rare in other populations. The disorder results from abnormal changes (mutations) of a gene on the long arm (q) of chromosome 7 (7q31.2). More than 400 different mutations of the CF gene have been identified.

In infants, children, and adults with cystic fibrosis, mucus-secreting glands within the air passages of the lungs (bronchi) produce unusually thick secretions, clogging and obstructing the airways and promoting the growth of certain bacteria. As a result, affected individuals may experience chronic obstruction and infection of the airways. In addition, the pancreas lacks sufficient digestive enzymes to break down food materials (malabsorption). Other exocrine gland abnormalities may also be present. For example, the sweat glands produce secretions containing abnormally high levels of salt; glands of the neck of the uterus (cervix) in affected females may produce abnormally increased, thickened secretions of mucus; and certain ducts of the male reproductive system (e.g., epididymis, ductus [vas] deferens, seminal vesicles) may be absent (atretic).

During the first or second day of life, some newborns with cystic fibrosis may experience bloating of the abdomen (abdominal distension), vomiting (emesis), and abnormal blockage of the lower region of the small intestine with meconium (meconium ileus). Meconium is the thick, sticky, darkish green material that accumulates in the fetal intestines and forms a newborn's first stools. Infants with cystic fibrosis also usually fail to grow and gain weight at the expected rate (failure to thrive). Additional symptoms and findings may include abnormally decreased muscle mass; a protruding abdomen; and loose, foul-smelling stools that contain an excessive amount of fat (steatorrhea). Children with cystic fibrosis often have respiratory abnormalities including wheezing; a chronic cough that may be accompanied by gagging and vomiting; recurrent inflammation of the air passages (bronchiolitis); and an increased susceptibility to lower respiratory infections (e.g., pneumonia). Affected adolescents may experience abnormally slow growth and delayed sexual development (i.e., average delay of two years); in addition, affected males may be infertile due to lack of sperm development (azoospermia). As the disease progresses, individuals with cystic fibrosis tend to experience increasingly severe respiratory abnormalities that may result in life-threatening complications.

Cystic fibrosis may be diagnosed based upon characteristic physical findings (e.g., chronic obstructive pulmonary disease, exocrine pancreatic insufficiency), specialized laboratory tests (e.g., sweat testing), and a positive family history (including DNA analysis). The treatment of cystic fibrosis is symptomatic and supportive and includes early intervention, ongoing monitoring, preventive measures, the use of certain medications, and other specialized treatment techniques. Approaches to treatment may include physical therapy, a high protein, high calorie diet, pancreatic enzyme replacement therapy, vitamin supplementation, specialized respiratory therapy, medications to help clean mucus from the airways and prevent or treat respiratory infections (e.g., antibiotic therapy). Median survival is about 31 years of age.

National Associations & Support Groups

2240 American Academy of Pediatrics
141 Northwest Point Boulevard
Elk Grove Village, IL 60007   847-434-4000
                                     800-433-9016
                                     Fax: 847-434-8000
                                     www.aap.org

The American Academy of Pediatrics and its member pediatricians are committed to the attainment of optimal physical, mental and social health and well-being for all infants, children, adolescents, and young adults.

Sandra Hassink, MD, FAAP, President

2241 American Lung Association
1301 Pennsylvania Ave, Suite 800
Washington, DC 20004   202-785-3355
                              800-548-8252
                              Fax: 202-452-1805
                              www.lungusa.org

The American Lung Association fights lung disease in all its forms, with special emphasis on asthma, tobacco control and environmental health. The American Lung Association is funded by contributions from the public, along with gifts and grants from corporations, foundations and government agencies. The association achieves its many successes through the work of thousands of committed volunteers and staff.

Harold P Wimmer, President/CEO

2242 Cystic Fibrosis Foundation
6931 Arlington Road
Bethesda, MD 20814   301-951-4422
                            800-344-4823
                            Fax: 301-951-6378
                            e-mail: info@cff.org
                            www.cff.org

The mission of CF Foundation is to assure the development of means to cure and control CF and to improve the quality of life for those with the disease. It funds medical research and care programs which are improving the length and quality of life for people with cystic fibrosis.

Robert J Beall, CEO

2243 Cystic Fibrosis Research, Inc.
2672 Bayshore Parkway, Suite 520
Mountain View, CA 94043   650-404-9975
                                 855-237-4669
                                 Fax: 650-404-9981
                                 e-mail: cfri@cfri.org
                                 www.cfri.org

Cystic Fibrosis Research Inc.'s mission is to fund CF research, to provide educational and personal support and to spread awareness of Cystic Fibroses, a life threatening genetic disease.

Carroll P Jenkins, Executive Director
David Sohoo, Director of Program
Mary Convento, Programme Associate

2244 Genetic Alliance
4301 Connecticut Avenue NW
Washington, DC 20008   202-966-7955
                             800-336-4363
                         Fax: 202-966-8553
                    e-mail: info@geneticalliance.org
                         www.geneticalliance.org

A coalition of voluntary genetic support groups, consumers and professionals addressing the needs of individuals and families affected by genetic disorders from a national perspective.

Sharon Terry, President
Natasha Bonhomme, Vice President
Vaughn Edelson, Assistant Director of Health Commun

2245 March of Dimes Birth Defects Foundation
1275 Mamaroneck Avenue
White Plains, NY 10605   914-997-4488
                              888-663-4637
                          Fax: 914-997-4763
                   e-mail: answers@marchofdimes.com
                         www.marchofdimes.com

Partnership of volunteers and professionals dedicated to improving the health of babies by preventing birth defects and infant mortality. Over 100 chapters are located across the country and can be located through the National Office.

Jennifer L Howse, President

Libraries & Resource Centers

2246 National Digestive Diseases Information Clearinghouse
31 Center Drive
Bethesda, MD 20892   301-496-3583
                           800-891-5389
                       Fax: 301-907-8906
                e-mail: nddic@info.niddk.nih.gov
                        www.niddk.nih.gov

The National Institute of Diabetes and Digestive and Kidney Diseases conducts and supports research on many of the most serious diseases affecting public health. The Institute supports much of the clinical research on the diseases of internal medicine and related subspecialty fields as well as many basic science disciplines.

Kathy Kranzfelder, Project Officer

Research Centers

Alabama

2247 Gregory Fleming James Cystic Fibrosis Cent er
790 McCallum Basic Health Sciences Bldg
Birmingham, AL 35294   205-934-9640
                         Fax: 205-934-7593
                    e-mail: sorscher@uab.edu
                        www.cfcenter.uab.edu

Eric J Sorscher MD, Director

Arizona

2248 Cystic Fibrosis Center: Phoenix Children's Hospital
1919 E Thomas Road
Phoenix, AZ 85016   602-546-0985
                          888-908-5437
                      www.phxchildrens.com

Wayne J Morgan MD, Director

California

2249 Brian Wesley Ray Cystic Fibrosis Center
San Bernadino County Medical Center
780 E Gilbert Street
San Bernardino, CA 92415   909-387-8111
Gerald Greene, MD

2250 Children's Hospital of Los Angeles
4650 W Sunset Boulevard
Los Angeles, CA 90027   323-660-2450
                              888-631-2452
                    e-mail: webmaster@chla.usc.edu
                            www.chla.org

Elisabeth L Raab, Contact

2251 Children's Hospital of Orange County: Depa rtment of Pulmonology - Cystic Fibrosis
1201 W. La Veta Ave
Orange, CA 92868   714-997-3000
                     Fax: 714-516-4348
                 e-mail: mail@choc.org
                       www.choc.org

Ivan I Kirov

2252 Children's Hospital: Pediatric Pulmonary Center
747 52nd Street
Oakland, CA 94609   510-428-3259
Kevan McCarten-Gibbs

2253 Cystic Fibrosis Center: Cedars-Sinai Medical Center
8700 Beverly Boulevard, N Tower, Fourth Floor
Los Angeles, CA 90048   800-233-2771
                          Fax: 310-423-1402

2254 Cystic Fibrosis Center: University of California at San Francisco
8700 Beverly Boulevard, N Tower, Fourth Floor
San Francisco, CA 94143   800-233-2771
                            Fax: 310-423-1402

2255 Cystic Fibrosis Research, Inc.
2672 Bayshore Parkway, Suite 520
Mountain View, CA 94043   650-404-9975
                                855-237-4669
                            Fax: 650-404-9981
                       e-mail: cfri@cfri.org
                             www.cfri.org

Cystic Fibrosis Research Inc.'s mission is to fund CF research, to provide educational and personal support and to spread awareness of Cystic Fibroses, a life threatening genetic disease.

Carroll P Jenkins, Executive Director
David Sohoo, Director of Program
Mary Convento, Programme Associate

2256 Cystic Fibrosis and Pediatric Respiratory Diseases Center
University of California at Davis
2315 Stockton Boulevard
Sacramento, CA 95817   800-282-3284
                          Fax: 916-734-0491
                   e-mail: children@ucdavis.edu
                 www.ucdmc.ucdavis.edu/children

2257 Kaiser Permanente Medical Center
Kaiser Permanente Oakland Medical Center
280 W MacArthur Boulevard
Oakland, CA 94611   510-752-1000
                      www.kaiserpermanente.org

Linda C Armstrong

2258 Memorial Miller Children's Hospital Cystic Fibrosis Center
2801 Atlantic Avenue
Long Beach, CA 90806   562-933-2000
                          Fax: 562-933-8539
                        www.memorialcare.org

Barry Arbuckle, President

2259 Pulmonary Care and Cystic Fibrosis Center
Lucille Packard Children's Hospital
725 Welch Road, Suite 350
Palo Alto, CA 94304   650-497-8000
                         Fax: 650-498-4209
                           www.lpch.org

Deals with children's breathing in all its aspects.
Richard B Boss MD, Director

2260 Stanford CF Center
Packard Children's Hospital At Stanford
730 Welch Road
Palo Alto, CA 94304
650-725-9302
e-mail: jkirby@leland.stanford.edu
cfcenter.stanford.edu

Kim Standridge, Manager

Colorado

2261 Denver Children's Hospital
1056 E 19th Avenue
Denver, CO 80218
303-837-2680
Fax: 303-837-2924

Martin A Koyle, Pulmonology Pediatrics

Connecticut

2262 University of Connecticut Health Center
282 Washington Street
Hartford, CT 06106
860-545-9440
Fax: 860-545-9445
e-mail: kdaigle@ccmckids.org
Karen Daigle MD, Pediatric Pulmonary Division

2263 Yale University Cystic Fibrosis Research Center
School of Medicine Department
333 Cedar Street, PO Box 208064
New Haven, CT 06520
203-785-4648
Fax: 203-688-7864
www.med.yale.edu

Respiratory Medicine in the Department of Pediatrics at Yale University and Yale-New Haven Hospital is a multi-disiplinary section that has developed considerably since the early 90's and continues to develop and refine its clinical and research activities. We have also reorganized our Cystic Fibrosis Care Center, increased the clinical research activities pertaining to the care of CF patients and organized a number of CF family group meetings to dissimenate new knowledge of care of patients.

Marie E Egan MD, Cystic Fibrosis Center

Florida

2264 CF & Pediatric Pulmonary Disease Center
University of Florida
PO Box 100225
Gainesville, FL 32610
352-392-3261
Fax: 352-392-0821
Eric L Olson, Director Adult CF Program

2265 Cystic Fibrosis Center - All Children's Hospital
801 6th Street S
St Petersburg, FL 33701
727-898-7451
800-456-4543

2266 Miami Children's Hospital, Division of Pulmonology
3100 SW 62nd Street
Miami, FL 33155
305-666-6511
800-432-6837
www.mch.com

Deise Granado-Villar, Director

2267 Pulmonary Wellness Program
Orlando Regional Medical Center
92 W. Miller St.
Orlando, FL 32806
321-841-4194
www.arnoldpalmerhospital.org

Our staff is trained in all diagnostic tests as well as a variety of Cystic Fibrosis therapies, including therapy vest treatments. Our professionals will work with your child and your family to create a more enriched diet including vitamin and enzyme supplements to help counteract the effects of Cystic Fibrosis. We also administer antibiotics in pill form as well as intravenously and through medicated vapors.

Georgia

2268 Department of Pediatrics, Medical College of Georgia
1120 15th Street, BT-1852
Augusta, GA 30912
706-721-2809
Fax: 706-721-7311
e-mail: kcooper@ gru.edu
www.georgiahealth.edu

Tracy Chavous, Manager

2269 Egleston Cystic Fibrosis Center: Departmen t of Pediatrics
Emory University
201 Dowman
Atlanta, GA 30322
404-727-6123
Fax: 404-727-4828
www.emory.edu

Daniel Caplan MD, Director

Illinois

2270 Cystic Fibrosis Center: Children's Memoria l Hospital
Northwestern University
2300 N Children's Plaza, #43
Chicago, IL 60614
773-880-4382
e-mail: cf@childrensmemorial.org
Susanna McColley MD, Head, Pulmonary Medicine

2271 Loyola University Medical Center/ Department of Pediatrics
2160 S First Avenue
Maywood, IL 60153
708-216-8563
888-584-7888
www.loyolamedicine.org
Sergio L Gonzalez, Pediatric Pulmonary

2272 Park Ridge, Cystic Fibrosis Center
Advocate Lutheran General Hospital
1775 Dempster Street
Park Ridge, IL 60068
423-622-6848
800-242-5662
www.parkridgemedicalcenter.com
Darell Moore, CEO

2273 Saint Francis Medical Center Specialty Clinics, CF Center
Hillcrest Medical Plaza
530 NE Glen Oak Avenue
Peoria, IL 61637
309-655-7171
www.childrenshospitalofil.org

2274 University of Chicago Children's Hospital, Department of Pediatrics
University of Chicago Hospitals and Clinics
5721 S Maryland Avenue
Chicago, IL 60637
773-702-6176
888-824-0200
Fax: 773-702-4753
www.uchicagokidshospital.org

Provides comperhensive, innovative medical care to children of all social and economic backgrounds. Dedicated to enhancing the health and wellness through patient care, education and research into the causes and cure of childhood diseases. Immediate access to the full resources of The University of Chicago Hospitals and to faculty of the division of Biological Sciences. The hospital sees children from the Chicago area, the Midwest and around the world who have the most complex medical problems.

Shannon Smith, Manager

Indiana

2275 Cystic Fibrosis and Chronic Pulmonary Disease Clinic
Saint Joseph's Regional Medical Center
801 E LaSalle Avenue
South Bend, IN 46617
574-239-6126
800-206-0879
Fax: 574-472-6067

2276 Riley Cystic Fibrosis Center
Riley Hospital for Children
702 Barnhill Drive
Indianapolis, IN 46202   317-274-5000

Iowa

2277 Blank Children's Hospital: Department of P ulmonology
1212 Pleasant Street, Suite 300
Des Moines, IA 50309   515-241-8336
                                         Fax: 515-241-6465

Carissa Schneider, Manager

2278 University of Iowa Hospitals & Clinics
Allergy and Pulmonary Division: Cystic Fibrosis Ct
200 Hawkins Drive
Iowa City, IA 52242   319-356-1616
                                       www.uihealthcare.org

Ronald Strauss, Director

Kansas

2279 Kansas University Medical Center: Departme nt of Pulmonology
Department of Pediatrics
3901 Rainbow Boulevard
Kansas City, KS 66160   913-588-5000
                                      TDD: 913-588-7963
                                        www.kumc.edu

Raymond Franklin, Manager

2280 Via Christi Specialty Clinics: Cystic Fibr osis, Adult and Pediatrics
St Joseph Campus
3600 E Harry Street
Wichita, KS 67218   316-689-5735
                                      Fax: 316-291-7963

Kentucky

2281 University of Kentucky: Pediatric Pulmonar y Medicine
Department of Pediatrics
740 S Limestone
Lexington, KY 40536   859-323-6426
                                      Fax: 859-257-7706

Michael I Anstead MD, Director

Louisiana

2282 Louisiana State University Health Sciences Center
Department of Pediatrics: Critical Care/Pulmonary
200 Henry Clay Avenue
New Orleans, LA 70118   504-896-2723
                                       Fax: 504-896-2720
                                  e-mail: dhoppe@lsuhsc.edu

Robert Hopkins MD, Professor of Clinical Pediatrics

Maine

2283 Central Maine Medical Center
Department of Pediatrics
300 Main Street
Lewiston, ME 04240   207-795-0111
                                       Fax: 207-797-7241
                                         www.cmmc.org

Focuses special attention on the services that it provides to Cystic Fibrosis patients. In microbiology, for example, the lab employs a number of techniques supporting the special needs of CF patients. The CMMC pathology departments's chemistry section provides quantitative sweat analysis for the diagnosis of patients to other laboratories in the region, thereby assisting in diagnosis.

Marly L Larrabee, Special Interst: Cystic Fibrosis

2284 Eastern Maine Medical Center: Cystic Fibrosis Center
489 State Street
Bangor, ME 04401   207-973-7000
                                        www.emmc.org

Shad Deering

2285 Pediatric Cystic Fibrosis Center
Maine Medical Center: Dept. of Resp. Care
22 Bramhall Street
Portland, ME 04102   207-662-0111
                                     Fax: 207-775-6024
                                        www.mmc.org

Services offered: pediatric pulmonary consultation, flexible bronchoscopy of the pediatric airway, full pediatric and infant pulmonary function testing, including exercise testing, bronchopulmonary challenge, and accredited sleep lab. Also offered, full-time inpatient consultation service for neonates through adolesence, a bimonthly Cystic Fibrosis Clinic, and a biweekly outpatient pulmonary clinic.

Maryland

2286 John Hopkins Children's Hospital
Division of Pulmonary
600 N Wolfe Street
Baltimore, MD 21287   410-955-5089
                                      Fax: 410-955-0761
                                    www.hopkinschildren.org

Edward Chambers, Administrator

Massachusetts

2287 Baystate Medical Center
280 Chestnut Street
Springfield, MA 01199   413-794-0000
                                      Fax: 413-794-7408
                                    www.baystatehealth.com

Gordon M Saperia, Chief, Pediatric Pulmonary

2288 Children's Hospital Boston
Pulmonary and Critical Care Unit
300 Longwood Avenue
Boston, MA 02115   617-355-6000
                                       800-355-7944
                                     Fax: 617-724-9948
                                     TTY: 617-730-0152
                                   www.childrenshospital.org

James Mandell, CEO
Sandra Fenwick, President & COO
Dick Argys, Chief Administrative Officer

2289 Massachusetts General Hospital
Pulmonary and Critical Care Unit
55 Fruit Street
Boston, MA 02114   617-726-2000
                                     TDD: 617-724-8800
                                        www.umass.org

Mass General aims to deliver the very best health care in a safe, compassionate environment; to advance that care through innovative research and education; and to improve the health and well-being of the diverse communities we serve.

Cathy Minehan, Chair
Peter Slavin, President & Trustee
Ronald Kleinman, Physician-in-Chief, Hospital for Ch

2290 Tufts New England Medical Center Floating Hospital for Children
Division of Pulmonary, Critical Care and Sleep
755 Washington Street
Boston, MA 02111   617-636-5000
                                   www.tuftsmedicalcenter.org

Joseph Campanelli, Chairman
Richard Freeman, Chair, Organ Transplantation
Brien Barnewolt, Chairman, Chief of Emergency Medici

Michigan

2291 Butterworth Hospital, Cystic Fibrosis Center
426 Michigan Street NE
Grand Rapids, MI 49503   616-454-1509
John Schuen, MD, Director

2292 Children's Hospital of Michigan Cystic Fibrosis Care, Teaching & Resource
Children's Hospital of Michigan
3901 Beaubien Boulevard
Detroit, MI 48201   313-745-5437
                                          888-362-2500
                                          www.childrensdmc.org
Herman Gray, Jr., President
Shawn Levitt, COO
Joseph Scallen, Jr., VP Finance

2293 Cystic Fibrosis Center/Pediatric Pulmonary and Sleep Medicine
330 Barclay Avenue NE, Suite 200
Grand Rapids, MI 49503   616-391-2125
                                          Fax: 616-391-2131
John Schuen, MD, Director
Susan Millard, MD, Director

2294 Kalamazoo Center for Medical Studies
Michigan State University
1000 Oakland Drive
Kalamazoo, MI 49008   269-337-4400
                                          www.kcms.msu.edu/
Robert Carter, CEO
Peter Ziemkowski, Family Practitioner

2295 University of Michigan, Cystic Fibrosis Center
1500 E. Medical Center Drive
Ann Arbor, MI 48109   734-936-4000
                                          800-962-3555
                                          Fax: 734-936-7635
                          www.med.umich.edu/mott/cysticfibrosiscenter/

The University of Michigan Cystic Fibrosis Program mission is to provide excellence and leadership in patient care, services, research and education.

Samya Z. Nasr, MD, Director, Cystic Fibrosis Center

Minnesota

2296 Minnesota Cystic Fibrosis Center
Fairview University Medical Center
420 Delaware Street SE, MMC 742
Minneapolis, MN 55455   612-624-0962
                                          Fax: 612-624-0696
                                          www.med.umn.edu/peds/cfcenter/

Comprehensive and coordinated care approach that is designed to prevent and slow the rate of disease progression. Since 1961, this care approach used by the University of Minnesota physicians has led to an increase in the average age of survival for patients with Cystic Fibrosis from 2 1/2 to 39 years.

Warren E. Regelmann, Co-Director, Ped CF Program
Carlye Tomczyk, CF Educator

Mississippi

2297 University of Mississippi Medical Center
2500 N State Street
Jackson, MS 39216   601-984-5820
                                          www.umc.edu/
Thomas H. Fortner, Chief Public Affairs and Communicat
John E. Hall, Associate Vice Chancellor for Resea
James M. Lightsey, Chief Financial Officer

Missouri

2298 Children's Mercy Hospital, University of Missouri
Kansas City School of Medicine
2401 Gillham Road
Kansas City, MO 64108   816-234-3000
                                          866-512-2168
                                          TTY: 816-234-3816
                                          e-mail: webmaster@cmh.edu
                                          www.childrensmercy.org
Ed Connolly, Jr., Chairman
Randall O'Donnell, President, CEO, and Director

2299 Cystic Fibrosis, Pediatric Pulmonary and Pediatric Gastrointestinal Center
Cardinal Glennon Memorial Hospital for Children
1465 S Grand
Saint Louis, MO 63104   314-577-5600
Anthony J Rejent, MD, Center Director

2300 University of Missouri-Columbia Cystic Fibrosis Center
University of Missouri/Department of Child Health
404 Keene Street
Columbia, MO 65203   573-875-9000
                                          www.muhealth.org

University of Missouri Children's Hospital seves patients from every county in Missouri. With over 30 pediatric subspecialties, a pediatric ICU, adolescent unit and child life therapy, MU Children's Hospital is mid-Missouri's largest and most comprehensive pediatric health care facility.

James Ross, Chief Executive Officer
Anita Larsen, Chief Operating Officer
Jeri Doty, Chief Planning Officer

2301 Washington University Cystic Fibrosis Center
Saint Louis Children's Hospital
1 Childrens Place
Saint Louis, MO 63110   314-454-2694
                                          888-503-2237
                                          Fax: 314-454-2515
                          peds.wustl.edu/pulmonary/CysticFibrosisCenter/tabid/
Thomas Ferkol, MD, Director

Nebraska

2302 University of Nebraska at Omaha Pediatric Pulmonary/Cystic Fibrosis Center
42nd and Emile
Omaha, NE 68198   402-559-6400
                                          Fax: 402-559-7062
                                          www.unmc.edu/pediatrics/
John W. Sparks, MD, Chairman

Nevada

2303 Children's Lung Specialists
3820 Meadows Lane
Las Vegas, NV 89107   702-598-4411
                                          Fax: 702-598-1988
Kris Hissung, Manager
Brian Woo, Pediatric Pulmonologist

New Hampshire

2304 New Hampshire Cystic Fibrosis Care and Teaching Center
Dartmouth Hitchcock Medical Center
1 Medical Center Drive
Lebanon, NH 03756   603-650-6244
                                          Fax: 603-650-8601
William Boyle Jr, MD, Director

2305 Monmouth Medical Center, Cystic Fibrosis & Pediatric Pulmonary Center
300 Second Avenue
Long Branch, NJ 07740   732-222-5200
Fax: 908-222-4472
http://www.saintbarnabas.com/hospitals/monmouth_medi
Carol Foster, Manager

2306 New Jersey Medical School
185 S Orange Avenue
Newark, NJ 07103   973-972-4871
800-482-3627
Fax: 201-982-7597
njms.umdnj.edu

Robert Wieder, Director

2307 University of New Mexico School of Medicine
2400 Tucker Ne 4th Fl
Albuquerque, NM 87131   505-272-0518
Fax: 505-272-0329
e-mail: somadmin@salud.unm.edu
www.som.unm.edu

The School of Medicine is committed to remain a world-leading institution in three equally valued and inter-related missions of patient care, education, and research.

Paul Roth, MD, Dean, School of Medicine
David Sklar, Emergency Medicine

2308 Albany Medical College Pediatric Pulmonary & Cystic Fibrosis Center
Department of Pediatrics
47 New Scotland Avenue
Albany, NY 12208   518-262-6008
Fax: 518-262-6472
www.amc.edu

Vincent P Verdile, Exec Vp

2309 Armond V. Mascia CF Center
NY Medical College
Munger Pavillion, Room 106
Valhalla, NY 10595   914-493-7585
Fax: 914-594-4336
e-mail: pedpulm@nymc.edu
www.nymc.edu/depthome/peds/pedspulm/CFCenter.asp

The mission of our CF Center is to enable our patients with cystic fibrosis to fulfill their maximal potential with the support of their families by providing state-of-the-art clinical care. To further this goal, our center is dedicated to the education of all patients, their families, healthcare professionals and the community, the pursuit of rigorous research and continuous quality improvement.

Allen Dozer, MD, Director

2310 CF & Pediatric Pulmonary Care Center
Mt. Sinai School of Medicine
5th Avenue at 100th Street
New York, NY 10029   212-241-7788
Richard J Bonforte, MD, Director

2311 CF, Pediatric Pulmonary & GI Center
Saint Vincent's Hospital & Medical Center of NY
36 7th Avenue
New York, NY 10011   212-604-8895
Joan DeGelie-Germana, MD, Director

2312 Children's Lung and Cystic Fibrosis Center
Children's Hospital of Buffalo
219 Bryant Street
Buffalo, NY 14222   716-878-7524
Fax: 716-888-3945
www.wchob.org/services/services_display.asp?PType=L

Services for infants, children and teenagers with cystic fibrosis and other chronic respiratory conditions.

Drucy Borowitz, MD, Director
David Sheehan, Medical Director

2313 Long Island College Hospital
350 Henry Street
Brooklyn, NY 11201   718-780-1071
www.futurenurselich.org/

Robert Giusti, MD, Director

2314 Pediatric Pulmonary Center
Babies Hospital & Columbia Presbyterian Med Center
750 East Adams Street
Syracuse, NY 13210   315-464-6323
Fax: 212-805-6103

Ran D Anbar, Medical Director
Mary Ann Russo, Dietician
Karen Watkins, Secretary

2315 Schneider Children's Hospital of Long Island
Albert Einstein College of Medicine
New Hyde Park, NY 14040   716-470-3250
Jack D Gorvoy, MD

2316 State University Hospital/Upstate Medical University
750 E Adams Street
Syracuse, NY 13210   315-464-8668
877-464-5540
Fax: 315-464-5158
www.upstate.edu/uh/

David Smith, President
Steven Brady, SVP Finance & Administration
Teresa Wagner, CIO

2317 University of Rochester Medical Center
Strong Memorial Hospital/Division of Pediatrics
601 Elmwood Avenue
Rochester, NY 14642   585-275-2838
www.urmc.rochester.edu/

Karen Z Voter, MD, Director

2318 Duke University Medical Center/ CF Center
350 Hanes House
Durham, NC 10236   919-684-3364
Fax: 919-684-2292
www.pediatrics.duke.edu

Marc Majure, MD, Director

2319 UNC CF Center
Department of Pediatrics
509 Burnett-Womack Building
Chapel Hill, NC 27599   919-966-1055
Gerald W Fernald, MD, Director

2320 Saint Alexius Medical Center/CF Center
311 N 9th Street
Bismarck, ND 58501   701-224-7500
Fax: 701-224-7560

Allan Stillerman, MD, Director

The Stanley Medical Research Institute (SMRI) is a nonprofit organization supporting research on the causes of, and treatments for, schizophrenia and bipolar disorder. Since it began in 1989, SMRI has supported more than $550 million in research in over 30 countries.

Maree J. Webster, Ph.D., Executive Director
Wendy Simmons, Research Assistant
Jana Bowcut, M.P.H., Treatment Trials Administrator

State Agencies & Support Groups

2478 Depressive and Manic-Depressive Assocation of Mount Sinai
100 LaSalle Street, Suite 5A
New York, NY 10027   917-445-2399
e-mail: jgg17@columbia.edu
www.columbia.edu

The NYC Depressive and Manic-Depressive Group is a support group for persons with mood disorders, depression and bipolar disorder, as well as their family members and friends.

Research Centers

2479 National Alliance for Research on Schizophrenia & Depression
60 Cutter Mill Road, Suite 404
Great Neck, NY 11021   516-829-0091
Fax: 516-487-6930
e-mail: info@bbrfoundation.org
www.narsad.org

The Brain and Behavior Research Foundation (formerly NARSAD, the National Alliance for Research on Schizophrenia and Depression) is committed to alleviating the suffering of mental illness by awarding grants that will lead to advances and breakthroughs in scientific research.

Benita Shobe, President & CEO

2480 University of Pennsylvania, Depression Research Unit
School of Medicine, Department of Psychiatry
3600 Spruce Street
Philadelphia, PA 19104   215-349-5979
Fax: 215-662-6443
www.med.upenn.edu

The mission of the Depression Research Unit (DRU) at Penn is to foster a greater understanding and knowledge of the causes, diagnosis, and treatment of mood disorders.

Adam I Rubin, Director

2481 University of Texas, Mental Health Clinical Research Center
5323 Harry Hines Boulevard
Dallas, TX 75235   214-648-2951

UT Southwestern Medical Center is home to one of the premier centers in the world for the study, diagnosis and treatment of mental health and addictive disorders.

A John Rush, MD, Director

2482 Yale University, Behavioral Medicine Clinic
Yale School of Medicine
333 Cedar Street
New Haven, CT 06510   203-785-4231

Focuses on mental disorders including schizophrenia and depression.

Henry M Rinder, Director

2483 Yale University, Ribicoff Research Facilities
CT Medical Health Center
34 Park Street
New Haven, CT 06519   203-764-9765
Fax: 203-688-2491

Clinical research in the areas of schizophrenia, depression and mental disorders.

George Heninger, MD, Director

Conferences

2484 ADAA Annual Conference
Anxiety Disorders Association of America
8701 Georgia Avenue, Suite 412
Silver Spring, MD 20910   240-485-1001
Fax: 240-485-1035
e-mail: information@adaa.org
www.adaa.org

Focusing exclusively on advancing science and treatment of anxiety and related disorders in children and adults.

April

Alies Muskin, Executive Director

2485 DSBA National Conference
Depression and Bipolar Support Alliance
730 N Franklin Street, Suite 501
Chicago, IL 60654   800-826-3632
Fax: 312-642-7243
www.dbsalliance.org

Offers a unique peer-centered conference for individuals living with depression or bipolar disorder, as well as for family members or health care providers looking for ways to best help their loved ones, patients, or clients by partnering with them on their path to recovery. The conference consists of compelling keynote presentations, educational workshops, and pre-conference institutes.

May

Allen Doederlein, President
Lisa Goodale, Vice President, Training
Charlene Knox, Coordinator, Human Resources

2486 FFCMH Annual Conference
Federation of Families for Childrens Mental Health
9605 Medical Center Drive, Suite 280
Rockville, MD 20850   240-403-1901
Fax: 240-403-1909
e-mail: ffcmh@ffcmh.org
www.ffcmh.org

Address the complex issue of trauma; the impact it has on children and families; the promotion of healing and prevention strategies; knowledge about how to address trauma through resiliency-based interventions, utilizing a familydriven, youth guided approach; and examples of how family organizations and the partners they work with are raising awareness and improving trauma-focused services and supports.

November

Sandra Spencer, Executive Director

2487 NADD Conference & Exhibit Show
National Association for the Dually Diagnosed
132 Fair Street
Kingston, NY 12401   845-331-4336
800-331-5362
Fax: 845-331-4569
e-mail: info@thenadd.org
www.thenadd.org

November

Dr Robert Fletcher, CEO

2488 NAMI Convention
National Alliance on Mental Illness
3803 N. Fairfax Dr.Suite 100
Arlington, VA 22203   703-524-7600
800-950-6264
Fax: 703-524-9094
TDD: 703-516-7227
e-mail: info@nami.org
www.nami.org

The NAMI Convention is packed with information, chances to network, leadership development opportunities, and lots more

July

Suzanne Vogel-Scibilia MD, President

Audio Video

2489 Coping with Depression
New Harbinger Publications
5674 Shattuck Avenue
Oakland, CA 94609   510-652-2002
                                     800-748-6273
                                Fax: 510-652-1613
       e-mail: customerservice@newharbinger.com
                                   newharbinger.com

60 minute videotape that offers a powerful message of hope for
anyone struggling with depression.
ISBN: 1-879237-62-8

**2490 Cry for Help - How to Help a Friend Who is Depressed or
Suicidal**
Aquarius Health Care Videos
36 Southern Eagle Cartway
Brewster, MA 2631   508-255-4685
                                     800-451-5006
                                Fax: 508-255-5705
       e-mail: customerservice@paracletepress.com
                                   www.paracletepress.com

Most suicidal young people don't really want to die; they just
want their pain to end. Teen sucide is often preventable if young
people know the signs to look for and the steps to take when they
suspect a friend is suicidal. This video teaches young people to
recognize the warning signs and to take specific actions to help a
friend.
22 Minutes
Donna Kaufman

2491 Day for Night: Recognizing Teenage Depression
DRADA-Depression and Related Affective Disorders
600 N Wolfe Street
Baltimore, MD 21287   410-955-4647
                                Fax: 410-614-3241

2492 Living with Depression and Manic Depression
New Harbinger Publications
5674 Shattuck Avenue
Oakland, CA 94609   510-652-2002
                                     800-748-6273
                                Fax: 510-652-1613
       e-mail: customerservice@newharbinger.com
                                   newharbinger.com

Describes a program based on years of research and hundreds of
interviews with depressed persons. Warm, helpful, and engaging,
this tape validates the feelings of people with depression while it
encourages positive change.
ISBN: 1-879237-63-6

**2493 Why Isn't My Child Happy? A Video Guide About Childhood
Depression**
ADD WareHouse
300 Northwest 70th Avenue, Suite 102
Plantation, FL 33317   954-792-8100
                                     800-233-9273
                                Fax: 954-792-8545
       e-mail: websales@addwarehouse.com
                                   addwarehouse.com

The first of its kind, this new video deals with childhood depression. Informative and frank about this common problem, this
book offers helpful guidance for parents and professionals trying
to better understand childhood depression. 110 minutes.

Web Sites

2494 AACAP
3615 Wisconsin Avenue, N.W.
Washington, DC 20016   202-966-7300
                                Fax: 202-966-2891
                                   www.aacap.org

Assisting parents and families in understanding developmental,
behavioral, emotional and mental disorders affecting children and
adolescents.
Paramjit T. Joshi, M.D., President
David G Fassler, M.D., Treasurer
Aradhana Bela Sood, M.D., Secretary

2495 Anxiety Disorders Association of America

Offers resources and information for persons with anxiety and
stress-related disorders.

2496 Dr. Ivan's Depression Central
www.psycom.net/depression.central.html

This site is the Internet's central clearinghouse for information
on all types of depressive disorders and on the most effective
treatments for individuals suffering from Major Depression, Manic
Depression (Bipolar Disorder), Cyclothymia, Dysthymia and
other mood disorders.
Ivan Goldberg, MD, Founder
Satish Reddy, M.D., Editor

2497 Internet Mental Health
www.mentalhealth.com/

                    e-mail: internetmentalhealth@shaw.ca
                                   www.mentalhealth.com/

Our goal is to improve understanding, diagnosis, and teatment of
meantal illness throughout the world.
Phillip W. Long, M.D., Psychiatrist

2498 Mental Health Net
Po Box 20709
Columbus, OH 43220   614-448-4055
       e-mail: info@centersite.net, editor@centersite.n
                                   www.mentalhelp.net

We wish to provide the following: to discuss, develop and debate
in an open forum the future of the mental health field in America
and throughout the world. To help coordinate various components of the mental health field so as to bring about greater communication between them. To educate the public about mental
health issues, to promote active collaboration between professionals in all segments of mental health development,
implementation and policy.

2499 NADD: National Association for the Dually Diagnosed
132 Fair Street
Kingston, NY 12401   845-331-4336
                                     800-331-5362
                                Fax: 845-331-4569
                       e-mail: info@thenadd.org
                                   www.thenadd.org

Nonprofit organization designed to promote the interests of professional and care providers for individuals who have the coexistence of mental illness and mental retardation. NADD provides
conferences, educational services and training materials to professionals, parents, concerned citizens and service organizations.
Donna McNelis, Ph.D., President
Don Baker, Ph.D., Vice President
Robert J. Fletcher, DSW, CEO

2500 Online Mendelian Inheritance in Man
U.S. National Library of Medicine, 8600 Rockville
Bethesda, MD 20894   888-346-3656
                       e-mail: info@ncbi.nlm.nih.gov
                                   www.ncbi.nlm.nih.gov

This database is a catalog of human genes and genetic disorders.
Christine E. Seidman, M.D., Chair
David J. Lipman, M.D., Executive Secretary
Michael Boehnke, Ph.D., Board Member

2501 Seasonal Affective Disorder
www.alt.support.depression.seasonal

The SAD Association is a voluntary organization and registered
charity which informs the public and health professions about
SAD and supports and advises sufferers of the illness.

2502 Understanding and Treating Depression
www.couns.uiuc.edu/depression.htm

Offers an understanding of depression, causes, how to help yourself, things to do, what to avoid while in the depression state, and
treatments of the depression.

2503 Wing of Madness: A Depression Guide
www.wingofmadness.com

Is a nonprofit organization dedicated to disseminating information about depression to consumers.

Book Publishers

2504 Anxiety & Depression In Adults & Children
Sage Publications
2455 Teller Road
Newbury Park, CA 91320   805-499-0721

1994 304 pages Softcover
ISBN: 0-803970-21-8

2505 Ask the Doctor: Depression
Andrews McMeel Publishing
PO Box 419150
Kansas City, MO 64141   816-932-6700
                               800-233-2336
                               Fax: 212-698-7336

A look at depression, its symptoms, what causes it, and what you
can do about it. Learn the difference between mood problems and
genuine depression, and how to read warning signs such as sleep
abnormalities, nervousness, and suicidal thoughts. Information on
chemicals, genetics, and medical solutions.

128 pages Softcover
ISBN: 0-836227-11-5

2506 Coping with Depression
Rosen Publishing Group
29 E 21st Street
New York, NY 10010   800-237-9932
                            Fax: 888-436-4643
                            e-mail: rosenpub@tribeca.ios.com
                            www.rosenpublishing.com

With an emphasis on life's myriad difficulties, the authors help
teens find practical ways to cope with depression.

ISBN: 0-823919-51-0

2507 Dealing with Depression: Five Ways to Help
Haworth Press
10 Alice Street
Binghamton, NY 13904   607-722-8277
                              Fax: 607-722-1424

1995
ISBN: 1-560249-33-1

2508 Depression and Its Treatment
Warner Books
1271 Avenue of the Americas
New York, NY 10020   212-522-7200

A layman's guide to help one understand and cope with America's number one mental health problem.

157 pages

2509 Depression, the Mood Disease
Johns Hopkins University Press
2715 N Charles Street
Baltimore, MD 21218   410-516-6900
                             800-537-5487
                             Fax: 410-516-6998
                             www.highbeam.com/doc/1G1-159331264.html

This book explores the many faces of an illness that will affect as
many as 36 million Americans at some point in their lives. Updated to reflect state-of-the-art treatment.

1993 240 pages
ISBN: 0-801851-84-X

2510 Depressive Illnesses: Treatments Bring New Hope
Superintendent of Documents
PO Box 371954
Pittsburgh, PA 15250   202-512-2250

Offers the general public an overview of the various depressive
illnesses. Topics include causes, symptoms and types of depression, clinical evaluation and treatment, helpful suggestions for
family and friends, and other sources of information.

28 pages

2511 Encyclopedia of Depression
Facts on File
Department M274, 11 Penn Plaza
New York, NY 10001   212-290-8090
                            800-322-8755
                            Fax: 212-678-3633

This volume defines and explains all terms and topics relating to
depression.

170 pages Hardbound

2512 Essential Guide to Psychiatric Drugs
Saint Martin's Press
175 5th Avenue
New York, NY 10010   212-674-5151
                            800-221-7945
                            Fax: 212-420-9314

Basic information on 123 drugs used for depression, anxiety and
bipolar illness.

2513 Everything You Need To Know About Depression
Rosen Publishing Group
29 E 21st Street
New York, NY 10010   212-777-3017
                            800-237-9932
                            Fax: 212-436-4643
                            e-mail: rosenpub@tribeca.ios.com
                            www.rosenpublishing.com

An important resource for teens who are looking for help with depression.

Grades 7-12
ISBN: 0-823926-06-0

2514 Handbook of School-Based Interventions
Courage to Change
PO Box 1268
Newburgh, NY 12551   800-440-4003
                            Fax: 800-772-6499

Comprehensive volume that describes interventions for virtually
every major problem behavior students may exhibit from K-12.
All interventions are research-based and guidance is given for
practical application of the techniques. Topics range from dishon-
esty, academic performance, procrastination and low self-esteem
to obsessive-compulsive behavior, substance abuse, AIDS and
depression.

512 pages Hardcover

2515 Help Me, I'm Sad
Penguin Putnam
PO Box 999
Bergenfield, NJ 07621   800-526-0275
                               Fax: 800-227-9604

Helping and understanding a child with depression.

**2516 Helping Your Child Cope with Depression and Suicidal
Thoughts**
Jossey-Bass
111 River Street
Hoboken, NJ 07030   201-748-6000
                           800-956-7739
                           Fax: 201-748-6088
                           www.josseybass.com

Shows parents how to learn to talk, listen, and communicate effectively with a depressed child; signs to watch for and situations which may cause a wish to commit suicide.

192 pages
ISBN: 0-787908-44-4

2517 Helping Your Depressed Child
Prima Publishing
PO Box 1260
Rocklin, CA 95677 916-624-5718

Reasurring guide to the causes and treatment of childhood and adolescent depression.

284 pages

2518 Kid Power Tactics for Dealing with Depression & Parent's Survival Guide
Childs Work/Childs Play
135 Dupont Street
Plainville, NY 11803 800-962-1141
Fax: 800-262-1886
e-mail: info@Childswork.com
www.Childswork.com

2 volume set was wriiten by a child who suffered from depression and his mother. Plain language and a wealth of information for children ages 8 and over, plus their parents and teachers.

2519 Mood Apart
Basic Books
10 E 53rd Street
New York, NY 10022 212-207-7057

An overview of depression and manic depression and the available treatments for them.

363 pages

2520 Overcoming Depression
Harper & Row
10 E 53rd Street
New York, NY 10022 212-207-7000
1987 318 pages Softcover

2521 Panic Disorder in the Medical Setting
Superintendent of Documents
PO Box 371954
Pittsburgh, PA 15250 202-512-2250

This book serves the primary care physicians as a helpful guide in recognizing and treating panic disorder in patients and in identifying those who need psychiatric consultation or referrals.

1993 135 pages

2522 Prozac Nation: Young & Depressed in America, A Memoir
Houghton Mifflin Company
222 Berkeley Street
Boston, MA 02116 617-351-3698
800-225-3362

Struck with depression at 11, now 27, Wurtzel chronicles her struggle with the illness. Witty, terrifying and sometimes funny, it tells the story of a young life almost destroyed by depression.

317 pages

2523 Psychotherapy of Severe and Mild Depression
Jason Aronson
400 Keystone Industrial Park
Dunmore, PA 18521 800-782-0015
Fax: 201-840-7242
www.aronson.com

464 pages Softcover
ISBN: 1-568211-46-5

2524 Report of the Secretary's Task Force on Youth Suicide
Superintendent of Documents
PO Box 371954
Pittsburgh, PA 15250 202-512-2250

A comprehensive review of information about youth suicide. The task force recommendations are presented in Volume 1.

110 pages

2525 Sad Days, Glad Days
National Alliance for the Mentally Ill
PO Box 753
Waldorf, MD 20604 703-524-7600
www.NIMF.org

Helps five to nine-year-olds understand a parent's depression.

1995

2526 Suicide, Why?
National Alliance for the Mentally Ill
PO Box 753
Waldorf, MD 20604 703-524-7600
www.NAMI.org

An authoritative book, noting that suicide is usually caused by brain disorders.

1989

2527 Surprising Truth About Depression: Medical Breakthroughs That Can Work
Zondervan
5300 Patterson SE
Grand Rapids, MI 49530 616-698-6900
Fax: 616-698-3439
www.zondervan.com

1994 224 pages Softcover
ISBN: 0-310401-01-1

2528 Treating Depressed Children
New Harbinger Publications
5674 Shattuck Avenue
Oakland, CA 94609 800-748-6273
Fax: 510-652-5472
e-mail: customerservice@newharbinger.com
www.newharbinger.com

This book explains a 12-session treatment program to help children change their negative thoughts, gain confidence and recognize their emotions. These actions are achieved with the help of cartoons and role-playing games.

160 pages Hardcover
ISBN: 1-572240-61-X

Laseu Pfaff, Publicist

2529 Treating Depression
Jossey-Bass
111 River Street
Hoboken, NJ 07030 201-748-6000
800-956-7739
Fax: 201-748-6088
www.josseybass.com

Offers guidelines and specific models for intervention in the treatment of numerous types and subtypes of depression. Also will assist you in deciding if it is appropriate to prescribe medication, if psychotherapy is the proper course of action, or if it is best to use a combination of medication and psychotherapy.

1997 223 pages
ISBN: 0-787915-85-8

2530 Understanding Depression
University Press of Mississippi
3825 Ridgewood Road
Jackson, MS 39211 601-432-6205
800-737-7788
Fax: 601-432-6217
e-mail: press@ihl.state.ms.us
www.upress.state.ms.us

A clear explanation for those who know the illness personally and for those who want to understand them.

120 pages Hardcover/Ppbck
ISBN: 1-578061-68-7

2531 Understanding Your Teenager's Depression
Berkley Books
200 Madison Avenue
New York, NY 10016 212-951-8800

1994 352 pages Softcover
ISBN: 0-399518-56-8

2532 When Nothing Matters Anymore: A Survival Guide for Depressed Teens
Free Spirit Publishing
217 5th Avenue N
Minneapolis, MN 55401

612-338-2068
800-735-7323
Fax: 612-337-5050
e-mail: help4kids@freespirit.com
www.freespirit.com

Written for teens with depression and those who feel despondent, dejected or alone. This powerful book offers help, hope, and potentially lifesaving facts and advice.

176 pages
ISBN: 1-575420-36-8

Penne Post, Tradesales Associate

2533 Working with Children and Adolescents in Groups
Courage to Change
PO Box 1268
Newburgh, NY 12551

800-440-4003
Fax: 800-772-6499

Step-by-step guide that discusses how to effectively treat problem behavior in children and adolescents using small groups. Based on empirical research and their own work with groups, the authors show how a variety of approaches can be effectively combined to help resolve such problem behaviors as fighting and low self-esteem.

384 pages Hard Cover

2534 Yesterday's Tomorrow
Hazelden
15251 Pleasant Valley Road
Center City, MN 55012

612-257-4010
800-328-9000
Fax: 917-339-0325
www.hazelden.org

A meditation book that shows why and how recovery works, from the author's own experiences.

432 pages Softcover
ISBN: 1-568381-60-3

Magazines

2535 EA Message
Emotions Anonymous
PO Box 4245
Saint Paul, MN 55104

651-647-9712
Fax: 651-647-1593
e-mail: info@emotionsanonymous.org
www.emotionsanonymous.org

Quarterly magazine.

Electronic

Karen Mead, Executive Director

Newsletters

2536 National Foundation for Depressive Illness
PO Box 2257
New York, NY 10116

212-268-4260
800-248-4344
Fax: 212-268-4434
www.depression.org

Information on the myths and misconceptions surrounding the illness. Informs the public, health care providers, healthcare professionals and corporations about depression and manic depression, and provides the information about correct diagnosis and treatment and the availability of qualified doctors and support groups.

4 pages Quarterly

Amy C Russell, Editor

2537 Outreach
Depression and Bipolar Support Alliance
55 E. Jackson Blvd, Suite 490
Chicago, IL 60604

800-826-3632
Fax: 312-642-7243
www.dbsalliance.org

Quarterly publication serving members and constituents of the organization. National DMDA educates patients, families, professionals, and the public concerning the nature of depressive and manic-depressive illnesses as treatable medical diseases; fosters self-help for patients and families; eliminates discrimination and stigma; improves access to care; advocates for research toward the elimination of these illnesses.

Karen Kraft, Publications Manager

2538 Smooth Sailing
Depression & Related Affective Disorders Assoc.
Meyer 3-181, 600 N Wolfe Street
Baltimore, MD 21287

410-955-4647
Fax: 410-614-3241
e-mail: drada@jhmi.edu
www.drada.org

Contains a variety of information including medical, educational and first hand experiences about mood disorders. Newsletter is free with membership.

Quarterly

Pamphlets

2539 Depression Is a Treatable Illness: A Patients Guide
Department of Health & Human Services
2101 E Jefferson Street, Suite 501
Rockville, MD 20852

301-217-1245

Tells about major depressive disorder, which is only one form of depressive illness. This booklet answers important questions regarding this disorder and gives information on where to go for more help.

2540 Depression in Children and Adolescents: A Fact Sheet for Physicians
National Institute of Mental Health
6001 Executive Boulevard, Room 6200, MSC 9663
Bethesda, MD 20892

301-443-4536
866-615-6464
Fax: 301-443-4279
TTY: 301-443-8431
e-mail: nimhinfo@nih.gov
www.nimh.nih.gov

Discusses the scope of the problem and the screening tools used in evaluating children with depression.

8 pages

Dr. Francis S. Collins, Director

2541 Let's Talk About Depression
Superintendent of Documents
PO Box 371954
Pittsburgh, PA 15250

202-512-2250

Targeted especially for inner-city youth. The colorful design will capture attention and focus on depression in a way that young people will understand and identify with.

2542 Let's Talk Facts About Childhood Disorders
American Psychiatric Association
1400 K Street NW
Washington, DC 20005

202-682-6220

Offers information on depression and depressive disorders including the causes, symptoms, treatments, anxiety, and various other phobias.

2543 Living Without Depression & Manic Depression: A Workbook
National Alliance for the Mentally Ill
3803 N. Fairfax Drive, Suite 100
Arlington, VA 22203 703-524-7600
800-950-6264
Fax: 703-524-9094
e-mail: info@nami.com
www.NAMI.org

Workbook offering checklists and helpful advice targeted for individuals whose depressive illness is stabilized.

1994

Jim Payne, J.D., President
Ralph E. Nelson, Jr., M.D., First Vice President
Marilyn Ricci, M.S., R.D., Second Vice President

2544 Major Depression in Children and Adolescents
Center for Mental Health Services
PO Box 42490
Washington, DC 20015 800-789-2647
Fax: 301-984-8796
e-mail: ken@mentalhealth.org
mentalhealth.org

This fact sheet defines depression and its signs, identifies types of help available, and suggests what parents or other caregivers can do.

2 pages

2545 Now We Can Successfully Treat the Illness Called Depression
National Foundation for Depressive Illness (NAFDI)
PO Box 2257
New York, NY 10116 212-268-4260
800-248-4344
Fax: 212-268-4434
www.depression.org

Basic information on depression and manic depression, gives symptoms, encourages persons who have symptoms to seek medical treatment. Tips on managing depressive illness.

Amy C Russell, Editor

2546 Panic Disorder
National Institutes of Health
5600 Fishers Lane, Room 7C-02
Rockville, MD 20857 301-443-4707
Fax: 301-443-6000

Written for the lay public, this pamphlet contains a description of panic disorder, gives the symptoms, describes treatment methods, and encourages the person who has the symptoms to seek treatment.

2547 Plain Talk About Depression
Superintendent of Documents
PO Box 371954
Pittsburgh, PA 15250 202-512-2250

A flyer discussing types of depression, major depression; symptoms and causes.

2548 Understanding Panic Disorder
National Institutes of Health
5600 Fishers Lane, Room 7C-02
Rockville, MD 20857 301-443-4707
Fax: 301-443-6000

Offers information on what panic disorder is, symptoms, causes, treatment, medications and therapy.

2549 Useful Information on Phobias and Panic
Superintendent of Documents
PO Box 371954
Pittsburgh, PA 15250 202-512-2250

This booklet provides information on both phobias and panic. Symptoms, causes and treatments of these disorders are referred to. If you know someone who is excessively fearful, this booklet will be of great help to them in understanding their problem.

40 pages 50 copies

2550 What to Do When a Friend Is Depressed: Guide for Students
Superintendent of Documents
PO Box 371954
Pittsburgh, PA 15250 202-512-2250

Offers information on depression and its symptoms and suggests things a young person can do to guide a depressed friend in finding help.

Description

2551 DIABETES MELLITUS
Involves the following Biologic System(s):
Endocrinologic Disorders

Diabetes mellitis refers to an inability of the body to utilize glucose. There are two types of DM: Insulin-dependent diabetes mellitus, referred to as Type I diabetes, is a disorder in which insufficient production of insulin by the pancreas results in abnormally high levels of the sugar glucose in the blood. Insulin is a hormone that regulates and stabilizes blood glucose levels by promoting the movement of energy-rich glucose into body cells for energy production or into the liver and fat cells for storage. Type I diabetes may also cause impaired fat metabolism and long-term complications affecting certain large and small blood vessels (angiopathy), the nerve-rich membranes at the back of the eyes (retinas), skin, kidneys, nerves, or other tissues of the body. The exact cause of Type I diabetes is unknown. However, researchers speculate that certain environmental factors, such as a viral infection, may inappropriately trigger the immune system to destroy insulin-producing cells within the pancreas (beta cells), resulting in severe insulin deficiency. Genetic factors are also thought to play some role in causing a predisposition for the disorder.

Type I diabetes is the major form of diabetes affecting children. It affects 1 million patients in the United States, most often in young people, 10-14 years of age. The other major type of diabetes, Type II diabetes, may be characterized by a resistance to the effects of insulin. Although this type of diabetes may occur at any age, it most commonly becomes apparent in middle-aged or older people, but is increasingly common during childhood and adolescence. It is most common in obese patients. In some children, various forms of diabetes may occur secondary to certain genetic multisystemic disorders that affect the pancreas, such as cystic fibrosis; other endocrine disorders, such as Cushing's syndrome; the administration of particular drugs; or exposure to certain poisons.

In most children with Type I diabetes, associated symptoms and findings may appear to occur suddenly and may include excessive urine production by the kidneys, causing increased urination (polyuria) and excessive thirst (polydipsia); weight loss; and abnormally increased hunger (polyphagia). Additional abnormalities may include exhaustion, blurred vision, abnormal sensations (paresthesias) in the hands and feet, and increased irritability. Without prompt diagnosis and treatment, symptoms may rapidly progress to a metabolic condition known as ketoacidosis. Because of deficient insulin production, the body's cells begin to rely on sources of energy other than glucose, causing an excessive breakdown of fats and an abnormal accumulation of certain chemical compounds (ketones) in body tissues and fluids. Early symptoms associated with ketoacidosis may be relatively mild, including increased urination, vomiting and dehydration but, without appropriate treatment, coma and potentially life-threatening complications may occur. The treatment of ketoacidosis may include the immediate administration of intravenous fluids; replacement of electrolytes, such as sodium and potassium; initiation of intravenous insulin therapy; measures to prevent or appropriately treat increased fluid pressure within the brain; and other therapies as required.

Patients with either Type I or Type II diabetes may eventually develop certain long-term complications associated with the disease. Complications may include thickening and leaking of the walls of certain small blood vessels, narrowing of medium and large-size arteries due to plaque development (atherosclerosis), abnormally high blood pressure (hypertension), poor blood circulation, and problems affecting the eyes, kidneys, nerves, and skin. For example, kidney damage may result in impaired kidney function and kidney failure; damage to blood vessels within the nerve-rich membranes at the back of the eyes (diabetic retinopathy) may lead to visual impairment; and nerve damage may cause weakness or the loss of certain sensations, such as changes in temperature or pressure, increasing the risk of injury. In addition, impaired blood supply to certain skin areas may increase the risk of developing skin sores (ulcers). Poor wound healing and susceptibility to infected foot ulcers may lead to localized loss of tissue (necrosis), potentially requiring amputation. Diet is central to management of diabetes and must be individualized according to the patient's activity level, food preferences, and need to attain and maintain ideal weight. Regular exercise is also correlated with better glucose control. Individuals with Type I diabetes take insulin, delivered either by injection or by insulin pump. Type II diabetics can take oral blood-sugar lowering (hypoglycemic) drugs that potentiate insulin secretion. Other drugs help regulate glucose storage or release.

National Associations & Support Groups

2552 American Academy of Pediatrics
141 Northwest Point Boulevard
Elk Grove Village, IL 60007

847-434-4000
800-433-9016
Fax: 847-434-8000
www.aap.org

The American Academy of Pediatrics and its member pediatricians are committed to the attainment of optimal physical, mental and social health and well-being for all infants, children, adolescents, and young adults.

Sandra Hassink, MD, FAAP, President

2553 American Association of Diabetes Educators
200 W Madison St, Suite 800
Chicago, IL 60606

312-424-2426
800-338-3633
Fax: 312-424-2427
e-mail: aade@aadenet.org
www.diabeteseducator.org

Founded in 1973, AADE is a multidisciplinary association of healthcare professionals dedicated to integrating self-management as a key outcome in the care of people with diabetes and related chronic conditions.

Donna Tomky, President
Tami Ross, Vice President
Cecilia Sauter, Treasurer

2554 American Autoimmune Related Diseases Association, Inc.
22100 Gratiot Avenue
East Detroit, MI 48021

586-776-3900
Fax: 586-776-3903
www.aarda.org

The American Autoimmune Related Diseases Association is dedicated to the eradication of autoimmune diseases and the alleviation of suffering and the socioeconomic impact of autoimmunity through fostering and facilitating collaboration in the areas of education, public awareness, research, and patient services in an effective, ethical and efficient manner.

Stanley M Finger, PhD, Chairman of the Board
Noel R Rose, MD, PhD, Chairman Emeritus

2555 American Diabetes Association
1701 North Beauregard Street
Alexandria, VA 22311
703-549-1500
800-342-2383
Fax: 703-836-7439
e-mail: askada@diabetes.org
www.diabetes.org

The nation's leading voluntary organization concerned with diabetes and its complications. The mission of the organization is to prevent and cure diabetes and to improve the lives of persons with diabetes. Offers a network of 52 affiliates with over 55,000 volunteers, including a professional membership of more than 10,000 physicians, social workers, nutritionists, educators and nurses.

Larry Hausner, MBA, Chief Executive Officer
Mary Vaneeda Bennett, Executive Vice President
Shereen Arent, EVP, Government Affairs & Advocacy

2556 Center for Disabilities and Development
University of Iowa Hospitals and Clinics
100 Hawkins Drive
Iowa City, IA 52242
319-353-6900
877-686-0031
Fax: 319-356-8284
e-mail: cdd-webmaster@uiowa.edu
www.uiowa.edu

A trusted resource for healthcare, training, research and information for people with disabilities that include: behavior disorders, brain injury, cerebral palsy, diabetes, down syndrome, learning disabilities, mental retardation, sleep disorders and spina bifida.

Judy Stephenson, Administrator
Amy Mikelson, Supervisor Info Resource Service

2557 Juvenile Diabetes Foundation International
26 Broadway, 14th Floor
New York, NY 10004
212-785-9500
800-533-2873
Fax: 212-785-9595
e-mail: info@jdrf.org
www.jdrf.org

Focuses energies on fund-raising, referrals, educational materials and information pertaining to juvenile diabetes.

Jeffrey Brewer, President & CEO
Frank Ingrassia, Chairman, Board of Directors
Mary Tyler Moore, International Chairman

2558 National Diabetes Action Network for the Blind
National Federation of the Blind
3101 NE 87th Avenue
Vancouver, WA 98662
360-576-5965
Fax: 410-685-5653
e-mail: k7uij@panix.com
www.nfb.org.com

Leading support and information organization of persons losing vision due to diabetes. Provides personal contact and resource information with other blind diabetics about non-visual techniques of independently managing diabetes, monitoring glucose levels, measuring insulin and other matters concerning diabetes. Publishes Voice of the Diabetic, the leading publication about diabetes and blindness.

Michael Freeman, President

Libraries & Resource Centers

2559 National Diabetes Information Clearinghouse
1 Information Way
Bethesda, MD 20892
301-654-3327
800-860-8747
Fax: 703-738-4929
TTY: 866-569-1162
e-mail: ndic@info.niddk.nih.gov
www.diabetes.niddk.nih.gov

Offers various materials, resources, books, pamphlets and more for persons and families in the area of diabetes.

Research Centers

2560 Center for the Partially Sighted
6101 W Centinela Ave, Suite 150
Culver City, CA 90230
310-988-1970
Fax: 310-458-8179
e-mail: info@low-vision.org
www.low-vision.org

Provides professional, comprehensive vision rehabilitation services to visually impaired people of all ages. For those whose sight is severely limited due to macular degeneration, diabetic retinopathy, glaucoma, retinal detachment, stroke or other conditions not correctable medically or surgically.

Sidney Machtinger, Chairman
Linnae M Anderson, Secretary

2561 Joslin Diabetes Center
One Joslin Place
Boston, MA 02215
617-309-2400
800-567-5461
e-mail: diabetes@joslin.harvard.edu
www.joslin.org

Joslin Diabetes Center, a teaching a research affiliate of Harvard Medical School, is a one-of-a-kind institution on the front lines of the world epidemic of diabetes - leading the battle to conquer diabetes in all of its forms through cutting-edge research and innovative approaches to clinical care and education.

John L Brooks III, President & CEO
Martin J Abrahamson, MD, Senior Vice President, Director
George L King, MD, SVP & Research Director

Audio Video

2562 Not So Sweet: Living With Diabetes
Fanlight Productions
32 Court Street, 21st Floor
Brooklyn, NY 11201
718-488-8900
800-876-1710
Fax: 718-488-8642
e-mail: info@fanlight.com, orders@fanlight.com
www.fanlight.com

Exciting new approaches to the prevention and control of diabetes, and a look at its prevalence in Native American communities in particular.

47 minutes VHS

Web Sites

2563 Mediconsult
A13/5/5 One Ampang Business Avenue, Jalan Ampang U
Selangor, Ma
6-3 -253
Fax: 6- 3 -253
e-mail: info@mediconsult.com.my
www.mediconsult.com.my

We are committed to provide excellent and professional services to our business partners. Through a team approach we will develop, provide and continuously improve our knowledge and competency. We work towards the betterment of healthcare delivery systems for the community.

Sharif Lough Abdullah, Director
Dieter Nassler, Director
Nguyen Thi Dung, Director

2564 National Diabetes Information Clearinghouse
3 Information Way
Bethesda, MD 20892
800-891-5390
Fax: 703-738-4929
TTY: 866-569-1162
e-mail: nkudic@info.niddk.nih.gov
www.kidney.niddk.nih.gov

The National Kidney and Urologic Diseases Information Clearinghouse is an information dissemination service of the National Institute of Diabetes and Digestive and Kidney Diseases.

Book Publishers

2565 Diabetes 101
Wiley
1 Wiley Drive
Somerset, NJ 08875
732-469-4400
800-225-5945
Fax: 732-302-2300
e-mail: bookinfo@wiley.com
www.wiley.com

Revised and expanded second edition. A layman's guide to everything you need to know to live healthfully with diabetes.

175 pages
ISBN: 1-565610-24-5

2566 Diabetes Dictionary
National Diabetes Information Clearinghouse
2 Information Way
Bethesda, MD 20892
301-654-3810
Fax: 301-907-8906
e-mail: nddic@info.niddk.nih.gov
www.niddk.nih.gov

Illustrated glossary of more than 300 diabetes-related terms.

2567 Diabetes Medical Nutition Therapy
American Diabetes Association
1701 North Beauregard Street
Alexandria, VA 22311
800-232-3472
Fax: 703-549-6995
www.diabetes.org

A professional guide to management and nutrition education resources. Provides in-depth coverage of nutrition assessment, goal setting, intervention, and outcome evaluation. Information is provided on specific resources and case studies are cited for practical examples.

2568 Diabetes Teaching Guide for People Who Use Insulin
Joslin Diabetes Center
1 Joslin Place
Boston, MA 02215
617-732-2400

Discusses the causes of diabetes, the role of diet and exercise, meal planning and complications. Also provides information on drawing blood, mixing and injecting insulin.

2569 Endocrine & Metabolic Disorders Sourcebook
Omnigraphics
PO Box 625
Holmes, PA 19043
800-234-1340
Fax: 800-875-1340
e-mail: info@omnigraphics.com
www.omnigraphics.com

Basic information for the lay person about pancreatic and insulin-related disorders such as pancreatitis, diabetes and hypoglycemia; adrenal gland disorders such as Cushing's syndrome, Addison's disease and congenital adrenal hyperplasia; pituitary gland disorders such as growth hormone deficiency, acromegaly and pituitary tumors; and thyroid disorders such as hypothyroidism, Grave's disease, Hashimoto's disease and goiter.

574 pages
ISBN: 0-780802-07-1

2570 Even Little Kids Get Diabetes
Albert Whitman & Company
6340 Oakton Street
Morton Grove, IL 60053
847-531-0033
800-255-7675
Fax: 847-531-0039
www.awhitmanco.com

A preschooler tells how when she was only two, that she was diagnosed with this common disease and describes her daily treatment and the precautions her family must observe.

ISBN: 0-807521-58-2

Joseph Boyd, President
Joe Campbell, Customer Service

2571 Everyone Likes to Eat
Wiley
1 Wiley Drive
Somerset, NJ 08875
732-469-4400
800-225-5945
Fax: 732-302-2300
e-mail: custserv@wiley.com
www.wiley.com

Revised and up-to-date second edition. How children can eat most of the foods they enjoy and still take care of their diabetes. Intended for elementary-school-age children, this guide is filled with activities, puzzles, and problem-solving exercises.

ISBN: 1-565610-26-1

2572 Grilled Cheese
American Diabetes Association
1701 North Beauregard Street
Alexandria, VA 22311
800-232-3472
Fax: 703-549-6995
www.diabetes.org

Story designed to ease children's fears and frustrations of having diabetes.

2573 If Your Child Has Diabetes: An Answer Book for Parents
Putnam Publishing Group
200 Madison Avenue
New York, NY 10016
212-951-8400

Provides information and recommendations for parents of children with diabetes on subjects such as school, recreation, medical and life insurance and employment as well as general information about diabetes.

2574 In Control: Guide for Teens with Diabetes
Wiley
1 Wiley Drive
Somerset, NJ 08875
732-469-4400
800-225-5945
Fax: 732-302-2300
e-mail: custserv@wiley.com
www.wiley.com

Dispels myths and tackles the real issues that teens with diabetes face. Teaches how to care for their diabetes without letting it get in the way of their lives.

ISBN: 1-565610-61-X

Mari Baker, Former Chief Executive Officer
Jean-Lou Chameau, President

2575 Kiss the Candy Days Good-Bye
Delacorte Press
1540 Broadway
New York, NY 10036
212-354-6500

This book focuses on Jimmy who is surprised to learn he has diabetes after seeming so healthy and fit. The story contains information on symptoms and the dangers of untreated diabetes.

2576 Let's Talk About Diabetes
Rosen Publishing Group's PowerKids Press
29 E 21st Street
New York, NY 10010
212-777-3017
800-237-9932
Fax: 888-436-4643
e-mail: rosenpub@tribeca.ios.com
www.powerkidspress.com

Defines diabetes and shows how a child can live a very normal life with the disease. Grades K-5.

24 pages
ISBN: 0-823951-96-0

2577 Life with Diabetes: A Series of Teaching Outlines
American Diabetes Association
1701 North Beauregard Street
Alexandria, VA 22311
800-342-2383
Fax: 703-549-6995
www.diabetes.org

Presents a comprehensive curriculum for diabetes education. Each outline includes a statement of purpose, pre-requisites for attending the session, materials needed for teaching the session, recommended teaching method, a content outline, instructor notes, and evaluation and documentation plan, and suggested readings related to each topic.

Larry Hausner, Chief Executive Officer
Shereen Arent, Executive Vice President

2578 Raising a Child with Diabetes: A Guide for Parents
American Diabetes Association
1701 North Beauregard Street
Alexandria, VA 22311　　　　　　　　　800-342-2383
　　　　　　　　　　　　　　　　　　Fax: 703-549-6995
　　　　　　　　　　　　　　　　　　www.diabetes.org

You'll learn how to help your child adjust to insulin, to allow for favorite foods, have a busy schedule and still feel healthy and strong, negotiate the twists and turns of being different, and much more.

Larry Hausner, Chief Executive Officer
Shereen Arent, Executive Vice President

Magazines

2579 Countdown
Juvenile Diabetes Foundation International
432 Park Avenue S
New York, NY 10016　　　　　　　　　212-889-7575
　　　　　　　　　　　　　　　　　　Fax: 212-532-7891

Offers the latest news and information in diabetes research and treatment to everyone from an international arena of diabetes investigators to parents of small children with diabetes, from physicians to school teachers, from pharmacists to corporate executives.

Sandy Dylak, Editor

2580 Diabetes Forecast
American Diabetes Association
1701 North Beauregard Street
Alexandria, VA 22311　　　　　　　　　800-342-2383
　　　　　　　　　　　　　　　　　　Fax: 703-549-6995
　　　　　　　　　　　　　　　　　　www.diabetes.org

The monthly lifestyle magazine for people with diabetes, featuring complete, in-depth coverage of all aspects of living with diabetes.

Janel Wright, JD, Chair, Anchorage,AK
David G. Marrero, PhD, President, Health Care
Suzanne Berry, MBA, CAE, Interim CEO

2581 Voice of the Diabetic
National Federation of the Blind
200 East Wells Street at Jernigan Place
Baltimore, MD 21230　　　　　　　　　410-659-9314
　　　　　　　　　　　　　　　　　　Fax: 410-685-5653
　　　　　　　　　　　　　　　　　　e-mail: nfb@nfb.org
　　　　　　　　　　　　　　　　　　nfb.org/voice-diabetic

The leading publication in the diabetes field. Each issue addresses the problems and concerns of diabetes, with a special emphasis for those who have lost vision due to diabetes. Available in print and on cassette.

Journals

2582 Diabetes
American Diabetes Association
1701 North Beauregard Street
Alexandria, VA 22311　　　　　　　　　800-342-2383
　　　　　　　　　　　　　　　　　　Fax: 703-549-6995
　　　　　　　　　　　　　　　　　　www.diabetes.org

A peer-reviewed journal focusing on laboratory research.

Janel Wright, JD, Chair, Anchorage,AK
David G. Marrero, PhD, President, Health Care
Suzanne Berry, MBA, CAE, Interim CEO

2583 Diabetes Care
American Diabetes Association
1701 North Beauregard Street
Alexandria, VA 22311　　　　　　　　　800-342-2383
　　　　　　　　　　　　　　　　　　Fax: 703-549-6995
　　　　　　　　　　　　　　　　　　www.diabetes.org

A peer-reviewed journal emphasizing reviews, documentaries and original research on topics of interest to clinicians.

Janel Wright, JD, Chair, Anchorage,AK
David G. Marrero, PhD, President, Health Care
Suzanne Berry, MBA, CAE, Interim CEO

2584 Diabetes Spectrum: From Research to Practice
American Diabetes Association
1701 North Beauregard Street
Alexandria, VA 22311　　　　　　　　　800-342-2383
　　　　　　　　　　　　　　　　　　Fax: 703-549-6995
　　　　　　　　　　　　　　　　　　www.diabetes.org

A journal translating research into practice and focusing on diabetes education and counseling.

Janel Wright, JD, Chair, Anchorage,AK
David G. Marrero, PhD, President, Health Care
Suzanne Berry, MBA, CAE, Interim CEO

Newsletters

2585 Clinical Diabetes
American Diabetes Association
1701 North Beauregard Street
Alexandria, VA 22311　　　　　　　　　800-342-2383
　　　　　　　　　　　　　　　　　　Fax: 703-549-6995
　　　　　　　　　　　　　　　　　　www.diabetes.org

A bimonthly newsletter providing practical treatment information for primary care physicians.

Janel Wright, JD, Chair, Anchorage,AK
David G. Marrero, PhD, President, Health Care
Suzanne Berry, MBA, CAE, Interim CEO

2586 Diabetes Advisor
American Diabetes Association
1701 North Beauregard Street
Alexandria, VA 22311　　　　　　　　　800-342-2383
　　　　　　　　　　　　　　　　　　Fax: 703-549-6995
　　　　　　　　　　　　　　　　　　www.diabetes.org

Offers informative articles and research in the area of diabetes for professionals and patients. Offers facts and research on diagnosis, symptoms, technology and the newest devices for persons with diabetes, as well as referral and hotline numbers.

Janel Wright, JD, Chair, Anchorage,AK
David G. Marrero, PhD, President, Health Care
Suzanne Berry, MBA, CAE, Interim CEO

2587 Diabetes Dateline
National Diabetes Information Clearinghouse
9000 Rockville Pike
Bethesda, MD 20892　　　　　　　　　301-496-3583
　　　　　　　　　　　　　　　　　　Fax: 301-907-8906
　　　　　　　　　　　　　　　　　　e-mail: nddic@info.niddk.nih.gov
　　　　　　　　　　　　　　　　　　www.niddk.nih.gov

Griffin P. Rodgers, MD, MACP, Director
Dr. Gregory Germino, Deputy Director
Kevin Abbott, Program Director

2588 Diabetes Educator
American Association of Diabetes Educators
444 N Michigan Avenue, Suite 1240
Chicago, IL 60611　　　　　　　　　　312-424-2426
　　　　　　　　　　　　　　　　　　800-338-3633
　　　　　　　　　　　　　　　　　　Fax: 312-424-2427
　　　　　　　　　　　　　　　　　　www.aadenet.org

Offers information to health professionals working with persons with diabetes.

James J Balija, Executive Director

2589 Kid's Corner
American Diabetes Association
1701 North Beauregard Street
Alexandria, VA 22311   800-342-2383
                                  Fax: 703-549-6995
                                  www.diabetes.org

A mini-magazine for kids that offers word searches, puzzles and jokes-plus an encouraging story in each issue about kids with diabetes.

Janel Wright, JD, Chair, Anchorage,AK
David G. Marrero, PhD, President, Health Care
Suzanne Berry, MBA, CAE, Interim CEO

Pamphlets

2590 Children with Diabetes
9000 Rockville Pike
Bethesda, MD 20892   301-496-3583
                                  Fax: 301-907-8906
                                  e-mail: nddic@info.niddk.nih.gov
                                  www.niddk.nih.gov

Griffin P. Rodgers, MD, MACP, Director
Dr. Gregory Germino, Deputy Director
Kevin Abbott, Program Director

2591 Complementary and Alternative Therapies for Diabetes Treatment
9000 Rockville Pike
Bethesda, MD 20892   301-496-3583
                                  Fax: 301-907-8906
                                  e-mail: nddic@info.niddk.nih.gov
                                  www.niddk.nih.gov

Griffin P. Rodgers, MD, MACP, Director
Dr. Gregory Germino, Deputy Director
Kevin Abbott, Program Director

2592 Diabetes Insipidus
9000 Rockville Pike
Bethesda, MD 20892   301-496-3583
                                  Fax: 301-907-8906
                                  e-mail: nddic@info.niddk.nih.gov
                                  www.niddk.nih.gov

Griffin P. Rodgers, MD, MACP, Director
Dr. Gregory Germino, Deputy Director
Kevin Abbott, Program Director

2593 Diabetes Overview
9000 Rockville Pike
Bethesda, MD 20892   301-496-3583
                                  Fax: 301-907-8906
                                  e-mail: nddic@info.niddk.nih.gov
                                  www.niddk.nih.gov

Griffin P. Rodgers, MD, MACP, Director
Dr. Gregory Germino, Deputy Director
Kevin Abbott, Program Director

2594 Diabetes in African Americans
9000 Rockville Pike
Bethesda, MD 20892   301-496-3583
                                  Fax: 301-907-8906
                                  e-mail: nddic@info.niddk.nih.gov
                                  www.niddk.nih.gov

Griffin P. Rodgers, MD, MACP, Director
Dr. Gregory Germino, Deputy Director
Kevin Abbott, Program Director

2595 Diabetes in Hispanic Americans
9000 Rockville Pike
Bethesda, MD 20892   301-496-3583
                                  Fax: 301-907-8906
                                  e-mail: nddic@info.niddk.nih.gov
                                  www.niddk.nih.gov

Griffin P. Rodgers, MD, MACP, Director
Dr. Gregory Germino, Deputy Director
Kevin Abbott, Program Director

2596 Diabetic Neuropathy: the Nerve Damage of Diabetes
9000 Rockville Pike
Bethesda, MD 20892   301-496-3583
                                  Fax: 301-907-8906
                                  e-mail: nddic@info.niddk.nih.gov
                                  www.niddk.nih.gov

Griffin P. Rodgers, MD, MACP, Director
Dr. Gregory Germino, Deputy Director
Kevin Abbott, Program Director

2597 Diabetics Control and Complications Trial
9000 Rockville Pike
Bethesda, MD 20892   301-496-3583
                                  Fax: 301-907-8906
                                  e-mail: nddic@info.niddk.nih.gov
                                  www.niddk.nih.gov

Griffin P. Rodgers, MD, MACP, Director
Dr. Gregory Germino, Deputy Director
Kevin Abbott, Program Director

2598 Financial Help for Diabetics Care
Information Clearinghouse
9000 Rockville Pike
Bethesda, MD 20892   301-496-3583
                                  Fax: 301-907-8906
                                  e-mail: nddic@info.niddk.nih.gov
                                  www.niddk.nih.gov

Griffin P. Rodgers, MD, MACP, Director
Dr. Gregory Germino, Deputy Director
Kevin Abbott, Program Director

2599 Gastoparesis in Diabetes
Information Clearinghouse
9000 Rockville Pike
Bethesda, MD 20892   301-496-3583
                                  Fax: 301-907-8906
                                  e-mail: nddic@info.niddk.nih.gov
                                  www.niddk.nih.gov

Griffin P. Rodgers, MD, MACP, Director
Dr. Gregory Germino, Deputy Director
Kevin Abbott, Program Director

2600 I Have Diabetes: How Much Should I Eat?
9000 Rockville Pike
Bethesda, MD 20892   301-496-3583
                                  Fax: 301-907-8906
                                  e-mail: nddic@info.niddk.nih.gov
                                  www.niddk.nih.gov

Griffin P. Rodgers, MD, MACP, Director
Dr. Gregory Germino, Deputy Director
Kevin Abbott, Program Director

2601 I Have Diabetes: What Should I Eat?
9000 Rockville Pike
Bethesda, MD 20892   301-496-3583
                                  Fax: 301-907-8906
                                  e-mail: nddic@info.niddk.nih.gov
                                  www.niddk.nih.gov

Griffin P. Rodgers, MD, MACP, Director
Dr. Gregory Germino, Deputy Director
Kevin Abbott, Program Director

2602 I Have Diabetes: When Should I Eat?
9000 Rockville Pike
Bethesda, MD 20892   301-496-3583
                                  Fax: 301-907-8906
                                  e-mail: nddic@info.niddk.nih.gov
                                  www.niddk.nih.gov

Griffin P. Rodgers, MD, MACP, Director
Dr. Gregory Germino, Deputy Director
Kevin Abbott, Program Director

2603 Kidney Disease of Diabetes
Information Clearinghouse
9000 Rockville Pike
Bethesda, MD 20892   301-496-3583
                                  Fax: 301-907-8906
                                  e-mail: ndoc@info.niddk.nih.gov
                                  www.niddk.nih.gov

Griffin P. Rodgers, MD, MACP, Director
Dr. Gregory Germino, Deputy Director
Kevin Abbott, Program Director

Camps

2604 American Diabetes Association
Center for Information, 1701 North Beauregard
Alexandria, VA 22311
                                            800-342-2383
                        e-mail: askada@diabetes.org
                                        www.diabetes.org

The American Diabetes Association provides research, and provides information and advocacy for people with diabetes and their families. The Asssociation also provides seminars for health care professionals.

Lynne Perry

2605 Camp Discovery American Diabetes Association
1168 K-157 Highway
Junction City, KS 66441
                                            316-684-6091
                                      Fax: 316-941-5699
                        e-mail: lgiles@diabetes.org
                                        www.diabetes.org

Offers young people with diabetes a week of fun at rock springs 4-H Center. Special attention to diabetes makes Camp Discovery a safe environment for active youth while providing valuable diabetes management education. Call the American Diabetes Association-Kansas area office for more information.

Lindsay Giles, District Manager

2606 Camp Hodia
1701 N 12th St
Boise, ID 83702
                                            208-891-1023
                                      Fax: 208-454-2841
                          e-mail: matt@hodia.org
                                          www.hodia.org

Camp for children with Type 1 Diabetes. Campers learn self care, good nutrition and blood-sugar control.

Don Scott, Director

2607 Camp Joslin
The Barton Center for Diabetes Education, Inc.
150 Richardson Corner Road
Charlton, MA 01507
                                            507-987-2056
                                      Fax: 508-987-2002
                        e-mail: info@bartoncenter.org
                                          www.joslin.org

Camp Joslin's programs combine camping, sports and fun with diabetes education and support to give children with diabetes, and their families, the tools they need to live happy, healthy, balanced lives.

Michael Kasparian, Camp Director
Sarah Gorman, Camp Coordinator

2608 Camp Kudzu
5885 Glenridge Drive, Suite 160
Atlanta, GA 30328
                                            404-250-1811
                                      Fax: 404-250-1812
                        e-mail: info@campkudzu.org
                                        www.campkudzu.org

Provides education, recreation and peer-networking for Georgia's children with Type 1 Diabetes.

2609 Camp Kushtaka
801 W. Fireweed Lane, Suite 103
Anchorage, AK 99503
                                            907-272-1428
                                            888-342-2383
                        e-mail: skamahele@diabetes.org
                http://www.childrenwithdiabetes.com/camps/

Camp for children with diabetes and, space permitting, their siblings.

2610 Camp de los Ninos - Diabetes Society
1165 Lincoln Avenue, Ste 300
San Jose, CA 95125
                                            408-287-3785
                                            800-800-989
                                      Fax: 408-287-2701
                        e-mail: campt@diabetessociety.org
                        www.childrenwithdiabetes.com/camps

Since 1974, the Diabetes Society of Santa Clara Valley has sponsored Camp de los Ninos, a resident camp for children 6 through 14. This camp provides an opportunity for children with diabetes to go to camp, meet other children and gain a better understanding of their diabetes. The total experience can help campers develop more confidence in their abilities to control their diabetes effectively while enjoying the traditional camp experience.

Sharon Ogbor, Executive Director

2611 Clara Barton Camp
PO Box 356
North Oxford, MA
                                            508-987-2056
                                      Fax: 508-987-2002
                          e-mail: bcdecamp@aol.com
                                      www.bartoncenter.org

Girls, ages 6-17, with diabetes participate in a well-rounded camp program with special education in diabetes, health and safety. Activities include swimming, boating, sports, dance, music and arts and crafts. Two week adventure camp for high school girls offering camping, hiking, canoeing, etc. Also a minicamp (one week) for girls 6-12. Day camps are offered in Worcester, Boston and New York City.

Brooke Beverly, Resident Camp Director
Kerry Packard, Day Camp Director
Beth Sayers, Adventure Camp Director

2612 Des Moines YMCA Camp
1192 166th Drive
Boone, IA 50036
                                            515-432-7558
                                      Fax: 515-432-7558
                          e-mail: ycamp@dmymca.org
                                          www.y-camp.org

For boys and girls with cancer, diabetes, asthma, cystic fibrosis, hearing impaired and other disabilities.

Dan Breitbach, Executive Director

2613 EDI
1020 Madison 9570
Fredericktown, MO 63645   e-mail: chartmann@diabetes.org
                                                www.diabetes.org

Youngsters with diabetes learn how to care for themselves while participating in a wide variety of outdoor activities and trips. The camp, managed and financed by the American Diabetes Association Greater St. Louis Affiliate, offers camperships to children from the Greater St. Louis area, ages 7-16, but nonresidents may also apply.

Fred Schaljo

2614 Easter Seal Kysoc
9810 Bluegrass Pkwy
Louisville, KY 40299
                                            502-584-9781
                                      Fax: 502-732-0783
                        e-mail: ek1@cardinalhill.org
                                        www.cardinalhill.org

Designed for the fullest camping experience for children or adults with physical disabilities, blind, deaf, behavior disorders, mental retardation, diabetes and multiple handicaps, ages 7 and up.

Heide Miller, CCD, CTRS, Director

2615 Florida Camp for Children and Youth
1701 SW 16th Ave
Gainesville, FL 32608
                                            352-334-1321
                                      Fax: 352-334-1326
                        e-mail: fccyd@floridadiabetescamp.org

An adventure camp for children and youth with diabetes.

Rhonda Rogers

2616 Floyd Rogers
PO Box 31536
Omaha, NE 68131
402-341-0866
www.campfloydrogers.com

A camp for diabetic children, ages 8 to 18

Sherman Poska

2617 Hickory Hill
PO Box 1942
Columbia, MO 65205
573-698-2510
e-mail: camphickoryhill@gmail.com
www.camphicoryhill.com

Educates diabetic children concerning diabetes and its care. In addition to daily educational sessions on some aspects of diabetes, campers participate in swimming, sailing, arts and crafts and overnight camping.

William Mees

2618 John Warvel
American Diabetes Association
Camp Crosley YMCA, 165 EMS T2 Land
North Webster, IN 46555
317-352-9226
Fax: 317-913-1592
e-mail: bookorders@diabetes.org

Provides an enjoyable, safe and educational out-of-doors experience for children with insulin-dependent diabetes. A unique learning atmosphere for children to acquire new skills in caring for their disease. The camp experience instills confidence for the child's self-management of diabetes. Offers one-week sessions and can accommodate 200 campers.

Carol Helming, Executive Director

2619 Makemie Woods Camp Conference Center
PO Box 39
Barhamsville, VA 23011
757-566-1496
800-566-1496
Fax: 757-566-8003
www.makwoods.org

Counselors serve as teachers, friends and activity leaders. The individual is important within the small group. No camper is lost in the crowd, but is an integral partner in the group process. Residential Christian Camp and conference center. Summer camp for children 8-18 special camp for children with diabetes.

Michelle Burcher, Director

2620 Sweeney
PO Box 918
Gainesville, TX 76241
940-665-2011
Fax: 940-665-9467
e-mail: info@campsweeney.org
www.campsweeney.org

Teaches self-care and self-reliance to children with diabetes. Campers participate in such activities as swimming, fishing, horseback riding, arts and crafts while learning about diabetes and how to cope with it.

T. Milton Dickson, Jr. DDS, Chairman
Robert D. Vandermeer, MD, Vice Chairman
Ernie M. Fernandez, MD, Secretary

Description

2621 DIGEORGE SYNDROME

Synonyms: DiGeorge sequence, Thymic agenesis
immunodeficiency

Involves the following Biologic System(s):
Genetic/Chromosomal/Syndrome/Metabolic Disorders,
Immunologic and Rheumatologic Disorders

DiGeorge syndrome is a disorder present at birth (congenital)
that is characterized by some combination of absence
(aplasia) or underdevelopment (hypoplasia) of the thymus
gland and the parathyroid glands, malformations of the heart
and its major blood vessels (cardiovascular abnormalities),
and characteristic malformations of the head and facial
(craniofacial) area. Due to absence or underdevelopment of
the thymus gland, affected children may have abnormalities
of the immune system, causing impaired resistance to certain
infections. DiGeorge syndrome occurs as the result of abnormal development of certain embryonic structures (third and
fourth pharyngeal pouches) that later develop into the thymus
and parathyroid glands. In some cases, other embryonic structures that are forming during the same approximate period
may also be affected, resulting in certain cardiovascular,
craniofacial, or other malformations. The thymus, a lymphoid
tissue organ located in the upper portion of the chest, plays
an essential role in the immune system beginning at approximately the 12th week of fetal development and lasts until puberty. It serves as a source of certain white blood cells
(lymphocytes) before birth and then promotes the development of certain specialized lymphocytes, known as T lymphocytes, through secretion of particular hormones (e.g.,
thymosin). The actions of the T lymphocytes help to defend
the body against certain microorganisms (i.e., cell-mediated
immunity). The parathyroid glands, which are two pairs of
small glands on the sides of the thyroid gland, produce
parathyroid hormone, which helps to maintain normal levels
of calcium in the blood.

DiGeorge syndrome usually occurs randomly and is caused
by spontaneous, minute deletions of material from the long
arm of chromosome 22 (22q11.2). DiGeorge syndrome may
also occur in association with certain chromosomal abnormalities (e.g., chromosome 10, monosomy 10p; chromosome 22,
monosomy 22q). In addition, there have been some cases in
which DiGeorge syndrome affected individuals within certain
families (kindreds) yet did not appear to result from known
chromosome syndromes. In some familial cases, DiGeorge
syndrome may have autosomal dominant inheritance. The disorder is thought to affect approximately one in 20,000 newborns.

In infants and children with DiGeorge syndrome, associated
symptoms and findings may be extremely variable. Patients
who have absence or severe underdevelopment of the thymus
gland are prone to frequent infections from fungi, viruses,
and certain bacteria (such as Pneumocystis jiroveci, previously knowns as Pneumocystis carinii). These patients often
experience chronic inflammation of the mucous membranes
of the nose (rhinitis), recurrent inflammation of the lungs
(pneumonia), fungal infection of the mucous membranes of
the mouth (oral candidiasis), recurrent diarrhea, or systemic
infections in which invading microorganisms or their toxins

are present inthe blood circulation (septicemia). In some
cases of serious infection, life-threatening complications may
result. Infants and children with mild underdevelopment
(hypoplasia) of the thymus are said to have partial DiGeorge
syndrome and may have little difficulty with recurring infections. Because of absence or underdevelopment of the
parathyroid glands (hypoparathyroidism), many affected infants experience certain symptoms and findings during the
first days of life, including abnormally low calcium levels in
the blood (hypocalcemia) and muscle twitching, tremors and
cramps, (neonatal tetany) and even seizures. Such symptoms
and findings can be treated with calcium supplementation and
are usually temporary but may recur later in life.

Some newborns with DiGeorge syndrome may also have defects of the heart and its great arteries. Some of these may be
simple defects while others may be more complex, such as in-
terrupted aortic arch, ventricular septal defects, and tetralogy
of Fallot.

Infants with DiGeorge syndrome may have an unusually narrow or blind-ending esophagus (esophageal atresia) that does
not form a passageway into the stomach. In addition, affected
newborns may have characteristic malformations of the head
and facial (craniofacial) area, such as widely spaced eyes (ocular hypertelorism); downwardly slanting eyelid folds
(palpebral fissures); a small mouth; an unusually short, vertical groove in the center of the upper lip (philtrum); and
low-set, notched ears. Some patients may also have mild to
moderate mental retardation.

The treatment of infants and children with DiGeorge syndrome is symptomatic and supportive. Treatment measures
may include the administration of calcium in those with
hypoparathyroidism and hypocalcemia, therapies to help prevent and aggressively treat infections (e.g., antiviral,
antifungal, and antibiotic agents) in patients with
immunodeficiency, medical and surgical measures for
cardiovascular malformations, or other measures as required.
If patients with immunodeficiency require blood transfusions,
donor blood must be exposed to high levels of radiation
(irradiated) to kill the donor lymphocytes and thus prevent
the occurrence of graft-versus-host disease, a serious disease
caused by an immune response of donor cells against the
recipient's tissues.

National Associations & Support Groups

2622 22Q and You Center
34th Street and Civic Center Boulevard
Philadelphia, PA 19104

215-590-1000
Fax: 215-590-3298
e-mail: lunny@email.chop.edu
www.chop.edu/service/22q-and-you-center/home.html

Services offered by the Department of Clinical Genetics in the
Children's Hospital of Philadelphia, include literature, support
groups and referrals.

Beverly Emmanuel, Chief, Human Genetics
Elaine Zackai, MD, Director, Clinical Genetics
Donna McDonald-McGinn, Program Director

2623 American Academy of Pediatrics
141 Northwest Point Boulevard
Elk Grove Village, IL 60007

847-434-4000
800-433-9016
Fax: 847-434-8000
www.aap.org

The American Academy of Pediatrics and its member pediatricians are committed to the attainment of optimal physical, mental and social health and well-being for all infants, children, adolescents, and young adults.

Sandra Hassink, MD, FAAP, President

2624 Genetic Alliance
4301 Connecticut Avenue NW, Suite 404
Washington, DC 20008   202-966-5557
                                        800-336-4363
                                   Fax: 202-966-8553
               e-mail: info@geneticalliance.org
                       www.geneticalliance.org

A coalition of voluntary genetic support groups, consumers and professionals addressing the needs of individuals and families affected by genetic disorders from a national perspective.

Sharon Terry, President
Kristen Baxter, Assistant Director Translational Re
Natasha Bonhomme, VP Strategic Development

2625 Immune Deficiency Foundation
40 W Chesapeake Avenue, Suite 308
Towson, MD 21204   410-321-6647
                                        800-296-4433
                                   Fax: 410-321-9165
               e-mail: IDF@primaryimmune.org
                       www.primaryimmune.org

The only national charitable organization aimed at fighting the primary immune deficiency diseases. The founders included parents of children with primary immune deficiency, immunologists who treat immune deficient patients and other individuals with an interest in helping others. The Foundation's main goal is to improve the care and treatment of adults and children with primary immune deficiency diseases and to promote public education and awareness about the diseases.

Marcia Boyle, CEO
Barbara Ballard, Secretary
John Boyle, Chair

2626 March of Dimes Birth Defects Foundation
1275 Mamaroneck Avenue
White Plains, NY 10605   914-997-4488
                                        888-663-4637
                                   Fax: 914-997-4763
                                   TDD: 914-997-4764
               e-mail: answers@marchofs.com
                       www.marchofdimes.com

A national not-for-profit organization that was established in 1938. The mission of the Foundation is to improve the health of babies by preventing birth defects and infant mortality.

Jennifer L Howse, President

Conferences

2627 Genetic Alliance Annual Conference
Genetic Alliance
4301 Connecticut Avenue NW, Suite 404
Washington, DC 20008   202-966-5557
                                        800-336-4363
                                   Fax: 202-966-8553
               e-mail: info@geneticalliance.org
                       www.geneticalliance.org

Consistently inspirational and enables partnership among all stakeholders: advocates and community leaders, health and industry professionals, policymakers, and academicians.

July

Sharon Terry, President/CEO
Tetyana Murza, Programs/Events Manager

2628 Immune Deficiency Foundation National Conference
Meetings Manager
40 W Chesapeake Avenue, Suite 308
Towson, MD 21204   410-321-6647
                                        800-296-4433
                                   Fax: 410-321-9165
               e-mail: info@primaryimmune.org
                       www.primaryimmune.org

Annual conference hosted by an organization aimed at fighting the primary immune deficiency diseases. The founders included parents of children with primary immune deficiency, immunologists who treat immune deficient patients and other individuals with an interest in helping others. The Foundation's main goal is to improve the care and treatment of adults and children with primary immune deficiency diseases and to promote public education and awareness about the diseases.

June

John Seymour, Chairman
Robert LeBien, Vice Chairman
Steve Fietek, Founder/Secretary

Web Sites

2629 International Patient Organization for Primary Immunodeficiencies
Av. Aida, Bloco 8, escritòrio 821
Estoril, 2765-   35- 21-407
                                   e-mail: info@ipopi.org
                                        ipopi.org

IPOPI is an international organization whose members are national patient organizations for the primary immunodeficiencies (PID's). It was formed to benefit and serve its members and patients with expertise and resources and influence of members in order to achieve worlwide improvement in the care and treatment of patients with PID's.

Jose Drabwell, Chairman
Martine Pergent, Vice Chairman
Johan Prevot, Executive Director

2630 Jeffrey Modell Foundation
www.jmfworld.com

The foundation is dedicated to the early and precise diagnosis, meaningful treatment, and ultimate cure of Primary Immunodeficiencies.

2631 Kansas University Medical Center
www.kumc.edu/gec/support/velo.html

                                   e-mail: dcollins@kumc.edu
                              www.kumc.edu/gec/support/velo.html

Offers information for genetic professionals, information on genetic conditions and support groups, and genetic educational information.

Debra Collins, MS, CGC, Genetic Counselor

2632 Online Mendelian Inheritance in Man
U.S. National Library of Medicine, 8600 Rockville
Bethesda, MD 20894   888-346-3656
                                   e-mail: info@ncbi.nlm.nih.gov
                                        www.ncbi.nlm.nih.gov

This database is a catalog of human genes and genetic disorders.

Christine E. Seidman, M.D., Chair
David J. Lipman, M.D., Executive Secretary
Michael Boehnke, Ph.D., Board Member

Book Publishers

2633 Let's Talk About Going to the Hospital
Rosen Publishing Group's PowerKids Press
29 E 21st Street
New York, NY 10010   212-777-3017
                                        800-237-9932
                                   Fax: 888-436-4643
               e-mail: rosenpub@tribeca.ios.com
                       www.powerkidspress.com

If a child has to check into the hospital, chances are he or she is already upset about being ill. Knowing how a hospital functions and what the procedures are, such as when family members can visit, will help in what is already a stressful situation. Grades K-5.

24 pages
ISBN: 0-823950-36-0

Description

2634 DOWN SYNDROME

Synonyms: Chromosome 21, trisomy 21, Trisomy 21 syndrome

Covers these related disorders: Trisomy 21 mosaicism, Trisomy 21 translocation

Involves the following Biologic System(s):
Genetic/Chromosomal/Syndrome/Metabolic Disorders

Down syndrome, also known as trisomy 21, is a chromosomal disorder that affects approximately one in 660 newborns, making it the most common genetic syndrome. Cells of the body (with the exception of reproductive cells) typically contain 23 pairs of chromosomes that are numbered from 1 to 22. The 23rd pair consists of one X chromosome from the mother and an X or Y chromosome from the father. However, in infants with Down syndrome, all or a portion of chromosome 21 is present three times rather than twice in cells of the body (trisomy). In rare cases, a certain percentage of cells contain the extra chromosome 21, whereas other cells have the normal two. This finding is known as chromosomal mosaicism.

The symptoms and physical findings associated with Down syndrome vary in range and severity and depend in part on the exact location and the percentage of body cells containing the extra chromosome 21.

Down syndrome is usually the result of errors during the division of a parent's reproductive cells. Increased maternal age (over 35) presents additional risk. The disorder may also result due to a chromosome 21 translocation that is transmitted by a parent or occurs sporadically. Translocations are chromosomal abnormalities in which pieces of two or more chromosomes break off and are rearranged, resulting in an altered set of chromosomes.

Many infants with Down syndrome have abnormally diminished muscle tone (hypotonia), a tendency to keep the mouth open, protrusion of the tongue, excessive mobility of the joints, absence of certain reflexes, and excessive skin on the back of the neck. Other abnormalities may include a small, short head, flattened facial features, upwardly slanting eyelid folds, vertical skin folds over the eyes' inner corners, a highly arched roof of the mouth, a small nose and depressed nasal bridge, and small, misshapen ears. Abnormalities of the limbs may also be present, including unusually short arms and legs; short, broad hands; improper positioning of the fifth fingers (clinodactyly); abnormal skin ridge patterns on the fingers, hands, toes, and feet (dermatoglyphics); and a wide gap between the first and second toes. Infants with Down syndrome have an increased frequency of intestinal narrowing or obstruction (atresia) at birth. Patients also tend to have relatively short stature, progressive delays in the acquisition of skills requiring the coordination of physical and mental activities (psychomotor delays), poor coordination, an awkward manner of walking (gait), and varying levels of mental retardation.

Approximately 40 percent of infants with Down syndrome have heart defects at birth (congenital heart defects). In some patients, such heart defects may require surgical repair. In addition, some individuals with Down syndrome are prone to recurrent respiratory infections and chronic inflammation of the membranes that line the eyes and eyelids (conjunctivitis) or the nasal cavity (rhinitis). Treatment of individuals with Down syndrome includes symptomatic and supportive measures, such as possible surgical correction of congenital heart defects, and special education.

Government Agencies

2635 NIH/National Institute of Child Health and Human Development
31 Center Drive, Building 31
Bethesda, MD 20892
301-496-1333
Fax: 301-496-1104
www.nichd.nih.gov

Established in 1962 by congress, today the institute conducts and supports research on topics related to the health of children, adults, families and populations. Some of these topics include: developmental disabilities, growth and development, infant death, reproductive health and birth defects.

Jay H Hoofnagle, Director
Lisa Kaeser, Program & Public Liaison

National Associations & Support Groups

2636 ARC of the United States
1825 K Street, NW, Suite 1200
Washington, DC 20006
202-534-3700
800-433-5255
Fax: 202-534-3731
e-mail: info@thearc.org
www.thearc.org

The ARC of the United States advocates for the rights and full participation of all children and adults with intellectual and developmental disabilities. Together with our network of members and affiliated chapters, we improve systems of supports and services; connect families; inspire communities an influence public policy.

Mohan Mehra, President
Nancy Webster, Vice President
Michael Mack, Secretary

2637 Aleh Foundation
Aleh Institutions USA
PO Box 4911
New York, NY 10185
866-717-0252
Fax: 212-517-3293
e-mail: dov@aleh-israel.org
www.aleh.org

The Aleh Rehabilitation Center in Bnei Break has served as a residential facility to close to 200 children with multiple, physical and mental disabilities. These children and their families have benefitted from our wide range of services in an atmosphere of warmth and love.

Yehuda Marmorstein, Executive Director
Shlomit Grayevsky, Director, Aleh Jerusalem Center

2638 American Academy of Pediatrics
141 Northwest Point Boulevard
Elk Grove Village, IL 60007
847-434-4000
800-433-9016
Fax: 847-434-8000
www.aap.org

The American Academy of Pediatrics and its member pediatricians are committed to the attainment of optimal physical, mental and social health and well-being for all infants, children, adolescents, and young adults.

Sandra Hassink, MD, FAAP, President

2639 American Association for Pediatric Opthalmology and Strabismus
655 Beach Street
San Francisco, CA 94109
415-561-8505
Fax: 415-561-8531
e-mail: aapos@aao.org
www.aapos.org

AAPOS is the American Association for Pediatric Ophthalmology and Strabismus. The organization's goals are to advance the quality of children's eye care, support the training of pediatric ophthalmologists, support research activities in pediatric ophthalmology, and advance the care of adults with strabismus.

Jennifer Hull, Client Services Manager
Brooke Lyon, Client Services Coordinator
Maria A. Schweers, CO, Scientific Program Coordinator

2640 American School Counselor Association
1101 King Street, Suite 310
Alexandria, VA 22314 703-683-2722
800-306-4722
Fax: 703-997-7572
e-mail: asca@schoolcounselor.org
www.schoolcounselor.org

The mission of ASCA is to represent professional school counselors and to promote professionalism and ethical practices.

Richard Wong, Executive Director
Jeff Broderson, Information Technology Admin.
Kathleen M Rakestraw, Director of Communications

2641 Arc of Montgomery County
11600 Nebel Street
Rockville, MD 20852 301-984-5777
Fax: 301-816-2429
e-mail: info@arcmontmd.org
www.arcmontmd.org

Aims to provide support, advocacy and choices for people who have mental retardation and related developmental disabilities and their families.

Joyce Taylor, Executive Director
Clyde Agnew, Jr., Director, Human Resources

2642 Association for Children with Down Syndrome
4 Fern Place
Plainview, NY 11803 516-933-4700
Fax: 516-933-9524
e-mail: information@acds.org
www.acds.org

Dedicated to providing lifetime resources of exceptional quality, innovation and inclusion for individuals with Down syndrome and other developmental disabilities and their families.

Michael Smith, Executive Director
Jane Shimkin, Educational Coordinator
Judith Anderson, Director of Student Services

2643 Birth Defects Research for Children
976 Lake Baldwin Lane, Suite 104
Orlando, FL 38214 407-895-0802
e-mail: staff@birthdefects.org
www.birthdefects.org

An organization that provides parents and expectant parents with information about birth defects and support services for their children. BDRC has a parent-matching program that links families who have children with similar birth defects.

Betty Mekdeci, Executive Director

2644 Center for Disabilities and Development
University of Iowa Hospitals and Clinics
200 Hawkins Drive
Iowa City, IA 52242 319-353-6900
888-573-5437
Fax: 319-356-8284
e-mail: cdd-webmaster@uiowa.edu
www.uichildrens.org

A trusted resource for healthcare, training, research and information for people with disabilities that include: behavior disorders, brain injury, cerebral palsy, diabetes, down syndrome, learning disabilities, mental retardation, sleep disorders and spina bifida.

Judy Stephenson, Administrator
Amy Mikelson, Supervisor Info Resource Service

2645 Down Syndrome Affiliates in Action
5010 Fountainblue Drive
Bismarck, ND 58503 701-425-7129
e-mail: info@dsaia.org
www.dsaia.org

To support and advance the growth and service capabilities of the local and regional Down syndrome organizations we serve, to be the conduit of value-driven training, programs, best practices and support for our members.

Sterling Lynk, President
Amy Van Bergen, Vice President
Deanna Tharpe, Executive Director

2646 Down Syndrome Community
www.downsyndromecommunity.org
206-257-7191
e-mail: contact@downsyndromecommunity.org
www.downsyndromecommunity.org

The Down Syndrome Community is a registered 501(c)(3) organization whose mission is to improve the lives of individuals with Down syndrome and their families by focusing on education, communication, and advocacy.

Linda Michael, Co-Chair
Lynne Palmisano, Co-Chair
Sean King, President

2647 Down Syndrome Guild of Greater Kansas City
10200 W 75th Street, Suite 281
Shawnee Mission, KS 66204 913-384-4848
Fax: 913-384-4949
e-mail: info@kcdsq.org
www.kcdsg.org

Provides new baby/parent hospital visits, monthly newsletter, support and encouragement for individuals with Down Syndrome and their families. Bi-lingual group. Job coaching scholarships.

Amy Allison, Executive Director

2648 Down Syndrome Information Alliance
5098 Foothills Boulevard, Suite 3, #464
Roseville, CA 95747 916-658-1686
Fax: 916-914-1875
e-mail: info@downsyndromeinfo.org
downsyndromeinfo.org

The Down Syndrome Information Alliance provides support and resources to empower individuals with Down syndrome, their families, and our community.

Heather Green, President
Jaoanna Heichlinger, Secretary
Trevor Stapleton, Treasurer

2649 Genetic Alliance
4301 Connecticut Avenue NW, Suite 404
Washington, DC 20008 202-966-5557
800-336-4363
Fax: 202-966-8553
e-mail: info@geneticalliance.org
www.geneticalliance.org

A coalition of voluntary genetic support groups, consumers and professionals addressing the needs of individuals and families affected by genetic disorders from a national perspective.

Sharon Terry, President & CEO
Tara Biagi, Maternal, Child Health Coordinator

2650 Global Down Syndrome Foundation
3300 East First Ave., Suite 390
Denver, CO 80206 303-321-6277
e-mail: info@globaldownsyndrome.org
www.globaldownsyndrome.org

The Global Down Syndrome Foundation is dedicated to significantly improving the lives of people with Down syndrome through Research, Medical Care, Education and Advocacy.

Michelle Sie Whitten, President
David Charmatz, Senior Vice President
Martha Cronen, Project Manager

2651 International Mosaic Down Syndrome Association
PO Box 354
Trenton, OH 45067 513-988-6817
888-MDS-LINK
Fax: 775-295-9373
e-mail: JACKSONC@HSC.VCU.EDU
www.imdsa.org

IMDSA is designed to support any family or individual whose life has been touched by mosaic Down syndrome by continuously pursuing research opportunities and increasing awareness in the medical, educational and public communities throughout the world

Brandy Hellard, President
Dr. Colleen Jackson-Cook, Member, Advisory Board
Lauren Vanner-Nicely,MS, Member, Advisory Board

2652 March of Dimes Birth Defects Foundation
1275 Mamaroneck Avenue
White Plains, NY 10605   914-997-4488
                                        888-663-4637
                                   Fax: 914-997-4763
                     e-mail: answers@marchofdimes.com
                                 www.marchofdimes.com

Partnership of volunteers and professionals dedicated to improving the health of babies by preventing birth defects and infant mortality. Over 100 chapters are located across the country and can be located through the National Office.

Jennifer L Howse, President

2653 National Association for Child Development
549 25th Street
Ogden, UT 84401   801-621-8606
                                   Fax: 801-621-8389
                              e-mail: prachi@nacd.org
                         downsyndrome.nacd.org/index.php

NACD has created an approach to human development, the achievement of human potential, and the remediation of developmental, educational, and neurological problems that is based upon the gestalt of the individual.

Robert J. Doman Jr., Founder and Director
Laird Doman, COO/ Family Liaison
Julian Neil, Dir. Of Health

2654 National Association for Down Syndrome (NADS)
PO Box 206
Wilmette, IL 60091   630-325-9112
                                  e-mail: info@nads.org
                                         www.nads.org

Established by parents of children with Down syndrome who felt a need to create a better environment and bring about understanding and acceptance of people with Down syndrome.

Jackie Rotondi, President
Patrick Crawford, First Vice President
Michael Walther, Treasurer

2655 National Dissemination Center for Children with Disabilities
1825 Connecticut Avenue, Suite 700
Washington, DC 20009   202-884-8200
                                        800-695-0285
                                   Fax: 202-884-8441
                                   TTY: 800-695-0285
                              e-mail: nichcy@aed.org
                                       www.nichcy.org

A national information and referral center that provides information on disabilities and disability-related issues for families, educators and other professionals.

Suzanne Ripley, Executive Director

2656 National Down Syndrome Adoption Network
4623 Wesley Avenue, Suite A
Cincinnati, OH 45212   513-213-9615
                                         www.ndsan.org

The mission of the NDSAN is to ensure that every child with Down syndrome has the opportunity to grow up in a loving family.

2657 National Down Syndrome Coalition
P.O. Box 725
Roseville, CA 95661   916-532-4773
                                   Fax: 916-663-1151
                     e-mail: heather@ndscoalition.org
                                     ndscoalition.org

The mission is to demonstrate to society the positive impacts of Down syndrome with various forms of media, parent support groups, parent counseling, provision of resources, community outreach, and with the education and training of parents and professionals.

Heather M. Haskin, President / CEO

2658 National Down Syndrome Congress
1370 Center Drive, Suite 102
Atlanta, GA 30338   770-604-9500
                                        800-232-6372
                                   Fax: 770-604-9898
                           e-mail: info@ndsccenter.org
                                    www.ndsccenter.org

It is the mission of the National Down Syndrome Congress to be the national advocacy organization for Down syndrome and to provide leadership in all areas of concern related to persons with Down syndrome. In that capacity, NDSC will function as a major source of support and empowerment to persons with down syndrome and their families.

David Tolleson, Executive Director
Sue Joe, Resource Specialist
Betty Totten, Office Manager

2659 National Down Syndrome Society
666 Broadway, 8th Floor
New York, NY 10012   800-221-4602
                                   Fax: 212-979-2873
                              e-mail: info@ndss.org
                                         www.ndss.org

The mission is to be the national advocate for the value, acceptance and inclusion of people with Down Syndrome. The NDSS envisions a world in which people with Down Syndrome have the opportunity to enhance their quality of life, realize their life aspirations, and become valued members of welcoming communities.

Jon Colman, President

2660 National Down Syndrome Society Hotline
666 Broadway, 8th Floor
New York, NY 10012   212-460-9330
                                        800-221-4602
                                   Fax: 212-979-2873
                              e-mail: info@ndss.org
                                         www.ndss.org

800-221-4602. Through its toll-free helpline and e-mail service, NDSS receives more than 32,000 requests a year for information on Down Syndrome. The professionally staffed Goodwin Family Information and Referral Center responds to questions from parents, professionals, self-advocates, and other interested individuals. Hours: 9 a.m to 5 p.m. EST, Monday thru Friday, in over 150 languages.

Jon Colman, President

2661 National Early Childhood Technical Assistance System
University of North Carolina, Chapel Hill
Campus Box 8040, UNC-CH
Chapel Hill, NC 27599   919-962-2001
                                   Fax: 919-966-7463
                                   TDD: 919-843-3269
                              e-mail: nectac@unc.edu
                                       www.nectac.org

Supports the national implementation of the early childhood provisions of the Individuals with Disabilities Education Act (IDEA). The mission is to strengthen systems at all levels to ensure that children (birth through five) with disabilities and their families receive and benefit from high quality, culturally appropriate and family centered supports and services.

Lynne Kahn, Director & Principal Investigator
Joan Danaher, Associate Director
Joicey Hurth, Associate Director Technical Assist

State Agencies & Support Groups

California

2662 Down Syndrome Association of Los Angeles
16461 Sherman Way, Suite 180
Van Nuys, CA 91406
818-786-0001
Fax: 818-786-0004
e-mail: info@dsala.org
www.dsala.org

Offers information on Down syndrome, counseling, resources, facts, laws and other forms of information.

Gail Williamson, Executive Director
Jim Hodgson, Senior Director

Colorado

2663 Mile High Down Syndrome Association
3515 South Tamarac Drive, Suite 320
Denver, CO 80237
303-756-6144
Fax: 303-756-6144
e-mail: info@mhdsa.org
www.mhdsa.org

Serves families of children and adults with Down syndrome, and interested professionals in the Mountain States region. Provides education, resources and support in partnership with individuals, families, professionals, and the community.

Mac Macsovits, Executive Director
Laurie Herrera, Family/Outreach Programs Director

Connecticut

2664 Connecticut Down Syndrome Congress
C/O: A.J. Pappanikou, University of Connecticut
200 Research Parkway
Meriden, CT 06450
860-563-9114
888-486-8537
e-mail: manager@ctdownsyndrome.org
www.ctdownsyndrome.org/

Established as a special interest group to advocate for persons with Down syndrome in the State of Connecticut. The mission is to advocate for the realization and enhancement of the full spectrum of human and civil rights for persons with Down syndrome, gather and disseminate accurate information regarding Down syndrome, provide support to families of children with Down syndrome, and to encourage quality services for persons with Down syndrome.

Walter Glomb, President
Karen Zbierski, Executive VP
Chris McAuliffe, Secretary/Director

Florida

2665 Gold Coast Down Syndrome Organization
2255 Glades Road, 342W
Boca Raton, FL 33431
561-912-1231
Fax: 561-912-1232
e-mail: gcdso@bellsouth.net
www.goldcoastdownsyndrome.org

Gold Coast Down Syndrome Organization is a private, nonprofit corporation dedicated to making the future brighter for people with Down syndrome in Palm Beach County, Florida.

Terri Harmon, Executive Director

2666 Goodwill Industries-Suncoast
10596 Gandy Boulevard
St. Petersburg, FL 33702
727-523-1512
888-279-1988
Fax: 727-563-9300
TDD: 727-579-1068
e-mail: gw.marketing@goodwill-suncoast.com
www.goodwill-suncoast.org

Nonprofit organization that helps people achieve their full potential through the dignity and power of work. The agency offers a variety of employment and training services to promote self-sufficiency, and contribute to community conservation through recycling.

Lee Waits, President
R Lee Waits, President/CEO

Georgia

2667 Down Syndrome Association of Atlanta
2221 Peachtree Road NE, Ste 226
Atlanta, GA 30339
404-320-3233
Fax: 404-228-7475
e-mail: contactus@atlantadsaa.org
www.atlantadsaa.org

A source of information and support to families, as well as working to promote public awareness and encouraging a better understanding of Down syndrome and individuals with Down syndrome.

Michelle Norweck, Executive Director

Hawaii

2668 Hawaii Down Syndrome Congress
419 Keoniana Street, Suite 804
Honolulu, HI 96815
808-949-1999
e-mail: Conkay@AOL.com
www.hawaiidownsyndrome.com

An organization of families and professionals concerned with all aspects of Down Syndrome. We provide outreach to parents of newborns to foster fellowship and social interaction, educational opportunities and resources, public relation activities to inform the general public about Down syndrome, monthly meetings that provide emotional and psychological support, and serve as activists and advocates on behalf of children with special needs.

Connie Smith, President

Indiana

2669 Down Syndrome Association of NWI
2927 Jewett Avenue
Highland, IN 46322
219-838-3656
Fax: 219-838-6959
e-mail: dsa@dsaofnwi.org
www.dsaofnwi.org

Provides informational and emotional support to parents who have a child, adolescent, or adult family member with special needs. Program offers an important connection for a parent who is seeking support for a special disability issue, by matching him or her with a trained veteran parent.

Christine Gill, President
Randy Sassano, Vice President
Dawn Weiler, Treasurer

2670 Down Syndrome Support Association of Southern Indiana (DSSASI)
1939 State Street
New Albany, IN 47150
812-725-1416
e-mail: support@dssasi.org
www.dssasi.org

Provides informational and emotional support to parents who have a child, adolescent, or adult family member with special needs. Program offers an important connection for a parent who is seeking support for a special disability issue, by matching him or her with a trained veteran parent.

Kelley Jacquay, President
Michelle Engle, Vice President
Gina DeWilde, Treasurer

2671 Parents of Children with Down Syndrome Arc of Montgomery County
PO Box 10416
Rockville, MD 20849   301-916-4985
Fax: 301-816-2429
e-mail: firemom31@yahoo.com
www.downsyndromehelp.boomja.com

Aims to provide support, advocacy and choices for people who have mental retardation and related developmental disabilities and their families.

Peter Holden, Executive Director
John Slavcoff, President

2672 Massachusetts Down Syndrome Congress (MDSC)
20 Burlington Mall Road, Ste 261
Burlington, MA 01803   781-221-0024
800-664-6372
Fax: 781-221-0011
e-mail: mdsc@mdsc.org
www.mdsc.org

An all-volunteer, non-profit organization made up of parents, professionals and anyone interested in gaining a better understanding of Down syndrome. The mission is to enhance on a continuous basis the lives of individuals with Down syndrome through the education and support of people with Down syndrome, their families, their friends, their teachers, and the community as a whole. To ensure individuals are valued, included, and live fulfilling lives in the community.

Suzanne Boudrot Shea, President
Jonathan Fee, Vice President
Leo Hogan, Secretary

2673 Down Syndrome Association of Minnesota
656 Transfer Road
St. Paul, MN 55114   651-603-0720
800-511-3696
e-mail: dsamn@dsamn.com
www.dsamn.org

A nonprofit organization composed of some 3,000 members; more than 900 people with Down syndrome, their families and friends, plus health-care, education and developmental professionals. We are the only organization in our region devoted exclusively to the needs of people with Down syndrome and their families.

Kathleen Forney, Executive Director
Connie Gunderson Warner, Program Coordinator
Jim Belka, Resource Coordinator

2674 Center for Family Support
2811 Zulette Avenue
Bronx, NY 10461   718-518-1500
Fax: 718-518-8200
www.cfsny.org

The Center for Family Support (CFS) is a not-for-profit human service agency providing support and assistance to individuals with developmental disabilities and traumatic brain injuries throughout New York City, Long Island, the lower Hudson Valley region and New Jersey.

Steven Vernikoff, Executive Director

2675 Miami Valley Downs Syndrome Association
1133 Edwin C Moses Boulevard, Suite 190
Dayton, OH 45408   937-222-0744
Fax: 937-222-0396
www.mvdsa.org

Informational and emotional support to parents who have a child, adolescent, or adult family member with special needs.

2676 Down Syndrome Association of Middle Tennessee
111 N Wilson Boulevard
Nashville, TN 37205   615-386-9002
Fax: 615-386-9754
e-mail: dsamt@bellsouth.net
www.dsamt.org

A nonprofit organization that is affiliated with the National Down Syndrome Society and the National Down Syndrome Congress. DSAMT works closely with The Arc of Tennessee and other disability organizations locally and throughout the state to provide support for individuals with Down syndrome.

Sheila Moore, Executive Director

2677 Down Syndrome Guild of Dallas
701 N Central Expressway, Building I
Richardson, TX 75080   214-267-1374
e-mail: dsged@sbcglobal.net
www.downsyndromedallas.org

Aims to impact the community so that everyone will acknowledge the inherent dignity and abilities of people with Down syndrome with full participation in society.

Becky Slakman, Executive Director
Kelly Drablos, Vice President
Minnie Blackwell, Membership Committee Chairperson

2678 Texas Association on Mental Retardation
PO Box 28076
Austin, TX 78755   512-349-7470
Fax: 512-349-2117
e-mail: pat.holder@tamr-web.com

An organization made up of professionals, parents, consumers and advocates. The goal is to create an accessible system of services and resources which support personal choice and promotes lives of dignity and self-determination. An Annual Convention is a forum for sharing ideas and research, offering opportunities for exchanging information, and developing an understanding for other perspectives.

Pat Holder, Executive Director
Robert Welsh, President
Kimberly Littlejohn, President-Elect

Research Centers

2679 Down Syndrome Clinic, Children's Hospital of Alabama
1600 7th Avenue S
Birmingham, AL 35233   205-368-9585
Fax: 205-975-6330
www.childrensal.org

Dr. Diane K Donley

California

2680 Children's Hospital & Research Center of Oakland
747 52nd Street
Oakland, CA 94609   510-428-3259
www.childrenshospitaloakland.org

Scientific research is an important part of the work that goes on at
Children's Hospital & Research Center Oakland. Researchers are
making significant progress in such areas as diagnosing and treating pediatric cancers, sickle cell disease, AIDS and HIV, hemophilia, cystic fibrosis, developing prenatal techniques for
diagnosing mental retardation and birth defects, and improving
infant nutrition.

Kevan McCarten-Gibbs, Senior VP/Chief Medical Officer
Nancy Shibata, RN, Nursing VP
Donald Livsey, VP/Chief Information Officer

2681 Pediatric Disabilities Clinic, Down Syndrome Clinic
University of California Medical Center
400 Parnassus, Box 0374
San Francisco, CA 94143   415-476-3276
www.ucsfhealth.org

Dorothy Pang

Georgia

2682 Pediatric Neurodevelopmental Center at Marcus Institute
Marcus Institute
1920 Briarcliff Road
Atlanta, GA 30329   404-419-5300
Fax: 404-419-5410
e-mail: ccoles@emory.edu
www.marcus.org

Provides an array of evaluation and treatment services for individuals from infancy through adolescence. As well as providing
individual evaluations, we feature a number of unique
multispecialty programs. Once a child is evaluated, the proper
course of treatment and/or therapy can be determined. The evaluation may result in a recommendation for further treatment at the
Marcus Institute, or may involve other programs and services in
the child's community.

Howard S Schub, MD, Medical Director

Illinois

2683 Adult Down Syndrome Center of Lutheran General Hospital
1999 Dempster Street
Park Ridge, IL 60068   847-318-2303
Fax: 847-318-2377
www.advocatehealth.com

A comprehensive medical resource providing multidisciplinary
medical and psychosocial care for adults with Down syndrome,
with an emphasis on health promotion.

Brian Chicoine, MD, Medical Director
Jenny Lobough-Howard, Outreach Specialist
Ann Jonaitis, Resource Coordinator

**2684 Advocate Lutheran General Children's Hospital, Pediatric
Research**
1775 Dempster Street
Park Ridge, IL 60068   847-318-9330
e-mail: denise.angst@advocatehealth.com
www.advocatehealth.com

An organization of physicians and health care professionals dedicated to serving the health needs of individuals, families and
communities in Northern Illinois. Ongoing research on Pediatric
disorders are being conducted and finding new procedures and
medicines.

Marissa Lowenthal, Medical Director
Denise B Angst, DNSc, Research Director
Sandy Maki, MAT; CCRP, Research Operations Manager

2685 LaRabida Children's Hospital, Down Syndrome Clinic
E 65th Street @ Lake Michigan
Chicago, IL 60649   773-753-8646
Fax: 773-363-7160
e-mail: info@larabida.org
www.larabida.org

Recognized as a leader in the diagnosis and treatment of children
with developmental disabilities and delays. La Rabida provides
comprehensive care and services for children with Down syndrome. The Down syndrome program at La Rabida is designed to
provide medical and developmental evaluations and be a resource
for both parents and pediatricians caring for children with this
chronic condition.

Paula Jaudas, Executive Director

Indiana

2686 Ann Whitehill Down Syndrome Program
Riley Hospital for Children
702 Barnhill Drive
Indianapolis, IN 46202   317-274-4846
Fax: 317-274-4471
www.rileychildrenshospital.com

Brings together specialists from many areas to address the medical and psychosocial needs of children with Down Syndrome. A
developmental pediatrician, pediatric nurse practitioner, pediatric
social worker, pediatric occupational therapist, physical therapist
and certified speech pathologist work closely with the primary
care physician to help each child achieve his or her optimal potential. We also refer the family to local resources for therapy and
developmental programs.

Marilyn Bell, MD

Maryland

**2687 Behavioral and Developmental Pediatrics Division, University
of Maryland**
22 S Greene Street
Baltimore, MD 21201   410-328-2214
800-492-5538
Fax: 410-328-3981
www.umm.edu

Offers comprehensive consultation, evaluation and treatment for
children, birth to age 21, with developmental and behavioral
problems.

Linda Grossman, MD, Associate Professor

2688 Kennedy Krieger Institute, Down Syndrome Clinic
1750 E Fairmount Avenue
Baltimore, MD 21231   443-923-9140
Fax: 410-550-9292
e-mail: koller@kennedykrieger.org
www.kennedykrieger.org/

Develop and conduct clinical research studies into the
neurobiologic basis of cognitive impairment and co-morbid psychiatric disorders in Down syndrome; to study potential therapies
for safety and efficacy; and to investigate genetic and environmental factors relevant to AV Canal defect.

George Capone, Director
Char Koller, Research Contact

Massachusetts

2689 Down Syndrome Program, Children's Hospital Boston
300 Longwood Avenue
Boston, MA 02115   617-355-6000
Fax: 617-735-7429
TTY: 617-730-0152
e-mail: CROCKER_A@A1.TCH.Harvard.edu
www.childrenshospital.org/

Medical and developmental monitoring for children from birth to 3 years of age. Evaluations are provided every 4 to 6 months by an interdisciplinary team comprised of a developmental pediatrician, physical therapist, nutritionist, audiologist, speech pathologist, and social worker. Individual support is available for families, along with information, referral, and case management assistance.

Dr. Allen Crocker, Director

Minnesota

2690 Down Syndrome Clinic of Minneapolis Children's Medical Center
2525 Chicago Avenue
Minneapolis, MN 55404
612-813-7800
Fax: 612-813-6100
e-mail: dmcconn606@aol.com

Mission of the clinic is to improve the quality of life for children and adolescents with Down syndrome and to help them reach their full potentials. A multi-disciplinary team of professionals provide care to the children and adolescents who come to the clinic. Because of the full spectrum of services available, the program can provide consultation for specific medical and developmental problems, developmental assessments, management of behavioral difficulties, and family support.

Dr. Kim McConnell, Director
Mary Bergs, Social Worker

Missouri

2691 Children's Mercy Hospital, Down Syndrome Clinic
2401 Gillham Road
Kansas City, MO 64108
816-234-3041
Fax: 816-842-6107
e-mail: webmaster@cmh.edu
www.childrens-mercy.org

Medical staff of nearly 600 pediatric specialists with a comprehensive range of programs and services, representing more than 40 pediatric specialities.

Erica Molitor-Kirsch, Executive Medical Director/SVP
Barbara Mueth, Community Relations VP
Davoren Tempel, Resource Development VP

2692 Down's Syndrome Medical Clinic
Washington University Medical Center
400 S Kingshighway Boulevard
Saint Louis, MO 63110
314-454-5437
800-678-5437
www.stlouischildrens.org
Dr. Arnold Strauss

New Hampshire

2693 Medical Genetics Clinic
Dartmouth-Hitchcock Medical Center
1 Medical Center Drive
Lebanon, NH 03756
603-653-6044
Fax: 603-650-8268
www.dhmc.org

Provides specialty consultations for diagnosis and treatment of suspected inherited conditions or syndromes.

John Moeschler, MD, Program Director
Mary Beth Dinulos, MD, Medical Geneticist
Susan Berg, MS, Genetic Counselor

New York

2694 Child Development Clinical Services
Westchester Institute for Human Development
Cedarwood Hallÿ
Valhalla, NY 10595
914-285-8178
Fax: 914-285-1973
e-mail: info@WIHD.org
www.wihd.org

Diagnostic evaluation and treatment services are provided for children with developmental concerns, communication disorders, attention deficit disorders (including ADHD) and learning disabilities, as well as cerebral palsy and other neuromotor disorders, spina bifida, mental retardation, and autism.

Mark Bertin, MD, Director
Karen Edwards, MD, Pediatrics Director

2695 Institute for Basic Research in Developmental Disabilities
1050 Forest Hill Road
Staten Island, NY 10314
718-494-0600
Fax: 718-698-3803
e-mail: ÿibr@opwdd.ny.gov
www.omr.state.ny.us

Research arm of the New York State Office of Mental Retardation and Developmental Disabilities (OMRDD). IBR conducts basic and clinical research into the causes, treatment, and prevention of mental retardation and other developmental disabilities. It also provides specialized biomedical, psychological, and laboratory services to individuals with developmental disabilities and their families, and educates the public and professionals regarding the causes, diagnosis, prevention, and treatment.

W Ted Brown, Manager

North Dakota

2696 Children's Hospital Merit Care Down Syndrome Service
737 Broadway
Fargo, ND 58102
701-234-2568
Fax: 701-234-6965

Dr. Guy Carter

Ohio

2697 Down Syndrome Clinic, Rainbow Babies and Children's Hospital
11100 Euclid Avenue
Cleveland, OH 44106
216-844-8447
888-844-844
Fax: 216-844-8444
www.uhhospitals.org/rainbow
Dr. Joanne Mortimer

2698 Jane and Richard Thomas Center for Down Syndrome
Cincinnati Children's Hospital Medical Center
3333 Burnet Avenue
Cincinnati, OH 45229
513-636-4561
800-344-2462
Fax: 513-636-7173
e-mail: development@cchmc.org
www.cincinnatichildrens.org

Conducts research and offers interdisciplinary evaluations and intervention for infants, children, adolescents and young adults with Down syndrome. By providing a range of comprehensive services within one center, families can now spend less time pursuing services through multiple agencies and professionals.

Richard T Strait, Division Head

2699 Pediatric Clinical Trials International
10 Winthrop Square, Fifth Floor
Boston, MA 02110
617-948-5100
866-219-3440
Fax: 617-948-5101
e-mail: marketing@centerwatch.com
www.centerwatch.com/

Consists of inpatient and outpatient capabilities. The inpatient facility includes research beds, a psychophysiological recording and observation/recording center. The latter, located on the neuromonitoring unit, consists of a subject testing room equipped with video cameras and psychological recording systems, and the second is the monitoring room equipped with computer programming and audio-video monitoring, etc.

Daniel R Boue, Medical Director
John P Niles, CEO
Karen Miller, RN, Affiliate Operations Manager

2700 Children's Hospital of Pittsburgh General Clinical Research Center
401 Penn Avenue
Pittsburgh, PA 15224   412-692-6438
                                        Fax: 412-692-5723
                               e-mail: linda.cherok@chp.edu
                                       www.chp.edu/research

Established to increase medical knowledge about childhood diseases and to improve the management and treatment of these diseases. Participation is of great importance and value to medical research. We have a dedicated staff of physicians, nurses and health care professionals experienced in health care delivery and research who will ensure your comfort and safety as you participate in medical studies.

Pamela Murray, Program Director
Diane E Cline, Administrative Manager

2701 Children's Seashore House
Children's Hospital in Philadelphia
3405 Civic Center Boulevard
Philadelphia, PA 19104   215-590-1734
                               e-mail: rac@email.chop.edu
                                            www.chop.edu

Leading research institution quickly bringing scientific discoveries into the clinical setting and community to improve care. Some current research studies include: cognitive studies of the development of mathematical competence in normal children and in those with congenital defects, studies of language development in children with inherited syndromes, and development of novel strategies to prevent violence in the school setting.

Marc Yudkoff, MD, Division Chief
Nathan Blum, MD, Behavioral Pediatrics

2702 Dr. Gertrude A. Barber National Institute
100 Barber Place
Erie, PA 16507   814-45- 766
                                        Fax: 814-455-1132
                            e-mail: BNIerie@barberinstitute.org
                                        www.barbercenter.org

Committed to remaining on the cutting-edge of breakthrough technologies and practices. We seek out research opportunities that will enhance our services and will provide the most current proven information to present to the public.

John J Barber, President
Maureen Barber-Carey, Executive VP
Karen Hahn Berry, RN, Health Services Director

2703 International Foundation for Genetic Research/Michael Fund
4371 Northern Pike
Pittsburgh, PA 15146   412-374-0111
                                       www.michaelfund.org

Research is directed toward preventing and treating the harmful consequences of the extra chromosome in Down's Syndrome. Also; dedicated to reversing this destructive universal trend by opening up new doors of therapy in the field of mental retardation associated with chromomal disorders such as Down Syndrome and continuing the curative research program.

Dr. Paddy Jim Baggot, Executive Director

2704 Children's Neurodevelopment Center at Hasbro Children's Hospital
Rhode Island Hospital
593 Eddy Street
Providence, RI 02903   401-444-4000
                                        Fax: 401-444-6115
                              e-mail: sigpueschel@aol.com
                                 www.lifespan.org/hch/services/

A site for the evaluation and treatment of children with neurological, genetic, developmental, metabolic and behavioral disorders.

Lee V Wesner, Director

2705 Down Syndrome Specialty Clinic
Children's Medical Center
1935 Medical District Dr.
Dallas, TX 75235   214-456-6388
                                        Fax: 214-456-2567
                                        www.childrens.com

Comprehensive care for children with Down syndrome and their families including; medical management, genetic counseling, speech and oral motor developmental evaluation and recommendations, psychosocial support, screening and referral for behavioral or psychiatric problems, and referrals to community agencies for educational intervention or therapies.

Mary Esther Carlin MD, Clinical Medical Doctor
Joanna Spahis, RN, Clinical Nurse Specialist

2706 University of Washington: Experimental Education Unit
University of Washington
Columbia Road, Gate #6
Seattle, WA 98195   206-543-2100
                                  www.depts.washington.edu/

Provide clinical services to children and their families, and conduct interdisciplinary research.

Rick Neel, Director
Kate Ahern, Admissions Coordinator

2707 Center for the Study of Bioethics
Medical College of Wisconsin
8701 Watertown Plank Road
Milwaukee, WI 53226   414-527-8191
                             e-mail: centerbioethics@mcw.edu
                                      www.mcw.edu/bioethics

Center for the Study of Bioethics is a leader in the field of bioethics. The Center has conscientiously served the functions of a typical institution of higher learning; research, education, and service.

Robyn S Shapiro, Director
Kristen Tym, Assistant Director

Conferences

2708 ARC Annual National Convention
The ARC
1825 K Street NW,Suite 1200
Washington, DC 20006   202-534-3700
                                             800-433-5255
                                        Fax: 202-534-3731
                                   e-mail: info@thearc.org
                                            www.thearc.org

Held in cities throughout the U.S. each fall which attracts nearly 1000 people for educational sessions, business meetings and social events.

Nancy Webster, President
Ronald Brown, Vice President
Elise McMillan, Secretary

2709 Genetic Alliance Annual Conference
Genetic Alliance
4301 Connecticut Avenue NW, Suite 404
Washington, DC 20008   202-966-5557
                                             800-336-4363
                                        Fax: 202-966-8553
                             e-mail: info@geneticalliance.org
                                      www.geneticalliance.org

Consistently inspirational and enables partnership among all stakeholders: advocates and community leaders, health and industry professionals, policymakers, and academicians.

July

Sharon Terry, President/CEO
Tetyana Murza, Programs/Events Manager

2710 NDSC Annual Convention
National Down Syndrome Congress
30 Mansel Court,Suite 108
Roswell, GA 30076
770-604-9500
800-232-6372
Fax: 770-604-9898
e-mail: info@ndsccenter.org
www.ndsccenter.org

offers parents and professionals an opportunity to learn from the best speakers from around the world and share experiences with one another.

August

David Tolleson, Executive Director
Sue Joe, Resource Specialist
Betty Totten, Office Manager

2711 National Down Syndrome Society Annual National Conference
666 Broadway,8th Floor
New York, NY 10012
212-763-4365
800-221-4602
e-mail: jnfo@ndss.org
www.ndss.org

The focus is on working together to improve the lives of individuals with Down syndrome, enabling them to enjoy the benefits of, and contribute to, their communities.

Jennifer Falik, Special Events Director
Elizabeth F Goodwin, Founder

Audio Video

2712 A Promising Future Together
National Down Syndrome Society
666 Broadway, 8th Floor
New York, NY 10012
800-221-4602
Fax: 212-979-2873
e-mail: info@ndss.org
www.ndss.org

A guide for new and expectant parents; available in video or print.

52 pages

CAPT Robert P. Taishoff USN (ret), Chairman
Stephen Beck, Jr., Vice Chairman
Sara Weir, President

2713 A Special Love
Association for Children with Down Syndrome
2616 Martin Avenue
Bellmore, NY 11710
516-221-4700
Fax: 516-221-4311

A candid video of a ten-year-old brother playing with his six-year-old sister with Down Syndrome. The brother describes his perceptions of mental retardation and his feelings towards his sister.

4 minutes, b/w

DB Shalom, Editor

2714 Boy in the World
Fanlight Productions
32 Court Street, 21st Floor
Brooklyn, NY 11201
718-488-8900
800-876-1710
Fax: 718-488-8642
e-mail: info@fanlight.com, orders@fanlight.com
www.fanlight.com

Following four-year-old Ronen, a young boy with down syndrome, this intimate documentary concretely demonstrates that inclusive preschool classrooms benefit both children with special needs and their typical peers. It examines the nuts and bolts of successful inclusion as well as the challenges of educationsl practices that help all children to learn - and find their place in the world. ISBN: DVD: 1-57295-944-4; VHS: 1-57295-488-4

44 minutes DVD of VHS

2715 Congratulations? An Introduction to Down Syndrome for Parents/Family/Friends
New Challenges
96 Ogden Avenue
White Plains, NY 10605
914-287-0723

A film for parents which addresses some of the most commonly asked questions about raising a child with Down syndrome.

57 mins.

2716 Daddy's Girl
Carle Media
110 W Main Street
Urbana, IL 61801
217-384-4838

Dina Lev, a 12-year-old actress with Down syndrome, portrays Nancy, a girl trying to deal with her divorced father's inability to accept the fact that his daughter has Down syndrome.

28 mins.

Bruce Postman, Producer
Regina Conroy, Writer/Director

2717 Educating Peter
State of the Art Production
2470 Fox Hill Road
State College, PA 16803
814-355-8004
800-458-3401
Fax: 814-355-2714
e-mail: sales@resistor.com, marketing@resistor.c
www.resistor.com

Thought-provoking film follows a child with Down syndrome through a year of inclusion in a public school in Mrs. Stallings' third grade class. The film raises many questions about inclusion by honestly presenting the reactions to, and methods of, dealing with Peter's behavior problems.

30 Minutes

Thomas C Goodwin, Producer/Director
Gerardine Wurzburg, Producer/Director

2718 Infant Motor Development: A Look at the Phases
Therapy Skill Builders
San Antonio, TX 78283
732-441-0404

Shows normal infant motor development from birth to 12 months. Identifies components of movement and specific skills that are acquired during 4 phases of motor development: infantile, preparation, modification, and refinement. Transitional movement patte rns and their relationship to skill acquisition are also described.

20 Minutes

Kerry Goudy, Producer
Joan Winger, Producer

2719 New Expectations
Altschul Group Corporation
1560 Sherman Avenue, Suite 100
Evanston, IL 60201
800-421-2363
e-mail: agcmedia@starnetinc.com

Focuses on the emotional and technical aspects of Down syndrome. Highlights four persons at various life stages from infancy to adulthood in the areas of education and employment.

Web Sites

2720 ARC of the United States
1825 K Street, NW, Suite 1200
Washington, DC 20006
202-534-3700
800-433-5255
Fax: 202-534-3731
e-mail: tnguyen@thearc.org
www.thearc.org

The ARC is the national organization of and for people with mental retardation and related developmental disabilities and their families. Devoted to promoting and improving supports and services for people with mental retardation and their families. The association also fosters research and education regarding the prevention of mental retardation in infants and young children. The ARC was founded in 1950 by a small group of parents and other concerned individuals.

Ronald Brown, President
Elise McMillan, Vice President
Peter V. Berns, CEO

2721 Aleh Foundation
PO Box 4911
New York, NY 10185
866-717-0252
Fax: 212-517-3293
e-mail: dov@aleh-israel.org
www.aleh.org

Aleh is a nonprofit organization that believes that every child, no matter how severe his/her disability, has potential. We are committed to providing severely disabled children through Israel with the high-level medical and rehabilitative care they need to grow beyond the boundaries of their prognoses.

Prof. Joehoshua Shemer, Chair, Board of Assuta
Avner Broker, Operations Manager, ALEH Negev
Dov Hirth, Marketing & Development

2722 Association for Children with Down Syndrome
4 Fern Place
Plainview, NY 11803
516-933-4700
www.acds.org

Dedicated to providing lifetime resources of exceptional quality, innovation and inclusion for individuals with Down syndrome and other developmental disabilities and their families.

Liz Lawlor Campbell, Chair, Advisory Committee
Gene Kirley, President
Thomas DeMaggio, Vice President

2723 Birth Defects Research for Children
976 Lake Baldwin Lane, Suite 104
Orlando, FL 32814
407-895-0802
e-mail: staff@birthdefects.org
www.birthdefects.org

An organization that provides parents and expectant parents with information about birth defects and support services for their children. BDRC has a parent-matching program that links families who have children with similar birth defects.

2724 Down Syndrome Guild
www.downsyndromedallas.com

Provides new baby/parent hospital visits, monthly newsletter, support and encouragement for individuals with Down Syndrome and their families. Bi-lingual group. Job coaching scholarships.

2725 Health Answers
410 Horsham Road
Horsham, PA 19044
215-422-9010
e-mail: Michael.tague@healthanswers.com
www.healthanswers.com

HealthAnswers offers a breadth of services in medical education, sales force training, patient support, solutions, professional promotion and consumer solutions.

Michael Tague, Managing Director

2726 National Association for Down Syndrome (NADS)
1460 Renaissance Drive, Suite #405
Park Ridge, IL 60068
630-325-9112
e-mail: info@nads.org
www.nads.org

Established by parents of children with Down syndrome who felt a need to create a better environment and bring about understanding and acceptance of people with Down syndrome.

Steve Connors, President
Jeni Friedland, First Vice President
Deb Mirabelli, Second Vice President

2727 National Down Syndrome Congress
30 Mansell Court, Suite 108
Roswell, GA 30076
770-604-9500
800-232-NDSC
Fax: 770-604-9898
e-mail: info@ndsccenter.org
www.ndsccenter.org

It is the mission of the National Down Syndrome Congress to be the national advocacy organization for Down syndrome and to provide leadership in all areas of concern related to persons with Down syndrome. In that capacity, NDSC will function as a major source of support and empowerment to persons with down syndrome and their families.

Marilyn Tolbert, Ed.D., President
Bret Bowerman, First Vice President
Andy Bean, Second Vice President

2728 National Down Syndrome Society
666 Broadway, 8th Floor
New York, NY 10012
800-221-4602
Fax: 212-979-2873
e-mail: info@ndss.org
www.ndss.org

Our mission is to benefit people with Down Syndrome and their families through national leadership in education research and advocacy.

CAPT Robert P. Taishoff USN (ret), Chairman
Stephen Beck, Jr., Vice Chairman
Sara Weir, President

2729 Online Mendelian Inheritance in Man
U.S. National Library of Medicine, 8600 Rockville
Bethesda, MD 20894
888-346-3656
e-mail: info@ncbi.nlm.nih.gov
www.ncbi.nlm.nih.gov

This database is a catalog of human genes and genetic disorders.

Christine E. Seidman, M.D., Chair
David J. Lipman, M.D., Executive Secretary
Michael Boehnke, Ph.D., Board Member

Book Publishers

2730 Adolescents with Down Syndrome
University of Victoria
3800 Finnerty Road
Victoria, BC, V8P
Canada
250-721-7211
www.uvic.ca

Adolescents with Down syndrome: International perspectives on research and programme development: Implications for parents, researchers, and practitioners.

165 pages
ISBN: 0-919955-16-9

Carey Denholm, Editor

2731 Babies with Down Syndrome
Woodbine House
6510 Bells Mill Road
Bethesda, MD 20817
301-897-3570
800-843-7323
Fax: 301-897-5838

Praised as the finest book ever written for new parents, this book covers everything they need to know about rearing these beautiful and special children in a loving environment.

340 pages Paperback
ISBN: 0-933149-64-6

Karen Stray-Gundersen, Editor

2732 Biomedical Concerns in Persons with Down's Syndrome
Brookes Publishing Company
PO Box 10624
Baltimore, MD 21285
410-337-9580
800-638-3775
Fax: 410-337-8539
www.brookespublishing.com

Written by leading authorities and spanning many disciplines and specialties, this comprehensive resource provides vital information on biomedical issues concerning individuals with Down's syndrome.

336 pages Hardcover
ISBN: 1-557660-89-1

Siegfried M Pueschel, Editor
Jeanette K Pueschel, Editor

2733 Cara: Growing with a Retarded Child
Temple University Press
1801 N.Broad Street
Philadelphia, PA 19122   215-204-8787
www.temple.edu/templepress/

Despite the fact that Cara Jablow was born with Down's syndrome, formerly known as mongolism, she was reading before she was five. Her mother, a journalist, dramatically recounts Cara's development from birth to age seven, revealing how a family reacts to the news that their baby is retarded, how they now can make use of early intervention programs, and what Cara's prospects are for the future.

210 pages Paperback
ISBN: 0-877222-69-X

Martha Moraghan Jablow, Editor

2734 Communication Skills in Children with Down Syndrome: A Guide for Parents
Woodbine House
6510 Bells Mill Road
Bethesda, MD 20817   301-468-8800
800-843-7323
Fax: 301-897-5838
e-mail: info@woodbinehouse.com
www.woodbinehouse.com

Offers parents a chance to learn what to expect as communication skills progress from infancy through early teenage years. Discussions are included on speech and language therapy, hearing problems, school performance and intelligibility issues.

241 pages Paperback
ISBN: 0-933149-53-0

Libby Kumin, Editor

2735 Count Us In: Growing up with Down Syndrome
Harvest Book Company
185 Commerce Drive
Fort Washington, PA 19034   215-619-0307
877-512-3022
e-mail: webservice@Harvestbooks.com
www.harvestbooks.com/

Mitchell Levitz and Jason Kingsley share their innermost thoughts, feelings, hopes and dreams, their lifelong friendship and their experiences of growing up with Down Syndrome.

1994 208 pages Paperback
ISBN: 0-156226-60-X

Jason Kingsley, Editor
Mitchell Levitz, Editor

2736 Current Approaches to Down's Syndrome
Greenwood Publishing Group
88 Post Road W, Suite 5007
Westport, CT 06880   203-226-3571
www.greenwood.com

An exploration of current initiatives relating to Down syndrome in the medical, educational and social fields.

447 pages Hardcover
ISBN: 0-275902-12-9

David Lane, Editor
Brian Stratford, Editor

2737 Differences in Common: Straight Talk on Mental Retardation/Down Syndrome & Life
Woodbine House
6510 Bells Mill Road
Bethesda, MD 20817   301-468-8800
800-843-7323
Fax: 301-897-5838
e-mail: info@woodbinehouse.com
www.woodbinehouse.com

A collection of essays by the mother of an adult son who has Down syndrome. Focuses on mainstreaming, terminology, parent groups and advocacy.

231 pages Paperback
ISBN: 0-933149-40-9

Marilyn Trainer, Editor

2738 Down Sydrome: Living and Learning in the Community
Wiley & Sonecial Children
10475 Crosspoint Boulevard
Indianapolis, IN 46256   877-762-2974
Fax: 800-597-3299
www.wiley.com

Four parents' personal observations. Challenges of people with DS as they become integrated into community, family role, cognitive development and acquisition of language, education, health care, independent living arrangement.

1995 312 pages Hardcover
ISBN: 0-471022-01-2

Lynn Nadel, Editor
Donna Rosenthal, Editor

2739 Down Syndrome: Birth to Adulthood: Giving Families an Edge
Love Publishing Company
9101 E Kenyon Evenue
Denver, CO 80237   303-221-7333
Fax: 303-221-7444
e-mail: lpc@lovepublishing.com
www.lovepublishing.com

Provides a collection of longitudinal perspectives on experiences of individuals with Down Syndrome, from birth to adulthood.

1995 356 pages Paperback
ISBN: 0-891082-36-0

John R Rynders, Editor

2740 Down Syndrome: The Facts
Oxford University Press
2001 Evans Road
Cary, NC 27513   212-726-6000
800-451-7556
Fax: 919-677-1303
www.oup-usa.org

A book for parents who have a child with Down Syndrome, written by a pediatrician who works with Down syndrome children.

208 pages Paperback
ISBN: 0-192626-62-0

Mark Selikowitz, Editor

2741 Let's Talk About Down Syndrome
Rosen Publishing Group's PowerKids Press
29 E 21st Street
New York, NY 10010   212-777-3017
800-237-9932
Fax: 888-436-4643
e-mail: rosenpub@tribeca.ios.com
www.rosenpublishing.com

By stressing that children with Down syndrome are wonderful, viable members of society, this book lessens the stigma attached to this rather common genetic condition.

Ages: 4-8 24 pages Library Binding
ISBN: 0-823951-97-9

Melanie Apel Gordon, Editor

2742 Medical and Surgical Care for Children with Down Syndrome
Woodbine House
6510 Bells Mill Road
Bethesda, MD 20817   301-897-3570
                                                      800-843-7323
                                                Fax: 301-897-5838
                              e-mail: info@woodbinehouse.com
                                         www.woodbinehouse.com

Provides detailed and easy-to-understand information for parents
on a wide range of medical conditions and treatments including:
heart disease, recurrent infections, thyroid problems, eye problems, skin conditions, ear, nose and throat problems, orthopedic
conditions, leukemia, facial and dental concerns and neurological
problems.

395 pages Paperback
ISBN: 0-933149-54-9

Philip Matheis, MD, Editor
Don Van Dyke, MD, Editor

**2743 Our Brother Has Down's Syndrome: An Introduction for
Children**
Annick Press
15 Patricia Avenue
Toronto, ON, M2M
Canada   416-221-4802
                                                Fax: 416-221-8400
                                           www.annickpress.com

Two young sisters tell about their little brother Jai, who has
Down's Syndrome. The text stresses the ways in which he is like
all children, although he needs extra help to walk, use a spoon,
stack blocks, etc. The color photographs show an engaging little
boy going about his daily activities, often with other family
members.

24 pages Paperback
ISBN: 0-920303-31-5

Shelly Cairo, Editor
Jasmine Cairo, Editor
Irene McNeil, Editor

2744 Parent's Guide to Down Syndrome: Toward a Brighter Future
Brookes Publishing Company
PO Box 10624
Baltimore, MD 21285   410-337-9580
                                                      800-638-3775
                                                Fax: 410-337-8539
                        e-mail: custserv@brookespublishing.com
                                      www.brookespublishing.com

A comprehensive reference book especially for new parents, but
useful and informative to seasoned parents as well. Range of topics include a history of Down syndrome, physical characteristics,
developmental expectations, early intervention, feeding the young
child and the school years.

352 pages Paperback
ISBN: 1-557664-52-8

Siegfried M Pueschel, Editor

2745 Perceptual-Motor Behavior in Down Syndrome
Human Kinetics Publishing
1607 N Market Street
Champaign, IL 61825   217-351-5076
                                                      800-747-4457
                                                Fax: 217-351-2674
                                           www.humankinetics.com

A comprehensive collection of contemporary research and provides readers a window into the life of someone with Down
Syndrome.

365 pages Hardcover
ISBN: 0-880119-75-6

Daniel J Weeks, Editor
Romeo Chua, Editor
Dibgy Elliott, Editor

2746 Screening for Down Syndrome
Cambridge University Press
32 Avenue of the Americans
New York, NY 10013   212-337-5000
                                                Fax: 212-691-3239
                              e-mail: newyork@cambridge.org
                                         www.cambridge.org

Summarises the recent exciting advances in screening for Down's
syndrome. It addresses important clinical questions such as; risk
assessment, whom to screen, when to screen, which techniques to
use and the organisation of screening programmes nationally and
internationally.

1995 358 pages Hardcover
ISBN: 0-521452-71-6

J G Grudzinskas, Editor
T Chard, Editor
M Chapman, Editor

**2747 Shattered Dreams - Lonely Choices: Birth Parents of Babies
with Disabilities**
Bergin & Garvey/Greenwood Publishing
88 Post Road W, PO Box 5007
Westport, CT 06880   203-226-3571
                                                      800-225-5800
                                                Fax: 203-222-1502
                              e-mail: custserv@greenwood.com
                                         www.greenwood.com

Joanne Finnegan shares her personal experience and that of several families she interviewed who, like herself, explored options
other than raising their child with a disability. Parents express
with candor the overwhelming pain they felt when receiving the
news, the frustration when searching for options, the no-win feeling of decision making, the resolve with a final decision, and
finally, life after the decision.

208 pages Hardcover
ISBN: 0-897892-86-0

Joanne Finnegan, Editor

**2748 Show Me No Mercy: Compelling Story of Remarkable
Courage**
Abingdon Press
201 8th Avenue South, P.O. Box 801
Nashville, TN 37202   800-251-3320
                              e-mail: orders@abingdonpress.com
                                         www.abingdonpress.com

A father of a young adult man with Down syndrome relates the
experience of his attempt to be reunited with his son after a family tragedy separates them.

144 pages Paperback
ISBN: 0-687384-35-4

Robert Perske, Editor

2749 Since Owen
Johns Hopkins University Press
2715 N Charles Street
Baltimore, MD 21218   410-516-6900
                                                      800-537-5487
                                                Fax: 410-516-6968
                              e-mail: webmaster@jhupress.jhu.edu
                                         www.press.jhu.edu

A well written book displaying understanding from a veteran parent communicating with other parents of children with disabilities.

488 pages Paperback
ISBN: 0-801839-64-5

Charles R Callanan, Editor
Alfred R. Berkeley, Chairman

2750 Special Kids Make Special Friends
Association for Children with Down Syndrome
4 Fern Place
Plainview, NY 11803   516-933-4700
                                                Fax: 516-933-9524
                              e-mail: information@acds.org
                                         www.acds.org

Written to assist young children, new parents, siblings, and professionals in developing a better understanding of Down syndrome. Photographs depict children in preschool, emphasizing similarities and strengths of youngsters with Down syndrome rather than their differences.

1995 Paperback
ISBN: 9-995007-64-9

Debra Shalom, Editor
Michael M. Smith, Executive Director

2751 To Give An Edge: A Guide for New Parents of Children with Down's Syndrome
Colwell Systems
1031 Mendola Heights Road
St. Paul, MN 55120 651-232-7800

A guide for new parents designed to provide information about the disorder and how other parents of children with Down syndrome have coped.

Paperback
ISBN: 9-993370-55-X

JM Horrobin, Editor

2752 Understanding Down Syndrome
Brookline Books
8 Trumbull Rd,Suite B-001
Northampton, MA 01060 413-584-0184
800-666-2665
Fax: 413-584-6184
e-mail: brbooks@yahoo.com
www.brooklinebooks.com

The author provides answers and explanations to the countless questions directed to him during his twenty years' involvement with Down syndrome individuals and their families.

243 pages Paperback
ISBN: 1-571290-09-5

Cliff Cunningham, Editor

2753 Where's Chimpy?
Albert Whitman & Company
250 South Northwest Highway,Suite 320
Park Ridge, IL 60068 847-581-0033
800-255-7675
Fax: 847-581-0039
e-mail: mail@awhitmanco.com
www.awhitmanco.com

Text and photographs show Misty, a little girl with Down syndrome and her father reviewing her day's activities in their search for her stuffed monkey.

32 pages Paperback
ISBN: 0-807589-27-6

Berniece Rabe, Editor
Diane Schmidt, Illustrator

Magazines

2754 Down Syndrome News
National Down Syndrome Congress
30 Mansell Court, Suite 108
Roswell, GA 30076 770-604-9500
800-232-6372
Fax: 770-604-9898
e-mail: info@ndscenter.org
www.ndsccenter.org

Down Syndrome News provides advocacy news and information to parents and family members of individuals with Down syndrome and those working with them.

6x/year

Marilyn Tolbert, Ed.D., President
Bret Bowerman, First Vice President
Andy Bean, Second Vice President

2755 Upbeat
National Down Syndrome Society
666 Broadway, 8th Floor
New York, NY 10012 800-221-4602
Fax: 212-979-2873
e-mail: info@ndss.org
www.ndss.org

For and by people with Down syndrome that comes out three times a year.

CAPT Robert P. Taishoff USN (ret), Chairman
Stephen Beck, Jr., Vice Chairman
Sara Weir, President

Newsletters

2756 About NDSS
National Down Syndrome Society
666 Broadway, 8th Floor
New York, NY 10012 800-221-4602
Fax: 212-979-2873
e-mail: info@ndss.org
www.ndss.org

Offers information on the society, stats, goals, mission, activities, affiliates, and governing body.

16 pages

CAPT Robert P. Taishoff USN (ret), Chairman
Stephen Beck, Jr., Vice Chairman
Sara Weir, President

2757 Communicating Together
PO Box 6395
Columbia, MD 21045 408-253-0246
Fax: 408-253-7391
e-mail: karen@kidsource.com
www.kidsource.com

An excellent resource for parents and professionals. Each issue includes a feature article, a question and answer section and home activities.

6x/year

Dr. Libby Kumin, Editor
Karen Dillon, Media Inquiries

Pamphlets

2758 About Down Syndrome
National Down Syndrome Society
666 Broadway, 8th Floor
New York, NY 10012 800-221-4602
Fax: 212-979-2873
e-mail: info@ndss.org
www.ndss.org

An overview of Down Syndrome produced by The Goodwin Family Information & Referral Center arm of NDSS.

18 pages

CAPT Robert P. Taishoff USN (ret), Chairman
Stephen Beck, Jr., Vice Chairman
Sara Weir, President

2759 Down Syndrome
National Down Syndrome Congress
30 Mansell Court, Suite 108
Roswell, GA 30076 770-604-9500
800-232-6372
Fax: 770-604-9898
e-mail: info@ndsccenter.org
www.ndsccenter.org

Pertinent information ranging from education to medicine to legal or legislative issues.

Marilyn Tolbert, Ed.D., President
Bret Bowerman, First Vice President
Andy Bean, Second Vice President

2760 Heart and Down Syndrome
National Down Syndrome Society
666 Broadway, 8th Floor
New York, NY 10012
800-221-4602
Fax: 212-979-2873
e-mail: info@ndss.org
www.ndss.org

1995

CAPT Robert P. Taishoff USN (ret), Chairman
Stephen Beck, Jr., Vice Chairman
Sara Weir, President

2761 Life Planning and Down Syndrome
National Down Syndrome Society
666 Broadway, 8th Floor
New York, NY 10012
800-221-4602
Fax: 212-979-2873
e-mail: info@ndss.org
www.ndss.org

CAPT Robert P. Taishoff USN (ret), Chairman
Stephen Beck, Jr., Vice Chairman
Sara Weir, President

2762 Neurology of Down Syndrome
National Down Syndrome Society
666 Broadway, 8th Floor
New York, NY 10012
800-221-4602
Fax: 212-979-2873
e-mail: info@ndss.org
www.ndss.org

1995

CAPT Robert P. Taishoff USN (ret), Chairman
Stephen Beck, Jr., Vice Chairman
Sara Weir, President

2763 New Parents
Association for Children with Down Syndrome
2616 Martin Avenue
Bellmore, NY 11710
516-221-4700
Fax: 516-221-4311
e-mail: info@acds.org
www.acds.org

A bibliography compiled for parents who have just given birth to a child with Down syndrome.

Liz Lawlor Campbell, Chair, Advisory Committee
Gene Kirley, President
Thomas DeMaggio, Vice President

Camps

2764 Camp Friendship
Friendship Ventures
10509 108th Street NW
Annandale, MN 55302
952-852-0101
800-450-8376
Fax: 952-852-0123
e-mail: info@friendshipventures.org
www.friendshipventures.org

Camp Friendship offers kids, teens, and adults the chance to have the time of their lives. The program focuses on building self-esteem and independence, and practicing social skills; and we nurture each person's strengths and abilities and encourage participation in activies at their own pace. Specially designed for persons with developmental, physical or multiple disabilities, special medical conditions, Down syndrome, autism or other conditions. Weekend camps and longer available.

Georgann Rumsey, Vice President, Programs
Laurie Tschetter, Program Director

2765 Camp Hawkins
800 Rudeseal Road
Mt. Airy, GA 30563
706-894-1678; e-mail: ksewell@gbchfm.org
www.gbchfm.org

Summer residential camp for children ages 8 to 21 with varying disabilities such as Cerebral Palsy, Down Syndrome, brain injuries and/or developmental delays.

Chris Hobbs, VP of Communications
Alice Bagley, Public Relations
Kendra Sewell, Director

2766 Camp Huntington
56 Bruceville Road
High Falls, NY 12440
845-687-7840
855-707-2267
Fax: 845-213-4313
e-mail: mbednarz@camphuntington.com
www.camphuntington.com

Summer activities include recreational, academic and vocational programs for the learning disabled, neurologically impaired and mildly ADA to mild/moderately retarded. An Olympic pool, horse riding and a special work training program are featured. Programs are tailored to meet individual needs, ages 6-21, and campers may enroll for 4 to 8 weeks.

Michael Bednarz, Executive Director, MS, MBA
Alex Mellor, Program Director, MA
Dr. Bruria Bodek, Consultant, Executive Director

2767 Camp Merrimack
3320 Triana Boulevard
Huntsville, AL 35805
256-534-6455
e-mail: ksimari@merrimackhall.com
www.merrimackhall.com

A unique arts half-day camp for children ages 3 through 12; open to children with special needs including Cerebral Palsy, Down Syndrome, autism and others.

Ashley Dinges, Executive Director
Kim Simari, Managing Director

2768 Camp New Hope
Friendship Ventures
53035 Lake Avenue
McGregor, MN 55760
952-852-0101
800-450-8376
Fax: 952-852-0123
e-mail: fv@friendshipventures.org
www.friendshipventures.org

Camp New Hope is a great place for children, teens, and adults to have the time of their lives. The program provides a unique opportunity for having fun, learning skills, boosting confidence, and making friends. Services are specifically designed for persons with developmental, phyisical or multiple disabilities, special medical needs, Down syndrome, autism, or other conditions. Weekend camps and longer available. Other services available throughout the year.

Georgann Rumsey, Vice President, Programs
Laurie Tschetter, Program Director

2769 Camp PALS
4368 Farmington Circle
Allentown, PA 18104
215-501-7157
e-mail: jenni@palsprograms.org
www.camppals.org

One-week summer camp for young adults with Down syndrome held at Cabrini College in PA.

Jason Toff, Board Chair
Jenni Newbury Ross, Executive Director
Sarah Barnes, Program Coordinator

2770 Eden Wood Center
Friendship Ventures
16165 Hillcrest Lane
Eden Prairie, MN 44346
952-852-0101; Fax: 952-934-5656
e-mail: fbiw.info@gmail.com
fbiw.net/old_site/JoinIn/meetings.htm

Offers resident camp programs for children, teenagers and adults with developmental, physical or multiple disabilities, Down Syndrome, special medical conditions, Williams Syndrome, autism and/or other conditions. Fishing, creative arts, golf, sports and other activities are available. Creative Options Respite Care offers weekend camps year round for children, teenagers and adults. Ventures Travel offers guided vacations for teens and adults with developmental disabilities or other unique needs.

Vicky Miller, President
Roger Person, Vice President
Marcus Johnson, Director

Description

2771 DYSLEXIA

Involves the following Biologic System(s):

Neurologic Disorders

Dyslexia refers to a specific learning disability characterized by the impaired ability to process written symbols. Although individuals with dyslexia are able to see and recognize letters, this disorder impairs their ability to read, write, and spell. Affected individuals typically have no problems with the correct recognition of pictures and objects.

No definition of dyslexia is universally accepted, thus incidence is difficult to determine. An estimated 15% of public school children receive special education for reading problems of whom 3 to 5% are probably dyslexic. Young children with dyslexia may have difficulty remembering the correct names of letters and numbers. Articulating proper speech may be difficult. Some children of school age may reverse letters and words when writing. For example, affected children may substitute the letter p for q or the word was for saw, while transposing letters so that bets may become best. Children with dyslexia may also have difficulty reading due to an impaired ability to determine the sequence of letters within words and to distinguish right from left. The hallmark of this learning disability is the fact that, despite the difficulties associated with dyslexia, affected children are of average or above average intelligence as evidenced by I.Q. testing as well as their success in other scholastic achievements.

Early diagnosis of dyslexia is an important factor in treating this learning disability. Children nearing the end of first grade who exhibit difficulties with word skills or any children whose reading and writing ability is not commensurate with that of their other scholastic abilities may be tested for dyslexia. Although dyslexia is not related to eye defects, an ophthalmologic evaluation is beneficial in determining if ocular abnormalities may be eliminated as a cause of symptoms. Also, eye irregularities may be present in addition to dyslexia and, therefore, may be diagnosed and corrected at that time. Treatment for dyslexia is geared toward remedial teaching techniques specific to this disability.

Dyslexia is thought to be a familial disorder that may be inherited through an autosomal dominant trait. Boys are more frequently affected than girls.

Government Agencies

2772 NIH/National Institute of Child Health and Human Development
31 Center Drive, Building 31
Bethesda, MD 20892

301-496-1333
Fax: 301-496-1104
www.nichd.nih.gov

Established in 1962 by congress, today the institute conducts and supports research on topics related to the health of children, adults, families and populations. Some of these topics include: developmental disabilities, growth and development, infant death, reproductive health and birth defects.

Jay H Hoofnagle, Director
Lisa Kaeser, Program & Public Liaison

National Associations & Support Groups

2773 American Academy of Pediatrics
141 Northwest Point Boulevard
Elk Grove Village, IL 60007

847-434-4000
800-433-9016
Fax: 847-434-8000
www.aap.org

The American Academy of Pediatrics and its member pediatricians are committed to the attainment of optimal physical, mental and social health and well-being for all infants, children, adolescents, and young adults.

Sandra Hassink, MD, FAAP, President

2774 American School Counselor Association
1101 King Street, Suite 310
Alexandria, VA 22314

703-683-2722
800-306-4722
Fax: 703-997-7572
e-mail: asca@schoolcounselor.org
www.schoolcounselor.org

The mission of ASCA is to represent professional school counselors and to promote professionalism and ethical practices.

Richard Wong, Executive Director
Jeff Broderson, Information Technology Admin.
Kathleen M Rakestraw, Director of Communications

2775 American Speech Language Hearing Association (ASHA)
10801 Rockville Pike
Rockville, MD 20852

301-897-5700
800-638-8255
Fax: 301-571-0457
e-mail: productsales@asha.org
www.asha.org

The mission of the American Speech-Language-Hearing Association is to promote the interests of and provide the highest quality services for professionals in audiology, speech-language pathology, speech and hearing science, and to advocate for people with communication disabilities.

Arlene A Pietranton, Executive Director
Maureen E Thompson, Director Governance Operations

2776 Center for Disabilities and Development
University of Iowa Hospitals and Clinics
100 Hawkins Drive
Iowa City, IA 52242

319-353-6900
877-686-0031
Fax: 319-356-8284
e-mail: cdd-webmaster@uiowa.edu
www.uiowa.edu

A trusted resource for healthcare, training, research and information for people with disabilities that include: behavior disorders, brain injury, cerebral palsy, diabetes, down syndrome, learning disabilities, mental retardation, sleep disorders and spina bifida.

Judy Stephenson, Administrator
Amy Mikelson, Supervisor Info Resource Service

2777 Davis Dyslexia Association International
1601 Bayshore Highway, Suite 245
Burlingame, CA 94010

650-692-7141
888-805-7216
Fax: 650-692-7075
e-mail: info@davislearn.com
www.davislearn.com

Offers books, materials, workshops and certification in the Davis Dyslexia Correction method.

Ron Davis, Manager

2778 Genetic Alliance
4301 Connecticut Avenue NW, Suite 404
Washington, DC 20008

202-966-5557
800-336-4363
Fax: 202-966-8553
e-mail: info@geneticalliance.org
www.geneticalliance.org

A coalition of voluntary genetic support groups, consumers and professionals addressing the needs of individuals and families affected by genetic disorders from a national perspective.

Sharon Terry, President

2779 International Dyslexia Association
40 York Road, Suite 400
Baltimore, MD 21204

410-296-0232
800-222-3123
Fax: 410-321-5069
e-mail: info@interdys.org
www.interdys.org

Our mission is to pursue and provide the most comprehensive range of information and services that address the full scope of dyslexia and related difficulties in learning to read and write.

Steve Peregoy, Executive Director
Gerri Morris, Coordinator Information/Referral
Robert Hott, Director of Development

2780 Learning Disabilities Association of Ameri ca
4156 Library Road
Pittsburgh, PA 15234

412-341-1515
888-300-6710
Fax: 412-344-0224
e-mail: info@LDAAmerica.org
www.ldaamerica.org

Helps families of the affected individual through information and referral to professionals in their area. A membership organization with affiliates across the country.

Sheila Buckley, Executive Director

2781 March of Dimes Birth Defects Foundation
1275 Mamaroneck Avenue
White Plains, NY 10605

914-997-4488
888-663-4637
Fax: 914-997-4763
e-mail: answers@marchofdimes.com
www.marchofdimes.com

Partnership of volunteers and professionals dedicated to improving the health of babies by preventing birth defects and infant mortality. Over 100 chapters are located across the country and can be located through the National Office.

Jennifer L Howse, President

2782 Option Institute: Son Rise Program
Autism Treatment Center of America
2080 S Undermountain Road
Sheffield, MA 01257

413-229-2100
877-766-7473
Fax: 413-229-3202
e-mail: information@son-rise.org
www.son-rise.org

Describes an effective, loving and respectful method for treating children with autism. It teaches parents and healing professionals how to set up a home based program using the child's motivation to reach their special child.

Barry Neil Kaufman, Co-Founder/Co-Creator
Samahria Lyte Kaufman, Co-Founder/Co-Creator

Research Centers

2783 Dyslexia Research Institute
5746 Centerville Road
Tallahassee, FL 32309

850-893-2216
Fax: 850-893-2440
e-mail: dri@talstar.com
www.dyslexia-add.org

Searching for new and better methods to deal with the unique needs of Dyslexics.

Pat Hardman, Executive Director
Robyn A Rennick, MS, Director

Conferences

2784 ASHA Convention
American Speech-Language-Hearing Association
10801 Rockville Pike
Rockville, MD 20852

301-897-5700
800-638-8255
Fax: 301-571-0457
e-mail: productsales@asha.org
www.asha.org

The premier annual professional education event for speech-language pathologists, audiologists, and speech, language, and hearing scientists. Bringing together more than 12,000 attendees, the Convention provides unparalleled opportunities to hear the latest evidence-based research and gain new skills and resources to advance your career.

November

Arlene A Pietranton, Executive Director
Maureen E Thompson, Director Governance Operations

2785 Genetic Alliance Annual Conference
Genetic Alliance
4301 Connecticut Avenue NW, Suite 404
Washington, DC 20008

202-966-5557
800-336-4363
Fax: 202-966-8553
e-mail: info@geneticalliance.org
www.geneticalliance.org

Consistently inspirational and enables partnership among all stakeholders: advocates and community leaders, health and industry professionals, policymakers, and academicians.

July

Sharon Terry, President/CEO
Tetyana Murza, Programs/Events Manager

2786 International Dyslexia Association Conference
40 York Road, Suite 400
Baltimore, MD 21204

410-296-0232
800-222-3123
Fax: 410-321-5069
e-mail: info@interdys.org
www.interdys.org

Focuses on the latest advances in dyslexia, related language difficulties and related fields. Individual sessions are geared towards educators and educational administrators, educational diagnosticians and therapists, parents, speech and language pathologists and of course, individuals with dyslexia and their families.

Kristen Penczek, Conference Director
Darnella Parks, Conference Coordinator

2787 LDA Annual Conference
Learning Disabilities Association of America
4156 Library Road
Pittsburgh, PA 15234

412-341-1515
888-300-6710
Fax: 412-344-0224
e-mail: info@LDAAmerica.org
www.ldaamerica.org

Meeting on learning disabilities, featuring over 200 workshops and exhibits.

February

Sheila Buckley, Executive Director

Audio Video

2788 Dyslexia
Fanlight Productions
32 Court Street, 21st Floor
Brooklyn, NY 11201

718-488-8900
800-876-1710
Fax: 718-488-8642
e-mail: info@fanlight.com, orders@fanlight.com
www.fanlight.com

Looks at the experiences of people with these learning disabilities as well as the potential value to society of their alternative ways of learning. Dartmouth Hitchcock Medical Center Series, The Doctor is In...

28 minutes VHS

Nicole Johnson, Publicity Coordinator

Web Sites

2789 American Speech Language Hearing Associati on (ASHA)
2200 Research Boulevard
Rockville, MD 20850   301-296-5700
                                            800-498-2071
                                      Fax: 301-296-8580
                                      TTY: 301-296-5650
                              e-mail: nsslha@asha.org
                                          www.asha.org

An organization working to promote a better quality of life for children and adults with communication disorders. Our mission is to advance knowledge about the causes and treatment of hearing, speech, and language problems.

Judith L. Page, PhD, CCC-SLP, President
Howard Goldstein, PhD, CCC-SLP, VP for Science & Research
Arlene A. Pietranton, PhD, CAE, CEO

2790 British Dyslexia Association
Unit 8 Bracknell Beeches, Old Bracknell Lane
Bracknell, RG12   033- 40- 455
                              www.bdadyslexia.org.uk

The BDA offers a range of practical help for dyslexic children, dyslexic adults, parents and professionals in education.

Margaret Malpas, Chair of Trustees
Diana Baring, Vice President
Kevin Morley, Vice President

2791 Davis Dyslexia Association International Dyslexia: The Gift
1601 Bayshore Highway 260
Burlingame, CA 94010   650-692-7141
                                            888-999-3324
                                      Fax: 650-692-7075
            e-mail: ddai@dyslexia.com, orders@dyslexia.com
                                        www.dyslexia.com

Offers information and training in methods for overcoming learning problems developed by Ron Davis, author of 'The Gift of Dyslexia,' listings of Davis Dyslexia Correction providers worldwide, a forum for networking and articles and reports on learning styles and educational approaches.

2792 International Dyslexia Association
40 York Rd., 4th Floor
Baltimore, MD 21204   410-296-0232
                                      Fax: 410-321-5069
        e-mail: info@interdys.org, members@interdys.org
                                        www.interdys.org

Dyslexia is a neurological disorder that impairs reading. If undetected in children, it can create major learning problems. Contact the IDA for free information. Publications are available for a range of fees.

Hal Malchow, President
Ben Shifrin, M.Ed., Vice President
Elsa Cÿrdenas-Hagan, Ed.D., C, Vice President

2793 Learning Disabilities Association of Ameri ca
www.ldaamerica.org

Helps families of the affected individual through information and referral to professionals in their area. A membership organization with affiliates across the country.

2794 Mental Health Net
P.O. Box 20709
Columbus, OH 43220   614-448-4055
                                            800-232-TALK
        e-mail: info@centersite.net, editor@centersite.n
                                        www.mentalhelp.net

We wish to provide the following: to discuss, develop and debate in an open forum the future of the mental health field in America and throughout the world. To help coordinate various components of the mental health field so as to bring about greater communication between them.

2795 NIH/National Institute of Child Health and Human Development
31 Center Drive, Building 31, Room 2A32
Bethesda, MD 20892   301-496-5133
                                            800-370-2943
                                      Fax: 866-760-5947
                                      TTY: 888-320-6942
        e-mail: NICHDInformationResourceCenter@mail.nih.
                                        www.nichd.nih.gov

Established in 1962 by congress, today the institute conducts and supports research on all stages of human dveelopment to better understand the health of children, adults, families and communities. Topics of research include: birth defects, mental retardation, developmental disabilities, reproductive health, growth and development, and infant death.

Alan Guttmacher, M.D., Director

2796 Option Institute
www.son-rise.org

Describes an effective, loving and respectful method for treating children with autism. It teaches parents and healing professionals how to set up a home based program using the child's motivation to reach their special child.

Barry Neil Kaufman, Co Founder/ Senior Teacher/ Trainer
Becky Damgaard, Program Teacher
Raun K. Kaufman, Program Group Facilitator

Book Publishers

2797 Let's Talk About Dyslexia
Melanie Apel Gordon, author

Rosen Publishing Group's PowerKids Press
29 E 21st Street
New York, NY 10010   212-777-3017
                                            800-237-9932
                                      Fax: 888-436-4643
                    e-mail: rosenpub@tribeca.ios.com
                                    www.powerkidspress.com

Children will learn what dyslexia is and how to tell if they have it. This book stresses that children with dyslexia are just as smart as their classmates. Tells about Albert Einstein and other well known people who were dyslexic. Grades K-5.

24 pages
ISBN: 0-823951-99-5

2798 Misunderstood Child
Larry B Silver, MD, author

Active Parenting Publishers
1220 Kennestone Circle,Suite 130
Marietta, GA 30066   770-429-0565
                                            800-825-0060
                                      Fax: 770-429-0334
                e-mail: cservice@activeparenting.com
                                    www.activeparenting.com

The fully revised and updated must-have resource to help you become a supportive and assertive advocate for your child. The Misunderstood Child, Fourth Edition has become the go-to reference guide for families of children with learning disorders. Item #8825.

432 pages

2799 Overcoming Dyslexia in Children, Adolescents, and Adults

Dale R Jordan, author

Pro-Ed
8700 Shoal Creek Boulevard
Austin, TX 78757

512-451-3246
800-897-3202
Fax: 800-397-7633
www.proedinc.com

The third edition summarizes what science knows today about what causes the forms of dyslexia that are related to left-brain language processing. This book also discusses in detail nonverbal types of learning disabilities (LD) and social and emotional types of LD. All forms of dyslexia are described in detail with graphic illustrations of how dyslexia impacts classroom learning, social behavior, emotional maturity and development.

432 pages Softcover
ISBN: 0-890796-42-4

2800 Straight Talk about Psychological Testing for Kids

Ellen Braaten PhD, Gretcen Felopulos PhD, author

Active Parenting Publishers
1220 Kennestone Circle,Suite 130
Marietta, GA 30066

770-429-0565
800-825-0060
Fax: 770-429-0334
e-mail: cservice@activeparenting.com
www.activeparenting.com

This authoritative guide gives parents the inside scoop on how psychological testing works and how to use testing to get the best help for their children. Item #8670.

260 pages Softcover

Camps

2801 Camp Dunnabeck at Kildonan

425 Morse Hill Road
Amenia, NY 12501

845-373-8111
Fax: 845-373-2004
e-mail: info@kildonanadmissions.org
www.kildonan.org

Specializes in helping intelligent children with specific reading, writing and spelling disablities. Provides Orton-Gillingham tutoring with camp activities, including swimming, sailing, waterskiing, horseback riding, ceramics, tennis and woodworking.

Ages 9-15

Christina Lang, Chair
Richard S. Berg, Vice Chair
Kevin F. Pendergast, Headmaster

2802 Landmark School

429 Hale Street, PO Box 227
Prides Crossing, MA 1965

978-236-3010
Fax: 978-927-7268
e-mail: admission@landmarkschool.org
www.landmarkschool.org

Offers academic skill development and exciting activities for boys and girls in grades 1-12, who have been diagnosed with a language-based learning disability.

Moira M. James, Chair
Martin P. Slark, Vice Chair
Robert J. Broudo, President & Headmaster

2803 Marvelwood Summer

Marvelwood School
476 Skiff Mountain Road, PO Box 3001
Kent, CT 6757

860-927-0047
800-440-9107
Fax: 860-927-5325
e-mail: summerschool@marvelwood.org
www.themarvelwoodschool.com

The emphasis in this summer program is on diagnosis and remediation of individual reading, spelling, writing, mathematics and study problems. Participants are boys and girls entering grades 6-10.

Scott E Pottbecker, Head of School
Katherine Almquist, Summer Admissions

Description

2804 DYSTONIA

Covers these related disorders: Dopa-responsive dystonia (DRD) or Segawa syndrome, Drug-induced dystonia, Dystonia musculorum deformans (DMD) or torsion, Fecal dystonia

Involves the following Biologic System(s):

Neurologic Disorders, Orthopedic and Muscle Disorders

Dystonia is a neurologic movement disorder characterized by relatively slow, involuntary, writhing motions that may result in twisting or distorted posturing of affected muscles. The abnormal motions associated with dystonia result from unusually increased muscle rigidity due to simultaneous contractions of certain muscles termed agonists and antagonists. In unaffected individuals, when voluntary movements occur, there are usually coordinated contractions and simultaneous relaxations of several muscles. Muscles known as agonists are primarily responsible for producing a particular movement, and other muscles, called synergists, contract to assist the agonist muscles. While these muscles contract, other muscles known as antagonists normally simultaneously relax, helping to ensure smooth rather than jerky, uncoordinated motions. However, in patients with dystonia, agonist and antagonist muscles simultaneously contract, resulting in abnormally distorted movements. Depending upon the form of dystonia present, abnormal motions may vary greatly in severity and may be limited to one muscle group or may affect many muscles of the body, causing severely distorted postures and significantly interfering with activities of daily living.

Dystonias that are limited to certain specific muscle groups may be referred to as focal dystonias. Focal dystonias may be confined to muscles of the neck (cervical dystonia or spasmodic torticollis); the eyelids, causing near or complete closure of the eyelids (blepharospasm) and functional blindness; the mouth and jaw (buccomandibular dystonia); the hand (writer's cramp); or certain other areas of the body. Although such conditions are considered the most prevalent forms of dystonia, they occur much more commonly in adults than children. The main causes of dystonia during childhood include certain genetic disorders, such as dystonia musculorum deformans, dopa-responsive dystonia, Wilson disease, or Hallervorden-Spatz disease; lack of oxygen during labor, delivery, or immediately after birth (perinatal asphyxia), causing brain damage (hypoxicischemic encephalopathy); or exposure to particular medications.

The most pronounced form of dystonia is observed in a group of genetic disorders known as dystonia musculorum deformans (DMD) or torsion dystonia. One form of the disorder is thought to most commonly affect individuals of Eastern European Ashkenazi Jewish descent. Symptoms typically become apparent between the ages of six to 14 years and initially include involuntary movement or posturing of one area of the body, particularly the foot. Most patients first experience abnormal periodic bending of one foot with the toes downward (plantar flexion), potentially causing tip-toe walking. Such posturing of the foot gradually becomes constant, and muscles in other areas of the body, such as the shoulders, pelvis, and spine, begin to develop periodic, involuntary, spasmodic, twisting movements. With disease progression, spasms become frequent and, eventually, are ongoing, causing contortion and severely distorted posturing of affected muscles. Although dystonic movements may initially subside during sleep, they may eventually be present at all times, severely restricting activities of daily living and causing a high level of functional disability. Treatment may include administration of the drug trihexyphenidyl or certain other medications, such as carbamazepine, bromocriptine, levodopa, or diazepam.

Dopa-responsive dystonia (DRD), also known as Segawa syndrome, is a genetic disorder that is thought to be transmitted as an autosomal dominant trait. The disorder more commonly affects females and usually becomes apparent between four to eight years of age. Initial symptoms often include periodic, involuntary stiffening and abnormal posturing of the foot. As the disease progresses, dystonia may also eventually affect muscles of the arms, torso, and, in some patients, the neck. Within about four to five years, all areas of the body are usually affected. Some patients may also have unusually slow movements (bradykinesia) and involuntary, rhythmic movements (tremors) of certain muscles while at rest. Symptoms usually subside with sleep and gradually worsen during the day. Administration of the medication levodopa, a biological forerunner or precursor of the neurotransmitter dopamine, typically causes a dramatic improvement of symptoms.

Wilson disease is an autosomal recessive disorder in which copper metabolism causes an abnormal accumulation of copper in the liver, brain, kidneys, corneas, and other tissues of the body. The disorder is often characterized by progressive liver disease, degenerative changes of the brain, kidney failure, and the presence of characteristic grayish-green or reddish-gold rings at the outer margins of the corneas (Kayser-Fleischer rings). Neurologic symptoms, which rarely become apparent before age 10, are thought to result from progressive involvement of a region of the brain that assists in regulating muscular movements (basal ganglia). Such symptoms usually initially include progressive dystonia that is characterized by abnormalities of muscle tone, muscle stiffness and rigidity, muscle spasms, and abnormal movement patterns and fixed postures, such as a fixed smile due to drawing back of the upper lip. Patients also experience involuntary, rhythmic, quivering movements of the extremities on one side of the body (unilateral) that eventually become generalized and disabling. The treatment of patients with Wilson disease often consists of administration of penicillamine, a medication that binds with copper and enables it to be excreted from the body; supplementation of vitamin B6; and a diet that is low in copper intake (less than one mg/day).

Hallervorden-Spatz disease is a rare autosomal recessive disorder characterized by an abnormal accumulation of iron pigment in certain areas of the brain. Symptoms usually develop during childhood and may include progressive dystonia characterized by muscle stiffness, rigidity, and relatively slow, involuntary, twisting and distorted posturing of affected muscles. By adolescence, patients may have restricted movements of certain muscles due to increased muscle rigidity (spasticity); an inability to coordinate voluntary movements (ataxia); difficulty speaking (dysarthria); and progressive confusion, disorientation, and deterioration of intellectual abilities (dementia). The treatment of patients with Hallervorden-Spatz disease is symptomatic and supportive.

In some children, the administration of certain drugs may

Award-winning video presentation explores the causes and effects of bulimia. Addresses the fact that many high school and college women view this type of behavior as routine aspect of their everyday lives.

Videotape

Carolyn Baxley, President

2919 Eating Disorder Video
Library Video
PO Box 580
Wynnewood, PA 19096   610-645-4000
                             800-843-3620
                        Fax: 610-645-4040
        e-mail: comments@libraryvideo.com
                    www.libraryvideo.com

Features compelling interviews with several young people who have suffered from anorexia nervosa, bulimia and compulsive eating. Discusses the treatments, causes, and techniques for prevention with field experts.

2920 Inside Out: Stories of Bulimia
Fanlight Productions
32 Court Street, 21st Floor
Brooklyn, NY 11201   718-488-8900
                            800-876-1710
                       Fax: 718-488-8642
   e-mail: info@fanlight.com, orders@fanlight.com
                       www.fanlight.com

Bulimia can affect women and men from all walks of life, and it kills nearly 20 percent of its victims every year. This moving documentary profilesindividuals and families affected by this eating disorder. ISBN: DVD: 1-57295-856-1; VHS: 1-57295-366-7

56 minutes DVD or VHS

Ben Achtenberg, President
Sandy St. Louis, Marketing Director
Nicole Johnson, Publicity Coordinator

2921 It Only Takes One Bite: Food Allergy and Anaphylaxis
Food Allergy Network
7925 Jones Branch Dr., Suite 1100
McLean, VA 22102   703-691-3179
                          800-929-4040
                     Fax: 703-691-2713
      e-mail: faan@foodallergy.org
               www.foodallergy.org/

Nonprofit organization dedicated to bringing about a clearer understanding of the issues surrounding food allergies and providing helpful resources. Explains food induced anaphylaxis and how to live with it. An excellent resource for training parents, teachers, caregivers and patients.

18 mins.

Janet Atwater, Chair
Robert Nichols, Vice Chair
James R. Baker, Jr., MD, CEO & Chief Medical Officer

Web Sites

2922 Anorexia Nervosa and Related Eating Disorders
www.anred.com

We are a nonprofit organization that provides information about anorexia nervosa, bulimia nervosa, binge eating disorder, and other less-well-known food and weight disorders. Our material includes self-help tips and information about recovery and prevention.

2923 Eating Disorders Online.com: 15 Styles of Distorted Thinking
www.eatingdisordersonline.com/specific/disthink.php

Reference useful for cognitive therapy.

2924 Food Allergy Network
7925 Jones Branch Dr., Suite 1100
McLean, VA 22102   703-691-3179
                          800-929-4040
                     Fax: 703-691-2713
               www.foodallergy.org

Mission is to raise public awareness, to provide advocacy and education, and to advance research on behalf of all those affected by food allergies and anaphylaxis.

Janet Atwater, Chair
Robert Nichols, Vice Chair
James R. Baker, Jr., MD, CEO & Chief Medical Officer

2925 Gurze Bookstore
www.bulimia.com

                          888-920-1501
                          www.bulimia.com

Specializes in information about eating disorders including anorexia nervosa, bulimia nervosa, and binge eating, plus related topics such as body image and obesity. We offer books at discounted prices, many free articles about eating disorders, newsletters, links to treatment facilities, organizations, other websites and much more.

2926 Health Answers
410 Horsham Road
Horsham, PA 19044   215-422-9010
        e-mail: Michael.tague@healthanswers.com
                    www.healthanswers.com

HealthAnswers offers a breadth of services in medical education, sales force training, patient support, solutions, professional promotion and consumer solutions.

Michael Tague, Managing Director

2927 Mental Help Net- Eating Disorders
P.O. Box 20709
Columbus, OH 43220   614-448-4055
                            800-232-TALK
   e-mail: info@centersite.net, editor@centersite.n
        www.mentalhelp.net/guide/eating.htm

We wish to provide the following: to discuss, develop and debate in an open forum the future of the mental health field in America and throughout the world. To help coordinate various components of the mental health field, so as to bring about greater communication between them and to educate the public about mental health issues.

2928 Mirror, Mirror
www.mirror-mirror.org/eatdis.htm

Helps with eating disorders, like how to get help, myths and realities, other websites, and about recovery.

Scott Mogul, Director
Dr. Lauren Muhlheim, Clinical Director
Dr. Elisha Carcieri, Editor

2929 National Association for Anorexia Nervosa and Associated Disorders (ANAD)
750 E Diehl Road #127
Naperville, IL 60563   630-577-1330
                     e-mail: anadhelp@anad.org
                              www.anad.org

We provide hotline counseling, a national network of free support groups, referrals to health care professionals, and education and prevention programs to promote self-acceptance and health lifesyles. All of our services are free of charge. ANAD also lobbies for state and national health insurance parity, undertakes and encourages advocacy campaigns to protect potential victims of eating disorders. ANAD stands with individuals and families and helps them win.

Patricia Santucci, MD, President
Kimberly Dennis, MD, Member, Scientific & Medical Board
Nomi Fredricks, MD, Member, Scientific & Medical Board

2930 Something Fishy
www.something-fishy.org

Dedicated to raising awareness, emphasizing always that Eating Disorders are NOT about food and weight, they are just the symptoms of something deeper going on, inside. We are determined to remind each and every sufferer that they are not alone, and that complete recovery is possible.

Book Publishers

2931 Anorexia Nervosa & Recovery: A Hunger for Meaning
The Haworth Press
10 Alice Street
Binghamton, NY 13904 607-771-0012
800-895-0582
e-mail: getinfo@haworthpress.com
www.haworthpress.com/

Anorexia Nervosa and Recovery lets the reader hear the personal struggles of women who have fought this powerful disease. They describe how anorexia controlled their lives and how, once they overcame their obsessions with food, weight, and thinness, they were able to lead fulfilling lives.

1993 142 pages Paperback
ISBN: 0-918393-95-7

William Cohen, President/Publisher
Al Horowitz, Chief Financial Officer
Sandra Jones Sickels, VP Marketing

2932 Billy's Story
Overeaters Anonymous World Service Office
PO Box 44020
Rio Rancho, NM 87174 505-891-2664
Fax: 505-891-4320
e-mail: info@oa.org
www.oa.org/

An inspirational story written for younger children suffering from eating disorders and weight problems.

Naomi Lippel, Managing Director
Sarah Armstrong, Associate Director
Rebbie Garza, Board Administrator

2933 Body Betrayed
Gurze Books
5145 B Avenida Encinas, PO Box 2238
Carlsbad, CA 92008 760-434-7533
800-756-7533
Fax: 760-434-5476
e-mail: leigh@gurze.net
www.gurze.com

Covers the most important aspects of diagnosis and treatment for eating disorders. Particularly appropriate for parents and loved ones who want a deeper, more thorough understanding of eating disorders.

447 pages Paperback

Kathryn J Zerbe, Author
Leigh Cohn, Publisher
Lindsey Hall Cohn, Editor in Chief

2934 Bulimia Nervosa & Binge Eating: A Guide to Recovery
New York University Press
838 Broadway, Third Floor
New York, NY 10003 212-998-2575
800-996-6987
Fax: 212-995-3833
e-mail: information@nyupress.org
www.nyupress.nyu.edu

Book offers guidance and advice for the understanding of the eating disorder bulimia and inspiring hope for change and regaining control of one's life.

1995 170 pages
ISBN: 0-814715-23-0

Steve Maikowski, Director
Ilene Kalish, Executive Editor
Eric Zinner, Editor-in-Chief

2935 Bulimia: A Guide to Recovery
Gurze Books
5145 B Avenida Encinas, PO Box 2238
Carlsbad, CA 92008 760-434-7533
800-756-7533
Fax: 760-434-5476
e-mail: leigh@gurze.net
www.gurze.com

This intimate guidebook offers a complete understanding of bulimia and a plan for recovery. Contains updated information from previous editions, and has added material on men and bulimia, sexual trauma, body image, relationships and much more.

285 pages Paperback

Lindsey Hall, Author
Leigh Cohn, Author

2936 Conversation with Anorexics: A Compassionate & Hopeful Journey
Rowman & Littlefield Publisher
4501 Forbes Blvd, Suite 200
Lanham, MD 20706 301-459-3366
Fax: 301-429-5748
e-mail: custserv@rowman.com
www.rowmanlittlefield.com/aronsonp/

Book is a collection of case studies on anorexia more aptly geared toward the professional as it does not provide guidance but more of an overview on the treatment of the eating disorder.

1994 238 pages Paperback
ISBN: 1-568212-61-5

Jonathan Sisk, Publisher
Christopher Anzalone, Washington Editor
Jack Meinhardt, Acquisitions Editor

2937 Coping with Eating Disorders
Rosen Publishing Group
29 East 21st Street
New York, NY 10010 212-777-3017
800-237-9932
Fax: 888-436-4643
e-mail: rosenpub@tribeca.ios.com
www.rosenpublishing.com/

This book offers practical suggestions on coping with eating disorders, explaining how to set positive goals, and briefly discusses where to go for additional help.

ISBN: 0-823929-74-4

Miriam Gilbert, Sales and Marketing Director

2938 Cult of Thinness
Oxford University Press
198 Madison Avenue
New York, NY 10016 212-726-6000
800-445-9714
Fax: 919-677-1303
e-mail: custserv.us@oup.com
www.oup.com/usa

Examining the testimonies of young women concerning the practice of body rituals, the author Hesse-Biber observes the extent to which these women sacrifice their bodies and minds to the pursuit of the ultra-slender ideal. Hesse-Biber provides new frameworks for envisioning femininity and personal power, overcoming body insecurity, strengthening the inner self, and changing the cultural environment itself.

1996 256 pages
ISBN: 0-195178-78-5

Joan Bossert, Psych/Behavioral Sciences Editor
Catharine Carlin, Health Psychology Editor

2939 Deadly Diet: Recovering From Anorexia and Bulimia
New Harbinger Publications
5674 Shattuck Avenue
Oakland, CA 94609 510-652-0215
800-748-6273
Fax: 800-652-1613
e-mail: customerservice@newharbinger.com
www.newharbinger.com

This book provides the reader with a great discussion of the use of cognitive-behavioral therapy in the treatment of eating disorders. The author also provides the reader with a step-by-step guide to implementing this approach in his or her own life during recovery from an eating disorder.

1993 248 pages Paperback
ISBN: 1-879237-42-3

Matthew McKay, Ph.D, Publisher
Earlita Chenault, Publicist

2940 Do I Look Fat in This?: Life Doesn't Begin Five Pounds From Now
Simon & Schuster Free Press
866 3rd Avenue
New York, NY 10022
877-989-0009
Fax: 800-943-9831
www.simonsays.com

For any woman who has bonded with a stranger by complaining about how fat she feels, here is a thoughtful and inspiring guide to breaking the cycle of body criticism and creating a powerful and healthy self-image.

2006 200 pages
ISBN: 1-416913-57-2

Jack Romanos, President/CEO
David England, SVP/Chief Financial Officer
Anne Lloyd Davies, SVP/Chief Information Officer

2941 Eating Disorder Sourcebook
Gurze Books
5145 B Avenida Encinas, PO Box 2238
Carlsbad, CA 92008
760-434-7533
800-756-7533
Fax: 760-434-5476
e-mail: leigh@gurze.net
www.gurze.com

This third edition is a welcomed revision and update of this popular reference guide for both the lay public and professionals.

328 pages Paperback

Carolyn Costin, Author

2942 Eating Disorders
Thomson Gale
PO Box 95501
Chicago, IL 60694
800-877-4253
Fax: 800-414-5043
e-mail: gale.galeord@cengage.com
www.gale.com/lucent/index.htm

This book examines how eating disorders can be identified, who is affected by them, and how they can be treated.

1991
ISBN: 1-560061-29-4

Andrew Becker, Director
John Barnes, EVP Strategic Business Development

2943 Eating Disorders & Obesity, 2nd Ed.
Guilford Press
72 Spring Street
New York, NY 10012
212-431-9800
800-365-7006
Fax: 212-966-6708
e-mail: info@guilford.com
www.guilford.com

Presents and integrates virtually all that is currently known about eating disorders and obesity in one authorative, accessible, and eminently practical volume. A comprehensive handbook for medical and social service professionals. Hard- or paperback.

2005 633 pages Paperback
ISBN: 1-593852-36-8

Robert Matloff, President
Seymoure Weingarten, Editor-in-Chief
Marian Robinson, Marketing Director

2944 Eating Disorders Resource Catalogue
Gurze Books
5145 B Avenida Encinas, PO Box 2238
Carlsbad, CA 92008
760-434-7533
800-756-7533
Fax: 760-434-5476
e-mail: leigh@gurze.net
www.gurze.com/

This catalogue of resources contains over 140 books, videos, and audiotapes, lists of national organizations and treatment facilities, and basic facts about eating disorders. It is widely distributed by individuals who are suffering, their loved-ones, the health care professionals who treat them, and educators who are working towards prevention.

24 pages Annually

Lindsey Hall, Editor in Chief
Leigh Cohn, Publisher

2945 Eating Disorders: When Food Turns Against You
Franklin Watts c/o Grolier
90 Old Sherman Turnpike
Danbury, CT 06816
203-797-3500
Fax: 203-797-3197
www.grolier.com

Anorexia nervosa and bulimia are specifically examined, including a listing of the danger signals of each. A final chapter suggests places to secure help.

1993 96 pages
ISBN: 0-531111-75-0

Richard Robinson, President/Chairman/CEO
Mary Winston, EVP/Chief Financial Officer
Jeffrey Mathews, VP/Investor Relations

2946 Encyclopedia of Obesity and Eating Disorders
Facts on File
132 West 31st Street, 17th Floor
New York, NY 10001
212-967-8800
800-322-8755
Fax: 800-678-3633
e-mail: custserv@factsonfile.com
www.factsonfile.com/

This revised and expanded edition includes more than 450 entries, more than 140 of them new. Complete with a history of obesity and eating disorders; chronology of key events, research, and breakthroughs; tables listing key facts and statistics; and a directory of resources and Web sites, this single-volume reference is the first stop in any serious research of these troubling health afflictions.

2006 384 pages Hardcover
ISBN: 0-816061-97-1

Laurie Katz, Publicity Director
Coreena Schultz, Library Sales Director
T J Mancini, Production Director

2947 Endorphins: Eating Disorders & Other Addictive Behavior
WW Norton & Company
500 5th Avenue
New York, NY 10110
212-354-5500
Fax: 212-869-0856
www.wwnorton.com

Dr. Huebner discusses anorexia nervosa and bulimia as addictions to endorphins, and presents a treatment model involving education about the addictive process, cognitive/behavioral strategies, and psychotherapy. He then reveals the role of endorphin addiction in other compulsive behaviors such as obsessive exercise, religious fanaticism, and cult involvement.

1993 320 pages
ISBN: 0-393701-56-5

William Drake McFeely, President

2948 Fear of Being Fat
Rowman & Littlefield Publishers
4501 Forbes Blvd, Suite 200
Lanham, MD 20706
301-459-3366
Fax: 301-429-5748
www.rowmanlittlefield.com/aronsonj/

This book, which presents one psychoanalytic approach to the treatment of anorexia nervosa, has been written by a number of authors, all members of the Psychosomatic Study Group of the Psychoanalytic Association of New York. The theoretical positions and therapeutic approaches are, consequently, conclusions based on extensive clinical experience acquired over many years. Geared more for the professional.

366 pages
ISBN: 0-876688-99-7

Thomas Koerner, Ph.D, VP/Editorial Director
Wanda Mathews, Marketing Manager

2949 Food for Recovery
Crown Publishing Group/Random House
280 Park Avenue
New York, NY 10017
212-572-6117
Fax: 212-940-7868
e-mail: crownpublicity@randomhouse.com
www.randomhouse.com/

Written for those in recovery from alcohol and drug abuse and eating disorders, this is an excellent basic book on nutrition. Beasley, director of a clinic that focuses on addictive diseases and nutritional medicine, and Knightly, a faculty member of Manhattan's Natural Gourmet Cooking School, discuss nutrition basics and explain how to select wholesome, unprocessed food.

1994 374 pages
ISBN: 0-517586-94-0

Jenny Frost, President/Publisher
Tina Constable, VP/Publicity Executive Director

2950 Getting Better Bit(e) by Bit(e)
Gurze Books
5145 B Avenida Encinas, PO Box 2238
Carlsbad, CA 92008
760-434-7533
800-756-7533
Fax: 760-434-5476
e-mail: leigh@gurze.net
www.gurze.com

Written by specialists from London, the author's addresses the day-to-day problems faced by bulimia and binge eating sufferers and key behavior changes for progress.

143 pages Paperback

Ulrike Schmidt, Author
Janet Treasure, Author

2951 Group Psychotherapy for Eating Disorders
American Psychiatric Press
1000 Wilson Boulevard, Suite 1825
Arlington, VA 22209
703-907-7322
800-368-5777
Fax: 703-907-1091
e-mail: appi@psych.org
www.appi.org/

The first book to fully explore the use of group therapy in the treatment of eating disorders.

353 pages Hardcover
ISBN: 0-880484-19-5

Robert E Hales, MD, Editor-in-Chief
Ron McMillen, Chief Executive Officer
John McDuffie, Editorial Director

2952 Hope and Recovery: A Mother-Daughter Story About Anorexia Nervosa & Bulimia
Franklin Watts
90 Old Sherman Turnpike
Danbury, CT 06816
800-621-1115
e-mail: custserv@scholastic.com
www.scholastic.com/aboutscholastic/

Mother and daughter tell a story of a young woman's recovery from the horror of an eating disorder. This compelling account shows how anorexia and bulimia can affect an entire family.

192 pages
ISBN: 0-531111-40-7

Richard Robinson, Chairman/President/CEO
Mary A Winston, EVP/Chief Financial Officer
Lisa Holton, EVP/Book Fairs and Trade Shows

2953 How to get Your Kid to Eat...
Bull Publishing
PO Box 1377
Boulder, CO 80306
800-676-2855
Fax: 303-545-6354
e-mail: bullpublishing@msn.com
www.bullpub.com

Touches on the various reasons for a child not wanting to eat, as well as continuos snacking, and not eating vegetables.

408 pages
ISBN: 0-915950-83-9

Jim Bull, Publisher

2954 I Was a Fifteen-Year-Old Blimp
Harper & Row
10 East 53rd Street
New York, NY 10022
212-207-7000
www.harpercollins.com/

This story focuses on Gabby, a teenage girl who overhears others discuss her weight and takes radical steps to become popular.

Grades 6-9

Jane Friedman, President/CEO
Lisa Herling, SVP/Corporate Communications
Brian Murray, Group President

2955 Insights in the Dynamic Psychotherapy of Anorexia And Bulimia
Rowman & Littlefield Publishers
4501 Forbes Blvd, Suite 200
Lanham, MD 20706
301-459-3366
Fax: 301-429-5748
www.rowmanlittlefield.com/

Discusses the eating disorders of anorexia and bulimia providing an overview of the dynamics in diagnosing the disease in addition to developmental and sociocultural issues, therapy and hospitalization.

320 pages Hardcover
ISBN: 0-876685-68-8

Shiela Burnett, Vice President/Marketing Director
Christopher Anzalone, Washington Editor/Director
Jack Meinhardt, Acquisitions Editor

2956 Life Beyond Your Eating Disorder
Johana S. Kandel, author

Harlequin
PO Box 5190
Buffalo, NY 14240
888-432-4879
e-mail: cutomerservice@harlequin.com
www.harlequin.com

With the collaboration of professionals in the field of eating disorders, the author developed a set of practical tools to address the everyday challenges of recovery.

ISBN: 0-373892-26-6

2957 Making Peace with Food
Gurze Books
5145 B Avenida Encinas, PO Box 2238
Carlsbad, CA 92008
760-434-7533
800-756-7533
Fax: 760-434-5476
e-mail: leigh@gurze.net
www.gurze.com

Filled with ideas, workbook pages, exercises, and resources, Kano's book is an excellent aid to clarifying and overcoming your personal diet/weight struggle.

224 pages Paperback

Susan Kano, Author

2958 Management of Eating Disorders and Obesity
Humana Press Scientific and Medical Publishers
999 Riverview Drive, Suite 208
Totowa, NJ 07512
973-256-1699
Fax: 973-256-8341
e-mail: humana@humanapr.com
www.humanapress.com/

Stressing human physiology, treatment, and disease prevention, the authors take advantage of the new molecular understanding of the biological regulation of energy. Updated chapters review specific evidence-based and future treatment modalities, present an objective evaluation of the treatment, and identify the positives and negatives that have been seen during clinical studies, as well as cumulative data derived from clinical practice.

2004 448 pages Hardcover
ISBN: 1-588293-41-6

Paul Dolgert, Editorial Director
Ellie Shaw, Developmental Editor
Robin Weisberg, Director Editorial Services

2959 Meals Without Squeals Sense
Bull Publishing
PO Box 1377
Boulder, CO 80306   800-676-2855
                                    Fax: 303-545-6354
                      e-mail: bullpublishing@msn.com
                                      www.bullpub.com

Straightforward information on childrens, growth accompanies
age-specific, child-tested recipes. Explained is how common feeding problems can be solved and show ways to offer children positive experiences with food.

288 pages
ISBN: 0-923521-39-9

Jim Bull, Publisher/President

2960 Overeaters Anonymous
World Service Office
PO Box 44020
Rio Rancho, NM 87174   505-891-2664
                                    Fax: 505-891-4320
                            e-mail: nlippel@oa.org
                                        www.oa.org/

World Service Office offers literature, provides information or
meetings world wide. Free sample of Lifeline Magazine available.

204 pages Hardcover

Naomi Lippel, Managing Director
Sarah Armstrong, Associate Director
Rebbie Garza, Board Administrator

2961 Practice Guidelines for Eating Disorders
American Psychiatric Publishing
1000 Wilson Boulevard, Suite 1825
Arlington, VA 22209   703-907-7322
                                       800-368-5777
                                    Fax: 703-907-1091
                         e-mail: appi@psych.org
                              www.appi.org/books.cfx

Designed for health care professionals, this guideline includes information on all aspects of anorexia nervosa and bulimia nervosa,
including self-induced vomiting, use of laxatives and vigorous
exercise to prevent weight gain.

38 pages Paperback
ISBN: 0-890423-00-8

Robert S Pursell, Marketing
John McDuffie, Product Information
Aimee Aponte, Technology/Webmaster

**2962 Self-Starvation: from Individual to Family Therapy in the
Treatment of Anorexia Ne**

rvosa, author

Rowman & Littlefield Publishers
4501 Forbes Blvd, Suite 200
Lanham, MD 20706   301-459-3366
                                    Fax: 301-429-5748
                        e-mail: custserv@rowman.com
                             www.rowmanlittlefield.com/

Discusses the eating disorder anorexia nervosa and how it affects
both the individual and family members alike, including information on possible treatment options.

1978 296 pages Hardcover
ISBN: 0-876683-10-3

Sheila Burnett, Marketing
Jack Meinhardt, Acquisitions Editor
Christopher Anzalone, Washington Editor/Director

2963 Starving to Death in a Sea of Objects
Rowman & Littlefield Publishers
4501 Forbes Blvd, Suite 200
Lanham, MD 20706   301-459-3366
                                    Fax: 301-429-5748
                         e-mail: custserv@rowan.com
                              www.rowmanlittlefield.com

How emanciation becomes security for anorexics.

464 pages Softcover
ISBN: 0-876684-35-5

Sheila Burnett, Marketing
Jack Meinhardt, Acquisitions Editor
Christopher Anzalone, Washington Editor/Director

2964 Surviving an Eating Disorder
Gurze Books
5145 B Avenida Encinas, PO Box 2238
Carlsbad, CA 92008   760-434-7533
                                       800-756-7533
                                    Fax: 760-434-5476
                             e-mail: leigh@gurze.net
                                       www.gurze.com

Discusses the psychological and behavioral aspects of eating disorders, pharmacology, and family therapy, with an emphasis on
bringing eating disorders out in the open, seeking help, coping
with anger and denial, developing a healthier relationship, and
guidance for making the situation better - now.

222 pages Paperback

Michelle Siegel PhD, Author
Judith Brisman PhD, Author
Margot Weinshel PhD, Author

2965 Treating Bulimia: A Psychoeducational Approach
American Anorexia/Bulimia Association
4200 Monument Avenue
Philadelpha, PA 19131   215-877-2000
                            e-mail: jbsmje@epix.net
                               www.aabaphila.org/

Book discusses the eating disorder bulimia focusing on utlizing
the multifaceted treatment approach through the incorporation of
education, self-monitoring, goal setting, assertion training, relaxation, and cognitive restructuring.

ISBN: 0-080323-99-5

Randi E Wirth, Ph.D, Executive Director

2966 Twelve Steps of Overeaters Anonymous
Overeaters Anonymous World Service Office
PO Box 44020
Rio Rancho, NM 87174   505-891-2664
                                    Fax: 505-891-4320
                            e-mail: nlippel@oa.org
                                        www.oa.org/

The ideas expressed in the Twelve Steps, which originated in Alcoholics Anonymous, reflect practical experience and application
of spiritual insights recorded by thinkers throughout the ages.
Their greatest importance lies in the fact that they work! They enable compulsive overeaters and millions of other Twelve-Step-
pers to lead happy, productive lives. They represent the
foundation upon which Overeaters Anonymous is built.

Naomi Lippel, Managing Director
Sarah Armstrong, Associate Director
Rebbie Garza, Board Administrator

2967 When Food is Love
Gurze Books
5145 B Avenida Encinas, PO Box 2238
Carlsbad, CA 92008   760-434-7533
                                       800-756-7533
                                    Fax: 760-434-5476
                             e-mail: leigh@gurze.net
                                       www.gurze.com

Roth's personal sharing in this book is both courageous and un-
forgettable. Explores similarities between eating and loving by
exploring topics such as fantasizing, wanting the forbidden, creating drama, control issues, being strong in the broken places,
and relationships.

205 pages Paperback
Geneen Roth, Author

2968 Withering Child
University of Georgia Press
320 South Jackson Street
Athens, GA 30602
404-542-2830
Fax: 706-542-6770
e-mail: books@ugapress.uga.edu
www.uga.edu/ugapress

Non-fiction book of a parents' struggle with their son and his diagnosis of borderline attention deficit disorder, therapy and his eventual return to school.
1993 288 pages
ISBN: 0-820315-60-5
Nicole Mitchell, Administrative Director
Lane Stewart, Development Director
John McLeod, Marketing Director

Journals

2969 BASH Magazine
Bulimia Anorexia Self-Help/Behavior Adaptation
6125 Clayton Avenue, Suite 215
Saint Louis, MO 63139
314-567-4080
800-227-4785
www.caringonline.com/eatdis/treatment.htm

A journal of eating and mood disorders.
Monthly

2970 Internal Journal of Eating Disorders
Wiley
350 Main Street
Malden, MA 02148
781-388-8598
800-835-6770
e-mail: cs-journals@wiley.com
www.onlinelibrary.wiley.com

In an effort to advance the scientific knowledge needed for understanding, treating and preventing eating disorders, the IJED publishes rigorously evaluated, high-quality manuscripts for distribution through print and electronic platforms.

2971 Journal of the American Dietetic Associati On
Elsevier Inc.
1600 John F. Kennedy Blvd. - Suite 1800
Philadelphia, PA 19103
215-239-3362
800-654-2452
Fax: 314-447-8029
e-mail: journalcustomerservice-usa@elsevier.com
www.adajournal.org

The American Dietetic Association is a source for accurate, credible and timely food and nutrition information.

Newsletters

2972 AABA Newsletter
American Anorexic and Bulimia Association
PO Box 27156
Philadelphia, PA 19118
215-221-1864
e-mail: mail.aabaphila@yahoo.com
www.aabaphila.org/

The American Anorexia Bulimia Association is a national, non-profit organization dedicated to the prevention and treatment of eating disorders. Publishes a monthly newsletter.
Randi E Wirth, Ph.D, Executive Director

2973 Eating Disorders Review
Gurze Books
PO Box 2238
Carlsbad, CA 92018
760-434-7533
800-756-7533
Fax: 760-434-5476
e-mail: leigh@gurze.net
www.gurze.com

Presents current clinical information for the professional treating eating disorders. Review features summaries of relevant research of journals and unpublished studies
8 pages Bimonthly
Joel Yager MD, Editor-in-Chief
Leigh Hall, Co Founder
Leigh Cohn, Co Founder

2974 Food Allergy News
Food Allergy & Anaphylaxis Network
7925 Jones Branch Dr., Suite 1100
McLean, VA 22102
703-691-3179
800-929-4040
Fax: 703-691-2713
e-mail: faan@foodallergy.org
www.foodallergy.org/

Contains tips for parents, including notices on ingredients in various foods, and recipes are published annually.
Bimonthly
Janet Atwater, Chair
Robert Nichols, Vice Chair
James R. Baker, Jr., MD, CEO & Chief Medical Officer

2975 Working Together
Anorexia Nervosa and Associated Disorders
750 E Diehl Road #127
Naperville, IL 60563
630-577-1330
Fax: 847-433-4632
e-mail: anadhelp@anad.org
www.anad.org

Designed for individuals, families, group leaders and professionals concerned with eating disorders. Provides updates on treatments, resources, conferences, programs, articles by therapists, recovered victims, group members and leaders.
Quarterly
Patricia Santucci, MD, President
Kimberly Dennis, MD, Member, Scientific & Medical Board
Nomi Fredricks, MD, Member, Scientific & Medical Board

Pamphlets

2976 Applying New Attitudes & Directions
Anorexia Nervosa and Associated Disorders
750 E Diehl Road #127
Naperville, IL 60563
630-577-1330
Fax: 847-433-4632
e-mail: anadhelp@anad.org
www.anad.org

Self-help booklet offering an eight-step program to recovery with suggestions, information and recovery stories.
Patricia Santucci, MD, President
Kimberly Dennis, MD, Member, Scientific & Medical Board
Nomi Fredricks, MD, Member, Scientific & Medical Board

2977 Body Image
ETR Associates
100 Enterprise Way, Suite G300
Scotts Valley, CA 95066
800-620-8884
Fax: 831-438-4284
e-mail: customerservice@etr.org
www.etr.org

Discusses the difference between healthy and disorted body image; the link between poor body image and low self esteem; five point list to help people check out their own body image.
Dan McCormick, CEO
David Kitchen, MBA, CFO
Matt McDowell, BS, Director, Marketing

Description

2978 ECTODERMAL DYSPLASIAS
Synonyms: Christ-Siemens-Touraine Syndrome, Clouston
Syndrome
Involves the following Biologic System(s):
Dental Disorders, Dermatologic Disorders

Ectodermal dysplasia is the term used to describe a large
group of hereditary disorders in which there are defects in
two or more body structures or organs derived from the
body's outermost later of cells, known as the ectoderm. These
body structures include the central nervous system, consisting
of the brain and spinal cord, and the eyes, ears, lips, teeth,
hair, sweat glands of the skin (sebaceous glands), nails, and
mucous membranes that line the mouth and nose.

There are more than 150 different kinds of ectodermal
dysplasia, all of which stem from aberrations or mutations in
genes. Because they originate in genes, the conditions included by the term ectodermal dysplasia are typically transmitted from parents to their offspring, and inherited.
However, they may also arise directly, from gene mutations
occurring prenatally in an individual's own cells. Each of the
various kinds of ectodermal dysplasia is present at birth, and
although their effects are not usually seen in newborn infants,
and may not become apparent until later in infancy or childhood, none of the different kinds of ectodermal dysplasia progresses or becomes more severe with growth. Ectodermal
dysplasia may also occur as an integral part of syndromes in
which it is accompanied by other disorders.

The manifestations and symptoms of a particular kinds of
ectodermal dysplasia depend on the body structures it affects
and the degree to which it affects them. Diminished tear flow
(xerophthalmia) and conjunctivitis, diminished salivation
(xerostomia), irritation and soreness of the nose and throat
from deficient production of mucus, high body temperatures
and fever from deficient sweat loss, cleft palate or cleft lip,
missing fingers or toes, and webbings of skin between fingers
and toes are among the effects of various ectodermal
dysplasias and of syndromes of which these dysplasias are a
part.

The two most common types of ectodermal dysplasia are
X-linked recessive anhydrotic or hypohidrotic ectodermal
dysplasia (Christ-Siemens-Touraine syndrome) and hidrotic
ectodermal dysplasia (Clouston syndrome). The first of these
syndromes is usually inherited as an X-linked recessive trait
that is transmitted along with the X or female sex chromosome and is fully expressed in boys; however, some children
may inherit anhidrotic or hypohidrotic ectodermal dysplasia
as an autosomal recessive trait that affects boys and girls in
equal numbers. This type of ectodermal dysplasia is characterized by absent (aplastic) or underdeveloped (hypoplastic)
sweat glands, dental irregularities such as absent or
widely-spaced, cone-shaped teeth, and sparse, light-colored
hair (hypotrichosis). Facial features of this condition may include a large chin; thick lips; bulging forehead (frontal bossing); flat nasal bridge; prominent, low-set ears; and wrinkled,
dark skin around the eyes. Children with this form of
ectodermal dysplasia may be at increased risk for gastrointestinal infections as well as potentially life-threatening respiratory infections.

The second most common form of ectodermal dysplasia,
hidrotic ectodermal dysplasia, also known as Clouston's syndrome, is inherited as an autosomal dominant trait, and is
characterized by defective or absent nails, thickening of the
skin on the palms of the hands and soles of the feet (pal-
mar/plantar hyperkeratosis), and sparse hair. Other findings
may include abnormally increased coloration of the skin over
major joints and the development of unusually small teeth
that are prone to decay. Treatment is symptomatic and supportive.

Prominent among syndromes of which ectodermal dysplasia
is a part is EEC (ectrodactyly-ectodermal dysplasia-clefting)
syndrome (EEC), which is inherited as an autosomal dominant trait. Symptoms and physical findings associated with
this disorder are variable and may include lightly-pigmented
skin, sparse hair and eyebrows, absent eyelashes, a split or
opening (cleft) in the lip and palate, defective nails, tear duct
irregularities, and absence of all or part of one or more fingers or toes (ectrodactyly). Other findings may include deafness and irregularities of the teeth, eyes, and urinary tract.

The treatment of ecotdermal dysplasia is focused on the
structures its affects. Parents and caregivers are counseled to
protect children from high environmental temperatures to
avoid excessive loss of body water. Consumption of fluids
and air conditioning are useful to patients who do not sweat
or have deficient sweating. Artificial tears and nasal sprays
may be used to ease drying of the membranes of the eyes and
nose. Ointments and creams may be useful for relieving drying or scaling of the skin or scalp, as may antibiotic ointments to prevent or treat infection. Dentures and dental
implants may be used to replace teeth affected by ectodermal
dysplasia, and surgery may be done to correct cleft palate and
deformities of the feet and hands. Genetic counseling is
recommended for advising the parents of children with
ectodermal dysplasia about the chance of the condition
recurring in subsequent children.

Government Agencies

**2979 NIH/National Institute of Arthritis and Mu sculoskeletal and
Skin Diseases**
1 AMS Circle
Bethesda, MD 20892   301-402-4484
                                                         877-226-4267
                                                    Fax: 301-718-6366
                                                    TDD: 301-565-2966
                                         e-mail: niamsinfo@mail.nih.gov
                                                     www.niams.nih.gov

The mission of the NIAMS, a part of the NIH, is to support research into the causes, treatment and prevention of arthritis and
musculoskeletal and skin diseases, the training of basic and clinical scientists to carry out this research, and the dissemination of
information on research progress in these diseases.
Stephen I Katz MD PhD, Director
Robert H Carter MD, Deputy Director

2980 NIH/National Institute of Dental and Crani ofacial Research
National Institutes of Health
31 Center Drive, MSC 2290, Building 31
Bethesda, MD 20892   301-496-4261
                                                    Fax: 301-402-2185
                                         e-mail: nidcrinfo@mail.nih.gov
                                                      www.nidcr.nih.gov

Provides leadership for a national research program designed to
understand, treat and prevent the infectious and inherited
craniofacial-oral-dental diseases and disorders.

327

Dr Lawrence A Tabak, Director
Thomas G Murphy, Acting Executive Director

National Associations & Support Groups

2981 American Academy of Pediatrics
141 Northwest Point Boulevard
Elk Grove Village, IL 60007 847-434-4000
800-433-9016
Fax: 847-434-8000
www.aap.org

The American Academy of Pediatrics and its member pediatricians are committed to the attainment of optimal physical, mental and social health and well-being for all infants, children, adolescents, and young adults.

Sandra Hassink, MD, FAAP, President

2982 American Dental Association
211 E Chicago Avenue
Chicago, IL 60611 312-266-7255
Fax: 312-266-9867
e-mail: ÿinfo@aae.org
www.aae.org

Professional association of dentists committed to the public's oral health, ethics, science and professional advancement; leading a unified profession through initiatives in advocacy, education, research and the development of standards.

James Drinan, Executive Director

2983 Genetic Alliance
4301 Connecticut Avenue NW
Washington, DC 20008 202-966-7955
800-336-4363
Fax: 202-966-8553
e-mail: info@geneticalliance.org
www.geneticalliance.org

A coalition of voluntary genetic support groups, consumers and professionals addressing the needs of individuals and families affected by genetic disorders from a national perspective.

Sharon Terry, President

2984 March of Dimes Birth Defects Foundation
1275 Mamaroneck Avenue
White Plains, NY 10605 914-997-4488
888-663-4637
Fax: 914-997-4763
e-mail: answers@marchofdimes.com
www.marchofdimes.com

Partnership of volunteers and professionals dedicated to improving the health of babies by preventing birth defects and infant mortality. Over 100 chapters are located across the country and can be located through the National Office.

Jennifer L Howse, President

2985 National Foundation for Ectodermal Dysplasias
410 E Main Street, PO Box 114
Mascoutah, IL 62258 618-566-2020
Fax: 618-566-4718
e-mail: info@nfed.org
www.nfed.org

Seeks to enrich the lives of individuals affected by all forms of the ectodermal dysplasia syndromes.

Mary K Richter, Founder/Executive Director

2986 Society for Pediatric Dermatology
8365 Keystone Crossing, Suite 107
Indianapolis, IN 46240 317-202-0224
Fax: 317-205-9841
e-mail: spd@hp-assoc.com
www.pedsderm.net

National organization dedicated to promote, develop and advance edcuation, research and care of skin disease in all pediatric age groups.

Kent Lindeman, Executive Director

State Agencies & Support Groups

2987 National Foundation for Ectodermal Dysplasias- Regional Office
PO Box 2069
Auburn, WA 98071 253-735-5195
Fax: 253-735-5195
TTY: 800-688-4889
e-mail: nfed3@aol.com
www.nfed.org

Disseminates information on this and related disorders for people of any age to access and use in everyday life situations.

Judy Woodruff, Executive Director
Kelley Atchison, Director of Supportÿ
ÿÿGale Hoedebeck, ÿÿDirector of Administration

Libraries & Resource Centers

2988 International Center for Skeletal Dysplasia Registry
St. Joseph Hospital
7620 York Road
Townson, MD 21204 310-423-9915
Fax: 310-423-9939

Provides patient services for those with skeletal dysplasia; does s research in dwarfism.

Dr. Steven Kopitis, Director

Conferences

2989 Genetic Alliance Annual Conference
Genetic Alliance
4301 Connecticut Avenue NW, Suite 404
Washington, DC 20008 202-966-5557
800-336-4363
Fax: 202-966-8553
e-mail: info@geneticalliance.org
www.geneticalliance.org

Consistently inspirational and enables partnership among all stakeholders: advocates and community leaders, health and industry professionals, policymakers, and academicians.

July

Sharon Terry, President/CEO
Tetyana Murza, Programs/Events Manager

2990 National Foundation for Ectodermal Dysplasias Annual Conference
National Foundation for Ectodermal Dysplasias
410 E Main Street
Mascoutah, IL 62258 618-566-2020
Fax: 618-566-4718
e-mail: info@nfed.org
www.nfed.org

Where individuals affected by ectodermal dysplasias and their families gather to receive information and support. Experts provide medical and dental presentations to explain the various symptoms and how to best treat them.

Mary K Richter, Founder/Executive Director

2991 Society for Pediatric Dermatology Annual M eeting
Society for Pediatric Dermatology
8365 Keystone Crossing, Suite 107
Indianapolis, IN 46240 317-202-0224
Fax: 317-205-9481
e-mail: spd@hp-assoc.com
www.pedsderm.net

July

Kent Lindeman, Executive Director

Web Sites

2992 American Dental Association
211 East Chicago Avenue
Chicago, IL 60611
312-440-2500
e-mail: affiliates@ada.org
www.ada.org

The ADA foundation enhances health by securing contributions
and providing grants for sustainable programs in dental research,
education, access to care and assistance for dentists and their
families in need.

2993 Dental Resources on the Web
www.dental-resources.com

Dental sites for education, practices, laboratories, office supplies,
dental care and associations.

2994 Online Mendelian Inheritance in Man
U.S. National Library of Medicine, 8600 Rockville
Bethesda, MD 20894
888-346-3656
e-mail: info@ncbi.nlm.nih.gov
www.ncbi.nlm.nih.gov

This database is a catalog of human genes and genetic disorders.

Christine E. Seidman, M.D., Chair
David J. Lipman, M.D., Executive Secretary
Michael Boehnke, Ph.D., Board Member

Description

2996 ECZEMA

Synonym: Eczematous dermatitis

Covers these related disorders: Allergic contact dermatitis, Atopic dermatitis, Dyshidrosis, Irritant contact dermatitis, Seborrheic dermatitis

Involves the following Biologic System(s):

Dermatologic Disorders

Eczema is a common inflammatory condition of the skin (dermatitis) characterized by redness, itching, blistering, and oozing of affected areas. As the condition progresses, the skin often becomes abnormally dry and may scale, crust over, thicken, or develop increased or decreased areas of coloration. There are several different types of eczema that may be caused by various internal or external factors. Children are mainly affected by certain forms of the condition, including atopic dermatitis, irritant and allergic contact dermatitis, seborrheic dermatitis, or dyshidrosis.

Approximately 2-8% of children develop atopic dermatitis, which is the most common form of childhood eczema. Also known as infantile eczema when it occurs during childhood, this form of eczema is characterized by an excessive immune response to particular substances (sensitizing antigens) that the body perceives as foreign. This excessive response, known as an allergic or hypersensitivity reaction, occurs upon exposure to previously encountered, usually environmental substances (allergens). Patients with atopic dermatitis are thought to have an inherited tendency toward allergy. This may be supported by the finding that many infants and children with this type of dermatitis later develop additional conditions caused by exposure to certain allergens. These additional conditions particularly include inflammation of the mucous membranes of the nose (allergic rhinitis) and inflammation and narrowing of the airways (asthma).

Atopic dermatitis usually begins during the first year of life, and up to 90% of affected patients have symptoms by five years of age. The disorder often occurs with the introduction of particular foods into a child's diet, such as wheat, cow's milk, soy, eggs, or peanuts. Although atopic dermatitis tends to subside with advancing age, the condition may recur over a period of many years before completely disappearing. Atopic dermatitis is characterized by the development of reddish, inflamed, intensely itchy (pruritic) patches that rapidly begin to ooze and crust over. During infancy, the condition usually initially affects the skin of the cheeks and gradually extends to involve the rest of the face; the neck, abdomen, wrists, and hands; the insides of the elbows; the areas behind the knees; or other areas. In response to intense itching, infants with atopic dermatitis may rub affected areas against their cribs, clothes, or other surfaces in an attempt to obtain relief. The repeated rubbing or scratching of affected areas may lead to their infection by bacteria on the skin, on clothing, or from other sources. With the passage of time, skin areas affected by atopic dermatitis may become dry and scaly and develop changes in color. In addition, the skin may thicken, accentuating skin lines and causing an unusual, "bark-like" skin appearance (lichenification).

The treatment of atopic dermatitis may include measures to eliminate or avoid certain factors that might worsen the condition, such as certain foods, extremes of humidity and temperature, detergents or soaps, or potentially abrasive textures, such as wool. Affected children should be dressed in garments with smooth textures, such as cotton; their fingernails should be kept as short as possible to discourage scratching; and excessive bathing should be avoided. Adding bath oil to bath water and applying moisturizing lotions and creams to damp skin after bathing may help to ease some symptoms of atopic dermatitis. At locations where inflammation is severe, the application of wet dressings may reduce inflammation and associated itching. Treatment may also include the direct (topical) application of medicated skin creams and ointments, such as corticosteroid preparations, as well as medications such as oral antihistamines to help reduce itching. Bacterial infections of skin affected by atopic dermatitis are treated with appropriate antibiotics.

Contact dermatitis, another common form of eczema, is a skin inflammation that is typically confined to a particular area and may have clearly defined boundaries. This disorder is often subdivided into irritant and allergic contact dermatitis. Irritant contact dermatitis is a skin inflammation caused by repetitive or prolonged exposure to certain substances that damage the skin. Allergic contact dermatitis is an inflammatory response of the skin caused by subsequent exposure to an allergen to which the skin has previously become sensitized.

Irritant contact dermatitis may be caused by repetitive or prolonged exposure to certain soaps or detergents, citrus juices, bubble bath preparations, or other substances. In many infants, saliva from drooling may cause inflammation of the skin of the face and neck folds. Diaper dermatitis is another common form of irritant contact dermatitis. Affected infants may develop a reddish, scaling, blistering skin inflammation and secondary bacterial infections from prolonged contact with waste materials, diaper soaps, and topical skin lotions. The treatment of irritant contact dermatitis includes removal or avoidance of the responsible irritants and topical application of corticosteroid creams or ointments. Affected areas of skin should also be carefully and regularly washed with warm water and a mild soap. To help prevent diaper dermatitis, physicians may recommend frequent changing of diapers; gentle, thorough cleansing of genitals with warm water and mild soaps, and application of mild protective topical preparations during the diaper changes; or the use of disposable diapers made with absorbent materials.

Allergic contact dermatitis is characterized by a hypersensitive or allergic response to previously encountered allergens. Common causes of this form of dermatitis include metal compounds in jewelry; particular plants, such as poison ivy, poison oak, or poison sumac; medications in skin creams, such as certain antibiotic- or antihistamine-containing creams; shoes; or clothing. Patients with allergic contact dermatitis may experience intensely itchy, reddish, blistering skin inflammations, with the affected areas of skin later developing scaling, cracking, (fissuring), changes in color, or an abnormal, thickened, bark-like appearance. Treatment includes the removal or avoidance of allergens responsible for the condition and the application of cool compresses, corticosteroid ointments or oral medications, antihistamine medications, and antibiotic therapy for secondary bacterial infections.

Seborrheic dermatitis is a chronic inflammatory disorder of unknown cause that may occur at any age and may appear to follow the distribution of sebaceous glands in skin tissue. These relatively small glands, which open into hair follicles, produce an oily secretion known as sebum that helps to lubricate the hair and skin and protect the skin from drying. In children, seborrheic dermatitis most commonly occurs during infancy. Affected infants may initially develop localized or widespread crusting and scaling of the scalp, known as cradle cap. In some patients, this may be the only effect of the this form of dermatitis. Other infants may develop reddish, greasy, scaling patches that may be localized or may spread to affect most of the body. Affected areas often include the face, the regions behind the ears, the neck, the diaper region, or the armpits and underarm areas. Patients with seborrheic dermatitis may experience associated itching, hair loss, or changes in skin color. Treatment may include the use of special anti-seborrheic shampoos or the application of wet compresses or topical corticosteroid creams or ointments.

Dyshidrotic eczema, also known as dyshidrosis or pompholyx, is another form of eczema that may occur during childhood. It is a recurrent, potentially seasonal blistering condition that affects the palms of the hands and soles of the feet. The condition is initially characterized by recurrent crops of severely itchy blisters. Affected skin areas gradually become abnormally thickened and may have cracking or fissuring. Many patients with dyshidrotic eczema also experience excessive sweating (hyperhidrosis) in affected areas, and may develop secondary bacterial infections from scratching of such areas. Because dyshidrotic eczema is typically a recurrent condition, appropriate measures should be taken to protect the hands and feet of infants and children with this condition from harsh soaps, chemicals, the effects of excessive sweating or adverse weather, or other factors that may trigger the condition. Treatment of dyshidrotic eczema may include the application of wet dressings, topical corticosteroid ointments or creams, or mild topical preparations that promote skin softening and peeling (keratolytic agents), and the administration of antibiotics to treat secondary bacterial infections.

Government Agencies

2997 NIH/National Institute of Allergy and Infectious Diseases
6610 Rockledge Drive, MSC 6612
Bethesda, MD 20892
301-496-5717
866-284-4107
Fax: 301-402-3573
TDD: 800-877-8339
e-mail: ocposfoffice@niaid.nih.gov
www.niaid.nih.gov

Conducts and supports basic and applied research to better understand, treat, and ultimately prevent infectious, immunologic, and allergic diseases.

Anthony S Fauci MD, Director

2998 NIH/National Institute of Arthritis and Mu sculoskeletal and Skin Diseases
1AMS Circle
Bethesda, MD 20892
301-402-4484
877-226-4267
Fax: 301-718-6366
TDD: 301-565-2966
e-mail: niamsinfo@mail.nih.gov
www.niams.nih.gov

The mission of the NIAMS, a part of the NIH, is to support research into the causes, treatment and prevention of arthritis and musculoskeletal and skin diseases, the training of basic and clinical scientists to carry out this research, and the dissemination of information on research progress in these diseases

Stephen I Katz MD PhD, Director
Robert H Carter MD, Deputy Director

National Associations & Support Groups

2999 American Academy of Pediatrics
141 Northwest Point Boulevard
Elk Grove Village, IL 60007
847-434-4000
800-433-9016
Fax: 847-434-8000
www.aap.org

The American Academy of Pediatrics and its member pediatricians are committed to the attainment of optimal physical, mental and social health and well-being for all infants, children, adolescents, and young adults.

Sandra Hassink, MD, FAAP, President

3000 National Eczema Association
4460 Redwood Highway, Suite 16-D
San Rafael, CA 94903
415-499-3474
800-818-7546
Fax: 415-472-5345
e-mail: info@nationaleczema.org
www.nationaleczema.org

Works to improve the health and the quality of life of persons living with atopic dermatitis/eczema, including those who have the disease as well as their loved ones.

3001 Society for Pediatric Dermatology
8365 Keystone Crossing, Suite 107
Indianapolis, IN 46240
317-202-0224
Fax: 317-205-9841
e-mail: spd@hp-assoc.com
www.pedsderm.net

National organization dedicated to promote, develop and advance education, research and care of skin disease in all pediatric age groups.

Kent Lindeman, Executive Director

Libraries & Resource Centers

California

3002 University of California, San Francisco Dermatology Drug Research
515 Spruce
San Francisco, CA 94143
415-476-2001
Fax: 415-476-6014
cc.ucsf.edu/people

Conducts clinical testing of new or existing pharmalogic agents used in the treatment of skin disorders.

John Koo, MD, Director

Delaware

3003 Delaware Division of Libraries for the Blind and Physically Handicapped
43 S Dupont Highway
Dover, DE 19901
302-736-4748
800-282-8676
Fax: 302-736-6787
TDD: 302-739-4748
e-mail: bedpg@lib.de.us
www.nfb.org/libraries-for-the-blind

Braille readers receive service from Philadelphia and Pennsylvania, summer reading program, braille writer and cassettes.

Beth Landon, Librarian

Illinois

3004 Dermatology Information Network (DERMINFONET)
American Academy of Dermatology
PO Box 4014
Schaumburg, IL 60168
847-330-0230
Fax: 847-330-0050
www.meddermsociety.org/Resource_Links.asp

Consists of a collection of dermatologic databases that are available to members on a subscription and/or purchase basis. These databases are designed to run on a wide variety of personal computers.

3005 National Library of Dermatologic Teaching Slides
American Academy of Dermatology
930 E Woodfield Road
Schaumburg, IL 60173
847-330-0230
Fax: 847-330-0050
www.aad.org

A collection of dermatologic teaching slides offering the most comprehensive series ever assembled. Each set offers a realistic presentation of classic clinical skin conditions encountered by the dermatologist.

New York

3006 Laboratory of Dermatology Research
Memorial Sloan-Kettering Cancer Center
1275 York Avenue
New York, NY 10065
212-639-2000
Fax: 212-639-3576
www.mskcc.org

Specific studies on the identification of skin disorders and dermatology.

Biijan Safai, MD, Head

3007 Rockefeller University Laboratory for Investigative Dermatology
1230 York Avenue
New York, NY 10065
212-327-8000
Fax: 212-327-7459
www.rockefeller.edu/research/faculty/labheads/JamesK

Research into skin disorders and the whole specialty of dermatology in general.

Barry Coller, Head

Research Centers

3008 University of California, San Francisco Dermatology Drug Research
515 Spruce
San Francisco, CA 94143
415-476-2001
Fax: 415-221-4751

Conducts clinical testing of new or existing pharmacologic agents used in the treatment of skin disorders.

John Koo, MD, Director

Conferences

3009 Society for Pediatric Dermatology Annual Meeting
Society for Pediatric Dermatology
8365 Keystone Crossing, Suite 107
Indianapolis, IN 46240
317-202-0224
Fax: 317-205-9841
e-mail: spd@hp-assoc.com
www.pedsderm.net

July

Kent Lindeman, Executive Director

Audio Video

3010 National Library of Dermatologic Teaching Slides
American Academy Of Dermatology
PO Box 94020
Palatine, IL 60094
847-330-0230
Fax: 847-330-0050

A collection of dermatologic teaching slides offering the most comprehensive series ever assembled. Each set offers a realistic presentation of classic clinical skin conditions encountered by the dermatologist.

Magazines

3011 International Journal of Dermatology
International Society of Dermatology
138 Palm Coast Parkway, NE No 333
Palm Coast, FL 32137
386-437-4405
Fax: 386-437-4427
e-mail: info@intsocdermatol.org
www.intsocderm.org

Focuses on information for dermatologists and the whole specialty of dermatology research and education.

10 times a year

3012 Journal of Dermatologic Surgery and Oncology
International Society for Dermatologic Surgery
930 N Meachan Road
Schaumburg, IL 60173
847-330-9830
Fax: 847-330-1135
onlinelibrary.wiley.com/journal/10.1111/(ISSN)1524-4

Focuses on medical updates and information on dermatology.

Monthly

Newsletters

3013 Awareness
NAPVI
PO Box 317
Watertown, MA 2471
617-972-7441
800-562-6265
Fax: 617-972-7444
www.spedex.com/napvi

Newsletter offering regional news, sports and activities, conferences, camps, legislative updates, book reviews, audio reviews, professional question and answer column and more for the visually impaired and their families.

Quarterly

3014 DVH Quarterly
University of Arkansas at Little Rock
2801 S University Avenue
Little Rock, AR 72204
Fax: 501-663-3536

Offers information on upcoming events, conferences and workshops on and for visual disabilities. Book reviews, information on the newest resources and technology, educational programs, want ads and more.

Quarterly

Bob Brasher, Editor

3015 Dermatology Focus
Dermatology Foundation
1560 Sherman Avenue, Suite 870
Evanston, IL 60201
847-328-2256
Fax: 847-328-0509
dermatologyfoundation.org

Includes membership activities, research articles and lists recipients of foundation awards.

Quarterly

Bruce U. Wintroub, MD, Chair
Michael D. Tharp, MD, President
Stuart R. Lessin, MD, Vice President

3016 Dermatology World
American Academy of Dermatology
PO Box 94020
Palatine, IL 60094   847-330-0230
                                  Fax: 847-330-0050

Offers Academy members information outside the clinical realm.
It carries news of government actions, reports of socioeconomic
issues, societal trends and other events which impinge on the
practice of dermatology.

Monthly

3017 Progress in Dermatology
Dermatology Foundation
1560 Sherman Avenue, Suite 870
Evanston, IL 60201   847-328-2256
                                  Fax: 847-328-0509
                          dermatologyfoundation.org

Bulletin offering information on research reports and clinical
trials.

Quarterly

Bruce U. Wintroub, MD, Chair
Michael D. Tharp, MD, President
Stuart R. Lessin, MD, Vice President

Pamphlets

3018 Eczema/Atopic Dermatitis
American Academy of Dermatology
PO Box 4014
Schaumburg, IL 60168   847-240-1280
                                       866-503-7546
                                  Fax: 847-240-1859
                          e-mail: president@aad.org
                                       www.aad.org

Explains how to recognize and treat dermatitis.

1995

Brett M. Coldiron, MD, President
Elise A. Olsen, MD, Vice President
Suzanne M. Olbricht, MD, Secretary-Treasurer

3019 Hand Eczema
American Academy of Dermatology
PO Box 4014
Schaumburg, IL 60168   847-240-1280
                                       866-503-7546
                                  Fax: 847-240-1859
                          e-mail: president@aad.org
                                       www.aad.org

Shows examples of hand rashes, explains causes, lists protective
measures and treatments.

1993

Brett M. Coldiron, MD, President
Elise A. Olsen, MD, Vice President
Suzanne M. Olbricht, MD, Secretary-Treasurer

Camps

3020 Camp Discovery
American Academy of Dermatology
930 E Woodfield Road
Schaumburg, IL 60173   847-240-1280
                                       866-503-7546
                                  Fax: 847-240-1859
                          e-mail: president@aad.org
                              www.campdiscovery.org

A camp for young people with chronic skin conditions. There is
no fee and transportation is provided. Three locations: Camp Horizon in Millville, PA, Camp Knutson in Crosslake, MN, and
Camp Dermadillo in Burton, TX.

Brett M. Coldiron, MD, President
Elise A. Olsen, MD, Vice President
Suzanne M. Olbricht, MD, Secretary-Treasurer

Description

3021 EHLERS-DANLOS SYNDROME
Involves the following Biologic System(s):

Connective Tissue Disorders

Ehlers-Danlos syndrome is a group of hereditary connective tissue disorders characterized by abnormalities of collagen, the major structural protein in the body. At least 10 forms of the disorder have been identified based upon underlying bio-chemical and genetic abnormalities and associated symptoms and findings. Although such subtypes were previously indentified by Roman numerals (e.g., I to X), different classi-fication systems have since been proposed. Most forms of Ehlers-Danlos syndrome are thought to have autosomal domi-nant inheritance. However, other subtypes have been identi-fied that may be inherited as an autosomal recessive or an X-linked recessive trait. Although certain symptoms and find-ings are commonly associated with Ehlers-Danlos syndrome, other abnormalities may be variable in range and severity, de-pending upon the form of the disorder present.

Although infants with Ehlers-Danlos syndrome often appear normal at birth, associated symptoms and findings soon be-come apparent. The main symptoms associated with the disor-der may include abnormally thin, elastic skin that is excessively fragile and unusually loose, flexible (hyperextensible) joints that may be prone to recurrent dislo-cation. Due to abnormal fragility of the skin, blood vessels, and other tissues, patients may be prone to tearing or splitting of the skin, be susceptible to easy bruising and bleeding, and tend to heal slowly. Healing of skin wounds may leave dis-tinctive, cigarette paper-like scars, such as over the knees, shins, elbows, and forehead. In addition, due to abnormal ac-cumulations of scar tissue, patients may develop small, rounded skin growths that resemble tumors (molluscoid pseudotumors). In some cases, small, round, hard lumps (cal-cified spheroids) may also develop under the skin.

Depending upon the form of the disorder present, affected children may have additional, variable symptoms, such as cer-tain skeletal, blood vessel, or eye (ocular) abnormalities. As-sociated skeletal malformations may include front-to-back and sideways curvature of the spine (kyphoscoliosis); short, wide collarbones (clavicles); bowing of bones of the arms and legs; bone fragility; short stature; or other abnormalities. Fragility of certain blood vessels may lead to ballooning of the wall of the major artery in the body (aortic aneurysm) or spontaneous rupture of certain intermediate- or large-sized ar-teries, potentially causing life-threatening complications. In addition, in some patients, ocular abnormalities may include fragility of the front, transparent region of the eye (cornea); noninflammatory protrusion of the cornea (keratoconus); rup-ture of the cornea or the tough, fibrous, outer coating of the eye (sclera); or detachment of the nerve-rich membrane at the back of the eye (retina). Additional symptoms and findings may include diminished muscle tone (hypotonia); abnormal prominence of blood vessels under the skin; protrusion of one of the heart valves back into the left upper chamber (atrium) of the heart during contraction of the left lower heart chamber (mitral valve prolapse); severe inflammation of the tissues that surround and support the teeth (periodontitis), leading to premature tooth loss; rupture of the intestine; or other abnor-malities.

The treatment of children with Ehlers-Danlos syndrome is symptomatic and supportive. Appropriate measures must be taken to avoid trauma and injuries, such as those that may occur in contact sports. Wearing protective clothing and padding may be beneficial. In addition, appropriate precautions must be taken during dental or surgical procedures.

Government Agencies

3022 NIH/National Institute of Arthritis and Mu sculoskeletal and Skin Diseases
1AMS Circle
Bethesda, MD 20892

301-402-4484
877-226-4267
Fax: 301-718-6366
TDD: 301-565-2966
e-mail: niamsinfo@mail.nih.gov
www.niams.nih.gov

The mission of the NIAMS, a part of the NIH, is to support re-search into the causes, treatment, and prevention of arthritis and musculoskeletal and skin diseases, the training of basic and clini-cal scientists to carry out this research, and the dissemination of information on research progress in these diseases.

Stephen I Katz MD PhD, Director
Robert H Carter MD, Deputy Director

National Associations & Support Groups

3023 American Academy of Pediatrics
141 Northwest Point Boulevard
Elk Grove Village, IL 60007

847-434-4000
800-433-9016
Fax: 847-434-8000
www.aap.org

The American Academy of Pediatrics and its member pediatri-cians are committed to the attainment of optimal physical, mental and social health and well-being for all infants, children, adoles-cents, and young adults.

Sandra Hassink, MD, FAAP, President

3024 Ehlers-Danlos National Foundation
1760, Old Meadow Road, Ste 500
McLean, VG 22102

703-506-2892
Fax: 213-427-0057
e-mail: ednfstaff@ednf.org
www.ednf.org

Provides emotional support and updated information to the indi-viduals and their families who are affected by the disease. The foundation produces educational and support pamphlets, bro-chures, audiovisual aids, journal article reprints, newsletter, and a referral service.

Cynthia Lauren, Ceo
Edzel Lejano, Member Services Coordinator

3025 Genetic Alliance
4301 Connecticut Avenue NW, Suite 404
Washington, DC 20008

202-966-7955
800-336-4363
Fax: 202-966-8553
e-mail: info@geneticalliance.org
www.geneticalliance.org

A coalition of voluntary genetic support groups, consumers and professionals addressing the needs of individuals and families af-fected by genetic disorders from a national perspective.

Sharon Terry, President

3026 March of Dimes Birth Defects Foundation
1275 Mamaroneck Avenue
White Plains, NY 10605

914-997-4488
888-663-4637
Fax: 914-997-4763
e-mail: answers@marchofdimes.com
www.marchofdimes.com

Partnership of volunteers and professionals dedicated to improving the health of babies by preventing birth defects and infant mortality. Over 100 chapters are located across the country and can be located through the National Office.

Jennifer L Howse, President

Conferences

3027 Ehlers-Danlos National Foundation Learning Conference
Ehlers-Danlos National Foundation
1760 Old Meadow Road, Suite 500
McLean, VA 22102

703-506-2892
Fax: 703-506-3266
e-mail: ednstaff@ednf.org
www.ednf.org

July

Shane Robinson, Executive Director

3028 Genetic Alliance Annual Conference
Genetic Alliance
4301 Connecticut Avenue NW, Suite 404
Washington, DC 20008

202-966-5557
800-336-4363
Fax: 202-966-8553
e-mail: info@geneticalliance.org
www.geneticalliance.org

Consistently inspirational and enables partnership among all stakeholders: advocates and community leaders, health and industry professionals, policymakers, and academicians.

July

Sharon Terry, President/CEO
Tetyana Murza, Programs/Events Manager

Web Sites

3029 Wheeless' Textbook of Orthopaedics
www.wheelessonline.com

Derives from a variety of sources, including journals, articles, national meetings lectures and other textbooks.

Clifford R. Wheeless III, MD, Editor-in-Chief
James A. Nunley, II, Managing Editor
James R. Urbaniak, MD, Managing Editor

Pamphlets

3030 Ehlers-Danlos Syndrome
Arthritis Foundation
PO Box 7669
Atlanta, GA 30357

404-872-7100
800-283-7800
Fax: 404-872-0457
www.arthiritis.org

Description

3031 ENCEPHALOCELE

Involves the following Biologic System(s):

Neurologic Disorders

Encephalocele is an abnormality that is present at birth (congenital)and belongs to a group of birth defects known as neural tube defects. These defects develop during the early stages of pregnancy at which time a specialized layer of tissue forms and extends along the back portion of the developing embryo. As the embryo grows, this tissue, known as the neural plate, forms a groove that is bordered by folds. This groove eventually deepens and closes to form the neural tube. Later in development, the neural tube gives rise to tissue that later forms the brain and spinal cord. The neural tube is surrounded and protected by the bones of the back (vertebrae). Failure in this sequence of developmental events results in a neural tube defect.

In newborns with encephalocele, a portion of the brain protrudes through a defect in the skull. This defect may be located at the back of the head (occipital region), the forehead (frontal region), or the area of the forehead and nose (nasofrontal region). Affected children may experience visual abnormalities, mental retardation, an abnormally small head (microcephaly), and seizures. Affected newborns may also have an increase in the volume of fluid surrounding the brain (hydrocephalus), possibly resulting in increased pressure within the skull, enlargement of the head, and convulsions.

Encephalocele may occur as the result of different genetic and environmental factors (multifactorial), alone or in combination. Such factors may include vitamin deficiencies or toxic factors. Genetic transmission in some children is supported by the fact that multiple cases of this neural tube defect have been reported in some families. In addition, encephalocele may sometimes be associated with other disorders. For example, physical characteristics of Meckel-Gruber syndrome, a rare, life-threatening disorder inherited as an autosomal recessive trait, include encephalocele in the back of the head; an abnormal ridge (cleft) or opening in the lip or palate; a sloping forehead, extra fingers or toes (polydactyly); and enlarged kidneys that contain multiple cysts (polycystic kidneys).

Treatment of encephalocele may often involve a team of medical specialists working together to determine the best course of therapy or management. Such treatment may include surgery, medication, or the insertion of a tube known as a shunt into the brain. This shunt diverts fluid away from the brain into the abdominal cavity where it is harmlessly absorbed into the systemic circulation.

The risk of neural tube defects is significantly reduced when supplemental folic acid is consumed in addition to a healthful diet prior to and during the first month following conception. Women who could become pregnant, especially those at risk who may have previously delivered a child with a neural tube defect, are advised to eat foods fortified with folic acid or take a folic acid supplement in addition to eating folate-rich foods to reduce the risk of some serious birth defects.

Government Agencies

3032 NIH/National Institute of Child Health and Human Development

31 Center Drive, Building 31
Bethesda, MD 20892

301-496-1333
Fax: 301-496-1104
www.nichd.nih.gov

Established in 1962 by congress, today the institute conducts and supports research on topics related to the health of children, adults, families and populations. Some of these topics include: developmental disabilities, growth and development, infant death, reproductive health and birth defects.

Jay H Hoofnagle, Director
Lisa Kaeser, Program & Public Liaison

National Associations & Support Groups

3033 AmeriFace

PO Box 75112
Las Vegas, NV 89130

702-301-5351
888-486-1209
Fax: 702-341-5351
e-mail: info@ameriface.org
www.ameriface.org

Provides information, services, emotional support and educational programs for and on behalf of individuals with facial differences and their families. Working to increase understanding through public awareness and education.

3M members

Debbie Oliver, Executive Director

3034 American Academy of Pediatrics

141 Northwest Point Boulevard
Elk Grove Village, IL 60007

847-434-4000
800-433-9016
Fax: 847-434-8000
www.aap.org

The American Academy of Pediatrics and its member pediatricians are committed to the attainment of optimal physical, mental and social health and well-being for all infants, children, adolescents, and young adults.

Sandra Hassink, MD, FAAP, President

3035 Birth Defect Research for Children

930 Woodcock Road, Suite 225
Orlando, FL 32803

407-895-0802
Fax: 407-895-0824
e-mail: staff@birthdefects.org
www.birthdefects.org

Organization that helps families with free birth defect information, parent matching that links families of children with similar defects and research through the National Birth Defect Registry to discover the causes of birth defects. Support group information and newsletter on Internet.

Betty Mekdeci, Executive Director

3036 Children's Craniofacial Association

13140 Coit Road, Suite 307
Dallas, TX 75240

214-570-9099
800-535-3643
Fax: 214-570-8811
e-mail: contactCCA@ccakids.com
www.ccakids.com

Devoted to the dispersion of medical knowledge of this and similar disorders, along with providing emotional support for the sufferers and their families.

Char Smith, Executive Director

3037 Fighters for Encephalocele Support Group

332 Brereton Street
Pittsburgh, PA 15219

412-261-5363

3038 Forward Face
317 E 34th Street, Suite 901A
New York, NY 10016
212-684-5860
Fax: 212-684-5864
e-mail: info@forwardface.org
www.forwardface.org

Founded in 1978 by parents of children with facial differences; helps children and their families find immediate support to manage the medical and social effects of facial differences.

Camille Walsh, Manager

3039 Guardians of Hydrocephalus Research Foundation
2618 Avenue Z
Brooklyn, NY 11235
718-743-4473
800-458-8655
Fax: 718-743-1171
e-mail: ghrf2618@aol.com
www.ghrforg.org

Nonprofit group dedicated to research into the cause and treatment of hydrocephalus. Guardians operate a laboratory in the Department of Neurology at New York University Medical Center, in which information from clinical and research facilities is integrated to provide for better diagnosis and treatment of hydrocephalus, a frequently occuring congenital disorder that can also occur shortly after birth. Hydrocephalus accounts for a large propotion of adult patients with a diagnosis of dementia.

Kathy Soriano

3040 Hydrocephalus Association
4340 East West Highway, Suite 905
Bethesda, MDÿ 20814, MD 20814
301- 20- 381
888-598-3789
Fax: 301-202-3813
e-mail: info@hydroassoc.org
www.hydroassoc.org

A national nonprofit organization devoted exclusively to hydrocepahalus. We provide support, education and an extensive range of resources to families and professionals dealing with the complex issues of hydrocephalus, the abnormal accumulation of cerebrospinal fluid within the brain. Our resources cover all age groups, from prenatal to adults with normal pressure hydrocepahalus. Our office is staffed daily from 10 AM to 4 PM Pacific time.

Dawn Mancuso,, CEO
Randi Corey, Director of Special Events
Aisha Heath, Director of Development

3041 Hydrocephalus Support Group
9245 Sky Park Court, Suite 130
San Diego, CA 92123
619-268-8252
Fax: 619-268-4275
e-mail: efrc@mail.sdsu.edu

Provides education and support for hydrocephalus patients and their families. The HSG puts out a quarterly newspaper, gives parent referrals and has a library with articles and tapes about hydrocephalus.

3042 March of Dimes Birth Defects Foundation
1275 Mamaroneck Avenue
White Plains, NY 10605
914-997-4488
888-663-4637
Fax: 914-997-4763
e-mail: answers@marchofdimes.com
www.marchofdimes.com

Partnership of volunteers and professionals dedicated to improving the health of babies by preventing birth defects and infant mortality. Over 100 chapters are located across the country and can be located through the National Office.

Jennifer L Howse, President

3043 National Craniofacial Foundation
PO Box 11082
Chattanooga, TN 37401
800-332-2373
e-mail: faces@faces-cranio.org
www.faces-cranio.org

Provides information to affected individuals; families of affected individuals; the public or media and professionals. We also provide peer support; professional counseling; medical referrals; referrals for non-medical services and to local chapters or groups. We offer pamphlets; fact sheets; newsletter; booklets; video's and movies.

Lynne Mayfield, Director

3044 National Hydrocephalus Foundation
12413 Centralia Road
Lakewood, CA 90715
562-924-6666
888-857-3434
e-mail: debbifields@nhfonline.org
www.nhfonline.org

Promotes information and educational assistance. Establishes and facilitates a communication network and works to increase public awareness. Promote and support research. Also has brochures, help sheets, and more. Quarterly newsletter with annual membership fee of $35.00.

Debbie Fields, Executive Director
Michael Fields, President
Jaynie Dunn, Secretary

Conferences

3045 North American Craniofacial Family Confere nce
AmeriFace
PO Box 751112
Las Vegas, NV 89136
702-769-9264
888-486-1209
Fax: 702-341-5351
e-mail: info@ameriface.org
www.ameriface.org

July

Debbie Oliver, Executive Director

Web Sites

3046 National Hydrocephalus Foundation
www.nhfonline.org

Promotes information and educational assistance. Establishes and facilitates a communication network and works to increase public awareness. Promote and support research. Also has brochures, help sheets and more. Quarterly newsletter included with annual membership fee of $35.00.

3047 Rare Genetic Diseases in Children (NYU)
550 First Avenue
New York, NY 10016
212-263-7300
www.med.nyu.edu/rgdc/homenow.htm

We target issues arising from rare genetic diseases affecting children. Also, to assist in the endeavor to bring knowledge and hope to those for whom there is, at present, so little.

Laurence D. Fink, Co Chair
Kenneth G. Langone, Co Chair
Robert I. Grossman, MD, Dean & CEO

Book Publishers

3048 Congenital Disorders Sourcebook
Omnigraphics
PO Box 8002
Aston, PA 19014
800-234-1340
Fax: 800-875-1340
e-mail: info@omnigraphics.com
www.omnigraphics.com

Basic consumer health information on disorders aquired during gestation, including spina bifida, hydrocephalus, cerebral palsy, heart defects, craniofacial abnormalities and fetal alcohol syndrome.

650 pages
ISBN: 0-780809-45-9

Newsletters

3049 AmeriFace Newsletter
AmeriFace
PO Box 75112
Las Vegas, NV 89136   702-769-9264
                                             888-486-1209
                                        Fax: 702-341-5351
                                 e-mail: info@ameriface.org
                                        www.ameriface.org

A free newsletter.

8 pages

David Reisberg, DDS, President
Christina Corsigla, Vice President
Debbie Oliver, Executive Director

3050 National Hydrocephalus Foundation Newsletter
12413 Centralia Road
Lakewood, CA 90715   562-924-6666
                                             888-857-3434
                                        Fax: 415-732-7044
           e-mail: debbifields@nhfonline.org, info@nhfonlin
                                        www.nhfonline.org

The Foundation is a national organization whose purpose is to
provide information and education, along with peer support newsletter quarterly.

12-15 pages Quarterly

Michael Fields, President/ Treasurer
Debbie Fields, Executive Director
Jaynie Dunn, Secretary

Description

3051 ENCOPRESIS

Involves the following Biologic System(s):

Developmental/Behavioral/Psychiatric Disorders, Gastrointestinal Disorders

Encopresis refers to the passage of feces in inappropriate or unacceptable places by children who have no detectable disorder or organic abnormality and who are past the age when toilet training is typically completed. This type of soiling may be considered primary encopresis, in which fecal incontinence persists from birth, or secondary encopresis, a regressive form of this disorder in which fecal incontinence occurs in children who were previously toilet trained. Children with this disorder may refuse to use a commode, may soil their clothing, or may defecate in secret places. Other associated findings may include chronic constipation leading to the presence of large, hardened fecal masses in the colon or rectum (fecal impaction) that, in turn, may result in an abnormally enlarged or dilated colon (megacolon). Encopresis occurs in approximately one percent of school children and is much more common in boys than it is in girls.

The causes of encopresis may sometimes be linked to anger, defiance, resistance, or fear of toilet training and, as such, may indicate the need for psychotherapeutic intervention that includes parents or caregivers, as well as the affected child. Treatment is often supportive. For example, a reward system may be established so that the child has an incentive to cooperate. In addition, the affected child may be encouraged to use the bathroom at specific times (e.g., after meals) and for specified periods of time. Parents are advised to remain nonjudgmental and nonretaliatory, so that consequences for noncompliance are minor. Additional treatment for primary encopresis may initially include the carefully monitored, short-term use of laxatives and enemas to relieve constipation and subsequent complications. Affected children may sometimes benefit from biofeedback, during which individuals learn how to control certain involuntary physiologic functions such as, in this case, the anal sphincter muscle. In addition, the careful administration of mineral oil, together with a high fiber diet, may be effective in relieving constipation and associated complications in children with secondary encopresis. Other treatment is symptomatic and supportive.

Government Agencies

3052 NIH/National Institute of Child Health and Human Development
31 Center Drive, Building 31
Bethesda, MD 20892
301-496-1333
Fax: 301-496-1104
www.nichd.nih.gov

Established in 1962 by congress, today the institute conducts and supports research on topics related to the health of children, adults, families and populations. Some of these topics include: developmental disabilities, growth and development, infant death, reproductive health and birth defects.

Jay H Hoofnagle, Director
Lisa Kaeser, Program & Public Liaison

National Associations & Support Groups

3053 American Academy of Pediatrics
141 Northwest Point Boulevard
Elk Grove Village, IL 60007
847-434-4000
800-433-9016
Fax: 847-434-8000
www.aap.org

The American Academy of Pediatrics and its member pediatricians are committed to the attainment of optimal physical, mental and social health and well-being for all infants, children, adolescents, and young adults.

Sandra Hassink, MD, FAAP, President

3054 International Foundation for Functional Gastrointestinal Disorders
700 W. Virginia St., #201
Milwaukee, WI 53204
414-964-1799
888-964-2001
Fax: 414-964-7176
e-mail: iffgd@iffgd.org
www.iffgd.org

The organization offers responses to those commonly asked questions for families and individuals whose lives have been touched with the disorder.

Nancy J Norton, Founder
William Norton, VP

3055 March of Dimes Birth Defects Foundation
1275 Mamaroneck Avenue
White Plains, NY 10605
914-997-4488
888-663-4637
Fax: 914-997-4763
e-mail: answers@marchofdimes.com
www.marchofdimes.com

Partnership of volunteers and professionals dedicated to improving the health of babies by preventing birth defects and infant mortality. Over 100 chapters are located across the country and can be located through the National Office.

Jennifer L Howse, President

Conferences

3056 IFFGD Professional Symposia
Int'l Foundation for Functional Gastrointestinal
700 W. Virginia St, Suite 201
Milwaukee, WI 53204
414-964-1799
888-964-2001
Fax: 414-964-7176
e-mail: iffgd@iffgd.org
www.iffgd.org

Aimed at promoting education and awareness among professionals from multiple disciplines who treat gastrointestinal disorders and incontinence.

April

Nancy J Norton, President

Web Sites

3057 Mental Help Net
P.O. Box 20709
Columbus, OH 43220
614-448-4055
800-232-TALK
e-mail: info@centersite.net, editor@centersite.n
mentalhelp.net

We wish to provide the following: to develop and debate in an open forum the future of the mental health field in America and throughout the world; to help coordinate various components of the mental health field, so as to bring about greater communication between them; also to educate the public about mental health issues.

Book Publishers

3058 What I Need to Know About Constipation
Nat'l Digestive Diseases Information Clearinghouse
31 Center Drive
Bethesda, MD 20892   301-496-3583
                                      Fax: 301-907-8906
                          e-mail: nddic@info.niddk.nih.gov
                                      www.niddk.nih.gov

Defines constipation and includes a list of steps for prevention, as
well as a list of additional resources

Pamphlets

3059 Constipation
NDDIC
9000 Rockville Pike
Bethesda, MD 20892   301-496-3583
                                      800-891-5389
                                      Fax: 301-907-8906
                          e-mail: nddic@info.niddk.nih.gov
                                      www.niddk.nih.gov

Includes a definition of constipation and information on how it
develops, how it is diagnosed, and how it can be treated. Also
provides details on misconceptions about constipation.

8 pages

Griffin P. Rodgers, MD, MACP, Director
Dr. Gregory Germino, Deputy Director
Kevin Abbott, Program Director

3060 Constipation in Children
Nat'l Digestive Diseases Information Clearinghouse
9000 Rockville Pike
Bethesda, MD 20892   301-496-3583
                                      Fax: 301-907-8906
                          e-mail: nddic@info.niddk.nih.gov
                                      www.niddk.nih.gov

Griffin P. Rodgers, MD, MACP, Director
Dr. Gregory Germino, Deputy Director
Kevin Abbott, Program Director

3061 Fecal Incontinence
NDDIC
9000 Rockville Pike
Bethesda, MD 20892   301-496-3583
                                      800-891-5389
                                      Fax: 301-907-8906
                          e-mail: nddic@info.niddk.nih.gov
                                      www.niddk.nih.gov

8 pages

Griffin P. Rodgers, MD, MACP, Director
Dr. Gregory Germino, Deputy Director
Kevin Abbott, Program Director

Description

3062 EPIDERMOLYSIS BULLOSA

Covers these related disorders: Epidermolysis bullosa dystrophica, Epidermolysis bullosa simplex, Junctional epidermolysis bullosa

Involves the following Biologic System(s):
Dermatologic Disorders

Epidermolysis bullosa is a group of inherited diseases that are often apparent at birth (congenital) and characterized by blistering of the skin after minor injury or trauma. In addition, blistering tends to worsen in warm temperatures. These disorders vary in severity, specific features, and mode of inheritance, and are classified under one of three groupings.

Epidermolysis bullosa simplex is a relatively mild, non-scarring form of this disorder that is inherited as an autosomal dominant trait. Epidermolysis bullosa simplex is further categorized as generalized or localized. The generalized type is usually apparent at birth or soon thereafter. The blisters, also known as bullae, are usually located on areas of the body that are prone to injury such as the hands, feet, elbows, knees, etc. Blistering tendencies usually lessen with advancing age with no long-term effects or scarring. The localized form of this disorder, known as Weber-Cockayne syndrome, affects the hands and feet and may not become apparent until walking commences or, in some cases, adolescence or adulthood. Blistering may be mild, but may severely worsen with such activities as extended walking. Treatment is symptomatic and supportive and may be directed toward prevention and treatment of secondary infections.

Junctional epidermolysis bullosa is inherited as an autosomal recessive trait and is also apparent at birth or soon thereafter. Characteristic findings and symptoms associated with this|potentially life-threatening form of the disorder may include severe blistering around the mouth and on the scalp, trunk, diaper area, and legs. In addition, slow-healing lesions may develop in the mucous membranes of the respiratory, gastrointestinal, and genitourinary tracts. Affected infants are also at increased risk for infections such as septicemia, a life-threatening condition in which harmful bacteria multiply in the bloodstream. In addition, the nails may appear defective and teeth may decay easily. Other findings may include growth retardation and abnormally low levels of circulating red blood cells (anemia). Treatment for junctional epidermolysis bullosa may include the administration of antibiotics to treat infections and blood transfusions to treat anemia. In addition, nutritional supplementation may be beneficial. Other treatment is symptomatic and supportive.

Epidermolysis bullosa dystrophica may be inherited as an autosomal dominant trait, an autosomal recessive trait, or it may appear sporadically. Findings associated with autosomal dominant inheritance are less severe than those of autosomal recessive transmission. This form of epidermolysis bullosa may be further categorized as the albopapuloid Pasini variant and the Cockayne-Touraine variant. The albopapuloid Pasini variant may first appear as early as infancy or as late as adolescence and is characterized by extensive, scarring-type blistering of the skin on the joints, arms, and legs; the appearance during adolescence of flesh-colored (albopapuloid) lesions on the trunk; and involvement of certain mucuous memberanes. The Cockayne-Touraine variant of this disorder develops during infancy or early childhood and is characterized by blisters that most commonly appear on the arms and legs.

Epidermolysis bullosa dystrophica that is inherited as an autosomal recessive trait is a severe form of this disorder that may be characterized at birth by extensive blistering and erosions of the body surfaces and mucous membranes. As the lesions heal, scarring may result in deformity and limited mobility. In addition, healing of the mucous membranes of the esophagus may cause narrowing of this structure, leading to difficulties in feeding and eating. Treatment may include the implementation of a special diet or use of special feeding devices necessitated by scarring or narrowing of the esophagus. Additional treatment may be directed toward the prevention or care of associated secondary infections. Other treatment is symptomatic and supportive.

Government Agencies

3063 NIH/National Institute of Arthritis and Mu sculoskeletal and Skin Diseases
1AMS Circle
Bethesda, MD 20892

301-402-4484
877-226-4267
Fax: 301-718-6366
TDD: 301-565-2966
e-mail: niamsinfo@mail.nih.gov
www.niams.nih.gov

The mission of the NIAMS, a part of the NIH, is to support research into the causes, treatment, and prevention of arthritis and musculoskeletal and skin diseases, the training of basic and clinical scientists to carry out this research, and the dissemination of information on research progress in these diseases.

Stephen I Katz MD PhD, Director
Robert H Carter MD, Deputy Director

National Associations & Support Groups

3064 American Academy of Pediatrics
141 Northwest Point Boulevard
Elk Grove Village, IL 60007

847-434-4000
800-433-9016
Fax: 847-434-8000
www.aap.org

The American Academy of Pediatrics and its member pediatricians are committed to the attainment of optimal physical, mental and social health and well-being for all infants, children, adolescents, and young adults.

Sandra Hassink, MD, FAAP, President

3065 DebRA: Dystrophic Epidermolysis Bullosa Research Association of America
16 East 41st Street
New York, NY 10017

212-868-1573
866-332-7276
Fax: 212-513-4099
e-mail: staff@debra.org
www.debra.org

Committed to providing referrals, patient advocacy and lobbying, offers networking services, and engages in patient and professional education.

Suzanne J Cohen, Executive Director
Abby Meadows, Development Manager

3066 Genetic Alliance
4301 Connecticut Avenue NW
Washington, DC 20008

202-966-5557
800-336-4363
Fax: 202-966-8553
e-mail: info@geneticalliance.org
www.geneticalliance.org

A coalition of voluntary genetic support groups, consumers and professionals addressing the needs of individuals and families affected by genetic disorders from a national perspective.

Sharon Terry, President

3067 March of Dimes Birth Defects Foundation
1275 Mamaroneck Avenue
White Plains, NY 10605   914-997-4488
                                888-663-4637
                           Fax: 914-997-4763
                e-mail: answers@marchofdimes.com
                        www.marchofdimes.com

Partnership of volunteers and professionals dedicated to improving the health of babies by preventing birth defects and infant mortality. Over 100 chapters are located across the country and can be located through the National Office.

Jennifer L Howse, President

Conferences

3068 Genetic Alliance Annual Conference
Genetic Alliance
4301 Connecticut Avenue NW, Suite 404
Washington, DC 20008   202-966-5557
                              800-336-4363
                         Fax: 202-966-8553
              e-mail: info@geneticalliance.org
                      www.geneticalliance.org

Consistently inspirational and enables partnership among all stakeholders: advocates and community leaders, health and industry professionals, policymakers, and academicians.

July

Sharon Terry, President/CEO
Tetyana Murza, Programs/Events Manager

Web Sites

3069 EB Medical Research Foundation
2757 Anchor Ave
Los Angeles, CA 90064   www.ebkids.org

The EBMRF is a nonprofit, whose sole purpose is dedicated to the support of medical research of epidermolysis bullosa — its causes, its cure, and the development of successful treatments.

Jerry J. Joseph, Chair
Lynn Anderson, President & Founder
Paul J. Joseph, CFO

3070 Family Village
www.familyvillage.wisc.edu

A global community that integrates information, resources and communication opportunities on the Internet for persons with cognitive and other disabilities, for their families and for those that provide them services and support.

3071 Online Mendelian Inheritance in Man
U.S. National Library of Medicine, 8600 Rockville
Bethesda, MD 20894   888-346-3656
                 e-mail: info@ncbi.nlm.nih.gov
                        www.ncbi.nlm.nih.gov

This database is a catalog of human genes and genetic disorders.

Christine E. Seidman, M.D., Chair
David J. Lipman, M.D., Executive Secretary
Michael Boehnke, Ph.D., Board Member

Newsletters

3072 DebRA Currents
DebRA
75 Broad Street, Suite 300
New York, NY 10004   212-868-1573
                            866-332-7276
                       Fax: 212-868-9296
                   e-mail: staff@deba.org
                          www.debra.org

Brett Kopelan, Executive Director
Rita Garson, Finance Director
Gabrielle Sedor, Program Manager

Description

3073 ERB'S PALSY

Synonym: Erb-Duchenne paralysis

Involves the following Biologic System(s):

Neurologic Disorders

Erb's palsy is a form of paralysis in newborns resulting from injury to certain nerves (i.e., fifth and sixth cervical nerves of upper brachial plexus) that supply specific muscles of the shoulder and arm. Nerve injury may be the result of a difficult delivery (e.g., breech presentation, delivery of an unusually large newborn, etc.). During delivery, lateral traction of the head and neck may occur and lead to stretching of these nerves, potentially resulting in such injury.

Newborns with Erb's palsy typically experience swelling and inflammation of the affected nerves and paralysis of the affected shoulder and arm muscles (e.g., deltoid, biceps, brachialis). This causes the arm to hang loosely with the elbow extended and inwardly rotated. Newborns with the condition are unable to move the affected arm away from the shoulder or rotate the arm away from the body. In addition, although they may extend the forearm, affected newborns lack a startle reflex known as Moro's reflex on the affected side. Moro's reflex, which is usually present at birth, involves stretching of the arms and legs forward and out and extension of the fingers when startled. In some severe cases, paralysis and associated loss of the muscle mass (atrophy)in the shoulder area (deltoid muscle) may cause drop shoulder, which is characterized by depression of the affected shoulder below the level of the other. Some infants may experience impairment of sensation in affected areas. Movements of the hand are typically not affected.

The effectiveness of certain treatments for Erb's palsy may vary, depending upon whether affected nerves (i.e., fifth and sixth cervical nerves) were torn or injured in a manner that allows a return of function within a few months. Treatment measures may include initial immobilization of the affected arm and shoulder with braces or splints and physical therapy including range of motion exercises, massage, and active and passive corrective exercises. Such therapy may help to improve muscle function and prevent permanent bending of affected joints in a fixed posture (flexion contractures). If paralysis continues at three to six months of age, surgical measures may be considered in some cases.

National Associations & Support Groups

3074 American Academy of Pediatrics
141 Northwest Point Boulevard
Elk Grove Village, IL 60007   847-434-4000
                                     800-433-9016
                                 Fax: 847-434-8000
                                      www.aap.org

The American Academy of Pediatrics and its member pediatricians are committed to the attainment of optimal physical, mental and social health and well-being for all infants, children, adolescents, and young adults.

Sandra Hassink, MD, FAAP, President

3075 Brachial Plexus Palsy Foundation
210 Springhaven Circle
Royersford, PA 19468   610-792-0974
          e-mail: contact@brachialplexuspalsyfoundation.or
                  www.brachialplexuspalsyfoundation.org

A non profit organizaztion designed to raise funds for activities in support of families with children who have suffered brachial plexus injuries. The Foundation also provides information about a brachial plexus injury ti better educate families who do not have the time or resources.

3076 March of Dimes Birth Defects Foundation
1275 Mamaroneck Avenue
White Plains, NY 10605   914-997-4488
                               888-663-4637
                          Fax: 914-997-4763
          e-mail: answers@marchofdimes.com
                  www.marchofdimes.com

Partnership of volunteers and professionals dedicated to improving the health of babies by preventing birth defects and infant mortality. Over 100 chapters are located across the country and can be located through the National Office.

Jennifer L Howse, President

3077 National Brachial Plexus/Erb's Palsy Association
PO Box 23
Larsen, WI 54947   920-836-9955
                     Fax: 920-836-9587
          e-mail: erbspalsy@usa.net
                  www.nbpepa.org

Provides support, promotes public awareness, serves as a resource to families and professionals and provides a network of information to incerase the understanding of Brachial Pelxus injuries and to discover new and better way to treat children with the injury.

3078 United Brachial Plexus Network
1610 Kent Street
Kent, OH 44240   781-315-6161
                        866-877-7004
                   Fax: 866-877-7004
          e-mail: info@ubpn.org
                  www.ubpn.org

A registered non-profit organization devoted to providing information, support, and leadership for families and those concerned with brachial plexus injuries worldwide. Also provided is an on-line registry, various outreach and awareness programs and publications.

Nancy Birk, President

Libraries & Resource Centers

3079 National Rehabilitation Information Center
4200 Forbes Blvd, Suite 202
Lanham, MD 20706   301-459-5900
                          800-346-2742
                     Fax: 301-562-2401
                     TTY: 301-459-5984
          e-mail: naricinfo@heitechservices.com
                  www.naric.com

Committed to providing direct, personal and high quality information services to anyone interested in disability and rehabilitation issues. We are committed to serving customers, researchers, family members, health professionals, educators, counselors and students throughout the country.

Mark Odum, Director

Web Sites

3080 Texas Children's Hospital
6621 Fannin Street
Houston, TX 77030   832-824-1000
                  www.texaschildrenshospital.org

Is an internationally recognized full-care prediatric hospital located in the Texas Medical Center in Houston. The largest pediatric hospital in the United States, Texas Children's is nationaly ranked in the top 5 among children's hospitals.

Mark A. Wallace, President & CEO
Dr. Mark Kline, Physician-in-Chief
Dr. Charles D. Fraser, Jr., Surgeon-in-Chief

Newsletters

3081 Outreach
United Brachial Plexus Network
1610 Kent Street
Kent, OH 44240

781-315-6161
866-877-7004
Fax: 866-877-7004
e-mail: info@ubpn.org
www.ubpn.org

Brachial Plexus/Erb's Palsy newsletter.

Description

3082 ERYTHEMA INFECTIOSUM

Synonyms: EI, Fifth disease, Sticker's disease, Parvovirus, Slapped Cheek

Involves the following Biologic System(s):

Infectious Disorders

Erythema infectiosum, or Fifth disease, is a contagious infection caused by the human parvovirus B19. It is characterized by a three-stage rash. First, there is the sudden appearance of a red rash on the face that may look as if the cheeks had been slapped. Then the rash progresses to a reddish, raised-spot, blotchy eruption that spreads to the trunk, buttocks, arms, and legs. When it begins to fade, the rash takes on a lacy-type appearance. The rash usually subsides within five to 10 days, but may reappear within a month's time, especially after exercise, stress, skin irritation, or exposure to sunlight. Transmission of this virus is through inhalation of droplets exhaled or coughed into the air by infected individuals. The incubation period for erythema infectiosum is approximately four to 14 days.

Erythema infectiosum occurs most commonly in preschool and young school-age children. The first symptoms may be low-grade fever and headache. Once the rash appears or shortly thereafter, fever and other signs of illness may be absent. However, some older children and adults may develop mild itching (pruritus), joint pain (arthralgia), and inflammation of the joints (arthritis). In addition, under certain circumstances, exposure to human parvovirus B19 may result in more severe complications. For example, individuals with certain blood disorders such as thalessemia or sickle cell anemia may develop a temporary inability to produce red blood cells, resulting in a decrease in the body's capacity to supply oxygen to the tissues of the body (anemia). Symptoms associated with severe anemia may include weakness, discomfort, pale skin (pallor), rapid breathing (tachypnea), and rapid heartbeat (tachycardia). In addition, those who have impaired immune function may experience severe consequences upon exposure to human parvovirus B19. For example, individuals undergoing certain types of chemotherapy, those with acquired immunodeficiency syndrome (AIDS), or those with certain types of primary, inherited immune defects may experience recurrent or prolonged infections, anemia, or other blood abnormalities.

Pregnant women infected with parvovirus B19 may transmit it to their unborn children, resulting, in rare cases, in miscarriage or stillbirth; however, most of those exposed in utero are born with no apparent consequences. Other viral-exposed infants may have abnormal accumulations of fluid in the tissues or cavities of the body (hydrops). If this condition is diagnosed before birth, special blood transfusions delivered by way of the umbilical vein may be of benefit to the affected fetus. Treatment for this viral infection is symptomatic.

Government Agencies

3083 NIH/National Institute of Allergy and Infectious Diseases
6610 Rockledge Drive, MSC 6612
Bethesda, MD 20892   301-496-5717; 866-284-4107
Fax: 301-402-3573; TDD: 800-877-8339
e-mail: ocpsfoffice@niaid.nih.gov; www.niaid.nih.gov

Conducts and supports basic and applied research to better understand, treat, and ultimately prevent infectious, immunologic, and allergic diseases.

Anthony S Fauci MD, Director

National Associations & Support Groups

3084 American Academy of Pediatrics
141 Northwest Point Boulevard
Elk Grove Village, IL 60007   847-434-4000, 800-433-9016
Fax: 847-434-8000; www.aap.org

The American Academy of Pediatrics and its member pediatricians are committed to the attainment of optimal physical, mental and social health and well-being for all infants, children, adolescents, and young adults.

Sandra Hassink, MD, FAAP, President

3085 March of Dimes Birth Defects Foundation
1275 Mamaroneck Avenue
White Plains, NY 10605   914-997-4488, 888-663-4637
Fax: 914-997-4763
e-mail: answers@marchofdimes.com; www.marchofdimes.com

Partnership of volunteers and professionals dedicated to improving the health of babies by preventing birth defects and infant mortality. Over 100 chapters are located across the country and can be located through the National Office.

Jennifer L Howse, President

3086 World Health Organization
Avenue Appia 20
Geneva, SL
Switzerland   122-791-2111; Fax: 122-791-3111
www.who.int

WHO is the directing and coordinating authority for health within the United Nations system.

Dr Margaret Chan, Director General

Web Sites

3087 Kid's Health
kidshealth.org

Kids health is the largest and most visited site on the web providing doctor-approved health information about children from before birth through adolescence. Kids health provides families with accurate, up to date and jargon free health information they can use.

Neil Izenberg, MD, Editor-in-Chief & Founder

3088 Med Help International
www.medhelp.org

800-522-5006; www.medhelp.org

Is dedicated to helping patients find the highest quality medical information in the world today. We offer patients the tools necessary to make informed treatment decisions within the short time lines dedicated by their illness or disease.

3089 New York State Department of Health
www.medhelp.org/lib/fifth.htm

800-522-5006; www.medhelp.org/lib/fifth.htm

Information on erythema infectiosum, like how does anyone get it, what is the treatment, and what can be done to prevent this disease from occuring.

Description

3090 ESOPHAGEAL ATRESIA

Synonyms: Tracheo-esophageal fistula, Vacterl, Vater

Involves the following Biologic System(s):

Gastrointestinal Disorders

Esophageal atresia is a defect that is present at birth (congenital). The esophagus, which is a muscular tube, is that portion of the digestive system that connects the throat and the stomach. In infants with esophageal atresia, the channel (lumen) within the tubular esophagus fails to develop properly, resulting in an esophagus that ends in a blind pouch, failing to provide a continuous passage to the stomach. In some infants, the upper section of the esophagus may be dramatically narrowed or it may be closed at its lower end. In others, the closed-end lower portion extends upward from the stomach and there is no through connection between the two. Most affected infants also have an abnormal tube-like connection or opening between the windpipe (trachea) and either the upper or lower portion of the esophagus. This is known as a tracheoesophageal fistula. In some children, there is a double connection in which there is an abnormal passage between the trachea and part of the esophagus, as well as between the trachea and a lower region of the esophagus.

Infants with esophageal atresia cannot swallow at all and therefore salivate and regurgitate excessively. If a tracheoesophageal fistula exists between the windpipe and upper portion of the esophagus, fluid may enter the lungs, resulting in coughing, choking, a bluish discoloration (cyanosis) of the nail beds, lips, and mucous membranes, and possibly pneumonia. The presence of an abnormal passage between the trachea and the lower section of the esophagus may allow air to enter the abdomen, resulting in excessive abdominal swelling (distension) that may interfere with normal breathing. In addition, contents of the abdomen may enter the lungs and severe inflammation may occur. If esophageal atresia is present without a fistula, characteristic findings may include a boat-shaped abdomen that is devoid of air.

Treatment includes surgery to join or connect the two sections of the esophagus. This procedure is known as an esophageal anastomosis. Tracheoesophageal fistulas may be surgically corrected by ligation, a procedure in which the passageway is tied off. Before surgery, special care is taken to ensure the infants do not draw fluid (aspirate) into their lungs through the esophagus.

As many as 50 percent of infants with esophageal atresia have associated structural malformations of other organs. For example, if a tracheoesophageal fistula is present, other abnormalities of the trachea may also be apparent. In addition, approximately half of all affected infants have a complex of congenital anomalies (VACTERL syndrome) characterized by additional malformations involving the heart, skeleton, kidneys, and urinary and genital systems. Treatment for esophageal atresia includes management or correction of associated anomalies. Esophageal atresia occurs in approximately one in 3,500 births in the United States. About 33 percent of these infants are born prematurely.

National Associations & Support Groups

3091 American Academy of Pediatrics
141 Northwest Point Boulevard
Elk Grove Village, IL 60007

847-434-4000
800-433-9016
Fax: 847-434-8000
www.aap.org

The American Academy of Pediatrics and its member pediatricians are committed to the attainment of optimal physical, mental and social health and well-being for all infants, children, adolescents, and young adults.

Sandra Hassink, MD, FAAP, President

3092 American College of Gastroenterology
PO Box 342260
Bethesda, MD 20827

301-263-9000
www.acg.gi.org

Founded to advance the scientific study and medical practice of diseases of the gastrointestinal (GI) tract.

Jack A DiPalma, President
Amy E Foxx-Orenstein, VP

3093 Digestive Disease National Coalition
507 Capitol Court NE, Suite 200
Washington, DC 20002

202-544-7497
Fax: 202-546-7105
www.ddnc.org

Advocacy organization comprised of 22 voluntary and professional societies concerned with the many diseases of the digestive tract and liver.

Dale Dirks, Administrator
Dr. Maurice Cerulli, President
Dr. Peter Banks, VP

3094 International Foundation for Functional Gastrointestinal Disorders
PO Box 170864
Milwaukee, WI 53217

414-964-1799
888-964-2001
Fax: 414-964-7176
e-mail: iffgd@iffgd.org
www.iffgd.org

Nonprofit education and research organization founded in 1991. IFFGD addresses the issues surrounding life with gastrointestinal (GI) functional and mobility disorders and increases the awareness about these disorders among the general public, researchers and the clinical care community.

Nancy J Norton, Founder
William Norton, VP

3095 North American Society for Pediatric Gastroenterology/Hepatology/Nutrition
PO Box 6
Flourtown, PA 19031

215-233-0808
Fax: 215-233-3918
e-mail: naspghan@naspghan.org
www.naspghan.org

Strives to improve the care of infants, children and adolescents with digestive disorders by promoting advances in clinical care of children with chronic abdominal pain, diarrhea, constipation, vomiting, bleeding from the GI tract, inflammatory bowel disease, liver diseases, diseases of the pancreas, poor weight gain and nutritional problems.

Philip Sherman, President
Margaret K Stallings, Executive Director

Libraries & Resource Centers

3096 National Digestive Diseases Information Clearinghouse
2 Information Way
Bethesda, MD 20892

301-654-3810
800-891-5389
Fax: 301-907-8906
e-mail: nddic@info.niddk.nih.gov
www.niddk.nih.gov

The National Institute of Diabetes and Digestive and Kidney Diseases conducts and supports research on many of the most serious diseases affecting public health. The Institute supports much of the clinical research on the diseases of internal medicine and related subspecialty fields as well as many basic science disciplines.

Kathy Kranzfelder, Project Officer

Conferences

3097 IFFGD Professional Symposia
Int'l Foundation for Functional Gastrointestinal
PO Box 170864
Milwaukee, WI 53217

414-964-1799
888-964-2001
Fax: 414-964-7176
e-mail: iffgd@iffgd.org
www.iffgd.org

Aimed at promoting education and awareness among professionals from multiple disciplines who treat gastrointestinal disorders and incontinence.

April
Nancy J Norton, President

3098 NASPGHAN Annual Meeting and Postgraduate Course
NASPGHAN
PO Box 6
Flourtown, PA 19031

215-233-0808
Fax: 215-233-3918
e-mail: naspghan@naspghan.org
www.naspghan.org

October
Margaret K Stallings, Executive Director

Web Sites

3099 National Digestive Diseases Information Clearinghouse
9000 Rockville Pike
Bethesda, MD 20892

301-496-3583
Fax: 301-907-8906
e-mail: nddic@info.niddk.nih.gov
www.digestive.niddk.nih.gov

The National Institute of Diabetes and Digestive and Kidney Diseases conducts and supports research on many of the most serious diseases affecting public health. The Institute supports much of the clinical research on the diseases of internal medicine and related subspecialty fields as well as many basic science disciplines.

Griffin P. Rodgers, MD, MACP, Director
Dr. Gregory Germino, Deputy Director
Kevin Abbott, Program Director

Journals

3100 Journal of Pediatric Gastroenterology and Nutrition
NASPGHAN, author

Lippincott Williams & Wilkins
530 Walnut Street
Philadelphia, PA 19106

215-521-8300
Fax: 215-521-8902
www.lww.com

Publication of the North American Society for Pediatric Gastroenterolgy, Hepatology and Nutrition, which strives to improve the care of infants, children and adolescents with digestive disorders by promoting advances in clinical care of children with chronic abdominal pain, diarrhea, constipation, vomiting, bleeding from the GI tract, inflammatory bowel disease, liver diseases, diseases of the pancreas, poor weight gain and nutritional problems.

Newsletters

3101 NASPGHAN News
PO Box 6
Flourtown, PA 19031

215-233-0808
Fax: 215-233-3939
e-mail: naspghan@naspghan.org
www.naspgn.org

Publication of the North American Society for Pediatric Gastroenterolgy, Hepatology and Nutrition, which strives to improve the care of infants, children and adolescents with digestive disorders by promoting advances in clinical care of children with chronic abdominal pain, diarrhea, constipation, vomiting, bleeding from the GI tract, inflammatory bowel disease, liver diseases, diseases of the pancreas, poor weight gain and nutritional problems.

3102 TEF/VATER International Support Network
9005 N Van Houten
Portland, OR 97203

301-535-7185
Fax: 301-952-9152
e-mail: info@tefvater.org
www.tefvater.org

Provides support to children and adults born with esophageal atresia.

Description

3103 EWING'S SARCOMA

Synonym: Ewing's tumor

Involves the following Biologic System(s):

Hematologic and Oncologic Disorders, Orthopedic and Muscle Disorders

Ewing's sarcoma is a malignant tumor that typically occurs in individuals under the age of 20 years. The tumor most often arises in the long bones of the shin (tibia), thigh (femur), or upper arm (humerus) or the flat bones of the pelvis, vertebrae, or chest wall. Ewing's sarcoma often invades surrounding soft tissues and tends to spread (metastasize) to other bones, the lungs, and, less frequently, to the bone marrow or other organs. In some cases, the primary tumor may develop in soft tissue. Approximately 75 percent of these tumors occur in the legs or arms as well as the bones of the shoulders.

The most common symptoms of Ewing's sarcoma include fever, as well as pain, tenderness, and swelling in the area of the tumor. Some children may also experience weight loss, low levels of circulating red blood cells (anemia), and elevated levels of circulating white blood cells (leukocytosis). In addition, the tumor may weaken the surrounding bone and thus increase vulnerability to bone fracture. The diagnosis of Ewing's tumor is established through the use of x-rays along with examination of tissue samples obtained through biopsy. In addition, other procedures such as bone scanning, computed tomography (CT), and magnetic resonance imaging (MRI) may be used to confirm the presence of lung, bone, or other metastases.

Ewing's sarcoma develops most frequently between the ages of 10 and 20 years of age and affects boys more often than girls by a ratio of two to one. These tumors rarely occur in black children. Treatment of Ewing's sarcoma may include the use of chemotherapy and radiation. Patients are also evaluated for possible surgical removal of the tumor. Other treatment is symptomatic and supportive. Outcome (prognosis) for children with Ewing's sarcoma depends on several factors that include the extent of the disease, the size and location of the tumor, presence or absence of metastases, the tumor's response to therapy, and the age and overall health of the child. Prompt medical attention and aggressive therapy are important for the best prognosis.

Government Agencies

3104 NIH/National Cancer Institute

6116 Executive Boulevard, Room 3036A
Bethesda, MD 20892

800-422-6237
www.cancer.gov

The National Cancer Institute coordinates the National Cancer Program, which conducts and supports research, training, health information dissemination, and other programs with respect to the cause, diagnosis, prevention, and treatment of cancer, rehabilitation from cancer, and the continuing care of cancer patients and the families of cancer patients.

John E Niederhuber MD, Director

National Associations & Support Groups

3105 American Academy of Pediatrics

141 Northwest Point Boulevard
Elk Grove Village, IL 60007

847-434-4000
800-433-9016
Fax: 847-434-8000
www.aap.org

The American Academy of Pediatrics and its member pediatricians are committed to the attainment of optimal physical, mental and social health and well-being for all infants, children, adolescents, and young adults.

Sandra Hassink, MD, FAAP, President

3106 American Cancer Society

Brain Tumor Support Group
ACS Building, 8900 Carpenter Freeway
Dallas, TX 75247

214-819-1200
800-227-2345
Fax: 214-631-3869
www.cancer.org

Attacks the support aspect of this disease from every angle including data on lowering risks to dealing with grief.

Maria Clark, Executive Director

3107 B.A.S.E. Camp Children's Cancer Foundation

7501 Glenmoor Lane
Winter Park, FL 32792

407-673-5060
Fax: 407-673-5095
e-mail: email@basecamp.org
basecampcf.org

Provides a year round base of support for children and families facing the challenge of living with cancer, hemophilia and other blood related illnesses.

Terri Jones, Executive Director

3108 Believe In Tomorrow National Children's Foundation

6601 Fredrick Road
Baltimore, MD 21228

410-744-1032
800-933-5470
Fax: 410-744-1984
e-mail: info@believeintomorrow.org
www.believeintomorrow.org

Provides exceptional hospital and retreat housing services to critically ill children and their families. The Foundation also provides a unique Hands On adventures program that allows children to experience unique once in a lifetime opportunities.

Brian Morrison, Ceo

3109 CancerCare

275 7th Avenue, Floor 22
New York, NY 10001

212-712-8400
800-813-4673
Fax: 212-712-8495
e-mail: info@cancercare.org
www.cancercare.org

CancerCare is a national nonprofit, 501(c)(3) organization that provides free, professional support services to anyone affected by cancer: people with cancer, caregivers, children, loved ones, and the bereaved. CancerCare programs - including counseling and support groups, education, financial assistance and practical help - are provided by professional oncology social workers and are completely free of charge.

Helen Miller, LCSW, Chief Executive Officer
Susan Smirnoff, Board President

3110 Candlelighters Childhood Cancer Foundation

PO Box 498
Kensington, MD 20895

301-962-3520
800-366-2223
Fax: 310-962-3521
e-mail: staff@candlelighters.org
www.candlelighters.org

The Candlelighters Childhood Cancer Foundation National Office was founded in 1970 by concerned parents of children with cancer. Today our membership of over 50,000 members of the national office and more than 100,000 members across the across the country, including Candlelighters affiliate groups, includes, parents of children who are being treated or have been treated for cancer.

Ruth Hoffman, Executive Director

3111 Hair Club for Kids: Hair Club for Men
270 Farmington Avenue, Suite 232
Farmington, CT 06032
860-674-0202
888-888-8986
Fax: 860-676-0805
www.hairclub.com/kids

If your child expresses an interest in wearing a wig, send pictures prior to hair loss with snippets of hair for a good match of original color and texture. The cost of the wig may be covered by insurance.

3112 Just In Time
PO Box 27693
Philadelphia, PA 19118
215-247-8777
Fax: 215-247-0956
www.softhats.com

100% cotton hat, turbans and caps designed for women with hair loss due to cancer, chemotherapy, alopecia or trichotillomania.

Verlay Platt, President

3113 National Childhood Cancer Foundation
4600 East West Highway, Suite 600
Bethesda, MD 20814
301-718-0042
Fax: 301-718-0047
e-mail: info@curesearch.org
www.curesearch.org

CureSearch unites the world's largest childhood cancer research organization, the Children's Oncology Group, and the National Childhood Cancer Foundation through our mission to cure childhood cancer. Research is the key to the cure.

Stacy Haller, Executive Director

3114 National Coalition for Cancer Survivorship
1010 Wayne Road, Suite 770
Silver Spring, MD 20910
301-650-9127
877-622-7937
Fax: 301-565-9670
e-mail: info@canceradvocacy.org
www.canceradvocacy.org

Furnishes information about legal rights and advocacy services for cancer survivors of all ages. Publications include: Health Insurance and Cancer: What You Need to Know; Working It Out: Your Employment Rights As a Cancer Survivor; and Charting the Journey: An Almanac of Practical Resources for Cancer Survivors.

Ellen Stovall, President
Michael Bergin, Chief Operating Officer

Web Sites

3115 CancerCare
275 Seventh Avenue
New York, NY 10001
212-712-8400
800-813-4673
Fax: 212-712-8495
e-mail: info@cancercare.org
www.cancercare.org

CancerCare is a national nonprofit, 501(c)(3) organization that provides free, professional support services to anyone affected by cancer: people with cancer, caregivers, children, loved ones, and the bereaved. CancerCare programs - including counseling and support groups, education, financial assistance and practical help - are provided by professional oncology social workers and are completely free of charge.

Michael Parisi, President
Patricia J. Goldsmith, CEO
John Rutigliano, COO

3116 Children's Cancer Web
www.cancerindex.org/ccw

An independent nonprofit site, established to provide a directory of childhood cancer resources.

3117 Ewing's Sarcoma Support Group Resources Page
www.cureourchildren.org
310-355-6046
Fax: 310-454-9592
www.cureourchildren.org

3118 OncoLink: The University of Penslyvania Cancer Center Resource
www.oncolink.upenn.edu

Book Publishers

3119 Let's Talk About Going to the Hospital
Rosen Publishing Group's PowerKids Press
29 E 21st Street
New York, NY 10010
212-777-3017
800-237-9932
Fax: 888-436-4643
e-mail: rosenpub@tribeca.ios.com
www.powerkidspress.com

If a child has to check into the hospital, chances are he or she is already upset about being ill. Knowing how a hospital functions and what the procedures are, such as when family members can visit, will help in what is already a stressful situation. Grades K-5.

24 pages
ISBN: 0-823950-36-0

3120 Let's Talk About when Kids Have Cancer
Rosen Publishing Group's PowerKids Press
29 E 21st Street
New York, NY 10010
212-777-3017
800-237-9932
Fax: 888-436-4643
e-mail: customerservice@rosenpub.com
www.powerkidspress.com

In a straightforward yet comforting way, this book explains what cancer is, what kinds of treatments surround the disease and how to cope if a child or the friend of a child has cancer.

24 pages
ISBN: 0-823951-95-2

3121 Pediatric Cancer Sourcebook
Omnigraphics
PO Box 8002
Aston, PA 19014
800-234-1340
Fax: 800-875-1340
e-mail: info@omnigraphics.com
www.omnigraphics.com

Basic consumer health information about leukemias, brain tumors, sarcomas, lymphomas and other cancers in infants, children and adolescents.

587 pages
ISBN: 0-780802-45-4

Camps

3122 Arizona Camp Sunrise
PO Box 27872
Tempe, AZ 85285
602-952-7550
Fax: 602-404-1118
e-mail: melissa@azcampsunrise.org
www.azcampsunrise.org

The camp is dedicated to provide an exciting, medically safe camp program for children who have or have had cancer and their siblings.

Melissa Lee, Camp Director

3123 Camp Catch-A-Rainbow
American Cancer Society
1205 E Saginaw Street
Lansing, MI 800-A
                              248-302-8985
e-mail: kwilson@ymcastorercamps.org
www.ymcastorercamps.org/ccar/camp-catch-a-rainbow/

Open to any child who has, or has had, cancer.

3124 Camp Sunshine Dreams
PO Box 28232
Fresno, CA 93729   www.campsunshinedreams.com

Summer camp for children with cancer.

3125 Okizu Foundation Camps
16 Digital Drive, Suite 130
Novato, CA 94949
                              415-382-8383
Fax: 415-382-8384
e-mail: info@okizu.org
www.okizu.org

This foundation runs family camp programs for children who
have cancer and their families, and for children who have or had a
parent with cancer.

Suzie Randall, Executive Director

Description

3126 FAMILIAL DYSAUTONOMIA

Synonyms: FD, HSAN-III, Riley-Day syndrome

Involves the following Biologic System(s):

Genetic/Chromosomal/Syndrome/Metabolic Disorders, Neurologic Disorders

Familial dysautonomia (FD) is a rare inherited disorder of that part of the nervous system responsible for regulating various essential involuntary functions (autonomic nervous system). This disorder is characterized in infants by feeding difficulties, including excessive salivation and poor swallowing and sucking reflexes. The breathing in of liquid or other substances into the lungs (aspiration) may lead to repeated episodes of bronchial pneumonia. Other associated symptoms and findings include skin blotching, sweating, fluctuating extremes in body temperature, and defective tear secretion (lacrimation). Affected children develop an reduced sensitivity to temperature and pain. This may lead to frequent injuries such as irritation of the corneas of the eyes. Corneal injury may also occur as the result of decreased tear production. In addition, slurred speech and drooling may become evident. Children with familial dysautonomia typically have weak reflex responses (hyporeflexia) and experience delays in walking accompanied by the inability to coordinate voluntary movements (motor incoordination). After three years of age, affected children often develop severe vomiting episodes (hyperemesis) that may occur three or four times an hour and, in some cases, may last for three days or more. These episodes may sometimes be accompanied by elevated blood pressure (hypertension), abdominal pain and swelling, increased irritability, or breathing difficulties (dyspnea). As children with this disorder reach adolescence, a sideward curvature of the spine (scoliosis) may become evident along with leg cramping and weakness. In addition, some children may experience a delay in the onset of puberty. Older children may develop emotional and behavioral changes, such as irritability and depression. Intolerance for anesthetics is a common finding among children with FD.

Treatment for familial dysautonomia is symptomatic and supportive. Artificial tears, drops, or ointments may be placed in the eyes to prevent injury to corneas. Certain medications known as antiemetics may be prescribed to help control episodes of vomiting. In addition, replacement fluids and electrolytes may be administered to prevent excessive fluid loss (dehydration) resulting from vomiting episodes. Other treatment may include surgery or the use of orthopedic aids to correct scoliosis.

Familial dysautonomia is inherited as an autosomal recessive trait and occurs most commonly among certain individuals of eastern European descent, particularly Ashkenazi Jews at a rate of one out of 10,000 to 20,000 births. The disease gene for this disorder is located on the long arm of chromosome 9 (9q31-33).

National Associations & Support Groups

3127 American Academy of Pediatrics
141 Northwest Point Boulevard
Elk Grove Village, IL 60007
847-434-4000
800-433-9016
Fax: 847-434-8000
www.aap.org

The American Academy of Pediatrics and its member pediatricians are committed to the attainment of optimal physical, mental and social health and well-being for all infants, children, adolescents, and young adults.

Sandra Hassink, MD, FAAP, President

3128 Dysautonomia Foundation
315 West 39th Street, Suite 701
New York, NY 10018
212-279-1066
Fax: 212-279-2066
e-mail: info@familialdysautonomia.org
www.familialdysautonomia.org

Provides parents the knowledge regarding both national and international facilities that specialize in the treatment of the disorder.

David Drenner, Executive Director

3129 Familial Dysautonomia Hope Foundation
605 5th Avenue
Conover, NC 28613
828-695-1060
Fax: 828-695-1060
e-mail: info@fdhope.org
www.fdvillage.org

To find a cure and new treatment options for Familial Dysautonomia by funding relevant research programs, to provide a support network aimed at addressing the needs of patients and families and to promote Familial Dysautonomia education and awareness programs in the medical community.

3130 Genetic Alliance
4301 Connecticut Avenue NW
Washington, DC 20008
202-966-7955
800-336-4363
Fax: 202-966-8553
e-mail: info@geneticalliance.org
www.geneticalliance.org

A coalition of voluntary genetic support groups, consumers and professionals addressing the needs of individuals and families affected by genetic disorders from a national perspective.

Sharon Terry, President

3131 March of Dimes Birth Defects Foundation
1275 Mamaroneck Avenue
White Plains, NY 10605
914-997-4488
888-663-4637
Fax: 914-997-4763
e-mail: answers@marchofdimes.com
www.marchofdimes.com

Partnership of volunteers and professionals dedicated to improving the health of babies by preventing birth defects and infant mortality. Over 100 chapters are located across the country and can be located through the National Office.

Jennifer L Howse, President

Conferences

3132 Genetic Alliance Annual Conference
Genetic Alliance
4301 Connecticut Avenue NW, Suite 404
Washington, DC 20008
202-966-5557
800-336-4363
Fax: 202-966-8553
e-mail: info@geneticalliance.org
www.geneticalliance.org

Consistently inspirational and enables partnership among all stakeholders: advocates and community leaders, health and industry professionals, policymakers, and academicians.

July

Sharon Terry, President/CEO
Tetyana Murza, Programs/Events Manager

Web Sites

3133 Family Village
www.familyvillage.wisc.edu

A global community that integrates information, resources and communication opportunities on the Internet for persons with cognitive and other disabilities, for their families and for those that provide them services and support.

3134 NYU
530 First Avenue
New York, 10016   212-263-7225
                                          www.med.nyu.edu/fd/fdcenter.html

Offers information about Familial Dysautonomia.

Horacio Kaufman, MD, FAAN, Director
Felicia Axelrod, MD, FAAP, Co Director
Jose Martinez, MA, Research Faculty

3135 Online Mendelian Inheritance in Man
U.S. National Library of Medicine, 8600 Rockville
Bethesda, MD 20894   888-346-3656
                           e-mail: info@ncbi.nlm.nih.gov
                                    www.ncbi.nlm.nih.gov

This database is a catalog of human genes and genetic disorders.

Christine E. Seidman, M.D., Chair
David J. Lipman, M.D., Executive Secretary
Michael Boehnke, Ph.D., Board Member

Description

3136 FETAL ALCOHOL SYNDROME

Synonyms: FAS, Fetal alcohol effect (FAE), Alcohol-related neurodevelopmental, Alcolol-related birth defects

Involves the following Biologic System(s):

Genetic/Chromosomal/Syndrome/Metabolic Disorders

Fetal alcohol syndrome, or FAS, is a condition that is present at birth and the result of persistent maternal alcohol consumption during pregnancy. This condition is characterized by various birth defects such as low birth weight, short birth length, and an unusually small head (microcephaly) that may be associated with slowed development of the brain. Infants with FAS may also have several abnormalities of the face and skull including an unusually short opening between the margins of the upper and lower eyelids (palpebral fissures), vertical folds of skin that extend from the inner corners of the upper eyelids to the sides of the nose (epicanthal folds), an abnormally small lower jaw (micrognathia), or a poorly developed upper jaw (maxillary hypoplasia). Additional unusual features may include an abnormal opening in the roof of the mouth (cleft palate), a prominent forehead (frontal bossing), a flattened nasal bridge, and a thin, smooth upper lip. Other characteristic findings may include heart defects, abnormalities of the limbs and joints (e.g., dislocated hip, etc.), and irregular skin crease patterns on the palms of the hands. Within the first day of life, affected newborns may also exhibit characteristic symptoms of alcohol withdrawal such as tremor, increased irritability, muscle spasms, vomiting, or other problems. The development of the brain may also be impaired resulting in moderate to severe mental retardation. Approximately 20 percent of newborns with fetal alcohol syndrome risk life-threatening symptoms and complications within the first few weeks of life.

Alcohol consumption during pregnancy affects the growth and development of the fetus within the uterus and may result not only in birth defects but, in some cases, miscarriage or stillbirth. Although it is believed that fetal alcohol syndrome results from persistent moderate or heavy drinking, no safe levels of alcohol intake during pregnancy have been established; therefore, pregnant women are counseled to avoid alcohol consumption. It has, however, been determined that the more alcohol consumed, the greater the chances of giving birth to children with associated abnormalities. Therefore, treatment is directed toward identification, counseling, and education of women at risk. Other treatment is symptomatic and supportive.

Government Agencies

3137 NIH/National Institute of Child Health and Human Development
31 Center Drive, Building 31
Bethesda, MD 20892
301-496-1333
Fax: 301-496-1104
www.nichd.nih.gov

Established in 1962 by congress, today the institute conducts and supports research on topics related to the health of children, adults, families and populations. Some of these topics include: developmental disabilities, growth and development, infant death, reproductive health and birth defects.

Jay H Hoofnagle, Director
Lisa Kaeser, Program & Public Liaison

3138 NIH/National Institute of Mental Health
6001 Executive Boulevard, Room 8184, MSC 9663
Bethesda, MD 20892
301-443-4513
866-615-6464
Fax: 301-443-4279
TTY: 301-443-8431
e-mail: nimhinfo@nih.gov
www.nimh.nih.gov

Conducts strategic planning for specific research areas as well as for the Institute as a whole.

Dr Thomas R Insel, Director

3139 NIH/National Institute on Alcohol Abuse an d Alcoholism
5635 Fishers Lane, MSC 9304
Bethesda, MD 20892
301-443-3885
877-266-4267
Fax: 301-443-7043
www.niaaa.nih.gov

Established in 1970, NIAAA conducts research focused on improving the treatment and prevention of alcoholism and alcohol-related problems to reduce the enormous health, social, and econmic consequences of this disease.

Dr Kenneth R Warren, Acting Director

National Associations & Support Groups

3140 ARC of the United States
1010 Wayne Avenue, Suite 650
Silver Spring, MD 20910
301-565-3842
Fax: 301-565-5342
e-mail: info@thearc.org
www.thearc.org

The ARC is the national organization of and for people with mental retardation and related developmental disabilities and their families. Devoted to promoting and improving supports and services for people with mental retardation and their families. The association also fosters research and education regarding the prevention of mental retardation in infants and young children. The ARC was founded in 1950 by a small group of parents and other concerned individuals.

Steven M Eidelman, Ceo
Adam Aaronson, Public Inquiries Director

3141 American Academy of Pediatrics
141 Northwest Point Boulevard
Elk Grove Village, IL 60007
847-434-4000
800-433-9016
Fax: 847-434-8000
www.aap.org

The American Academy of Pediatrics and its member pediatricians are committed to the attainment of optimal physical, mental and social health and well-being for all infants, children, adolescents, and young adults.

Sandra Hassink, MD, FAAP, President

3142 American Association for Pediatric Opthalmology
655 Beach Street
San Francisco, CA 94109
415-561-8505
Fax: 415-561-8531
e-mail: aapos@aao.org
www.aapos.org

AAPOS is the American Association for Pediatric Ophthalmology and Strabismus. The organization's goals are to advance the quality of children's eye care, support the training of pediatric ophthalmologists, support research activities in pediatric ophthalmology, and advance the care of adults with strabismus.

Jennifer Hull, Client Services Manager
Brooke Lyon, Client Services Coordinator
Maria A. Schweers, CO, Scientific Program Coordinator

3143 American Pregnancy Association
1425 Greenway Drive, Suite 440
Irving, TX 75038
e-mail: info@americanpregnancy.org
americanpregnancy.org

The American Pregnancy Association is a 501(c)(3) nonprofit organization committed to promoting pregnancy wellness through education, advocacy and community awareness.

3144 Association of Reproductive Health Professionals
1330 Broadway, Suite 1100
Oakland, CA 96412
202-466-3825
e-mail: ARHP@arhp.org
www.arhp.org

It is a multidisciplinary association of professionals who provide reproductive health services or education, conduct reproductive health research, or influence reproductive health policy.

Nerys Benfield, Medical Director
Alayna Florman, Associate Director of Development
Megan A. Henszey, Program Manager

3145 Families Affected by Fetal Alcohol Spectrum Disorder
P.O. Box 427
Pittsboro, NC 27312
919-360-7073
e-mail: adrienne@fafasd.org
fafasd.org

It seeks to spread information, awareness, and hope for caregivers of people with FASD.

Becky Brantley, President
Janet Schanzenbach, Vice-President
Tina Andrews, Treasurer

3146 Family Empowerment Network: Supporting Families Affected by FAS/FAE
777 South Mills Street
Madison, WI 53715
608-262-6590
800-462-5254
Fax: 608-263-5813
e-mail: fen@fammed.wisc.edu
www.fammed.wisc.edu/fen/index.html

Provides education, resources and referrals to families affected by Fetal Alcohol Synadrome (FAS/FAE) and other professionals involved with them.

Georgiana Wilton, PhD, Director
Patricia Cameron, BS/FAS, Family Advocacy Specialist

3147 Fetal Alcohol Education Program
7 Kent Street
Brookline, MA 02445
617-739-1424
Fax: 617-566-4019

Works to educate the professional and community on the affects of alcohol consumption during pregnancy.

3148 Fetal Alcohol Syndrome Family Resource Institute
PO Box 2525
Lynwood, WA 98036
253-531-2878
800-999-3429
Fax: 253-531-2668
e-mail: vicky@fetalalcoholsyndrome.org
www.fetalalcoholsyndrome.org

Provides information packets, a statewide hotline for information, crisis and referral and a newsletter. Parents are available to give talks throughout the United States and Canada.

3149 March of Dimes Birth Defects Foundation
1275 Mamaroneck Avenue
White Plains, NY 10605
914-997-4488
888-663-4637
Fax: 914-997-4763
e-mail: answers@marchofdimes.com
www.marchofdimes.com

Partnership of volunteers and professionals dedicated to improving the health of babies by preventing birth defects and infant mortality. Over 100 chapters are located across the country and can be located through the National Office.

Jennifer L Howse, President

3150 National Alliance on Mental Illness
3803 N. Fairfax Drive, Suite 100
Arlington, VA 22203
703-524-7600
800-950-6264
Fax: 703-524-9094
e-mail: info@nami.org
www.nami.org

Grassroots mental health organization dedicated to building better lives for the millions of Americans affected by mental illness.

Jim Payne, J.D., President
David Levy, Chief Financial Officer
Mary Giliberti, J.D., Executive Director

3151 National Mental Health Association
2000 N Beauregard Street, 6th Floor
Alexandria, VA 22311
703-684-7722
800-969-6642
Fax: 703-684-5968
TTY: 800-433-5959
www.mentalhealthamerica.net

Addresses all aspects of mental health and mental illness. NMHA with over 340 affiliates works to improve the mental health of all Americans.

David Shern, Ceo

3152 National Mental Health Consumers' Self-Help Clearinghouse
1211 Chestnut Street, Suite 1207
Philadelphia, PA 19107
215-751-1810
800-553-4539
Fax: 215-636-6312
e-mail: info@mhselfhelp.org
www.mhselfhelp.org

Offers information, support and appropriate referrals; and promotes public and professional education. Provides networking for those with special interests related to albinism. Promotes and supports research and funding that will improve diagnosis and management of albinism and hypopigmentation.

Joseph Rogers, Executive Director & Founder

3153 National Organization on Fetal Alcohol Syndrome
200 Eton Court, NW , Third Floor
Washington, DC 20007
202-785-4585
800-666-6327
Fax: 202-466-6456
www.nofas.org

Dedicated to eliminating birth defects caused by alcohol consumption during pregnancy and to improving the quality of life for those affected individuals and families.

Tom Donaldson, President
Kathleen Tavenner Mitchell, MHS/LCADC, VP/National Spokesperson
Kelly Raiser, MPH, Program Associate

3154 National Resource Center for Prevention of Perinatal Abuse of Alcohol
CSAP Division of Communications Programs
5600 Fishers Lane, Building 2
Rockville, MD 20857
301-443-9936

Offers information and resources to pregnant women on substance abuse, alcoholism and drugs pertaining to their unborn child's health.

3155 The Arc
1825 K Street, NW, Suite 1200
Washington, DC 20006
202-534-3700
800-433-5255
Fax: 202-534-3731
e-mail: tnguyen@thearc.org.
www.thearc.org

An organization advocating for and serving people with intellectual and developmental disabilities and their families. They encompass all ages and all spectrums from autism, Down syndrome, Fragile X and various other developmental disabilities.

Ronald Brown, President
Elise McMillan, Vice President
M.J. Bartelmay, Jr., Secretary

Conferences

3156 ARC National Convention
1825 K Street NW, Suite 1200
Washington, DC 20006
202-534-3700
800-433-5255
Fax: 202-534-3731
e-mail: info@thearc.org
www.thearc.org

Each year hundreds of members, staff, volunteers, professionals, experts, self advocates and their families gather for a dynamic convention to meet each other, learn from each other, and tackle the tough issues facing the intellectual and developmental disability (I/DD) community together.

Peter V Berns, CEO

Book Publishers

3157 Alcohol, Tobacco and Other Drugs May Harm the Unborn
National Clearinghouse for Alcohol and Drug Info.
PO Box 2345
Rockville, MD 20847
800-729-6686

Presents the most recent findings of basic research and clinical studies conducted on the effects of alcohol, drugs and tobacco on the unborn.

3158 Congenital Disorders Sourcebook
Omnigraphics
PO Box 625
Holmes, PA 19043
800-234-1340
Fax: 800-875-1340
e-mail: info@omnigraphics.com
www.omnigraphics.com

Basic consumer health information on disorders aquired during gestation, including spina bifida, hydrocephalus, cerebral palsy, heart defects, craniofacial abnormalities and fetal alcohol syndrome.
650 pages
ISBN: 0-780809-45-9

3159 Drugs and Pregnancy: It's Not Worth The Risk
American Council On Drug Education
204 Monroe Street, Suite 110
Rockville, MD 20850
800-488-3784

A scientific monograph for health care providers which teaches them to identify alcohol and drug problems in their patients.
48 pages

3160 Pregnancy and Exposure to Alcohol and Other Drug Use
National Clearinghouse for Alcohol and Drug Info.
PO Box 2345
Rockville, MD 20849
800-729-6686
www.health.org

This report is for health care professionals presenting state-of-the-art information about preventing alcohol use among women of childbearing age.

3161 Prevention Resource Guide: Pregnant, Postpartum Women and Their Infants
National Clearinghouse for Alcohol and Drug Info.
PO Box 2345
Rockville, MD 20849
800-729-6686
www.health.org

This resource guide targets health care providers, prevention program planners and counselors of pregnant and postpartum women between the ages of 15 and 44.

Pamphlets

3162 Effects of Alcohol on Pregnancy National Clearinghouse for Alcohol Information
PO Box 2345
Rockville, MD 20847
301-468-2600

Free publications are available that discuss the effects of alcohol on pregnancy: Fetal Alcohol Syndrome; and The Fact Is Alcohol and Other Drugs Can Harm an Unborn Baby.

3163 Fetal Alcohol Syndrome
Hazelden
PO Box 11
Center City, MN 55012
651-213-4200
800-257-7810
Fax: 612-257-1331
e-mail: info@hazeldenbettyford.org
www.hazelden.org

A source of information about the effects of drinking while pregnant.

Mark Mishek, President & CEO
Sharon Birnbaum, Director of Human Resources
Jim Blaha, VP, CFO & CAO

3164 Fight Drug Abuse at Home, Work, School and in the Community
American Council for Drug Education
204 Monroe Street, Suite 110
Rockville, MD 20850
800-488-3784

A catalog of print and video materials pertaining to substance abuse, alcoholism and drugs.

3165 How to Take Care of Your Baby Before Birth
National Clearinghouse for Alcohol and Drug Info.
PO Box 2345
Rockville, MD 20849
800-729-6686
www.health.org

A low-literacy brochure aimed at pregnant women that describes what they should and should not do during pregnancy.

3166 Things To Avoid During Pregnancy
March of Dimes Pregnancy & Newborn Health Edu Ctr
1275 Mamaroneck Avenue
White Plains, NY 10605
914-997-4488
Fax: 914-997-4763
e-mail: answers@marchofdimes.com
www.marchofdimes.com/pnhec/pnhec.asp

Information about the effects of certain drugs, stress, pets, abuse, and hazardous materials. Each topic is an online article available under the link: During Your Pregnancy.
2008

Description

3167 **FETAL RETINOID SYNDROME**

Covers these related disorders: Etretinate embryopathy, Isotretinoin embryopathy, Retinol embryopathy

Involves the following Biologic System(s):
Neonatal and Infant Disorders

Fetal retinoid syndrome is a characteristic pattern of birth defects caused by exposure to vitamin A (retinol) or its derivatives during early pregnancy. The term retinoid refers to retinol or any natural or artificially created derivative of vitamin A. In newborns with fetal retinoid syndrome, characteristic symptoms and findings include small, low-set ears or complete absence of the outer ears and external ear canals (microtia); an abnormally small head (microcephaly); enlargement of the cavities (ventricles) within the brain; and underdevelopment (hypoplasia) of the thymus, a small gland in the upper portion of the chest that functions as an essential part of the immune system during infancy and childhood.

Several studies have reported fetal retinoid syndrome in newborns as a result of maternal use of vitamin A derivatives such as isotretinoin during early pregnancy. In addition, an increasing number of studies reveal the occurrence of such birth defects due to maternal use of other vitamin A derivatives, particularly the medication etretinate, or large doses of vitamin A (e.g., greater than 15,000 units daily) during early embryonic development. Although the frequency of fetal retinoid syndrome is unknown, reported cases represent only a small percentage of actual occurrences of the syndrome. Moreover, there is ongoing concern that increasing use of high dose vitamin A preparations and of vitamin A derivatives to treat certain common skin conditions, such as cystic acne or psoriasis, may result in additional cases of fetal retinoid syndrome. The most well known retinoid is isotretinoin. Because it can cause severe birth defects, including mental retardation and physical malformations, a woman must not become pregnant while taking it. If a woman of childbearing age requests isotretinoin, her doctor will ask her to sign a detailed consent form before presribing it. If a woman accidentally becomes pregnant while taking the medication, she should immediately consult her doctor. Dosage levels and the stage of embryonic development during which retinoid exposure occurs are thought to be the major factors influencing the occurrence of fetal retinoid syndrome. The period of greatest risk may occur between approximately two to five weeks after conception. The specific underlying abnormality that causes fetal retinoid syndrome is not known. Studies indicate that retinoid exposure may cause disrupted development in the embryonic region that later becomes the brain and spinal cord (neural crest). The role that genetic influences or other environmental factors may have in contributing to fetal retinoid syndrome is unknown.

Although the symptoms and findings associated with fetal retinoid syndrome vary somewhat from case to case, affected newborns typically have a characteristic pattern of malformations. Affected newborns may have abnormalities of the head and face, including premature closure of the fibrous joint between the bones forming the forehead (metopic craniosynostosis); downslanting eyelid folds (palpebral fissures); widely spaced eyes (ocular hypertelorism) that may be abnormally small (microphthalmia); a short or broad nose; a small jaw (micrognathia); or incomplete closure of the roof of the mouth (cleft palate) and a groove in the upper lip (cleft lip). Abnormalities of the brain and spinal cord (central nervous system) are also common and include obstruction of the flow of cerebrospinal fluid around the brain, causing the fluid to accumulate under increasing pressure within the cavities of the brain (hydrocephalus); loss of vision; or other abnormalities (e.g., holoprosencephaly [failure of the forebrain (prosencephalon) to grow as two separate hemispheres in the first few weeks of fetal life], posterior fossa cyst). Additional neurologic problems may include paralysis of the nerves that supply muscles responsible for eye movements (oculomotor paralysis) or weakness or paralysis of the nerve that supplies the forehead, scalp, eyelids, cheeks, jaws, and muscles of facial expression (facial nerve palsy).

Newborns with fetal retinoid syndrome may also have clouding of the lenses of the eyes (congenital cataracts); malformations of the heart and its major blood vessels (e.g., ventricular septal defects, hypoplastic aortic arch, transposition of the great arteries); underdevelopment (hypoplasia) of the kidneys and tubes (ureters) that carry urine from the kidneys into the bladder; and ab normalities of the liver. Many affected newborns may also have malformations of the arms, legs, hands, and feet, such as webbing or fusion of the fingers and toes (syndactyly); malformations of the bone on the thumb side of the forearm (radial defects); a defect in which the foot is twisted out of shape or position (clubfoot or talipes); or fusion of the lower legs and absence of the feet (sirenomelia). In some patients, life-threatening complications may occur soon after birth. Treatment of newborns with fetal retinoid syndrome includes symptomatic and supportive measures.

Government Agencies

3168 **NIH/National Institute of Child Health and Human Development**
31 Center Drive, Building 31
Bethesda, MD 20892
　　　　　　　　　　　　　　　　301-496-1333
　　　　　　　　　　　　　　Fax: 301-496-1104
　　　　　　　　　　　　　　www.nichd.nih.gov

Established in 1962 by congress, today the institute conducts and supports research on topics related to the health of children, adults, families and populations. Some of these topics include: developmental disabilities, growth and development, infant death, reproductive health and birth defects.

Jay H Hoofnagle, Director
Lisa Kaeser, Program & Public Liaison

National Associations & Support Groups

3169 **American Academy of Pediatrics**
141 Northwest Point Boulevard
Elk Grove Village, IL 60007
　　　　　　　　　　　　　　　　847-434-4000
　　　　　　　　　　　　　　　　800-433-9016
　　　　　　　　　　　　　　Fax: 847-434-8000
　　　　　　　　　　　　　　www.aap.org

The American Academy of Pediatrics and its member pediatricians are committed to the attainment of optimal physical, mental and social health and well-being for all infants, children, adolescents, and young adults.

Sandra Hassink, MD, FAAP, President

3170 Association of Children's Prosthetic/ Orthotic Clinics
6300 N River Road, Suite 727
Rosemont, IL 60018
847-698-1637
Fax: 847-823-0536
e-mail: raymond@aaos.org
www.acpoc.org

The Association of Children's Prosthetic Clinics is an association of professionals who are involved in clinics providing prosthetic-orthotic care for children with limb loss or orthopaedic disabilities.

Melody Raymond, Contact

3171 March of Dimes Birth Defects Foundation
1275 Mamaroneck Avenue
White Plains, NY 10605
914-997-4488
888-663-4637
Fax: 914-997-4763
e-mail: answers@marchofdimes.com
www.marchofdimes.com

Partnership of volunteers and professionals dedicated to improving the health of babies by preventing birth defects and infant mortality. Over 100 chapters are located across the country and can be located through the National Office.

Jennifer L Howse, President

3172 National Rehabilitation Information Center
4200 Forbes Blvd, Suite 202
Lanham, MD 20706
301-459-5984
800-364-2742
Fax: 301-459-4263
TTY: 301-459-5984
e-mail: naricinfo@heitechservices.com
www.naric.com

NARIC is a library and information center focusing in disability and rehabilitation research. Information specialists provide quick information and referrals free of charge. Other sevices include customized searches of REHABDATA, the premier database of disability and rehabilitation literature.

Mark Odum, Director

Conferences

3173 ACPOC Annual Meeting
Assoc of Children's Prosthetic-Orthotic Clinics
6300 N River Road, Suite 727
Rosemont, IL 60018
847-698-1637
Fax: 847-823-0536
e-mail: acpoc@aaos.org
www.acpoc.org

April

Web Sites

3174 Association of Children's Prosthetic/ Orthotic Clinics
9400 West Higgins Road, Suite 500
Rosemont, IL 60018
847-698-1637
Fax: 847-268-9560
e-mail: acpoc@aaos.org
www.acpoc.org

An association of professionals who are involved in clinics which provide prosthetic-orthotic care for children with limb loss or orthopaedic disabilities.

David B. Rotter, CPO, President
Jorge Amelio Fabregas, MD, Vice President
Hank White, PT, PhD, Secretary-Treasurer

3175 March of Dimes Birth Defects Foundation
www.marchofdimes.com

Partnership of volunteers and professionals dedicated to improving the health of babies by preventing birth defects and infant mortality. Over 100 chapters are located across the country and can be located through the National Office.

3176 National Rehabilitation Information Center
8400 Corporate Drive, Suite 500
Landover, MD 20785
800-346-2742
Fax: 301-459-4263
TTY: 301-459-5984
www.naric.com/naric

NARIC is a library and information center focusing in disability and rehabilitation research. Information specialists provide quick information and referrals free of charge. Other sevices include customized searches of REHABDATA, the premier database of disability and rehabilitation literature.

Description

3177 FRAGILE X SYNDROME

Synonyms: Marker X Syndrome, Martin-Bell Syndrome

Involves the following Biologic System(s):

Genetic/Chromosomal/Syndrome/Metabolic Disorders

Fragile X Syndrome, a disorder that results from an inherited defect of the X chromosome, is the most common cause of mental retardation in males. The disorder is thought to affect approximately one in 2,000 to 4,000 males and to be slightly less frequent in females. Although symptoms may be variable, the most common feature associated with fragile X syndrome is mental retardation.

Most males with fragile X syndrome have mild to profound mental retardation (e.g., an intelligence quotient or I.Q. ranging from approximately 30 to 55.) However, some may have an I.Q. that is considered borderline normal. Affected males with mild mental retardation may have a distinctive speech pattern characterized by rapid speech with a variable rhythm (cluttering). Those with more severe retardation typically communicate in bursts of repetitive speech. Affected males with severe or profound mental retardation may lack the ability to speak. In addition, most males with fragile X syndrome may have poor eye contact or experience emotional difficulties. Some may have poor concentration associated with hyperactivity or engage in autistic-like behaviors, such as hand biting or hand flapping.

In many cases, affected males may also have physical abnormalities. For example, many males with fragile X syndrome may have unusually large testes (macroorchidism), a finding that is most apparent after puberty; however, testicular function is normal. Affected males may also typically have characteristic facial features, such as a large head (macrocephaly) and forehead, a relatively long face and prominent jaw, thick lips, and prominent ears. Other findings may include crowding of the teeth, excessive flexibility of the finger joints, or flat feet (pes planus). In addition, approximately 50 percent of affected females have varying degrees of mental retardation or learning difficulties. In some cases, females with fragile X syndrome may also have physical abnormalities, such as irregular teeth or unusually flexible finger joints. The treatment of children with fragile X syndrome includes symptomatic and supportive measures, such as special education, speech therapy, and, in some cases, multidisciplinary techniques such as behavioral therapies to help manage hyperactivity or autistic-like behaviors.

Individuals with fragile X syndrome inherit a fragile area or site on the long arm (q) of the X chromosome (Xq27.3). Chromosomal analysis reveals that the genetic material on the end of this arm appears to be broken off. In reality, this genetic material is actually dangling from the end of the long arm. The diseased gene within this area is known as the FRAXA gene. This region (locus) of the X chromosome contains abnormally long repeats (e.g., over 200 repeats) of coded DNA instructions (CGG trinucleotide repeat expansion). Males have only one X chromosome; therefore, if they inherit a fragile X locus containing more than 200 CGG repeats, they generally express the symptoms associated with this syndrome and are typically more severely affected than females. However, because females have two X chromosomes, certain disease traits may be masked by the presence of a normal gene on the other X chromosome, resulting in lower frequency and decreased severity of the disease among females.

Government Agencies

3178 NIH/National Institute of Child Health and Human Development
31 Center Drive, Building 31
Bethesda, MD 20892
301-496-1333
Fax: 301-496-1104
www.nichd.nih.gov

Established in 1962 by congress, today the institute conducts and supports research on topics related to the health of children, adults, families and populations. Some of these topics include: developmental disabilities, growth and development, infant death, reproductive health and birth defects.

Jay H Hoofnagle, Director
Lisa Kaeser, Program & Public Liaison

National Associations & Support Groups

3179 ARC of the United States
1825 K Street, NW, Suite 1200
Washington, DC 20006
301-565-3842
800-433-5255
Fax: 301-565-5342
e-mail: info@thearc.org
www.thearc.org

The ARC is the national organization of and for people with mental retardation and related developmental disabilities and their families. Devoted to promoting and improving supports and services for people with mental retardation and their families. The association also fosters research and education regarding the prevention of mental retardation in infants and young children. The ARC was founded in 1950 by a small group of parents and other concerned individuals.

Steven M Eidelman, Ceo
Adam Aaronson, Public Inquiries Director

3180 American Academy of Pediatrics
141 Northwest Point Boulevard
Elk Grove Village, IL 60007
847-434-4000
800-433-9016
Fax: 847-434-8000
www.aap.org

The American Academy of Pediatrics and its member pediatricians are committed to the attainment of optimal physical, mental and social health and well-being for all infants, children, adolescents, and young adults.

Sandra Hassink, MD, FAAP, President

3181 FRAXA Research Foundation
10 Prince Place
Newburyport, MA 01950
978-462-1866
Fax: 978-463-9985
e-mail: info@fraxa.org
www.fraxa.org

FRAXA supports research on fragile X syndrome, a genetic disorder which is the most common inherited cause of mental retardation.

2,500 members

Katie Clapp, Co-Founder & President
Megan Massey, RN, Vice President
Michael Tranfaglia, MD, Co-Founder/Medical Director

3182 Genetic Alliance
4301 Connecticut Avenue NW
Washington, DC 20008
202-966-7955
800-336-4363
Fax: 202-966-8553
e-mail: info@geneticalliance.org
www.geneticalliance.org

A coalition of voluntary genetic support groups, consumers and professionals addressing the needs of individuals and families affected by genetic disorders from a national perspective.

Sharon Terry, President

3183 National Fragile X Foundation
1615 Bonanza Street, Suite 202
Walnut Creek, CA 94596   925-938-9300
                                          800-688-8765
                                          Fax: 925-938-9315
                                          e-mail: natlfx@fragilex.org
                                          www.fragilex.org

Unites the Fragile X community with support, education, awareness, research and advocacy.

Michael Kelly, President
Robert M Miller, Executive Director

State Agencies & Support Groups

California

3184 Fragile X Association of Southern California
PO Box 6924
Burbank, CA 91510   818-754-4227
                                          Fax: 310-276-9251
                                          e-mail: info@fraxsocal.org
                                          www.fraxsocal.org

Promotes awareness of Fragile X syndrome with special emphasis on educators and health professionals; provides a forum for families of children with fragile X to meet and share their ideas, concerns and problems; and supports scientific research on fragile X syndrome.

Naomi Star, President
Diane Bateman, Vice President

3185 Fragile X Center of San Diego
4653 Carmel Mountain Rd, Ste 308-515
San Diego, CA 92130   760-434-6290
                                          877-300-7143
                                          e-mail: info@fragilesandiego.org
                                          www.fragilexsandiego.org

Provides information for families and professionals. Activities include: family support, improving awareness of fragile X syndrome, increasing the identification for affected families, promoting research into fragile X syndrome.

Nicole Schweizer, Secretary

Ohio

3186 Fragile X Alliance of Ohio
6790 Ridgecliff Drive
Solon, OH 44139   440-519-1517
                                          Fax: 440-519-1518
                                          e-mail: fraxohio@adelphia.org
                                          www.fragilexohio.org

Promotes awareness of Fragile X syndrome with special emphasis on educators and health professionals; provides a forum for families of children with fragile X to meet and share their ideas, concerns and problems; and supports scientific research on fragile X syndrome.

Leslie A. Bagdasarian, President

Conferences

3187 ARC Annual National Convention
The ARC
1825 K Street NW, Suite 1200
Washington, DC 20006   202-534-3700
                                          800-433-5255
                                          Fax: 202-534-3731
                                          e-mail: info@thearc.org
                                          www.thearc.org

held in cities throughout the U.S. each fall which attracts nearly 1000 people for educational sessions, business meetings and social events.

Mohan Mehra, President
Nancy Webster, Vice President
Michael Mack, Secretary

3188 Genetic Alliance Annual Conference
Genetic Alliance
4301 Connecticut Avenue NW, Suite 404
Washington, DC 20008   202-966-5557
                                          800-336-4363
                                          Fax: 202-966-8553
                                          e-mail: info@geneticalliance.org
                                          www.geneticalliance.org

Consistently inspirational and enables partnership among all stakeholders: advocates and community leaders, health and industry professionals, policymakers, and academicians.

July

Sharon Terry, President/CEO
Tetyana Murza, Programs/Events Manager

Web Sites

3189 ARC of the United States
1825 K Street, NW, Suite 1200
Washington, DC 20006   202-534-3700
                                          800-433-5255
                                          Fax: 202-534-3731
                                          e-mail: tnguyen@thearc.org
                                          www.thearc.org

The ARC is the national organization of and for people with mental retardation and related developmental disabilities and their families. Devoted to promoting and improving supports and services for people with mental retardation and their families. The association also fosters research and education regarding the prevention of mental retardation in infants and young children.

Ronald Brown, President
Elise McMillan, Vice President
Peter V. Berns, CEO

3190 American College of Medical Genetics
7220 Wisconsin Ave., Suite 300
Bethesda, MD 20814   301-718-9603
                                          Fax: 301-718-9604
                                          e-mail: acmg@acmg.net
                                          www.acmg.net

Offers information about fragile X syndrome.

3191 FRAXA Research Foundation
10 Prince Place, Suite 203
Newburyport, MA 1950   978-462-1866
                                          e-mail: info@fraxa.org
                                          www.fraxa.org

FRAXA supports research on fragile X syndrome, a genetic disorder which is the most common inherited cause of mental retardation.

Debbie Stevenson, Chair
Katie Clapp, MS, President & Co Founder
Sasa Zorovic, PhD, Vice President

3192 National Fragile X Foundation
2100 M St., NW, Suite 170, Box 302
Washington, DC 20037   202-747-6210
                                          800-688-8765
                                          Fax: 202-747-6208
                                          e-mail: natlfx@fragilex.org
                                          www.fragilex.org

Provides a wide variety data for people suffering from the disorder to acces at any time with ease.

Jennifer Silverton, President
Brian Silver, Vice President
Tony Ferlenda, CEO

Book Publishers

3193 Children With Fragile X Syndrome

Jayne Dixon Weber, author

Peytral Publications
PO Box 1162
Minnetonka, MN 55345

952-949-8707
877-739-8725
Fax: 952-906-9777
www.peytral.com

A complete, sensitive introduction to Fragile X Syndrome, covering diagnosis, parental emotions, therapies and medications, early intervention, education, daily care, legal rights and more. Item #WP-307X.

472 pages

3194 Educating Boys with Fragile X Syndrome

Gail Spiridigliozzi, PhD, author

FRAA Research Foundation
10 Prince Place,Suite 203
Newburyport, MA 01950

978-462-1866
Fax: 978-463-9985
e-mail: info@fraxa.org
www.fraxa.org

Guide for parents, teachers and therapist to give specific strategies for education.

20 pages

3195 Fragile X - A to Z: Guide for Families by Families

Sally Nantais, Mary Beth Langan, Wendy Dillworth, author

FRAA Research Foundation
10 Prince Place,Suite 203
Newburyport, MA 01950

978-462-1866
Fax: 978-463-9985
e-mail: info@fraxa.org
www.fraxa.org

Intended to help families cope with many daily challenges of living with a child or adult who has fragile X syndrome.

100 pages

3196 My Brother has Fragile X

Charles Stieger, author

FRAA Research Foundation
10 Prince Place,Suite 203
Newburyport, MA 01950

978-462-1866
Fax: 978-463-9985
e-mail: info@fraxa.org
www.fraxa.org

Suitable for young children and for reading in an elementary school classroom to educate children about what it's like to have fragile X.

23 pages

Newsletters

3197 FRAXA Research Foundation Newsletter
10 Prince Place, Suite 203
Newburyport, MA 1950

978-462-1866
Fax: 978-463-9985
e-mail: info@fraxa.org
www.fraxa.org

FRAXA supports research on fragile X syndrome, a genetic disorder which is the most common inherited cause of mental retardation.

Quarterly

Debbie Stevenson, Chair
Katie Clapp, MS, President & Co Founder
Sasa Zorovic, PhD, Vice President

Description

3198 GALACTOSEMIA

Covers these related disorders: Classic galactosemia, Galactokinase deficiency, Deficiency of uridyl diphosphogalactose-4-epimerase

Involves the following Biologic System(s):

Gastrointestinal Disorders,

Genetic/Chromosomal/Syndrome/Metabolic Disorders

Galactosemia is a disorder in which the body cannot use the sugar known as galactose, which is an important component of the sugar in milk (lactose) and an important source of nutrition for infants and children. Because of this inability, this sugar accumulates in the blood, and substances produced by the partial breakdown of galactose build up in the body, where they can damage the kidneys, liver, brain, and eyes.

Galactosemia is a hereditary genetic disorder, caused by mutations in genes that carry the structural codes for three enzymes that normally break down or digest galactose. As a result, there are three forms of galactosemia, each stemming from a deficiency of one of the three galactose-digesting enzymes. The most frequent and severe form of galactosemia, named classic galatosemia, results from deficiency of galactose-1 phosphate uridyl transferase. A second form of galactosemia stems from deficiency of galactose kinase, and the third form comes from deficiency of galactose epimerase. All three forms of galactosemia are transmitted in an autosomal recessive manner, meaning that each parent of an affected child must carry a copy of the gene responsible for the same form of galactosemia.

Symptoms of galactosemia may include a yellowish discoloration of the skin, eyes, and mucous membranes (jaundice); opacity of the lenses of the eyes (cataracts); vomiting; convulsions; increased irritability; sluggishness; difficulty in feeding; and failure to gain weight. Characteristic findings may include enlargement of the liver and spleen (hepatosplenomegaly), low blood sugar (hypoglycemia), the presence of amino acids in the urine (aminoaciduria), an abnormal accumulation of fluid in the abdomen (ascites), the formation of scar tissue in the liver (cirrhosis), and mental retardation.

If infants with classic galactosemia are not treated promptly with a low-galactose diet, life-threatening complications appear within a few days after birth. Affected infants typically develop feeding difficulties, a lack of energy (lethargy), a failure to gain weight and grow (failure to thrive), yellowing of the skin and whites of the eyes (jaundice), liver damage, and bleeding. Affected children are also at increased risk of delayed development, clouding of the lens of the eye (cataract), speech difficulties, and intellectual disability. Complications of galactosemia can include severe infection and shock. Women with classic galactosemia, caused by deficiency of the enzyme galactose-1 phosphate uridyl transferase, may have disorders of the reproductive system.

The most effective treatment for galactosemia is the complete elimination of milk and milk products from the diet. Women who carry any of the three genes responsible for galactosemia should avoid lactose-containing foods during pregnancy, to prevent galactose from crossing the placenta and causing disease in the fetus. Although a completely lactose-free diet may prevent the complications of galactosemia, some affected children and adults may experience delays in growth and development, speech irregularities, and difficulties with motor function.

National Associations & Support Groups

3199 American Academy of Pediatrics
141 Northwest Point Boulevard
Elk Grove Village, IL 60007
847-434-4000
800-433-9016
Fax: 847-434-8000
www.aap.org

The American Academy of Pediatrics and its member pediatricians are committed to the attainment of optimal physical, mental and social health and well-being for all infants, children, adolescents, and young adults.

Sandra Hassink, MD, FAAP, President

3200 American Liver Foundation
39 Broadway, Suite 2700
New York, NY 10006
212-668-1000
800-465-4837
Fax: 212-483-8179
e-mail: info@liverfoundation.org
www.liverfoundation.org

Nonprofit, national voluntary health organization dedicated to the prevention, treatment and cure of hepatitis and other liver diseases through research, education, and advocacy on behalf of those affected by or at risk of liver disease.

Gina Parziale, Executive Director
James L Boyer MD, Chair

3201 Genetic Alliance
4301 Connecticut Avenue NW
Washington, DC 20008
202-966-7955
800-336-4363
Fax: 202-966-8553
e-mail: info@geneticalliance.org
www.geneticalliance.org

A coalition of voluntary genetic support groups, consumers and professionals addressing the needs of individuals and families affected by genetic disorders from a national perspective.

Sharon Terry, President

3202 March of Dimes Birth Defects Foundation
1275 Mamaroneck Avenue
White Plains, NY 10605
914-997-4488
888-663-4637
Fax: 914-997-4763
e-mail: answers@marchofdimes.com
www.marchofdimes.com

Partnership of volunteers and professionals dedicated to improving the health of babies by preventing birth defects and infant mortality. Over 100 chapters are located across the country and can be located through the National Office.

Jennifer L Howse, President

3203 Parents of Galactosemic Children
1519 Magnolia Bluff Drive, PO Box 2401
Mandeville, LS ÿ7047
228-497-5886
ÿ86- 90- 742
e-mail: president@galactosemia.org
www.galactosemia.org

National nonprofit, volunteer organization whose misssion is to provide information, support and networking opportunities to families affected by galactosemia.

Michelle Fowler, President & Treasurer
Nishkala Rao, Secretary

Libraries & Resource Centers

3204 National Digestive Diseases Information Clearinghouse
31 Center Drive
Bethesda, MD 20892
301-496-3583
800-891-5389
Fax: 301-907-8906
e-mail: nddic@info.niddk.nih.gov
www.niddk.nih.gov

The National Institute of Diabetes and Digestive and Kidney Diseases conducts and supports research on many of the most serious diseases affecting public health. The Institute supports much of the clinical research on the diseases of internal medicine and related subspecialty fields as well as many basic science disciplines.

Kathy Kranzfelder, Project Officer

Conferences

3205 Genetic Alliance Annual Conference
Genetic Alliance
4301 Connecticut Avenue NW, Suite 404
Washington, DC 20008
202-966-5557
800-336-4363
Fax: 202-966-8553
e-mail: info@geneticalliance.org
www.geneticalliance.org

Consistently inspirational and enables partnership among all stakeholders: advocates and community leaders, health and industry professionals, policymakers, and academicians.

July

Sharon Terry, President/CEO
Tetyana Murza, Programs/Events Manager

Web Sites

3206 American Liver Foundation
39 Broadway, Suite 2700
New York, NY 10006
212-668-1000
800-465-4837
Fax: 212-483-8179
www.liverfoundation.org

Nonprofit, national voluntary health organization dedicated to the prevention, treatment, and cure of hepatitis and other liver diseases through research, education and advocacy on behalf of those affected by or at risk of liver disease.

Thomas F. Nealon III, Chair
David Ticker, CFO
Lynn Seim, COO

3207 Disability Information and Resource Center
www.dircsa.org.au/pub/docs/galac.txt

DIRC provides a professional and friendly information and referral service to the people of South Australia.

3208 Galactosemia Resources and Information
PO Box 1512
Deerfield Beach, FL 33443
866-900-7421
www.galactosemia.com

Information about galactosemia.

Scott Shepard, President
Scott Saylor, Vice President
Paul Fowler, Treasurer

3209 Online Mendelian Inheritance in Man
U.S. National Library of Medicine, 8600 Rockville
Bethesda, MD 20894
888-346-3656
e-mail: info@ncbi.nlm.nih.gov
www.ncbi.nlm.nih.gov

This database is a catalog of human genes and genetic disorders.

Christine E. Seidman, M.D., Chair
David J. Lipman, M.D., Executive Secretary
Michael Boehnke, Ph.D., Board Member

3210 Parents of Galactosemic Children
www.galactosemia.com

National nonprofit, volunteer organization whose mission is to provide information, support and networking opportunities to families affected by galactosemia.

Scott Shepard, President
Scott Saylor, Vice President
Paul Fowler, Treasurer

3211 Rare Genetic Diseases in Children (NYU)
550 First Avenue
New York, NY 10016
212-263-7300
www.med.nyu.edu/rgdc/homenow.htm

We target issues arising from rare genetic diseases affecting children. Also, to assist in the endeavor to bring knowledge and hope to those for whom there is, at present, so little.

Robert I. Grossman, MD, Dean & CEO
Michael T. Burke, SVP, CFO, Vice Dean
Annette Johnson, JD, PhD, SVP & Vice Dean, General Counsel

3212 Save Babies Through Screening Foundation
PO Box 42179
Cincinnati, OH 45242
888-454-3383
e-mail: email@savebabies.org
www.savebabies.org

Is a national, nonprofit, public charity run by volunteers. Its mission is to improve the lives of babies by working to prevent disabilities and early death resulting from disorders detectable through newborn screening.

Jill Levy-Fisch, President
Micki Gartzke, Vice President
Anne Rugari, Treasurer

Description

3213 GAUCHER'S DISEASE

Synonyms: Gaucher disease, Glucosylceramide lipidosis, Glucosyl cerebroside lipidosis

Covers these related disorders: Chronic Gaucher's disease (Adult or Classic Gaucher's disease), Infantile Gaucher's disease, Juvenile Gaucher's disease

Involves the following Biologic System(s): Genetic/Chromosomal/Syndrome/Metabolic Disorders

Gaucher's disease is an inherited metabolic disorder characterized by a deficiency of the enzyme glucocerebrosidase (glucosylceramidase), which assists in the metabolism of certain fats (lipidosis). This deficiency results in the accumulation of certain fatty substances (glucocerebroside or glucosylceramide) throughout the body. Although uncommon, Gaucher's disease is the lipidosis seen most often by physicians. Gaucher's disease is subdivided into three main types. The first, known as chronic, adult, or classic Gaucher's disease, may develop at any age from birth to 80 years old. This form of the disease is common among eastern European Jews, with an incidence rate of as many as one in 500 births. Findings associated with chronic Gaucher's disease include enlargement of the spleen (splenomegaly) or liver (hepatomegaly), or both (hepatosplenomegaly); a decrease in levels of hemoglobin in the blood (anemia); decreased numbers of circulating white blood cells (leukopenia); and abnormally low levels of circulating platelets (thrombocytopenia), which may lead to easy bruising or bleeding. Symptoms may include a brownish-pigmented skin; yellow spots in the eyes resulting from accumulation of fatty substances; and bone pain resulting from accumulations in the bone marrow. Treatment for chronic Gaucher's disease includes enzyme replacement therapy.

Infantile Gaucher's disease, a life-threatening form of this disorder, affects the central nervous system of the newborn. Symptoms and findings may include enlargement of the spleen, crossed eyes (strabismus); muscle spasms in the jaw (trismus or lockjaw); seizures; backward bending of the head; or a rigid, arched back. Additional abnormalities of the central nervous system may become apparent.

Juvenile Gaucher's disease may appear at any time during childhood. Characteristic findings may include enlargement of the liver and spleen (hepatosplenomegaly), bone abnormalities resulting in pain and swelling of the joints, anemia, and abnormally low levels of circulating white blood cells and platelets. Affected children may be pale, weak, and particularly susceptible to bleeding and recurring infection. Symptoms related to nervous system involvement include lack of motor coordination and loss of balance, inflammation of the nerves in the arms and legs accompanied by abnormal sensations and discomfort, muscle spasms, paralysis of the nerves of the eye (ophthalmoplegia), and impairment of mental function.

Enzyme replacement therapy is usually not effective in the treatment of the infantile and juvenile forms of Gaucher's disease. Alternative treatment may include removal of the spleen (splenectomy). Other treatment is symptomatic and supportive.

Gaucher's disease is inherited as an autosomal recessive trait. The gene responsible for the regulation of the enzyme glucocerebrosidase is located on the long arm of chromosome 1 (1q21-q31).

National Associations & Support Groups

3214 ARC of the United States
1010 Wayne Avenue, Suite 650
Silver Spring, MD 20910

301-565-3842
Fax: 301-565-5342
e-mail: info@thearc.org
www.thearc.org

The ARC is the national organization of and for people with mental retardation and related developmental disabilities and their families. Devoted to promoting and improving supports and services for people with mental retardation and their families. The association also fosters research and education regarding the prevention of mental retardation in infants and young children. The ARC was founded in 1950 by a small group of parents and other concerned individuals.

Steven M Eidelman, Ceo
Adam Aaronson, Public Inquiries Director

3215 American Academy of Pediatrics
141 Northwest Point Boulevard
Elk Grove Village, IL 60007

847-434-4000
800-433-9016
Fax: 847-434-8000
www.aap.org

The American Academy of Pediatrics and its member pediatricians are committed to the attainment of optimal physical, mental and social health and well-being for all infants, children, adolescents, and young adults.

Sandra Hassink, MD, FAAP, President

3216 National Gaucher Foundation
2227 Idlewood Road, Suite 6ÿ
Tucker, GA 30084

301-816-1515
800-504-3189
Fax: 301-816-1516
e-mail: ngf@gaucherdisease.org
www.gaucherdisease.org

A nonprofit organization whose primary objective is to assist in perfecting a treatment program and discovering a cure for Gaucher disease. The Foundation supports medical research and clinical programs which enhance the current understanding of Gaucher disease.

Robin A. Ely, MD, President
Rhonda P. Buyers, Executive Director
Cyndi Frank, Director Development

3217 National Tay-Sachs and Allied Diseases Association
2001 Beacon Street, Suite 204
Boston, MA 02135

617-277-4463
800-906-8723
Fax: 617-277-0134
e-mail: info@ntsad.org
www.ntsad.org

Direct, fund and promote research to develop treatments and cures; provides comprehensive support services to affected families and individuals; guides prevention, education, awareness and screening through effective grassroots collaborations with chapters and affiliates; lead advocacy efforts as the recognized authority for this family of genetic diseases.

Diana Pangonis, Interim Executive Director

Conferences

3218 Genetic Alliance Annual Conference
Genetic Alliance
4301 Connecticut Avenue NW, Suite 404
Washington, DC 20008
202-966-5557
800-336-4363
Fax: 202-966-8553
e-mail: info@geneticalliance.org
www.geneticalliance.org

Consistently inspirational and enables partnership among all stakeholders: advocates and community leaders, health and industry professionals, policymakers, and academicians.

July

Sharon Terry, President/CEO
Tetyana Murza, Programs/Events Manager

Web Sites

3219 ARC of the United States
1825 K Street, NW, Suite 1200
Washington, DC 20006
202-534-3700
800-433-5255
Fax: 202-534-3731
e-mail: tnguyen@thearc.org
www.thearc.org

The ARC is the national organization of and for people with mental retardation and related developmental disabilities and their families. Devoted to promoting and improving supports and services for people with mental retardation and their families.

Ronald Brown, President
Elise McMillan, Vice President
Peter V. Berns, CEO

3220 Children's Gaucher Research Fund
8110 Warren Court
Granite Bay, CA 95746
916-797-3700
Fax: 916-797-3707
e-mail: research@childrensgaucher.org
www.childrensgaucher.org

We are a nonprofit organization, that raises funds to coordinate and support research to find a cure for type 2 and type 3 Gaucher disease.

Roscoe Brady, MD, Member, Scientific Advisory Board
Gregory Grabowski, MD, Member, Scientific Advisory Board
Kondi Wong, MD, USAF, MC, Member, Scientific Advisory Board

3221 Gaucher Registry
Genzyme Corporation, 500 Kendall Street
Cambridge, MA 2142
617-591-5500
800-745-4447
e-mail: help@gaucherregistry.com
www.registrynxt.com

Our goal is to significantly contribute to the medical understanding of Gaucher disease and to improve the quality of care for Gaucher patients worldwide through active publication of Registry findings and disease management approaches.

3222 Health Answers
410 Horsham Road
Horsham, PA 19044
215-422-9010
e-mail: Michael.tague@healthanswers.com
www.healthanswers.com

HealthAnswers offers a breadth of services in medical education, sales force training, patient support, solutions, professional promotion and consumer solutions.

Michael Tague, Managing Director

3223 National Gaucher Foundation
61 Gneral Early Drive
Harpers Ferry, WV 25425
800-504-3189
e-mail: ngf@gaucherdisease.org
www.gaucherdisease.org

The mission of the NGF is to find a cure for Gaucher Disease by funding vital research programs, to meet the ever-increasing needs of patients and families, as well as to promote community/physician awareness and educational programs.

3224 Rare Genetic Diseases in Children (NYU)
550 First Avenue
New York, NY 10016
212-263-7300
www.med.nyu.edu/rgdc/homenow.htm

We target issues arising from rare genetic diseases affecting children. Also, to assist in the endeavor to bring knowledge and hope to those for whom there is, at present, so little.

Robert I. Grossman, MD, Dean & CEO
Michael T. Burke, SVP, CFO, Vice Dean
Annette Johnson, JD, PhD, SVP & Vice Dean, General Counsel

Newsletters

3225 Gaucher Disease Newsletter
National Gaucher Foundation
61 Gneral Early Drive
Harpers Ferry, WV 25425
301-816-1515
800-504-3189
Fax: 301-816-1516
e-mail: ngf@gaucherdisease.org
www.gaucherdisease.org

Offers information on the latest research, treatments and technology for persons affected by Gaucher Disease. Also includes legislative and medical information.

Quarterly

Robin A. Ely, MD, President
Rhonda P. Buyers, Executive Director
Cyndi Frank, Director Development

Pamphlets

3226 Gaucher Disease Fact Sheet
National Gaucher Foundation
61 Gneral Early Drive
Harpers Ferry, WV 25425
301-816-1515
800-504-3189
Fax: 301-816-1516
e-mail: ngf@gaucherdisease.org
www.gaucherdisease.org

Offers information on what Gaucher Disease is, the symptoms, risks, treatments and the workings of the National Gaucher Foundation.

Robin A. Ely, MD, President
Rhonda P. Buyers, Executive Director
Cyndi Frank, Director Development

3227 Living with Gaucher Disease
National Gaucher Foundation
61 Gneral Early Drive
Harpers Ferry, WV 25425
301-816-1515
800-504-3189
Fax: 301-816-1516
e-mail: ngf@gaucherdisease.org
www.gaucherdisease.org

A guide for parents, families and relatives that teach them how to deal with and cope with a diagnosis of Gaucher Disease.

24 pages

Robin A. Ely, MD, President
Rhonda P. Buyers, Executive Director
Cyndi Frank, Director Development

Description

3228 GROWTH HORMONE DEFICIENCY

Synonym: GH deficiency

Involves the following Biologic System(s):

Endocrinologic Disorders

Growth hormone deficiency is a condition characterized by deficient production or an impaired response to growth hormone (GH), resulting in growth impairment and short stature with normal proportions of the head, limbs, hands, and feet (pituitary dwarfism). Secreted by the pituitary gland in the brain. GH, also known as somatotropin, stimulates body growth and development by promoting the production of protein in cells, releasing energy through the breakdown of fats, and performing other vital functions. Also known as the master gland, the pituitary gland is connected, through a bundle of nerve fibers known as the pituitary stalk, to a region of the brain known as the hypothalamus, which controls the functioning of the pituitary gland through direct stimulation by nerves as well as through the actions of proteins known as hormone-releasing and hormone-inhibiting factors that the hypothalamus releases into the bloodstream for transport to the pituitary gland. The forward or anterior region of the pituitary gland secretes GH in response to the particular hormone-releasing factor known as growth hormone releasing factor (GHRF), which is carried by the blood from the hypothalamus to the pituitary gland.

Depending upon the underlying cause of GH deficiency, some patients with this condition may also have deficiencies of other hormones produced by the anterior pituitary gland, such as thyroid-stimulating hormone (TSH), which stimulates the production of thyroid hormones, or adrenocorticotropic hormone (ACTH), which promotes the growth and production of hormones by cells in the outer region (cortex) of the adrenal gland. Inadequate functioning of the pituitary gland is known as hypopituitarism.

GH deficiency may have many different causes, including absence, underdevelopment, or malformation of the pituitary gland or hypothalamus at birth; tumors of the anterior pituitary gland, pituitary stalk, or hypothalamus, particularly the type of pituitary tumors known as craniopharyngiomas; or radiation given for the treatment of certain cancers of the brain or other organs in the head. GH deficiency may also result from trauma affecting the pituitary gland or hypothalamus, such as injury during birth or interruption of the oxygen supplied to the brain (anoxia) by the lungs and red cells of the blood. Other causes of GH deficiency include some abnormalities affecting the genes or chromosomes that carry the structural plans for GH and the body's other substances, and some conditions that occur randomly for unknown reasons (idiopathic hypopituitarism). Moreover, some genetically caused types of hypopituitarism may result in GH deficiency alone or accompanied by deficiencies of other hormones produced by the anterior pituitary gland.

There are several genetic subtypes of isolated growth hormone deficiency (IGHD), including those that may be inherited as an autosomal recessive, autosomal dominant, or X-linked trait. Autosomal recessive IGHD may be caused by the complete absence of a gene known as the GH1 gene, located on chromosome 17. This form of IGHD is typically

characterized by marked growth delays after birth and severe shortness of stature. Other types of autosomal recessive IGHD are caused by various other abnormalities (mutations) of the GH1 gene, causing varying degrees of growth failure and short stature. Some patients with autosomal dominant IGHD may also have mutations of the GH1 gene. The gene responsible for X-linked IGHD, so named because this gene is located on the X chromosome, has not yet been identified. The genetic form of growth impairment known as Laron syndrome is caused by deficient function of the pituitary gland, (hypopituitarism) and is thought to result from an impaired response to GH. This condition is characterized by abnormally increased levels of GH in the blood.

Most children with GH deficiency are of normal weight and length at birth. By the first year of life, children with severe GH deficiency or Laron syndrome may be significantly shorter than would be expected for their age and sex. Patients with less severe GH deficiency experience regular growth spurts that alternate with periods during which no growth occurs. Patients with GH deficiency may continue to experience growth beyond the age when most individuals attain their adult height. This is due to abnormal delays in the fusion of the growing ends (epiphyseal plates) and shafts of the long bones of the legs and arms. If children with GH deficiency do not receive treatment, their adult height may range from moderately to severely below the average height for a mature adult.

Children with GH deficiency typically have normally proportioned arms and legs, but they may have relatively small hands and feet. Many also have a characteristic facial appearance, including a short, broad face and relatively round head; an undeveloped upper and lower jaw; a small, saddle-shaped nose with a depressed nasal bridge; a small neck; delayed eruption and crowding of the teeth; and fine, sparse scalp hair. Because of abnormal smallness of the voice box (larynx), many patients with GH deficiency have a high-pitched voice. Other findings may include underdeveloped genitals, delayed or absent sexual development, and abnormally low concentrations of the sugar known as glucose (hypoglycemia).

Children with GH deficiency caused by tumors of the pituitary gland or hypothalamus may experience effects beyond growth deficiency, depending upon the location, nature, and growth of the tumor. In some patients, invasion and destruction of the pituitary gland cause degeneration (atrophy) of the thyroid gland, sex glands (gonads), and outer regions of the adrenal glands (adrenal cortex). Associated findings may include absence of sweating, weight loss, abnormal sensitivity to cold, delayed or absent sexual maturation, lack of response to certain stimuli (torpor), or other abnormalities. Tumors in the pituitary gland or hypothalamus may also cause total growth failure, abnormally increased urination (polyuria), vomiting, headaches, visual disturbances, episodes of abnormally increased electrical activity in the brain (seizures), and other abnormalities.

The treatment of GH deficiency depends on its underlying cause and nature. If GH deficiency is caused by a tumor, its treatment may include surgery, radiation therapy, or other appropriate measures to eliminate the tumor. Pituitary function should be carefully evaluated after such measures, in order to determine the appropriate treatment for pituitary abnormalities caused by the tumor or its treatment. The treatment of children with IGHD includes early replacement therapy with synthetic GH, which is continued until there is no further growth in response to the treatment. The maximum response usually occurs during the first year of treatment, with further treatment producing slower growth. Because such therapy may cause abnormally decreased activity of the thyroid gland (hypothyroidism), thyroid function should be regularly evaluated. Children with deficiencies of other anterior pituitary hormones in association with GH deficiency may receive additional hormone replacement therapies as required. Other treatment for GH deficiency is symptomatic and supportive.

Government Agencies

3229 NIH/National Institute of Child Health and Human Development
31 Center Drive, Building 31
Bethesda, MD 20892   301-496-1333
Fax: 301-496-1104
www.nichd.nih.gov

Established in 1962 by congress, today the institute conducts and supports research on topics related to the health of children, adults, families and populations. Some of these topics include: developmental disabilities, growth and development, infant death, reproductive health and birth defects.

Jay H Hoofnagle, Director
Lisa Kaeser, Program & Public Liaison

National Associations & Support Groups

3230 American Academy of Pediatrics
141 Northwest Point Boulevard
Elk Grove Village, IL 60007   847-434-4000
800-433-9016
Fax: 847-434-8000
www.aap.org

The American Academy of Pediatrics and its member pediatricians are committed to the attainment of optimal physical, mental and social health and well-being for all infants, children, adolescents, and young adults.

Sandra Hassink, MD, FAAP, President

3231 Dwarf Athletic Association of America
708 Gravenstein Hwy, North, #118
Sebastopol,, CA 95472   972-317-8299
888-598-3222
Fax: 972-966-0184
e-mail: daaa@flash.net
www.daaa.org

The DAAA mission is to encourage people with dwarfism to participate in sports regardless of their level of skills. We promote and provide quality amateur level athletic opportunities for dwarf athletiecs in the US.

Jimmy Loyless, President
Gerry Graff, Vice President
Janet Brown, Executive Director

3232 Genetic Alliance
4301 Connecticut Avenue NW
Washington, DC 20008   202-966-7955
800-336-4363
Fax: 202-966-8553
e-mail: info@geneticalliance.org
www.geneticalliance.org

A coalition of voluntary genetic support groups, consumers and professionals addressing the needs of individuals and families affected by genetic disorders from a national perspective.

Sharon Terry, President

3233 Human Growth Foundation
997 Glen Cove Avenue, Suite 5
Glen Head, NY 11545   516-671-4041
800-451-6434
Fax: 516-671-4055
e-mail: hgfl@hgfound.org
www.hgfound.org

A nonprofit, national organization committed to expanding and accelerating research into growth and growth disorders, provides education and support to those affected by growth disorders and their families, and fosters the exchange of information with the medical community.

Patricia D Costa, Executive Director

3234 Lawson Wilkins Pediatric Endocrine Society
6728 Old McLean Village Dr.
McLean, VA ÿ2210   703-556-9222
Fax: 703-556-8729
e-mail: secretary@lwpes.org
www.lwpes.org

To promote the acquisition and dissemination of knowledge of endocrine and metabolic disorders from conception through adolescence.

Kenneth Copeland, President
Ronald Rosenfield, President-Elect
John Kirkland, Treasurer

3235 Little People of America
250 El Camino Real, Suite 201
Tustin, CA 92780   714-368-3689
888-572-2001
Fax: 714-368-3367
e-mail: info@lpaonline.org
www.lpaonline.org

A nonprofit organization that provides support and information to people of short stature and their families.

Lois Gerage-Lamb, President
Bill Bradford, Senior Vice President
Jon North, Vice President, Finance

3236 MAGIC Foundation: Major Aspects of Growth in Children
6645 W North Avenue
Oak Park, IL 60302   708-383-0808
800-362-4423
Fax: 708-383-0899
e-mail: ÿContactUs@magicfoundation.org
www.magicfoundation.org

A national nonprofit organization providing support and education regarding growth disorders in children and related adult disorders. Provides educational information, networking, a national conference, a kids' program and an extensive medical library.

Mary Andrews, Ceo
Dianne Tamburrino, Executive Director

3237 March of Dimes Birth Defects Foundation
1275 Mamaroneck Avenue
White Plains, NY 10605   914-997-4488
888-663-4637
Fax: 914-997-4763
e-mail: answers@marchofdimes.com
www.marchofdimes.com

A unique partnership of volunteers and professionals that provides leadership in the treatment and prevention of birth defects and prematurity. It is funded by voluntary contributions from individuals and a variety of organizations.

Jennifer L Howse, President

State Agencies & Support Groups

Arkansas

3238 Little People of America - District 7
250 El Camino Real, Suite 201
Tustin, CA 92780

714-368-3689
888-572-2001
Fax: 714-368-3367
e-mail: info@lpaonline.org
www.lpaonline.org

District 7 of the Little People of America represents short stature individuals from the states of Arkansas, Kansas, Missouri and Oklahoma.

Karen Shelby, Director
Jack Dohr, Vice Director
Cyndy Dohr, Treasurer

California

3239 Little People of America - San Francisco Bay Area Chapter
National Headquarters
250 El Camino Real, Suite 201
Tustin, CA 92780

714-368-3689
888-572-2001
Fax: 714-368-3367
e-mail: info@lpaonline.org
www.lpaonline.org

A nonprofit organization that provides support and information to people of short stature and their families.

Lee Uniacke, President
Keren Stronach, Co-Vice President
Caroline Jones, Co-Vice President

Colorado

3240 Little People of America - Front Range Chapter
7117 E Euclid Drive
Englewood, CO 80111

303-740-8555
e-mail: ebennettebennett@netscape.net
www.curesearch.org

Little People of America, Inc. (LPA), will assist dwarfs with their physical and developmental concerns resulting from short stature. By providing medical, environmental, educational, vocational, and parental guidance, short-stature individuals and their families may enhance their lives and lifestyles with minimal limitations. Through peer support and personal example, members will be supportive of all those who reach out to LPA.

Chris & Bob Kotzian, President
Souda Bell, Vice President
Brandi VanAnne, Treasurer

Kansas

3241 Little People of America - District 7
250 El Camino Real, Suite 201
Tustin, CA 92780

714-368-3689
888-572-2001
Fax: 714-368-3367
e-mail: info@lpaonline.org
www.lpaonline.org

District 7 of the Little People of America represents short stature individuals from the states of Arkansas, Kansas, Missouri and Oklahoma.

Karen Shelby, Director
Jack Dohr, Vice Director
Cyndy Dohr, Treasurer

Missouri

3242 Little People of America - District 7
250 El Camino Real, Suite 201
Tustin, CA 92780

714-368-3689
888-572-2001
Fax: 714-368-3367
e-mail: info@lpaonline.org
www.lpaonline.org

District 7 of the Little People of America represents short stature individuals from the states of Arkansas, Kansas, Missouri and Oklahoma.

Karen Shelby, Director
Jack Dohr, Vice Director
Cyndy Dohr, Treasurer

New Jersey

3243 Little People of America - District 2
National Headquarters
250 El Camino Real, Suite 201
Tustin, CA 92780

714-368-3689
888-572-2001
Fax: 714-368-3367
e-mail: info@lpaonline.org
www.lpaonline.org

A nonprofit organization that provides support and information to people of short stature and their families.

Joe Zrinski, District Director
Patty Ott, Assistant District Director
Jim Davis, District Treasurer

New York

3244 Little People of America - District 2
National Headquarters
250 El Camino Real, Suite 201
Tustin, CA 92780

714-368-3689
888-572-2001
Fax: 714-368-3367
e-mail: info@lpaonline.org
www.lpaonline.org

A nonprofit organization that provides support and information to people of short stature and their families.

Joe Zrinski, District Director
Patty Ott, Assistant District Director
Jim Davis, District Treasurer

Oklahoma

3245 Little People of America - District 7
250 El Camino Real, Suite 201
Tustin, CA 92780

714-368-3689
888-572-2001
Fax: 714-368-3367
e-mail: info@lpaonline.org
www.lpaonline.org

District 7 of the Little People of America represents short stature individuals from the states of Arkansas, Kansas, Missouri and Oklahoma.

Karen Shelby, Director
Jack Dohr, Vice Director
Cyndy Dohr, Treasurer

3246 Little People of America - District 2
National Headquarters
250 El Camino Real, Suite 201
Tustin, CA 92780 714-368-3689
888-572-2001
Fax: 714-368-3367
e-mail: info@lpaonline.org
www.lpaonline.org

A nonprofit organization that provides support and information to people of short stature and their families.

Joe Zrinski, District Director
Patty Ott, Assistant District Director
Jim Davis, District Treasurer

Utah

3247 Little People of America - Utah Seagulls
250 El Camino Real, Suite 201
Tustin, CA 92780 714-368-3689
888-572-2001
Fax: 714-368-3367
e-mail: info@lpaonline.org
www.utahlittlepeople.org

A nonprofit organization that provides support and information to people of short stature and their families.

Steve Hatch, President

Research Centers

3248 Case Western Research University, Bolton Brush Growth Study Center
10900 Euclid Ave.
Cleveland, OH 44106 216-368-0592
Fax: 216-368-3204
e-mail: mgh4@cwru.edu
www.case.edu

Investigations and research into the growth and development of the human body.

Kate Chapman, Manager

3249 Jackson Laboratory
600 Main Streeet
Bar Harbor, ME 04609 207-288-6000
800-474-9880
Fax: 207-288-6079
www.jax.org

Studies focusing on growth disorders and human genetics.

Rick Woychik, Executive Director

3250 New Jersey Institute of Technology Center for Biomedical Engineering
323 Martin Luther King Jr Boulevard
Fenster Hall, Sixth Floor, University Heights
Newark, NJ 07102 973-596-5268
Fax: 973-596-5222
www.njit.edu

Offers research into facial and bone disorders.

Richard Foulds, Director, Masters Program
Judith D. Redling, Coordinator, Undergraduate Program

3251 W.M. Krogman Center for Research In Child Growth and Development
University of Pennsylvania
3451 Walnut Street
Philadelphia, PA 19104 215-898-1470

Focuses research and studies on growth disorders and birth defects.

Solomon Katz, MA, PhD, Director

Conferences

3252 Genetic Alliance Annual Conference
Genetic Alliance
4301 Connecticut Avenue NW, Suite 404
Washington, DC 20008 202-966-5557
800-336-4363
Fax: 202-966-8553
e-mail: info@geneticalliance.org
www.geneticalliance.org

Consistently inspirational and enables partnership among all stakeholders: advocates and community leaders, health and industry professionals, policymakers, and academicians.

July

Sharon Terry, President/CEO
Tetyana Murza, Programs/Events Manager

3253 LPA National Conference
Little People of America
250 El Camino Real, Suite 201
Tustin, CA 92780 714-368-3689
888-572-2001
Fax: 714-368-3367
e-mail: info@lpaoline.org
www.lpaonline.org

July

Joanna Campbell, Executive Director
Lois Gerage-Lamb, President

Web Sites

3254 Alliance of Genetic Support Groups
4301 Conneticut Ave. NW, Suite 404
Washington, DC 20008 202-966-5557
Fax: 202-966-8553
www.geneticalliance.org

Is an international coalition comprised of millions of individuals with genetic conditions and more than 600 advocacy, research and health care organizations that represent their interests. As a broad-based coalition of key stakeholders, the Alliance builds partnerships to promote healthy lives for all those living with genetic condtions.

3255 Dwarf Athletic Association of America
www.daaa.org

The DAAA mission is to encourage people with dwarfism to participate in sports regardless of their level of skills. We promote and provide quality amateur level athletic opportunities for dwarf athletiecs in the US.

3256 Health Answers
410 Horsham Road
Horsham, PA 19044 215-422-9010
e-mail: Michael.tague@healthanswers.com
www.healthanswers.com

HealthAnswers offers a breadth of services in medical education, sales force training, patient support solutions, professional promotion and consumer solutions.

Michael Tague, Managing Director

3257 Human Growth Foundation
www.hgfound.org

Information regarding disorders related to growth or growth hormone.

3258 Little People of America
250 El Camino Real, Suite 211
Tustin, CA 92780 www.lpaonline.org

Offers resources pertaining to dwarfism and Little People of America, medical data, instructions on how to join an e-mail discussion group, and links to numerous other dwarfism-related sites.

Gary Atrbold, President
April Brazier, Senior Vice President
Clinton Brown, Finance Director

3259 OHSU Homepage Search
www.ohsu.edu

Educates health and high-technology professionals, scienists and enviromental engineers, and it undertakes the indispendible functions of patient care, community service and biomedical research.

3260 Online Mendelian Inheritance in Man
U.S. National Library of Medicine, 8600 Rockville
Bethesda, MD 20894   888-346-3656
e-mail: info@ncbi.nlm.nih.gov
www.ncbi.nlm.nih.gov

This database is a catalog of human genes and genetic disorders.

Christine E. Seidman, M.D., Chair
David J. Lipman, M.D., Executive Secretary
Michael Boehnke, Ph.D., Board Member

3261 Society for Endocrinology
22 Apex Court, Woodlands, Bradley Stoke
Bristol, UK BS32   145-464-2200
TTY: 145-464-2210
www.endocrinology.org

Aims to advance education and research in endocrinology for the public benefit.

G R Williams, Chair, Finance Committee
C J McCabe, Chair, Program Committee
D W Ray, Chair, Publications Committee

Book Publishers

3262 Endocrine & Metabolic Disorders Sourcebook
Linda M. Shin, author

Omnigraphics
PO Box 8002
Aston, PA 19014   800-234-1340
Fax: 800-875-1340
e-mail: info@omnigraphics.com
www.omnigraphics.com

Basic information for the lay person about pancreatic and insulin-related disorders such as pancreatitis, diabetes and hypoglycemia; adrenal gland disorders such as Cushing's syndrome, Addison's disease and congenital adrenal hyperplasia; pituitary gland disorders such as growth hormone deficiency, acromegaly and pituitary tumors; and thyroid disorders such as hypothyroidism, Grave's disease, Hashimoto's disease and goiter.

574 pages Hardcover
ISBN: 0-780802-07-1

3263 Growing Children: A Parent's Guide
Human Growth Foundation
977 Glen Cove Avenue, Suite 5
Glen Head, NY 11545   516-671-4041
800-451-6434
Fax: 516-671-4055
e-mail: hgfl@hgfound.org
www.hgfound.org

Offers parents information on the normal pattern of their child's growth, growth charts, recognition of growth problems, evaluation of growth problems and resources for more information. Available to members.

Frank Diamond, MD, President
Emily Germain-Lee, MD, Vice President
Patricia D. Costa, Executive Director

3264 Short and OK
Patricia Rieser, Heino FL Mayer-Bahlbug, author

Human Growth Foundation
977 Glen Cove Avenue, Suite 5
Glen Head, NY 11545   516-671-4041
800-451-6434
www.hgfound.org

This is a guide for parents of short children offering information on behavior issues, medical issues and psychological warning signs.
54 pages

Newsletters

3265 MAGIC Foundation: Major Aspects of Growth in Children
6645 W North Avenue
Oak Park, IL 60302   708-383-0808
800-362-4423
Fax: 708-383-0899
TTY: 123-019-99
e-mail: contactus@magicfoundation.org
www.magicfoundation.org

A national nonprofit organization providing support and education regarding growth disorders in children and related adult disorders. Provides educational information, networking, a national conference, a kids' program and an extensive medical library.

36 pages Quarterly

Rich Buckley, Chairman
Ken Dickard, Vice Chairman
Mary Andrews, CEO

3266 Orphan Disease Update
National Organization for Rare Disorders
55 Kenosia Avenue
Danbry, CT 6810   203-744-0100
800-999-6673
Fax: 203-798-2291
e-mail: orphan@rarediseases.org
www.rarediseases.org

It provides updates on research, advocacy, and special events, as well as advice and sources of help for caregivers, Web sites of interest, current clinical trials, and funding opportunities.

16 pages 3/year

Sheldon M. Schuster, Chair
Peter L Saltonstall, President & CEO
Pamela Gavin, COO

Pamphlets

3267 Dental Problems with Growth Hormone Deficiency
Human Growth Foundation
997 Glen Cove Avenue, Suite 5
Glen Head, NY 11545   516-671-4041
800-451-6434
Fax: 516-671-4055
e-mail: hgfl@hgfound.org
www.hgfound.org

Growth hormone has a strong effect on bone growth, including the bones of the upper and lower jaws.

Pisit (Duke) Pitukcheewanont, MD, President
Emily Germain-Lee, MD, Vice President
Patricia (Patti) D. Costa, Executive Director

3268 Growth Hormone Deficiency
Human Growth Foundation
997 Glen Cove Avenue, Suite 5
Glen Head, NY 11545   516-671-4041
800-451-6434
Fax: 516-671-4055
e-mail: hgfl@hgfound.org
www.hgfound.org

Causes and control of growth hormone deficiency.

Pisit (Duke) Pitukcheewanont, MD, President
Emily Germain-Lee, MD, Vice President
Patricia (Patti) D. Costa, Executive Director

3269 Growth Hormone Testing
Human Growth Foundation
997 Glen Cove Avenue, Suite 5
Glen Head, NY 11545

516-671-4041
800-454-6434
Fax: 516-671-4055
e-mail: hgfl@hgfound.org
www.hgfound.org

Describes how growth hormone testing is used, when growth hormone test is ordered, and what growth hormone test results might mean.

Pisit (Duke) Pitukcheewanont, MD, President
Emily Germain-Lee, MD, Vice President
Patricia (Patti) D. Costa, Executive Director

3270 Intrauterine Growth Retardation
Human Growth Foundation
977 Glen Cove Avenue, Suite 5
Glen Head, NY 11545

516-671-4041
800-451-6434
Fax: 516-761-4055
e-mail: hglf@hgfound.org
hgfound.org

Offers information on how to understand this growth disorder and how to cope with it.

Pisit (Duke) Pitukcheewanont, MD, President
Emily Germain-Lee, MD, Vice President
Patricia (Patti) D. Costa, Executive Director

3271 Most Frequently Asked Questions with Growth Hormone Deficiency
Human Growth Foundation
977 Glen Cove Avenue, Suite 5
Glen Head, NY 11545

516-671-4041
800-451-6434
Fax: 516-671-4055
e-mail: hgfl@hgfound.org
www.hgfound.org

Discusses the consequences of growth hormone deficiency in chidlren and adults.

Pisit (Duke) Pitukcheewanont, MD, President
Emily Germain-Lee, MD, Vice President
Patricia (Patti) D. Costa, Executive Director

Description

3272 GUILLAIN-BARRE SYNDROME

Synonyms: Acute ascending polyneuritis, Acute febrile polyneuritis, Acute idiopathic polyneuritis, Acute postinfectious polyneuropathy, GBS, Landry's paralysis

Involves the following Biologic System(s):
Neurologic Disorders

Guillain-Barre syndrome (GBS) (pronounced gE-Ian-ba-rA) is a progressive neurologic disorder that affects many nerves (polyneuropathy) and is characterized by unusual sensations (paresthesias) in the arms, legs, or both. GBS generally causes progressive muscle weakness over days and, in some cases, paralysis accompanied by lack of muscle tone. Guillain-Barre syndrome is thought to be an autoimmune disorder and may occur as a reaction to a previous viral infection, immunization, or bacterial infection (e.g., Lyme disease). Autoimmune disorders involve the body's inappropriate immune response to its own healthy tissues.e symptoms of GBS typically begin approximately one to three weeks following the triggering event.

Symptoms associated with Guillain-Barre syndrome range from mild to severe and may include numbness, tingling, muscle weakness, and sometimes paralysis that begins in the legs and then usually spreads upward toward the trunk, arms, muscles of the chest, and sometimes the face (ascending paralysis). Affected children may become irritable and unable or unwilling to walk. As weakness spreads to the chest and facial areas, muscles required for speech, breathing, and eating may become affected. In addition, if the nerves of the autonomic nervous system which control vital involuntary functions are affected, individuals with GBS may develop fluctuations in blood pressure and heart rate as well as other heart irregularities. A rare form of Guillain-Barreyndrome called the Miller-Fisher syndrome is characterized by paralysis of the nerves and muscles of the eyes (ophthalmoplegia), an absence of normal reflexes (areflexia), and an inability to coordinate voluntary movement (ataxia).

Most children with Guillain-Barre syndrome recover completely within two to three weeks. Some may experience ongoing muscular weakness. In addition, in rare cases, affected individuals may experience prolonged or recurring episodes of GBS that may last for months or years. These uncommon manifestations are referred to as chronic unremitting polyradiculoneuropathy and chronic relapsing polyradiculoneuropathy.

Guillain-Barre syndrome may be diagnosed through specialized tests of the fluid that surrounds the brain and spinal cord (cerebrospinal fluid) and other clinical findings. Early diagnosis and hospitalization allow for observation and monitoring of affected individuals. If the progression of muscle weakness or paralysis is very slow and limited, treatment may include observation and supportive care until recovery is complete. If, however, paralysis progresses to involve breathing and swallowing, appropriate support is necessary. Other treatment may include plasma exchange (plasmapheresis), a procedure during which blood is withdrawn and the liquid portion (plasma) removed in order to filter out harmful substances. A plasma substitute is then mixed with the blood, and the reconstituted blood is then returned to the body. Alternative treatment may include the intravenous administration of immunoglobulin (IVIG). In some cases, certain immunosuppressive drugs or corticosteroids may be effective. Physical therapy may aid in the maintenance of joint and muscle function. Other treatment is symptomatic and supportive.

National Associations & Support Groups

3273 American Academy of Pediatrics
141 Northwest Point Boulevard
Elk Grove Village, IL 60007
847-434-4000
800-433-9016
Fax: 847-434-8000
www.aap.org

The American Academy of Pediatrics and its member pediatricians are committed to the attainment of optimal physical, mental and social health and well-being for all infants, children, adolescents, and young adults.

Sandra Hassink, MD, FAAP, President

3274 American Autoimmune Related Diseases Association
22100 Gratiot Avenue
Eastpointe, MI 48021
586-776-3900
800-598-4668
Fax: 586-776-3903
e-mail: aarda@aarda.org
www.aarda.org

Dedicated to the eradication of autoimmune diseases and the alleviation of suffering and the socio-economic impact of autoimmunity through fostering and facilitating collaboration in the areas of education, public awareness, research and patient services in an effective, ethical and efficient manner.

Virginia Ladd, Executive Director

3275 GBS/CIDP Foundation International
Holly Bldg, 104 1/2 Forrest Avenue
Narberth, PA 19072
610-667-0131
866-224-3301
Fax: 610-667-7036
e-mail: info@gbsfi.com
www.gbs-cidp.org

Provides emotional support and assistance to people affected by this rare disease. Arranges personal visits to affected individuals in hospitals and rehabilitation centers. Fosters research into the cause, treatment, and other aspects of the disorder and directs affected individuals with long-term disabilities to resources for vocational, financial, and other aspects of the disorder.

Sara Voorhees, PMP, President
Estelle L. Benson, Executive Director
Barbara Katzman, Associate Director

Web Sites

3276 American Autoimmune Related Diseases Association
22100 Gratiot Ave.
Eastpointe, MI 48021
586-776-3900
800-598-4668
Fax: 586-776-3903
www.aarda.org

Dedicated to the eradication of autoimmune diseases and the alleviation of suffering and the socio-economic impact of autoimmunity through fostering and facilitating collaboration in the areas of education, public awareness, research and patient services in an effective, ethical and efficient manner.

Rev. Herbert G. Ford, D. Min., Chair
Stanley M. Finger, PhD, Vice Chair
Virginia T. Ladd, R.T., President & Executive Director

3277 GBS Support Group of the UK
Woodholme House, Heckingt, Li NG34
152-946-9910
080-037-4803
Fax: 152-946-9915
www.gbs.org.uk/

Objectives are to: provide emotional support to patients, families and friends; provide, when possible, personal visits by former patients to those currently in hospitals and rehabilitation centres and those recovering; supply a comprehensive short guide for patients, relatives and friends, and other literature, so that patients and their families can learn what to expect during the illness; and to educate the public and medical community about the Support Group.

Caroline Morrice, Director
Lesley Dimmick, Charity Officer
Chris Fuller, Trustee

Book Publishers

3278   Immune System Disorders Sourcebook

Joyce Brennfleck Shannon, author

Omnigraphics
PO Box 8002
Aston, PA 19014

800-234-1340
Fax: 800-875-1340
e-mail: info@omnigraphics.com
www.omnigraphics.com

Basic information about lupus, multiple sclerosis, guillain-barre syndrome and more.

671 pages Hardcover
ISBN: 0-780807-48-0

Pamphlets

3279   Fact Sheet: Guillain-Barre Syndrome

National Inst. of Neurological Disorders/Stroke
PO Box 5801
Bethesda, MD 20824

301-496-5751
800-352-9424

Information about Guillain-Barren Syndrome, what causes Guillain-Barren Syndrome, how is it diagnosed and treated, etc. Also available in Spanish.

Description

3280 HIV INFECTION

Synonyms: Fetal AIDS, Acquired Immune Deficiency Syndrome
Involves the following Biologic System(s):
Immunologic and Rheumatologic Disorders, Infectious Disorders

HIV Infection destroys the body's ability to fight infections, resulting in Acquired Immune Deficiency, or AIDS. T-cells, which are responsible for responding to infections, are destroyed by the virus. The process is slow and silent, which means that HIV can be contracted unwittingly years before any symptoms appear. As the T-cells are destroyed, organisms that are usually defeated by a normal immune system, infect the body. Patients suffer from one infection after another. HIV is usually spread from an infected person to a non-infected person by unprotected sexual intercourse, or by sharing needles. Most young children with AIDS contract the disease through in utero transmission; however, infants may occasionally acquire the infection through mother's milk. In addition, children with hemophilia and others who may have received transfusions of blood or blood products before HIV blood-screening became standard in 1985 may have become infected by contaminated blood.

Some children with HIV infection develop symptoms in the first or second year of life, while the majority may not show signs of infection for several years. AIDS is diagnosed in about 50 percent of HIV-infected children by three years of age. Early signs may include chronic or recurrent fevers and diarrhea, rashes, swollen lymph glands (lymphadenopathy), enlarged liver and spleen (hepatosplenomegaly), and delays in growth and nervous system development. Some infants and young children are anemic, experience weight and appetite loss, decreased energy, and irregularities of the heart and kidneys. Early symptoms may include chronic or recurrent bacterial infections and uncommon viral, fungal, and other types of infections caused by microorganisms that do not ordinarily cause disease or infections. As the immune system continues to weaken, children may develop lung inflammations and potentially life-threatening pneumocystis pneumonia. Children with AIDS are also at increased risk for certain types of malignant diseases such as non-Hodgkin's lymphoma.

Most infants born to mothers with HIV show antibodies in their blood for approximately 12 to 14 months. In infants who are not infected with the virus, these passive antibodies disappear. For this reason, standardized HIV testing is not conclusive in children younger than 18 months. However, HIV infection in these children may often be detected through the use of virus cultures and a specialized DNA-copying technique called polymerase chain reaction or| PCR.

Prevention of HIV and subsequent AIDS infection in infants may be directed toward counseling of at-risk women of child-bearing age who may be advised to avoid becoming pregnant. The strictly prescribed administration of the drug AZT during the last six months of pregnancy, as well as during labor and delivery, has been shown to greatly improve the chances of an HIV-infected mother delivering an infant who is not infected with HIV. In fact, congenitally acquired HIV has been reduced dramatically in recent years. Delivery by Cesarean section may also reduce risk of transmission to the newborn. In addition, mothers with HIV should refrain from breast-feeding their infants, as there is some evidence of HIV transmission from mother to child in women who may have contracted the virus after pregnancy.

Infants and children with HIV may be treated with antibiotics to prevent pneumocystis pneumonia. Intravenous gamma globulin therapy may be used to maintain or increase the ability of the immune system to fight the effects of secondary infections. In addition, certain steroidal drugs may be administered to treat lymphoid interstitial pneumonitis, while AZT, alone or in combination, is often used to treat children and has been found to be particularly effectiv|e against neurologic irregularities. Additional therapies are also being tested in children. Other treatment is symptomatic and supportive.

Government Agencies

3281 NIH/National Institute of Allergy and Infectious Diseases
6610 Rockledge Drive, MSC 6612
Bethesda, MD 20892
301-496-5717
866-284-4107
Fax: 301-402-3573
TDD: 800-877-8339
e-mail: ocposfoffice@niaid.nih.gov
www.niaid.nih.gov

Conducts and supports basic and applied research to better understand, treat, and ultimately prevent infectious, immunologic, and allergic diseases.
Anthony S Fauci MD, Director

National Associations & Support Groups

3282 AIDS Healthcare Foundation
6255 W. Sunset Blvd. 21st Fl.
Los Angeles, CA 90028
323-860-5200
e-mail: info@aidshealth.org
www.aidshealth.org

It is a nonprofit, tax-exempt 501(c)(3) organization, is a global organization providing cutting-edge medicine and advocacy to over 350,000 patients in 36 countries.
Michael Weinstein, President
Peter Reis, Senior Vice President
Laura Boudreau, Chief Counsel for Operations

3283 AIDS Research Alliance
1400 South Grand Avenue, Suite 701
Los Angeles, CA 90015
310-358-2423
Fax: 310-358-2431
e-mail: info@aidsresearch.org
aidsresearch.org

The mission is to develop a cure for HIV/AIDS, medical strategies to prevent new infections, and better treatments for people living with HIV.
W. David Hardy, M.D., Chairman
Cary D. Stevens, Treasurer
Kenneth "Cam" Davis, Jr., Secretary

3284 AIDS United
1424 K Street, N.W., Suite 200
Washington, DC 20005
202-408-4848
Fax: 202-408-1818
www.aidsunited.org
Katy Caldwell, Executive Director
Tim Armitage, Brand & Marketing Strategy
Rick Gomez, Senior Vice President, Marketing

3285 American Academy of HIV Medicine
1705 DeSales Street NW, Suite 700
Washington, DC 20036
202-659-0699
Fax: 202-659-0976
www.aahivm.org

3286 American Academy of Pediatrics
141 Northwest Point Boulevard
Elk Grove Village, IL 60007   847-434-4000
                                             800-433-9016
                                             Fax: 847-434-8000
                                             www.aap.org

The American Academy of Pediatrics and its member pediatricians are committed to the attainment of optimal physical, mental and social health and well-being for all infants, children, adolescents, and young adults.

Sandra Hassink, MD, FAAP, President

3287 American College of Preventive Medicine
455 Massachusetts Avenue NW, Suite 200
Washington, DC 20001   202-466-2044
                                             Fax: 202-466-2662
                                             e-mail: info@acpm.org
                                             www.acpm.org

The mission is to improve the health of individuals and populations through evidence-based health promotion, disease prevention, and systems-based approaches to improving health and health care.

Haydee Barno, Contact
Michael Barry, Contact
Paul Bonta, Contact

3288 American Foundation for Children with AIDS
6221 Blue Grass Avenue?
Harrisburg, PA 17112   888-683-8323
                                             e-mail: info@afcaids.org
                              www.americanfoundationforchildrenwithaids.org

It is a non-profit organization providing critical support to infected and affected HIV and children and their caregivers.

Tanya Weaver, Executive Director
Michelle Miller, Executive Assistant
Betsy Dorsey, Warehouse Manager

3289 American Nurses Association
8515 Georgia Avenue, Suite 400
Silver Spring, MD 20910   800-274-4262
                                             Fax: 301-628-5001
                                             e-mail: anf@ana.org
                                             www.nursingworld.org

The American Nurses Association (ANA) is the only full-service professional organization representing the interests of the nation's 3.1 million registered nurses through its constituent and state nurses associations and its organizational affiliates.

Pamela F. Cipriano, PhD, President
Marla J. Weston, PhD, RN, FAAN, Chief Executive Officer
Cindy R. Balkstra, Vice President

3290 American Psychiatric Association
1000 Wilson Boulevard, Suite 1825
Arlington, VA 22209   703-907-7300
                                             888-35 -7924
                                             e-mail: apa@psych.org
                                             www.psychiatry.org

It is a medical specialty society representing growing membership of more than 36,000 psychiatrists.

3291 American Psychological Association
750 First St. NE
Washington, DC 20002   202-336-5500
                                             800-374-2721
                                             TTY: 202-336-6123
                                             www.apa.org

The mission is to advance the creation, communication and application of psychological knowledge to benefit society and improve people's lives.

Norman B. Anderson, PhD, CEO/ EVP
L. Michael Honaker, PhD, Deputy Chief Executive Officer
Ellen G. Garrison, PhD, Senior Policy Advisor

3292 American Public Health Association
800 I Street, NW
Washington, DC 20001   202-777-2742
                                             Fax: 202-777-2534
                                             TTY: 202-777-2500
                                             www.apha.org

APHA champions the health of all people and all communities. They aim to strengthen the public health profession and speak out for public health issues and policies backed by science.

Georges C. Benjamin, MD, Executive Director
Kemi Oluwafemi, MBA, CPA, Chief Financial Officer
Susan Polan, PhD, Associate Executive Director

3293 American Social Health Association
PO Box 13827
Research Triangle Park, NC 27709   919-361-8400
                                             800-783-9877
                                             Fax: 919-361-8425
                                             www.ashastd.org

Dedicated to improving the health of individuals, families, and communities with a focus on preventing sexually transmitted diseases and their harmful consequences.

Lynn Barclay, President/CEO
Deborah Arrindell, VP Health Policy
David Allen, MBA, CPA, Vice President/CFO

3294 American Society for Microbiology
1752 N Street, N.W.
Washington, DC 20036   202-737-3600
                                             Fax: 202-942-9333
                                             e-mail: service@asmusa.org
                                             www.asm.org

he American Society for Microbiology is a life science membership organization. Membership has grown from 59 scientists in 1899 to more than 39,000 members today, with more than one third located outside the United States. The members represent 26 disciplines of microbiological specialization plus a division for microbiology educators.

Nancy Sansalone, Interim Executive Director
Timothy Donohue, President
Joseph M. Campos, Secretary

3295 American Society of Clinical Oncology
2318 Mill Road, Suite 800
Alexandria, VA 22314   571-483-1300
                                             www.asco.org

With the number of cancer patients projected to grow dramatically in the years ahead in the U.S. and worldwide, we must do everything possible to ensure that we are well-positioned to deliver the care they will need.

Peter Paul Yu, President
Julie M. Vose, President-Elect
Susan L. Cohn, Treasurer

3296 Association of Nurses in AIDS Care
3538 Ridgewood Road
Akron, OH 44333   330-670-0101
                                             800-260-6780
                                             Fax: 330-670-0109
                                             e-mail: anac@anacnet.org
                                             www.nursesinaidscare.org

The mission of the Association is to promote the individual and collective professional development of nurses involved in the delivery of health care to persons infected or affected by the Human Immunodeficiency Virus (HIV) and to promote the health and welfare of infected persons.

Suzanne Willard, President
Jason Farley, President-Elect
Don Kurtyka, Treasurer

3297 Association of State and Territorial Health Officials
2231 Crystal Drive, Suite 450
Arlington, VA 22202   202-371-9090
                                             Fax: 571-527-3189
                                             www.astho.org

The mission is to transform public health within states and territories to help members dramatically improve health and wellness.

Jewel Mullen, President
Edward Ehlinger, President-Elect
Brenda Fitzgerald, Secretary-Treasurer

3298 Black AIDS Institute
1833 West 8th Street #200
Los Angeles, CA 90057
213-353-3610
Fax: 213-989-0181
www.blackaids.org

It is the only national HIV/AIDS think tank focused exclusively on Black people. The Institute's Mission is to stop the AIDS pandemic in Black communities by engaging and mobilizing Black institutions and individuals in efforts to confront HIV.

Grazell R. Howard, J.D, Chair
Vanessa Williams, 1st Vice Chair
Gerard McCallum II, 2nd Vice Chair

3299 Elizabeth Glazer Pediatric AIDS Foundation
1140 Connecticut Avenue, N.W, Ste 200
Washington,, DC 20036
ÿ20- 29- 916
888-499-4673
Fax: 202-296-9185
e-mail: info@pedsaids.org
www.pedsaids.org

A national nonprofit organization dealing with medical problems unique to children infected with HIV/AIDS. The foundation is focused specifically on creating a future that will offer hope, finding effective therapies and issues of pregnancy and HIV. The foundation encourages students to enter the world of pediatric AIDS through a student intern program and more.

Pamela Barnes, President/CEO
Trish Carlin, Vice President Programs
Diane Thompson, VP Policy/Communications

3300 HIV Medicine Association
1300 Wilson Boulevard,ÿSuite 300
Arlington, VA 22209
703-299-1215
Fax: 703-299-8766
e-mail: info@hivma.org
www.hivma.org

The HIV Medicine Association is an organization of medical professionals who practice HIV medicine.

Adaora Adimora, Chair
Carlos del Rio, Chair Elect
Wendy Armstrong, Vice Chair

3301 Hemophilia Federation of America
820 First Street NE, Suite 720
Washington, DC 20002
202-675-6984
800-230-9797
Fax: 972-616-6211
e-mail: info@hemophiliafed.org
www.hemophiliafed.org

Hemophilia Federation of America (HFA) is a community based organization that serves people with bleeding disorders and their families in the USA. With a broad mission to assist and advocate, HFA provides programs, services and policy education and support through its Member Organization affiliations as well as direct to consumers.

Tracy Cleghorn, Board President
Scott Boling, Co-Vice President
Douglas Hartsough, Board Treasurer

3302 Immune Deficiency Foundation
Immune Deficiency Foundation
40 W Chesapeake Avenue, Suite 308
Towson, MD 21204
410-321-6647
800-296-4433
Fax: 410-321-9165
e-mail: idf@primaryimmune.org
www.primaryimmune.org

The only national charitable organization aimed at fighting the primary immune deficiency diseases. The founders included parents of children with primary immune deficiency, immunologists who treat immune deficient patients and other individuals with an interest in helping others. The Foundation's main goal is to improve the care and treatment of adults and children with primary immune deficiency diseases and to promote public education and awareness about the diseases.

Marcia Boyle, Ceo
Katherine Antilla, Vice Chair
Carol Ann Demaret, Secretary

3303 Infectious Diseases Society of America
1300 Wilson Blvd, Suite 300
Arlington, VA 22209
703-299-0200
Fax: 703-299-0204
www.idsociety.org

The Infectious Diseases Society of America (IDSA) represents physicians, scientists and other health care professionals who specialize in infectious diseases. IDSA's purpose is to improve the health of individuals, communities, and society by promoting excellence in patient care, education, research, public health, and prevention relating to infectious diseases.

Stephen B. Calderwood, MD, FIDSA, President
Johan S. Bakken, MD, PhD, FIDSA, President-Elect
William G. Powderly, MD, FIDSA, Vice President

3304 International Antiviral Society-USA
425 California Street, Suite 1450
San Francisco, CA 94104
415-544-9400
Fax: 415-544-9401
e-mail: info@iasusa.org
www.iasusa.org

TheÿIAS-USAÿis a not-for-profit professional education organization that has been sponsoring continuing medical education (CME) programs for physicians since 1992 and is accredited by the Accreditation Council for Continuing Medical Education (ACCME).

Paul A. Volberding, MD, Chair, Board of Directors
Donna M. Jacobsen, Executive Director/President
Constance A. Benson, MD, Board of Director

3305 International Association of Providers of AIDS Care
1990 M Street, NW, Suite 380
Washington, DC 20036
202-808-2754
Fax: 202-315-3651
e-mail: iapac@iapac.org
www.iapac.org

IAPAC envisions a world in which people at risk for and those living with HIV/AIDS may access the best prevention, care, and treatment services delivered by clinicians and allied health workers armed with cutting-edge knowledge and expertise.

Ian Sparks, CEO
Benjamin Young, MD, PhD, SVP/ CMO
Michael S. Glass, MA, EVP/ Chief of Staff

3306 National AIDS Hotline
American Social Association
PO Box 13827
Research Triangle Park, NC 27709
919-361-8400
800-342-2437
Fax: 919-361-8425
TDD: 800-243-7889
www.ashastd.org

Information and advocacy resources for families and professionals. Includes listings of organizations providing general information and organizations focusing on more specific areas of concern to families and young adults who have disabilities.

Lynn Barclay, President/CEO
Deborah Arrindell, VP Health Policy
David Allen MBA, CPA, Vice President/CFO

3307 National Abandoned Infants Assistance Resource Center
University of California, Berkeley
1950 Addison Street, Suite 104, #7402
Berkeley, CA 94720
510-643-8390
Fax: 510-643-7019
e-mail: aia@berkeley.edu
www.aia.berkeley.edu

The Center's vision is to enhance the quality of social and health services delivered to drug and HIV-affected children and their families. Its strategy is to provide state-of-the-art training, technical assistance, research, and information to professionals who serve these families. Services include a national newsletter, telephone seminars, conferences, monographs, guides and reports.

Jeanne Pietrzak, Director
Neil Gilbert PhD, Principal Investigator
Amy Price MPA, Associate Director

3308 National Alliance of State & Territorial AIDS Directors
444 North Capitol Street, NWÿÿSuite 339
Washington, DC 20001 202-434-8090
e-mail: nastad@nastad.org
www.nastad.org

The National Alliance of State and Territorial AIDS Directors
(NASTAD) represents the nation's chief state health agency staff
who have programmatic responsibility for administering
HIV/AIDS and viral hepatitis healthcare, prevention, education,
and supportive service programs funded by state and federal governments. NASTAD is dedicated to reducing the incidence of
HIV/AIDS and viral hepatitis infections in the U.S. and its territories, providing comprehensive, compassionate, and high-quality
ca

Kevin Trotter, Manager, Operations
Lucy Slater, Director, Global Programÿ
Mark Griswold, Senior Manager, Global Program

3309 National Association of Community Health Centers
7501 Wisconsin Ave, Suite 1100W
Bethesda, MD 20814 301-347-0400
www.nachc.com

To address the widespread lack of access to basic health care,
Community Health Centers serve over 23 million people at more
than 9,000 sites located throughout all 50 states and U.S. territories.

Gary Wiltz, MD, Chair of the Board
Ricardo Guzman, Chair Elect
Kauilaÿ Clark, Immediate Past Chair

3310 National Association of People with AIDS
8041 Colesville Road, Suite 750
Silver Spring, MD 20910 240-247-0880
Fax: 240-247-0574
e-mail: info@napwa.org
www.napwa.org

Advocates on behalf of all people with HIV and AIDS in order to
end the pandemic and the human suffering caused by HIV/AIDS.

Frank Oldham, Jr, Executive Director
Vanessa Johnson, Deputy Executive Director
Andrew Spieldenner, Director Programs

3311 National Black Leadership Commission on AIDS, Inc.
215 W. 125th Street, 2ndÿFloor
New York, NY 10027 212-614-0023
Fax: 212-614-0508
e-mail: info@nblca.org
www.nblca.org

The National Black Leadership Commission on AIDS, Inc.
(NBLCA) is a non-profit organization in the United States. There
mission is to educate, mobilize, and empower black leaders to
meet the challenge of fighting HIV/AIDS and other health disparities in their local communities.

C. Virginia Fields, President and CEO
Felecia Webb, Vice President of Development
Leatrice Wactor, Program Coordinator

3312 National Medical Association
8403 Colesville Road, Suite 820
Silver Spring, MD 20910 202-347-1895
Fax: 202-347-0722
www.nmanet.org

The National Medical Association (NMA) is the collective voice
of African American physicians and the leading force for parity
and justice in medicine and the elimination of disparities in
health.

Garfield Clunie, M.D., Chairman of the Board
Lawrence Sanders, President
Martin Hamlette, J.D., M.H.A., Executive Director

3313 National Minority AIDS Council
1931 13th Street NW
Washington, DC 20009 202-483-6622
Fax: 202-483-1135
e-mail: communications@nmac.org
nmac.org

NMAC represents a coalition of faith based and community based
organizations as well as AIDS Service organizations advocating
and delivering HIV/AIDS services in communities of color
nationwide.ÿÿ

Paul Kawata, Executive Director
Kim Ferrell, Director of Facilities Management
Kim Johnson, Director

3314 Physician's Research Network
39 West 19th Street, Suite 605
New York, NY 10011 212-924-0857
Fax: 212-924-0759
www.prn.org

The Physicians' Research Network (PRN) is a not-for-profit,
peer-support and educational organization serving clinicians
working in the fight against HIV/AIDS and viral hepatitis.

James F. Braun, DO, President
Edward Vladich, Office Manager

3315 Support for Children with AIDS
1222 T Street NW, Grandma's House
Washington, DC 20009 202-234-4128
Fax: 202-234-8145
e-mail: terrific03@aol.com
www.grandmashouse-terrific.org

A support organization that provides service, care, and preventive
education for children and adults with AIDS. It provides housing
for children with AIDS (e.g. Grandma's House® in Washington,
DC).

Susan McCarley, Vice President

3316 World Health Organization
Avenue Appia 20
CH-1211 Geneva 27,
Switzerland www.who.int

WHO is the directing and coordinating authority for health within
the United Nations system.

Dr Margaret Chan, Director General

3317 anfAR
120 Wall Street, 13th Floor
New York, NY 10005 212-806-1600
Fax: 212-806-1601
www.amfar.org

With the freedom and flexibility to respond quickly to emerging
areas of scientific promise, amfAR plays a catalytic role in accelerating the pace of HIV/AIDS research and achieving real
breakthroughs.

Kenneth Cole, Chairman
Mathilde Krim, Ph.D., Founding Chairman
Wallace Sheft, C.P.A., Treasurer

Research Centers

3318 American Foundation for AIDS Research
120 Wall Street, 13th Floor
New York, NY 10005 212-806-1600
800-392-6327
Fax: 212-806-1601
www.amfar.org

Dedicated to the support of HIV/AIDS research, HIV prevention,
treatment education, and the advocacy of sound AIDS related
public policy.

Kevin Frost, Ceo
Deborah C. Hernan, VP Public Information
Monica S. Ruiz PhD, MPH, Acting Director, Public Policy

3319 Children's Clinical Research Center
New York Hospital, Cornell Medical Center
525 E 68th Street, Box 149
New York, NY 10065　　　　　　　212-746-4745
Fax: 212-746-8922
www.ccrc.med.cornell.edu

Offers research into the study of pediatric AIDS and other disorders.

Julianne Imperato-McGinley, MD, Program Director
Patricia Giardina, MD, Associate Program Director

3320 Developmental Medicine Center
Children's Hospital
300 Longwood Avenue
Boston, MA 02115　　　　　　　617-355-6000
800-355-7944
Fax: 617-735-7429
TTY: 617-730-0152
e-mail: webteam@tch.harvard.edu
www.childrenshospital.org

The Developmental Medicine Center (DMC) at Children's Hospital Boston provides developmental evaluation and treatment services for children aged birth to adolescence with a wide range of developmental, behavioral and learning difficulties. The Center was founded for the purpose of enhancing the coordination of services for children and families with special needs.,

Leonard A. Rappaport MD, MS, Program Director

Conferences

3321 Immune Deficiency Foundation National Conference
40 West Chesapeake Avenue, Suite 308
Towson, MD 21204　　　　　　　410-321-6647
800-296-4433
Fax: 410-321-9165
e-mail: info@primaryimmune.org
www.primaryimmune.org

Annual conference hosted by an organization aimed at fighting the primary immune deficiency diseases. The founders included parents of children with primary immune deficiency, immunologists who treat immune deficient patients and other individuals with an interest in helping others. The Foundation's main goal is to improve the care and treatment of adults and children with primary immune deficiency diseases and to promote public education and awareness about the diseases.

June

Marcia Boyle, Founder/Chairman/President
Katherine Antilla, Vice Chair
Carol Ann Demaret, Secretary

Web Sites

3322 AEGIS
10866 Washington Blvd., #309
Culver City, CA 90232　　　　　　　310-838-2787
e-mail: info@aegis.com
www.aegis.com/

Web based reference for HIV/AIDS-related information.

Jeff Zisner, President & CEO

3323 AIDS Knowledge Base
hivinsite.ucsf.edu/InSite

415-476-9000
e-mail: webdev@pubaff.ucsf.edu
hivinsite.ucsf.edu/InSite

A comprehensive, on-line textbook of HIV disease from the University of California San Francisco and San Francisco Hospital.

Sam Hawgood, MBBS, Chancellor
Daniel Lowenstein, MD, Executive Vice Chancellor & Provost
Bruce Wintroub, Interim Dean, School of Medicine

3324 American Social Health Association
www.ashastd.org

Dedicated to improving the health of individuals, families, and communities with a focus on preventing sexually transmitted diseases and their harmful consequences.

3325 Children with AIDS Project
PO Box 23778
Tempe, AZ 85285　　　　　　　480-774-9718
www.aidskids.org/

The mission is to transform the silenct that surrounds HIV infected, children and AIDS orphans into an audible sound. This sound must be amplified until the needs are met for all children in the nation and globally affected by the AIDS epidemic.

3326 Elizabeth Glazer Pediatric AIDS Foundation
1140 Connecticut Avenue NW, Suite 200
Washington, DC 20036　　　　　　　202-296-9165
888-499-4673
Fax: 202-296-9185
e-mail: info@pedaids.org, research@pedaids.org
www.pedaids.org/

The foundation created a future of hope for children and families worldwide by eradicating pediatric AIDS, providing care and treatment to people with HIV/AIDS, and accelerating the discovery of new treatments for other serious and life-threatening pediatric illnesses.

Russ Hagey, Chair
Charles Lyons, President & CEO
Brad Kiley, COO

3327 Food and Drug Administration
10903 New Hampshire Avenue
Silver Spring, MD 20903　　　　　　　301-796-8240
888-463-6332
e-mail: webmail@oc.fda.gov
www.fda.gov

The FDA is responsible for protecting the public health by assuring the safety, efficacy, and security of human and veterinary drugs, biological products, medical devices, our nation's food supply, cosmetics, and products that emit radiation. The FDA is also responsible for advancing the public health by helping to speed innovations that make medicines and foods more effective, safer, and more affordable and helping the public get accurate, science-based information they need to improve health.

Margaret A. Hamburg, Commissioner
Walter S. Harris, MBA, PMP, Deputy Commissioner
James Tyler, CFO

3328 Immune Deficiency Foundation
110 West Road, Suite 300
Towson, MD 21204　　　　　　　800-296-4433
Fax: 410-321-9165
www.primaryimmune.org

The only national charitable organization aimed at fighting the primary immune deficiency diseases. The founders included parents of children with primary immune deficiency, immunologists who treat immune deficient patients and other individuals with an interest in helping others.

John Seymour, Phd, LMFt, Chair
Steve Fietek, Vice Chair
Marcia Boyle, President & Founder

3329 National Association of People with AIDS
8401 Colesville Road, Suite 505
Silver Spring, MD 20910　　　　　　　240-247-0880
866-846-9366
Fax: 240-247-0574
www.napwa.org

Advocates on behalf of all people with HIV and AIDS in order to end the pandemic and the human suffering caused by HIV/AIDS.

3330 National Pediatric & Family HIV Resource Center
www.womenchildrenhiv.org

e-mail: editor@WomenChildrenHIV.org
www.womenchildrenhiv.org

The goal of this site is to contribute to an improvement in the scale and quality of international HIV/AIDS prevention care and treatment programs for women and children by increasing access to authoritative HIV/AIDS information.

Arthur Ammann, MD, President
Heather Dron, MPH, Project Manager
Robert Grey, Programmer

3331 National Pediatric AIDS Network
PO Box 1507
Nevada City, CA 95959   e-mail: gary@npan.org
                                         www.npan.org/

Is a nonprofit organization, that works collaboratively with a number of other HIV/AIDS information providers.

Gary Gale, Director

3332 Parents Helping Parents
1400 Parkmoor Ave., Suite 100
San Jose, CA 95126   408-727-5772
                                         855-727-5775
                                         Fax: 408-286-1116
                                         www.php.com

Mission is to help children with special needs receive the resources, love, hope, respect, health care, education, and other services they need to reach their full potential by providing them with strong families, dedicated professionals, and responsive systems to serve them.

Hitesh Shah, Chair
Mary Ellen Peterson, MA, Executive Director/ CEO
Paul Schutz, CFO

3333 Pediatric AIDS Clinical Trials Group
pactg.s-3.com

Goals are: to optimize strategies to maintain or improve mother to infant transmission at less than 2% without long termn toxicity to exposed infants or treated pregnant women in the United States; and to enable more than 90% of children perinatally infected with HIV to achieve normal growth and development, and more than 20 years survival in the United States.

3334 Sunshine for HIV Kids
www.sunshinesite.com

Is a nonprofit tax exempt organization that identifies and raises funds for charities who directly deliver care to children afficted with HIV/AIDS and their familes.

3335 Wayne State University
42. West Warren Ave.
Detroit, MI 48202   315-577-2424
                                         www.research.wayne.edu

Advances in therapy to prevent HIV transmission from mothers to infants have brought hope to thousands, but transmission of HIV continues to increase in developing countries. We must identify effective intervention strategies usable by all nations if we are to reduce the incidence of mother to infant HIV transmission worldwide.

Debbie Dingell, Chair
Gary S. Pollard, Vice Chair
M. Roy Wilson, President

Book Publishers

3336 AIDS Awareness Library

Anna Forbes, MSS, author

Rosen Publishing Group
29 E 21st Street
New York, NY 10010   212-777-3017
                                         800-237-9932
                                         Fax: 888-436-4643
                                         e-mail: info@rosenpub.com
                                         www.rosenpublishing.com

This series of eight 24-page books for grades K-5, speaks to children in nonthreatening langauge that provides vital information without graphic detail. This series is meant to be a gentle introduction to this frightening epidemic. Titles in series: Heroes Against AIDS, Kids with AIDS, Living in a World with AIDS, Myths and Facts About AIDS, What is AIDS?, What You Can Do About AIDS, When Someone You Know Has AIDS, Where Did AIDS Come From?.
24 pages
ISBN: 0-823974-06-5

3337 AIDS and the Education of Our Children
Consumer Information Center
US Department of Education
Pueblo, CO 81009   719-948-3334
                                         888-878-3256
                                         www.pueblo.gsa.gov

A guide for parents and teachers offering helpful information on the topic of AIDS education.
28 pages

3338 Heroes Against AIDS

Anna Forbes, MSS, author

Rosen Publishing Group
29 E 21st Street
New York, NY 10010   212-777-3017
                                         800-237-9932
                                         Fax: 888-436-4643
                                         e-mail: info@rosenpub.com
                                         www.rosenpublishing.com

Ryan White and Magic Johnson are just two of the heroes in this book who demonstrate through their courage and kindness their strength in adversity.
K-5 24 pages
ISBN: 0-823923-71-1

3339 Kids with AIDS

Anna Forbes, MSS, author

Rosen Publishing Group
29 E 21st Street
New York, NY 10010   212-777-3017
                                         800-237-9932
                                         Fax: 888-436-4643
                                         e-mail: info@rosenpub.com
                                         www.rosenpublishing.com

This book is written so as not to scare kids but teach compassion for their peers who might have AIDS. It stresses the importance of eliminating blame from this disease.
K-5 24 pages
ISBN: 0-823923-72-X

3340 Let's Talk About Going to the Hospital
Rosen Publishing Group's PowerKids Press
29 E 21st Street
New York, NY 10010   212-777-3017
                                         800-237-9932
                                         Fax: 888-436-4643
                                         e-mail: rosenpub@tribeca.ios.com
                                         www.powerkidspress.com

If a child has to check into the hospital, chances are he or she is already upset about being ill. Knowing how a hospital functions and what the procedures are, such as when family members can visit, will help in what is already a stressful situation. Grades K-5.

24 pages
ISBN: 0-823950-36-0

3341 Living in a World with AIDS
Anna Forbes, MSS, author

Rosen Publishing Group
29 E 21st Street
New York, NY 10010
212-777-3017
800-237-9932
Fax: 888-436-4643
e-mail: info@rosenpub.com
www.rosenpublishing.com

AIDS is a reality. Kids hear about it on TV, at school, and on the streets. This introductory volume reassures kids about their basic safety and provides gentle preventative advice that is age appropriate.

K-5 24 pages
ISBN: 0-823923-67-3

3342 Myths and Facts About AIDS
Rosen Publishing Group's PowerKids Press
29 E 21st Street
New York, NY 10010
212-777-3017
800-237-9932
Fax: 888-436-4643
e-mail: rosenpub@tribeca.ios.com
www.powerkidspress.com

In a simple and reassuring manner, the author demystifies this disease and puts to rest many misconceptions. Grades K-5.

K-5 24 pages
ISBN: 0-823923-66-5

3343 What Is AIDS?
Rosen Publishing Group's PowerKids Press
29 E 21st Street
New York, NY 10010
212-777-3017
800-237-9932
Fax: 888-436-4643
e-mail: rosenpub@tribeca.ios.com
www.powerkidspress.com

Accessible scientific look at AIDS puts it in the context of other diseases, teaching about the human organism in an age-appropriate manner. Grades K-5.

K-5 24 pages
ISBN: 0-823923-68-1

3344 What You Can Do About AIDS
Anna Forbes, MSS, author

Rosen Publishing Group
29 E 21st Street
New York, NY 10010
212-777-3017
800-237-9932
Fax: 888-436-4643
e-mail: info@rosenpub.com
www.rosenpublishing.com

It's never too early to teach kids about social responsibility. This book emphasizes community participation.

K-5 24 pages
ISBN: 0-823923-70-3

3345 When Someone You Know Has AIDS
Anna Forbes, MSS, author

Rosen Publishing Group
29 E 21st Street
New York, NY 10010
212-777-3017
800-237-9932
Fax: 888-436-4643
e-mail: info@rosenpub.com
www.rosenpublishing.com

This unique volume helps kids who might know someone with AIDS to approach that person with love and compassion as one would any sick person.

K-5 24 pages
ISBN: 0-823923-69-X

3346 Where Did AIDS Come From?
Anna Forbes, MSS, author

Rosen Publishing Group
29 E 21st Street
New York, NY 10010
212-777-3017
800-237-9932
Fax: 888-436-4643
e-mail: info@rosenpub.com
www.rosenpublishing.com

AIDS is frightening, especially to young children who sense the secrecy around it. This is a gentle introduction to the topic. It treats AIDS like any other epidemic.

K-5 24 pages
ISBN: 0-823923-65-7

Pamphlets

3347 Hope for Children with AIDS
Elizabeth Glazer Pediatric AIDS Foundation
1140 Connecticut Avenue NW, Suite 200
Washington, DC 20036
202-296-9165
888-499-4693
Fax: 202-296-9185
e-mail: info@pedaids.org, research@pedaids.org
www.pedaids.org

The Elizabeth Glaser Pediatric AIDS Foundation creates a future of hope for children and families worldwide by eradicating pediatric AIDS, providing care and treatment to people with HIV/AIDS, and accelerating the discovery of new treatments for other serious and life-threatening pediatric illnesses. In working toward our mission the foundation is committed to ensuring that the vast majority of every dollar raised goes directly into our research education and outreach program.

Russ Hagey, Chair
Charles Lyons, President & CEO
Brad Kiley, COO

Camps

3348 Camp Heartland
1845 N Farwell Avenue, Suite 310
Millwaukee, WI 53202
414-272-1118
800-724-4673
Fax: 414-272-9916
e-mail: webmaster@campheartland.org
www.campheartland.org

Set up to provide children impacted by HIV/AIDS with the best week of their lives. Provides children forever affected by the isolation and tragedy of the disease the opportunity to experience - sometimes for the first time - the pure joys of being a kid.

Neil Willenson, Founder/CEO
Jeffrey Maiken, President
Patrick Kindler, Program Manager

3349 Camp Kindle
PO Box 81147
Lincoln, NE 81147
661-257-1901
877-800-2267
Fax: 702-995-9186
e-mail: info@projectkindle.org
www.campkindle.org

Camp with the purpose to enhance the overall well-being of children and young people infected with or affected by HIV and AIDS.

Eva Payne, Founder & Executive Director
Mandy Nickolite, VP & Psychosocial lead
Erin Fitzgerald, Program Coordinator

3350 Camp Kindle- Project Kindle
28245 Ave Crocker, Ste 104
Santa Clarita, CA 91355

661-257-1901
877-800-2267
Fax: 702-995-9186
e-mail: info@projectkindle.org
www.campkindle.org

Camp for youth ages 7-18 who are infected with or affected by
HIV and AIDS.

Eva Payne, Founder & Executive Director
Alison Boring, Co-Camp Director

3351 Hole in the Wall Gang Camp
565 Ashford Center Road
Ashford, CT 6278

860-429-3444
Fax: 860-429-7295
e-mail: ashford@holeinthewallgang.org
www.holeinthewallgang.org

Nonprofit organization that provides a recreational camp experience for children ages 7-15 with cancer, genetic blood diseases
and HIV/AIDS.

Raymond Lamontagne, Chair
James Canton, CEO
Kevin Magee, CFO

Description

3352 HEAD INJURIES

Synonyms: Closed head injury, Concussion, Traumatic brain injury

Involves the following Biologic System(s):

Neurologic Disorders

Head injuries describe trauma to the head that results in damage to the scalp, skull, or brain and associated membranes, nerves, or blood vessels. Every year in the United States, approximately 100,000 children require hospitalization because of head injuries. Many of these injuries are the result of motor vehicle and bicycle accidents. The risk of sustaining head or brain injury during a vehicular or bicycle accident is reduced by the proper use of restraint systems such as approved car seats, seat belts, or helmets. There are different types of head injuries, some of which are minor and, after healing, of no further significance; however, certain injuries that impact upon the brain may have severe complications and be potentially life-threatening. These include skull fractures, concussions, brain contusions and lacerations, and bleeding in the brain (e.g., subdural or epidural hematomas). Brain injury may result in mild, moderate, or severe functional disabilities, depending upon the particular area of brain tissue that is damaged or destroyed. Disabilities may affect physical, emotional, or intellectual development and include impairment in the comprehension or production of speech and language (aphasia); the inability to remember or perform certain familiar tasks requiring sequential movements (apraxia); the failure to remember past events or experiences (amnesia); the lack of ability to recognize familiar persons or objects (agnosia); and the development of episodes of uncontrolled electrical activity in the brain (posttraumatic epilepsy), usually within two years of the initial head injury.

In children with skull fractures or an open-head injury, there is an actual break in the skull bone (cranium). Many skull fractures do not interfere with normal brain function and will heal with no complications. However, in some patients, fractures may damage blood vessels or the membranes surrounding the brain (meninges), resulting in leakage of the fluid that surrounds the brain and spinal cord (cerebrospinal fluid). The break in the skull may also serve as an entry point for bacteria that may subsequently cause serious infection. A thorough evaluation is necessary to determine the extent of the injury. Surgical intervention may sometimes be necessary.

Concussions are closed-head injuries that occur as a result of a jarring of the brain within the skull. Symptoms and findings associated with this type of injury in children may include a temporary loss of consciousness, lack of muscle tone, poor or absent reflexes (areflexia), dilated pupils, blurred vision, irritability, or restlessness. These signs of concussion may be followed by rapid heartbeat (tachycardia), vomiting, listlessness, drowsiness, apathy, a pale skin color, or confusion. Treatment for concussion always involves observation. Although most children recover completely, hospitalization may be required for those whose level of consciousness continues to drop or those who appear listless, drowsy, or confused. Those who vomit excessively or experience seizures or other neurological symptoms may also require hospitalization.

Other closed-head injuries may include contusions, character-ized by bruises on the brain; lacerations, characterized by tears in the brain tissue; subdural hematomas, characterized by accumulations of blood under the outermost membrane layer surrounding the brain (dura mater); and epidural hematomas, characterized by blood between the dura mater and the skull. Hematomas may result from ruptures or lacerations in certain blood vessels. Contusions and hematomas may cause the brain to swell with an accompanying buildup of fluid (edema). Increasing pressure within the skull may result in brain damage. Symptoms and findings may include headache; seizures; altered levels of consciousness sometimes leading to coma; loss of strength; numbness; paralysis; confusion; amnesia; or life-threatening complications such as respiratory distress and heart irregularities. Treatment is aimed at the maintenance of respiratory and cardiovascular function in order to prevent further injury. If necessary, the upper spine (cervical spine) is stabilized. The monitoring and management of brain swelling and fluid accumulation may include the careful administration of intravenous fluids and medications, bed elevation, and the use of supplemental oxygen. In addition, surgical intervention may be required to relieve intracranial pressure, remove blood clots, or control bleeding around the brain. Further treatment may include medication for the control of seizures. Recovery from major head or brain trauma may be a very slow, progressive process and, as such, may require the assistance of a team of specialists who will work with the family or caregivers of the child to coordinate symptomatic and supportive care.

Government Agencies

3353 NIH/National Institute of Neurological Disorders and Stroke (NINDS)
PO Box 5801
Bethesda, MD 20824

301-496-5751
800-352-9424
Fax: 301-496-0296
TTY: 301-468-5981
www.ninds.nih.gov

The mission of NINDS is to reduce the burden of neurological disease, a burden borne by every age group, by every segment of society, by people all over the world.

Story C Landis PhD, Director
Audrey S Penn MD, Deputy Director

National Associations & Support Groups

3354 Acoustic Neuroma Association
600 Peachtree Parkway, Suite 108
Cumming, GA 30041

770-205-8211
877-200-8211
Fax: 770-205-0239
e-mail: info@anausa.org
www.anausa.org

The Acoustic Neuroma Association provides information and support to patients who have been diagnosed with or experienced an acoustic neuroma or other benign problem affecting the cranial nerves. The ANA is an incorporated, nonprofit organization, and is supported by contributions from its members. The association also furnishes information on patient rehabilitation to physicians and health care personnel, promotes research on acoustic neuroma, and educates the public.

Jeffrey D. Barr, President
Alan Goldberg, VP
Steven M. Houghton, Secretary

3355 American Academy of Pediatrics
141 Northwest Point Boulevard
Elk Grove Village, IL 60007
847-434-4000
800-433-9016
Fax: 847-434-8000
www.aap.org

The American Academy of Pediatrics and its member pediatricians are committed to the attainment of optimal physical, mental and social health and well-being for all infants, children, adolescents, and young adults.

Sandra Hassink, MD, FAAP, President

3356 Association for Neurologically Impaired Brain Injured Children
61-35 220th Street
Oakland Gardens, NY 11364
718-423-9550
Fax: 718-423-9838
e-mail: mail@anibic.org
www.anibic.org

ANIBIC is a voluntary, multi-service organization that is dedicated to serving individuals with severe learning disabilities, neurological impairments and other developmental disabilities. Services include: residential, vocational, family support services, recreation (children and adults), respite (adult), summer day camp, counseling, and tramatic brain injury services (adults).

Michael Steward, President
Phyllis Kaye, VP
Jerry Smith, Executive Director

3357 Brain Injury Association of America Helpli ne
8201 Greensboro Drive, Suite 611
McLean, VA 22102
703-761-0750
800-444-6443
Fax: 703-761-0755
e-mail: familyhelpline@biausa.org
www.biausa.org

The mission of the Brain Injury Association is to create a better future through brain injury prevention, research, education and advocacy. This national number can link people to local BIA affiliates.

Susan H Connors, President/CEO
Mary S Reitter, CAE, Executive VP/COO
Gregory J. O'Shanick, Managing Director

3358 Brain Injury Association of America Nation al Office
1608 Spring Hill Road, Suite 110
Vienna, VA 22182
703-761-0750
800-444-6443
Fax: 703-761-0755
e-mail: info@biausa.org
www.biausa.org

Our mission is to create a better future through brain injury prevention, research, education and advocacy.

Susan H Connors, President/CEO
Mary S Reitter, CAE, Executive VP/COO
Gregory J. O'Shanick, Managing Director

3359 Brain Injury Association of Michigan
7305 Grand River, Suite 100
Brighton, MI 48114
810-229-5880
800-444-6443
Fax: 810-229-8947
e-mail: info@biami.org
www.biami.org

The mission of BIAMI is to enhance the lives of those affected by brain injury through education, advocacy, research, and local support groups; and to reduce the incidence of brain injury through prevention.

Michael F Dabbs, President
Cheryl A Burda, VP of Operations & Programs
Helena Dinqeldey, Office Coordinator

3360 Brain Trauma Foundation
7 World Trade Center, 34th Floor, 250 Greenwich St
New York, NY 10007
212-772-0608
Fax: 212-772-0357
e-mail: info@braintrauma.org
www.braintrauma.org

The Brain Trauma Foundation mission is to improve the outcome of Traumatic Brain Injury (TBI) patients nationwide.

Jamshid Ghajar, President
Alan Quasha, Chairman
Pamela J. Newman, Executive Director

3361 Center for Disabilities and Development
University of Iowa Hospitals and Clinics
100 Hawkins Drive
Iowa City, IA 52242
319-353-6900
877-686-0031
Fax: 319-356-8284
e-mail: cdd-scheduling@uiowa.edu
www.uichildrens.org/cdd

A trusted resource for healthcare, training, research and information for people with disabilities that include: behavior disorders, brain injury, cerebral palsy, diabetes, down syndrome, learning disabilities, mental retardation, sleep disorders and spina bifida.

Judy Stephenson, Administrator
Amy Mikelson, Supervisor Info Resource Service

3362 Coma Recovery Association
8300 Republic Airport, Suite 106
Farmingdale, NY 11735
631-756-1826
Fax: 631-756-1827
e-mail: office@comarecovery.org
www.comarecovery.org

Our purpose is to help families of coma and head injury survivors by providing information and referrals, enabling them to make informed choices regarding treatment, rehabilitation and socialization alternatives as well as support from others who struggle with similar concerns.

3363 Head Injury Hotline
212 Pioneer Building
Seattle, WA 98104
206-621-8558
Fax: 206-329-4355
e-mail: brain@headinjury.com
www.headinjury.com

Sponsors public information seminars designed to bring together survivors of head injuries, their families and professionals for networking and information sharing, as well as operating a national helpline for people suffering from a head injury.

Constance Miller, MA, Founder
Paul M. Kuroiwa, PH.C., Performance management consultant
Bill Levinger, Managing Director

3364 Perspectives Network
PO Box 121012
W Melbourne, FL 32912
770-844-6898
800-685-6302
Fax: 770-844-6898
e-mail: TPN@tbi.org
www.tbi.org

Primary focus is positive communication between persons with brain injury, family members, caregivers and friends of persons with brain injury, the many professionals who treat persons with brain injury and community members in order to create positive changes and enhance public awareness and knowledge of acquired and traumatic brain injury.

State Agencies & Support Groups

Alabama

3365 Alabama Head Injury Foundation
3100 Lorna Road, Suite 200
Hoover, AL 35216
205-823-3818
800-433-8002
Fax: 205-823-4544
e-mail: ahif1@bellsouth.net
www.ahif.org

Our mission is to improve the quality of life for survivors of traumatic brain injury and for their families and to increase public awareness of (TBI).

Keith T. Belt, Jr., President
Kim F. Hooks, VP
Charles D Priest, Executive Director

Arizona

3366 Brain Injury Association of Arizona
5025 E Washington St., Suite 108
Phoenix, AZ 85034

602-508-8024
888-500-9165
Fax: 602-508-8285
e-mail: info@biaaz.org
www.biaaz.org

A non-profit membership organiation of people with brain injuries, their families, friends and service providers working together since 1983 to provide information and referrels, education, advocacy and support for those affected by brain injury.

Lisa Counters, President
Rebecca Armendariz, VP
Mattie Cummins, Executive Director

Arkansas

3367 Brain Injury Association of Arkansas
PO Box 26236
Little Rock, AR 72221

501-374-3585
866-610-4841
Fax: 501-918-6595
e-mail: info@BIA-AR.org
www.brainassociation.org

Creating a better future through brain injury prevention, research, education and advocacy.

Dana Austen, President
Kortney E Gold, VP
Tessa Davis, Secretary

California

3368 California Brain Injury Association
1800 30th St., Suite 250
Bakersfield, CA 93301

661-872-4903
888-662-4222
Fax: 661-873-2508
e-mail: calbiainfo@yahoo.com
www.biacal.org

Our mission is to serve and empower the community of many thousands of persons living in California with brain injuries and to enable them to live with dignity and to access all therapy, hospitalization, long term care, and all possible means for recovery and rehabilitation and to support their families.

Paula Daoutis, Administrative Director
Ursula Pesta, Project Coordinator
Elaine Solan, Community Liaison

3369 Jodi House
1235 C Veronica Springs Road
Santa Barbara, CA 93105

805-563-2882
Fax: 805-593-3982
e-mail: info@jodihouse.org

The mission of Jodi House is to create a nurturing place of order, caring, acceptance and motivation for people with acquired brain injury,and to provide opportunities for each person to discover new paths to regain responsible independence and effective interdependence to the best of our ability, in order to achieve worthwhile purposes in our community.

Jim Cook, President
Andrew Chung, VP
Tracy Cohn, Treasurer

Colorado

3370 Brain Injury Association of Colorado
1385 South Colorado Boulevard, Ste 606, Building A
Denver, CO 80204

303-355-9969
800-955-2443
Fax: 303-355-9968
e-mail: informationreferralbiacolorado.org
www.biacolorado.org

The Brain Injury Association of Colorado began in April 1980. BIAC was formed by a group of family members and professionals in Denver and Colorado Springs who were concerned with the lack of support services for survivors and family members affected by head injury.The mission is to improve the quality of life for survivors of brain injury and their families, and to support programs that prevent brain injury.

Dannis Schanel, President
Helen Kellogg, Executive Director
Peggy Spaulding, Executive Director

Connecticut

3371 Brain Injury Association of Connecticut
200 Day Hill Road, Suite 250
Windsor, CT 06095

860-219-0291
800-278-8242
Fax: 860-219-0568
e-mail: general@biact.org
www.biact.homestead.com

Supports persons with brain injuries and their families by promoting services to facilitate full inclusion within their local community, and to increase awareness and understanding of brain injury and its prevention through community education.

500 Members

Paul A. Slager, Esq., President
Dr. Johnny Magwood, BSME, MBA, DBA, Vice President
Julie Peters, Executive Director

3372 TBI Support Group for Families & Survivors
Gaylord Hospital Conference Room
Wallingford, CT 06492

203-284-2800
TDD: 203-284-2700

Our mission is to preserve and enhance a person's health and function. We offer people a comprehensive continuum of care ranging from our Medically Complex Program and inpatient rehabilitation programs to outpatient services and sleep services.

Delaware

3373 Brain Injury Association of Delaware
840 Walker Rd
Dover, DE 19904

302-346-2083
800-411-0505
Fax: 302-678-3183
e-mail: biadresources@cavtel.net
www.biausa.org

A nonprofit organization whose mission is to advocate for and with people who survive traumatic brain injury; to secure and develop community-bases services for survivors and their families; to support research leading to better outcomes that enhance the lives of those who sustain brain injuries; and to promote prevention of brain injury through awareness, education and legislation.

Elizabeth Furber, President
Timothy J. Walker, VP
Esther J. Curtis, Executive Director

District of Columbia

3374 Brain Injury Association of Washington DC
1232 17th St, N.W.
Washington, DC 20036

202-659-0122
Fax: 202-291-5366
e-mail: info@biadc.org
www.biadc.org

Provide support to survivors of brain injury and their families, education to those who are being effected by brain injury, including the general public, and advocacy, to give the many suffering from this silent epidemic a public voice.

Joseph Cammarata, President/Treasurer
Ira Sherman, VP
Michael Yochelson, M.D., Board of Director

Florida

3375 Brain Injury Association of Florida
1637 Metropolitan Blvd, Suite B
Tallahassee, FL 32308
850-410-0103
800-992-3442
Fax: 954-786-2437
e-mail: admin@biaf.org
www.biaf.org

A non profit organization founded in 1985, with the mission to improve the quality of life for persons with brain injury and their families by creating a better future through brain injury prevention, research, education, suport services and advocacy.

Mark Todd, PhD, President
Elynor Kazuk, Executive Director
Marilyn Ronshausen, Admin Secretary

3376 Family/Community Support Group of the Brain Injury Association of Florida
North Broward Medical Center
201 E Sample Road
Pompano Beach, FL 33064
954-786-2400
800-992-3442
www.biaf.org

Helping individuals with traumatic brain injuries and their families find practical solutions to the difficult problems faced when living with the long-term consequences of a traumatic brain injury (TBI).

Gary Clarke, Chairman
Johny Jallad, Chair-Elect
Larry Baxter, Secretary

3377 Goodwill Industries-Suncoast: Choices for Work Program
Goodwill Industries-Suncoast
10596 Gandy Boulevard
St. Petersburg, FL 33702
727-523-1512
888-297-1988
Fax: 727-579-1068
www.goodwill-suncoast.org

Provides short-term, light-duty work options for individuals recovering from on-the-job injuries. Participants are sponsored by a referring insurance company. This service is available in Hillsborough, Pinellas, Pasco and Polk counties through Suncoast Business Solutions.

Deborah A. Passerini, President
Oscar J. Horton, Chair
Martin W. Gladysz, Vice Chair

Georgia

3378 Brain Injury Resource Foundation
1841 Montreal Road, Suite 220
Tucker, GA 30084
678-937-1555
888-334-2424
Fax: 678-937-1557
e-mail: info@birf.info
www.birf.info/index.shtml

A nonprofit charitable orginazation working together with families and professionals since 1982 to provide education, advocacy and support for those effected by brain injury. Our mission is to empower individuals with brain injury by making available resources that may improve the quality of their lives.

Karen Parsley, Executive Director

Hawaii

3379 Brain Injury Association of Hawaii
420 Kuwili Street, Suite 103
Honolulu, HI 96817
808-436-8977
Fax: 808-454-1975
e-mail: biahi@verizon.net
www.biausa.org/Hawaii

Dedicated to improving the quality of life of persons with brain injury and the families of such persons in Hawaii and other areas of the Pacific Basin. The goals of BIA-HI include promoting the rights of individuals experiencing disability caused by brain injury, io increase public awareness of brain injury, and to provide education for individuals who have sustained a brain injury and their families.

Mary Isley-Wilson, President
Angie Enoka, VP
Lyna Burian, Secretary

3380 Special Education Center of Hawaii
708 Palekaua Street
Honolulu, HI 96816
808-734-0233
Fax: 808-734-0391
e-mail: info@secoh.org
www.secoh.org

Committed to providing individual and family supports that promote successful community living in the lifestyle of choice. Services and supports are provided to people with developmental disabilities, or acquired disabilities due to aging or head injury. Services include day care, respite care, and supported employment.

Jon McKenna, President
Douglas Inouye, VP
Debbie Hiraoka, Treasurer

Idaho

3381 Brain Injury Association of Idaho
1055 North Curtis Road, PO Box 414
Boise, ID 83706
208-367-2747
800-444-6443
Fax: 208-333-0026
e-mail: info@biaid.org
www.biaid.org

A non-profit organization helping persons with brain injuryand their familiy members.

Michelle Featherson, President

Illinois

3382 Brain Injury Association of Illinois
PO Box 64420
Chicago, IL 60664
312-726-5699
800-699-6443
Fax: 312-630-4011
e-mail: info@biail.org
www.biail.org

A not-for-profit statewide membership organization comprised of people with brain injuries, family members, friends and professionals, with the mission to create a better future through brain injury awareness, prevention, education and advocacy.

Ginny Lazzara, President
Philicia Deckard, Executive Director
Irene Pedersen, Founder

Indiana

3383 Brain Injury Association of Indiana
9531 Valparaiso Court, Suite A
Indianapolis, IN 46268
317-356-7722
866-854-4246
Fax: 317-808-7770
e-mail: info@BIAI.org
www.biai.org

A nonprofit service organization comprised of people with brain injury, their families, and concerned stakeholders who are dedicated to creating a better future by reducing the incidence and effects of brain injury through public and professional education, advocacy, support, and by facilitating inter-agency commitment and collaboration.

Nancy Ritter, Chairman
Tom John, VP
Scott Branam, Secretary

Iowa

3384 Brain Injury Association of Iowa
7025 Hickman Road, Suite 7
Urbandale, IA 50322
319-233-3235
855-444-6443
Fax: 319-272-2109
e-mail: info@biai.org
www.biaia.org

Founded in 1980, exists to support, assist, and advocate for persons with acquired brain damage and for their families; advocates for and with people with brain injury and family members by responding to their challenges and representing their concerns through legislative efforts and active support of programs created for their needs.

Jackie Preston, Manager
Geoffrey Lauer, MA, LOC, Executive Director
Natasha Retz, BS, CBIS, Director of Programs and Services

Kansas

3385 Brain Injury Association of Kansas & Greater Kansas City
6701 W. 64th St., Suite 120
Overland Park, KS 66202
913-754-8883
800-783-1356
Fax: 816-842-1531
e-mail: Lliggett@biaks.org
www.biaks.org

Offers support services to individuals and their families in the greater Kansas City area and throughout the state of Kansas who are recovering from traumatic brain injury.

Terrie Price, President
Whitney Sunderland, VP
Bonnie Stephens, Secretary

Kentucky

3386 Brain Injury Association of Kentucky
7321 New LaGrange Road, Suite 100
Louisville, KY 40222
502-493-0609
800-592-1117
Fax: 502-426-2993
e-mail: dir@braincenter.org
www.biak.us

Serves those affected by brain injury through advocacy, education, injury prevention, research, service and support.

Andrew Horne, President
Eileen Edlin, Treasurer
Ben Ruiz, Secretary

Louisiana

3387 Brain Injury Association of Louisiana
8325 Oak Street, PO Box 57527
New Orleans, LA 70118
504-982-0685
800-500-2026
www.biala.org

A non-profit organization that serves the needs of persons with brain injury, their families, and care providers. The focus is to create a better future for individuals who have survived brain injury through brain injury prevention awareness, promotion of research, public education, and advocacy.

Janet Clark, Chairman
Paul Genco, Vice Chairman
William E Moak, President/Executive Director

Maine

3388 Brain Injury Association of Maine
109 North State Street, Suite 2
Concord, NH 03301
603-225-8400
800-773-8400
Fax: 603-228-6749
e-mail: mail@biame.org
www.biame.org

A nonprofit organization that looks to create a better future for the people of Maine, through brain injury awareness, prevention, education and advocacy.

Bev Bryant, President
John Bott, Executive Director

Maryland

3389 Brain Injury Association of Maryland
2200 Kernan Drive
Baltimore, MD 21207
410-448-2924
800-221-6443
Fax: 410-448-3541
e-mail: info@biamd.org
www.biamd.org

Our mission is to create a better future through brain injury prevention, research, education and advocacy.

Diane Triplett, Executive Director
Diane Triplett, Executive Director

Massachusetts

3390 Brain Injury Association of Massachusetts
30 Lyman Street
Westborough, MA 01581
508-475-0032
800-242-0030
Fax: 508-475-0040
e-mail: biama@biama.org
www.biama.org

Our mission is to serve as an information and resource center for persons with brain injury, their families and friends, and providers and professionals in the field of brain injury treatment and rehabilitation.

Teresa Hayes, President
Harold Wilkinson, Secretary
Matthew Martino, Executive Board Member

Michigan

3391 Brain Injury Association of Michigan
7305 Grand River, Suite 100
Brighton, MI 48114
810-229-5880
800-444-6443
Fax: 810-229-8947
e-mail: info@biami.org
www.biami.org

The mission of BIAMI is to enhance the lives of those affected by brain injury through education, advocacy, research, and local support groups; and to reduce the incidence of brain injury through prevention.

Michael F Dabbs, President
Cheryl A Burda, VP of Operations & Programs
Helena Dinqeldey, Office Coordinator

3392 Rehabilitation Institute of Michigan
261 Mack Avenue
Detroit, MI 48201
313-745-1203
Fax: 313-745-9863
www.rimrehab.org

Providing quality patient care, academic excellence and cutting-edge research in physical medicine and rehabilitation.

Mildred Matlock, Ceo
William H. Restum, PhD, President

Minnesota

3393 Brain Injury Association of Minnesota
34 13th Avenue NE, Suite B001
Minneapolis, MN 55413
612-378-2742
800-669-6442
Fax: 612-378-2789
e-mail: info@braininjurymn.org
www.braininjurymn.org

The only non-profit organization in the state devoted solely to serving the needs of the 100,000 Minnesotans who live with a disability due to brain injury. Providing hope, help and a voice for brain injured persons for over 20 years.

quaterly 20-24 pages

Ardis Sandstrom, Executive Director
Ardis Sandstrom, Executive Director

Mississippi

3394 Brain Injury Association of Mississippi
2727 Old Canton Road, Suite 191
Jackson, MS 39216
601-981-1021
800-444-6443
Fax: 601-981-1039
e-mail: biaofms@aol.com
www.msbia.org

Enhances the quality of life for Traumatic Brain Injury survivors and their families, and to develop and support programs that prevent brain injury.

Lee Jenkins, Executive Director
Paul Gospodarski, EdD, Executive Director
Dana C. Pierce, Associate Director

Missouri

3395 Brain Injury Association of Missouri
2265 Schuetz Road
Saint Louis, MO 63146
314-426-4024
800-444-6443
Fax: 314-426-3290
e-mail: info@biamo.org
www.biamo.org

Founded in 1982, a community based organization serving persons with brain injury, their families, caregivers, physicians, therapists, case managers, and others throught the state of Missouri.

Eric Hart, President
Scott Gee, Executive Director
Scott Gee, Executive Director

Montana

3396 Brain Injury Association of Montana
1280 S 3rd West, Suite 4
Missoula, MT 59801
406-541-6442
800-241-6442
Fax: 406-541-4360
e-mail: biam@biamt.org
www.biamt.org

To create a better future through brain injury prevention, research, education and advocacy.

Kristen Morgan, Program Director
Christien Morgan, Manager
Stacy Rye, Executive Director

New Hampshire

3397 Brain Injury Association of New Hampshire
109 N State Street, Suite 2
Concord, NH 03301
800-773-8400
800-444-8400
Fax: 603-228-6749
e-mail: mail@bianh.org
www.bianh.org

Founded in 1983, a private, non-profit family and consumer run organization representing over 5000 New Hamphire residents with acquired brain disorders and stroke.

Steven D. Wade, Executive Director
Laura Flashman, Ph.D, President
Amy Messer, Vice-President

New Jersey

3398 Brain Injury Association of New Jersey
825 Georges Road, Second Floor
North Brunswick, NJ 08902
732-745-0200
732-745-0211
Fax: 732-738-1132
e-mail: info@bianj.org
www.bianj.org

A nonprofit organization that brings together people with brain injury, their families and friends, and concerned allied health professionals to improve the quality of life people experience after brain injury.

Edward Kim, Chairperson
Anthony G. Cuzzola, Vice-Chairperson
Michael H. Greenwald, Secretary

New Mexico

3399 Brain Injury Association of New Mexico
3232 Candelaria NE
Albuquerque, NM 87107
505-292-7414
888-292-7415
Fax: 505-271-8983
e-mail: info@braininjurynm.com
www.braininjurynm.org

Actively supports progressive public policy for persons with traumatic brain injury on both state and federal levels.

John Tiwald, Board President
Clara Holguin, Executive Director

New York

3400 Brain Injury Association of New York State
10 Colvin Avenue
Albany, NY 12206
518-459-7911
800-228-8201
Fax: 518-482-5285
e-mail: info@bianys.org
www.bianys.org

A statewide non-profit membership organization that advocates on behalf of individuals with brain injury and their families, and promotes prevention. Established in 1982, provides education, advocacy, and community support services that lead to improved outcomes for children and adults with brain injuries and their families.

Debbie Berenda, Manager
Judy Avner, Executive Director
Jutith Sandman, Director Membership/Development

3401 Hy Feinstein Clubhouse
Long Island Head Injury Association
300 Kennedy Drive
Hauppauge, NY 11788
631-543-2245
Fax: 631-543-2261
e-mail: club@lihia.org
www.lihia.org

A non-profit organization whose primary mission is to provide a place for people with head injuries to participate in meaningful work; to have the opportunity to meet and build friendships; and ulimately seek employment within the community.

3402 Mount Sinai Traumatic Brain Injury
Mt Sinai Medical Center
5 E. 98th Street, B-15
New York, NY 10029

212-241-7911
888-241-5152
e-mail: margaret.brown@mssm.edu
www.icahn.mssm.edu

Specializing not only in helping patients regain mastery over their physical environment, but also in addressing the cognitive and emotional aftermaths, including anxiety and depression, which are frequently triggered by such injuries. The program contains different treatment levels to address the very specific needs of this population.

David Vandergoot, President
Wayne A. Gordon, Director
Joshua Cantor, Co-Director

North Carolina

3403 Brain Injury Association of North Carolina
2113 Cameron Street, Bryan Bldg, Suite 242, PO Box
Raleigh, NC 27605

919-833-9634
800-377-1464
Fax: 919-833-5415
e-mail: bianc@bianc.net
www.bianc.net

Founded in 1982 by families and concerned professionals. The Association is an affiliate of the Brain Injury Association of America. Today, the Association has Family and Community Support Centers in Raleigh, Greenville, and Charlotte and 29 local chapters and support groups across the state.

Marylin Lash, President
Pam Gutherie, Vice President
Karen L. McCulloch, Co-Chair Elect

North Dakota

3404 Brain Injury Association of North Dakota
Open Door Center
1225 South 12th Street
Bismarck, ND 58504

701-845-1124
877-525-2724
Fax: 701-845-1175
www.braininjurynd.com

Mary Simonson, President
Richard Ott, Executive Director
Rebecca Quinn

Ohio

3405 Brain Injury Association of Ohio
855 Grandview Avenue, Suite 225
Columbus, OH 43215

614-481-7100
800-444-6443
Fax: 614-481-7103
e-mail: help@biaoh.org
www.biaoh.org

The Brain Injury Association of Ohio aims to improve community services, supports, and awareness for the life-long challenges presented by brain injury and to increase the independence of those coping with its impact. There are five core services designed to achieve this: information & resource coordination; education & training for professionals; support groups for Ohio residents; prevention initiatives; advocacy for policies and funding that address service system gaps.

Stephanie Ramsey, President
Anthon Brooks, Vice President
Julie Robbins, Vice President

Oklahoma

3406 Brain Injury Association of Oklahoma
3015 E Skelly Dr.
Tulsa, OK 74105

918-789-0406
800-765-6809
Fax: 918-712-9019
e-mail: braininjuryoklahoma@gmail.com
www.braininjuryoklahoma.org

Adam Sherman, President
Mary Dobbs, Vice President
Joan Gass, Treasurer

Oregon

3407 Brain Injury Association of Oregon
Po Box 549
Molalla, OR 97038

503-413-7707
800-544-5243
Fax: 503-961-8730
e-mail: biaor@biaoregon.org
www.biaoregon.org

To improve the quality of life of persons with brain injury and their families; and to prevent brain injury.

Ralph Wiser, President
Chuck McGilvrary, Vice President
Carol Altman, Treasurer

3408 Oregon Brain Injury Resource Network
345 N Monmouth Avenue, PO Box 1329
Monmouth, OR 97361

541-346-0593
877-872-7246
Fax: 541-346-0599
e-mail: tbi@wou.edu
www.tr.wou.edu/tbi/

Aims to improve access to information and services for individuals with brain injuries, their families, and the professionals who serve them. The Resource Network houses information on all aspects of brain injury, from the point of initial injury throughout the life span of the individual.

Pennsylvania

3409 Pittsburgh Area Brain Injury Alliance
630 Bascom Avenue
Pittsburgh, PA 15212

412-481-0443
e-mail: jp@pabia.org
www.pabia.org

Dedicated to the people recovering from Brain Injury and who live with the consequences of Traumatic Brain Injury. The purpose is to provide a forum for peer-to-peer support and to assist in the development of peer-to-peer support groups in Western Pennsylvania.

Ed Crinnion, President

Rhode Island

3410 Brain Injury Association of Rhode Island
935 Park Avenue, Suite 8, PO Box 2743
Cranston, RI 02910

401-461-6599
Fax: 401-461-6561
e-mail: braininjuryctr@biaofri.org
www.biausa.org/RI

To improve the quality of life for people with brain injuries and their families, and to develop and support programs that prevent brain injuries.

Sharon Brinkworth, Executive Director
Michael L. Baker, Co-President
Jean E. Cassiere, Secretary

South Carolina

3411 Brain Injury Alliance of South Carolina
Po Box 21523
Columbia, SC 29221
803-731-9823
800-290-6461
Fax: 803-731-0589
e-mail: scbraininjury@bellsouth.net
www.biausa.org/SC/

Mission is to create a better future through brain injury prevention, research, education and advocacy.

Jeremy Hertza, President
Joyce Davis, Executive Director
Lyman Whitehead, Consultant

3412 Brain Injury Association of South Carolina
5605 Bush River Road
Columbia, SC 29212
803-731-9823
877-TBI-FACT
Fax: 803-731-4804
e-mail: scbraininjury@bellsouth.net
www.biausa.org/SC/

To create a better future through brain injury prevention, education, and advocacy.

Jeremy Hertza, President
Joyce Davis, Executive Director
Lyman Whitehead, Consultant

Tennessee

3413 Brain Injury Association of Tennessee
955 Woodland St
Nashville, TN 37206
615-248-2541
800-444-6443
Fax: 615-383-1176
e-mail: biaoftn@yahoo.com
www.braininjurytn.com

The mission is to improve the quality of life for persons with brain injuries and their families and to reduce the incidence of brain injury.

Guynn Edwards, President
Pam Bryan, Executive Director
Brian Webb, Treasurer

Texas

3414 Brain Injury Association of Texas
316 W 12th Street, Suite 405
Austin, TX 78701
512-326-1212
800-392-0040
Fax: 512-478-3370
e-mail: info@biatx.org
www.texasbia.org

A non-profit public service organization, strives to meet the urgent need to develop programs for public awareness and education, to support research and rehabilitation and to provide family guidance.

San Marcos, President
Amy Santus, Vice President
Erin Garrison, Admin Director

Utah

3415 Brain Injury Association of Utah
5280 Commerce Dr., Suite E-190
Murray, UT 84107
801-716-4993
800-281-8442
Fax: 801-716-4995
e-mail: info@biau.org
www.biau.org

Created in 1984, the only non-profit organization dedicated exclusively to education and support for the issues of prevention and recovery of brain injury in the state of Utah. The mission of the Brain Injury Association of Utah is to create a better future through brain injury prevention, research, education and advocacy.

Antonietta Anna Rosso, President
Pauline Fontaine, Treasurer
Ron S. Roskos, Executive Director

Vermont

3416 Brain Injury Association of Vermont
92 South Main Street, PO Box 482
Waterbury, VT 05676
802-244-6850
877-856-1772
Fax: 802-244-4005
e-mail: support1@biavt.org
www.biavt.org

To create a better future through brain injury, prevention, research, education, and advocacy.

Trevor Squirrell, Executive Director
Barb Winters, Program Manager
Christy Opuszynski, Office Administrator

Virginia

3417 Brain Injury Association of Virginia
1506 Willow Lawn Dr., Suite 212
Richmond, VA 23230
804-355-5748
800-444-6443
Fax: 804-355-6381
e-mail: infoa@biav.net
www.biav.net

Nonprofit organization Creating a better future through brain injury education, awareness, advocacy, and support.

Irv Cantor, President
Anne McDonnell, Executive Director
Theresa Alonso, Data Coordinator

Washington

3418 Brain Injury Association of Washington
PO Box 3044
Seattle, WA 98114
206-388-0900
877-982-4292
Fax: 206-388-0901
e-mail: admin@braininjurywa.org
www.braininjurywa.org

The mission, which begins with prevention, is to provide support to survivors of brain injury and their families, education to those who are being effected by brain injury, including the general public, and advocacy, to give the many suffering from this silent epidemic a public voice.

Mark T. Long, President
David A. Butters, Chair
Patrice Roney, Co-Chair Elect

3419 Head Injury Hotline
Brain Injury Resource Center
PO Box 84151
Seattle, WA 98124
206-621-8558
Fax: 206-624-4961
e-mail: brain@headinjury.com
www.headinjury.com

Disseminates head injury information and provides referrals to facilitate adjustment to life following head injury. Organizes seminars for professionals, head injury survivors, and their families. Our intention is to help you avoid much of the greif and loss of brain injury, and perhaps to inspire you to get involved.

Constance Miller, Founder

West Virginia

3420 Brain Injury Association of West Virginia
PO Box 574
Institute, WV 25112   304-400-4506
                                       800-356-6443
                                    Fax: 304-205-7915
                                 e-mail: biawv@aol.com
                                 www.biawestvirginia.org

A nonprofit agency dedicated to providing support, advocacy, education and training on behalf of survivors of brain injuries, their families and those who provide services or care for them.

Michael W Davis, President
Sharon McKenny Lord
Jennifer Rhule Stockton

Wisconsin

3421 Brain Injury Association of Wisconsin
N63 W23583 Main Street, Suite A
Sussex, WI 53089   262-790-9660
                                       800-882-9282
                                    Fax: 262-790-9670
                                 e-mail: lschultz@biaw.org
                                       www.biaw.org

Established in 1980 by a group of individuals with brain injury, their families, friends, and professionals. BIAW is a chartered member affiliate of the national Brain Injury Association, Inc. BIAW provides services in these 5 core areas: information and resources, education, prevention, advocacy, and support services

Audrey Nelson, President
Lori Schultz, Executive Director
Patricia David, Operations Director

Wyoming

3422 Brain Injury Association of Wyoming
111 W 2nd Street, Suite 106
Casper, WY 82601   307-473-1767
                                       800-643-6457
                                    Fax: 307-237-5222
                                 e-mail: director@wybia.org
                                       www.wybia.org

The mission is to create a better future through brain injury prevention, research, education, and advocacy.

Dorothy Cronin, Executive Director
Dorothy Cronin, Executive Director

Libraries & Resource Centers

3423 Brain Injury Association of Michigan
7305 Grand River, Suite 100
Brighton, MI 48114   810-229-5880
                                       800-772-4323
                                    Fax: 810-229-8947
                                 e-mail: info@biami.org
                                       www.biami.org

The mission of BIAMI is to enhance the lives of those affected by brain injury through education, advocacy, research, and local support groups; and to reduce the incidence of brain injury through prevention.

Michael F Dabbs, President
Cheryl A Burda, VP of Operations & Programs

3424 University of Illinois at Chicago, Craniofacial Center
College of Medicine
808 S Wood Street
Chicago, IL 60612   312-996-7870
                                    Fax: 312-413-1526
                                    www.medicine.uic.edu

Richard M Novak, Director

Research Centers

California

3425 Brain Imaging Center at the University of California, Irvine
University of California, Irvine
Irvine, CA 92697   949-824-7872
                                    Fax: 949-824-7873
                                 e-mail: bic@msx.hsis.uci.edu
                                       www.bic.uci.edu

Performs clinical assessment of regional brainmetabolism for Parkinson's disease, epilepsy, brain tumor evaluation, Alzheimer'sdisease, and head injury. Other neuropsychiatric illnesses that are assessed with PETscans at UCI include stroke, psychotic disorders, and movement disorders.

Steven L Small, Director
David B. Keator, Technical Director
Jill Upton, Research Coordinator

3426 Brain Research Institute
Brain Research Institute UCLA
1506 Gonda, PO Box 951761
Los Angeles, CA 90095   310-825-5061
                                    Fax: 310-206-5855
                                 e-mail: lmaninger@mednet.ucla.edu
                                       www.bri.ucla.edu

An organization research unit within the School of Medicine at the University of California , Los Angeles.

Christopher J. Evans, Director
J David Jentsch, Associate Director for Research
Michael S Levine, PhD, Associate Director for Education

3427 Brain and Spinal Injury Center (BASIC) Research at University of California
UCSF Department of Neurological
505 Parnassus Avenue, Room 779 M, PO Box 0112
San Francisco, CA 94143   415-353-7500
                                    Fax: 415-353-2889
                                 www.neurosurgery.medschool.ucsf.edu

Established to promote collaborative basic, translational, and clinical studies on injuries to the brain and spinal cord. BASIC is a joint effort between the Departments of Neurological Surgery and Neurology. Both departments bring their particular areas of expertise to a multidisciplinary effort centered on translational research.

Mitchel S. Berger, Managing Director
Manish Aghi, Managing Director
Christopher P. Ames, Managing Director

Louisiana

3428 Tulane University, US-Japan Biomedical Research Laboratories
Herbert Research Center
6823 St. Charles Avenue
New Orleans, LA 70118   504-862-8000
                                    Fax: 504-394-7169
                                 e-mail: pr@tulane.edu
                                       www.tulane.edu

Focuses research efforts on neuroendocrinology and neurosciences.

Yvette M. Jones, Vice President
Michael A. Bernstein, Provost/Vice President
Benjamin P. Sachs, Senior Vice President/Dean

389

Massachusetts

3429 Harold Goodglass Aphasia Research Center
150 S Huntington Avenue (12A), PO Box 4817
Boston, MA 02130
617-232-9500
857-364-4774
Fax: 617-739-8926
e-mail: aphasia@bu.edu
www.bu.edu/aphasia

Research done into cognitive and language impairment following brain damage and closely related topics.

Harold Goodglass, MD, Director
Martin L. Albert, Managing Director
Lena Maskowich, Managing Director

Michigan

3430 Bioengineering Center of Wayne State University
Wayne State University
818 W Hancock
Detroit, MI 48201
313-577-1345
Fax: 313-577-8333
e-mail: bmeinfo@eng.wayne.edu
www.engineering.wayne.edu

A leading laboratory doing research work in the areas of impact trauma, low back pain and orthopedic biomechanics. Current projects in impact trauma include research on side impact, rear end collisions, head injury and lower extremity injuries.

Albert I King, Director
Farshad Fotouhi, Dean of Engineering
Michael A. Anderson, Research Support Officer

3431 Rehabilitation Institute of Michigan
Detroit Medical Center/Wayne State University
261 Mack Avenue
Detroit, MI 48201
313-745-1203
Fax: 313-745-9863
www.rimrehab.org

Our dedicated group of board certified physicians are committed to improving the lives of their patients by providing quality, compassionate medical care and contributing to the science of rehabilitation medicine.

Mildred Matlock, Ceo
William H. Restum, PhD, President

New York

3432 Brady Institute for Traumatic Brain Injury
Jamaica Hospital Medical Center
8900 Van Wyck Expressway
Jamaica, NY 11418
718-206-6000
e-mail: hr@jhmc.org
www.jamaicahospital.org

Provides general medical, pediatric,and psychiatric emergency services, ambulatory care, on and off campus ambulatory surgery, a broad spectrum of diagnostic and treatment services, and home health services.

3433 Dana Alliance for Brain Initiatives
505 5th Avenue, 6th Floor
New York, NY 10017
212-223-4040
Fax: 212-317-8721
e-mail: dabiinfo@dana.org
www.dana.org

A nonprofit organization of more than 250 pre-eminent scientists dedicated to advancing education about the progress and promise of brain research.

Edward F Rover, President
Barbara E. Gill, Vice President
Burton M. Mirsky, Vice President-Finance

3434 Rehabilitation Research and Training Center on Traumatic Brain Injury
Mt. Sinai School of Medicine, Dept. Rehabilitation
155 Washington Ave, Suite 410, PO Box 2332
New York, NY 12210
518-449-2976
Fax: 518-426-4329
TDD: 518-449-2993
e-mail: wayne.gordon@mssm.edu
www.rrti.org

Research to improve mood in people with TBI; analyze the content and quality of recently published post-TBI intervention studies; development of new measures of rehabilitation outcomes that incorporates both objective and subjective perspectives on participation in home and community activities; and a capacity building program to better educate professionals in identifying, assessing and providing appropriate interventions, treatments and accommodations for people with TBI.

Jacqueline A. Negri, Interim CEO
Stacie Muscolino-Benfer, Directors of Event & Administration
Lisa Zimmermann, HRSA Program Assisstant

3435 Stroke Rehabilitation & Traumatic Brain Injury Research
Ruft Institute at NYU Medical Center
400 E 34th Street
New York, NY 10016
212-263-6519
Fax: 212-263-8510
e-mail: yehuda.ben-yishay@med.nyu.edu
www.med.nyu.edu/rusk/research

Ways of improving problem-solving behavior in individual with acquired brain damage are being investigated and instruments measuring problem solving in interpersonal situations are being developed.

Joan T Gold, Medical Director

Ohio

3436 Ohio State University Laboratory of Psychobiology
225 Psychology Bldg., 1835 Neil Avenue
Columbus, OH 43210
614-292-8185
Fax: 614-292-4537
www.psy.ohio-state.edu

Studies done on recovery of function after brain damage.

Karissa Basey, Fiscal/HR Associate
Stephanie Fowler, CCBBI Business Manager
Blanche Hollingshead, Fiscal/HR Associate

Pennsylvania

3437 Institutes for Achievement of Human Potential
8801 Stenton Avenue
Wyndmoor, PA 19038
215-233-2050
800-344-8322
Fax: 215-233-9312
e-mail: institutes@iahp.org
www.iahp.org

A teaching institute that focuses on home-based neurological training for brain-injured children. Commited to the significant increases of the ability of all children to perform in the physical, intellectual and social realms. Our work has led to powerful insights about the brain and, especially, about its development in the neonate and very young children. We have developed exciting concepts and practices applied by parents at home, to mulitply the intelligence of tiny children.

500 members

Janet Doman, President
Glenn Doman, Founder
Dr. Ralph Pelligra, Chairman

3438 Thomas Jefferson University Brain Injury Rehabilitation Program
Thomas Jefferson University Hospital
111 South 11th Street
Philadelphia, PA 19107
215-955-6000
www.jeffersonhealth.org

Provides coordinated, multidisciplinary acute medical and surgical care for all levels of brain injury. The program delivers care for the acute phases of injury at Jefferson and shifts follow-up care to Magee Rehabilitation Hospital.

Thomas J Lewis, Ceo

Tennessee

3439 University of Memphis Neuropsychology Lab
Department of Psychology
202 Psychology Building, Room 126
Memphis, TN 38152
901-678-2000
Fax: 901-678-2579
www.memphis.edu

Evaluation and development of assessment and treatment procedures for neurologically impaired persons.

Shirley C. Raines, President
Rosie Phillips Bingham, Vice President for Student Affairs
Linda Bonnin, Vice President for Communications,

Texas

3440 Brain Injury Research Center of the Institute for Rehabilitation & Research
1333 Moursund Avenue
Houston, TX 77030
713-799-5000
e-mail: tirrreferrals@tirr.tmc.edu
www.tirr.memorialhermann.org

Brings together world-renowned researchers to study the many complicated facets of recovery from brain injury. BIRC has been able to leverage resources from the US Department of Education's National Institute for Rehabilitation and Research (NIDRR) and from NIH to conduct its research in a manner that facilitates the greatest progress in identifying effective treatments.

Carl Josehart, CEO
Gerard E. Francisco, MD/Chief Medical Officer
Mary Ann Euliarte, CNO/COO

Virginia

3441 Virginia Commonwealth University Department of Neurosurgery Research
417 North 11th Street, 6th Floor, PO Box 980631
Richmond, VA 23298
804-828-9165
Fax: 804-828-0374
www.neurosurgery.vcu.edu

Studies include work on cerebral blood flow, subarachnoid hemorrhage, vasospasm, ischemia, metabolism, cerebral edema, elevated intracranial pressure, trauma, secondary neural insults, CNS tumor biology, clinical trials for new brain tumor therapies, spinal biomechanics, computer imaging on the CNS and immunology of the nervous system.

Stuart P Adler, Research Director
Paul Dent, Vice Chair/Professor
Andrey Budanov, Asst. Professor

Conferences

3442 ANA Symposium
Acoustic Neuroma Association
600 Peachtree Parkway, Suite 108
Cumming, GA 30041
770-205-8211
877-200-8211
Fax: 770-205-0239
e-mail: info@anausa.org
www.anausa.org

For pre-and post-treatment acoustic neuroma patients, family members, friends and health care professionals for a weekend of educational lectures, workshops and panel discussions-all with leading acoustic neuroma medical professionals.

June
Jeffrey D Barr, President
Alan Goldberg, Vice President
Scott Van Ells, Secretary

Audio Video

3443 Face First
Fanlight Productions
32 Court Street, 21st Floor
Brooklyn, NY 11201
718-488-8900
800-876-1710
Fax: 718-488-8642
e-mail: info@fanlight.com, orders@fanlight.com
www.fanlight.com

Profiles of several people born with facial deformities; they chronicle both physical pain and the pain of rejection, as well as the strengths that have enabled them to achieve successful adult lives. ISBN: DVD: 1-57295-886-3; VHS: 1-572952-59-8

29 minutes DVD or VHS

Nicole Johnson, Publicity Coordinator

3444 Surviving Coma: the Journey Back
Brain Injury Association of Mississippi
2727 Old Canton Road
Jackson, MS 39296
601-981-1021
Fax: 601-981-1039
e-mail: biaofms@aol.com

A realistic presentation about coma survival and the problems encountered during the long journey through rehabilitation.

19 Minutes

Paul Gospodarski, Ed.D, Executive Director

Web Sites

3445 Brain Injury Association
1608 Spring Hill Rd. Suite 110
Vienna, VA 22182
703-761-0750
800-444-6443
Fax: 703-761-0755
www.biausa.org

Founded in 1980, the leading national organization serving and representing individuals, families and professionals who are touched by a life-altering, often devastating, traumatic brain injury (TBI).

Daniel S. Chamberlain, Esq, Chair
Brant A. Elkind, MS, CBIST, Vice Chair
Susan H. Connors, President & CEO

3446 Brain Research Institute (BRI) School of Medicine University of California LA
PO Box 951761
Los Angeles, CA 90095
310-825-5061
Fax: 310-206-5855
e-mail: bri@mednet.ucla.edu
www.bri.ucla.edu

BRI's mission is to increase understanding of how the brain works, how it dvelops, and how it responds to experience, injury and disease, and to help make UCLA the preeminent center for translating basic knowledge into medical interventions and new technologies.

Dr. Christopher Evans, Director
Rafael Romero, Asst Director for Outreach
Baljit Khakh, Assoc. Dir. For Research

3447 Centre for Neuro Skills
5215 Ashe Rd.
Bakersfield, CA 93313
661-872-3408
800-922-4994
Fax: 661-872-5150
e-mail: cns@neuroskills.com, spersel@neuroskills.com
www.neuroskills.com

391

The TBI Resource Guide is the internet's central source of information, services, and products relating to traumatic brain injury, brain injury recovery, and post-acute rehabilitation.

Mark J. Ashley, ScD, CCM, President & CEO/ Co Founder

3448 Dana Alliance for Brain Initiatives
505 Fifth Ave., 6th Floor
New York, NY 10017
212-223-4040
Fax: 212-317-8721
www.dana.org/brainweb

Is a nonprofit organization of more then 200 neuroscientists, formed to help provide information about the personal and public benefits of brain research. Today one out of five Americans suffers from a brain-related disease or disorder, ranging from cocain addiction to learning diabilities from Alzheimer's disease to spinal cord injuries.

Edward F. Rover, Chair & President
Burton M. Mirsky, EVP, Finance
Barbara E. Gill, EVP, Public Affairs, Executive Dir.

3449 NIH/National Institute of Neurological Dis orders and Stroke (NINDS)
PO Box 5801
Bethesda, MD 20824
301-496-5751
800-352-9424
www.ninds.nih.gov

The mission of NINDS is to reduce the burden of neurological disease, a burden borne by every age group, by every segment of society, by people all over the world.

Walter J. Koroshetz, MD, Acting Director
Alan L. Willard, PhD, Acting Deputy Director
Caroline Lewis, Executive Officer

3450 Northeast Rehabilitation Health Network
70 Butler Street
Salem, NH 3079
603-893-2900
800-439-0183
TTY: 800-439-2370
e-mail: webmaster@northeastrehab.com
www.northeastrehab.com

We provide services within a continuum of care to individuals and families whos lives have been impcated by illness or injury in order to restore stability and maximize their potential for independence, functional abilites, and quality of life. In addition, we provide services that encourage well being. Our customers include: patients, families, physicians, referrers, payers, employees and the community.

John Prochilo, CEO & Administrator

3451 Perspectives Network
www.tbi.org

It's primary focus is positive communications between persons with brain injury, family members, caregivers, friends of persons with brain injury, those many professionals who treat persons with brain injury and community members in order to create positive changes and enhance public awareness and knowledge of acquired, traumatic brain injury.

3452 Traumatic Brain Injury Model Systems Natio nal Data and Statistical Center
www.tbindc.org

e-mail: tbindc@kmrrec.org
www.tbindc.org

The TBIMS program seeks to improve the lives of persons who experience traumatic brain injury, their families and their communities by creating and disseminating new knowledge about the course, treatment and outcomes relating to their condtion.

Book Publishers

3453 Children with Traumatic Brain Injury
Peytral Publications
PO Box 1162
Minnetonka, MN 55345
952-949-8707
877-739-8725
Fax: 952-949-8707
www.peytral.com

Comprehensive, must-have reference that provides parent with the support and information needed to help their child recover from a closed-head injury. Written by a team of medical specialists, therapists, educators and an attorney this publications covers medical concerns, rehabilitation, treatment, adjustment, effects on learning, thinking, language behavior and more.

482 pages

Lisa Schoenbrodt, EdD, Editor

3454 Cognitive Effects of Early Brain Injury
John's Hopkins University Press
2715 N Charles Street
Baltimore, MD 21218
410-516-6900
800-537-5487
Fax: 410-516-6968
e-mail: webmaster@jhupress.jhu.edu
www.press.jhu.edu

This book offers a detailed overview of the effects of genetic, prenatal, and perinatal brain disorders on cognitive development and learning in children. Summarizing the available data as well as presenting previously unpublished research, the book provides clinicians with practical information that will aid their diagnostic and therapeutic work with children who have sustained early brain injury.

1994 336 pages Hardcover
ISBN: 0-801848-56-3

Kathleen Keane, Director
Erik A Smist, Director
Timothy D Fuller, Chief Information Officer

3455 Cognitive Rehabilitation for Persons with Traumatic Brain Injury
Paul H Brookes Publishing/Brookes
PO Box 10624
Baltimore, MD 21285
410-337-9580
800-638-3775
Fax: 410-337-8539
e-mail: custserv@brookespublishing.com
www.brookespublishing.com

Virtually all persons with brain injury retain ability to learn. Cognitive rehab is a set of stategies to improve problems. Reports on theory, practices, research, consequences of brain trauma and assessment & intervention. Case studies.

1991 299 pages Hardcover
ISBN: 1-557660-71-9

Jeffrey S Kreutzer, Editor
Paul H Wehman, Editor

3456 From the Ashes
Brain Injury Resource Center
PO Box 84151
Seattle, WA 98124
206-621-8558
e-mail: brain@headinjury.com
www.headinjury.com/ashesord.htm

An enduring resource for survivors, families and the professionals serving them.

1987 108 pages
ISBN: 0-963659-40-5

Constance Miller, Editor
Kay Campbell, Editor

3457 **Handbook of Head Truma: Acute Care to Recovery**
Springer Publishing Company
11 W 42nd Street, 15th Floor
New York, NY 10036 877-687-7476
Fax: 212-941-7842
e-mail: contactus@springerpub.com
www.springerpub.com

Providing a thorough collection of information regarding clinical aspects of head injury from acute care to recovery, this treatise interrelates a variety of neural specialties and broadens the rehabilitation process to include the family

1992 472 pages
ISBN: 0-306439-47-6

Charles Long, Editor
Leslie Ross, Editor

3458 **Head Injury in Children and Adolescents: A Resource and Review for School**
John Wiley & Sons
10475 Crosspoint Boulevard
Indianapolis, IN 46256 877-762-2974
Fax: 800-597-3299
e-mail: consumers@wiley.com
www.wiley.com

Complex nature of traumatic brain injury and its implications are examined carefully from medical, neuropsychological, rehabilitative and educational perspectives. Contents are arranged in a spiraling manner to provide the reader with a progressive and practical appreciation of traumatic brain injury and its neurobehavioral effects.

260 pages Hardcover
ISBN: 0-884220-98-2

Vivian Begali, Editor

3459 **Head Trauma Sourcebook**
Omnigraphics
PO Box 8002
Aston, PA 19014 800-234-1340
Fax: 800-875-1340
e-mail: info@omnigraphics.com
omnigraphics.com

Basic consumer information for the layperson about open-head and closed-head injuries, treatment advances, recovery and rehabilitation.

414 pages
ISBN: 0-780802-08-X

Karen Bellenir, Editor

3460 **Let's Talk About Going to the Hospital**
Rosen Publishing Group's PowerKids Press
29 E 21st Street
New York, NY 10010 212-777-3017
800-237-9932
Fax: 888-436-4643
e-mail: rosenpub@tribeca.ios.com
www.powerkidspress.com

If a child has to check into the hospital, chances are he or she is already upset about being ill. Knowing how a hospital functions and what the procedures are, such as when family members can visit, will help in what is already a stressful situation. Grades K-5.

24 pages
ISBN: 0-823950-36-0

3461 **What To Do About Your Brain Injured Child**
National Book Network
8801 Stenton Avenue
Wyndmoor, PA 19038 215-233-2050
800-344-8322
Fax: 215-233-3940
e-mail: institutes@iahp.org
www.iahp.org

The author reveals life saving techniques to measure mobility, language, and manual, visual, auditory and tactile development.

318 pages
ISBN: 1-591170-23-0

Glen Doman, Editor

Magazines

3462 **Brain Injury Source**
Brain Injury Association of America
1608 Spring Hill Road, Suite 110
Vienna, VA 22182 703-761-0750
Fax: 703-761-0755
e-mail: Publications@biausa.org
www.biausa.org

Written for and by professionals in the field. Blends professionally written articles on information and research in brain injury with a user friendly format that incorporates graphics and charts to effectively deliver the messages. Full color.

50+ pages Quarterly

Susan H Connors, President/CEO
Pat Britz, Information Director
Marianna Abashian, Director of Professional Services

Journals

3463 **Journal of Head Trauma Rehabilitation**
Aspen Publishers
7201 McKinney Circle
Frederick, MD 21704 301-698-7100
800-234-1660
Fax: 800-901-9075
e-mail: customer.service@wolterskluwer.com
www.wklawbusiness.com

A leading, peer-reviewed resource that provides up-to-date information on the clinical management and rehabilitation of persons with traumatic brain injuries. The journal is comprised of feature articles, brief reports, pharmacological updates, legislative and public policy updates, columns on ethics, book reviews, abstracts of selected literature, and more.

Mitchell Rosenthal, MD, Editor

Newsletters

3464 **American Brain Tumor Association Message Line**
8550 W. Bryn Mawr Ave, Ste 550
Chicago, IL 60631 773-577-8750
800-886-2282
Fax: 773-577-8738
e-mail: info@abta.org
www.abta.org

Offers association news, events, fundraising and convention news, as well as medical and legislative updates for patients and their families.

Quarterly

Jeff Fougerousse, Chair
Barbara Dunn, Vice Chair
Brian Olson, Treasurer

3465 **Headlines**
Brain Injury Association of Minnesota
2277 Highway 36 West, Suite 200
Roseville, MN 55113 612-378-2742
800-669-6442
Fax: 612-378-2789
e-mail: info@braininjurymn.org
www.braininjurymn.org

Published for the families and professionals who are involved with brain injuries. We also have an e-mail newsletter that reaches several hundred.

Quarterly

Ardis Sandstrom, Executive Director
Brad Donaldson, Associate Director of Operations
Richard Bloom, Board Treasurer

3466 Headway
Brain Injury Association of Virginia
1506 Willow Lawn Dr., Suite 212
Richmond, VA 23230
804-355-5748
800-444-6443
Fax: 804-355-6381
e-mail: biav@visi.net
www.biav.net

Information and resources for individuals with brain injury, their family members and professionals dealing with brain injury.

16 pages Quarterly

Michelle Ward, Editor
Stephen Smith, President
Steve Hicks, Director of Development

3467 TBI Challenge
Brain Injury Association of America
1608 Spring Hill Road, Suite 110
Vienna, VA 22182
703-761-0750
Fax: 703-761-0755
e-mail: familyhelpline@biausa.org
www.biausa.org

Exclusively for and about persons with brain injury. Provides information to individuals with brain injury and their families. Professionals will benefit from the perspectives provided in Kid's Corner, Relatively Speaking, Ask the Lawyer, Information and Resources and Ask the Doctor.

Quarterly

Susan H Connors, President/CEO
Pat Britz, Information Director
Marianna Abashian, Director of Professional Services

3468 The Headliner
Brain Injury Association of Oregon
2145 NW Overton Street
Portland, OR 97210
503-413-7707
800-544-5243
Fax: 503-413-6849
e-mail: biaor@biaoregon.org
www.biaoregon.org

To improve the quality of life of persons with brain injury and their families; and to prevent brain injury.

16 pages Quarterly

Craig Nichols, JD, President
Chuck McGilvrary, Vice President
Sherry Stock, Executive Director

Pamphlets

3469 Brain Injury Glossary
HDI Publishers
2407 Waugh Drive, PO Box 131401
Houston, TX 77219
713-526-6900
800-321-7037
Fax: 713-526-7787
e-mail: sales@braininjurybooks.com
www.braininjurybooks.com

Contains special sections on terms relating to insurance, definitions relating to The Americans with Disabilities Act and descriptions of commonly prescribed medications. The Brain Injury Glossary is a must for all persons working or involved in brain injury rehabilitation.

1993 46 pages

L Don Lehmkuhl, Editor

3470 Brain Injury Update
HDI Publishers
2407 Waugh Drive, PO Box 131401
Houston, TX 77219
713-526-6900
800-321-7037
Fax: 713-526-7787
e-mail: sales@braininjurybooks.com
www.braininjurybooks.com

Monthly digest of news and information from the brain injury research and rehabilitation fields. Expanded summaries of journal articles, research papers, news releases and government reports are provided in a concise, time saving format. Brain Injury Update also provides information on grant opportunities, pharmacological intervention, calls for papers, people in the news, listings of upcoming conferences and symposia, legal and legislative developments and advances in prevention.

1991 Annual

Dr. Linda Thoi, Editor-in-Chief
Nathan D Zasler, MD, Contributing Editor

Camps

3471 Camp Barefoot
Brain Injury Association of Michigan
7305 Grand River, Suite 100
Brighton, MI 48114
810-229-5880
800-772-4323
Fax: 810-229-8947
e-mail: info@biami.org
www.biami.org

Primary goal of our recreational programming is to give people who have experienced a brain injury a normal camping experience. Dedicated to providing quality summer camping experiences for people who sustained a brain injury. Over six days, Camp Barefoot provides structured, enriching personal and recreational experiences for people with brain injury.

Michael F Dabbs, President
Thomas J. Constand, VP, Development and Marketing
Char Luttrell, Office Manager

3472 Camp Hickory Wood
Traumatic Brain Injury Program
425 5th Avenue N, Cordell Hull Building
Nashville, TN 37243
800-882-0611
health.state.tn.us/TBI/index.htm

Each year the TBI Program in collaboration with Easter Seals Tennessee Inc. sponsors a weekend and a weeklong camp for adult and youth survivors of brain injury. These camps focus on providing a unique social and recreational opportunity to persons with brain injury. Nestled between the banks of Old Hickory Lake and surrounded by protective woods, camp offers great outdoor fun.

3473 Crotched Mountain School & Rehabilitation Center
1 Verney Drive
Greenfield, NH 3047
603-547-3311
800-800-966
Fax: 603-547-3232
e-mail: info@crotchedmountain.org
www.cmf.org

Currently serves children ages 6-22 with multiple-handicaps including: Cerebral Palsy, Spina Bifida, visual and hearing impairments and neurological disabilities, developmental disorders, mental retardation, autism, behavioral and emotional disorders, seizure disorders, spinal cord and head injuries. Member of the National Association of Independent Schools and accredited with the NE Association of Schools and Colleges, Independent Schools of Northern NE.

Kathleen C. Brittan, Vice President of Development
William Cossaboon, MS, Director of Education
W. Carl Cooley, MD, Chief Medical Officer

3474 Oklahoma Brain Injury Camp
Oklahoma Brain Injury Association
3015 E. Skelly Dr.
Tulsa, OK 74105
405-928-1647
Fax: 918-712-9019
e-mail: braininjuryoklahoma@gmail.com
www.braininjuryoklahoma.org

An annual camp for brain injury survivors sponsored by the Brain Injury Association of Oklahoma. Great fun had by all with music, games, crafts, a hayride, cookout, bingo, fishing, and paddle boat rides.

Cathe Fox, Camp Director
Adam Sherman, Ph.D, President
Mary Dobbs, BSN, RN, CRRN, Vice President

Description

3475   HEARING IMPAIRMENT/DEAFNESS

Covers these related disorders: Conductive deafness or hearing loss, Mixed hearing loss, Sensorineural deafness or hearing loss, Noise Induced Hearing Loss

Involves the following Biologic System(s):
Neurologic Disorders

Hearing impairment may be defined as a loss of the ability to hear that is sufficient enough to impede the ability to communicate. Deafness refers to severe or profound hearing loss. Hearing loss or deafness may occur as the result of hereditary factors or birth defects. Hearing loss may also be acquired and occur after birth (e.g., from disease or physical damage to the hearing mechanism). However, genetic factors are thought to be responsible for moderate to severe hearing loss in about half of affected children. Hearing loss may be further categorized into three types: conductive, sensorineural, or mixed.

Conductive hearing loss occurs as a result of the faulty transmission of sound through the external or middle ear to the inner ear. This transmission problem may be due to infections of the middle ear (otitis media), damage to the eardrum or bones of the middle ear, the absence or the narrowing of the ear canal, impacted earwax (cerumen), foreign bodies in the ear canal, or other physical causes. In addition, conductive hearing loss is sometimes inherited as a feature of certain syndromes such as Klippel-Feil syndrome, Crouzon syndrome, osteogenesis imperfecta, and others. In children with sensorineural hearing loss, sounds are conducted to the inner ear through the external and middle ear, but are not transmitted from there to the brain. This occurs as the result of a defect in the structure of the inner ear or problems with the nerve that conveys impulses from the inner ear to the brain (auditory nerve; acoustic nerve; eighth cranial nerve). Sensorineural hearing loss that results from defects of inner ear structures is considered sensory and includes: the absence or underdevelopment of the snail shell-type tubular structure of the inner ear (cochlea); damage to hair cells or other inner ear structures from prolonged exposure to loud noise, certain drugs; viral infections or other diseases; and other irregularities.

Noise Induced Hearing Loss (NIHL) results from exposure to harmful noise levels that trigger the formation of molecules inside the ear that damage hair cells. The hair cells are small sensory cells that convert sound energy into electrical signals that travel to the brain. Damaged hair cells cannot grow back. These destructive molecules play an important role in hearing loss in children and adults who are exposed to loud noise for extended periods. Individuals of all ages, including children, can develop NIHL.

Sensorineural hearing loss that results from damage to the auditory nerve pathway is considered neural and may be due to brain lesions or tumors; childhood disorders such as German measles, mumps, inner ear infections, etc.; certain hereditary disorders (e.g., Waardenburg syndrome, Usher syndrome, etc.); diseases that affect the myelin sheath, which is the fatty, protective, insulating covering on certain nerve fibers (demyelinating diseases); or seizures. Mixed hearing loss refers to a combination of both conductive and sensorineural hearing loss.

Early screening for hearing loss is important in order to provide early intervention that will allow the best outcome for educational and social development. Treatment may require the cooperation of parents, caregivers, pediatricians, speech and language pathologists, and specialists in hearing loss (audiologists) who assess the extent of hearing loss through the use of specialized tests. Infant screening by specialists may include tests that gauge behavioral responses to noise through observation, such as a startle response to a sudden hand clap. Other tests may electronically assess hearing loss (audiometry); measure the head-turning response of an infant or toddler using animated aids in conjunction with sounds emitted through a loudspeaker (visual reinforcement audiometry or VRA); measure the lowest intensity at which certain words are heard or understood (speech recognition threshold or SRT); measure the ability of the middle ear to impede or resist sound energy (tympanometry); differentiate between sensory and neural hearing loss (auditory brain stem response); measure the integrity of the cochlea (otoacoustic emissions or OAEs).

According to the National Institute on Deafness and Other Communication Disorders, males are more likely to experience hearing loss than females. Two to three of every 1,000 children who are born deaf have hearing parents.

Treatment for conductive hearing loss may include theremoval of fluid, earwax, or foreign bodies through drainage or other means. Surgical intervention may be indicated for the correction of structural abnormalities. Children as well as infants with hearing loss may benefit from the use of certain types of hearing aids; however, repeat testing is necessary to provide more exact hearing aid specification.

In the United States, roughly 41,500 adults and 25,500 children receive cochlear implants per year. Hearing loss affects only one ear in nine out of 10 people who experience sudden deafness. Approximately 26 million Americans have Noise Induced Hearing Loss (NIHL). Recreational activities that can put someone at risk for NIHL include target shooting and hunting, snowmobile riding, woodworking and other hobbies, playing in a band, and attending rock concerts. Harmful noises at home may come from lawnmowers, leaf blowers, and shop tools.

In addition, cochlear implants are available to children with severe or profound hearing loss. Other treatment is directed toward the teaching of communication skills such as lip-reading, sign language, and speech. Cooperation and support of family, medical specialists, and educators is important in determining the best approach for the education and social development of the individual child.

Government Agencies

3476   National Institute on Deafness and Other C ommunication Disorders
31 Center Dr, MSC 2320
Bethesda, MD 20892

800-241-1055
Fax: 301-770-8977
TTY: 800-241-1055
e-mail: nidcdinfo@nidcd.nih.gov
www.nidcd.nih.gov

The NIDCD conducts and supports research in the normal and disordered processes of hearing, balance, tast, smell, voice, speech, and language.

3477 Office of Special Education and Rehabilita tion Services
550 12th St, SW - Rm 5133
Washington, DC 20004

202-245-7307
Fax: 202-245-7636
TTY: 202-205-5637
e-mail: carolyn.corlett@ed.gov
www.ed.gov/about/offices/list/osers/index.html

A service of the U.S. Department of Education, responds to people with disabilities and others who request information by conducting research and providing documents related to federal funding available for disability-related programs.

National Associations & Support Groups

3478 Academy of Rehabilitative Audiology
PO Box 2323
Albany, NY 12220

952-920-0484
Fax: 952-920-6098
e-mail: ara@audrehab.org
www.audrehab.org

The primary purpose of ARA is to promote excellence in hearing care through the provision of comprehensive rehabilitative and habilitative services.

350 Members

Kathleen Cienkowski, President
Linda Thibodeau, President-Elect
Kristin Vasil-Dilaj, Secretary

3479 Acoustical Society of America
2 Huntington Quadrangele - Ste 1N01
Melville, NY 11747

516-576-2360
Fax: 516-576-2377
e-mail: asa@aip.org
www.acousticalsociety.org

The ASA specializes in acoustics. They are dedicated to diffusing and increasing the knowledge of acoustics and its practical application.

3480 Alexander Graham Bell Association for the Deaf and Hearing Impaired
Alexander Graham Bell Association for the Deaf
3417 Volta Place NW
Washington, DC 20007

202-337-5220
800-432-7543
Fax: 202-337-8314
TTY: 202-337-5221
e-mail: info@agbell.org
www.listeningandspokenlanguage.org

The Alexander Graham Bell Association for the Deaf and Hard of Hearing (AG bell) is a lifelong resource,support network and advocate for listening,learning,talking and living independently with hearing loss. Through publications, advocacy,training,scholarships and financial aid,AG Bell promotes the use of spoken language and hearing technology.

Alexander T. Graham, Executive Director
Judy Harrison, Director of Programs
Robin Bailey, Programs Specialist

3481 American Academy of Audiology
11480 Commerce Park Drive, Suite 220
Reston, VA 20191

703-790-8466
800-222-2336
Fax: 703-790-8631
e-mail: info@audiology.org
www.audiology.org

A professional organization dedicated to providing high quality and balanced hearing care to the public. Provides professional development, education and research and provides increased public awareness of hearing disorders and audiologic services.

Deborah Carlson, President
Bettie Borton, President-Elect
Therese Walden, AuD, Past President

3482 American Academy of Pediatrics
141 Northwest Point Boulevard
Elk Grove Village, IL 60007

847-434-4000
800-433-9016
Fax: 847-434-8000
www.aap.org

The American Academy of Pediatrics and its member pediatricians are committed to the attainment of optimal physical, mental and social health and well-being for all infants, children, adolescents, and young adults.

Sandra Hassink, MD, FAAP, President

3483 American Association of the Deaf-Blind
PO Box 2831
Kensington, MD 20891

301-495-4403
Fax: 301-495-4404
TTY: 301-495-4402
e-mail: aadb-info@aadb.org
www.aadb.org

The American Association of the Deaf-Blind (AADB) is a nonprofit 501(c)(3) national consumer organization, of, by, and for the deaf-blind Americans and their supporters. 'Deaf-blind' includes all types and degrees of dual vision and hearing loss. Their mission is to ensure that all deaf-blind persons achieve their maximum potential through increased independence, productivity, and integration into the community.

600 Members

Jill Gaus, President
Lynn Jansen, Vice President
Debby Lieberman, Secretary

3484 American Cochlear Implant Alliance
P.O. Box 103
McLean, VA 22101

703-534-6146
e-mail: info@aciaalliance.org
www.aciaalliance.org

Theÿ American Cochlear Implant Allianceÿis a not-for-profit membership organization created with the purpose of eliminating barriers to cochlear implantation by sponsoring research, driving heightened awareness and advocating for improved access to cochlear implants for patients of all ages across the US.

John K. Niparko, MD, Founding Chairman
Craig A. Buchman, MD FACS, Chair, Board of Director
Jill B. Firszt, PhD, Treasurer

3485 American Deafness and Rehabilitation Assoc iation (ADARA)
PO Box 480
Myersville, MD 21773

501-868-8850
Fax: 501-868-8812
www.adara.org

A network of professionals who serve people who are deaf or hard of hearing

Barry Critchfield, President
Michelle Niehaus, President-Elect
Doug Dittfurth, Vice President

3486 American Hearing Impaired Hockey Association
4214 W. 77th Place
Chicago, IL 60652

978-922-0955
e-mail: kkmm2won@aol.com
www.usadeafhockey.org

Theÿ American Hearing Impaired Hockey Associationÿprovides deaf and hard of hearing hockey players the opportunity to learn about and improve their hockey skills through our program. We offer these hockey players the opportunity to be coached by a coaching staff with college, national and international experience.

Jeff Sauer, Head Coach/ President
Kevin Delaney, Coach - Power Skating
Michael Drew, Coach - Current player

3487 American Hearing Research Foundation
8 S Michigan Avenue, Suite 1205
Chicago, IL 60603

312-726-9670
Fax: 312-726-9695
e-mail: ahrf@american-hearing.org
www.american-hearing.org

As a not-profit organization, a major source of our income is through donations. We have received generous contributions from individuals, corporations, and institutions, and continue to rely on these donations to found future research.

Richard G. Muench, Chairman
Alan G. Micco, President
Mark R. Muench, Vice President

3488 American Sign Language Teachers Association
www.aslta.org

ASLTA is the only national organization dedicated to the improvement and expansion of the teaching of ASL and Deaf Studies at all levels of instruction. ASLTA is an individual membership organization of more than 1,000 ASL and Deaf Studies educators from elementary through graduate education as well as agencies. The mission of the American Sign Language Teachers Association (ASLTA) is to preserve the integrity of American Sign Language (ASL) and Deaf Culture.

Timothy Owens, M. Ed.ÿ, President
Arlene Gunderson, M.Ed., Vice President
Bill Newell, Ph.D., Treasurer

3489 American Society for Deaf Children
#2047, 800 Florida Avenue NE., PO Box 3695
Washington, DC 20002
202-644-9204
800-942-2732
Fax: 717-909-5599
e-mail: asdc@deafchildren.org
www.deafchildren.org

A nonprofit parent-helping-parent organization promoting a positive attitude toward signing and deaf culture. Also provides support, encouragement, and current information about deafness to families with deaf and hard-of-hearing children.

Roger Williams, Co-President
Sherry Williams, Co-President
Diana Poeppelmeyer, Executive Secretary

3490 American Speech Language Hearing Associati on (ASHA)
2200 Research Boulevard
Rockville, MD 20850
301-296-5700
800-638-8255
Fax: 301-571-0457
TTY: 301-296-5650
e-mail: actioncenter@asha.org
www.asha.org

ASHA is the professional, scientific and credentialling association for more than 123,000 members and affiliates who are speech-language pathologists, audiologists, and speech, language, and hearing scientists. Their mission is to promote the interests of and provide the highest quality services for proesstionals, and to advocate for people with communication disabilities.

Patriacia A. Prelock, President
Elizabeth S. McCrea, President-Elect
Donna Fisher Smiley, Vice President

3491 American Speech-Language-Hearing Foundatio n
2200 Research Blvd.
Rockville, MD 20850
301-296-8700
Fax: 301-296-8567
e-mail: foundation@asha.org
www.ashfoundation.org

An organization which promotes a better quality of life for children and adults with communication disorders.

3492 American Tinnitus Association
522 S.W. Fifth Avenue; Suite 825
Portland, OR 97204
503-248-9985
800-634-8978
Fax: 503-248-0024
e-mail: tinnitus@ata.org
www.ata.org

The American Tinnitus Association exists to cure tinnitus through the development of resources that advance tinnitus research.

Thomas J. Lobl, Ph.D., Chair
Marsha Johnson, Au.D.ÿ, Treasurer
Scott C. Mitchell, J.D., Secretary

3493 Auditory - Verbal International
2121 Eisenhower Avenue, Suite 402
Alexandria, VA 22314
703-519-7400
Fax: 703-739-0395
TTY: 703-739-0874
e-mail: audiverb@aol.com
www.rvjintl.com

Provides the choice of listening and speaking as the way of life for children and adults who are deaf or hard of hearing. Through the use of assistive technology such as digital hearing aids or cochlear implants and auditory-verbal therapy, many deaf and hard of hearing children can learn to listen and speak.

900 members

John Jones, President
Steven Rech JD, President

3495 BEGINNINGS for Parents of Children Who Are Deaf or Hard of Hearing
PO Box 17646
Raleigh, NC 27619
919-850-2746
800-541-HEAR
Fax: 919-715-4093
TTY: 800-541-HEAR
e-mail: raleigh@ncbegin.org
www.ncbegin.com

BEGINNINGS provides emotional support and access to as a central resource for families with deaf or hard of hearing children, age birth through 21. These services are also available to deaf parents who have hearing children. Their mission is to help parents to be informed, empowered and supported as they make decisions about their child. In addition, they are committed to providing technical assistance to professionals who work with these families.

Stephanie J. Sjoblad, President
Lekita Essa, Vice President
Joni Y Alberg, Executive Director

3496 Better Hearing Institute
Ste 700
Washington, DC 20005
202-449-1100
800-327-9355
Fax: 703-684-6048
TTY: 703-642-0580
e-mail: mail@betterhearing.org
www.betterhearing.org

A nonprofit educational organization that implements national public information programs on hearing loss and available medical, surgical, hearing aid, and rehabilitation assistance for millions with uncorrected hearing problems. Its award-winning series of television, radio, and print media public service messages include many celebrities who overcame hearing loss. BHI maintains a toll-free Hotline HelpLine telephone service that provides information on hearing loss and hearing help to callers.

Sergei Kochkin, PhD, Executive Director
Sasha Ward, Administrative Director

3497 Center for Early Intervention of Deafness (CEID)
1035 Grayson Street
Berkeley, CA 94710
510-848-4800
Fax: 510-848-4801
TTY: 510-848-5686
TDD: 510-527-5196
e-mail: ceid@ceid.org
www.ceid.org

A non-profit organization dedicated to providing a program of intensive and comprehensive early intervention services to young children up to five years old who have hearing losses or severe speech/language delays and their families. CEID uses 'Total Communication', which includes the simultaneous use of spoken English, audition, and literal representation of sign language (SEE signing), in a play based curriculum incorportating thematic active learning strategies and total family involvement.

Rosalie Streett, President
Warren Wincorn, VP
Alan Gould, Treasurer

3498 Children's Legal Advocacy Program (CLA)
Alexander Graham Bell Association for the Deaf
3417 Volta Place NW
Washington, DC 20007

202-337-5220
800-432-7543
Fax: 202-337-8314
TTY: 202-337-5221
e-mail: info@agbell.org
www.agbell.org

Supports families of children who are deaf or hard of hearing by providing legal representation and technical assistance to families who need help obtaining appropriate services in their communities.

Alexander T. Graham, Executive Director
Judy Harrison, Director of Programs
Robin Bailey, Programs Specialist

3499 Coalition for Global Hearing Health
www.coalitionforglobalhearinghealth.org

Works with the mission to promote and enhance hearing health services in low-resourced communities.

3500 Cochlear Implant Assocciation
5335 Wisconsin Avenue NW, Suite 440
Washington, DC 20015

202-895-2781
Fax: 202-895-2782
e-mail: C_I_A_I info@cici.org
www.cici.org

A non-profit organization dedicated to educating and supporting cochlear implant recipients and their familiies; advocating and promoting cochlear implants.

John McCelland, President
Lorie Singer, VP
Wayne L Roorda, Treasurer

3501 Cochlear Implant Awareness Foundation
130 South John Street
Rochester, IL 62563

e-mail: info@ciafonline.org
www.ciafonline.org

Connect people with the resources they need to make an educated decision about cochlear implant surgery.

Michelle Tjelmeland, Founder and Chairwoman
Sheryl Klemm, Director
Max Klemm, Director

3502 Council of the American Instructors of the Deaf
P.O. Box 377
Bedford, TX 76095

TTY: 817-354-8414
e-mail: caid@swbell.net
www.caid.org

The organization for all teachers, administrators, educational interpreters, residential personnel, and other concerned professionals involved in education of the deaf.

Larry Quinsland, Ph.D, President
Keith Mousley, President
Christina Yuknis, President Elect

3503 Council on Education of the Deaf
PO Box 976
North Kingstown, RI 2852

e-mail: executivedirector@councilondeafed.org
councilondeafed.org

The Council on Education of the Deaf (CED) is an organization sponsored by five major national organizations dedicated to quality education for all deaf and hard of hearing students.

Joseph E. Fischgrund, Executive Director
Trina Schooley, CED Office Manager

3504 Deaf Counseling, Advocacy & Referral Agency
14895 E. 14th Street, Suite #200ÿ
San Leandro, CA 94578

510-343-6670
Fax: 510-483-1790
e-mail: info@dcara.org
www.dcara.org

Deaf, Counseling, Advocacy & Referral Agency (DCARA), is a non-profit, community-based social service agency serving the Deaf, Hard of Hearing, Late-Deafened and Deaf-blind (D/HH/LD/DB)community.ÿ

Steve Longo, President
Lonnie Tanenberg, Vice President
David Martin, Treasurer

3505 Deaf REACH
3521 12th Street NE
Washington, DC 20017

202-832-6681
Fax: 202-832-8454
TTY: 202-832-6681
www.deaf-reach.org

Nonprofit organization: our mission is to maximize the self-sufficiency of deaf adults needing special services by providing referral, education, advocacy, counseling, and housing.

Annette Riechman, President
Jon Tomar, VP
Teresa Arcarl, Secretary

3506 Dial-a-Hearing Screening Test
300 S Chester Road
Swathmore, PA 19081

610-544-7700
800-222-3277
Fax: 610-543-2802
e-mail: dahst@aol.com
www.dialatest.com

National telephone hearing screening test service. Consumers receive a copy of their hearing screening test results and referral to a hearing health care center in the Dial A Hearing Screening Test network. Flexible participation plans for hearing health care providers.

George Biddle, President
James Biddle, Vice President
Joseph Rago, Controller

3507 Dogs for the Deaf, Inc.
10175 Wheller Road
Central Point, OR 97502

541-826-9220
800-990-3647
e-mail: info@dogsforthedeaf.org
www.dogforthedeaf.org

This organization rescues and professionally trains dogs to assist people with hearing loss, autism, and other challenges.

3508 EAR Foundation
Ste A
Nashville, TN 37201

615-627-2724
800-545-4327
Fax: 615-627-2728
TDD: 615-627-2724
e-mail: info@earfoundation.org
www.earfoundation.org

The EAR foundation has three basic purposes: to provide the general public support services promoting the integration of the hearing and balance impaired into mainstream society; to provide practicing ear specialists continuing medical education courses and related programs specifically regarding rehabilitation and hearing preservation; and to educate young people and adults about hearing preservation and early detection of hearing loss, enabling them to prevent hearing and balance disorders.

Michael E Glasscock, III, MD, Founder and President
Steve Masie, Chair
Suzanne Wyatt, Executive Director

3509 Educational Audiology Association
700 McKnight Park Drive, Suite 708
Pittsburgh, PA 15237

800-460-7322
Fax: 888-729-3489
e-mail: admin@edaud.org
edaud.org

The Educational Audiology Association is an international organization of audiologists and related professionals who deliver a full spectrum of hearing services to all children, particularly those in educational settings.

Mike Sharp, AuD, CCC-A, President
Gary Pillow, President-Elect
Susan Dillmuth-Miller, Past President

3510 Episcopal Conference of the Deaf
www.ecdeaf.org

The ECD is a central clearing house concerning all aspects of work among Deaf people in the Episcopal Church. Episcopal Conference of the Deaf spreads the Gospel of Christ among Deaf people.

Marianne Stuart, President
Erich Krengel, First Vice President
Steve Holst, Treasurer

3511 Friends of Libraries for Deaf Action
2930 Craiglawn Road
Silver Spring, MD 20904
e-mail: folda86@aol.com
www.folda.net

The Red Notebook is a loose-leaf binder containing fact sheets, library reprints, announcements and other printed informational materials that are related to both deaf and library issues.

Alice L. Hagemeyer, MLS, President
Merrie A. Davidson, MLS, Associate
Ricardo Lopez, MS, Associate

3512 Hands & Voices National
PO Box 3093
Boulder, CO 80307
303-492-6283
866-422-0422
e-mail: parentaladvocate@handsandvoices.org
www.handsandvoices.org

A nationwide non-profit organization dedicated to supporting families and their children who are deaf or hard-of-hearing as well as the professionals who serve them.

3513 Hands Organization
2501 W 103rd Street
Chicago, IL 60655
773-239-6632

Advocacy for the deaf and hard-of-hearing; information and referrals, educational events, sign language summer youth camps and newsletters.

Kate Kubey, Contact

3514 Hear Now
9745 E Hampden Avenue, Suite 300
Denver, CO 80231
303-695-7797
800-648-4327
Fax: 303-695-7789
TTY: 800-648-4327
e-mail: 76350.650@compuserve.com

Committed to making technology accessible to deaf and hard-of-hearing individuals throughout the United States. Also raises funds to provide hearing aids, cochlear implants and related services to children and adults who have hearing losses but do not have financial resources to purchase their own devices.

Bernice Dinner, MA, CCC, President/Founder
Elaine Hansen

3515 Hearing Health Foundation
363 Seventh Avenue, 10th Floorÿ
New York, NY 10001
212-257-6140
866-454-3924
e-mail: info@hearinghealthfoundation.org
hearinghealthfoundation.org

Hearing Health Foundation (HHF) is the largest private funder of hearing research,ÿwith a mission to prevent and cure hearing loss and tinnitus through groundbreaking research.

Shari Eberts, Chairman
Claire Schultz, CEO
Antonio Coppola, Director of Corporate Partnerships

3516 Hearing Impairments Better Hearing Institute
PO Box 1840
Washington, DC 20013
800-327-9355
Fax: 703-750-9302
TTY: 800-EAR-WELL

To educate the public and medical profession about hearing loss, its treatment and prevention.

3517 Hearing Loss Association of America
7910 Woodmont Ave, Suite 1200
Bethesda, MD 20814
301-657-2248
Fax: 301-913-9413
www.hearingloss.org

HLAA provides assistance and resources for people with hearing loss and their families to learn how to adjust to living with hearing loss. HLAA is working to eradicate the stigma associated with hearing loss and raise public awareness about the need for prevention, treatment, and regular hearing screenings throughout life.

Anna Gilmore Hall, Executive Director
Lise Hamlin, Director of Public Policy
Nancy Macklin, Director of Events and Marketing

3518 HearingPlanet
100 Westwood Place, Suite 300
Brentwood, TN 37027
615-248-5910
800-432-7669
Fax: 615-248-5903
www.hearingplanet.com

A hearing specialist is ready to answer questions about hearing aids, hearing loss and treatments.

3519 Hearts and Homes For Youth
1320 Fenwick Lane, Suite 800
Silver Spring, MD 20910
301-589-8444
Fax: 301-495-0923
e-mail: hhyinfo@heartsandhomes.org
www.hh4y.org

Helps troubled children and youth who are abused, neglected or runaways, become independent, productive adults. To fulfill this mission, HHY provides a broad specterum of educational, residential, independent living and mental health programs to a culturally diverse client population.

Rex Smith, President
Tammy O' Rourke, VP
Stephen Liggett-Creel, Administrator

3520 House Ear Institute
2100 W 3rd Street
Los Angeles, CA 90057
213-483-4431
800-388-8612
Fax: 213-483-8789
TDD: 213-484-2642
e-mail: info@hei.org
www.hei.org

A non-profit organization dedicated to advancing hearing science through research and education to improve the quality of life. HEI scientists explore the developing ear, hearing loss and ear disease at the cell and molecular level, as well as the complex relationship between the ear and the brain. They are also working to improve hearing aids and auditory implants, diagnostics, clinical treatments and intervention methods. HEI employs more than 180 staff members within 22 departments.

Catherine D. Meyer, Chair
David Z. D'Argenio, Vice Chair
William B. Witte, Treasurer

3521 International Deaf Education Association
P.O. Box 20715
Billings, MT 59104
406-656-2766
e-mail: info@ideadeaf.org
www.ideadeaf.org

IDEA is a USA non-profit foundation that is working to educate impoverished and neglected deaf children in the Philippines.

George Dennis Drake, President / CEO
Marilouÿ Drake, CFO
Rhonda Hillabush, Sponsorship Director

3522 International Hearing Society
16880 Middlebelt Road, Suite 4
Livonia, MI 48154
734-522-7200
800-521-5247
Fax: 734-522-0200
e-mail: chelms@ihsinfo.org
www.ihsinfo.org

IHS is the professional association that represents Hearing Instrument Speicalists worldwide. IHS members are engaged in the practice of testing human hearing and selecting, fitting and dispensing hearing instruments. The Society continues to recognize the need for promoting and maintaining the highest possible standards for its members in the best interest of the hearing impaired it serves.

3000 members

Thomas Higgins, President
Scott Beall, President-Elect
Todd Beyer, Secretary

3523 John Tracy Clinic
806 W Adams Boulevard, PO Box 2505
Los Angeles, CA 90007
213-748-5481
800-522-4582
Fax: 213-749-1651
TTY: 213-747-2924
e-mail: canguita@jtc.org
www.jtc.org

A private, non-profit education center whose mission is to offer hope, guidance and encouragement to families of infants and preschool children with hearing loss by providing free, parent-centered services worldwide. The center has over 60 years of expertise in the spoken language option.

Michael D. Barker, Chair
Speed Fry, Vice Chair
Nihar Shah, Treasurer

3524 Junior National Association of the Deaf
8630 Fenton Street, Suite 820
Silver Spring, MD 20910
301-587-1788
Fax: 301-587-1791
TTY: 301-587-1789
e-mail: nadinfo@nad.org
www.nad.org/jrnad

An organization of chapters from junior high and high schools across the United States whose motto is: Promoting the Tomorrow of All the Deaf by Working with the Deaf Youth of Today. Members learn and practice leadership, teamwork, and responsibility, and develop self-confidence.

Christopher D. Wagner, President
Melissa S. Draganac-Hawk, Vice President
Kirsten Poston, Secretary

3525 National Alliance of Black Interpreters
naobi2.org
e-mail: naobiincmembershipchair@gmail.com
naobi2.org

Theÿmission of NAOBIÿis to promote excellence and empowerment among African Americans/Blacks in the profession of sign language interpreting in the context of a multi-cultural, multi-lingual environment.

3526 National Association for Hearing and Speech Action
American Speech Language Hearing Association
2200 Research Blvd., PO Box 3289
Rockville, MD 20850
301-296-5700
800-478-2071
Fax: 301-296-5777
TDD: 301-296-5650
www.asha.org

Provides general information on speech, language and hearing disorders to members and the public. Provides referrals to speech/language pathologists and audiologists.

77,346 members

Patriacia A. Prelock, President
Elizabeth S. McCrea, President-Elect
Donna Fisher Smiley, VP for Audiology Practice

3527 National Association of Parents with Children in Special Education
3642 E Sunnydale Drive
Chandler Heights, AZ 85142
800-754-4421
Fax: 800-424-0371
e-mail: contact@napcse.org
www.napcse.org

NAPCSEÿis a national membership organization dedicated to rendering all possible support and assistance to parents whose children receive special education services, both in and outside of school.

Dr. George Giulianiÿ, President

3528 National Association of School Psychologists
4340 East West Highway, Suite 402
Bethesda, MD 20814
301-657-0270
866-331-NASP
Fax: 301-657-0275
www.nasponline.org

NASP empowers school psychologists by advancing effective practices to improve students' learning, behavior, and mental health.

Stephen E. Brock, President
Todd A. Savage, President-Elect
Sally Baas, Past President

3529 National Association of State Agencies of the Deaf and Hard of Hearing
4425 North Market Street
Wilmington, DE 19802
nasadhh.org

The National Association of State Agencies of the Deaf and Hard of Hearing is comprised of administrators of the state agencies serving deaf and hard of hearing.ÿ

Steve Florio, President, B.O.D.
Sherri Collins, Vice President
Virginia Moore, Treasurer

3530 National Association of the Deaf (NAD)
451 7th St. SW
Washington, DC 20410
301-587-1788
Fax: 301-587-1791
TTY: 301-587-1789
e-mail: nadinfo@nad.org
www.nad.org

Established in 1880, the vision of NAD is that the language, culture, and heritage of hard of hearing Americans will be aknowledged and respected in pursuit of life, liberty and equality. There efforts to realize the vision have been in preserving, protecting, and promoting civil, human and liguitis rights of deaf and hard of hearing persons in America.

Christopher D. Wagner, President
Melissa S. Draganac-Hawk, Vice President
Kirsten Poston, Secretary

3531 National Black Deaf Advocates
P.O. Box 502658
Indianapolis, IN 46250
e-mail: president@nbda.org
www.nbda.org

The National Black Deaf Advocates (NBDA) is the official advocacy organization for thousands of Black Deaf and hard of hearing people in the United States.ÿ

Patrick Robinson, President
Opeoluwa Sotonwa, Vice President
Betty Henderson, Treasurer

3532 National Captioning Institute
3725 Concorde Pkwy, Ste 100
Chantilly, VA 20151
703-917-7600
Fax: 703-917-9853
TTY: 703-917-7600
e-mail: mail@ncicap.org
www.ncicap.org

NCI was established in 1979 as a non-profit corporation with the mission of ensuring that deaf and hard of hearing people, as well as others who can benefit from the same service, have access to television's entertainment and news through the technology of closed captioning. NCI employs almost 200 individuals.

Gene Chao, President
Jack Gates, President
Drake Smith, Chief Technology Officer

3533 National Catholic Office for the Deaf
www.ncod.org

e-mail: info@ncod.org
www.ncod.org

There mission is to Spread God's message through the support of the Deaf and Hard of Hearing Pastoral Ministry so that we may all be one in Christ!

Kevin C. Rhoades, B.O.D.
Gregory Schott, Member at Large

3534   National Center On Deaf-Blindness
345 N. Monmouth Ave.
Monmouth, OR 97361
503-838-8754
Fax: 503-838-8150
e-mail: info@nationaldb.org
nationaldb.org

NCDB works to improve the quality of life for children who are deaf-blind and their families.

Brenda Baroncelli, Administrative Assistantÿ
Robbin Bull, Project Specialist
Megan Cote, Project Specialist

3535   National Center for Hearing Assessment & Management
Utah State University, 2615 Old Main Hill
Logan, UT 84322
435-797-3584
www.infanthearing.org

NCHAMÿserves as theÿNational Resource Centerÿfor the implementation and improvement of comprehensive and effective Early Hearing Detection and Intervention (EHDI) systems.

3536   National Center for Voice and Speech
University of Iowa
677 Phillips Hall
Iowa City, IA 52242
319-335-2238
Fax: 319-335-8851
e-mail: ASL-Program@uiowa.edu
www.uiowa.ude

This is a consortium of the following institutions focusing on voice and speech disorders: University of Iowa, Denver Center for Performing Arts, University of Wisconsin-Madison, University of Utah. NCVS trains scientists interested in careers in voice and speech research, provides continuing education for professionals, and conducts research on voice and speech production.

Ingo Titze, PhD, Director
Cynthia Kintigh, MA

3537   National Council of Hispano Deaf and Hard of Hearing
P.O. Box 22011
Santa Fe, NM 87502
www.nchdhh.org

The mission of the National Council of Hispano Deaf and Hard of Hearing is to ensure equal access of the Hispano Deaf and Hard of Hearing community in the areas of social, recreational, cultural, educational, and vocational welfare.

Rogelio Fern ndez, Jr., President
Milmaglyn Morales, Vice President
Paolina Ramirez, Treasurer

3538   National Cued Speech Association
1300 Pennsylvania Avenue, Suite 190-713
Washington, DC 20004
216-292-6213
800-459-3529
TTY: 216-292-6213
e-mail: cuedspdisc@aol.com
www.cuedspeech.org

A non-profit membership organization founded in 1982 to promote and support the effective use of Cued Speech. They raise awareness of Cued Speeck and its applications, provide educational services, assist local affiliate chapters, establish standards for Cued Speech and certify Cued Speech instructors and transliterators. Their mission and goals are to promote and support the effectue use of Cued Speech for communication, language acquistion and literacy.

Shannon Howell, President
Penny Hakim, VP
John Brubaker, VP

3539   National Family Association for Deaf-Blind
141 Middle Neck Road
Sands Point, NY 11050
800-255-0411
Fax: 516-883-9060
TTY: 516-944-8637
e-mail: nfadb@aol.com
www.nfadb.org

A nonprofit, volunteer based, family association that believes individuals who are deaf-blind are valued members of society and are entitled to the same opportunity and choices as other members of the community

Susan Green, President
Debbie Ethridge, VP
Cynthia Jackson-Glenn, Treasurer

3540   National Information Center on Deafness
Gallaudet Univ. Press c/o Chicago Distrib. Center
800 Florida Avenue NE
Washington, DC 20002
202-250-2474
800-995-0550
Fax: 202-651-5744
TTY: 202-651-5114
e-mail: admissions.office@gallaudet.edu
www.gallaudet.edu

Provides information or referrals on questions about deafness, including general information, education, research, legislation, assistive devices and more. Offers a bibliography of readings available on 30 topics relating to deafness.

Loraine DiPietro, Director
Vickie Whetstone, Executive Secretary
David King, Admissions Support

3541   National Rehabilitation Information Center
8201 Corporate Drive, Suite 600
Landover, MD 20785
301-459-5900
800-346-2742
Fax: 301-562-2401
TTY: 301-459-5984
e-mail: naricinfo@heitchservices.com
www.naric.com

Its mission is to generate, disseminate and promote new knowledge to improve the options available to disabled persons. The ultimate goal is to allow these individuals to perform their regular activities in the community and to bolster society's ability to provide full opportunities and appropriate supports for its disabled citizens.

Mark Odum, Director

3542   National Technical Institute for the Deaf
Rochester Institute of Technology
One Lomb Memorial Drive
Rochester, NY 14623
585-475-2411
Fax: 585-475-5978
TTY: 585-475-6400
e-mail: ntidmc@rit.edu
www.rit.edu

Technical college for students who are deaf or hard of hearing. Its mission is to provide these students with outstanding state-of-the-art technical and professional programs, complemented by a strong liberal arts and sciences curriculum, that prepare them to live and work in the mainstream of a rapidly changing global community and enhances their lifelong learning.

Alan Hurwitz, Vice President/Dean

3543   SEE Center for the Advancement of Deaf Chi ldren
PO Box 1181
Los Alamitos, CA 90720
562-430-1467
Fax: 562-795-6614
TTY: 562-430-1467
e-mail: seecenter@seecenter.org
www.seecenter.org

Established in 1984 as a nonprofit organization to work with parents and educators of hearing impared children. Their goals are to promote early identification and intervention; to promote development of improved English skills; to promote development and understanding of principles of Signing Exact English and its uses; to promote information to parents on deafness and related topics; and to foster the positive development of self concept in the deaf child.

Esther Zawolkow, Executive Director

3544 Self Help for Hard of Hearing People Hearing Loss Association of America
7910 Woodmont Avenue, Suite 1200
Bethesda, MD 20814   301-657-2248
                                      Fax: 301-913-9413
                                      TTY: 301-657-2248
                               e-mail: info@hearingloss.org
                                      www.hearingloss.org

The HLAA exists to open the world of communication for people with hearing loss through information, education, advocacy and support. They believe people with hearing loss can help themselves and one another to participate fully and successfully in society. HLAA promotes self-confidence; empowers individuals with skills to improve their lives; and provides an opportunity for affiliation among people with hearing loss and their friends, families, and professionals.

Barbara Kelley, Editor-In-Chief
Brenda Battat, Executive Director
Lise Hamlin, Director of Public Policy

3545 Telecommunications for the Deaf
8630 Fenton Street, Suite 604
Silver Spring, MD 20910   301-589-3786
                                      Fax: 301-589-3797
                                      TTY: 301-589-3006
                               e-mail: info@tdi-online.org
                                      www.tdi-online.org

An active national advocacy organization focusing its energies and resources to address equal access issues in telecommunications and media for four constituences in deafness and hearing loss, specifically people who are deaf, hard-of-hearing, late-deafened, or deaf-blind.

Miller Roy, President
Stout Claudd L., Executive Director
Jim House, Public Relations

3546 Telecommunications for the Deaf and Hard of Hearing
8630 Fenton Street, Suite 121
Silver Spring, MD 20910   301-563-9112
                                      www.tdiforaccess.org

TDI (formally known as Telecommunications for the Deaf and Hard of Hearing, Inc.) was established in 1968 originally to promote further distribution of TTYs in the deaf community and to publish an annual national directory of TTY numbers.

Claude Stout, Executive Director
Don Cullens, Public Relations Director
John Skjeveland, Business Manager

Libraries & Resource Centers

3547 AbleData
8630 Fenton Street - Suite 300 B
Lexington, KY 40513   301-608-8998
                                           800-227-0216
                                      Fax: 301-608-8958
                                      TTY: 301-608-8912
                         e-mail: abledata@macrointernational.com
                                      www.abledata.com

AbleData provides information on assistive technology and rehabilitation equipment available from international and domestic sources to consumers, professionals, organizations, and caregivers within the United States.

3548 Center for Hearing and Communication
50 Broadway - 6th Fl
New York, NY 10004   917-305-7700
                                      Fax: 917-305-7888
                                      TTY: 917-305-7999
                                         www.chchearing.org

This organization provides hearing health services to people of all ages who have a hearing loss.

3549 Communication Service for the Deaf, Inc.
102 North Krohn Place
Sioux Falls, SD 57103   800-642-6410
                                      TTY: 866-273-3323
                               e-mail: inquiry@c-s-d.org
                                         www.ceasd.org

CSD Relay is a telephone service which allows persons with hearing or speech disabilities to place and receive telephone calls.

3550 Dangerous Decibels Oregon Health & Science University
3181 SW Sam Jackson Park Road - NRC-04
Portland, OR 97239   503-494-0670
                                      Fax: 503-494-0670
                                      e-mail: dd@ohsu.edu
                                   www.dangerousdecibels.com

Through the creation of exhibits, education and research this organization helps to reduce the incidence and prevalence of Noise Induced Hearing Loss (NIHL) and tinnitus (ringing in the ear) by changing knowledge, attitudes, and behaviours of school-aged children.

3551 Hard of Hearing Advocates
245 Prospect St, PO Box 1184
Upton, MA 01701   e-mail: hoha@charter.net
                                         www.hohadvocates.org

This organization helps hard-of-hearing (HOH) people by creating and implementing programs and solutions where HOH people have undue problems.

3552 Hearing Education & Awareness for Rockers
PO Box 460847
San Francisco, CA 94146   415-409-3277
                                   e-mail: hear@hearnet.com
                                         www.hearnet.com

H.E.A.R. is a hearing information source for musicians and music lovers.

Alabama

3553 Alabama Institute for the Deaf & Blind
PO Box 698
Talladega, AL 35161   256-761-3331
                                      Fax: 256-761-3344
                                         www.aidb.org

Services include central directory, representatives of agencies, service providers, families, and coordinators of infant, toddler, and preschool special education programs.

Terry Graham, President

3554 University of Alabama Speech and Hearing Center
Deparment of Communicative Disorders
166 Rose Administration Building Box 870144
Tuscaloosa, AL 35487   205-348-5320
                                      Fax: 205-348-8320
                               e-mail: gculton@ed.ua.edu
                                   www.universityrelations.ua.edu

Enhancing the educational mission of the Department, the Speech and Hearing Center is further dedicated to reducing the impact of communicative disorders affecting diverse populations across a life-span.

Carl E Ferguson, Executive Director
Austin Dare, Director, Office of Design/Productio

California

3555 American Action Fund for Blind Children and Adults
18440 Oxnard Street
Tarzana, CA 91356
818-343-2022
Fax: 818-343-3219
e-mail: lucyabba@aol.com
www.actinfund.org

A lending library for the visually impaired. We send out a weekly Braille newspaper for the deaf-blind (worldwide), we also send out pocket-sized Braille calendars. Our lending library is for pre-school thru high school. All of our services are free.

Lucille Abbazia, Manager

3556 Hear Center
301 E Del Mar Boulevard
Pasadena, CA 91101
626-796-2016
Fax: 626-796-2320
e-mail: auditory@hearcenter.org
www.hearcenter.org

The Hear Center's mission is to help individuals with hearing loss or speech and language impairments integrate into the mainstream of the community by providing them with the means for developing auditory and oral communication skills.

Ellen Simon, Executive Director

District of Columbia

3557 Center for Auditory and Speech Sciences-Gallaudet University
800 Florida Avenue NE
Washington, DC 20002
202-651-5000
Fax: 202-651-5295
e-mail: clerc.center@gallaudet.edu
www.gallaudet.edu

The Hearing and Speech Center provides comprehensive speech, language, and audiology services to Gallaudet students, faculty, staff and to clients in the Washington, D.C. area. These services include hearing and hearing aid evaluations, hearing aid dispensing, assistive devices evaluations, speech-language evaluations and therapy, communication therapy, and speech reading classes.

I King Jordan, President
Jane K Fernandes, Provost
Paul Kelly, VP Administration and Finance

3558 District of Columbia Public Library/ Librarian for the Deaf Community
901 G Street NW, Room 215
Washington, DC 20001
202-727-2142
Fax: 202-727-1129
e-mail: lbphb_2000@yahoo.com
www.dclibrary.org

Offers reference services through TDD, portable TDD for public use at pay phones, signers for library programs, sign language classes, information about deafness, print and nonprint materials for persons who are deaf.

Vaneisha Denson, Manager

3559 Laurent Clerc National Deaf Education Center-Gallaudet Universty
800 Florida Avenue NE
Washington, DC 20002
202-651-5300
Fax: 202-651-5477
TTY: 202-651-5300
www.gallaudet.edu

Gallaudet University's Laurent Clerc National Deaf Education Center provides deaf and hard of hearing children through the Model Secondary School for the Deaf and the Kendall Demonstration Elementary School and also collects, evaluates and disseminates best practices in deaf education.

I King Jordan, President
Katherine Jankowski, Dean
Paul Kelly, VP Administration/Finance

3560 Volta Bureau Library
Alexander Graham Bell Association for the Deaf
3417 Volta Place NW
Washington, DC 20007
202-337-5220
866-337-5220
Fax: 202-337-8314
TTY: 202-337-5221
e-mail: agbell2@aol.com
www.agbell.org

Contains one of the world's largest historical collections of publications, documents and information on deafness. In addition to the main collection, which includes books, periodicals and indexed clipping files dating from the turn of the century, the library also houses a significant archival collection dealing with the history of deafness since the 16th century. Membership dues for professionals are $50.00.

4500 members

Rebecca Parlakian, Director Member Services

Illinois

3561 Loyola University of Children, Parmly Hearing Institute
6525 N Sheridan Road
Chicago, IL 60626
773-508-2766
Fax: 773-508-2719
e-mail: ssheft@luc.edu

The Parmly Hearing Institute is part of Loyola University Chicago.

Stanley Edward Sheft PhD, Director

Maine

3562 University of Maine, Conley Speech and Hearing Center
5724 Dunn Hall, Room 336
Orono, ME 04469
207-581-2006

The Madelyn E and Albert D Conley Speech, Language and Hearing Center is a center for clinical education and research as well as a facility for comprehensive state-of-the-art speech, language and hearing services. Both the Audiology Clinic and the Speech-Language Clinic provide services for individuals across the lifespan. The Speech-Language Clinic includes a Diagnostic Clinic, a Family-Based Treatment Clinic, and a Stuttering Clinic.

Susan K Riley MS, Clinic Director

Massachusetts

3563 Eaton-Peabody Laboratory of Auditory Physiology
Massachusetts Eye & Ear Institute
243 Charles Street
Boston, MA 02114
617-573-7900
Fax: 617-720-4408
TDD: 617-523-5498
www.meei.harvard.edu

A consortium between the Massachusetts Eye and Ear Infirmary, the Harvard Medical School, the Research Laboratory of Electronics at Massachusetts Institute of Technology, and the Massachusetts General Hospital. Research interests span the auditory system from peripheral to central, from normal to abnormal function, from neurophysiology to behavior, and from the molecular and genetic bases of deafness, to its treatment via hearing aids and cochlear implants.

Nelson YS Kiang, PhD, Director

Nebraska

3564 University of Nebraska, Lincoln Barkley Memorial Center
Barkley Center 301
Lincoln, NE 68583
402-472-2145
Fax: 402-472-7697
www.unl.edu.barkley/index.shtml

The University of Nebraska-Lincoln Barkley Memorial Center and Boys Town National Research Hospital have joined forces to offer an exciting future in the audiology profession.

John E Bernthal, Director

New York

3565 Wallace Memorial Library
Rochester Institute of Technology
90 Lomb Memorial Drive
Rochester, NY 14623   585-475-2562
                                www.library.rit.edu/collections/wallace.html

A multimedia resource center with a collection of more than
750,000 items. Resource materials include more than 350,000
books; 2900 print journals subscriptions; 380,000 microforms;
3,100 audio cassettes and recordings; 6,700 film and video titles.
They have an extensive web-based online collection which features over 150 research databases, 7,000+ eBooks, 16,000 electronic journal subscriptions and thousands of digital images in
various collections.

Melanie Norton, Reference Librarian

Oregon

3566 Regional Resource Center on Deafness
Western Oregon State University
345 N Monmouth Avenue
Monmouth, OR 97361   503-838-8444
                                               877-877-1593
                                          Fax: 503-838-8228
                                   e-mail: webmaster@wou.edu
                                               www.wou.edu

Prepares professionals in the Northwest to be qualified to serve
the unique communication, rehabilitation, and educational needs
of deaf and hard of hearing individuals. The Center offers graduate and undergraduate degree programs for professionals entering
fields that serve people who are deaf or hard of hearing, continuing education opportunities for currently practicing professionals,
and consultation and community service activities designed to
enhance the quality of life for all affected.

Cheryl Davis, Director
Hilda Rosselli PhD, Dean

South Carolina

3567 Described and Captioned Media Program
National Association of the Deaf
1447 E Main Street
Spartanburg, SC 29307   864-585-1778
                                               800-237-6213
                                          Fax: 864-585-2611
                                          TTY: 864-585-2617
                                      e-mail: info@cfv.org
                                               www.cfv.org

Renamed the Described and Captioned Media Program, CMP continues to provide all persons who are deaf or hard of hearing
awareness of and equal access to communication and learning
through the use of captioned educational media and supportive
collateral materials. They also act as a captioning information and
training center. Their ultimate goal is to permit media to be an integral part in the lifelong learning process for all stakeholders in
the deaf and hard of hearing community.

Bill Stark, Manager

Research Centers

**3568 Boston Children's Hospital Dept. of Otolaryngology &
Communication**
300 Longwood Ave
Boston, MA 02115   617-355-6000
                                          TTY: 617-730-0152
                                      www.childrenshospital.com

Provides diagnosis and surgical treatment for disorders of the
head and neck.

Arkansas

**3569 Arkansas Rehabilitation Research and Training Center for
Deaf Persons**
University of Arkansas
4601 W Markham Street
Little Rock, AR 72205   501-686-9691
                                          Fax: 501-686-9698
                                          TTY: 501-686-9698

The center focuses on issues affecting the employability of deaf
and hard-of-hearing rehabilitation clients.

Douglas Watson, PhD, Director

Massachusetts

**3570 National Temporal Bone, Hearing and Balanc e Pathology
Resource Registry**
Massachusetts Eye & Ear Infirmary
243 Charles Street, PO Box 3096
Boston, MA 02114   617-573-3711
                                             800-822-1327
                                          Fax: 617-573-3838
                                          TTY: 800-439-0183
                              e-mail: tbregistry@meei.harvard.edu
                                             www.tbregistry.org

The Registry, established by the National Institute on Deafness
and Other Communication Disorders, maintains a database of human temporal bone collections, responds to inquiries from the
public and researchers interested in temporal bone donation or research, disseminates information about temporal bone collection
and its importance, implements professional educational activities in the field of temporal bone and auditory brain cell stem
study and implements a national acquistion network.

Nicole Pelletier, Coordinator

Michigan

3571 University of Michigan, Kresge Hearing Research Institute
1301 E Ann Street, Room 5032
Ann Arbor, MI 48109   734-763-9600
                                          Fax: 734-764-0014
                                          TTY: 734-764-8110

Research programs include multi-disciplinary projects in behavior, morphology, physiology, molecular biology and genetics,
bioengineering, pharmacology and biochemistry. They include:
the genetics of hearing and deafness, mechanisms of auditory
processing, molecular otology, cochlear prosthesis and tissue
bioengineering, and training.

Jochen Schacht PhD, Scientific Director
Diana Gilham, Finance
Gary Dootz, Grant Administrator

Missouri

3572 Central Institute for the Deaf
825 S Taylor Ave
Saint Louis, MO 63110   314-977-0000
                                               888-444-4565
                                          Fax: 314-977-0223
                                          TTY: 314-997-0001
                                          TDD: 314-977-0037
                                   e-mail: rfeder@cid.wustl.edu
                                               www.cid.wustl.edu

Central Institute for the Deaf is a private, nonprofit institute composed of research laboratories in which scientists study the normal aspects as well as the disorders of hearing, language, and
speech; a school for children who have hearing impairments;
speech, language, and hearing clinics; and professionals with
hearing impairment, and communication sciences.

Robin Feder, Ceo

Nebraska

3573 Lied Learning and Technology Center for Ch ildhood Deafness and Vision Disorders
Boys Town National Research Hospital
555 North 30th Street
Omaha, NE 68131   402-498-6511
                                   800-448-3000
                              Fax: 402-498-1348
                              TTY: 402-498-6543
              e-mail: hotline@girlsandboystown.org
                        www.boystown.org/chlc

A not-for-profit corporation closely affiliated with the Boys Town National Research Hospital. The center houses Model Childhood Education Classrooms, a Cochlear Implant Clinic and Research Center, Educational Media Production Studios, Distance Learning and Family Outreach Center, Hearing and Vision Laboratories, Bio-informatics and Computer Center and a Communication Technology Development Center.

Patrick E Brookhouser MD, President
John K. Arch, Executive VP
Edward M. Kolb, Medical Director

New York

3574 Montifiore Medical Center
2475 St. Raymonds Avenue
Bronx, NY 10461   718-430-7300
                                   800-636-6683
                              Fax: 718-741-2033
                  e-mail: ruben@aecom.vu.edu
                             www.montefiore.org

Provides diagnosis, treatment and research of diseases of the ear, nose and throat.

Steven M. Safyer, MD, President/Chief Executive Officer
Philip O. Ozuah, MD, PhD, Executive Vice President/Chief Oper
Joel A. Perlman, Executive Vice President/Chief Fina

3575 State University College at Plattsburgh Auditory Research Laboratory
101 Broad Street
Plattsburgh, NY 12901   518-564-2040
                                   888-673-0012
                              Fax: 518-564-2045
              e-mail: hamernrp@plattsburgh.edu
                          www.plattsburgh.edu

The Auditory Research Laboratory (ARL) is home to several laboratories, including acoustics lab, anatomy lab, auditory evoked potential lab, and otoacoustic emissions lab. Facilities include: acoustics and vibrations laboratory, otoacoustic emmissions laboratory, middle ear analysis laboratory, auditory evoked potential laboratory, and cochlear anatomy laborator.

Roger Hamernik, MD, Director

3576 Syracuse University, Institute for Sensory Research
621 Skytop Road, PO Box 5290
Syracuse, NY 13244   315-443-4164
                              Fax: 315-443-1184
                    e-mail: rlsmith@syr.edu
                             www.isr.syr.edu

Research center dedicated to the discovery and application of knowledge of the sensory systems. Integration of engineering, life, and physical sciences, combining rigorous experimental methodology with mathematical analysis is stressed.

Robert Smith, MD, Director

Oregon

3577 Oregon Health Sciences University Research Center
3181 SW Sam Jackson Park Road, PO Box 3098
Portland, OR 97239   503-494-8311
                              Fax: 503-494-5656
              e-mail: contact@ohsuhealth.com
                          www.ohsuhealth.com

OSHU blends education, research, patient care and community outreach into one shared mission: to improve the well-being of people in Oregon and beyond. They incorporate the latest medical research, technology and innovation.

Michael Heinrich

Pennsylvania

3578 Temple University, Section of Auditory Research
1801 N. Broad Street
Philadelphia, PA 19122   215-707-3663
                              Fax: 215-707-7523
                  e-mail: anita@ent.temple.edu
                               www.temple.edu

The Auditory Research Section includes the Garfied Auditory Research Laboratory, the Hearing Science Research Program and the Electrophysiology Progject.

Anita Cilea, Departmental Administrator
Kate Haney, Financial Administrator
Neil D. Theobald, President

Tennessee

3579 Bill Wilkerson Center
1211 Medical Center Drive
Nashville, TN 37232   615-322-5000
                              Fax: 615-936-5013
            e-mail: kate.carney@vanderbilt.edu
                          www.mc.vanderbilt.edu

The Vanderbilt Bill Wilkerson Center for Otolaryngology and Communication Sciences is dedicated to serving persons with diseases of the ear, nose, throat, head and neck, and hearing, speech, language and related disorders.

Robert H Ossoff DMD MD, Director
Fred H Bess PhD, Associate Director

Texas

3580 Houston Ear Research Foundation
7737 SW Freeway, Suite 630
Houston, TX 77074   713-771-9966
                                   800-843-0807
                              Fax: 713-771-0546
                              TTY: 800-843-0807
              e-mail: info@houstoncochlear.org
                          www.houstoncochlear.org

The Foundation was incorporated in August, 1983 as a center to provide excellence in service dedicated to the cochlear implant.

Jan Gilden, Executive Director

Conferences

3581 AADB National Symposium
American Association of the Deaf-Blind
8630 Fenton Street, Suite 121
Silver Spring, MD 20910   301-495-4403
                              Fax: 301-495-4404
                              TTY: 301-495-4402
                  e-mail: aadb-info@aadb.org
                                 www.aadb.org

The symposium offers a training workshop, keynote speakers, full day exhibit hall, demonstration room, awards lunch and ceremony, talent show, Walk-A-Thon, and a banquet and dance.

Jill Gaus, President
Lynn Jansen, Vice President
Debby Lieberman, Secretary

3582 AG Bell Biennial Convention
Alexander Graham Bell Association for the Deaf
3417 Volta Place NW
Washington, DC 20007
202-337-5220
800-432-7543
Fax: 202-337-8314
TTY: 202-337-5221
e-mail: info@agbell.org
www.agbell.org

June

Alexander T Graham, Executive Director

3583 ANA National Symposium Acoustic Neuroma Association
600 Peachtree Pkwy, Ste 108
Cumming, GA 30041
770-205-8211
877-200-8211
Fax: 770-205-0239
e-mail: info@anausa.org
www.anausa.org

Biennial national symposium for pre-and post-treatment acoustic neuroma patients, family members, friends and health care professionals for a weekend of educational lectures, workshops and panel discussions with acoustic neuroma medical professionals.

3584 ASCD Biennial Conference
American Society for Deaf Children
800 Florida Ave NE, Suite 2047
Washington, DC 20002
800-942-2732
Fax: 410-795-0965
e-mail: asdc@deafchildren.org
www.deafchildren.org

Provides families with five days of information and fun. Daytime workshops captivates parents while children participate in educational and recreational activities. Evening events bring families together, providing the opportunity to form new friendships and peer support.

June

Beth S Benedict, President

3585 ASHA Annual Convention
American Speech-Language-Hearing Association
2200 Research Boulevard
Rockville, MD 20850
301-897-5700
800-638-8255
Fax: 301-296-8580
TTY: 301-296-5700
e-mail: productsales@asha.org
www.asha.org

Professional education event for speech-language pathologists, audiologists, and speech, language, and hearing scientists. Provides unparalleled opportunities to hear the latest evidence-based research and gain new skills and resources to advance your career.

12,000 November

Arlene A Pietranton, Executive Director

3586 Cued Speech Conference
National Cued Speech Association
1300 Pennsylvania Avenue
Washington, DC 20004
800-459-3529
e-mail: info@cuedspeech.org
www.cuedspeech.org

3587 IHS Annual Convention & Expo
International Hearing Society
16880 Middlebelt Road, Suite 4
Livonia, MI 48154
734-522-7200
800-521-5247
Fax: 734-522-0200
e-mail: chelms@ihsinfo.org
www.ihsinfo.org

September

Kathleen Mennillo, Executive Director

3588 NAD Biennial Conference
National Association of the Deaf
8630 Fention Street, Suite 820
Silver Spring, MD 20910
301-587-1788
Fax: 301-587-1791
TTY: 301-587-1789
e-mail: nadinfo@nad.org
www.nad.org

Held in the even numbered years, brings together deaf,hard of hearing, late-deafened, deaf-blind and hearing consumers, parents, youth, professionals, educators, organizational and corporate representatives for professional development, enrichment, training, networking, governance meetings, exhibits, receptions, and related evening.

2,000 July

Bobbie Beth Scoggins, President

Audio Video

3589 50th Anniversary Collection
Harris Communications
15155 Technology Drive
Eden Prairie, MN 55344
952-906-1180
800-825-6758
Fax: 952-906-1099
TTY: 800-825-9187
e-mail: info@harriscomm.com
www.harriscomm.com

Stories: A picture for Harold's Room; Corduroy; Danny and the Dinosaur; Harry the Dirty Dog; Click, clack moo, Cows that type. DVD-R, voiced; signed in ASL, no captions.

3590 A Few Errands
Modern Sign Press
10443 Los Alamitos Boulevard, PO Box 1181
Los Alamitos, CA 90720
562-596-8548
800-572-7332
Fax: 562-795-6614
TTY: 562-493-4168
e-mail: modsigns@modernsignspress.com
www.modernsignspress.com

Basic level videotape of signed story for Expressive and Receptive practice. Story is repeated three times for ease of use. Watch how the visual features are incorporated. Turn the sound off for receptive practice. Written script and tape use suggestions included. VHS

Esther Zawolkow, President

3591 A Lesson With Heart
American Sign Language Productions
4450 La Crosse Ave
San Diego, CA 92117
952-906-1180
800-767-4461
Fax: 952-906-1099
TTY: 952-906-1198
e-mail: SignEnhancers@iCloud.com
www.signenhancers.com

A skilled 4th grade teacher presents a lesson on Anatomy including the respiratory system, digestive system, and the heart that will increase your familiarity with this vocabulary and content. Improve your interpreting skills for this subject matter and grade level by accepting this assignment. You won't be alone...we provide two interpreters to demonstrate it for your. 55 minutes. DVD - $59.95; VHS - 49.95

3592 A Mother's Persepctive on the IEP Process
American Sign Language Productions
4450 La Crosse Ave
San Diego, CA 92117
952-906-1180
800-767-4461
Fax: 952-906-1099
TTY: 952-906-1198
e-mail: SignEnhancers@iCloud.com
www.signenhancers.com

Maxine Camvel is a parent of a Deaf daughter wanting to make it easier for other parents. She gives valuable insight into how to advocate for your children by maximizing parent input to the Individualized Education Plan (IEP) process. This program also provides an opportunity to interpret vocabulary and emotional content commonly expressed by parents. Your two team interpreters demonstrate how to interpret this sample. 1 hour. DVD - $59.95; VHS - $49.95

3593 A is for Access: Creating Full & Interacti ve Access for Students
Hands and Voices
PO Box 3093
Boulder, CO 80307   303-492-6283
                                                   866-422-0422
                   e-mail: parentadvocate@handsandvoices.org
                                   www.handsandvoices.org

This video is a source to generate greater awareness of communication access issues for students who are deaf or hard of hearing. DVD or VHS, captioned.

3594 ABC Stories DVD
Sign Media
4020 Blackburn Lane
Burtonsville, MD 20866   301-421-0268
                                                   800-475-4756
                                              Fax: 301-421-0270
                              e-mail: info@signmedia.com
                                           www.signmedia.com

You will marvel at the skill of these Deaf performers as they use every letter of the manual alphabet, in sequence, to tell a story. To capture the creativity and genius of the stories, the videotape uses slow motion and graphic displays. 1 hour

3595 ABCs of AVT: Analyzing Auditory-Verbal Therapy
Alexander Graham Bell Association for the Deaf
3417 Volta Place NW
Washington, DC 20007   202-337-5220
                                                   800-432-7543
                                              Fax: 202-337-8314
                                              TTY: 202-337-5221
                                  e-mail: info@agbell.org
                              listeningandspokenlanguage.org

An Educational Tool for Professionals. Developed for use in university classrooms and training environments; provides an overview of Auditory-Verbal techniques and guidance on appropriate intervention for children experiencing difficulties with language development.
2005 104 pages 46 Minute video
Warren Estabrooks MEd, Author
Rhonda Schwartz MA, Co-Author
Lisa Chutjian, Chief Development Officer

3596 ASL Stories: Christmas Stories
Harris Communications
15155 Technology Drive
Eden Prairie, MN 55344   952-906-1180
                                                   800-825-6758
                                              Fax: 952-906-1099
                                              TTY: 800-825-9187
                              e-mail: info@harriscomm.com
                                           www.harriscomm.com

This video is one in a collection of videotapes featuring classic fairy tales signed by Deaf storytellers, and is a wonderful way to get into the spirit of Christmas. This video also makes a welcome gift. Stories include: The Night Before Christmas, A Christmas Carol, The First Christmas Tree, The Birth of Christ, In the Great Walled City, and The Little Match Girl. For ages 10 and over. VHS: 80 minutes; signed in ASL; no captions; voice over.

3597 ASL Stories: Fairy Tales I
Harris Communications
15155 Technology Drive
Eden Prairie, MN 55344   952-906-1180
                                                   800-825-6758
                                              Fax: 952-906-1099
                                              TTY: 800-825-9187
                              e-mail: info@harriscomm.com
                                           www.harriscomm.com

This video is one of a collection of videotapes featuring classic fairy tales signed by Deaf storytellers. Stories include Rapunzel, Snow White and Rose Red, The Frog Prince, Hansel and Gretel, and The Brave Little Tailor. For ages 10 and over. VHS: 114 minutes; signed in ASL; no captions; voice-over.

3598 ASL Stories: Fairy Tales II
Harris Communications
15155 Technology Drive
Eden Prairie, MN 55344   952-906-1180
                                                   800-825-6758
                                              Fax: 952-906-1099
                                              TTY: 800-825-9187
                              e-mail: info@harriscomm.com
                                           www.harriscomm.com

This video is one of a collection of videotapes featuring classic fairy tales signed by Deaf storytellers. Stories include Sleeping Beauty, The Golden Goose, Little Red Riding Hood, The Princess and the Pea, and The Tinder Box. For ages 10 and over. VHS: 83 minutes; signed in ASL; no captions; voice-over.

3599 Acoustics, Audition and Speech Reception
Daniel Lind OC, PhD, author
Alexander Graham Bell Association for the Deaf
3417 Volta Place NW
Washington, DC 20007   202-337-5220
                                                   202-337-8314
                                              Fax: 202-337-8314
                                              TTY: 203-337-5221
                                  e-mail: info@agbell.org
                              listeningandspokenlanguage.org

This videotape of four professionals provides viewers with an overview of the properties of speech and the ways children can get the most from their hearing aids or cochlear implants. The tape is a practical how-to guide in which team members demonstrate how speech sounds are created in the vocal tract, how distance affects the intensity of spoken language and how patterns are distorted by profound hearing loss.
Lisa Chutjian, Chief Development Officer
Emilio Alonso-Mendoza, Chief Executive Officer
Judy Harrison, Director of Programs

3600 American Sign Language Handshape Dictionar y DVD
Gallaudet University Press
800 Florida Avenue NE
Washington, DC 20002   202-651-5448
                                              Fax: 202-651-5489
                                              TTY: 202-651-5444
                              e-mail: gupress@gallaudet.edu
                                           gupress.gallaudet.edu

A perfect complement to the dictionary, this new DVD features a diverse cast of native signers forming more than 1,400 ASL signs organized by 40 basic handshapes, with a complete list of English glosses and synonyms for each sign.
Richard Tennant, Co-Producer
Marianne Gluszak Brown, Co-Producer

3601 American Sign Language Video Series
DeBee Communications/TJ Publishers
P.O. Box 702701
Dallas, TX 75370   972-416-0800
                                                   800-999-1168
                                              Fax: 972-416-0944
                                              TTY: 972-416-0933
                       e-mail: customerservice@tjpublishers.com
              https://www388.safesecureweb.com/tjpublishers/store/

Learning ASL with the Deaf Robinson family. The family acts out scenes that occur in everyday life in this videotape series. Each situation is reviewed in an ASL classroom with a deaf teacher. This series also includes sections on Deaf culture and grammar, rounding off a complete and effective instructional tool. Work Day-VHS-90 minutes, School Day-VHS-90 minutes, Shopping-VHS-90 minutes, Softball Game-VHS-90 minutes. $39.95 each

3602   American Sign Language: Green Books Text a nd Tapes
Sign Media
4020 Blackburn Lane
Burtonsville, MD 20866
301-421-0268
800-475-4756
Fax: 301-421-0270
e-mail: info@signmedia.com
www.signmedia.com

The classic ASL series. This unique set of texts, written by Dennis Cokely and Charlotte Baker-Shenk, is complimented by DVDs. The DVDs explain difficult concepts and offer practice situations to improve your sign language skills. The series may be ordered as a complete set of books and DVDs, a complete set of DVDs only, individual books and DVDs, or a specific DVD and book combination set. Individual DVD $44.95, DVD set & books $379.95, DVD set $233.95

3603   Ancient Greece
American Sign Language Productions
4450 La Crosse Ave
San Diego, CA 92117
952-906-1180
800-767-4461
Fax: 952-906-1099
TTY: 952-906-1198
e-mail: SignEnhancers@iCloud.com
www.signenhancers.com

We often think about interpreting for Deaf children, but often need to understand the speech and thought patterns of their hearing classmates. Krisjana is a hearing child presenting a report on Ancient Greece. A great way to practice with vocabulary from the classroom before you have to sit in the hot seat. Is it all Greek to you? No need to worry. Two interpreters will show you how. 30 minutes. DVD - $59.95; VHS - $49.95

3604   Animals, Insects, School, Colors Spanish/E nglish Videos
Modern Signs Press
10443 Los Alamitos Boulevard, PO Box 1181
Los Alamitos, CA 90720
562-596-8548
800-572-7332
Fax: 562-795-6614
TTY: 562-493-4168
e-mail: modsigns@modernsignspress.com
www.modernsignspress.com

Entertaining sign language instructional videos in Spanish and English. Great tool to help bridge the gap between Spanish, English and Sign Language. The videos have a split screen - Connie and Merced teach you the sign and say the word in both Spanish and English. Vocabulary words are used in sentences to reinforce the signs. There are graphics showing the vocabulary they are reviewing. 10 titles available, either alone or in a complete package.

Esther Zawolkow, President

3605   Art Show
Modern Sign Press
10443 Los Alamitos Boulevard, PO Box 1181
Los Alamitos, CA 90720
562-596-8548
800-572-7332
Fax: 562-795-6614
TTY: 562-493-4168
e-mail: modsigns@modernsignspress.com
www.modernsignspress.com

Basic level videotape of signed story for Expressive and Receptive practice. Story is repeated three times for ease of use. Watch how the visual features are incorporated. Turn the sound off for receptive practice. Written script and tape use suggestions included. VHS

Esther Zawolkow, President

3606   Baby See 'n Sign
Harris Communications
15155 Technology Drive
Eden Prairie, MN 55344
952-906-1180
800-825-6758
Fax: 952-906-1099
TTY: 800-825-9187
e-mail: info@harriscomm.com
www.harriscomm.com

Features American Sign Language signs and real-life images in full color. They may be used as an educational tool for effectively promoting communication with people who are autistic, have Down Syndrome, or are ESL. For parents who have decided to sign to their children, this is a great video. Over 60 basic American Sign Language signs and real-life images are presented in full-color, making it enjoyable for parents and children to watch. A parental question and answer guide is included.

6 months + DVD 45 minutes

3607   Baby See 'n Sign II
Harris Communications
15155 Technology Drive
Eden Prairie, MN 55344
952-906-1180
800-825-6758
Fax: 952-906-1099
TTY: 800-825-9187
e-mail: info@harriscomm.com
www.harriscomm.com

This DVD shows over 100 real-life images that relate to your child's daily life, including animals, foods, toys and activities. Volume II has beginning abstract concepts and continues with object-word association. It is never too late to begin signing. Ages 6 months and up. DVD: 50 minutes.

3608   Baby Signing Time
Harris Communications
15155 Technology Drive
Eden Prairie, MN 55344
952-906-1180
800-825-6758
Fax: 952-906-1099
TTY: 800-825-9187
e-mail: info@harriscomm.com
www.harriscomm.com

Designed specifically for babies 3-36 months old, the DVD combines sign-along songs, playful animation and the positive reinforcement of signing babies - who are all ages 2 and under - to teach you and your baby to sign the easy way. Baby Signing Time sets your baby's day to music as you learn sign and sogns for everyday events in baby's life - eating, family, pets and more.

3609   Baby Signing Time DVD 2
Harris Communications
15155 Technology Drive
Eden Prairie, MN 55344
952-906-1180
800-825-6758
Fax: 952-906-1099
TTY: 800-825-9187
e-mail: info@harriscomm.com
www.harriscomm.com

This video sets your baby's day to music as you learn signs and sogns for everyday events in baby's life - eating, family, pets and more. Designed specifically for babies 3-36 months old, this DVD combines sign-along songs, playful animation and the positive reinforcement of signing babies - who are all ages 2 and under - to teach you and your baby to sign the easy way.

3610   Bachelor Father
Modern Sign Press
10443 Los Alamitos Boulevard, PO Box 1181
Los Alamitos, CA 90720
562-596-8548
800-572-7332
Fax: 562-795-6614
TTY: 562-493-4168
e-mail: modsigns@modernsignspress.com
www.modernsignspress.com

Basic level videotape of signed story for Expressive and Receptive practice. Story is repeated three times for ease of use. Watch how the visual features are incorporated. Turn the sound off for receptive practice. Written script and tape use suggestions included. VHS

Esther Zawolkow, President

32 pages Hardcover

3803 Medical Sign Language: Easily Understood D efinitions of Commonly Used Medical Term

W Joseph Garcia, author

Charles C Thomas Publishers
2600 South First Street
Springfield, IL 62704   217-789-8980
                                                          800-258-8980
                                        e-mail: books@ccthomas.com
                                                  www.ccthomas.com

In this glossary, a multitude of medical and dental terms are accurately defined and precisely translated, through description and illustration, into American Sign Language. The book easily lends itself to use at both ends of the chain of communication that links health care professionals with their deaf patients. Includes bibliography. Comes in both hardcover and softcover

726 pages

3804 Messy Monsters Jungle Joggers and Bubble B aths

Nehama Pluznik and Rochelle Sobel, author

Alexander Graham Bell Association for the Deaf
3417 Volta Place NW
Washington, DC 20007   202-337-5220
                                               Fax: 202-337-8314
                                               TTY: 202-337-5221
                                          e-mail: info@agbell.org
                                                    www.agbell.org

An illustrated book of poetry for children with hearing loss. Poems are organized according to the accepted group of speechreading phonemes which are classified by their appearance on the lips. Each poem emphasizes a particular phoneme which appears in the initial, medial, or final position of the word. Four worksheets accompany each poem: About the poem, Tell me more, Speech practice, and Language activities.

97 pages Softcover

3805 Nursery Rhymes from Mother Goose: Told in Signed English

Harry Bornstein and Karen L Saulnier, author

Gallaudet University Press
800 Florida Avenue NE
Washington, DC 20002   202-651-5488
                                               Fax: 202-651-5489
                                       e-mail: gupress@gallaudet.edu
                                               www.gupress.gallaudet.edu

More than a dozen favorite nursery rhymes are presented in this unique edition of Mother Goose. All of the rhymes are illustrated with full-color paintings accompanied by more than 389 drawings showing the verses in Signed English. Young readers, both hearing and deaf, will learn the special charm of rhyme while also discovering new vocabulary and new ways to experience English through signing. As they learn and memorize their favorite verses, children will also strengthen their language skills.

64 pages Hardcover
ISBN: 0-930323-99-8

3806 Operation SHHH

Self Help for Hard-of-Hearing People
7910 Woodmont Avenue, Suite 1200
Bethesda, MD 20814   301-657-2248
                                               Fax: 301-913-9413
                                               TTY: 301-657-2249
                                        e-mail: info@hearingloss.org
                                                 www.hearingloss.org

Features SHHHerman, the lion who does not roar. This program is designed for elementary school children. Includes video, posters, brochures and more.

Barbara Kelley, Editor-In-Chief
Brenda Battat, Executive Director

3807 Opposites

HEAR-MORE
42 Executive Boulevard
Farmingdale, NY 11735   800-881-4327
                                               Fax: 631-752-0689
                                               TTY: 800-281-4327
                                                   www.hearmore.com

The Early Sign Language Series: A fascinating and enjoyable way for children and adults to learn sign language. Opposites presents the early concepts of opposite relationships. It fosters both recptive and expressive language through signs and pictures, and it is perfect for young children whether hearing impaired, hearing, pre-verbal or verbal. Reviews 10 opposite items (20 in total).

3808 Out for a Walk: Baby's First Sign Book

Kim Votry and Curt Waller, author

Gallaudet University Press
800 Florida Avenue NE
Washington, DC 20002   202-651-5488
                                               Fax: 202-651-5489
                                       e-mail: gupress@gallaudet.edu
                                               www.gupress.gallaudet.edu

Offers toddlers their first look at signs for the world around them. As they follow our distinctively hatted youngster on a stroll, they encounter familiar animals and insect, among them a dog, cat, butterfly, and squirrel, and learn which ones can be pets. They'll enjoy imaginative images of senses, too - sight, smell, hearing, taste, and touch.

16 pages Board Book
ISBN: 1-563681-46-3

3809 Parent's Guide to Chochlear Implants

Patricia M Chute and Mary Ellen Nevins, author

Gallaudet University Press
800 Florida Avenue NE
Washington, DC 20002   202-651-5488
                                               Fax: 202-651-5489
                                       e-mail: gupress@gallaudet.edu
                                               www.gupress.gallaudet.edu

Now, parents of deaf children have at hand a complete guide to the process of cochlear implantation. It explains in a friendly easy-to-follow style each stage of the process. Parents will discover how to have their child evaluated to determine his or her suitability for an implant. They'll learn about implant device options, how to choose an implant center, and every detail of the surgical procedure. The initial 'switch-on' is described along with counseling about device maintainance.

208 pages Softcover
ISBN: 1-563681-29-3

3810 Parents and Their Deaf Children: The Early Years

Gallaudet University Press
800 Florida Avenue NE
Washington, DC 20002   202-651-5488
                                               Fax: 202-651-5489
                                       e-mail: gupress@gallaudet.edu
                                               http://gupress.gallaudet.edu

This book stems from a nationwide survey of parents with 6-7 year old deaf or hard of hearing children, followed up by interviews with 80 parents. The authors not only discuss the parents' communication choices for their children, but also provide how parents' experiences differ, especially for those whose children are hard of hearing, have additional conditions, or have cochlear implants. One chapter is devoted to minority cultures. Includes tables, figures, references and index.

272 pages Hardcover
ISBN: 1-563681-37-4

Kathryn P Meadow-Orlans, Co-Author
Donna M Mertens, Co-Author
Marilyn S Sass-Lehrer, Co-Author

3811 Police Officer Jones
HEAR-MORE
42 Executive Boulevard
Farmingdale, NY 11735

800-881-4327
Fax: 631-752-0689
TTY: 800-281-4327
www.hearmore.com

This beginning book describes a police officer and his exciting job. Use the signs when reading the book to your child and speak when you sign so the child will learn to associate the sign with sound and lip shape.

3812 Religious Signing: A Comprehensive Guide f or All Faiths
Elaine Costello, author

TJ Publishers
P.O Box 702701
Dallas, TX 75370

972-416-0800
800-999-1168
Fax: 972-416-0944
TTY: 972-416-0933
e-mail: customerservice@tjpublishers.com
www.tjpublishers.com

Contains over 500 religious signs and their meanings for all denominations. Clearly demonstrated and defined through illustrations that show movement of hands, body and face. Includes a special section on favorite verses, prayers and blessings.

219 pages Softcover
ISBN: 0-553342-44-4

3813 Rhode Island Test of Language Structure RITLS
Pro Ed
8700 Shoal Creed Boulevard
Austin, TX 78757

512-451-3246
800-897-3202
Fax: 800-397-7633
e-mail: info@proedinc.com
www.proedinc.com

The Rhode Island Test of Language Structure (RITLS) provides a measure of English language development and assessment data. It is designed primarily for use with children who are hearing impaired, but also useful in other areas where level of language development is of concern, including mental retardation, learning disability, and bilingual programs. The RITLS focuses on syntax, unlike other tests compared with other reading, language, intelligence, and achievement tests frequently used.

1983

3814 Schedules of Development for Hearing Impaired Infants and Their Parents
Alexander Graham Bell Association for the Deaf
3417 Volta Place NW
Washington, DC 20007

202-337-5220
Fax: 202-337-8314
TTY: 202-337-5221
e-mail: info@agbell.org
www.agbell.org

Written for parents and teachers, this assessment record of verbal learning will help to evaluate each child's language development.

1977 14 pages
Agnes Ling Philips PhD, Author

3815 Screening for Hearing Loss and Otitis Medi a in Children
Jackson Roush PhD, author

Alexander Graham Bell Association for the Deaf
3417 Volta Place NW
Washington, DC 20007

202-337-5220
Fax: 202-337-8314
TTY: 202-337-5221
e-mail: info@agbell.org
www.agbell.org

Provides a concise yet comprehensive guide to hearing and middle ear screening in children. From acoustic emissions and automated ABR in newborns to hearing screening of school-age children.

245 pages Softcover

3816 Sign Language for Babies
Walter Paul Kelly, author

Harris Communications
15155 Technology Drive
Eden Prairie, MN 55344

952-906-1180
800-825-6758
Fax: 952-906-1099
TTY: 800-825-9187
e-mail: info@harriscomm.com
www.harriscomm.com

A black and white illustrated story on how love and eventually the ILY handsign in American Sign Language got started.
Hardcover

3817 Sign Numbers
Nancy Bartusch, author

Modern Signs Press
PO Box 1181
Los Alamitos, CA 90720

562-596-8548
800-572-7332
Fax: 562-795-6614
TTY: 562-493-4168
e-mail: modsigns@modernsignspress.com
www.modernsignspress.com

Mandy helps Handy teach manual and written numbers. Includes printed numbers and easy-to-follow drawings of the number hand shapes. Also shows words and signs for the objects counted in a picture on each page. Black and white drawings make this a coloring book, too.

60 pages

3818 Sign With Kids Supplement
Modern Signs Press
PO Box 1181
Los Alamitos, CA 90720

562-596-8548
800-572-7332
Fax: 562-795-6614
TTY: 562-493-4168
e-mail: modsigns@modernsignspress.com
www.modernsignspress.com

The supplement contains easy to use illustrations for all the signs in every lesson of Sign With Kids. Both volumes together provide a comprehensive program for teaching sign language to hearing kids.

3819 Sign-Me-Fine
Gallaudet University Press
800 Florida Avenue NE
Washington, DC 20002

202-651-5488
Fax: 202-651-5489
TTY: 202-651-5488
e-mail: gupress@gallaudet.edu
www.gupress.gallaudet.edu

Written for young adults, this book introduces American Sign Language and how it differs from English.

1997 120 pages paperback
ISBN: 0-930323-76-9

3820 Signing Exact English Using Affixes
Modern Signs Press
PO Box 1181
Los Alamitos, CA 90720

562-596-8548
800-572-7332
Fax: 562-795-6614
TTY: 562-493-4168
e-mail: modsigns@modernsignspress.com
www.modernsignspress.com

A catalog of signed vocabulary extended by prefixes, suffixes, contractions and tenses.

3821 **Signing Family: What Every Parent Should K now About Sign Communication**

David A Stewart and Barbara Leutke-Stahlman, author

Gallaudet University Press
800 Florida Avenue NE
Washington, DC 20002
202-651-5488
Fax: 202-651-5489
e-mail: gupress@gallaudet.edu
www.gupress.gallaudet.edu

Parents of deaf children concerned with finding the best means of communication for their family will welcome the straightforward, reader-friendly information in this book. In a style both positive and pragmatic, the authors employ common-sense reasoning to establish the importance of teach deaf children language fundamentals as early as possible. This essential book for parents continues by explaining why the visual-gestural nature of signing is generally the best langue mode for deaf children

192 pages Softcover
ISBN: 1-563680-69-6

3822 **Signing Fun: American Sign Language Vocabu lary, Phrases, Games and Activities**

Penny Warner and Paula Gray, author

Gallaudet University Press
800 Florida Avenue NE
Washington, DC 20002
202-651-5488
Fax: 202-651-5489
e-mail: gupress@gallaudet.edu
www.gupress.gallaudet.edu

For young adults age 11 and up. Signing is visual, easy to learn, and fun to use. Offers 441 useful signs on a variety of favorite topics: activities, animals, fashion, food, holidays, home, out-doors, parties, people, places, play, emotions, school, shopping, travel, plus extra fun signs for especially popular words. Each chapter includes practice sentences using everyday phrases to help new signers learn in a fun way. Provides dozens of entertaining games and activities.

192 pages Softcover
ISBN: 1-563629-23-6

3823 **Signing: How to Speak With Your Hands, Sec ond Edition**

Elaine Costello, author

TJ Publishers
P.O Box 702701
Dallas, TX 75370
972-416-0800
800-999-1168
Fax: 972-416-0944
TTY: 972-416-0933
e-mail: customerservice@tjpublishers.com
www.tjpublishers.com

This book presents more than 1300 signs and their descriptions. Linguistic principles are described at the beginning of each chapter giving insight into the rules which govern American Sign Language.

248 pages Softcover
ISBN: 0-553375-39-3

3824 **Signs for Me**

Ben Bahan and Joe Dannis, author

Harris Communications
15155 Technology Drive
Eden Prairie, MN 55344
952-906-1180
800-825-6758
Fax: 952-906-1099
TTY: 800-825-9187
e-mail: info@harriscomm.com
www.harriscomm.com

Ideal for youngsters and other sign language beginners, a unique illustrated approach to presenting basic vocabulary. While the book provides a multidimensional sign vocabulary for pre-school and elementary school children, its appealing format makes it suitable for signers of all ages.

111 pages Softcover

3825 **Signs for Me: Basic Sign Vocabulary for Ch ildren, Parents and Teachers**

Ben Bahan and Joe Dannis, author

TJ Publishers
P.O Box 702701
Dallas, TX 75370
972-416-0800
800-999-1168
Fax: 972-416-0944
TTY: 972-416-0933
e-mail: customerservice@tjpublishers.com
www.tjpublishers.com

Sign language vocabulary for preschool and elementary school children introduces household items, animals, family members, actions, emotions, safety concerns and other concepts. Over 300 vocabulary words, pictures and sign illustrations.

112 pages Softcover
ISBN: 0-915035-27-8

3826 **Signs of Sharing: An Elementary Sign Language and Deaf Awareness Curriculum**

Charles C Thomas Publisher
2600 S 1st Street
Springfield, IL 62704
217-789-8980
800-258-8980
Fax: 217-789-9130
e-mail: books@ccthomas.com
www.ccthomas.com

A unique set of materials that provides educators whose responsi-bilities include the integration of hearing-impaired children, with a multifaceted tool to teach sign language and deaf awareness.

1993 380 pages
ISBN: 0-398058-51-2

Sue F V Rakow, Co-Author
Carol B Carpenter, Co-Author

3827 **Silent Garden**

Paul W Ogden, author

Gallaudet University Press
800 Florida Avenue NE
Washington, DC 20002
202-651-5488
Fax: 202-651-5489
e-mail: gupress@gallaudet.edu
www.gupress.gallaudet.edu

This completely rewritten edition presents parents of deaf chil-dren with more crucial information enhanced by the advances made in the general understanding of what it means to be deaf and the greater possibilities afforded deaf children today. Pro-vides parents with a firm foundation for making the difficult de-cisions necessary to begin their child on the road to realizing his or her full potential.

304 pages Softcover
ISBN: 1-563680-58-0

3828 **Silent Observer**

Christy MacKinnon, author

Gallaudet University Press
800 Florida Avenue NE
Washington, DC 20002
202-651-5488
Fax: 202-651-5489
e-mail: gupress@gallaudet.edu
www.gupress.gallaudet.edu

An affectionage, poignant memoir of childhood as seen through the eyes of a vivacious young girl. Teachers, parents, and chil-dren will share in their enjoyment of this beautiful, sensitive story of a harder but wonderful time that has passed.

48 pages Hardcover
ISBN: 1-563680-22-X

3829 Simple Signs

Cindy Wheeler, author

Harris Communications
15155 Technology Drive
Eden Prairie, MN 55344
        952-906-1180
        800-825-6758
        Fax: 952-906-1099
        TTY: 800-825-9187
        e-mail: info@harriscomm.com
        www.harriscomm.com

Children have a lot to say, whether through gestures, movement, pictures or words. American Sign Language incorporates all these natural skills. With pictures, clear diagrams, and hints, learn from these 28 signs. Ages 3-6 years.

30 pages Softcover

3830 Six-Sound Song

Warren Estabrooks MEd, author

Alexander Graham Bell Association for the Deaf
3417 Volta Place NW
Washington, DC 20007
        202-337-5220
        Fax: 202-337-8314
        TTY: 202-337-5221
        e-mail: info@agbell.org
        www.agbell.org

Based on the Six-Sound Tests developed by the late Daniel Ling, PhD. Used for both individual and group therapy sessions in auditory and oral environments. Children will enjoy the illustrations created by seven-year-old Hunter Jackson who received his cochlear implant while the Auditory-Verbal Centre of the Learning to Listen Foundation. Hardcover Book and CD set

3831 Songs in Sign

S Harold Collins, author

TJ Publishers
P.O Box 702701
Dallas, TX 75370
        972-416-0800
        800-999-1168
        Fax: 972-416-0944
        TTY: 972-416-0933
        e-mail: customerservice@tjpublishers.com
        www.tjpublishers.com

Presents six songs in Signed English. The easy-to-follow illustrations enable you to sign: Twinkle, Twinkle Litt Star; The Mullberry Bush; Row, Row, Row Your Boat; If You're Happy; Bingo and The Muffin Man.

16 pages Softcover
ISBN: 0-931993-71-7

3832 Speak to Me (Second Edition)

Marcia Calhoun Forecki, author

Gallaudet University Press
800 Florida Avenue NE
Washington, DC 20002
        202-651-5488
        Fax: 202-651-5489
        e-mail: gupress@gallaudet.edu
        www.gupress.gallaudet.edu

An engrossing, personal account of life with Charlie, an adorable, active, deaf seven-year-old. The story of an ordinary person confronted with an overwhelming reality - the fact that her son is deaf. Forecki's struggle as a single parent to care for her child, to find the right schools, and to establish communication with her son will strike a familiar chord in all hearing parents of deaf children. All readers will be touched by the mixture of pathos and humor in this account.

154 pages Softcover
ISBN: 0-930323-68-8

3833 Speech and the Hearing Impaired Child (Second Edition)

Daniel Ling, PhD, author

Alexander Graham Bell Association for the Deaf
3417 Volta Place NW
Washington, DC 20007
        202-337-5220
        Fax: 202-337-8314
        TTY: 202-337-5221
        e-mail: info@agbell.org
        www.agbell.org

An extension of the original text published by the late Daniel Ling in 1976. It looks much more closely at the development of speech in the context of spoken language. It incorporates informal strategies for promoting spoken language development that are appropriate for use with modern technology such as digital hearing aids and cochlear implants. Considerable emphasis is placed on the ongoing evaluation of speech in the context of spoken language.

440 pages Softcover

3834 Speechreading: A Way to Improve Understanding
Gallaudet University Press
800 Florida Avenue NE
Washington, DC 20002
        202-651-5488
        Fax: 202-651-5489
        TTY: 202-651-5488
        e-mail: gupress@gallaudet.edu
        www.gupress.gallaudet.edu

This useful guide for teachers and therapists approaches speechreading instruction with the help of context cues.

160 pages

3835 Student Study Guide to A Basic Course in A merican Sign Language

Frances DeCapite, author

TJ Publishers
P.O Box 702701
Dallas, TX 75370
        972-416-0800
        800-999-1168
        Fax: 972-416-0944
        TTY: 972-416-0933
        e-mail: customerservice@tjpublishers.com
        www.tjpublishers.com

Designed to supplement the text of A Basic Course in American Sign Language, the guide provides a wide array of supplemental practice materials for student and teacher. Exercises and practice sentences allow students to practice receptive and expressive skills.

197 pages Spiral bound
ISBN: 0-932666-33-7

3836 Talking Finger Series - At Grandma's House
Modern Signs Press
PO Box 1181
Los Alamitos, CA 90720
        562-596-8548
        800-572-7332
        Fax: 562-795-6614
        TTY: 562-493-4168
        e-mail: modsigns@modernsignspress.com
        www.modernsignspress.com

Pictures, signs and printed words tell the tale of April, a cuddly little rabbit who loves to play with her beloved Grandma. Uses 27-word vocabulary, includes manual alphabet and glossary of signs.

3837 Talking Finger Series - Little Green Monst er
Modern Signs Press
PO Box 1181
Los Alamitos, CA 90720
        562-596-8548
        800-572-7332
        Fax: 562-795-6614
        TTY: 562-493-4168
        e-mail: modsigns@modernsignspress.com
        www.modernsignspress.com

This storybook features Becky and Barry, two playful little bears who keep you in suspense. The 45-word vocabulary in signs and printed words introduces concept of directionality (here, there, behind, etc.). Includes manual alphabet and glossary of signs.

36 pages

3838 Teach Your Tot to Sign

Stacy A Thompson and Valerie Nelson-Metlay, author

Gallaudet University Press
800 Florida Avenue NE
Washington, DC 20002   202-651-5488
                                             Fax: 202-651-5489
                                   e-mail: gupress@gallaudet.edu
                                          www.gupress.gallaudet.edu

This book provides parents and teachers the opportunity to teach more than 500 basic American Sign Language signs to their infants, toddlers, and young children. It features fundamental signs of great appeal to young children and concise instructions on how to sign, including the critical importance of facial expression. Anticipates all of the common desires and interests of young children - food, pets, planes, trains, cars and boats, games, holidays, vegetables, family - nearly everything.

232 pages Softcover
ISBN: 1-563683-11-3

3839 The Book of Choice

Hands and Voices
PO Box 3093
Boulder, CO 80307   303-492-6283
                                                  866-422-0422
                          e-mail: parentadvocate@handsandvoices.org
                                        www.handsandvoices.org

Support for parents of a child who is deaf or hard of hearing. Also available in Spanish.

3840 The Development of Deaf Children: Academic Achievement Levels and Social Processes

Kerstin Heiling, author

Gallaudet University Press
800 Florida Avenue NE
Washington, DC 20002   202-651-5488
                                             Fax: 202-651-5489
                                   e-mail: gupress@gallaudet.edu
                                          www.gupress.gallaudet.edu

This revealing volume presents the research from a videotape study of the behavior of 20 deaf children for 14 years, and a comprehensive test at age 15 to assess their development.

280 pages Hardcover
ISBN: 3-927731-58-7

3841 The Handbook of Pediatric Audiology

Sanford E Gerber, Editor, author

Gallaudet University Press
800 Florida Avenue NE
Washington, DC 20002   202-651-5488
                                             Fax: 202-651-5489
                                   e-mail: gupress@gallaudet.edu
                                          www.gupress.gallaudet.edu

Presents 14 comprehensive chapters written by expert in each discipline. Clinicians and students now can refer to specific subjects in pediatric audiology for treating children from infancy through their elementary school years. Contributors include: Yash Pal Kapur, Franklin A. Katz, Robert J. Ruben, Allen O. Diefendorf, Judith S. Gravel, Jane R. Madell, Shlomo Silman, Carol A. Silverman, Herbert Jay Gold, and Maurice Mendel. Tables, figures, references, bibliography, author and subject index

478 pages Softcover
ISBN: 1-563680-99-7

3842 The Hearing Aid Handbook: Clinician's Guid e to Client Orientation

Donna S Wayner, author

Gallaudet University Press
800 Florida Avenue NE
Washington, DC 20002   202-651-5488
                                             Fax: 202-651-5489
                                   e-mail: gupress@gallaudet.edu
                                          www.gupress.gallaudet.edu

This handbook consists of three volumes for audiologists and other clinicians to help clients learn to use hearing aids. Planned for three classes, the guide explains exactly how to conduct the initial visit, fit ear molds, clean and maintain hearing aids and adjust amplification. Clinicians will also learn to encourage the use of visual cues, speechreading, and contextual clues to ensure a high rate of success for their clients. Users Guides feature information and worksheets.

172 pages Softcover
ISBN: 0-930323-56-4

3843 The Joy of Signing Second Edition

Lottie L Riekehof, author

TJ Publishers
P.O Box 702701
Dallas, TX 75370   972-416-0800
                                                  800-999-1168
                                             Fax: 972-416-0944
                                             TTY: 972-416-0933
                          e-mail: customerservice@tjpublishers.com
                                           www.tjpublishers.com

This popular dictionary of approximately 1500 known signs makes them easier to remember. Sentences present signs in proper context. Appendix gives information about the most effective way to add signs to spoken English.

352 pages Hardcover
ISBN: 0-882435-20-5

3844 The Listener

Warren Estabrooks, MEd, author

Alexander Graham Bell Association for the Deaf
3417 Volta Place NW
Washington, DC 20007   202-337-5220
                                             Fax: 202-337-8314
                                             TTY: 202-337-5221
                                          e-mail: info@agbell.org
                                               www.agbell.org

Subject material is centered around listening, speech, language, spoken communication, and cognitive, social and psychological development of children who are deaf or hard of hearing and their families. Articles address: Making sense of complex skills lesson planning, Morphosyntax: evidence-based AVT, Your young child's newly diagnosed hearing loss: knowing how to cope, What is Auditory-Verbal Therapy?, Teachers' perceptions of the integration of children with hearing loss.

64 pages Softcover

3845 The Night Before Christmas told in Signed english

Adapted By Harry Bornstein and Karen L Saulnier, author

Gallaudet University Press
800 Florida Avenue NE
Washington, DC 20002   202-651-5488
                                             Fax: 202-651-5489
                                   e-mail: gupress@gallaudet.edu
                                          www.gupress.gallaudet.edu

Now this wonderful, seasonal poem can be enjoyed in a new way by both hearing and deaf children. Accompanying the complete verses and full-color illustrations, line drawings show this holiday favorite in Signed English, the system that uses American Sign Language signs in English word order. Uses both rhyme and signing to help children practice their vocabulary and learn English grammar. Entertains at the same time that it teaches.

435

64 pages Hardcover
ISBN: 1-563680-20-3

Clement C Moore, Original Author

3846 The Rising of Lotus Flowers: Self-Educatin g Deaf Children in Thai Boarding Schools

Charles B Reilly and Nipapon Reilly, author

Gallaudet University Press
800 Florida Avenue NE
Washington, DC 20002   202-651-5488
                                      Fax: 202-651-5489
                              e-mail: gupress@gallaudet.edu
                              www.gupress.gallaudet.edu

In developed nations around the world, residential schools for deaf students are giving way to the trend of inclusion in regular classrooms. Nonetheless, deaf education continues to lag as students struggle to communicate. In the Bua School in Thialand, however, 400 residential deaf students ranging in age from 6 to 19 have met with great success in teaching each other Thai Sign Language and a world of knowledge once thought to be lost to them.

272 pages Hardcover
ISBN: 1-563682-75-3

3847 The Young Deaf Child

David Luterman, PhD, author

Alexander Graham Bell Association for the Deaf
3417 Volta Place NW
Washington, DC 20007   202-337-5220
                                      Fax: 202-337-8314
                                      TTY: 202-337-5221
                                   e-mail: info@agbell.org
                                          www.agbell.org

A valuable resource for audiologists, early interventionists and special educators who provide diagnostic or therapeutic services to parents of newborns and children with hearing loss. Discusses the history of deaf education in the United States and offers valuable information on the pros and cons of screening, elements essential to effective programming and therapy, a model for intervention centered on the parent-child connection, assistive hearing technologies and counseling techniques.

3848 Un Curso Basico de Lenguaje Americano de S enas
TJ Publishers
P.O Box 702701
Dallas, TX 75370   972-416-0800
                                          800-999-1168
                                      Fax: 972-416-0944
                                      TTY: 972-416-0933
                          e-mail: customerservice@tjpublishers.com
                                      www.tjpublishers.com

Features English and Spanish translations side by side. It is designed for teachers, parents and students working with Deaf Hispanic American children and adults learning English and American Sign Language.

356 pages Spiral bound
ISBN: 0-932666-35-3

3849 We Can Hear and Speak
Alexander Graham Bell Association for the Deaf
3417 Volta Place NW
Washington, DC 20007   202-337-5220
                                      Fax: 202-337-8314
                                      TTY: 202-337-5221
                                   e-mail: info@agbell.org
                                          www.agbell.org

Written by parents for families of children who are deaf or hard-of-hearing, this work describes auditory-verbal terminology and approaches and contains personal narratives written by parents and their children who are deaf or hard-of-hearing.

1998 184 pages Softcover

Carol Flexer PhD, Contributor
Catherine Richards, Contributor

3850 Winnie-the-Pooh's ABCs
HEAR-MORE
42 Executive Boulevard
Farmingdale, NY 11735   800-881-4327
                                      Fax: 631-752-0689
                                      TTY: 800-281-4327
                                          www.hearmore.com

In this special edition of Winnie-the-Pooh's ABC, both hearing and deaf children are introduced to the written and ASL alphabets, Hundred Acre Wood-Style. Inspired by A.A. Milne

32 pages

3851 Word Signs: A First Book of Sign Language

Debbie Slier, author

Gallaudet University Press
800 Florida Avenue NE
Washington, DC 20002   202-651-5488
                                      Fax: 202-651-5489
                              e-mail: gupress@gallaudet.edu
                              www.gupress.gallaudet.edu

Charming, full-cover photgraphs of basic animals plus illustrations of their corresponding signs offer children ages 1 to 4 a fun way to learn their first signs and vocabulary words.

164 pages Board book
ISBN: 1-563680-48-3

3852 You and Your Deaf Child
Gallaudet University Press
800 Florida Avenue NE
Washington, DC 20002   202-651-5488
                                      Fax: 202-651-5489
                                      TTY: 202-651-5489
                              e-mail: gupress@gallaudet.edu
                              www.gupress.gallaudet.edu

This guide for parents explores how families interact to deal with the special impact of a child who is hearing impaired.

1997 224 pages softcover
ISBN: 0-563680-60-2

3853 You and Your Deaf Child: A Self-Help Guide for Parents of Deaf and Hard of Hearing

John W Adams, author

Gallaudet University Press
800 Florida Avenue NE
Washington, DC 20002   202-651-5488
                                      Fax: 202-651-5489
                              e-mail: gupress@gallaudet.edu
                              www.gupress.gallaudet.edu

A guide for parents of deaf or hard of hearing children that explores how parents and their children interact. It examines the special impact of having a deaf child in the family. Eleven chapters focus on such topics as feelings about hearing loss, the importance of communication in the family, and effective behavior management. Many chapters contain practice activities and check their grasp of the material.

224 pages Softcover
ISBN: 1-563680-60-2

3854 Young Deaf Child
Alexander Graham Bell Association for the Deaf
3417 Volta Place NW
Washington, DC 20007   202-337-5220
                                      Fax: 202-337-8314
                                      TTY: 202-337-5221
                                   e-mail: info@agbell.org
                                          www.agbell.org

With a foreward by Mark Ross, Ph.D., this book is based on experience by the three authors and outlines the best approach for the child, early intervention, maximization of technology and strong family involvment.

1999 235 pages

David Luterman PhD, Author

Magazines

3855 Auditory - Verbal International
2121 Eisenhower Avenue, Suite 402
Alexandria, VA 22314
703-739-1049
Fax: 703-739-0395
TTY: 703-739-0874
e-mail: audiverb@aol.com

Magazine of the organization dedicated to helping children who have hearing losses learn to listen and speak. Promotes the Auditory-Verbal Therapy approach, which is based on the belief that the overwhelming majority of these children can hear and talk by using their residual hearing and hearing aids. Membership dues for Canada are $55, International, $60, US $50, and students are charged $30.

Quarterly

Sara Lake, Executive Director/CEO
Mary Benson, Executive Assistant

3856 Deaf Life
c/o MSM Productions, LTD
1095 Meigs Street
Rochester, NY 14620
716-442-6370
Fax: 716-442-6371
TTY: 716-442-6370
e-mail: deaflife@deaflife.com
www.deaflife.com

This magazine focuses on profiles, news, controversial issues, cultural topics and more relating to the deaf community, first published in 1988.

64 pages Monthly
ISSN: 0898-719x

Matthew Moore, Publisher

3857 Deaf USA
Eye Festival Communications
6917B Woodley Avenue
Van Nuys, CA 91406
Fax: 818-902-9840

Provides news coverage on all activities and issues of interest to deaf and hard-of-hearing readers as well as professionals and associates within this specialized market.

Monthly

David Rosenbaum, Editor

3858 Hearing Health
363 Seventh Avenue, 10th Floor
New York, NY 10001
212-257-6140
866-454-3924
Fax: 361-776-3278
e-mail: info@hhf.org
hearinghealthfoundation.org/hearing-health-magazine

A publication for deaf and hard-of-hearing people, as well as hearing health care professionals, libraries, agencies, schools and organizations.

Bimonthly

Paula Bartone-Bonillas, Editor
Shari Eberts, Chairman
Robert Boucai, Principal

3859 Perspectives in Education and Deafness
Gallaudet University Press
800 Florida Avenue NE
Washington, DC 20002
202-651-5488
800-621-2736
Fax: 800-621-8476
TTY: 202-651-5444
e-mail: gupress@gallaudet.edu
gupress.gallaudet.edu

A practical, reader-friendly magazine, offering help and advice in and beyond the classroom, tuned to the needs of today's students, teachers and families.

5 times a year

Mary Abrams Perica, Editor

3860 The Deaf-Blind American
American Association of the Deaf-Blind
PO Box 8064
Silver Spring, MD 20907
301-563-9064
Fax: 301-495-4404
TTY: 301-495-4402
e-mail: aadb-info@aadb.org
www.aadb.org

The Deaf-Blind American (DBA), the official quarterly magazine of the AADB, is available only to its members. It contains articles of interest to deaf-blind individuals, their families, and service providers who work with people who are deaf-blind. The DBA is available in large print, Braille, disk and email.

Timothy Jackson, President
Jill Gaus, Vice President
Debby Lieberman, Secretary

3861 Volta Voices
Alexander Graham Bell Association for the Deaf
3417 Volta Place NW
Washington, DC 20007
202-337-5220
800-432-7543
Fax: 202-337-8314
TTY: 203-337-5221
e-mail: info@agbell.org
listeningandspokenlanguage.org

A magazine highlighting inspirational stories from parents of children who are deaf, legislative news, technology update, and stories pertaining to speech, speech-reading, and the use of residual hearing.

Bimonthly

Brooke Rigler, Editor
Lisa Chutjian, Chief Development Officer
Emilio Alonso-Mendoza, Chief Executive Officer

Journals

3862 American Annals of the Deaf
Convention of American Instructors of the Deaf
800 Florida Avenue NE, Fowler Hall 409
Washington, DC 20002
202-651-5488
Fax: 202-651-5708
TTY: 202-651-5444
e-mail: gupress@gallaudet.edu
gupress.gallaudet.edu

Scholarly journal at the forefront of research related to the education of deaf people. Annual reference Issue identifies programs and services for deaf people nationwide.

5 times a year

Donald F Moores, Editor
Mary Ellen Carew, Managing Editor

3863 Hearing Loss Magazine
Self Help for Hard-of-Hearing People
7910 Woodmont Avenue, Suite 1200
Bethesda, MD 20814
301-657-2248
Fax: 301-913-9413
TTY: 301-657-2249
www.hearingloss.org

An educational journal about hearing loss for hard-of-hearing people.

Bimonthly

Barbara Kelley, Editor-In-Chief
Anna Gilmore Hall, Executive Director
Lisa Hamlin, Director of Public Policy

3864 Journal of Speech, Language, and Hearing Research
American Speech Language Hearing Association
2200 Research Blvd
Rockville, MD 20850
301-296-5700
800-478-2071
Fax: 301-296-8580
TTY: 301-296-5650
TDD: 301-296-5650
e-mail: productsales@asha.org
www.asha.org

Pertains broadly to studies of the processes and disorders of hearing, language, and speech and to the diagnosis and treatment of such disorders.

Bi-monthly

Dr Anne Smith, Editor, Speech
Dr Karla McGregor, Editor, Language
Dr Robert Schlauch, Editor, Hearing

3865 Language, Speech, and Hearing in Schools
American Speech Language Hearing Association
2200 Research Blvd
Rockville, MD 20850

301-296-5700
800-478-2071
Fax: 301-296-8580
TTY: 301-296-5650
TDD: 301-296-5650
e-mail: productsales@asha.org
www.asha.org

An archival journal for research and practice in educational settings. Publishes studies and articles that pertain to speech, language, and hearing disorders and differences in children and adolescents, as well as to professional issues affecting service delivery in educational setting.

Quarterly

Dr Kenn Apel, Editor
Judith L. Page, PhD, CCC-SLP, President
Margot L. Beckerman, AuD, CCC-A, Chair

Newsletters

3866 AADB E-News
American Association of the Deaf-Blind
PO Box 8064
Silver Spring, MD 20907

301-563-9064
Fax: 301-495-4404
TTY: 301-495-4402
e-mail: aadb-info@aadb.org
www.aadb.org

A free newsletter, the AADB E-News is available to anyone during the months when the DBA is not being published. It contains information about the latest events occurring within AADB and in the deaf-blind community. One does not need to be an AADB member to receive the free AADB E-News newsletter.

Timothy Jackson, President
Jill Gaus, Vice President
Debby Lieberman, Secretary

3867 Endeavor
American Society for Deaf Children
PO Box 3355
Gettysburg, PA 17325

717-334-7922
800-942-2732
Fax: 717-334-8808

Newsletter for parents of deaf children.

Quarterly

Barbara Aschembrenner, Editor

3868 Gallaudet Today
Gallaudet University Press
800 Florida Avenue NE
Washington, DC 20002

202-651-5488
800-621-2736
Fax: 800-621-8476
TTY: 202-651-5444
e-mail: gupress@gallaudet.edu
gupress.gallaudet.edu

A university alumni publication with both general and special issues on deafness-related topics.

44 pages Quarterly

Roz Prickett, Publications Manager

3869 Hear
Deafness Research Foundation
15 W 39th Street
New York, NY 10018

212-768-1181

Offers information on the Foundation's activities and events, technical updates on assistive devices, legislative and medical information on the latest breakthroughs and laws for the hearing impaired, book reviews and resources.

Monte H Jacoby, Executive Director

3870 NADezine
National Association of the Deaf
8630 Fenton Street, Suite 820
Silver Spring, MD 20910

301-587-1788
Fax: 301-587-1791
TTY: 301-587-1789
e-mail: nad.info@nad.org
www.nad.org

A biweekly, online web-zine providing up-to-date information about NAD advocacy, biennial conferences, workshops and training, youth happenings, community news and how you can become involved.

Internet

Christopher D. Wagner, President
Melissa S. Draganac-Hawk, Vice President
Joshua Beckman, Secretary

3871 Newsletter of American Hearing Research
American Hearing Research Foundation
275 N. York Street, Suite 401
Elmhurst, IL 60126

630-617-5079
Fax: 630-563-9181
american-hearing.org

Concerned with hearing research and education.

Richard G. Muench, Chairman
Alan G. Micco, M.D., President
Mark R. Muench, Vice President

3872 Newsline
Sertoma Foundation
1912 E Meyer Boulevard
Kansas City, MO 64132

816-333-8300
e-mail: infosertoma@sertomahq.org
www.sertoma.org

Reports on activities of the Sertoma Foundation in the field of speech and hearing impairments.

David Johnson, President
Don Bartelmay, Senior Vice President
Cheryl Cherny, Junior Vice President

3873 Signs for Me: Basic Sign Vocabulary for Children, Parents, & Teachers
TJ Publishers
817 Silver Spring Avenue, Suite 206
Silver Spring, MD 20910

301-585-4440
800-999-1168
Fax: 301-585-5930
TTY: 301-585-4440
TDD: 301-585-4441
e-mail: TJPubinc@aol.com

Sign language vocabulary for preschool and elementary school children introduces household items, animals, family members, actions, emotions, safety concerns and other concepts.

112 pages Softcover

3874 Speech and Deafness Newsletter
Hearing, Speech
1620 18th Avenue
Seattle, WA 98122

206-323-5770

Agency newsletter for membership and community.

8 pages

Patty Tumberg, Editor

3875 Volta Review
Alexander Graham Bell Association for the Deaf
3417 Volta Place NW
Washington, DC 20007
202-337-5220
800-432-7543
Fax: 202-337-8314
TTY: 203-337-5221
e-mail: info@agbell.org
listeningandspokenlanguage.org

Offers the latest theory, research, current perspectives and practical guidance from noted specialists in education, audiology, speech and language sciences and psychology. Each issue contains a Special Focus-a group of chapters exploring a specific topic in detail.

Quarterly

Lisa Chutjian, Chief Development Officer
Emilio Alonso-Mendoza, Chief Executive Officer
Judy Harrison, Director of Programs

Pamphlets

3876 25 Ways to Promote Spoken Language in Your Child with a Hearing Loss
Alexander Graham Bell Association for the Deaf
3417 Volta Place NW
Washington, DC 20007
202-337-5220
800-432-7543
Fax: 202-337-8314
TTY: 203-337-5221
e-mail: info@agbell.org
listeningandspokenlanguage.org

This pamphlet teaches twenty-five golden rules about preparing your child to listen and to speak.

1995 62 pages

Lisa Chutjian, Chief Development Officer
Emilio Alonso-Mendoza, Chief Executive Officer
Judy Harrison, Director of Programs

3877 Books for Parents of Deaf and Hard-of- Hearing Children
National Information Center on Deafness
800 Florida Avenue NE
Washington, DC 20002
202-651-5488
Fax: 202-651-5054
TTY: 202-651-5444
e-mail: gupress@gallaudet.edu
gupress.gallaudet.edu

Identifies books written for parents and everday experiences of deaf and hard-of-hearing children.

3878 Can Your Baby Hear?
Alexander Graham Bell Association for the Deaf
3417 Volta Place NW
Washington, DC 20007
202-337-5220
800-432-7543
Fax: 202-337-8314
TTY: 203-337-5221
e-mail: info@agbell.org
listeningandspokenlanguage.org

This simple card for parents lists risk indicators and warning signs of hearing loss in babies.

Lisa Chutjian, Chief Development Officer
Emilio Alonso-Mendoza, Chief Executive Officer
Judy Harrison, Director of Programs

3879 Care of the Ears and Hearing for Health
American Hearing Research Foundation
275 N. York Street, Suite 401
Elmhurst, IL 60126
630-617-5079
Fax: 630-563-9181
american-hearing.org

Offers information on ear infections relating to chronic progressive deafness.

Richard G. Muench, Chairman
Alan G. Micco, M.D., President
Mark R. Muench, Vice President

3880 Communicating with People who Have a Hearing Loss
Alexander Graham Bell Association for the Deaf
3417 Volta Place NW
Washington, DC 20007
202-337-5220
800-432-7543
Fax: 202-337-8314
TTY: 203-337-5221
e-mail: info@agbell.org
listeningandspokenlanguage.org

This brochure describes ways to communicate more effectively with people who have hearing losses.

1994

Lisa Chutjian, Chief Development Officer
Emilio Alonso-Mendoza, Chief Executive Officer
Judy Harrison, Director of Programs

3881 Deafness: A Fact Sheet
National Information Center On Deafness
800 Florida Avenue NE
Washington, DC 20002
202-651-5488
Fax: 202-651-5054
TTY: 202-651-5444
e-mail: gupress@gallaudet.edu
gupress.gallaudet.edu

3882 Developing Cognition in Young Children Who are Deaf
Hope
55 E 100 N
Logan, UT 84321
435-752-9533
Fax: 435-752-9533

Presents interesting, updated information on the importance of early cognition development in young children who are deaf. Contains many ideas for ways to promote early thinking skills, especially those that promote and enhance early communication and language development.

3883 Educating Deaf Children: An Introduction
National Information Center on Deafness
800 Florida Avenue NE
Washington, DC 20002
202-651-5488
Fax: 202-651-5054
TTY: 202-651-5444
e-mail: gupress@gallaudet.edu
gupress.gallaudet.edu

Describes the different settings in which deaf children are currently educated.

3884 Hearing Alert Informational Brochures
Alexander Graham Bell Association for the Deaf
3417 Volta Place NW
Washington, DC 20007
202-337-5220
800-432-7543
Fax: 202-337-8314
TTY: 203-337-5221
e-mail: info@agbell.org
listeningandspokenlanguage.org

These brochures encourage early detection of hearing loss in young children; for medical facilities, speech and hearing clinics, and schools.

Lisa Chutjian, Chief Development Officer
Emilio Alonso-Mendoza, Chief Executive Officer
Judy Harrison, Director of Programs

3885 Helping Your Hard-of-Hearing Child Succeed
Alexander Graham Bell Association for the Deaf
3417 Volta Place NW
Washington, DC 20007
202-337-5220
800-432-7543
Fax: 202-337-8314
TTY: 203-337-5221
e-mail: info@agbell.org
listeningandspokenlanguage.org

Offers information on how to help children succeed in school with speech and language development.

Lisa Chutjian, Chief Development Officer
Emilio Alonso-Mendoza, Chief Executive Officer
Judy Harrison, Director of Programs

3886 How Does Your Child Hear and Talk?
American Speech Language Hearing Association
2200 Research Blvd
Rockville, MD 20850

301-296-5700
800-478-2071
Fax: 301-296-8580
TTY: 301-296-5650
TDD: 301-296-5650
e-mail: productsales@asha.org
www.asha.org

Offers a chart to parents on children's growth pertaining to their hearing and speech.

Judith L. Page, PhD, CCC-SLP, President
Margot L. Beckerman, AuD, CCC-A, Chair
Barbara K. Cone, PhD, CCC-A, VP, Academic Affairs in Audiology

3887 Leading National Publications of and for Deaf People
National Information Center On Deafness
800 Florida Avenue NE
Washington, DC 20002

202-651-5488
Fax: 202-651-5054
TTY: 202-651-5444
e-mail: gupress@gallaudet.edu
gupress.gallaudet.edu

Identifies publications with national circulations to deaf audiences.

3888 Listen - Hear for Parents of Hearing Impaired Children
Alexander Graham Bell Association for the Deaf
3417 Volta Place NW
Washington, DC 20007

202-337-5220
800-432-7543
Fax: 202-337-8314
TTY: 203-337-5221
e-mail: info@agbell.org
listeningandspokenlanguage.org

Offers information that parents of deaf and hard-of-hearing children need to be aware of. Also includes information on hearing aids, hearing loss and the association in general.

Lisa Chutjian, Chief Development Officer
Emilio Alonso-Mendoza, Chief Executive Officer
Judy Harrison, Director of Programs

3889 National Information Center on Deafness Brochure
National Information Center on Deafness
800 Florida Avenue NE
Washington, DC 20002

202-651-5488
Fax: 202-651-5054
TTY: 202-651-5444
e-mail: gupress@gallaudet.edu
gupress.gallaudet.edu

A description of services offered by NICD.

3890 Parent Packets
Alexander Graham Bell Association for the Deaf
3417 Volta Place NW
Washington, DC 20007

202-337-5220
800-432-7543
Fax: 202-337-8314
TTY: 203-337-5221
e-mail: info@agbell.org
listeningandspokenlanguage.org

These educational packets for parents are specifically designed to address important age-related topics about your child with a hearing impairment.

Packet

Lisa Chutjian, Chief Development Officer
Emilio Alonso-Mendoza, Chief Executive Officer
Judy Harrison, Director of Programs

3891 Perspectives Folio: Parent-Child
Gallaudet University Press
800 Florida Avenue NE
Washington, DC 20002

202-651-5488
800-621-2736
Fax: 800-621-8476
TTY: 202-651-5444
e-mail: gupress@gallaudet.edu
gupress.gallaudet.edu

Seven articles emphasizing family communication while providing important information for parents about deafness and the deaf culture.

29 pages

3892 Publications From the National Information Center on Deafness
National Information Center on Deafness
800 Florida Avenue NE
Washington, DC 20002

202-651-5488
Fax: 202-651-5054
TTY: 202-651-5444
e-mail: gupress@gallaudet.edu
gupress.gallaudet.edu

Order form and explanations of NICD publications.

3893 Questions and Answers on Hearing Loss
Self Help for Hard-of-Hearing People
7910 Woodmont Avenue, Suite 1200
Bethesda, MD 20814

301-657-2248
Fax: 301-913-9413
TTY: 301-657-2249
e-mail: info@hearingloss.org
www.hearingloss.org

Barbara Kelley, Editor-In-Chief
Anna Gilmore Hall, Executive Director
Lisa Hamlin, Director of Public Policy

3894 Signs for Me: Basic Sign Vocabulary for Children, Parents, & Teachers
DawnSignPress
6130 Nancy Ridge Drive
San Diego, CA 92121

858-625-0600
800-549-5350
Fax: 858-625-2336
e-mail: info@dawnsign.com
www.dawnsign.com

ASL/English vocabulary primer. Young readers will associate a sign and picture with the English form of a word. Introduces more than 300 primary words arranged in thematic groupings. Captures students' interest through clearly illustrated signs and actions; includes an illustrated look at the English word for effective bilingual learning.

128 pages paperback
ISBN: 0-915035-27-8

Ben Bahan, Co-Author
Joe Dannis, Co-Author

3895 So You Have Had An Ear Operation...What Next?
American Hearing Research Foundation
275 N. York Street, Suite 401
Elmhurst, IL 60126

630-617-5079
Fax: 630-563-9181
american-hearing.org

Offers information on ear infections and surgery.

Richard G. Muench, Chairman
Alan G. Micco, M.D., President
Mark R. Muench, Vice President

3896 Speechreading: Methods and Materials
Self Help for Hard-of-Hearing People
7910 Woodmont Avenue, Suite 1200
Bethesda, MD 20814

301-657-2248
Fax: 301-913-9413
TTY: 301-657-2249
e-mail: info@hearingloss.org
www.hearingloss.org

Barbara Kelley, Editor-In-Chief
Anna Gilmore Hall, Executive Director
Lisa Hamlin, Director of Public Policy

3897 Statewide Services for Deaf and Hard of Hearing People
National Information Center on Deafness
800 Florida Avenue NE
Washington, DC 20002
202-651-5488
Fax: 202-651-5054
TTY: 202-651-5444
e-mail: gupress@gallaudet.edu
gupress.gallaudet.edu

A resource list of states that have established commissions and other offices to serve deaf people.

3898 World of Sound
International Hearing Society
16880 Middlebelt Road, Suite 4
Livonia, MI 48154
734-522-7200
Fax: 734-522-0200
www.hearingihs.org

The purpose of this booklet is to provide basic information for those with questions about hearing loss, hearing aids and hearing instrument specialists.

Camps

3899 Camp Civitan
12635 North 42nd Street
Phoenix, AZ 85032
602-953-2944
Fax: 602-953-2946
e-mail: info@campcivitan.org
www.campcivitan.org

A 501c3 non-profit organization, that has been providing multiple ever-changing programs to meet the needs of children and adults who are developmentally disabled.

Rob Adams, Camp Director
Charlie Riggs, Camp Maintenance
Mary Kellogg, Operations

3900 Camp Emanuel
PO Box 752343
Dayton, OH 45475
973-477-5504
e-mail: ginter.7@wright.edu
campemanuel.weebly.com

Camp Emanuel is a camp for children with and without disabilities. It is the only camp of its kind in southwestern Ohio. The camp is designed to promote decision-making, team building skills, self-esteem, and an understanding of acceptance between all children.

Stephanie Ackner, President
Brian Demarke, Vice President
Mary Foreman, Secretary

3901 Camp Grizzly
4708 Roseville Road, Suite 112
North Highlands, CA 95660
916-349-7500
Fax: 916-993-3048
TTY: 916-349-7500
e-mail: sfarinha@norcalcenter.org
www.norcalcenter.org

A one-week residential camp program for deaf and hard of hearing youth age 7 to 17.

Sheri Farinha, CEO
Cheryl Bella, Chair
Michael D. Wilson, Vice Chair

3902 Camp Juliena
4151 Memorial Dr, Suite 103-B
Decatur, GA 30032
404-292-5312
800-541-0710
Fax: 404-299-3642
e-mail: campjuliena@gmail.com
www.gachi.org

A weeklong residential summer camp for youths and teens who are deaf or hard of hearing. Through challanging, team-oriented activities, campers form lasting friendships and acquire valuable leadership, social and communication skills.

Pat Ford, President
Jeanette Lorch, Vice President
Martha Timms, Secretary

3903 Camp Shocco for the Deaf
PO Box 6569
Talladega, AL 35161
256-761-1100
e-mail: campshocco@albcdeaf.org
www.campshocco.org

Camp for deaf and hard of hearing students age 8 through high school. The campers will learn about Bible stories, teamwork, and have plenty of fun with various activities during recreation time.

Chad Fleming, Camp Director
Matthew Dixon, Co-Director
Linnea Elliott, Assistant Director

3904 Central Michigan University Summer Clinics
444 Moore
Mount Pleasant, MI
517-774-3803

Designed for children, ages 6 and up, with speech, language and hearing disorders who can benefit from intensive clinical work. A wide range of recreational and social activities form part of the clinical program and promote the social use of skills learned in class.

3905 Children's Beach House
100 W, 10th Street, Suite 411
Wilmington, DE 19801
302-655-4288
Fax: 302-655-4216
e-mail: childrens.beach.house@dol.net
www.cbhinc.org

Summer camp for children from Delaware of normal mental level, with speech, language and hearing disorders are accepted, ages 6-13. Activities include aquatics, art, music, nature and dramatics. Speech and language therapy are provided. Also school-year environmental education for Delaware students of all exceptionalities.

Richard T. Garrett, Executive Director
Jennifer A. Clement, Director
Nicholas Imhoff, Business Manager

3906 Des Moines YMCA Camp
1192 166th Drive
Boone, IA 50036
515-432-7558
Fax: 515-432-5414
e-mail: ycamp@dmymca.org
www.y-camp.org

For boys and girls with cancer, diabetes, asthma, cystic fibrosis, hearing impaired and other disabilities.

David Sherry, Executive Director
Mike Havlik, Program Director
Alex Kretzinger, Program Director- Summer Camp

3907 Easter Seal Kysoc
2050 Versailles Road
Lexington, KY 40504
859-254-5701
800-800-888
Fax: 502-732-0783
e-mail: ek1@cardinalhill.org
www.cardinalhill.org

Designed for the fullest camping experience for children or adults with physical disabilities, blind, deaf, behavior disorders, mental retardation, diabetes and multiple handicaps, ages 7 and up.

Heide Miller, CCD, CTRS, Director
Gary Payne, President/CEO

3908 Enchanted Hills Camp
Lighthouse
214 Van Ness Avenue
San Francisco, CA 94102   415-431-1481
                                      Fax: 415-863-7568
                                      TTY: 415-431-4572
                            e-mail: info@lighthouse-sf.org
                                        lighthouse-sf.org

For blind, deaf/blind children and adults, ages 5 and up. This program offers a basic camping experience. Activities include music, art, dance, hiking and riding. Camperships are available to California residents.

Joshua A. Miele, Ph.D., President
Chris Downey, 1st Vice President
Kathleen Knox, 2nd Vice President

3909 Florida School-Deaf and Blind Summer Camp
207 N. San Marco Avenue
Saint Augustine, FL 32084   904-827-2200
                                           800-800-344
                              e-mail: info@fsdb.k12.fl.us
                                        www.fsdb.k12.fl.us

The Florida School for the Deaf and the Blind hosts summer campers from all over teh state of Florida for a week of fun and adventure. FSDB's 80 acre campus is where campers participate in a variety of activities including rock climbing, archery, swimming, kayaking, team games, arts and crafts, dance music, and much more.

Jeanne Glidden Prickett, President
Nancy Bloch, Executive Director, Comm & PR
Tanya Rhodes, Executive Director, Advancement

3910 Indiana Deaf Camp
100 West 86th Street
Indianapolis, IN 46260   317-846-3404
                                      Fax: 317-844-1034
                         e-mail: deafcamp@hotmail.com
                                        www.indeafcamps.org

Camp dedicated to promoting the educational, social, spiritual, physical and personal development of individuals with a hearing loss, or who are related to individuals with a hearing loss.

Nunery, President

3911 Meadowood Springs Speech and Hearing Camp
PO Box 1025
Pendleton, OR 97801   541-276-2752
                                      Fax: 541-276-7227
                         e-mail: info@meadowoodsprings.org
                                        www.meadowoodsprings.org

On 143 acres in the Blue Mountains of Eastern Oregon, this camp is designed to help young people who have diagnosed clinical disorders of speech, hearing or language. A full range of activities in recreational and clinical areas is available. For cabin reservations 541-566-2191.

Rosemarie Atfield, Executive Director
Marie Story, Camp Manager
Cliff Story, Camp Manager

3912 NAD Youth Leadership Camp
National Association of the Deaf
8630 Fenton Street, Suite 820
Silver Spring, MD 20910   301-587-1788
                                      Fax: 301-587-1791
                                      TTY: 301-587-1789
                              e-mail: nad.info@nad.org
                                        www.nad.org

An annual 4-week summer program designed to foster leadership and teamwork skills in deaf and hard of hearing high school students. Campers have the opportunity to build and develop their knowledge, social interaction, and leadership skills through hands-on activities focusing on literacy, and often make life-long friends here. 2009 Dates & Location: June 25 - July 22, Camp Taloali at Stayton, Oregon.

Christopher D. Wagner, President
Melissa S. Draganac-Hawk, Vice President
Joshua Beckman, Secretary

3913 Texas Lions Camp
Lions Clubs of Texas
PO Box 290247
Kerrville, TX 78029   830-896-8500
                                           830-896-8500
                                      Fax: 830-896-3666
                                 e-mail: tlc@ktc.com
                                        www.lionscamp.com

The primary purpose of Texas Lions camp is to provide, without charge, a camp for physically disabled, hearing/vision impaired and diabetic children from the State of Texas, regardless of race, religion, or national origin. Our goal is to create an atmosphere wherein campers will learn the can do philosophy and be allowed to achieve maximum personal growth and self esteem. The camp welcomes boys and girls ages 7-16.

Stephen Mabry, CEO
Doug Parker, Business Manager
Steven King, Program/Client Service Director

3914 University of Iowa - Wendell Johnson Speech and Hearing Clinic
Wendell Johnson Speech And Hearing Center
Iowa City, IA 52242   319-335-1845
                                      Fax: 319-335-8851
                                        www.uiowa.edu

The clinic offers assessment and remediation for disordered communication in adults and children. The clinic also offers an Intensive Summer Residential Clinic for school age children needing intervention services because of speech, language, hearing and/or reading problems.

Richard Hurtig, Professor/Chair
Ann L Michael, Clinic Director

3915 Windsor Mountain Camp
One World Way
Windsor, NH 3244   603-478-3166
                         e-mail: jake@windsormountain.org
                                        www.windsormountain.org

Summer camp for deaf and hard of hearing students and for hearing campers who want to learn ASL.

Jake Labovitz, Director
Dianna Hahn, Student Travel Programs
Pam Butler, Administrative Assistant

3916 Wisconsin Lions Camp
3834 County Road A
Rosholt, WI 54473   715-677-4969
                                      Fax: 715-677-3297
                                      TTY: 715-677-6999
                                 e-mail: wlf@wlf.info
                                        www.wisconsinlionscamp.com

Serves children who have either a visual, hearing or mild cognitive disability. Many of the children also have multiple disabilities or medical conditions. Program activities include sailing, ropes course, bike and canoe trips, environmental education, swimming, camping, canoeing, outdoor living skills and handicrafts. ACA accredited, located in central Wisconsin, near Stevens Point.

Evett J. Hartvig, Executive Director
Dale Schroeder, Facility Director
Elizabeth Shelley, Administrative Assistant

Description

3917 HEMANGIOMAS AND LYMPHANGIOMAS

Covers these related disorders: Capillary hemangiomas, Cavernous hemangiomas, Cystic hygromas, Disseminated hemangiomatosis, Mixed hemangiomas, Port-wine stains (or salmon patches), Kasabach-merritt syndrome

Involves the following Biologic System(s):

Dermatologic Disorders

Hemangiomas are the most common benign tumors in infants. In addition, during childhood, lymphangiomas, also known as lymphatic malformations, are the second most common benign tumor affecting vessels of the body. Hemangiomas consist of an abnormal distribution of relatively small blood vessels (e.g., capillaries) due to malformation of developing fetal tissue from which the vessels arise. Lymphangiomas consist of masses of abnormally enlarged (dilated), newly formed lymph vessels, which are the channels that transport lymphatic fluid throughout the body. Lymph, a thin bodily fluid that consists of proteins, fats, and certain white blood cells (lymphocytes), accumulates in spaces between tissue cells and flows back into the bloodstream via lymph vessels.

Hemangiomas usually affect blood vessels of the skin (cutaneous hemangiomas). They most commonly develop in the head and neck regions and are rarely fully formed at birth. These tumors, which occur more frequently in females than males, are usually single growths that occur randomly for unknown reasons. However, some multigenerational families (kindreds) have been reported in which several individuals developed isolated hemangiomas. In such cases, the condition may be transmitted as an autosomal dominant trait. In addition, in rare cases, certain forms of hemangiomas may occur in association with particular underlying syndromes.

Cutaneous hemangiomas may be superficial (capillary hemangiomas), deep (cavernous hemangiomas), or both (mixed hemangiomas). Capillary hemangiomas are considered the most common type of hemangioma, affecting approximately 60 percent of patients. These hemangiomas include port-wine stains (a form of nevus flammeus) and strawberry hemangiomas (strawberry nevi). Port-wine stains are present at birth (congenital) and are typically permanent defects. These lesions consist of mature, abnormally widened capillaries; are flat (macular) with sharply defined borders; and are usually reddish purple in color. They may vary greatly in size and typically develop on the head, face, and neck areas. As patients reach adulthood, port-wine stains may darken and form elevated (papular) areas that may occasionally bleed. Port-wine stains must be differentiated from salmon patches, which are flat, salmon-colored lesions that are typically present during infancy on certain facial areas, such as over the eyelids, on the middle of the forehead, or between the eyes. Salmon patches typically fade completely over time. Port-wine stains may be an isolated condition or may occur in association with several rare underlying syndromes (e.g., Klippel-Trenaunay-Weber syndrome, Sturge-Weber syndrome, etc.). Treatment may include a variety of measures, such as laser therapy, destruction of affected tissue through the use of extreme cold (cryosurgery), surgical removal (excision), transplantation of skin tissues (grafting), or masking with cosmetics.

Strawberry hemangiomas are dull or bright red and elevated, have clearly defined borders, and consist of immature capillaries. The lesions, which may develop as single or multiple growths, may affect any area of the body; however, they are most common on the scalp, face, chest, or back. Strawberry hemangiomas usually appear within approximately two months after birth. In most patients, the hemangiomas initially grow rapidly, cease such growth (stationary phase), and then gradually begin to regress in size (involution). After the lesions have reduced in size, approximately 10 percent of patients have residual discoloration or puckering of affected skin. In rare cases, complications associated with strawberry hemangiomas may include infection; destruction of the skin's surface, resulting in open sores and inflammation (ulceration); bleeding (hemorrhaging); or extensive growth that interferes with necessary functions, such as breathing difficulties due to tumor growth affecting the airways. Because most strawberry hemangiomas spontaneously regress, treatment typically consists of careful, ongoing observation. However, if hemangiomas rapidly grow, potentially causing tissue destruction,removal, using elastic bandages or other measures, may be recommended in selected patients. If there is rapid growth that may ultimately cause life-threatening complications, treatment may include the administration of corticosteroids by injection or| mouth or therapy with an artificial (synthetic) form of interferon (interferon alpha-2a). Interferons are natural proteins that are produced by the body's immune system in response to certain invading viruses or other stimuli. In the most severe cases, radiation therapy may be necessary. Other treatment is symptomatic and supportive.

Cavernous hemangiomas may be firm or form cysts. The skin overlying such hemangiomas is often bluish in color. However, if physicians suspect that underlying structures may be affected, specialized imaging techniques, such as CT scanning or ultrasonography, are conducted to detect and characterize such involvement. Rarely, some patients develop multiple hemangiomas. In such cases, affected children may have numerous small, red or purplish, raised hemangiomas on the skin. In addition, internal hemangiomas may be present involving certain organs, particularly the liver, lungs, brain and spinal cord, and organs of the gastrointestinal tract. In such cases, affected children are said to have disseminated hemangiomatosis. Life-threatening complications may potentially arise due to hemorrhage, tissue compression (e.g., neural tissue compression), obstruction of the airways, or an inability of the heart to effectively pump blood to the lungs and throughout the body (heart failure). In some cases, multiple internal and cutaneous hemangiomas occur in association with certain rare, underlying syndromes (e.g., macrocephaly with pseudopapilledema).

Lymphangiomas may be localized or widely distributed growths that, in some cases, may have hemangioma-like components. In almost all affected children, lymphangiomas are apparent by approximately age three. Lymphangiomas most commonly develop in the neck and facial regions, in the chest area (thorax), or under the arms (axillae). For example, some affected children may have an abnormal cystic growth consisting of dilated lymph vessels beneath the skin in the neck area (cystic hygroma). Lymphangiomas, such as cystic hygroma, may occur as isolated findings or in association with certain underlying syndromes (e.g., Noonan syndrome). Unlike hemangiomas, lymphangiomas rarely spontaneously

443

regress. In some patients, they may expand in size and may obstruct the gastrointestinal tract or the airways, potentially causing life-threatening complications without appropriate treatment. Because most lymphangiomas are relatively widely distributed (diffuse), treatment often includes removal of the growths in several stages (staged surgical resection). Additional treatment includes symptomatic and supportive measures.

Government Agencies

3918 NIH/National Institute of Arthritis and Mu sculoskeletal and Skin Diseases
1AMS Circle, PO Box 3675
Bethesda, MD 20892

301-495-4484
877-226-4267
Fax: 301-718-6366
TTY: 301-565-2966
TDD: 301-565-2966
e-mail: niamsinfo@mail.nih.gov
www.niams.nih.gov

The mission of the NIAMS, a part of the NIH, is to support research into the causes, treatment, and prevention of arthritis and musculoskeletal and skin diseases, the training of basic and clinical scientists to carry out this research, and the dissemination of information on research progress in these diseases.

Stephen I Katz MD PhD, Director
Robert H Carter MD, Deputy Director

National Associations & Support Groups

3919 American Academy of Dermatology (AAD)
PO Box 4014
Schaumburg, IL 60168

866-503-7546
Fax: 847-240-1859
e-mail: MRC@aad.org
www.aad.org

To promote and advance the art of medicine and surgery of the skin; promote the highest possible standards in clinical practice , education and research in dermatology and related disciplines.

Dirk M. Elston, President
Lisa A. Garner, VP
Brett M. Coldiron, President-Elect

3920 American Academy of Pediatrics
141 Northwest Point Boulevard
Elk Grove Village, IL 60007

847-434-4000
800-433-9016
Fax: 847-434-8000
www.aap.org

The American Academy of Pediatrics and its member pediatricians are committed to the attainment of optimal physical, mental and social health and well-being for all infants, children, adolescents, and young adults.

Sandra Hassink, MD, FAAP, President

3921 American Skin Association
6 East 43rd Street, 28th Floor
New York, NY 10017

212-889-4858
800-499-7546
Fax: 212-889-4959
e-mail: info@americanskin.org
www.americanskin.org

The American Skin Association is the only volunteer led health organization dedicated through research, education and advocacy to saving lives and alleviating human suffering caused by the full spectrum of skin disorders.

Howard P. Milstein, Chairman
George W Hambrick, Jr, President/Founder
David R Bickers, MD, Executive VP

3922 Hemangioma Support System
C/O Cynthia Schumerth
1484 Sand Acres Drive
Depere, WI 54115

920-336-9399

Provides parent-to-parent support for families with children affected by hemangiomas.
1990

3923 Society for Pediatric Dermatology
8365 Keystone Crossing, Suite 107
Indianapolis, IN 46240

317-202-0224
Fax: 317-205-9841
e-mail: spd@hp-assoc.com
www.pedsderm.net

National organization dedicated to promote, develop and advance education, research and care of skin disease in all pediatric age groups.

Kent Lindeman, Executive Director

3924 Society for Pediatric Dermatology Annual Meeting
8365 Keystone Crossing, Suite 107
Indianapolis, IN 46240

317-202-0224
Fax: 317-205-9841
e-mail: spd@hp-assoc.com
www.pedsderm.net

July
Kent Lindeman, Executive Director

3925 Vascular Birthmarks Foundation
PO Box 106
Latham, NY 12110

518-782-9637
877-823-4646
e-mail: HVBF@aol.com
www.birthmark.org

A not for profit organization that provides support and informational resources for individuals affected by hemangiomas, port wine stains, and other vascular birthmarks and tumors.

Linda Rozell Shannon, Founder
Dr. Milton Waner, MD, Medical Chairman
Paige Salvador, Executive Director

Libraries & Resource Centers

3926 Children's Center for Cancer and Blood Disorders
University of South Carolina School of Medicine
5 Richland Memorial Park
Columbia, SC 29203

803-434-3533

Joint clinical and basic research of juvenile cancer and blood disorders.

Fauni Lowe, Manager

Conferences

3927 VBF Conference
Vascular Birthmarks Foundation
PO Box 106
Latham, NY 12110

518-782-9637
877-823-4646
e-mail: HVBF@aol.com
www.birthmark.org

November
Martin Mihm Jr MD, Director

Web Sites

3928 Vascular Anomalies Center
www.hemangioma.org/

Provide the most up-to-date information to parents and patients as well as give the resources to help understand vascular anomaly.

Book Publishers

3929 Sturge-Weber Syndrome: A Resource Guide for a Reason, a Season and a Lifetime

Sturge-Weber Foundation
PO Box 418
Mt. Freedom, NJ 07970   973-895-4445
                                          800-627-5482
                                     Fax: 973-895-4846
                              e-mail: swf@sturge-weber.com
                                      www.sturge-weber.com

Covers most of the issues and concerns of parents and individuals with SWS, PWS and KT in short essays and chapters that provide practical and helpful advice

95 pages Paperback
ISBN: 0-967048-40-0

Carol Buck, Patient/Family Services Director
Lauris Partizian, Information Services Manager

Description

3930 HEMOLYTIC DISEASE OF THE NEWBORN
Synonyms: Erythroblastosis fetalis, Erythroblastosis neonatorum
Involves the following Biologic System(s):
Hematologic and Oncologic Disorders, Neonatal and Infant
Disorders

Hemolytic disease of the newborn, also known as
erythroblastosis neonatorum or erythroblastosis fetalis, is
characterized by destruction of a newborn's red blood cells
by antibodies that crossed the placenta from the mother's
bloodstream during pregnancy. Antibodies are produced by
certain white blood cells in response to foreign proteins (antigens) that are present in some cells and invading microorganisms. In hemolytic disease of the newborn the mother's
immune system treats the baby's blood cells as foreign and
makes antibodies against them. In most cases, the condition
occurs when a developing fetus has Rh-positive blood (i.e.,
inherited from the father), but the mother has Rh-negative
blood.

In approximately 85 percent of individuals, red blood cells
contain an antigen called the Rh factor. Those with this antigen are said to have Rh-positive blood, whereas those without
the antigen have Rh-negative blood. The blood plasma does
not naturally contain antibodies to inactivate or destroy the
Rh antigen (anti-Rh antibodies). However, if a fetus has
Rh-positive blood and the mother is Rh negative, the presence of the Rh factor in the fetus' red blood cells causes the
mother's body to produce anti-Rh antibodies. If the woman
becomes pregnant again and the developing fetus has Rh-positive blood, the mother's antibodies may react with the fetus'
Rh-positive cells, resulting in hemolysis (breakdown of red
blood cells). In many cases, mothers who are known to have
Rh-negative blood may be treated with a protein to help prevent them from producing anti-Rh antibodies (e.g., injection
of human anti-D globulin), thereby lowering the risk of
erythroblastosis fetalis during future pregnancies.

In infants affected by hemolytic disease of the newborn, associated symptoms and findings may vary. These may range
from a mild breakdown of red blood cells to severely low levels of circulating red blood cells (anemia); paleness of the
skin (pallor); tiny reddish, purplish spots on the skin
(petechiae) due to abnormal bleeding under the skin's surface; enlargement of the liver and spleen
(hepatosplenomegaly); or development of abnormal yellowish
coloring of the mucous membranes, whites of the eyes, and
skin (jaundice). In extremely severe cases, affected newborns
may experience low levels of oxygen supply (hypoxia), difficulty breathing (respiratory distress), heart (cardiac) failure,
severe abnormal accumulations of fluid in body tissues and
cavities (hydrops), and potentially life-threatening complications. Depending upon the severity of the condition, treatment may include transfusions (e.g., partial or full exchange
transfusions with Rh-negative blood) and supportive measures, such as ventilation assistance.

Hemolytic disease of the newborn may also result due to
other blood type incompatibilities, primarily if the mother is
type O and the developing fetus is type A or B. However, the
condition develops in only about 10 percent of such cases of
ABO incompatibility. In addition, the condition is typically

less severe than that associated with Rh incompatibility. In
cases of ABO blood type incompatibility, the development of
jaundice approximately a day after birth may be the only
associated symptom.

Government Agencies

3931 NIH/National Heart, Lung and Blood Institu te
National Institute of Health
PO Box 30105
Bethesda, MD 20824
301-592-8573
Fax: 301-592-8563
TTY: 240-629-3255
e-mail: NHLBIinfo@nhlbi.nih.gov
www.nhlbi.nih.gov

Primary responsibility of this organization is the scientific investigation of heart, blood vessel, lung and blood disorders. Oversees research, demonstration, prevention, education, control and
training activities in these fields and emphasizes the prevention
and control of heart diseases.

Elizabeth G Nabel, MD, Director
Susan Shurin, MD, Deputy Director
Sheila Pohl, Chief of Staff

**3932 NIH/National Institute of Child Health and Human
Development**
31 Center Drive, Building 31, Room 2A32
Bethesda, MD 20892
301-496-1333
800-370-2943
Fax: 866-760-5947
TTY: 888-320-6942
e-mail: NICHDInformationResourceCenter@mail.nih.
www.nichd.nih.gov

Established in 1962 by congress, today the institute conducts and
supports research on topics related to the health of children,
adults, families and populations. Some of these topics include:
developmental disabilities, growth and development, infant death,
reproductive health and birth defects.

Jay H Hoofnagle, Director
Lisa Kaeser, Program & Public Liaison

National Associations & Support Groups

3933 American Academy of Pediatrics
141 Northwest Point Boulevard
Elk Grove Village, IL 60007
847-434-4000
800-433-9016
Fax: 847-434-8000
www.aap.org

The American Academy of Pediatrics and its member pediatricians are committed to the attainment of optimal physical, mental
and social health and well-being for all infants, children, adolescents, and young adults.

Sandra Hassink, MD, FAAP, President

3934 American Autoimmune Related Diseases Association
22100 Gratiot Avenue
Eastpointe, MI 48021
586-776-3900
800-598-4668
Fax: 586-776-3903
e-mail: aarda@aarda.org
www.aarda.org

Dedicated to the eradication of autoimmune diseases and the alleviation of suffering and the socio-economic impact of
autoimmunity through fostering and facilitating collaboration in
the areas of education, public awareness, research and patient services in an effective, ethical and efficient manner.

Virginia Ladd, Executive Director
Betty Diamond, Chair
Noel R. Rose, Chairman

Web Sites

3935 American Autoimmune Related Diseases Association
22100 Gratiot Ave.
Eastpointe, MI 48021
586-776-3900
800-598-4668
Fax: 586-776-3903
www.aarda.org

Dedicated to the eradiction of autoimmune diseases and the alleviation of suffering and the socio-economic impact of autoimmunity through fostering and facilitating collaboration in the areas of education, public awareness, research and patient services in an effective, ethical and efficient manner.

Betty Diamond, M.D., Chairperson
Stanley M. Finger, Ph.D., Vice Chairperson

3936 NIH/National Institutes of Health/Office o f Rare Diseases
6701 Democracy Boulevard, Suite 1001
Bethesda, MD 20892
301-402-4336
Fax: 301-480-9655
e-mail: ordr@nih.gov
rarediseases.info.nih.gov/

Provides information about ORD-sponsored scientific activites, and ORD cosponsored genetic and rare disease information center, and a portal to databases that provide information on major topics of interest in rare disease research.

Pamela M. McInnes, D.D.S., Acting Director
P.J. Brooks, Ph.D., Health Scientist Administrator
John H. Ferguson, M.D., Medical Advisor

3937 Online Mendelian Inheritance in Man
8600 Rockville Pike
Bethesda, MD 20894
888-346-3656
e-mail: info@ncbi.nlm.nih.gov
www.ncbi.nlm.nih.gov

This database is a catalog of human genes and genetic disorders.

Description

3938 HEMOPHILIA

Synonyms: AHF, Antihemophilic factor deficiency, Classic hemophilia, Factor VIII deficiency, Hemophilia A

Covers these related disorders: Hemophilia A, Hemophilia B (Christmas disease; Factor IX deficiency), Von Willebrand's disease (Factor VIIIR deficiency)

Involves the following Biologic System(s):
Hematologic and Oncologic Disorders

The term hemophilia refers to a group of bleeding disorders including hemophilia A, hemophilia B, and von Willebrand's disease. Each of these diseases is characterized by the deficiency of a specific blood-clotting protein (factor). Hemophilia A, the most common form of the disease, affects approximately 80 percent of people with hemophilia and is caused by a deficiency of factor VIII. Hemophilia B, accounting for approximately 12 to 15 percent of all cases, results from a deficiency in clotting factor IX. In both forms of hemophilia, the severity of the disease and associated symptoms depend upon the level of coagulating activity of the individual clotting factors; the lower the activity of these factors, the more severe the disease. The most common symptoms, usually appearing at about 18 months when the child becomes more physically active, include easy bruising and bleeding into the joints (hemarthrosis) and muscles. Pain and swelling in the ankles, knees, and elbows may follow and eventually lead to degenerative changes and limited range of motion. Bleeding episodes may occur after injury, trauma, minor surgery, and, in some cases, for no apparent reason (spontaneously). Von Willebrand's disease involves a deficiency of factor VIIIR and is characterized by easy bruising, nose bleeds and bleeding into the gastrointestinal tract. In affected females, excessive uterine bleeding may occur during menstruation or childbirth. In some patients, blood may be present in the urine (hematuria). Unlike hemophilia A or B, bleeding into the joints is rare and the disorder seems to improve with advancing age.

Treatment of hemophilia A and B includes transfusions of appropriate clotting factor when a bleeding episode occurs. These concentrates may also be regularly self-administered to prevent bleeds. Other preventive measures may include the administration of certain clot-aiding drugs before surgery, the avoidance of certain drugs that may exacerbate bleeding problems, and avoidance of participation in contact sports or other similar activities that could provoke a bleeding episode. The treatment of von Willebrand's disease may include the infusion of DDAVP or VW protein prior to surgery or childbirth.

Hemophilia A and hemophilia B are transmitted as x-linked recessive traits and affect males almost exclusively. Approximately 10 males out of every 100,000 are born with hemophilia A, while the rate of occurrence of hemophilia B is about two males out of every 100,000. For the most part, von Willebrand's disease is inherited as an autosomal dominant disorder. In rare instances, the disease may be inherited as a recessive gene. Children with hemophilia who may have received transfusions of blood or blood products before HIV blood-screening became standard in 1985 may have unwittingly become infected by receiving contaminated blood.

National Associations & Support Groups

3939 American Academy of Pediatrics
141 Northwest Point Boulevard
Elk Grove Village, IL 60007

847-434-4000
800-433-9016
Fax: 847-434-8000
www.aap.org

The American Academy of Pediatrics and its member pediatricians are committed to the attainment of optimal physical, mental and social health and well-being for all infants, children, adolescents, and young adults.

Sandra Hassink, MD, FAAP, President

3940 Baxter Healthcare Hyland Division
One Baxter Parkway
Deerfield, IL 60015

224-948-2000
800-422-9837
Fax: 800-568-5020
www.baxter.com/

Government affairs office that monitors and selectively lobbies on issues relating to Medicare, Medicaid, orphan drugs and other subjects relating to hemophilia.

Phillip L. Batchelor, Corporate Vice President - Quality
Jean-Luc Butel, Corporate Vice President - Presiden
Robert M. Davis, Corporate Vice President - Presiden

3941 Children's Blood Foundation
333 E 38th Street, Suite 830
New York, NY 10016

212-297-4336
Fax: 212-297-4340
e-mail: info@childrenscbf.org
www.childrenscbf.org

The foundation's major emphasis is on blood diseases affecting children: leukemia, thalassemia, hemophilia, sickle cell anemia, platelet disorders. retinoblastoma and AIDS.

John Calicchio, Chairman
Jennifer Zaleski, Executive Director
Alysse Brennan, Operations Associate

3942 Hemophilia Health Services
201 Great Circle Rd
Nashville, TN 37228

615-353-3814
866-712-5200
Fax: 800-330-0756
e-mail: info@HemophiliaHealth.com
www.hemophiliahealth.com

Specializes in providing pharmaceuticals, therapeutic supplies and disease management services for people with hemophilia and related bleeding disorders.

Kyle J Callahan, President

3943 National Hemophilia Foundation
116 W 23rd Street, 11th Floor
New York, NY 10011

212-328-3700
800-424-2634
Fax: 212-328-3777
e-mail: handi@hemophilia.org
www.hemophilia.org

Offers various information, articles, resources, books and more for the hemophilia and HIV/AIDS community.

Ken Trader, Chair
Jorge De La Riva, Vice Chair
Steve Helm, Secretary

State Agencies & Support Groups

Arkansas

3944 Hemophilia Center of Arkansas
Arkansas Children's Hospital
1 Children's Way, PO Box 3591
Little Rock, AR 72202
501-364-1100
TDD: 501-364-1184
www.archildrens.org

Patients with coagulation disorders can be diagnosed and evaluated by a group of physicians, physical therapists, dentists, psychologists and geneticists to provide education, prevention and continuity of care. The Hemophilia Center of Arkansas offers the latest diagnosis, prevention and treatment modalities for children and adults.

David Becton, MD, Medical Director

California

3945 Central California Chapter of the National Hemophilia Foundation
PO Box 163689
Sacramento, CA 95816
916-448-0370
Fax: 916-489-1569
e-mail: hubbert@newfactor.com
www.hemophilia.org

An organization devoted to improving the quality of life for persons affected with bleeding disorders and their complications. This is accomplished through outreach development, educational programs, informational literature, support services and patient referrals.

Ken Trader, Chair
Jorge De La Riva, Vice Chair
Steve Helm, Secretary

3946 Hemophilia Association of San Diego County
3550 Camino Del Rio N, Suite 105
San Diego, CA 92108
619-325-3570
Fax: 619-325-4350
e-mail: info@hasdc.org
www.hasdc.org

An organization devoted to improving the quality of life for persons affected with bleeding disorders and their complications. This is accomplished through outreach development, educational programs, informational literature, support services and patient referrals.

Michael Brown, Esq., President
Heather Masserly, Director at Large
Judy Faitek, Director at Large

3947 Hemophilia Foundation of Northern California
6400 Hollis St Suite 6
Emeryville, CA 94608
ÿ51- 65- 332
888-749-4362
Fax: 510-658-3384
e-mail: execadmin@hfnconline.org
www.hemofoundation.org

An organization devoted to improving the quality of life for persons affected with bleeding disorders and their complications. This is accomplished through outreach development, educational programs, informational literature, support services and patient referrals.

Bethane Deuel, President
Ben Martin, Secretary
Hari Young, Treasurer

3948 Hemophilia Foundation of Southern California
6720 Melrose Avenue
Hollywood, CA 90038
323-525-0440
800-371-4123
Fax: 323-525-0445
e-mail: hfsc@hemosocal.org
www.hemosocal.org

An organization devoted to improving the quality of life for persons affected with bleeding disorders and their complications. This is accomplished through outreach development, educational programs, informational literature, support services and patient referrals.

Tamara Kato, President
Judy Mangione, Secretary
Michael Franzen, Treasurer

Colorado

3949 Hemophilia Society of Colorado
2465 Sheridan Blvd.
Edgewater, CO 80214
720-626-1263
888-687-2568
Fax: 303-629-7035
e-mail: info@cohemo.org
www.cohemo.org

An organization devoted to improving the quality of life for persons affected with bleeding disorders and their complications. This is accomplished through outreach development, educational programs, informational literature, support services and patient referrals.

Larry Hoyle, Manager
Daniel Reilly, President
Sean Perkins, Development Coordinator

Florida

3950 Florida Hemophilia Association
915 Middle River Drive, Suite 421
Ft Lauderdale, FL 33304
305-235-0717
888-880-8330
e-mail: info@floridahemophilia.org
www.floridahemophilia.org

An organization devoted to improving the quality of life for persons affected with bleeding disorders and their complications. This is accomplished through outreach development, educational programs, informational literature, support services and patient referrals.

Barbie Arrebola, President
Jonathan Salk, VP
Janella Espinosa, Secretary/Treasurer

3951 Hemophilia Foundation of Greater Florida
1350 N Orange Avenue, Suite 227
Winter Park, FL 32789
407-629-0000
800-293-6527
Fax: 407-629-9600
e-mail: Hemofoundation@earthlink.net
www.hemophiliaflorida.org

An organization devoted to improving the quality of life for persons affected with bleeding disorders and their complications. This is accomplished through outreach development, educational programs, informational literature, support services and patient referrals.

Alan Apte, VP
Ron Sachs, President
Mike Berkman, Secretary

Georgia

3952 Hemophilia Foundation of Georgia
8800 Roswell Road, Suite 170, PO Box 1844
Atlanta, GA 30350
770-518-8272
800-866-4366
Fax: 770-518-3310
e-mail: mail@hog.org
www.hog.org

An organization devoted to improving the quality of life for persons affected with bleeding disorders and their complications. This is accomplished through outreach development, educational programs, informational literature, support services and patient referrals.

Andrew Maurer, Chief Governance Officer
Nick Blackmon, Vice CGO
Jonathan Lawrie, Secretary

Hawaii

3953 Hemophilia Foundation of Hawaii
1164 Bishop Street, Suite 1501
Honolulu, HI 96813
281-379-4600
Fax: 281-379-1450
e-mail: hemophiliafoundation@hawaii.rr.com
www.bleedingdisorders.org

An organization devoted to improving the quality of life for persons affected with bleeding disorders and their complications. This is accomplished through outreach development, educational programs, informational literature, support services and patient referrals.

Rita Gonzales, President

Idaho

3954 Hemophilia Foundation of Idaho
4696 Overland Road, Suite 234
Boise, ID 83705
208-344-4476
866-453-4476
Fax: 208-344-4476
e-mail: hfi@velocitus.net
www.idahoblood.org

An organization devoted to improving the quality of life for persons affected with bleeding disorders and their complications. This is accomplished through outreach development, educational programs, informational literature, support services and patient referrals.

Shane Bell, President
Ryan Hein, VP
Taryn Magrini, Executive Director

Illinois

3955 Hemophilia Foundation of Illinois
210 S. DesPlaines St, PO Box 5500
Chicago, IL 60661
312-427-1495
Fax: 312-427-1602
e-mail: info@bdai.org
www.hemophiliaillinois.org

An organization devoted to improving the quality of life for persons affected with bleeding disorders and their complications. This is accomplished through outreach development, educational programs, informational literature, support services and patient referrals.

Bill Eftax, President
Eric Sary, VP
Robert Stewart, Treasurer

Indiana

3956 Hemophilia Foundation of Indiana
5172 E. 65th Street, Suite 105
Indianapolis, IN 46220
317-570-0039
800-241-2873
Fax: 317-396-0058
e-mail: mrice@hemophiliaofindiana.org
www.hemophiliaofindiana.org.

An organization devoted to improving the quality of life for persons affected with bleeding disorders and their complications. This is accomplished through outreach development, educational programs, informational literature, support services and patient referrals.

Kasey Shade, President
Joseph McKamey, VP
Melissa Breedlove, Secretary

Kentucky

3957 Kentucky Hemophilia Foundation
1850 Taylor Avenue, Suite 2
Louisville, KY 40213
502-456-3233
800-582-2873
Fax: 502-456-3234
e-mail: info@kyhemo.org
www.kyhemo.org

An organization devoted to improving the quality of life for persons affected with bleeding disorders and their complications. This is accomplished through outreach development, educational programs, informational literature, support services and patient referrals.

Ursela Lacer, Executive Director

Louisiana

3958 Louisiana Hemophilia Foundation
3636 S Sherwood Forest Boulevard, Suite 450
Baton Rouge, LA 70816
225-291-1675
Fax: 225-291-1679
e-mail: lahemophilia@etigers.net
www.louisianahemophilia.org

An organization devoted to improving the quality of life for persons affected with bleeding disorders and their complications. This is accomplished through outreach development, educational programs, informational literature, support services and patient referrals.

Lori Keels, Executive Director
Tres Major, President

Maryland

3959 Hemophilia Foundation of Maryland
13 Class Court
Parkville, MD 21234
410-661-2307
800-964-3131
Fax: 410-661-2308
e-mail: Miller8043@comcast.net
www.hfmonline.org

An organization devoted to improving the quality of life for persons affected with bleeding disorders and their complications. This is accomplished through outreach development, educational programs, informational literature, support services and patient referrals.

Harvey Gates, President
Ryan Melton, VP
Annette Maurits, Secretary

Massachusetts

3960 Massachusetts, New England Hemophilia Association
347 Washington Street, Suite 402
Dedham, MA 02026
781-326-7645
Fax: 781-329-5122
e-mail: info@newenglandhemophilia.org
www.newenglandhemophilia.org

An organization devoted to improving the quality of life for persons affected with bleeding disorders and their complications. This is accomplished through outreach development, educational programs, informational literature, support services and patient referrals.

Kevin R Sorge, Executive Director
Patrick Mancini, President
William McCartney, Treasurer

3961 Hemophilia Foundation of Michigan
1921 W Michigan Avenue
Ypsilanti, MI 48197   734-544-0015
                                       800-482-3041
                                  Fax: 734-544-0095
                     e-mail: harner@hfmich.org
                                    www.hfmich.org

An organization devoted to improving the quality of life for persons affected with bleeding disorders and their complications. This is accomplished through outreach development, educational programs, informational literature, support services and patient referrals.

Ivan Harner, Executive Director
Calvin DeKuiper, President
Amy Denton, VP

Minnesota

3962 Hemophilia Foundation of Minnesota and the Dakotas
750 S Plaza Drive, Suite 207
Mendota Heights, MN 55120   651-406-8655
                                       800-994-4363
                                  Fax: 651-406-8656
                e-mail: hemophiliafoundation@visi.com
                                      www.hfmd.org

An organization devoted to improving the quality of life for persons affected with bleeding disorders and their complications. This is accomplished through outreach development, educational programs, informational literature, support services and patient referrals.

John Schulte, President
Mike Neubert, VP
Elizabeth Myers, Secretary

Mississippi

3963 Mississippi Hemophilia Foundation
36 Avery Circle, PO Box 13608
Jackson, MS 39236   601-957-2706
                        e-mail: patty8501@aol.com
                                www.mshemophilia.com

An organization devoted to improving the quality of life for persons affected with bleeding disorders and their complications. This is accomplished through outreach development, educational programs, informational literature, support services and patient referrals.

Haley Jones, President
Leslee Londen, VP
Patty Lyons, Treasurer

Missouri

3964 Gateway Hemophilia Association of Missouri
14248 F Manchester Road, PMB#310
Manchester, MO 63011   314-482-5973
                                       866-729-0233
                                  Fax: 314-729-7033
                   e-mail: hemophilia@sbcglobal.net
                              www.gatewayhemophilia.org

An organization devoted to improving the quality of life for persons affected with bleeding disorders and their complications. This is accomplished through outreach development, educational programs, informational literature, support services and patient referrals.

Nic Fahey, President
Brent Miller, VP
Andrea Metcalf, Treasurer

Nebraska

3965 Nebraska Chapter of the National Hemophilia Foundation
215 Centennial Mail South, Suite 512
Lincoln, NE 68508   402-742-5663
                                  Fax: 402-742-5677
                   e-mail: office@nebraskanhf.org
                                 www.nebraskanhf.org

An organization devoted to improving the quality of life for persons affected with bleeding disorders and their complications. This is accomplished through outreach development, educational programs, informational literature, support services and patient referrals.

Jason Everts, President
Karie Quintana, VP
Mollie Lovell, Secretary

New York

3966 Bleeding Disorders Association of Northeastern New York
BDANENY, PO Box 947
Rensselaer, NY 12144   518-782-9787
                                  Fax: 518-356-5612
                   e-mail: bdaneny@bdaneny.org
                                   www.bdaneny.org

Formerly known as the Upper Hudson Valley Chapter of the National Hemophilia Foundation. The Association endeavors to meet the diverse needs of a geographically dispersed community through a variety of programs, including; emergency financial support, scholarships, Camp High Hopes, Double Hole in the Woods Ranch, HIV/AIDS education, outreach and support, and recreational community activities.

Deborah Huskie, Co-Executive Director
Kevin Pelletier, Co-Executive Director
David Huskie, President

3967 Hemophilia Center of Western New York
936 Delaware Avenue, Suite 300
Buffalo, NY 14209   716-896-2470
                                       866-434-6551
                                  Fax: 716-218-4010
                                www.hemophiliawny.com

A nonprofit, licensed diagnostic and treatment center. It offers a variety of services for persons with hemophilia and other herditary blood disorders ensuring that the patient is cared for at all times whether at the hospital, at home, at the center at school or on the job.

Robert Long, Chairman
Marcia Gellin, VP
Mary Haggerty, VP

3968 Mary M Gooley Hemophilia Center of the National Hemophilia Foundation
1415 Portland Avenue, Suite 500
Rochester, NY 14621   585-922-5700
                                  Fax: 585-922-5775
                  e-mail: Robert.Fox@viahealth.org
                                 www.hemocenter.org

Specialized diagnostic testing, expert medical evaluation and diagnosis, personal counseling and support groups, home care treatment training, routine and urgent care, education of school and daycare personnel, research to advance knowledge, improve treatment and enhance quality of life for patients and families.

Robert Fox, President
Linda Magliocco, Sr. VP
Jennifer LaFranco, VP

North Carolina

3969 Hemophila Foundation of North Carolina
260 Town Hall Dr., Suite A
Morrisville, NC 27560   336-289-4446
                                          880-990-5557
                                    Fax: 336-725-4873
                          e-mail: rbrummett@triad.rr.com
                                  www.hemophilia-nc.org

An organization devoted to improving the quality of life for persons affected with bleeding disorders and their complications. This is accomplished through outreach development, educational programs, informational literature, support services and patient referrals.

Steven Peretti, President
Leonard Poe, VP
Kathy Register, Treasurer

Ohio

3970 Central Ohio Chapter of the National Hemophilia Foundation
PO Box 345
Worthington, OH 43085   614-457-0027
                                          800-847-0345
                              e-mail: steje08@aol.com
                                www.nhfcentralohio.org

An organization devoted to improving the quality of life for persons affected with bleeding disorders and their complications. This is accomplished through outreach development, educational programs, informational literature, support services and patient referrals.

Jeff Stewart, President
Tracy Kauffman, Treasurer
Anish Mistry, Secretary

3971 Northern Ohio Chapter of the National Hemophilia Foundation
One Independence Place
5000 Rockside Road, Suite 230
Independence, OH 44131   216-834-0051
                                          800-554-4366
                                    Fax: 216-834-0055
                       e-mail: lynnecapretto@nohf.org
                                           www.nohf.org

The mission is to enhance the quality of life for people with genetic bleeding disorders and their families, through advocacy, education, research and other constituency services.

Marlene Piatak, President
Michelle Zawadski, VP
Katey Vanderwyst, Treasurer

3972 Northwest Ohio Hemophilia Foundation
2121 Hughes Drive Harris-McIntosh Tower 2nd Floor
Toledo, OH 43606   419-291-5882
                                    Fax: 419-479-3269
                         e-mail: info@nwohemophilia.org
                                  www.nwohemophilia.org

A volunteer nonprofit organization that serves the bleeding disorders community in Northwest Ohio.

Carla Wells, Executive Director
Scott Newsom, President

3973 Southwestern Ohio Chapter of the National Hemophilia Foundation
82 Elva Court, Suite B
Dayton, OH 45377   937-415-0644
                                    Fax: 937-415-0604
                                  e-mail: SWOF@aol.com

Serving people with hemophilia and blood clotting disorders in an 11 county area. Dedicated to offering people and their families; educational opportunities about the physical, psychological and social aspects of these disorders. Workshops and seminars are regularly offered to address these issues. Offers support groups, volunteer services, telephone and walk-in education, information, counseling and referrals.

Dena M Shephard, President

3974 Tri-State Bleeding Disorders Chapter of the National Hemophilia Foundation
635 W 7th Street, Suite 407
Cincinnati, OH 45203   513-961-4366
                                    Fax: 513-961-1740
                           e-mail: hemophilia@fuse.net
                                           www.tsbdf.com

Formerly known as the Greater Cincinnati/Northern Kentucky Chapter of the National Hemophilia Foundation. An organization devoted to improve the quality of life for persons affected with bleeding disorders and their complications. This is accomplished through outreach development, educational programs, informational literature, support services and patient referrals.

Lisa Raterman, Executive Director
Jeff Reichert, President
Andy Proeschel, Secretary

Oklahoma

3975 Oklahoma Chapter of the National Hemophilia Foundation
720 West Wilshire Blvd., Suite 101-B
Okhlama, OK 73116   405-463-6634
                                          800-735-3855
                                    Fax: 405-879-9748
                               e-mail: ohf@dmgp.com
                                      www.hemophilia.org

An organization devoted to improving the quality of life for persons affected with bleeding disorders and their complications. This is accomplished through outreach development, educational programs, informational literature, support services and patient referrals.

Tom Ayers, President
Kerri Crabtree, Vice President
Bob Goodley, Executive Director

Oregon

3976 Hemophilia Foundation of Oregon
10940 SW Barnes Rd #129
Portland, OR 97225   503-297-7207
                                    Fax: 503-297-0127
                       e-mail: info@hemophiliaoregon.org
                                 www.hemophiliaoregon.org

An organization devoted to improving the quality of life for persons affected with bleeding disorders and their complications. This is accomplished through outreach development, educational programs, informational literature, support services and patient referrals.

Linda Charles, President
Dave Worthington, Vice President

Pennsylvania

3977 Delaware Valley Chapter of the National Hemophilia Foundation
14 E. 6th St. First Floor
Lansdale, PA 19446   215-393-3611
                                    Fax: 215-393-9419
                        e-mail: hemophilia@navpoint.com
                                 www.hemophiliasupport.org

An organization devoted to improving the quality of life for persons affected with bleeding disorders and their complications. This is accomplished through outreach development, educational programs, informational literature, support services and patient referrals.

Thomas Galvin, President
William Widerman, Vice President
Jon Worthington, Treasurer

3978 Western Pennsylvania Chapter of The National Hemophilia Foundation
532 S Aiken Avenue, Suite 102
Pittsburgh, PA 15232 412-683-2231
Fax: 412-683-2568
e-mail: wpcnhf@earthlink.net

Brings together and serves as a focal point for those segments of the community most concerned with hemophilia. They include medical and social service providers, people with hemophilia and their families, educators and the general public. This chapter combines service, education and advocacy programs.

Kerry Fatula, Executive Director
Ida McFarren, President

South Carolina

3979 Hemophilia Association of South Carolina
PO Box 3874
Sumter, SC 29151 864-350-9941
888-829-4849
Fax: 888-829-4849
e-mail: information@hemophiliaofsouthcarolina.ne
www.hemophiliaofsouthcarolina.net

An organization devoted to improving the quality of life for persons affected with bleeding disorders and their complications. This is accomplished through outreach development, educational programs, informational literature, support services and patient referrals.

Mark Eichelberger, President
Brandy Stewart, Vice President

Tennessee

3980 Tennesse Hemophilia & Bleeding Disorders Foundation
1819 Ward Drive, Suite 102
Murfreesboro, TN 37129 615-900-1486
888-703-3269
Fax: 615-900-1487
e-mail: mail@thbdf.org
www.thbdf.org

Offers a hemophilia clinic, social workers and consultants, a state hemophilia program, blood donor programs, counseling programs, genetic counseling, literature and resources, summer camp, grants and more for the hemophilia and HIV/AIDS community.

Kent Russ, President
John Snook, West-TN VP
Jerry Duntop, East-TN VP

Texas

3981 Lone Star Chapter of the National Hemophilia Foundation
10500 Northwest Freeway, Suite 226
Houston, TX 77092 713-686-6100
888-LSC-NHF1
Fax: 832-383-4601
e-mail: Director@LoneStarHemophilia.org
www.lonestarhemophilia.org

An organization devoted to improving the quality of life for persons affected with bleeding disorders and their complications. This is accomplished through outreach development, educational programs, informational literature, support services and patient referrals.

Nick Zasowski, President
Jennifer Borders, Vice President
Brian Crompton, Treasurer

3982 Texas Central Chapter of the National Hemophilia Foundation
12700 Hillcrest Road, Suite 191
Dallas, TX 75230 972-386-3865
Fax: 214-654-9954
e-mail: mail@texcen.org
www.texcen.org

A group of volunteers seeking solutions to the various aspects of the hemophilia problem. Supports blood drives, sponsors a summer camp for hemophiliac children, conducts educational member meetings, arranges for genetic counseling and sponsors group support meetings.

Shannon Brush, President
Jacob Banker, Vice President
David Simmons, Treasurer

Utah

3983 Utah Chapter of the National Hemophilia Foundation
772 East 3300 South, Suite 210
Salt Lake City, UT 84106 801-484-0325
877-INF- VWD
Fax: 801-484-2488
e-mail: smuir@hemophiliautah.org
www.hemophiliautah.org

Offers educational information, pamphlets, fundraising events and more for persons and families affected by hemophilia.

Scott Muir, Executive Director
Reg Ecker, President
Lynn Barker, VP

Virginia

3984 Hemophilia Association of the Capital Area
10560 Main Street, Suite 419
Fairfax, VA 22030 703-267-6502
Fax: 703-352-2145
e-mail: admin@hacacares.org
www.hacacares.org

A nonprofit organization serving persons with bleeding disorders and their families in northern Virginia, Washington, DC and Montgomery and Prince George's Counties in Maryland. The mission is to improve the quality of life for persons with hemophilia and Von Willebrand's disease and their families, to educate, to act as an advocate, to provide member services and to raise money to fulfill all these purposes.

Sandi Qualley, Executive Director
Miriam Goldstein, President
Paul Brayshaw, VP

3985 United Virginia Chapter of the National Hemophilia Foundation
PO Box 188
Midlothian, VA 23113 804-740-8643
800-266-8438
Fax: 804-740-8643
e-mail: vahemophiliaed@verizon.net
www.vahemophilia.org

An organization devoted to improving the qualit of life for persons affected with bleeding disorders and their complications. This is accomplished through outreach development, educational programs, informational literature, support servcies and patient referrals.

Kelly Waters, Executive Director
Kevin O'Connor, President
Erica George, President-Elect

Washington

3986 Bleeding Disorders Foundation of Washington
9639 Firdale Ave, Ste A
Edmunds, WA 98020 206-533-1660
Fax: 206-533-1686
e-mail: general@bdfwa.org
www.bdfwa.org

An organization devoted to improving the quality of life for persons affected with bleeding disorders and their complications. This is accomplished through outreach development, educational programs, informational literature, support services and patient referrals.

Regina Timmons, Executive Director
Reid Morgan, President
Caprice Sauter, Board President

3987 Hemophilia Foundation of Washington
PO Box 4565
West Richland, WA 99353
509-967-0203
e-mail: iebd4u@verizon.net

The Foundation's mission is to provide a conduit for education and information, advocate for excellent medical care, and support affected individuals and their families via peer outreach programs and special events

Jill McCary, President
Debbie Campeau, Executive Director

Wisconsin

3988 Great Lakes Hemophilia Foundation
638 N 18th Street, Suite 108
Milwaukee, WI 53233
414-257-0200
888-797-4543
Fax: 414-257-1225
e-mail: info@glhf.org
www.glfh.org

The only Wisconsin organization that addresses the physical, emotional, social and financial needs of individuals affected by hemophilia. This chapter supports high-quality, cost-effective programs for patient care, education, research and public awareness.

Bill Finn, President
Jeff Koopmeiners, VP
David Osswald, Secretary

Libraries & Resource Centers

Alabama

3989 Alabama Department of Rehabilitation Services
602 S Lawrence St.
Montgomery, AL 36104
334-293-7500
800-441-7607
Fax: 334-293-7383
e-mail: cboswell@rehab.state.al.us
www.rehab.state.al.us

Mission is to enable children and adolescents with special health needs and adults with hemophilia to achieve their maximum potential within a community-based, family-centered, comprehensive, culturally sensitive and coordinated system of services.

Cary Boswell, Ed.D, Director

Indiana

3990 Riley Hemophilia and Thrombophilia Center
702 Barnhill Drive, ROC 4270
Indianapolis, IN 46202
317-274-2153
800-769-2848
Fax: 317-278-3751
e-mail: anholcom@iupui.edu
www.rileypeds.org

We strive to improve the health and health care of children by developing and applying best scientific evidence and methods in health services research and informatics.

Richard Schreiner, MD, Chairman of Pediatrics
Anna Holcomb, Executive Director

Wisconsin

3991 Hemophilia Outreach Center
2060 Bellevue St
Green Bay, WI 54311
920-965-0606
800-992-6026
Fax: 920-965-0607
e-mail: info@hemophiliaoutreach.org
www.hemophiliaoutreach.org

A comprehensive treatment center serving individuals and families with bleeding disorders. A facility maintained and administered through the collaboration of lay people, professionals, medical providers, consumers and families. Offering a variety of programs and services in a family-oriented, safe environment directed toward a holistic approach to wellness and to living a full life, including coordinating comprehensive care, consumer advocacy and financial and emotional support.

Katie Kralovetz, Executive Director

Research Centers

3992 Albany New York Regional Comprehensive Hemophilia Treatment Center
Albany Medical College
43 New Scotland Avenue
Albany, NY 12208
518-262-3125
800-773-7080
Fax: 518-262-6320
e-mail: ALBANYHTC@mail.amc.edu
www.amc.edu/patient/services/hemophilia

Providing comprehensive health care for patients with mild to severe hemophilia A, hemophilia B, von Willebrand's disease and thrombophilia in the Albany, New York region.

Barbara Leckerling, Administrator
Joanne Porter, MD, Director

3993 Blood Research Institute of Saint Michael's Medical Center
Cathedral Healthcare System
111 Central Avenue
Newark, NJ 07102
973-877-5000
Fax: 973-877-5466
www.smmcnj.org

Dedicated to research and the treatment of blood-related disorders and cancers, the Blood Research Institute is a multi-disciplinary unit of the hematology/oncology departments.

Yale S Arkel, MD

3994 Boston Hemophilia Center
Children's Hospital Boston
300 Longwood Avenue, Fegan 7
Boston, MA 02115
617-355-4977
Fax: 617-730-0641
e-mail: international.center@childrens.harvard.e
www.childrenshosptial.org

A federally funded hemophilia treatment center, the program offers comprehensive care to people with hemophilia and their families. Services range from medical treatment, counseling and support to discounts on clotting-factor replacement and other products that people with hemophilia require.

Haroon Patel

3995 Cardeza Foundation Hemophilia Center
Thomas Jefferson University Hospital
705 Curtis Building, 1015 Walnut Street
Philadelphia, PA 19107
215-955-8544
www.jefferson.edu

Devoted to research into the causes of a wide v ariety of diseases of the blood and to the diagnosis and care of patients with blood and lymphatic diseases. Our members have competence in all areas of hematology, with particularly well recognized depth and experience in diseases affecting blood platelets, hemorrhagic (bleeding) and thrombotic (clotting) disorders, hematologic malignancies (leukemia, lymphoma and multiple myeloma) and other bone marrow disorders.

Jamie Siegel, MD, Director
Pamela Scruci, Admin Asst.
David Boligitz, Interim Business Manager

3996 Center for Cancer and Blood Disorders at Children's Medical Center in Dallas
1935 Medical District Drive
Dallas, TX 75235
214-456-7000
Fax: 214-456-6133
e-mail: CCBDinfo@childrens.com
www.childrens.com/ccbd

Comprehensive diagnostic and treatment program for patients with disorders of blood coagulation which results in increased risk of bleeding or clotting.

George Buchanan, MD, Director

3997 Children's Center for Cancer and Blood Disorders of Palmetto Health Richland
7 Richland Medical Park Drive
Columbia, SC 29203
803-434-3533
800-775-2287
Fax: 803-434-4598
www.palmettohealth.org

Diagnosis and treatment of cancer and blood disorders. The staff includes a nurse practitioner and a patient and family educator who provide complex nursing management, treatment and navigation through the healthcare system. The multidisciplinary team also includes skilled social workers, therapists, nutritionists and child-life specialists, all of whom play an active role in each child's care.

Fauni Lowe, Manager
Beth Blackmon, Public Relations Director

3998 Children's Hospital of Philadelphia Hemophilia Program
34th Street & Civic Center Boulevard
Philadelphia, PA 19104
215-590-1000
800-879-2467
Fax: 215-426-5480
www.chop.edu

Provides multidisciplinary comprehensive care for children and adolescents with inherited bleeding disorders. Services include diagnosis, acute and chronic medical management of hemophilia and its complications, genetic counseling, physical therapy, HIV care and counseling and coordination with other services.

A Michael Broennle, Program Director
Regina B Bulter, RN, Program Nurse Coordinator

3999 Comprehensive Bleeding Disorder Center
Children's Hospital of Illinois
4727 N. Sheridan Rd.
Peoria, IL 61614
309-655-7171
Fax: 309-688-0917
e-mail: CBDC@hemophilia-ctr-peoria.com
www.compbleed.com

Provides and facilitates state-of-the-art treatment for children and adults with hemophilia and related bleeding and thrombatic disorders. The staff includes a board-certified physician in pediatrics and pediatric hematology/oncology, nurses, social worker, rural outreach coordinator, reimbursement specialist/patient advocate, physical therapist and dentist.

Edward Hui, Executive Director
Sara Dill, Administration Director
John Redington, Executive Director

4000 Comprehensive Pediatric Hemophilia Treatment Center
University of Miami
1150 NW 14th Street
Miami, FL 33136
305-243-7570
www.pediatrics.med.miami.edu

Provided excellent medical and psychological care and emotional support for patients with bleeding disorders and their families since 1987. The HTC participates in national and regional research protocols dealing with various aspects of coagulation disorders. Orthopaedic and physical therapy are also offered at the monthly comprehensive clinic.

Maria Santaella, RN, Director
Steve E Lipshultz, MD, Chairman

4001 East Tennessee Comprehensive Hemophilia Center
University of Tennessee Medical Center
1924 Alcoa Highway 4 NW, Suite 180, Building E
Knoxville, TN 37920
865-454-9170
Fax: 865-544-9876
www.utmedicalcenter.org/hemophilia_services

Provides multidisciplinary comprehensive care to persons with bleeding disorders, including information, education and counseling to families affected by these disorders. The center's professional staff and consultants serve patients with hereditary bleeding disorders in Knoxville and surrounding counties.

William Rukeyser, Chairman
Renda Burkhart, Vice Chair
Bernard Bernstein, Secretary/Treasurer

4002 Eastern Michigan Hemophilia Center
Hurley Medical Center
1921 W. Michigan Avenue
Ypsilanti, MI 48197
734-544-0015
800-482-3041
Fax: 734-544-0095
www.hfmich.org/medical_resources

Provide and coordinate a broad range of treatment and prevention services provided by physicians who specialize in hematology and other relevant specialties such as orthopedics, social work, psychologists, nurses with extensive training and experience with hemophilia, genetic counselors, dentists, dental hygienists, and dieticians.

Calvin DeKuiper, President
Amy Denton, VP
Peter Deininger, Treasurer

4003 Federal Hemophilia Treatment Center Program of Los Angeles
Children's Hospital of LA
4650 Sunset Boulevard
Los Angeles, CA 90027
323-660-2450
Fax: 323-660-7128
www.chla.org

Provides continuing and comprehensive care to children and young adults with inherited bleeding disorders (in particular, hemophilia). The hemophilia treatment program is a federally funded resource which focuses on multidisciplinary management of bleeding disorders and collaborates with other programs in the United States to provide comprehensive care and teaching for patients and health care providers.

Wing-Yen Wong, MD, Director
Robert Miller, Coordinator

4004 Federal Hemophilia Treatment Center of Hawaii
Kapiolani Medical Center for Women and Children
1319 Punchou Street Pau
Honolulu, HI 96826
808-983-8551
Fax: 808-983-6000
e-mail: martha.smith@kapiolani.org
www.kapiolani.org

Part of a nation-wide network established to promote comprehensive hemophilia care and to prevent hemophilia complications.

Desiree Medeiros, MD, Director
Dee Ann Omatsu, RN, Coordinator

4005 First Regional Hemophilia Center
James H Quillen College of Medicine
400 N State of Franklin Road, 1st Floor
Johnson City, TN 37604
423-433-6206
Fax: 423-433-6220

Helping patients and families to manage every aspect of living with hemophilia, from providing information about the latest medical developments to organizing support groups for parents and teens.

Sheri Miller, RN

4006 Hemophilia Center of Arkansas
Arkansas Children's Hospital
1 Children's Way, PO Box 3591
Little Rock, AR 72202
501-364-1100
Fax: 501-364-4332
TDD: 501-364-1184
www.archildrens.org/

Patients with coagulation disorders can be diagnosed and evaluated by a group of physicians, physical therapists, dentists, psychologists and geneticists to provide education, prevention and continuity of care. The Hemophilia Center of Arkansas offers the latest diagnosis, prevention and treatment modalities for children and adults.

Nikki Shock

4007 Hemophilia Center of Western New York
936 Delaware Avenue, Suite 300
Buffalo, NY 14209
716-896-2470
866-434-6551
Fax: 716-218-4010
e-mail: hemoctr@pce.net
www.hemophiliawny.com

The center provides a variety of services to the hemophilia and HIV/AIDS community. Included among these services are diagnostics, registration, outpatient treatment, home care programs, home visits, school visits, dental services and counseling services. Offers an adult unit and a pediatric unit.

Thomas Long, President
Marcia Gellin, VP
Mary Haggerty, VP

4008 Hemophilia Center of Western Pennsylvania
3636 Boulevard of the Allies
Pittsburgh, PA 15213
412-209-7280
Fax: 412-683-4029
www.hcwp.net

Comprehensive care to all individuals who are diagnosed with Hemophilia residing in Western Pennsylvania.

Karen Saban, Manager
A. Kim Ritchey, MD, Vice Chair
Kim Goldby-Reffner, Co-Ordinator

4009 Hemophilia Center of the New England Medical Center
UMass Memorial Medical Center; Memorial Campus
119 Belmont Street
Worcester, MA 01605
508-334-1000
www.umassmemorial.org

Family-oriented, state-of-the-art medical and psychosocial services, education and research. Provides diagnostic and treatment services for individuals with bleeding disorders using a community-based, family centered and culturally sensitive approach. A hematologist is available 24 hours a day.

Doreen Brettler, MD, Director
Ann Forsberg, Program Administrator

4010 Hemophilia Program at Children's National Medical Center
Hematology/Oncology Department
111 Michigan Avenue NW
Washington, DC 20010
202-476-5000
www.childrensnational.org

Children's Hemophilia Program offers high quality, comprehensive care for children with hemophilia and thrombophilia. Children's is the only program in the Metropolitan DC are that is supported by the National Institutes of Health. Nearly 150 patients are treated here annually.

Anne Angiolillo, MD, Director
Kurt Newman, MD

4011 Hemophilia Treatment Center at the University of Iowa
UI Health Care Department of Pediatrics
200 Hawkins Drive
Iowa City, IA 52242
319-356-1616
Fax: 319-356-3862
e-mail: melinda-schultz@uiowa.edu
www.uihealthcare.com

Committed to provide the best care for individuals with bleeding disorders. To accomplish this mission we offer state of the art comprehensive clinical care, education to patients and their families and accessibility to clinical research projects that are oriented to improve the lives of people with these type of disorders.

Donna Katen-Bahensky, Ceo
Donald E McFarlane, MD, Co-Director
Mindy Schultz, Secretary

4012 Hemophilia and Coagulation Programs
Norris Cotton Cancer Center
1 Medical Center Drive
Lebanon, NH 03756
603-650-5000
Fax: 603-650-7791
www.cancer.dartmouth.edu/services/hemophilia

Provides complete clinical and laboratory diagnostic facilities for evaluation and treatment of patients with cogenital bleeding disorders and disorders of thrombosis and hemostasis.

Sophia Ouhilal, Program Director

4013 Hemophilia and Thrombosis Center at the University of Minnesota Medical Center
Phillips-Wangensteen Building, Sixth Floor, Clinic
Minneapolis, MN 55455
612-626-6455
800-688-5252
Fax: 612-625-4955
e-mail: htc@fairview.org
www.uofmmedicalcenter.org

Offers a wide range of services for patients with inherited bleeding and clotting disorders. We care for patients of all ages using a team approach. Hematologists and nurse clinicians are involved and provide services including diagnostic evaluations, treatment, education, research and care coordination.

Beverly Christie, Manager
Margaret Heisel Kurth, MD, Co-Director
Shannon Fabick, Administrative Secretary

4014 Hemophilia and Thrombosis Center of Nevada
2020 W Palomino Lane, Suite 110
Las Vegas, NV 89106
702-385-2702
Fax: 702-322-0158
www.htcnevada.org

Offers diagnosis and management for persons with inherited or acquired bleeding disorders including hemophilia, von Willebrand's Disease, and platelet disorders. Comprehensive care is administered using a team approach with input from social services, physical therapy, orthopedic specialists, dentist, nursing, laboratory support, and medical services.

Nancy Sewell, Manager

4015 Hemophilia and Thrombosis Center: Division of Blood Disease Center
Cincinnati Children's Hospital Medical Center
3333 Burnet Avenue, PO Box 3026
Cincinnati, OH 45229
513-636-4200
800-344-2462
Fax: 513-636-4900
e-mail: blood@cchmc.org
www.cincinnatichildrens.org

Aim is to improve the lives of children and adolescents with hemophilia and thrombophilia. This is achieved by offering compassionate, state-of-the-art clinical care to patients and their families, advancing our understanding of the disorder through research and educating future health care providers and leaders in the field.

Karen Kalinyak, MD, Director
Vinod V Balasa, Thrombosis Director

4016 Indiana Hemophilia and Thrombosis Center
8402 Harcourt Road, Suite 420
Indianapolis, IN 46260
317-871-0000
888-256-8837
Fax: 317-871-0010
e-mail: info@ihtc.org
www.ihtc.org

Multidisciplinary evaluation and treatment facility serving the people of Indiana who have bleeding disorders or thrombotic disease (known collectively as disorders of coagulation). The center aids local medical providers in the care of individuals of all ages with blood disorders and their families.

Phillip E. Himelstein, Founder
Ike G. Batalis, President
Edward R. Schmidt, President

4017 Kalamazoo Comprehensive Hemophilia Treatment Center
Michigan State University
1000 Oakland Drive, PO Box 8000
Kalamazoo, MI 49008
269-337-4400
e-mail: webmaster@med.wmich.edu
www.kcms.msu.edu

Offers diagnosis, management, and genetic counseling for these patients, as well.

Frank J. Sardone, President/CEO
John M. Dunn, Chairman of the Board
Hal B. Jenson, Dean

4018 Louisiana Comprehensive Hemophilia Care Center
Tulane University School of Medicine
6823 St. Charles Avenue
New Orleans, LA 70118

504-865-5000
Fax: 504-988-6808
e-mail: website@tulane.edu
www.tulane.edu

Provides diagnostic, evaluation and treatment services for individuals with hemophilia, von Willebrand disease and other coagulopathies throughout Louisiana and the Mississippi gulf coast. The Center provides comprehensive medical and psychosocial evaluations through a multi-disciplinary team of adult and pediatric hematologists, orthopedists, nurses, social workers, physical therapists and dentists.

Anthony Lorino, Senior Vice President for Operation
Frances Vickers, Executive Assistant to the Senior V

4019 Maine Hemophilia and Thrombosis Center
Maine Medical Center
22 Bramhall Street, PO Box 3175
Portland, ME 04102

207-662-0111
877-339-3107
Fax: 207-885-7687
TTY: 207-662-4900
www.mmc.org

Offers a wide range of services for patients with inherited bleeding and clotting disorders. We care for patients of all ages using a team approach. Hematologists and nurse clinicians are involved and provide services including diagnostic evaluations, treatment, education, research and care coordination. Also, a full-time social worker provides psychosocial assessment, counseling and resource information.

Glen Roy, RN, Contact

4020 Mayo Comprehensive Hemophilia Center
13400 E. Shea Blvd.
Scottsdale, AZ 85259

480-301-8000
800-446-2279
Fax: 507-284-0161
www.mayoclinic.org

Specializes in treating people with hemophilia and other bleeding disorders. The Center provides evaluation and care to approximately 200 patients per year. It also assists in the management and care of another 100 patients annually who come to Mayo Clinic for initial evaluation or consultation.

Denis Cortese, MD, CEO

4021 Miami Comprehensive Hemophilia Center
University of Miami, Department of Pediatrics
1601 N.W. 12th Ave
Miami, FL 33136

305-270-3400
Fax: 305-325-8387
e-mail: pedsinformation@med.miami.edu
www.pediatrics.med.miami.edu

The Comprehensive Pediatric Hemophilia Treatment Center has provided excellent medical and psychological care and emotional support for patients with bleeding disorders and their families since 1987. HTC participates in national and regional research protocols dealing with various aspects of coagulation disorders. The major goal of the HTC medical team is to improve the quality of life for patients and their families coping with the stress and discomfort of living with a chronic illness.

Luis Caldera-Nieves, Medical Director

4022 Michigan State University Comprehensive Center for Bleeding Disorders
138 Service Road, Suite A-225
East Lansing, MI 48824

517-353-4920
800-759-5595
Fax: 517-353-9421
www.healthteam.msu.edu/

Offering education and information to individuals and families affected by blood clots and blood clotting disorders, and to assist with research efforts relating to all aspects of thrombosis and thrombophilia.

Gerald R Aben, Director
Roshni Kulkarni, MD, Coordinator

4023 Nebraska Regional Hemophilia Center
Nebraska Medical Center
42nd and Emile
Omaha, NE 68198

402-559-4000
800-922-0000
Fax: 402-552-2410
e-mail: nmamdani@nebraskamed.com
www.unmc.edu/

Medical and educational support for those dealing with hemophilia, and their families.

Nizar Mamdani, Executive Director

4024 North Dakota Comprehensive Hemophilia and Thrombosis Treatment Center
Roger Maris Cancer Center/MeritCare Health System
820 4th Street N
Fargo, ND 58122

701-234-7544
800-437-4010
Fax: 701-234-7577
www.meritcare.com/specialties/more/hemophilia

Provides comprehensive care for people who have hemophilia, von Willebrand's disease and many other types of bleeding and clotting disorders. Using a team approach, professionals work together to provide evaluations, recommendations, treatment plans and follow-up care. They also offer a variety of services including assistance with clotting factors and home therapy.

Dr. Nathan Kobrinsky, MD, Director

4025 Northern Regional Bleeding Disorder Center
1105 6th Street
Traverse City, MI 49684

231-935-7227
800-468-6766
Fax: 231-935-6582
e-mail: contact@mhc.net
www.munsonhealthcare.org

A program which cares for patients with all types of bleeding disorders from 26 northern Michigan counties. Provides specialty treatment to patients with hemophilia with the goal of minimizing complications from bleeding episodes.

Dan Wolf, Chairman
John Pelizzari, Vice Chairman
Bob Sprunk, Secretary

4026 Northwest Ohio Hemophilia Treatment Center
Toledo Childrens Hospital
2142 N Cove Boulevard
Toledo, OH 43606

419-291-5437
888-291-5437
Fax: 419-479-3258
www.promedica.org

A full range of inpatient and outpatient services is provided for children and adolescents with blood conditions and cancer. The patient care program also offers support for the psychosocial needs of patients and their families.

Ann Gilbert, RN, Director

4027 Orthopaedic Hospital's Hemophilia Treatment Center
2400 S Flower Street
Los Angeles, CA 90007

213-742-1000
Fax: 213-741-8338
e-mail: info@orthohospital.org
www.orthohospital.org

Objective of the Center is the diagnosis and optimal management of bleeding disorders and their complications. Disorders treated include hemophilia A and B, von Willebrand's disease, and other inborn deficiencies of plasma clotting factors and platelets. Adolescents and adults who have acquired blood-borne infections, including chronic hepatitis and HIV infection, through prior treatment with blood products, are also treated at the Center.

Joseph Mirra, Director
Carol K Kasper, MD, Emeritus Director
James V Luck, Jr.; MD, Center's Surgeon

4028 Pediatric Hemophilia Program of Pennsylvania
Children's Hospital of Pittsburgh
4401 Penn Ave
Pittsburgh, PA 15224   412-692-5325
                                        www.chp.edu

Provides high quality, comprehensive care for children with hemophilia and thrombophilia through research and clinical programs.

Vincent Deeney, Director
Kim Ritchey, MD, Pediatric Program Director
Melanie Finnigan, Public Affairs Director

4029 Phoenix Center for Cancer and Blood Disorders
Phoenix Children's Hospital
1919 E Thomas Road
Phoenix, AZ 85016   602-546-1000
                                        888-908-5437
                                        www.phoenixchildrens.com

Largest program of its kind in Arizona and is making significant difference in the quality of life for pediatric and adult hemophilia patients. It is one of only two federally funded hemophilia treatment programs in the state. The Center treats children with sickle cell disease, hemophilia and other hematologic disorders, and it is a designated center for the treatment and study of Gaucher's disease, an inherited metabolic disorder that can cause multiple medical problems.

Mark Bonsall, Chairman of the Board
Jon Hulburd, Vice Chairman
Robert L Meyer, President/CEO

4030 Puget Sound Blood Center
921 Terry Avenue
Seattle, WA 98104   206-292-6500
            e-mail: HumanResources@psbc.org
                                        www.psbc.org

Puget provides all the blood and tissue services that people in our region need. It is this longstanding pledge to the community that has guided the Blood Center to more than sixty years of unparalleled success and to a leadership position in healthcare. In addition, our work in medical research is advancing medical care and making cures possible for patients around the world.

Jmaes P. AuBuchon, President/CEO
A. Kent Fisher, VP
Frederick R. Appelbaum, Executive Director

4031 Regional Hemophilia Program
Children's Hospital of Michigan
3901 Beaubien Street
Detroit, MI 48201   313-745-5437
                                        888-362-2500
                                        www.chmkids.org/

Clinical evaluations and recommendations by a team of experts, home treatment, training and educational programs, HIV/AIDS counceling and management, carrier detection and genetic counceling. Clinical trials provide our patients with the latest treatment modalities and in-depth surveillence of complications.

Lynne Thomas Gordon, COO
Herman Gray, MD, President

4032 Research at BloodCenter of Wisconsin
638 North 18th Street
Milwaukee, WI 53233   414-257-2424
                                        877-232-4376
                                        Fax: 414-937-6580
            e-mail: jeanne.mccabe@bcw.edu
                                        www.bcw.edu

Through basic, clinical and applied research programs, the center's scientists are enable to continue discoveries that enables to extend continuum of care.

Jeanne McCabe, Research Administration Director

4033 Rhode Island Hemostasis and Thrombosis Center
Rhode Island Hospital
593 Eddy Street, Hasbro Lower Level
Providence, RI 02903   401-444-7731
                                        Fax: 401-444-6104
                                        www.rhodeislandhospital.org

Formerly known as the Rhode Island Hemophilia Treatment Center, we have expanded our services to offer to persons with clotting disorders the same cutting edge, comprehensive program that has been extremely successful for our bleeding disorders community.

Timothy J. Babineau, President/CEO
Cathy Duquette, Executive Vice President
Mamie Wakefield, Executive VP/CFO

4034 SUNY Upstate Medical University Research Development
750 E Adams Street, PO Box 2375
Syracuse, NY 13210   315-464-5540
                                        Fax: 315-464-4318
                                        www.upstate.edu/research

In collaboration with Upstate faculty, the Center conducts research and executes data analyses designed to guide the improvement of patient care and associated patient outcomes.

William J Hardoby, Research VP

4035 South Dakota Center For Bleeding Disorders
Sioux Valley Hospital
1600 W. 22nd St
Sioux Falls, SD 57117   605-312-1000
            e-mail: info@siouxvalley.org
                                        www.glhf.org

Provides comprehensive care based on family centered/community based health care. Hemophilia specialists are available 24 hours a day.

Bill Finn, President
Jeff Koopmeiners, VP
David Osswald, Secretary

4036 South Texas Comprehensive Hemophilia and Thrombophilia Treatment Center
University of Texas Medicine
7703 Floyd Curl Drive
San Antonio, TX 78229   210-567-5200
                                        Fax: 210-567-6921
            e-mail: NAVAE@UTHSCSA.EDU
                                        www.pediatrics.uthscsa.edu

A federally funded program focusing on the evaluation, treatment, and prevention of complications from Hemophilia, Von Willebrand's disease, thrombophilia, and menorrhagia in adolescents and women.

Thomas C. Mayes, M.D., MBA, Chairman
Steven R. Neish, MD, SM, Vice Chairman
Dennis A. Conrad, MD, Associate Chairman for Continuing M

4037 Spectrum Health Research
DeVos Hospital/Spectrum Health
100 Michigan Street NE
Grand Rapids, MI 49503   616-391-9000
                                        866-989-7999
        e-mail: research.department@spectrum-health.org
                                        www.helendevoschildrens.org

Formerly known as the Cook Institute for Research and the Cook Research Department. The Spectrum Health research department has a reputation for selectively participating in clinical research that brings cutting-edge treatments to the people of West Michigan. Many of the diseases under study currently have limited or no treatment options.

David T Lock, President
Dominic Sanflippo, MD, Executive Medical Director

4038 Steele Children's Research Center
University of Arizona College of Medicine
1501 N Campbell Avenue, Suite 3301, PO Box 245073
Tucson, AZ 85724   520-626-2221
                                        Fax: 520-626-7176
                                        www.steelecenter.arizona.edu

At the University of Arizona College of Medicine, internationally known physicians and scientists, who also are professors in the UA Department of Pediatrics, work together to research causes and develop cures for childhood illnesses and diseases. Our goal is to advance medical knowledge to help improve the health of Arizona's children and children throughout the world.

Fayez Ghishan, MD, Director
Lori Stratton, MPH, Director of Development
Darci Slaten, MA, Director of Communications and Mark

4039 Ted R. Montoya Hemophilia Program
University of New Mexico Health Sciences Center
2211 Lomas Blvd NE
Albuquerque, NM 87131   505-272-2111
                                        Fax: 505-272-6845
                            www.hospitals.unm.edu/outpt/trmhp/

Division program provides comprehensive care to the individual
(child and adult) with hemophilia and other hereditary bleeding
disorders.

Steve Mckernan, Chief Operations Officer
Carolyn Voss, Chief Operations Officer
David Pitcher, Chief Medical Officer

4040 UCD Hemophilia Treatment Center
2315 Stockton Boulevard
Sacramento, CA 95817   916-734-2011
                                         800-2 U- DAV
                                        TDD: 916-734-9230
                                      www.ucdmc.ucdavis.edu

Offers a variety of medical, educational and social services to
people with hemophilia or other inherited bleeding disorders and
their families across Northern California.

John Meyer, Vice Chancellor
Linda P.B. Katehi, Chancellor
Ralph Hexter, Provost and Executive Vice Chancell

4041 UCSD Hemophilia Treatment Center
Div of Hematology-Oncology, UCSD Med Ctr Hillcrest
9500 Gilman Dr., La Jolla
San Diego, CA 92093   858-534-2230
                                        Fax: 858-822-6288
                                  e-mail: kdherbst@ucsd.edu
                                            www.ucsd.edu

Part of the federal network of over 140+ specialty centers for
bleeding disorder diagnosis and management. These two HTCs
are funded, in part, by grants from the Maternal and Child Health
Bureau and Centers for Disease Control and Prevention. The purpose of the grants is to support a multidisciplinary team which
can provide comprehensive care and conduct research to prevent
hemophilia complications.

Amy Lovejoy, MD, Director
Catherine Glass, RN, Nurse Coordinator

**4042 UT Southwestern Medical Center at Dallas:
Hematology-Oncology Research**
5323 Harry Hines Boulevard
Dallas, TX 75390   214-648-3111
                                        Fax: 214-645-7999
                                  e-mail: utsouthwestern.org
                                      www.utsouthwestern.edu

Basic science research is enhanced by the world class investigative environment at UT Southwestern that includes 4 Nobel Prize
winners and other internationally known scientists with whom hematology-oncology faculty regular collaborate. Cutting edge clinical research in hemophilia/thrombophilia and ITP are also major
commitments.

Daniel K. Podolsky, President
Robin M. Jacoby, VP/Chief of Staff

4043 United Health Services Blood Disorder Center
Wilson Regional Medical Center
33-57 Harrison Street
Johnson City, NY 13790   607-763-6000
                                        Fax: 607-763-5514
                                            www.uhs.net/

Provides comprehensive care for those with blood disorders_from
diagnosis to treatment to home care and support services. Physicians, nurse specialists, dentists, orthopedists, physical therapists,
and social workers treat people diagnosed with hemophilia and
vWD at a dedicated site at Wilson Memorial Regional Medical
Center. They also assist family physicians throughout the region
in caring for persons with blood disorders.

Rajesh J Dave', President/CEO
Peter LoFaso, Chair
Roger Scott, Managing Director

4044 University of Cincinnati Adult Hemophilia Program
Division of Hematology & Oncology
Mail Location 11009, 3333 Burnet Avenue
Cincinnati, OH 45229   513-636-4269
                                        Fax: 513-636-5599
                                  e-mail: palascje@ucmail.uc.edu
                                  www.hemophilia-information.com

Patient care, teaching, and research in the area of hematology/on-
cology. Rapidly growing in all research, clinical, and educational
components. The division participates in investigator-initiated
protocols, pharmaceutical or industry-sponsored studies, as well
as cooperative groups, such as the Southwest Oncology Group
and Radiotherapy Oncology Group.

Joseph Palascak, MD, Director
Albert Muhleman, MD, Division Director
Madeline Heffner, RN, Nurse Coordinator

**4045 University of Michigan Adult Hemophilia and Cougulation
Disorders Program**
1500 E Medical Center Drive, Floor B1
Ann Arbor, MI 48109   734-936-6641
                                         800-211-8181
                                        Fax: 734-936-6666
                            www2.med.umich.edu/healthcenters

Provides comprehensive, coordinated assessments and management services for individuals with blood disorders. Disorders
may include disorders of blood coagulation (abnormal bleeding
and clotting), hematology, hematopoietic malignancies, coagulation disorders, Von Willebrand's disease, lupus anticoagulant and
thrombosis, and hemophilia.

Christine L Holland, Director

4046 University of Tennessee Hemophilia Clinic
UT Health Science Center
920 Madison Avenue, Suite 822
Memphis, TN 38163   901-448-1751
                                        Fax: 901-448-7929
                                        TDD: 901-448-7382
                                            www.uthsc.edu

Diagnosis, evaluation, management, and treatment. The Hemophilia Center uses a comprehensive model to deliver effective
care coordinated in the community. Emphasis is on educating
providers, educators, patients, and their families for successful
management. The center also manages a hemophilia factor
concentrate program.

Dr. Marion Dugdale, Director
Steve J. Schwab, CEO/MD

4047 University of Texas Department of Hematology Research
University of Texas Medical School at Houston
7000 Fannin, Suite 1200
Houston, TX 77030   713-500-4HSC
                                        Fax: 713-500-3026
                                         www.uthouston.edu

Major research activities include a multidisciplinary center for
vascular and thrombosis research and diversified hematologic and
oncologic research projects covering a wide scope of disciplines
from molecular biology to clinical trials.

Giuseppe N. Colasurdo, President
Kevin Dillon, Sr. VP
George M. Stancel, VP

4048 Vanderbilt Hemostasis-Thrombosis Clinic
Vanderbilt University Medical Center
2200 Children's Way, 6105 DOT, PO box 9830
Nashville, TN 37232   615-936-1765
                                         866-372-5663
                                        Fax: 615-936-8400
                                  e-mail: VHTCClinic@vanderbilt.edu
                                  www.vanderbiltchildrens.com

Comprehensive health promotion; preventive medical and dental
services; diagnostic testing; genetic testing and counseling; individual case management; specific and prompt treatments as
needed; education and training; options for home treatment; and
referrals, when necessary.

Anderson B Collier III, MD, Director
Mary G Hudson, RN, Nursing Coordinator
Kim Blittle, Administrative Assistant

4049 Vermont Regional Hemophilia Center
Fletcher Allen Health Care
UHC Campus, Old Hall Room 2106A, 1 South Prospect
Burlington, VT 05401   802-847-8041
                                            Fax: 802-847-8041
                            www.hemophilia-information.com

Miriam Grant, RN
Alan Homans, MD

4050 West Central Ohio Hemophilia Center
Children's Medical Center of Dayton
1 Childrens Plaza, PO Box 1815
Dayton, OH 45404   937-641-5877
                                            Fax: 937-641-5878
                            www.hemophilia-information.com

The center provides complete care for individuals and families
with hemophilia and related bleeding disorders. Some of the services offered include a comprehensive clinic, emergency treatment network, consultations, diagnostic coagulation laboratory,
home infusion programs, HIV/AIDS education and counseling
and more.

James French III, MD, Medical Director

4051 Yale Pediatric Hematology/Oncology Research Center
Yale School of Medicine
333 Cedar Street
New Haven, CT 06510   203-785-4640
                                            Fax: 203-737-2228
                        e-mail: diana.beardsley@yale.edu
                                        www.medicine.yale.edu

Oriented toward improving the lives of children with blood disorders and childhood cancer, while working toward future improved
treatments and outcomes.

Diana S Beardsley, MD; PhD, Research Director
Robert J. Alpern, MD
James E. Rothman, Chairman

Conferences

4052 National Hemophilia Foundation Annual Meet ing
National Hemophilia Foundation
116 W 23rd Street, 11th Floor
New York, NY 10001   212-328-3700
                                                  800-424-2634
                                            Fax: 212-328-3777
                            e-mail: handi@hemophilia.org
                                        www.hemophilia.org

A three-day conference that offers educational sessions, networking opportunities and social events for all ages.

Val Bias, CEO
Ken Trader, Chairman

Audio Video

4053 Song of Superman
National Hemophilia Foundation
116 W 32nd Street, 11th Floor
New York, NY 10001   212-328-3700
                                                  800-424-2634
                                            Fax: 212-328-3777
                            e-mail: handi@hemophilia.org
                                        www.hemophilia.org

Designed to help young people with bleeding disorders come to
terms with their HIV status, sexuality, and living with HIV. The
video explores issues of disclosure in relationships and safer sex
through dramatic scenes and frank testimonials by young people
living with hemophilia and/or HIV. The companion workbook
contains group exercises that follow each of the main topics of
the video and serve as a bridge to discussion.

1993 33 Mins

Val Bias, CEO
John Indence, VP, Marketing & Communications
Mary Ann Ludwig, Vice President for Development

Web Sites

4054 Health Answers
410 Horsham Road
Horsham, PA 19044   215-442-9010
                    e-mail: Michael.tague@healthanswers.com
                                        www.healthanswers.com

HealthAnswers offers a breadth of services in medical education,
sales force training, patient support solutions, professional promotion and customer solutions.

Michael Tague, Managing Director

4055 National Hemophilia Foundation
116 W 32nd Street, 11th Floor
New York, NY 10001   212-328-3700
                                                  800-424-2634
                                            Fax: 212-328-3777
                            e-mail: handi@hemophilia.org
                                        www.hemophilia.org

Devoted to improving the quality of life for persons affected with
bleeding disorders. This is accomplished through outreach development, educational programs, information literature, support
services and patient referrals.

Val Bias, CEO
John Indence, VP, Marketing & Communications
Mary Ann Ludwig, Vice President for Development

4056 Online Mendelian Inheritance in Man
8600 Rockville Pike
Bethesda, MD 20894   888-346-3656
                                e-mail: info@ncbi.nlm.nih.gov
                                        www.ncbi.nlm.nih.gov

This database is a catalog of human genes and genetic disorders.

Book Publishers

4057 Adventures of Maxx
Nova Factor
1620 Century Centery Parkway, Suite 109
Memphis, TN 38137   901-385-3600
                                                  800-235-8498
                                            Fax: 901-385-3778

An activity book for children with hemophilia, this publication is
intended to be both educational and entertaining.

1991 15 pages

4058 Genetics Coloring Book
Medical College of Virginia
P.O Box 980565
Richmond, VA 23298   804-828-9793
                                            Fax: 804-828-5115
                            e-mail: bodurtha@gems.vcu.edu
                                        www.medschool.vcu.edu/

Adventures of Gene coloring book for children ages 5-9. Two
coloring books, one dealing with cystic fibrosis and one with hemophilia.

1994-1995 Comic/Coloring

4059 Guide to Insurance Coverage for People With Hemophilia
Armour Pharmaceutical Company
500 Arcola Road
Collegeville, PA 19426   215-454-3720

An educational guide designed to assist with health insurance
concerns.

4060 Harold Talks About How He Inherited Hemophilia
Hemophilia Foundation
1850 Taylor Avenue,Suite 2
Louisville, KY 40213   502-456-3233
                                                  800-582-2873
                                            Fax: 502-456-3234
                                e-mail: info@kyhemo.org
                                        www.kyhemo.org

Children's brochure explaining hemophilia causes, symptoms and living a regular life.

4061 Harold's Secret: A Boy with Hemophilia
Bayer
400 Morgan Lane
West Haven, CT 06516   203-937-2765

A comic book for youngsters pertaining to children with hemophilia and understanding of the illness among school friends.

16 pages

4062 Hemophilia Camp Directory
National Hemophilia Foundation
116 W 32nd Street
New York, NY 10001   212-328-3700
                                      Fax: 212-328-3777
                            e-mail: handi@hemophilia.org
                                      www.hemophilia.org

Lists camps in the United States for children with hemophilia and other coagulation disorders.

16 pages

4063 Hemophilia Diseases and People
Enslow Publishers
40 Industrial Road
Berkeley Heights, NJ 07922   908-771-9400
                                      800-398-2504
                                 Fax: 908-771-0925
                  e-mail: CustomerService@enslow.com
                                      www.enslow.com

An excellent resource for basic research for personal or academic use. The disease is carefully described, with effective black-and-white graphics, charts, and photos, showing blood biology and the circulatory system and the various levels of severity (depending on what clotting factors the individual is missing).

Ages: 9-12 128 pages Library Binding
ISBN: 0-766016-84-6

Edward Willet, Editor

4064 Hemophilia Handbook
Hemophilia of Georgia
8800 Roswell Road, Suite 170
Atlanta, GA 30350   770-518-8272
                                Fax: 770-518-3310
                            e-mail: mail@hog.org
                                      www.hog.org

A comprehensive, easy-to-read resource for people with hemophilia and their families. The fourth edition of this handbook, contains up-to-date information on all important topics.

1988 348 pages

Hikie Allen, Director
Arthur Herman, Director

4065 Hemophilia Nursing Handbook
National Hemophilia Foundation
116 W 32nd Street
New York, NY 10001   212-328-3700
                                      Fax: 212-328-3777
                            e-mail: handi@hemophilia.org
                                      www.hemophilia.org

A revision and expansion of the 1995 Hemophilia Nursing Handbook. Now incorporating von Willebrand disease and other bleeding disorders. It is intended to provide comprehensive information as well as practical ideas to assist nurses at all levels in caring for patients with bleeding disorders. The guide is designed to be both an introduction to nurses new to coagulation and a resource for more experienced nurses.

1995 Members: $20

4066 Let's Talk About Going to the Hospital
Rosen Publishing Group's PowerKids Press
29 E 21st Street
New York, NY 10010   212-777-3017
                                      800-237-9932
                                 Fax: 888-436-4643
                  e-mail: rosenpub@tribeca.ios.com
                                      www.powerkidspress.com

If a child has to check into the hospital, chances are he or she is already upset about being ill. Knowing how a hospital functions and what the procedures are, such as when family members can visit, will help in what is already a stressful situation. Grades K-5.

24 pages
ISBN: 0-823950-36-0

4067 Passport: Global Treatment Centre Directory
World Federation of Hemophilia
1425 Rene Levesque Boulevard W, Suite 1010
Montreal, Quebec, H3G
Canada   514-875-7944
                                 Fax: 514-875-8916
                            e-mail: wfh@wfh.org
                                      www.wfh.org

Lists over 900 hemophilia treatment centres and national hemophilia organizations in more than 100 countries, including contact names, telephone and fax numbers, as well as e-mail and web site addresses. It is very useful for people with hemophilia who are travelling to other countries and as a directory of hemophilia treaters around the world.

1990 188 pages Members: $6

Magazines

4068 Bloodstone Magazine
Hemophilia Health Services
1640 Century Center Parkway
Memphis, TN 38134   877-222-7336
                     e-mail: info@hemophiliahealth.com
                                      www.hemophiliahealth.com

A premier magazine of the bleeding disorders community. Features of community news, The Adventures of Welligan Hugsley, ProToCall, and human interest stories. A must read for anyone interested in the latest hemophilia related information.

Quarterly

Kyle J Callahan, Publisher/President
Lydia Dixon Harden, Editor-in-Chief

4069 HEMALOG
Materia Medica
208 E 51st Street, Box 234
New York, NY 10022   212-725-5151
                                      Fax: 212-725-2794
                            e-mail: mmca@earthlink.net
                                      www.mmca.com

The purpose of Hemalog is to serve as a national forum for the hemophilia community, providing current news, information, opinion, and contact with others in the community. The material contained in this journal reflects the experience and opinion of a wide range of people connected with hemophilia, and encourages story and art contributions.

Quarterly

Barbara Robin Slonevsky, Publisher
Janet Spencer-King

4070 HemAware
National Hemophilia Foundation
116 W 32nd Street, 11th Floor
New York, NY 10001   212-328-3700
                                      800-424-2634
                                      Fax: 212-328-3777
                            e-mail: handi@hemophilia.org
                                      www.hemophilia.org

Packed with medical updates, analysis, professional news, and practical health information for people living with a bleeding disorder and for their care providers. This magazine showcases how custom publishing can deepen relationships within a community by providing useful information in a compelling format.

Bi-Monthly

Val Bias, CEO
John Indence, VP, Marketing & Communications
Mary Ann Ludwig, Vice President for Development

4180 March of Dimes Birth Defects Foundation
1275 Mamaroneck Avenue
White Plains, NY 10605   914-997-4488
                                                    888-663-4637
                                                 Fax: 914-997-4763
                              e-mail: answers@marchofdimes.com
                                           www.marchofdimes.com

Partnership of volunteers and professionals dedicated to improving the health of babies by preventing birth defects and infant
mortality. Over 100 chapters are located across the country and
can be located through the National Office.

Jennifer L Howse, President

Conferences

4181 Genetic Alliance Annual Conference
Genetic Alliance
4301 Connecticut Avenue NW, Suite 404
Washington, DC 20008   202-966-5557
                                                    800-336-4363
                                                 Fax: 202-966-8553
                                  e-mail: info@geneticalliance.org
                                            www.geneticalliance.org

Consistently inspirational and enables partnership among all
stakeholders: advocates and community leaders, health and industry professionals, policymakers, and academicians.

July

Sharon Terry, President/CEO
Tetyana Murza, Programs/Events Manager

Web Sites

4182 National Histicytosis Organizations
332 North Broadway
Pitman, NJ 8071   856-589-6606
                                                 Fax: 856-589-6614
                                          e-mail: info@histio.org
                                                www.histio.org/

Is an international partnership of patients, families, physicians
and friends. Is is a nonprofit organization whose goals are to promote scientific research into the hitiocytoses, seeking to develop
better means of control and management of the disease and
ultimatley seeking to develop scientific means to prevent and cure
them and to provide solutions to some of the problems which are
specific to patients suffering from this disease and to offer support to such patients and their families.

James Hassan, Esq., Chairman
Robert List, Treasurer
Tracy Brown, Trustee

4183 Online Mendelian Inheritance in Man
8600 Rockville Pike
Bethesda, MD 20894   888-346-3656
                                       e-mail: info@ncbi.nlm.nih.gov
                                              www.ncbi.nlm.nih.gov

This database is a catalog of human genes and genetic disorders.

4184 Texas Children's Cancer Center
P.O. Box 2659
Austin, TX 78768   512-474-1798
                                                      www.txcc.org

Offers innovative therapies for all forms of childhood cancer and
blood disorders. The Cancer Center is working to improve the
outcome for all patients afflicted with these diseases and to develop and perfect new treatment approaches that are born from
only the most extraordinary scientific insights.

Geanie Morrison, President
James Frank, Vice President
Jodie Laubenberg, Secretary

Book Publishers

4185 Let's Talk About Going to the Hospital
Rosen Publishing Group's PowerKids Press
29 E 21st Street
New York, NY 10010   212-777-3017
                                                    800-237-9932
                                                 Fax: 888-436-4643
                              e-mail: rosenpub@tribeca.ios.com
                                           www.powerkidspress.com

If a child has to check into the hospital, chances are he or she is
already upset about being ill. Knowing how a hospital functions
and what the procedures are, such as when family members can
visit, will help in what is already a stressful situation. Grades
K-5.
24 pages
ISBN: 0-823950-36-0

Description

4186 HODGKIN'S DISEASE

Synonym: Hodgkin's lymphoma

Covers these related disorders: Hodgkin's disease—lymphocyte depletion type, Hodgkin's disease—lymphocyte predominance type, Hodgkin's disease—mixed cellularity type, Hodgkin's disease—nodular sclerosing type

Involves the following Biologic System(s):
Hematologic and Oncologic Disorders

Hodgkin's disease is a malignant disorder (cancer) characterized by painless, progressive enlargement of the lymph nodes, spleen, and other lymphoid tissues (lymphoma). The lymphatic system includes a network of vessels that collect a fluid known as lymph from different areas of the body and drain this fluid into the bloodstream. As lymph moves through the lymphatic system, it is filtered by a network of lymph nodes, which are small structures located along the course of the lymphatic vessels. Most lymph nodes that can be felt (palpable) are located in the neck, mouth, and groin and under the arms (axillae). Lymph nodes store certain white blood cells and are thought to play a role in producing antibodies, thus functioning as part of the body's immune system.

Malignancies of lymph tissue, known as lymphomas, are the third most common form of cancer affecting children in the United States. Approximately 13 per one million children are affected by lymphoma in the U.S. each year. There are two main categories of lymphoma, including Hodgkin's disease and non-Hodgkin's lymphoma. Although Hodgkin's disease may affect individuals of any age, it usually occurs between the ages of 15 and 35 or after age 50. In children, the disease is most common during late childhood or early adolescence and rarely affects those younger than five years of age. About 6,000 to 7,000 cases of the disease occur in the U.S. annually. Epstein-Barr virus, a member of the herpesvirus family that causes mononucleosis 35-50 percent of the time, may play some role in the disease. In addition, some familial cases have been reported, suggesting possible genetic mechanisms.

Hodgkin's disease is characterized by the presence of relatively large, abnormal white blood cells that have more than one nucleus and a distinctive appearance under a microscope. These cancerous cells, known as Reed-Sternberg cells, may be seen during the microscopic examination of small tissue samples removed from affected lymph nodes or other lymphoid tissues. Hodgkin's disease is categorized into four main subtypes based upon the number and relative proportion of such cells as well as the proportions of certain other white blood cells (e.g., plasma cells, eosinophils, macrophages, etc.). The frequency of the different subtypes varies with age. For example, nodular sclerosing type is the most common form of the disease and affects approximately 50 percent of children and up to 70 percent of adolescents with Hodgkin's disease. Another subtype, known as the mixed cellularity type, affects about 40 to 50 percent of patients, and the lymphocyte predominance type of the disease primarily occurs in males and younger patients. The fourth subtype, called lymphocyte depletion type, is the rarest and most aggressive form of the disorder and occurs in fewer than 10 percent of patients.

Hodgkin's disease usually originates in the lymphatic vessels. As the disease progresses, the malignancy may spread from lymph nodes and infiltrate certain organs, particularly the spleen, lungs, liver, and bone marrow. Most patients initially experience painless swelling of lymph nodes in the neck or, in some cases, under the arm or in the groin area. Some may gradually develop generalized symptoms including fever, night sweats, fatigue, listlessness (lethargy), generalized itching (pruritus), loss of appetite (anorexia), and weight loss. Involvement of other organs or tissues may cause varying symptoms. For example, if the lungs are affected, patients may experience coughing and shortness of breath (dyspnea). Advanced involvement of the bone marrow may result in abnormally low levels of circulating red blood cells (anemia), platelets (thrombocytopenia), or certain white blood cells (neutropenia). Advanced disease may cause progressive impairment of the body's immune system, resulting in an increased susceptibility to certain infections. In patients with severe disease progression, infection with certain microorganisms that typically cause no or only minor symptoms in healthy individuals may result in severe or potentially life-threatening complications.

Treatment of patients with the disease varies, depending on the stage of the disease and other factors. For patients in early stages who have localized disease and have obtained full growth, radiation therapy alone may be effective; the 10-year survival rate exceeds 80 percent. However, up to 15 percent of such patients may experience recurrences, requiring therapy with certain anticancer drugs (combination chemotherapy). However, combination therapy cures more than 50 percent of patients, even those with advanced-stage disease. Combination chemotherapy may include the drugs doxorubicin (Adriamycin), bleomycin, vinblastine, and dacarbazine (known as ABVD) or a combination of mechlorethamine, vincristine (Oncovin), procarbazine, and prednisone (called MOPP). Physicians who specialize in the treatment of childhood cancers (pediatric oncologists) often select alternating therapy with MOPP and ABVD in combination with low-dose radiation therapy due to this treatment's high success and a reduction in certain long-term effects potentially associated with treatment for Hodgkin's disease. For example, such combination chemotherapy/radiation therapy may help reduce the risk of potential growth defects in affected children, damage to heart and lung tissue, infertility, or the development of certain secondary malignancies later in life, such as acute myeloid leukemia (AML) or certain solid tumors. Patients should receive ongoing monitoring throughout life to ensure prompt detection and treatment of possible recurrences or secondary malignancies.

Government Agencies

4187 NIH/National Cancer Institute
9609 Medical Center Drive, 7th Floor, West Tower,
Bethesda, MD 20892

240-276-6340
800-422-6237
www.cancer.gov

The National Cancer Institute coordinates the National Cancer Program, which conducts and supports research, training, health information dissemination, and other programs with respect to the cause, diagnosis, prevention, and treatment of cancer, rehabilitation from cancer, and the continuing care of cancer patients and the families of cancer patients.

John E Niederhuber MD, Director
Harold Varmus, M.D., Director

National Associations & Support Groups

4188 American Academy of Pediatrics
141 Northwest Point Boulevard
Elk Grove Village, IL 60007
847-434-4000
800-433-9016
Fax: 847-434-8000
www.aap.org

The American Academy of Pediatrics and its member pediatricians are committed to the attainment of optimal physical, mental and social health and well-being for all infants, children, adolescents, and young adults.

Sandra Hassink, MD, FAAP, President

4189 Candlelighters Childhood Cancer Foundation
PO Box 498
Kensington, MD 20895
301-962-3520
855-858-2226
Fax: 310-962-3521
e-mail: staff@candlelighters.org
www.acco.org

The Candlelighters Childhood Cancer Foundation National Office was founded in 1970 by concerned parents of children with cancer. Today our membership of over 50,000 members of the national office and more than 100,000 members across the across the country, including Candlelighters affiliate groups, includes, parents of children who are being treated or have been treated for cancer.

Ruth Hoffman, Executive Director
Amber Masso, Program Director
Liz Dicus, Administrative Co-Ordinator

4190 Leukemia & Lymphoma Society
1311 Mamaroneck Avenue, Suite 310
White Plains, NY 10605
914-949-5213
Fax: 914-949-0391
www.lls.org

Largest voluntary health organization dedicated to funding blood cancer research, education and patient services.

Timonthy S. Durst, Chairman
James H. Davis, Vice-Chair
Kenneth Schwartz, Secretary

4191 Lymphoma Research Foundation of America
115 Broadway 19th Floor, Suite 1301
New York, NY 10006
212-349-2910
800-500-9976
Fax: 212-349-2886
e-mail: Helpline@lymphoma.org
www.lymphoma.org

National nonprofit organization dedicated to eradicating lymphoma and serving those touched by this disease. LRF funds research to develop safer, more effective treatments and ultimately, a cure for lymphoma. LRF delivers a comprehensive slate of educational and support programs, services, and publications for lymphoma patients and their loved ones.

Steven J. Prince, Chairman
Jerry Freundlich, Secretary
Tom Condon, Treasurer

4192 National Childhood Cancer Foundation
4600 East West Highway, Suite 600
Bethesda, MD 20814
301-718-0042
800-458-6223
Fax: 301-718-0047
e-mail: info@curesearch.org
www.curesearch.org

CureSearch unites the world's largest childhood cancer research organization, the Children's Oncology Group, and the National Childhood Cancer Foundation through our mission to cure childhood cancer. Research is the key to the cure.

Stuart Siegal, Chairman
Timothy Harmon, Vice-Chair
Mary Payne, Treasurer

4193 National Foundation for Cancer Research
4600 East West Highway, Suite 525
Bethesda, MD 20814
301-654-1250
800-321-2873
Fax: 301-654-5824
e-mail: info@nfcr.org
www.nfcr.org

The National Foundation for Cancer Research (NFCR) was founded in 1973 to support cancer research and public education relating to the prevention, early diagnosis, better treatments and ultimately, a cure for cancer. NFCR promotes and facilitates collaboration among scientists to accelerate the pace of discovery from bench to bedside.

Franklin C Salisbury, President
Judith P. Barnhard, Chairman
Michael Burke, Treasurer

Web Sites

4194 Children's Cancer Web
www.cancerindex.org/ccw

An independent nonprofit site, established to provide a directory of childhood cancer resources.

Book Publishers

4195 Let's Talk About Going to the Hospital
Rosen Publishing Group's PowerKids Press
29 E 21st Street
New York, NY 10010
212-777-3017
800-237-9932
Fax: 888-436-4643
e-mail: rosenpub@tribeca.ios.com
www.powerkidspress.com

If a child has to check into the hospital, chances are he or she is already upset about being ill. Knowing how a hospital functions and what the procedures are, such as when family members can visit, will help in what is already a stressful situation. Grades K-5.

24 pages
ISBN: 0-823950-36-0

4196 Let's Talk About when Kids Have Cancer
Rosen Publishing Group's PowerKids Press
29 E 21st Street
New York, NY 10010
212-777-3017
800-237-9932
Fax: 888-436-4643
e-mail: rosenpub@tribeca.ios.com
www.powerkidspress.com

In a straightforward yet comforting way, this book explains what cancer is, what kinds of treatments surround the disease and how to cope if a child has cancer.

24 pages
ISBN: 0-823951-95-2

4197 Living with Childhood Cancer: A Practical Guide to Help Families Cope
Leigh A. Woznick, Carol D. Goodheart EdD, author

American Psychological Association
750 1st Street
Washington, DC 20002
202-336-5500
800-374-2721
TTY: 202-336-6123
www.apa.org

This book offers information for families faced with the shattering experience of having a child with cancer.

2001 359 pages Hardcover
ISBN: 1-557988-72-2

Donald N. Bersoff,PhD, JD, President
Norman B. Anderson, PhD, Chief Executive Officer & Executive
Bonnie Markham, PhD, Treasurer

4198 Surviving Childhood Cancer: A Guide for Families
New Harbinger Publications
5674 Shattuck Avenue
Oakland, CA 94609

510-652-0215
800-748-6273
Fax: 800-652-1613
e-mail: customerservice@newharbinger.com
www.newharbinger.com

Cancer in a child is an overwhelming experience for a family.
This book explains common medical procedures and offers readers practical advice about how to cope with emotions and stress
during this time.

1998 232 pages
ISBN: 1-572241-02-0

Pamphlets

4199 Hodgkin's Disease and Non-Hodgkin's Lymphomas
Leukemia and Lymphoma Society
1311 Mamaroneck Avenue, Suite 310
White Plains, NY 10605

914-949-5213
800-955-4572
Fax: 914-949-6691
e-mail: infocenter@lls.org
www.leukemia-lymphoma.org

Explanation of the disease, its symptoms, diagnosis, prognosis
and treatment, psychological responses to a confirmed diagnosis
and current research.

36 pages

Louis J. DeGennaro, Ph.D., President & CEO
Rosemarie Loffredo, Chief Administrative Officer & CFO
Mark Roithmayr, Chief Development Officer

Description

4200 HOMOCYSTINURIA

Covers these related disorders: Homocystinuria Type I (Classic homocystinuria), Homocystinuria Type II, Homocystinuria Type III

Involves the following Biologic System(s):
Genetic/Chromosomal/Syndrome/Metabolic Disorders

Homocystinuria is a metabolic disorder characterized by an inborn error in the metabolism of the amino acid methionine. There are three types of homocystinuria, each resulting from a deficiency or defect of a specific enzyme or compound that is essential in the processing of methionine.

Homocystinuria Type I (Classic homocystinuria) is caused by a deficiency of the enzyme cystathionine synthase. Although symptoms and physical findings are not apparent at birth, early symptoms may include delays in development and failure to thrive. Characteristic findings, which are often not apparent until after the age of three years, may include eye abnormalities such as dislocation of the lens of the eyes (ectopia lentis), followed by nearsightedness (myopia) and tremors of the iris (iridodonesis). Other physical findings may include skeletal abnormalities such as osteoporosis, sideways curvature of the spine (scoliosis), either a sunken or prominent chest (pectus deformity), and a condition known as genu valgum in which the legs curve inward causing the knees to touch (knock-knee) and the space between the feet to increase. Affected children often have a fair complexion, blue eyes, sparse blonde hair, and a characteristic flushed face (malar flush). In addition, there is a tendency to develop blood clots (thromboemboli) in the veins and arteries.These clots may occur at any time, and if they lodge in the brain can result in paralysis and seizures heart problems and high blood pressure may also occur. Laboratory findings may include elevated levels of both methionine and the sulfur compound homocystine in body fluids. Mental retardation is apparent in approximately 65 percent of affected people. It is estimated that about 50 percent of patients experience some form of psychiatric disorder.

Treatment for classic homocystinuria includes aggressive vitamin B6 supplementation. In addition, restriction of foods that contain methionine is recommended in conjunction with supplementation of cysteine, also a sulfur-containing amino acid. In some affected individuals who do not respond to vitamin B6 treatment, administration of betaine may be effective. Classic homocystinuria is inherited as an autosomal recessive trait and occurs in approximately one in 200,000 live births. The gene for cystathionine synthase is located on the long arm of chromosome 21 (21q22.3).

Homocystinuria Type II is transmitted as an autosomal recessive trait and results from a defect in the formation of methylcobalamin. Characteristic symptoms and findings depend on the particular underlying defect. Some children with homocystinuria type II may also have a condition called methylmalonic aciduria characterized by excessive methylmalonic acid in the urine. Symptoms usually develop in the early months of life and may include difficulty in feeding, listlessness, vomiting, diminished muscle tone (hypotonia), and delays in development. Treatment for this form of homo stinuria includes vitamin B12 supplementation (cobalamin).

Homocystinuria Type III, a very rare form of the disorder, results from a deficiency of the enzyme methylenetetrahydrofolate reductase (MTHFR), also essential to the maintenance of methionine. Symptoms and physical findings are extremely variable and depend upon the extent of the deficiency. Complete absence of this enzyme may result in life-threatening episodes of respiratory distress as well as seizure-like muscle contractions (myoclonus). A partial enzyme deficiency may cause convulsions, an abnormally small head (microcephaly), mental retardation, and muscular irregularities. Occasional findings may include psychiatric disturbances, abnormalities of certain blood vessels, and inflammation or degenerative changes of specific nerves. In addition, blood clot activity may be apparent in some affected individuals.

Treatment for homocystinuria type III may include supplementation with folic acid, vitamin B6 (pyridoxine), vitamin B12, methionine, and betaine (also known as trimethylglycine). Early intervention with betaine has a particularly effective outcome. Homocystinuria Type III is transmitted as an autosomal recessive trait. The gene for methylenetetrahydrofolate reductase is located on the short arm of chromosome 1 (1p36.3).

National Associations & Support Groups

4201 ARC of the United States
1825 K Street MW, Suite 1200
Washington, DC 20006

202-534-3700
800-433-5255
Fax: 202-534-3731
e-mail: info@thearc.org
www.thearc.org

The ARC is the national organization of and for people with mental retardation and related developmental disabilities and their families. Devoted to promoting and improving supports and services for people with mental retardation and their families. The association also fosters research and education regarding the prevention of mental retardation in infants and young children. The ARC was founded in 1950 by a small group of parents and other concerned individuals.

Nancy Webster, President
Ronald Brown, VP
Elise McMillan, Secretary

4202 American Academy of Pediatrics
141 Northwest Point Boulevard
Elk Grove Village, IL 60007

847-434-4000
800-433-9016
Fax: 847-434-8000
www.aap.org

The American Academy of Pediatrics and its member pediatricians are committed to the attainment of optimal physical, mental and social health and well-being for all infants, children, adolescents, and young adults.

Sandra Hassink, MD, FAAP, President

4203 Genetic Alliance
4301 Connecticut Avenue NW
Washington, DC 20008

202-966-7955
800-336-4363
Fax: 202-966-8553
e-mail: info@geneticalliance.org
www.geneticalliance.org

A nonprofit tax exempt organization founded in 1986 as a national coalition of consumers, professionals and genetic support groups to voice the common concerns of children and adults and families living with, and at risk of, genetic conditions. The Alliance builds partnerships among consumers and professionals and the private and public sectors to promote optimum healthcare and enhanced quality of life for individuals identified with genetic conditions.

Joan Oppenheimer Weiss, Founder
Sharon Terry, President

4204 March of Dimes Birth Defects Foundation
1275 Mamaroneck Avenue
White Plains, NY 10605   914-997-4488
888-663-4637
Fax: 914-997-4763
e-mail: answers@marchofdimes.com
www.marchofdimes.com

Partnership of volunteers and professionals dedicated to improving the health of babies by preventing birth defects and infant mortality. Over 100 chapters are located across the country and can be located through the National Office.

Jennifer L Howse, President

Conferences

4205 ARC Annual National Convention
The ARC
1825 K Street NW, Suite 1200
Washington, DC 20006
202-534-3700
800-433-5255
Fax: 202-534-3731
e-mail: info@thearc.org
www.thearc.org

held in cities throughout the U.S. each fall which attracts nearly 1000 people for educational sessions, business meetings and social events.

Nancy Webster, President
Ronald Brown, Vice President
Elise McMillan, Secretary

4206 Genetic Alliance Annual Conference
Genetic Alliance
4301 Connecticut Avenue NW, Suite 404
Washington, DC 20008
202-966-5557
800-336-4363
Fax: 202-966-8553
e-mail: info@geneticalliance.org
www.geneticalliance.org

Consistently inspirational and enables partnership among all stakeholders: advocates and community leaders, health and industry professionals, policymakers, and academicians.

July

Sharon Terry, President/CEO
Tetyana Murza, Programs/Events Manager

Web Sites

4207 ARC of the United States
1825 K Street, NW, Suite 1200
Washington, DC 20006
800-433-5255
www.thearc.org

The ARC is the national organization of and for people with mental retardation and related developmental disabilities and their families. Devoted to promoting and improving supports and services for people with mental retardation and their families. The association also fosters research and education regarding the prevention of mental retardation in infants and young children. The ARC was founded in 1950 by a small group of parents and other concerned individuals.

Ronald Brown, President
Elise McMillan, Vice President
M.J. Bartelmay, Jr., Secretary

4208 CLIMB: Children Living with Inherited Metabolic Disorders
www.climb.org.uk

800-652-3181
www.climb.org.uk

Official website for the organization, committed to fighting metabolic diseases through research, awareness and support, providing advice, information and support on all metabolic diseases to children, young adults, families, carers and professionals. Includes links to other sites.

4209 Genetic Alliance
4301 Connecticut Ave NW, Suite 404
Washington, DC 20008   www.geneticalliance.org

A nonprofit tax exempt organization founded in 1986 as a national coalition of consumers, professionals and genetic support groups to voice the common concerns of children and adults and families living with, and at risk of, genetic conditions. The Alliance builds partnerships among consumers and professionals and the private and public sectors to promote optimum healthcare and enhanced quality of life for individuals identified with genetic conditions.

Sharon Terry, MA, President & CEO
Natasha Bonhomme, VP, Strategic Development
Ruth Evans, Director of Accounting

4210 March of Dimes Birth Defects Foundation
1275 Mamaroneck Avenue
White Plains, NY 10605   914-997-4488; www.marchofdimes.com

Partnership of volunteers and professionals dedicated to improving the health of babies by preventing birth defects and infant mortality. Over 100 chapters are located across the country and can be located through the National Office.

4211 Maryland Department of Health
201 W. Preston Street
Baltimore, MD 21201   410-767-6500; 877-463-3464
e-mail: dhmh.healthmd@maryland.gov; dhmh.maryland.gov

Our mission is to protect, promote and improve the health and well being of all Maryland citizens in a fiscally responsible way.

4212 National Center for Biotechnology Information
8600 Rockville Pike
Bethesda, MD 20894   888-346-3656
e-mail: info@ncbi.nlm.nih.gov; www.ncbi.nlm.nih.gov

A national resource for biology information, the center creates public databases, conducts research in computational biology, develops software tools for analyzing genome data, and disseminated biomedical information, all for the better understanding of molecular processes affecting human health and disease.

4213 Online Mendelian Inheritance in Man
8600 Rockville Pike
Bethesda, MD 20894   888-346-3656; e-mail: info@ncbi.nlm.nih.gov
www.ncbi.nlm.nih.gov

This database is a catalog of human genes and genetic disorders.

4214 Rare Genetic Diseases in Children (NYU)
550 First Avenue
New York, NY 10016   212-263-7300; development.med.nyu.edu

We target issues arising from rare genetic diseases affecting children. Also, to assist in the endeavor to bring knowledge and hope to those for whom there is, at present, so little.

Robert I. Grossman, MD, Dean & CEO

4215 Save Babies Through Screening Foundation
P. O. Box 42197
Cincinnati, OH 45242   888-454-3383
e-mail: email@savebabies.org; www.savebabies.org

Is a national nonprofit public charity run by volunteers. Its mission is to improve the lives of babies by working to prevent disabilities and early death resulting from disorders detectable through newborn screening.

Jill Levry-Fisch, President
Micki Gartzke, Vice President
Anne Rugari, Treasurer

Description

4216 HYDROCEPHALUS

Synonym: Hydrocephaly

Covers these related disorders: Acute hydrocephalus, Occult tension hydrocephalus, Overt tension hydrocephalus, Communicating hydrocephalus, Non-communicating hydrocephalus, Obstructive hydrocephalus, Non-obstructive hydrocephalus

Involves the following Biologic System(s):

Neurologic Disorders

Hydrocephalus is a general term used to describe a group of conditions characterized by the accumulation of cerebrospinal fluid (CSF) around the brain. This fluid, which acts as a protective shock absorber for the brain and spinal cord, flows through the four cavities in the brain (ventricles); through the cavity containing the spinal fluid (spinal canal); and between layers of the membrane that surrounds the brain and spinal cord (subarachnoid space). Obstructed flow or impaired absorption of the CSF results in increasing fluid pressure within the brain. Hydrocephalus is thought to affect approximately one in 500 to 1,500 births. The condition may occur as a result of certain malformations that are present at birth, such as Arnold-Chiari malformation or Dandy-Walker syndrome, certain infectious diseases, head injuries, bleeding within the brain, or certain tumors.

Symptoms associated with hydrocephalus may vary, depending upon the nature of the underlying abnormality, the age of onset, and the rate and duration of increasing pressure within the brain. Hydrocephalus may be apparent at birth (congenital) or develop during the first few months or years of life. Because the fibrous joints of the skull (fontanels) have not fused or completely closed, rapid enlargement of the head may occur. The forehead appears abnormally prominent; the skin over the skull is thin with obvious scalp veins; and the face may appear relatively small. Additional symptoms and findings many include difficulties feeding, irritability, sluggishness, lack of interest in surroundings, lack of normal reflex responses, and downward turning of the eyes. Progression of the condition without treatment may result in extreme drowsiness, episodes of uncontrolled electrical disturbances in the brain (seizures), and potentially life-threatening complications.

In other children, hydrocephalus becomes apparent after the bones of the skull are fused (i.e., after two years of age). Some children may have no apparent symptoms, whereas others may have mild, intermittent, or progressive symptoms. These symptoms may include headaches, easy distractibility, poor memory, and progressively impaired walking and balance. Others may experience an acute form of hydrocephalus in which there is rapidly increasing intracranial pressure, causing severe headache, vomiting, visual disturbances, increasing drowsiness over the period of minutes or hours, potential coma, and possibly life-threatening complications.

Treatment of infants and children with hydrocephalus depends upon the underlying cause of the condition. Therapeutic measures may include use of certain medications, such as acetazolamide and furosemide, which are diuretics ("water pills") that help to reduce the build up of cerebrospinal fluid.

Other treatment options may include surgical removal of any obstruction or surgical implantation of a specialized device known as a shunt. Shunts allow excess fluid to drain away from the brain to another part of the body for absorption into the bloodstream. After treatment, many affected children may continue to have associated impairment, such as intellectual deficits, impaired memory, and visual abnormalities. Physicians may regularly monitor affected children and suggest a variety of multidisciplinary measures.

National Associations & Support Groups

4217 American Academy of Pediatrics
141 Northwest Point Boulevard
Elk Grove Village, IL 60007
847-434-4000
800-433-9016
Fax: 847-434-8000
www.aap.org

The American Academy of Pediatrics and its member pediatricians are committed to the attainment of optimal physical, mental and social health and well-being for all infants, children, adolescents, and young adults.

Sandra Hassink, MD, FAAP, President

4218 Birth Defect Research for Children
976 Lake Baldwin Lane, Suite 104
Orlando, FL 32814
407-895-0802
Fax: 407-895-0824
e-mail: staff@birthdefects.org
www.birthdefects.org

Organization that helps families with free birth defect information, parent matching that links families of children with similar defects and research through the National Birth Defect Registry to discover the causes of birth defects. Support group information and newsletter on Internet.

Betty Mekdeci, Executive Director

4219 Cerebrospinal Fluid Shunt Systems for the Management of Hydrocephalus
Hydrocephalus Association
4340 East West Highway, Suite 905
Bethesda, MD 20814
415-732-7040
888-598-3789
Fax: 415-732-7044
e-mail: info@hydroassoc.org
www.hydroassoc.org

The nations's largest and most repected nonprofit organization devoted exclusively to hydrocepalus. Our office is staffed daily from 10 AM to 4 PM Pacific time. We invite your inquiries.Our mission is to provide support, education and advocacy for individuals, families and professionals.

Dawn Mancuso, CEO
Randi Corey, Director
Aisha Heath, Director of Development

4220 Genetic Alliance
4301 Connecticut Avenue NW
Washington, DC 20008
202-966-7955
800-336-4363
Fax: 202-966-8553
e-mail: info@geneticalliance.org
www.geneticalliance.org

A coalition of voluntary genetic support groups, consumers and professionals addressing the needs of individuals and families affected by genetic disorders from a national perspective.

Joan Oppenheimer Weiss, Founder
Sharon Terry, President

4221 Guardians of Hydrocephalus Research Foundation
2618 Avenue Z
Brooklyn, NY 11235
718-743-4473
800-458-8655
Fax: 718-743-1171
e-mail: GHRF2618@aol.com
www.ghrforg.org

Nonprofit group dedicated to research into the cause and treatment of hydrocephalus. Guardians operate a laboratory in the Department of Neurology at New York University Medical Center, in which information from clinical and research facilities is integrated to provide for better diagnosis and treatment of hydrocephalus, a frequently occuring congenital disorder that can also occur shortly after birth. Hydrocephalus accounts for a large portion of adult patients with a diagnosis of dementia.

Michael Fischette, Founder
Katherine Soriano, National Vice President

4222 Hydrocephalus Association
Hydrocephalus Association
4340 East West Highway, Suite 905
Bethesda, MD 20814

301-202-3811
888-598-3789
Fax: 301-202-3813
e-mail: info@hydroassoc.org
www.hydroassoc.org

This is the nation's largest and most respected nonprofit organization devoted exclusively to hydrocephalus. We provide support, education and an extensive range of resources to families and professionals dealing with the complex issues of hydrocephalus, the abnormal accumulation of cerebrospinal fluid within the brain. Our resources cover all ages, from prenatal to adult normal pressure hydrocephalus. Our office is staffed daily, we invite your inquiries.

Dawn Mancuso, CEO
Randi Corey, Director
Aisha Heath, Director of Development

4223 Hydrocephalus Foundation
910 Rear Broadway, Rt. 1
Saugus, MA 01906

781-942-1161
Fax: 781-231-5250
e-mail: hyfll@nestcape.net
www.hydrocephalus.org

Foundation established to help assist patients and their families during the transition from their diagnosis to a resumption of their normal lifestyles. The primary focus is to contribute emotional support to patients of hydrocephalus and their families.

Dawn Mancuso, CEO
Randi Corey, Director
Aisha Heath, Director of Development

4224 March of Dimes Birth Defects Foundation
1275 Mamaroneck Avenue
White Plains, NY 10605

914-997-4488
888-663-4637
Fax: 914-997-4763
e-mail: answers@marchofdimes.com
www.marchofdimes.com

Partnership of volunteers and professionals dedicated to improving the health of babies by preventing birth defects and infant mortality. Over 100 chapters are located across the country and can be located through the National Office.

Jennifer L Howse, President

4225 National Conference on Hydrocephalus
Hydrocephalus Association
4340 East West Highway, Suite 905
Bethesda, MD 20814

415-732-7040
888-598-3789
Fax: 415-732-7044
e-mail: info@hydroassoc.org
www.hydroassoc.org

Dawn Mancuso, CEO
Randi Corey, Director
Aisha Heath, Director of Development

4226 National Foundation for Facial Reconstruction
333 East 30th Street, Lobby Unit
New York, NY 10016

212-263-6656
Fax: 212-263-7534
e-mail: info@nffr.org
www.nffr.org

To enable patients with facial deformities lead productive and fulfilling lives. The NFFR lends its support to the mulidisciplinary craniofacial team at the Institute of Reconstructive Plastic Surgery at NYU Medical Center. An assembly of world-renowned surgeons, mental health professionals, research specialists and staff, give their time and expertise, using the latest techniques.

1951

Eileen Newman, President
John R. Gordon, Chairman
Yoron Cohen, VP

4227 National Hydrocephalus Foundation
12413 Centralia Road
Lakewood, CA 90715

562-924-6666
888-857-3434
e-mail: debbifields@nhfonline.org
www.nhfonline.org

Promotes information and educational assistance. Establishes and facilitates a communication network and works to increase public awareness. Promote and support research. Also has brochures, help sheets, and more. Quarterly newsletter with annual membership fee of $35.00.

Debbie Fields, Executive Director
Michael Fields, President
Jaynie Dunn, Secretary

State Agencies & Support Groups

Arizona

4228 Injury Prevention Center
Phoenix Children's Hospital
1919 E Thomas Road
Phoenix, AZ 85016

602-933-1000
888-908-5437
e-mail: nquay@phxchildrens.com
www.phoenixchildrens.com

Their mission is to promote family-directed care through education and support of children and families with hydrocephalus. Biannual newsletter published, yearly educational conference.

Mark Bonsall, Chairman
Robert Meyer, President/CEO
Jon Hulburd, VP

California

4229 Hydrocephalus Support Group of Southern California
412 N Coast Highway, Suite 131
Laguna Beach, CA 92651

714-389-7465
Fax: 949-465-0550
e-mail: HydroBrat@earthlink.net
www.hydrowoman.com

This group was formed as a group of concerned families and patients with hydrocephalus to share information and experiences in dealing with this disease, locally and nationwide.

Jason Vandriel, Manager

Florida

4230 Hydrocephalus Family Support Group of Central Florida
22 Lake Beauty Drive, Suite 204, PO Box 2010
Orlando, FL 32806

407-649-7686
Fax: 407-649-7692
e-mail: mrssm1000@aol.com
www.oreilly.com

Their mission is to nurture understanding and increase awareness of hydrocephalus in their community.

Jogi V Pattisapu MD
Tim O'Reilly, Founder/CEO

Michigan

4231 Hydrocephalus Support Group
Children's Hospital of Michigan
PO Box 4236
Chesterfield, MO 63006

314-532-8228
Fax: 314-995-4108
e-mail: hydro@inlink.com
www.oreilly.com

Provides information to connect parents who have children with hydrocephalus in a mutual support group.

Mary Smellie-Decker RN, MSN, Clinical Nurse Specialist
Tim O'Reilly, Founder/CEO

4232 SW Michican Spina Bifida & Hydrocephalus Association
PO Box 212
Mattawan, MI 49071

269-385-3959
Fax: 269-342-9765

Provides support, education, and advocacy for families with spina bifida and/or hydrocephalus.

Richard Benthin, President

Missouri

4233 Hydrocephalus Support Group
PO Box 4236
Chesterfield, MO 63006

314-532-8228
Fax: 314-995-4108
e-mail: hydro@inlink.com
www.oreilly.com

Nonprofit organization providing education and support to individuals with hydrocephalus and their families.

Debby Buffa, Founder/Director
Tim O'Reilly, Founder/CEO

New Jersey

4234 Hydrocephalus Group - Children's Hospital of New Jersey
Children's Hospital of New Jersey
201 Lyons Avenue at Osborne Terrace
Newark, NJ 07112

973-926-7000
Fax: 973-325-2078
e-mail: info@sbhcs.com
www.sbhcs.com

Serves parents of infants and children in the local community and around the state.

Timothy S Yeh MD, FAAP, FAACM, Physician-in-Chief

New York

4235 New York University Medical Center Auxillary of Tisch Hospital
530 1st Avenue
New York, NY 10016

212-263-8122
www.nyukidshealth.org

Conducts national symposiums on hydrocephalus.

Ana Monteagudo, Co-President Auxillary Medical Ctr

North Carolina

4236 Lipomyelomeningocele Family Support
415 Webster Street
Cary, NC 27511

919-844-2043
Fax: 919-844-2044
e-mail: bborchert@mindspring.com
www.lfsn.org

Providing support services to families and individuals affected by Occult Spinal Dysraphisms.

Bonnie Borchert, Director

Ohio

4237 Cleveland Clinic
9500 Euclid Avenue
Cleveland, OH 44195

216-444-4508
800-223-2273
Fax: 216-444-9050
www.clevelandclinic.org

Provides education about hydrocephalus using speakers and parent-to-parent information.

Gene Altus, Executive Director

Rhode Island

4238 Hydrocephalus Association of Rhode Island
PO Box 343
Valley Falls, RI 02864

401-723-6065

The mission of this Association is to provide information, support and advocacy for individuals with hydrocephalus and for friends and family members.

Gabriella Halmi, Director

Texas

4239 Hydrocephalus Association of N Texas
PO Box 670552
Dallas, TX 75367

214-528-2877
Fax: 214-528-8097

The mission is to provide information and support to parents of children with hydrocephalus in the state of Texas and neighboring states.

Jana Dransfield, Director

Washington

4240 Hydrocephalus Support Group of Seattle
Po Box 14055
Tumwater, WA 98511

206-324-4084
e-mail: hydropr61@hotmail.com

The group of Seattle provides support to individuals with hydrocephalus.

Kim Anderson, Director

Wisconsin

4241 Fox Valley Hydrocephalus Support Group
W5929 Highway KK
Appleton, WI 54915

920-739-1751

The group provides referrals for parents and information to the community and throughout Wisconsin.

Donna Uitenbroek, Director

Research Centers

4242 New York University Medical Center Auxillary of Tisch Hospital
560 1st Avenue
New York, NY 10016

212-263-5800
e-mail: Stevenb.Abramson@nyumc.org
www.med.nyu.edu

Conducts national symposiums on hydrocephalus.

Steven B. Abramson, Sr. VP
Dianna Jacob, VP
Ramona Batra, Business Operations Manager

4243 Seeking Techniques Advancing Research in Shunts (STARS)
33006 Seven Mile Road, Suite 113
Livonia, MI 48152   313-384-3232
                                                     www.stars-kids.org

Offers support to patients with hydrocephalus and their families.
Judy Brady, President

Conferences

4244 Genetic Alliance Annual Conference
Genetic Alliance
4301 Connecticut Avenue NW, Suite 404
Washington, DC 20008   202-966-5557
                                                     800-336-4363
                                                     Fax: 202-966-8553
                                         e-mail: info@geneticalliance.org
                                                     www.geneticalliance.org

Consistently inspirational and enables partnership among all
stakeholders: advocates and community leaders, health and industry professionals, policymakers, and academicians.
July

Sharon Terry, President/CEO
Tetyana Murza, Programs/Events Manager

Audio Video

4245 Hydrocephalus, a Neglected Disease
Guardians of Hydrocephalus Research Foundation
2618 Avenue Z
Brooklyn, NY 11235   718-748-4473
                                                     Fax: 718-743-1171
                                           e-mail: ghrf2618@aol.com
                                                     www.ghrf.homestead.com/ghrf

Information on Hydrocephalus.

Michael Fischette, Founder
Katherine Soriano, National Vice President

Web Sites

4246 Beth Israel Medical Center-Hydrocephalus
330 Brookline Avenue
Boston, MA 2215   617-667-7000
                                                     800-667-5356
                                                     TDD: 800-439-0183
                                        e-mail: custserv@bidmc.harvard.edu
                                                     www.bidmc.org

Is a full tertiary teaching hospital that was originally dedicated to
serving a vulnerable population in that community.

Daniel J. Jick, Chair
Edward H. Ladd, Vice Chair
Margaret A. McKenna, Vice Chair

4247 Birth Defect Research for Children
976 Lake Baldwin Lane, Suite 104
Orlando, FL 32814   407-895-0802
                                          e-mail: staff@birthdefects.org
                                                     www.birthdefects.org

Organization that helps families with free birth defect information, parent matching that links families of children with similar
defects and research through the National Birth Defect Registry
to discover the causes of birth defects. Support group information
and newsletter on Internet.

4248 Guardians of Hydrocephalus Research Foundation
1101 Wootton Parkway, Suite LL100
Rockville, MD 20852   240-453-8282
                                             e-mail: odphpinfo@hhs.gov
                                                     www.health.gov

Nonprofit group dedicated to research into the cause and treatment of hydrocephalus. Guardians operate a laboratory in the Department of Neurology at New York University Medical Center,
in which information from clinical and research facilities is integrated to provide for better diagnosis and treatment of hydrocephalus, a frequently occuring congenital disorder that can also
occur shortly after birth. Hydrocephalus accounts for a large
portion of adult patients with a diagnosis of dementia.

4249 HYCEPH-L
www.geocities.com/HotSprings/Villa/2020/

The purpose of the list is to share information and support in
dealing with hydrocephalus.

4250 Hydrocephalus Association
4340 East West Highway, Suite 905
Bethesda, MD 20814   301-202-3811
                                                     888-598-3789
                                                     Fax: 301-202-3813
                                           e-mail: info@hydroassoc.org
                                                     www.hydroassoc.org

Our mission is to provide support, education and advocacy for individuals families and professionals.

Aseem Chandra, Chair
Craig Brown, Senior Vice Chair
David Browdy, Vice Chair

4251 Hydrohaven Chat Room
www.geocities.com/HotSprings/Villa/2020/hydrohav

Hydrocephalus support group for patients, family and friends.

4252 National Hydrocephalus Foundation
www.nhfonline.org

Promotes information and educational assistance. Establishes and
facilitates a communication network and works to increase public
awareness. Promote and support research. Also has brochures,
help sheets and more. Quarterly newsletter included with annual
membership fee of $35.00.

4253 Online Mendelian Inheritance in Man
8600 Rockville Pike
Bethesda, MD 20894   888-346-3656
                                          e-mail: info@ncbi.nlm.nih.gov
                                                     www.ncbi.nlm.nih.gov

This database is a catalog of human genes and genetic disorders.

4254 Pediatric Neurosurgery-Hydrocephalus
710 West 168 Street
New York, NY 10032   212-305-4118
                                                     Fax: 212-305-2026
                                                     www.columbianeurosurgery.org

This site is dedicated to providing families regarding various aspects of the field of pediatric neurosurgery.

4255 Rare Genetic Diseases in Children (NYU)
550 First Avenue
New York, NY 10016   212-263-7300
                                                     www.med.nyu.edu

We target issues arising from rare genetic diseases affecting children. Also, to assist in the endeavor to bring knowledge and hope
to those for whom there is, at present, so little.

Robert I. Grossman, MD, Dean & CEO
Steven B. Abramson, MD, Senior Vice President
Dafna Bar-Sagi, PhD, Senior Vice President

Book Publishers

4256 A Guide to Hydrocephalus
Spina Bifida Association of America
4590 MacArthur Boulevard NW, Suite 250
Washington, DC 20007   202-944-3285
                                                     800-621-3141
                                                     Fax: 202-944-3295
                                              e-mail: sbaa@sbaa.org
                                                     www.spinabifidaassociation.org

Information to help you understand the circumstances that surround you and make the job of advocacy an easier one.

Cindy Brownstein, President & CEO
Sara Struwe, Chief Operating Officer & Director
Christopher Vance, Director of Development

4257 Congenital Disorders Sourcebook
Omnigraphics
PO Box 8002
Aston, PA 19014
800-234-1340
Fax: 800-875-1340
e-mail: info@omnigraphics.com
www.omnigraphics.com

Basic consumer health information on disorders aquired during gestation, including spina bifida, hydrocephalus, cerebral palsy, heart defects, craniofacial abnormalities and fetal alcohol syndrome.

650 pages
ISBN: 0-780809-45-9

4258 Hydrocephalus: A Guide for Patients, Families, and Friends
Chuck Toporek, Kellie Robinson, author

O'Reilly & Associates
1005 Gravenstein Highway N
Sebastopol, CA 95472
707-827-7019
800-889-8969
Fax: 707-824-8268
e-mail: patientguides@oreilly.com
www.oreilly.com

This book educates families so they can select a skilled neurosurgeon, understand treatments, participate in care and know what symptoms need attention, keep records needed for follow-up treatments and make wise lifestyle choices.

1999 377 pages Softcover
ISBN: 1-565924-10-X

Tim O'Reilly, Founder & CEO

4259 Spina Bifida Association Insights into Spina Bifida
Spina Bifida Association
4590 MacArthur Boulevard NW, Suite 250
Washington, DC 20007
202-944-3285
800-621-3141
Fax: 202-944-3295
e-mail: sbaa@sbaa.org
www.spinabifidaassociation.org

News on medical, legislative and education topics relevant to individuals with spina bifida

Bimonthly

Cindy Brownstein, President & CEO
Sara Struwe, Chief Operating Officer & Director
Christopher Vance, Director of Development

Newsletters

4260 G. Advocacy
Genetic Alliance
4301 Connecticut Avenue NW, Suite 404
Washington, DC 20008
202-966-5557
800-336-4363
Fax: 202-966-8553
e-mail: info@geneticalliance.org
www.geneticalliance.org

Our e-newsletter features news about upcoming events, spotlights member organizations, and keeps you informed about legislation before Congress. We welcome your feedback on articles and suggestions on future topics.

Sharon F. Terry MA, President/CEO
Natasha Bonhomme, VP, Strategic Development
Ruth Evans, Director of Accounting

4261 Hydrocephalus Association Newsletter
Hydrocephalus Association
4340 East West Highway, Suite 905
Bethesda, MD 20814
301-202-3811
888-598-3789
Fax: 301-202-3813
e-mail: info@hydroassoc.org
www.hydroassoc.org

Offers information on association news, conference articles, meetings, support and educational groups.

12 pages Quarterly

Aseem Chandra, Chair
Craig Brown, Senior Vice Chair
David Browdy, Vice Chair

4262 Hydrocephalus Support Group Newsletter
PO Box 4236
Chesterfield, MO 63006
314-532-8228
Fax: 314-995-4108
e-mail: hydro@inlink.com

This group provides information, education and support to anyone dealing with hydrocephalus.

quarterly

Debby Buffa, Founder/Chairman

4263 LINK
Hydrocephalus Association
4340 East West Highway, Suite 905
Bethesda, MD 20814

Provides members with direct access to other families and individuals coping with the complexities of hydrocephalus with the goal being to develop a nationwide network of individuals supporting one another, sharing information and strategies which enable them to become educated and empowered advocates.

12 pages Quarterly

4264 National Hydrocephalus Foundation Newsletter
12413 Centralia Road
Lakewood, CA 90715
562-924-6666
888-857-3434
Fax: 415-732-7044
e-mail: debbifields@nhfonline.org
www.nhfonline.org

The Foundation is a national organization whose purpose is to provide information and education, along with peer support newsletter quarterly.

12-15 pages Quarterly

Michael Fields, President/Treasurer
Debbie Fields, Executive Director
Jaynie Dunn, Secretary

4265 Update
Spina Bifida and Hydrocephalus Association/Canada
Suite 647-167 av. Lombard Avenue
Winnipeg, MB R3B 0
Canada
204-925-3650
800-565-9488
Fax: 204-925-3654
e-mail: info@sbhac.ca
www.sbhac.ca

Newsletter dedicated to improving the quality of life of individuals with spina bifida and/or hydrocephalus and their families.

4 pages Quarterly

Colleen Talbot, President
Linda Randall, Vice President
Sarah Williams, Secretary

Pamphlets

4266 About Hydrocephalus - Book for Families
Hydrocephalus Association
4340 East West Highway, Suite 905
Bethesda, MD 20814

Booklet in either English or Spanish, detailing all aspects of hydrocephalus from diagnosis and treatment to complications and follow-up care.

36 pages Paperback

4267 Cephalic Disorders Fact Sheet
National Inst. of Neurological Disorders/Stroke
PO Box 5801
Bethesda, MD 20824
301-496-5751
800-352-9424
www.ninds.nih.gov

Fact sheet indexing the following: What are Cephalic Disorders?, What are the Different Kinds of Cephalic Disorders?, What are Other Less Common Cephalics?, What Research is Being Done?, Where Can I Get More Information?.

Walter J. Koroshetz, M.D., Acting Director
Audrey S. Penn MD, Special Advisor to the Director
Caroline Lewis, Executive Officer

4268 Cerebrospinal Fluid Shunt Systems for the Management of Hydrocephalus
Hydrocephalus Association
4340 East West Highway, Suite 905
Bethesda, MD 20814

Our resources cover hydrocephalus in all age groups from prenatal diagnosis to adult normal pressure hydrocephalus. Our office is staffed daily from 10 AM to 4 PM Pacific time. We invite your inquiries.

4269 Directory of Pediatric Neurosurgeons
Hydrocephalus Association
4340 East West Highway, Suite 905
Bethesda, MD 20814

Names and addresses of more than 200 neurosurgeons who specialize in pediatrics, listed alphabetically and geographically.

4270 Durable Power of Attorney for Health Care Decisions
Hydrocephalus Association
4340 East West Highway, Suite 905
Bethesda, MD 20814

Provided by The Hydrocephalus Association. Our resources cover hydrocephalus in all age groups from prenatal diagnosis to adult normal pressure hydrocepahlus. Our office is staffed daily from 10 AM to 4 PM Pacific time. We invite your inquiries.

4271 Endoscopic Third Ventriculoscopy
Hydrocephalus Association
4340 East West Highway, Suite 905
Bethesda, MD 20814

Provided by the Hydrocephalus Association. Our resources cover all age groups from prenatal diagnosis through normal pressure hydrocephalus in older adults. Our office is staffed daily from 10 AM to 4 PM Pacific time. We invite your inquiries.

4272 Eye Problems Associated with Hydrocephalus in Children
Hydrocephalus Association
4340 East West Highway, Suite 905
Bethesda, MD 20814

Provided by the Hydrocephalus Association. Our resources cover all age groups from prenatal diagnosis to normal pressure hydrocephalus in older adults. Our office is staffed daily from 10 AM to 4 PM Pacific time. We invite your inquiries.

4273 Fact Sheet: Hydrocephalus
Hydrocephalus Association
4340 East West Highway, Suite 905
Bethesda, MD 20814

Also available in Spanish, provided by the Hydrocephalus Association. Our resources cover all age groups from prenatal diagnosis to normal pressure hydrocephalus in older adults. Our office is staffed daily from 10 AM to 4 PM Pacific time. We invite your inquiries.

4274 Fact Sheet: Syringomyelia
National Inst. of Neurological Disorders/Stroke
PO Box 5801
Bethesda, MD 20892
301-496-5751
800-352-9424
www.ninds.nih.gov

Provided by the Hydrocephalus Association. Our resources cover all age groups, from prenatal diagnosis to normal pressure hydrocephalus in older adults. We welcome your inquiries.

Walter J. Koroshetz, M.D., Acting Director
Audrey S. Penn MD, Special Advisor to the Director
Caroline Lewis, Executive Officer

4275 Headaches and Hydrocephalus
Hydrocephalus Association
4340 East West Highway, Suite 905
Bethesda, MD 20814

Causes and tips for headache relief unique to hydrocephalus.

4276 Hospitalization Tips
Hydrocephalus Association
4340 East West Highway, Suite 905
Bethesda, MD 20814

Provided by the Hydrocephalus Association. Our resources cover all age groups, from prenatal diagnosis, to normal pressure hydrocephalus in older adults. Our office is staffed daily from 10 AM to 4 PM, Pacific time. We welcome your inquiries.
1997

4277 How to be an Assertive Member of the Treatment Team
Hydrocephalus Association
4340 East West Highway, Suite 905
Bethesda, MD 20814

Hydrocephalus information to ask involved treatment questions.

4278 Hydrocephalus: Fact Sheet
National Inst. of Neurological Disorders/Stroke
PO Box 5801
Bethesda, MD 20824
301-496-5751
800-352-9424
www.ninds.nih.gov

Our fact sheet covers all age groups, from prenatal diagnosis to normal pressure hydrocephalus in older adults. Also available in Spanish.

Walter J. Koroshetz, M.D., Acting Director
Audrey S. Penn MD, Special Advisor to the Director
Caroline Lewis, Executive Officer

4279 ID Card for Third Ventriculostomy Patients
Hydrocephalus Association
4340 East West Highway Suite 905
Bethesda, MD 20814

Patients with hydrocephalus managed by an ETV may request a free patient ID card from the Hydrocephaus Association. This card idenifies them as patients with hydrocephalus being managed by this procedure.

4280 Individualized Education Program (IEP) - Communication Skills for Parents
Hydrocephalus Association
4340 East West Highway Suite 905
Bethesda, MD 20814

Is a written education plan that describes the special education and related services a student will receive.

4281 LINK Directory Information
Hydrocephalus Association
4340 East West Highway Suite 905
Bethesda, MD 20814

A nationwide network of individuals listed in Directory format giving members direct access to others in similar circumstances.

4282 Learning Disabilities in Children with Hydrocephalus
Hydrocephalus Association
4340 East West Highway Suite 905
Bethesda, MD 20814

Also available in Spanish and English. Our offices are staffed daily from 10 AM to 4 PM, Pacific time. We welcome your inquiries.

4283 National Directory of Hydrocephalus Support Groups
Hydrocephalus Association
4340 East West Highway Suite 905
Bethesda, MD 20814

The Directory lists information on 16 hydrocephalus groups nationwide.

4284 Nonverbal Learning Disorder Syndrome
Hydrocephalus Association
4340 East West Highway Suite 905
Bethesda, MD 20814

Is a specific type of learning disability that affect's children's academic progress as well as their social and emotional development. This specific type of learning disability has been identified in some children with Hydrocephalus.

4285 Prenatal Hydrocephalus-Book for Parents
Hydrocephalus Association
4340 East West Highway Suite 905
Bethesda, MD 20814

Provides information about the diagnosis of prenatal-onset hydrocephalus.

16 pages

4286 Primary Care Needs of Children with Hydrocephalus
Hydrocephalus Association
4340 East West Highway Suite 905
Bethesda, MD 20814

Our office is staffed daily from 10 AM to 4 PM Pacific time. We welcome your inquiries.

28 pages

4287 Resource Guide
Hydrocephalus Association
4340 East West Highway Suite 905
Bethesda, MD 20814

A comprehensive listing of 450 articles on all aspects of hydrocephalus. Articles may be ordered from the Association for a small fee.

4288 Social Skills Development in Children with Hydrocephalus
Hydrocephalus Association
4340 East West Highway Suite 905
Bethesda, MD 20814

4289 Survival Skills for the Family Unit
Hydrocephalus Association
4340 East West Highway Suite 905
Bethesda, MD 20814

Our resources cover hydrocepahlus in all age groups from prenatal diagnosis through normal pressure hydrocephalus in older adults.

4290 Understanding Your Child's Education Needs /Individualized Education Program Packet
Hydrocephalus Association
4340 East West Highway Suite 905
Bethesda, MD 20814

From the Hydrocephalus Association the nations largest nonprofit group devoted exclusively to this disorder. Our offices are staffed daily from 10 AM to 4 PM, Pacific time. We welcome your inquiries.

Description

4291 HYPERTROPHIC CARDIOMYOPATHY
Involves the following Biologic System(s):
Cardiovascular Disorders

Hypertrophic cardiomyopathy is a genetic disease that occurs because of mutations in the contraction mechanisms in the muscles of the heart. Because of this genetic abnormality, the heart muscle fibers are arranged in a disorganized fashion. This leads to enlargement of the left ventricular muscle (hypertrophy). This hypertrophic muscle may lead to variable amounts of obstruction of blood flow out of the heart into the general circulation and a spectrum of clinical manifestations. There have been several genes that have been found to be abnormal in patients with hypertrophic cardiomyopathy. Depending on the different genetic abnormality there may be different clinical findings ranging from no symptomatology to severe disease.

Hypertrophic cardiomyopathy is most commonly inherited in an autosomal dominant pattern, meaning that a child inherits a copy of the gene from one of his or her parents.aAs a result, the majority of children and adolescents who are diagnosed with the disease have a parent who also suffers from the entity. Sporadic cases are also well documented where neither parent has the disease but the child has the disease. It is presumed that in these cases, there has been a spontaneous mutation in the gene in the earliest stages of embryonic development.

Hypertrophic cardiomyopathy may become clinically evident at any time during the first two decades of life, though typically it is not diagnosed until the adolescent years. It is important to note that the hypertrophic changes that are the hallmark of the disease may not develop until as late as the teens or early twenties. As a result, in families where a parent has the disease, children should undergo repeated interval examination by a pediatric cardiologist through their adolescence.

The diagnosis is hypertrophic cardiomyopathy relies heavily on good history taking from the primary care provider. There are several important questions to ask in order to assess for risk. A family history should be taken, asking about unexplained deaths, family members with frequent episodes of fainting, or cardiac arrhythmia (abnormal heart rhythm). Patients should be questioned about episodes of shortness of breath (dyspnea) and chest pain. Any recent change in exercise tolerance should be evaluated closely. Additionally, a known history of family members with documented hypertrophic cardiomyopathy should raise the concern of disease in other family members.

There are many patients with hypertrophic cardiomyopathy who are largely asymptomatic. When patients are symptomatic they usually exhibit a slow decline in function. Often, patients may not experience symptoms until they exert themselves. Symptoms may consist of shortness of breath with exertion or when lying down, chest pain, fainting (syncope) or lightheadedness, palpitations (racing heart), and fatigue. Although it is agreed that the thickened left ventricular muscle may cause some obstruction to blood flow out of the aora (the main blood vessel leading from the left side of the heart to the general circulation), this is not the only mechanism causing symptoms. In fact, there are some patients with a great deal of obstruction who have minimal symptoms, while other patients with minimal obstruction may have severe symptoms. Patients may also experience some of the above symptoms from decreased functioning of the heart muscle itself, or arrhythmia.

Hypertrophic cardiomyopathy is the most common cause of sudden death in young athletes who die during sports; clearly those individuals with HCM should be restricted from participating in sports.

The physical exam of patients with hypertrophic cardiomyopathy may be normal if there is no significant obstruction to blood flow. In some patients, findings may include a fourth heart sound or a systolic murmur heard best at the left lower sternal border. This murmur is often heard more easily during maneuvers that increase the amount of resistance in the body's tissues from muscular contraction, for example, when patients stand up after a sitting or squatting position, or when patients bear down (Valsalva maneuver). Additional findings may include increased carotid pulses, increased force of the heart beat felt near the left lower sternum or axilla (parasternal lift).

Patients with suspected hypertrophic cardiomyopathy should be referred to a pediatric cardiologist for further testing, which may consist of an echocardiogram (ultrasound imaging of the heart), electrocardiogram and perhaps an exercise stress test.

Treatment options are varied. Medical management may be difficult and surgical or catheter interventions may be recommended to decrease the amount of obstructing tissue in the heart. Mainstays of medical treatment include calcium channel blockers, beta blockers, and anti-arrhythmics. Most recently, the use of implantable defribrillators (small pacemaker-like devices that correct severe heart arrhythmias) have become common. It is critical that patients with confirmed hypertrophic cardiomyopathy be restricted from playing competitive sports. Additionally, patients should receive prophylactic antibiotics for prevention of endocarditis before dental or invasive procedures.

National Associations & Support Groups

4292 American Academy of Pediatrics
141 Northwest Point Boulevard
Elk Grove Village, IL 60007
847-434-4000
800-433-9016
Fax: 847-434-8000
www.aap.org

The American Academy of Pediatrics and its member pediatricians are committed to the attainment of optimal physical, mental and social health and well-being for all infants, children, adolescents, and young adults.

Sandra Hassink, MD, FAAP, President

4293 American Heart Association
7272 Greenville Avenue
Dallas, TX 75231
214-373-6300
800-242-8721
Fax: 214-706-1341
e-mail: inquire@amhrt.org
www.americanheart.org

Supports research, education and community service programs with the objective of reducing premature death and disability from cardiovascular diseases and stroke; coordinates the efforts of health professionals, and others engaged in the fight against heart and circulatory disease.

M Cass Wheeler, Ceo

4294 Hypertrophic Cardiomyopathy Association
322 Green Pond Road, PO Box 306
Hibernia, NJ 07842
973-983-7429
Fax: 973-983-7870
e-mail: support@4hcm.us
www.4hcm.org

A not-for-profit organization that provides information, support and advocacy to patients, their families and medical providers.

Lisa Salberg, Founder & President

4295 March of Dimes Birth Defects Foundation
1275 Mamaroneck Avenue
White Plains, NY 10605
914-997-4488
888-663-4637
Fax: 914-997-4763
e-mail: answers@marchofdimes.com
www.marchofdimes.com

Partnership of volunteers and professionals dedicated to improving the health of babies by preventing birth defects and infant mortality. Over 100 chapters are located across the country and can be located through the National Office.

Jennifer L Howse, President

Research Centers

4296 Hypertrophic Cardiomyopathy Program at St. Luke's-Roosevelt Hospital Center
University Medical Practice Associates
425 W 59th Street, Suite 9C
New York, NY 10019
212-492-5550
Fax: 212-492-5555
www.hcmny.org

We offer comprehensive diagnostic evaluation, a range of treatments and screening for relatives of affected patients.

Mark V Sherrid MD FACC FASE, Director

Web Sites

4297 American Heart Association
7272 Greenville Ave
Dallas, TX 75231
800-242-8721
www.heart.org/HEARTORG

Supports research, education and community service programs with the objective of reducing premature death and disability from cardiovascular diseases and stroke; coordinates the efforts of health professionals, and others engaged in the fight against heart and circulatory disease.

Bernie Dennis, Chairman
Alvin Royse, Chairman Elect
Elliott Antman, President

4298 Hypertrophic Cardiomyopathy Association
18 E. Main St - Suite 202
Denville, NJ 7834
973-983-7429
Fax: 973-983-7870
e-mail: support@4hcm.org
www.4hcm.org/WCMS/

A not-for-profit organization that provides information, support and advocacy to patients, their families and medical providers.

4299 Hypertrophic Cardiomyopathy: Heart Center Online for Patients
www.heartcenteronline.com

The mission of the HeartCenterOnline is to give our premier cardiovascular patients, their families and other site visiors with the tools they need to better understand the complex nature of heart-related conditions, treatments and preventive care, and to provide services and applications that deliver value to cardiovascular practices.

4300 Implantable Defibrillators in Preventing Sudden Death
www.findarticles.com

Article from American Family Physician magazine. Search by article name.

4301 MEDLINEplus
8600 Rockville Pike
Bethesda, MD 20894

www.nlm.nih.gov/medlineplus/ency/article/000192.htm

MedlinePlus has extensive information from the National Institutes of Health and other trusted sources on over 650 diseases and conditions. There are also lists of hospitals and physicians, a medical encyclopedia and a medical dictionary, health information in Spanish, extensive information on perscription and nonperscription drugs, health information from the media and links to thousands of clinical trials.

Dr. Donald A.B. Lindberg, Director

4302 March of Dimes Birth Defects Foundation
1275 Mamaroneck Avenue
White Plains, NY 10605
914-997-4488
www.marchofdimes.com

Partnership of volunteers and professionals dedicated to improving the health of babies by preventing birth defects and infant mortality. Over 100 chapters are located across the country and can be located through the National Office.

Franklin Roosevelt, President

4303 Sudden Death of Young Athletes Can Be Prevented (Hypertrophic Cardiomyopathy)
www.findarticles.com

Article from USA Today. Search by article name.

Book Publishers

4304 Let's Talk About Going to the Hospital
Rosen Publishing Group's PowerKids Press
29 E 21st Street
New York, NY 10010
212-777-3017
800-237-9932
Fax: 888-436-4643
e-mail: rosenpub@tribeca.ios.com
www.rosenpublishing.com

If a child has to check into the hospital, chances are he or she is already upset about being ill. Knowing how a hospital functions and what the procedures are, such as when family members can visit, will help in what is already a stressful situation. Grades K-5.

24 pages
ISBN: 0-823950-36-0

Roger Rosen, President

Newsletters

4305 HCMA - Heart Link Online
Hypertrophic Cardiomyopathy Association
18 E. Main St, Suite 202
Denville, NJ 7842
973-983-7429
Fax: 973-983-7870
e-mail: support@4hcm.us
www.4hcm.org/WCMS/

A newsletter that provides information, support and advocacy to patients, their families and medical providers.

Description

4306 HYPOPLASTIC LEFT HEART SYNDROME

Synonym: HLHS

Involves the following Biologic System(s):

Cardiovascular Disorders

Hypoplastic Left Heart Syndrome, also referred to as HLHS, is a severe and complex form of congenital heart disease, wherein the entire left side of the heart is underdeveloped and unable to pump blood to the body. Classically, this involves underdevelopment (hypoplasia) of the: 1). mitral valve, which connects the left atrium to the left ventricle, 2). left ventricle, which is the pumping chamber that delivers oxygenated blood to the body and 3). aortic valve and aorta, the valve and blood vessel, respectively, which carry oxygenated blood from the left ventricle to the organs and the tissues of the body.

Hypoplastic Left Heart Syndrome is the 4th most common congenital heart disorder diagnosed in the first year of life and almost always in the first few days of life. Typically, infants with HLHS are full term and tend to have normal birth weights and few non-cardiac defects. In those born with the disorder, males out number female. The cause of this HLHS remains unclear, but like many of the congenital heart diseases, it likely develops in most pregnancies early in the first trimester and may very well have a genetic component.

Because of the underdevelopment of the left side of the heart, infants born with Hypoplastic Left Heart Syndrome become gravely ill soon after birth. In the fetus, a specialized blood vessel, known as the ductus arteriosus, connects the aorta and the pulmonary artery. In normal fetal heart structure, the ductus arteriosus allows the deoxy genated (blue) blood pumped by the right ventricle to the pulmonary artery to avoid going to the lungs (which in the fetus are non-functioning and filled with fluid), delivering it to the placenta for oxygenation. After birth the lungs are inflated with air and the ductus arteriosus, which is no longer necessary, begins to undergo a natural closure process. In the infant with Hypoplastic Left Heart Syndrome, the ductus arteriosus is the only source of blood flow into the aorta, as the left heart is unable to pump adequate (if any) blood forward and, therefore, crucial to the survival of the infant; without it, inadequate blood flow to the organs and tissues leads to shock. Prior to the advent of specialized medications, such as prostaglandins, that prevent the closing process of the ductus arteriosus, patients with Hypoplastic Left Heart Syndrome would not be able to survive when the ductus underwent its natural closure.

Over the last two decades, congenital heart surgery techniques have been developed to surgically alter the path of blood leaving the right heart. Surgery for Hypoplastic Left Heart Syndrome typically involves three separate operations, the first being the most difficult and complicated, occurring in the first week or two of life. The second operation usually occurs between 4 and 6 months of life and the third may be undertaken between 18 and 36 months. Alternatively, some pediatric cardiac centers have promoted heart transplant for the patient with Hypoplastic Left Heart Syndrome. Children with Hypoplastic Left Heart Syndrome require lifelong follow-up by a cardiologist for repeated checks of how their heart is working. Virtually all the children will require heart

medicines. They also risk infection on the heart's valves (endocarditis) and will need antibiotics, such as amoxicillin, before dental work and certain surgeries to help prevent endocarditis.

National Associations & Support Groups

4307 American Academy of Pediatrics
141 Northwest Point Boulevard
Elk Grove Village, IL 60007
847-434-4000
800-433-9016
Fax: 847-434-8000
www.aap.org

The American Academy of Pediatrics and its member pediatricians are committed to the attainment of optimal physical, mental and social health and well-being for all infants, children, adolescents, and young adults.

Sandra Hassink, MD, FAAP, President

4308 Cincinnati Children's Hospital Medical Center
3333 Burnet Avenue, PO Box 3026
Cincinnati, OH 45229
513-636-4200
800-344-2462
TTY: 513-636-4900
www.cincinnatichildrens.org

Cincinnati Children's Heart Center is dedicated to serving the cardiac care needs of patients, fetus through young adult, and their families in a convenient, compassionate and high quality manner. The Heart Center is committed to providing research and teaching programs in an enviroment characterized by intergrity, innovation, excellence, and respect.

Murray Dock, Chairman
James M Anderson, President & CEO

4309 Congenital Heart Information Network
PO Box 3397
Margate City, NJ 08402
609-823-4507
Fax: 215-627-4036
e-mail: mb@tchin.org
www.tchin.org

An international organization that provides reliable information, support services and resources to families of children with congenital heart defects and acquired heart disease, adults with congenital heart defects, and the professionals who work with them.

Mano Barmash, President
Stuart Berger, Associate Professor of Pedriatics
Edward L. Bove, Director

State Agencies & Support Groups

Arizona

4310 Arizona HeartLight
University Medical Center
PO Box 286
Hallsville, TX 75650
903-668-2173
Fax: 903-668-3453
www.heartlightministries.org

Joe Crawford, Chairman
Jana Crawford, Chairman

Colorado

4311 Cardiac Kids/Association of Volunteers
13123 E. 16th Avenue, PO Box 465
Aurora, CO 80045
303-861-6259
e-mail: abbbybee@msn.com
www.childrenscolorado.org

Mark Erickson

Florida

4312 Pediatric Heart Foundation
PO Box 540354
Lake Worth, FL 33454
561-738-4554
e-mail: phfheart@aol.com
www.pediatricheartfoundation.org

Urquisa Fernandez, President
Reese Robinson
Laurie Bernat, Contact

Georgia

4313 Heart to Heart
401 S. Clairborne Rd., Suite 302
Olathe, KS 66062
913-764-5200
Fax: 913-764-0809
e-mail: info@hearttoheart.org
www.hearttoheart.org

Gary Morsch, Founder/President
Jim Kerr, Board Chair
Krystal Barr, Interim CEO

Hawaii

4314 Kardiac Kids
C/O Kapi'olani Medical Center for Women & Children
1319 Punahou Street
Honolulu, HI 96826
808-983-8166
e-mail: info@thekardiackids.com
www.thekardiackids.com

Lisa Rohr RN, Contact

Illinois

4315 Chilren's Heart Services
PO Box 8275
Bartlett, IL 60103
630-415-0282
e-mail: CHILDHRTSVC@aol.com

4316 Heart of the Matter
4760 Highland Drive, Suite 515
Salt Lake City, UT 84117
815-469-9146
888-868-4686
e-mail: CT875@aol.com
www.hotm.tv

Indiana

4317 Our Hearts
1738 N Shortridge Road
Indianapolis, IN 46219
317-322-1017
e-mail: ourhearts@iquest.net

Massachusetts

4318 Heart to Heart Fund
750 Washington Street, Suite 313
Boston, MA 02111
617-636-8101
e-mail: info@heart2heartfund.org

Michigan

4319 Families at Heart
100 Michigan Ave, MC117
Grand Rapids, MI 49503
616-391-4327
Rick Breon, Ceo

Minnesota

4320 Parents For Heart of Minnesota
Attention: 32-P190
2525 Chicgo Avenue S
Minneapolis, MN 55404
e-mail: mailinglist@parentsforheart.org
www.parentsforheart.org

Celeste Gebauer, Contact

Missouri

4321 Heart to Heart - St. Louis
St Louis Children's Hospital
One Children's Place
St Louis, MO 63110
314-454-6000
www.heart2heartstl.com

Elaine Wear, Contact
Nan Winters, Contact

New Hampshire

4322 Families with Heart
824 High Street
Candia, NH 03034
603-483-3025
Laura Briggs, Contact

New Jersey

4323 Young Hearts
791 Fredrick Court
Wyckoff, NJ 07481
201-848-9608
Barbara Mcfadden, Contact

New York

4324 Big Hearts for Little Hearts
34 Sintsink Drive West
Port Washington, NY 11050
516-883-4080
Ruth Maszrik, Contact

4325 Cardiac Kids
PO Box 154
Fishkill, NY 12524
845-896-7321
Cindy-Jean Dennis, Contact

4326 Helping Hearts
601 Elmwood Avenue, PO Box 631
Rochester, NY 14642
716-275-6108
e-mail: info@helpinghearts.org

Ohio

4327 Healing Hearts
PO Box 7890
Bonney Lake, WA 98391
253-268-0348
866-230-3463
Fax: 330-543-3084
e-mail: flemings249@aol.com
www.healinghearts.org

Provides participants with an opportunity to share their emotions and concerns.

Sue Liljenberg, Founder/President
Judy Hansen, Secretary
Dan Morton, Member

Pennsylvania

4328 Fontan Friends
482 Reginald Lane
Collegeville, PA 19426
610-831-9878

Barbara Lewis, Contact

South Dakota

4329 Thumpers
HC 58, Box 26
Fairburn, SD 57738
605-255-4377
e-mail: clsogge@cs.com

Tammy Sogge, Contact

Tennessee

4330 Tennessee Saving Little Hearts
5629 Barineau Lane, PO Box 52285
Knoxville, TN 37950
865-748-4605
e-mail: info@savinglittlehearts.com
www.savinglittlehearts.com

Provides emotional assistance, educational information,and fun experiences for children that will help them build friendship and confidence.

Karen Coulter, President
Brad Coulter, Vice President

Texas

4331 Heart to Heart
401 S. Clairborne Rd., Suite 302
Olathe, KS 66062
913-764-5200
Fax: 913-764-0809
e-mail: info@hearttoheart.org
www.hearttoheart.org

Gary Morsch, Founder/President
Jim Kerr, Board Chair
Krystal Barr, Interim CEO

4332 Texas Heart to Heart
Po Box 720072
Dallas, TX 75372
888-475-2787
www.heart-to-heart-tx.org

Offering hope, education, and support to families.

Sally Pearson, Contact

Vermont

4333 Heart to Heart
401 S. Clairborne Rd., Suite 302
Olathe, KS 66062
913-764-5200
Fax: 913-764-0809
e-mail: info@hearttoheart.org
www.hearttoheart.org

Gary Morsch, Founder/President
Jim Kerr, Board Chair
Krystal Barr, Interim CEO

Virginia

4334 Precious Hearts
144 Locust Avenue
Winchester, VA 22601
540-678-0654
e-mail: hurlbutK@aol.com

Washington

4335 Heart to Heart
401 S. Clairborne Rd., Suite 302
Olathe, KS 66062
913-764-5200
Fax: 913-764-0809
e-mail: info@hearttoheart.org
www.hearttoheart.org

Gary Morsch, Founder/President
Jim Kerr, Board Chair
Krystal Barr, Interim CEO

Wisconsin

4336 Kids With Heart
1578 Careful Drive
Green Bay, WI 54304
920-498-0058
800-538-5390
www.kidswithheart.org

Michelle Rintamaki, President
Dean Rintamaki, VP
Melody Burkard, Secretary/Treasurer

4337 Left Hearts
250 N 6th Street
DePere, WI 54115
920-403-1154
Dyan Larmay, Contact

Web Sites

4338 Children's Heart Society
www.childrensheart.org

Reliable information and resources to families of children with congenital heart defects and acquired heart disease.

4339 Cincinnati Children's Hospital Medical Center
3333 Burnet Avenue
Cincinnati, OH 45229
513-636-4200
800-344-2462
TTY: 513-636-4900
www.cincinnatichildrens.org

Cincinnati Children's Hospital is dedicated to serving the cardiac care needs of patiens, fetus through young adult, and is committed to providing research and teaching programs.

4340 Congenital Heart Information Network
http://tchin.org

Provides reliable information, support services and resources to families of children with congenital heart defects and acquired heart disease.

4341 Yale University School of Medicine
330 Cedar St, Boardman 110. P.O. Box 208056
New Haven, CT 06520
medicine.yale.edu/intmed/cardio/

Information on congential heart conditions, including Hypoplastic Left Heart Syndrome symptoms, treatments and support.

Henry Scott Cabin, Professor of Medicine
Joseph Akar, Associate Professor of Medicine
Henry Cabin, Acting Section Chief

Book Publishers

4342 Parent's Guide to Children's Congenital Heart Defects
Random House
280 Park Avenue (11-3)
New York, NY 10017
800-733-3000
Fax: 212-940-7381
www.crownpublishing.com

A practical and useful resource for families coping with a child who has CHD. An easy to read book uses personal stories and a question and answer format on a wide range of medical and daily living issues.

ISBN: 0-609807-75-7

4343 Young People and Chronic Illness: True Stories, Help and Hope
Congenital Heart Information Network
P.O. Box 3397
Margate City, NJ 08402
609-823-4507
e-mail: mb@tchin.org
www.tchin.org

Presents inspirational chapters based upon interviews of young people growing up with various chronic illnesses, including a chapter on Congenital Heart Disease.

ISBN: 1-575420-41-4

Mona Barmash, President

Pamphlets

4344 Congenital Heart Information Network
600 North 3rd Street, First Floor
Philadelphia, PA 19123

215-627-4034
Fax: 215-627-4036
http://tchin.org

Four color brochure includes information about the programs and services offered.

Description

4345 HYPOTHYROIDISM

Covers these related disorders: Acquired hypothyroidism, Congenital hypothyroidism, Hoishimoto's disease

Involves the following Biologic System(s):

Endocrinologic Disorders

Hypothyroidism is a condition characterized by decreased activity of the thyroid gland, an endocrine gland that consists of two lobes on either side of the windpipe (trachea). Certain specialized cells within the thyroid gland secrete the thyroid hormones thyroxine (T-4) and triiodothyronine (T-3), which assist in regulating the rate of metabolism. Metabolism refers to the chemical activities within cells that release energy from nutrients or consume energy to create certain substances. The thyroid hormones also play a vital role in the normal mental and physical development and growth of infants and children. Other specialized cells in the thyroid gland secrete the hormone calcitonin, which helps to regulate concentrations of calcium in the body by inhibiting the loss of bone.

Hypothyroidism may result from an underlying defect that is present at birth (congenital). In children with congenital hypothyroidism, associated symptoms may begin at birth or be delayed until later during childhood, depending upon the nature of the underlying abnormality. Congenital hypothyroidism may result from several underlying causes, such as abnormal development (dysplasia) or absence (aplasia) of the thyroid gland; abnormalities in the production of certain hormones due to particular biochemical defects; or fetal exposure to particular medications or therapies (e.g., radioiodine therapy) during pregnancy. In children with malformation of the thyroid gland or abnormalities in hormonal production, the condition may appear to occur randomly for unknown reasons (sporadically) or may be familial. Congenital hypothyroidism affects approximately one in 4,000 infants worldwide and is about twice as common in females as in males.

Hypothyroidism may also occur later during childhood (acquired hypothyroidism) due to an autoimmune disorder in which the immune system develops antibodies against cells of the thyroid gland (Hashimoto's disease) or in association with other underlying disorders (e.g., nephropathic cystinosis, histiocytosis). Acquired hypothyroidism may also develop due to the use of particular medications or surgical removal of all or a portion of the thyroid gland as a treatment for certain diseases or conditions (e.g., thyroid cancer, thyrotoxicosis).

In newborns and infants with congenital hypothyroidism, associated symptoms may vary in range, severity, and rate of progression, depending upon the degree of thyroid hormone deficiency. Some patients may have an abnormally enlarged thyroid gland (goiter), causing swelling in front of the neck. In addition, early symptoms may include yellowish discoloration of the skin, mucous membranes, and whites of the eyes (jaundice); sluggishness; and feeding difficulties, including choking episodes during nursing. Many patients also have a large abdomen; a weakening of the abdominal wall muscles through which an abdominal organ or fatty tissue may protrude (umbilical hernia); constipation; widely open soft spots (fontanels) under the front and back of the scalp; and respira-

tory difficulties, including episodes in which there is a temporary cessation of spontaneous breathing (apnea). Some patients may have progressive retardation of mental and physical development that becomes increasingly severe without early diagnosis and prompt treatment. Patients may experience delays in obtaining certain developmental milestones, such as sitting up and standing; may not learn to speak; and may be increasingly lethargic. Additional physical findings associated with severe hypothyroidism include delayed skeletal maturation; a short, thick neck; short fingers and broad hands; a thick, protruding tongue; delayed eruption of the teeth (dentition); dry, scaly skin; coarse, scanty hair; and an abnormal, progressive accumulation of fluid within body tissues and associated swelling, particularly in the genital area, eyelids, and backs of the hands (myxedema).

The symptoms and findings associated with acquired hypothyroidism may also vary, depending upon the underlying cause, the age at onset, and the degree of thyroid hormone deficiency. Children with acquired hypothyroidism may experience an abnormally decreased rate of growth, decreased energy, puffiness of the skin (myxedematous changes), constipation, cold intolerance, headaches, visual problems, or other abnormalities.

In the United States, thyroid hormone levels in the blood are routinely tested in all newborns shortly after birth. Early diagnosis and prompt treatment of congenital hypothyroidism are essential for normal brain development during infancy. Such treatment includes thyroid hormone replacement therapy (e.g., sodium-L-thyroxine by mouth). The treatment of children with acquired hypothyroidism also includes thyroid hormone replacement therapy. Additional treatment is symptomatic and supportive.

National Associations & Support Groups

4346 American Academy of Pediatrics
141 Northwest Point Boulevard
Elk Grove Village, IL 60007   847-434-4000
                                               800-433-9016
                                               Fax: 847-434-8000
                                               www.aap.org

The American Academy of Pediatrics and its member pediatricians are committed to the attainment of optimal physical, mental and social health and well-being for all infants, children, adolescents, and young adults.

Sandra Hassink, MD, FAAP, President

4347 American Association of Clinical Endocrinologists
1000 Riverside Avenue, Suite 205
Jacksonville, FL 32204   904-353-7878
                                               Fax: 904-353-8185
                                               e-mail: info@aace.com
                                               www.aace.com

A professional medical organization devoted to the enhancement of the practice of clinical endocrinology.

Donald C. Jones, CEO
Dan Kelsey, Deputy CEO
Michael Avallone, CFO

4348 Genetic Alliance
4301 Connecticut Avenue NW
Washington, DC 20008   202-966-7955
                                               800-336-4363
                                               Fax: 202-966-8553
                                               e-mail: info@geneticalliance.org
                                               www.geneticalliance.org

A coalition of voluntary genetic support groups, consumers and professionals addressing the needs of individuals and families affected by genetic disorders from a national perspective.

Joan Oppenheimer Weiss, Founder
Sharon Terry, President

4349 Lawson Wilkins Pediatric Endocrine Society
6728 Old McLean Village Drive
McLean, VA 22101　　　　　703-556-9222
　　　　　　　　　　　　Fax: 703-556-8729
　　　　　　　　e-mail: info@pedsendo.org
　　　　　　　　　　　www.lwpes.org

To promote the acquisition and dissemination of knowledge of endocrine and metabolic disorders from conception through adolescence.

Morey W. Haymond, President
Mitchell E. Geffiner, President-Elect
Karen Rubin, Treasurer

4350 March of Dimes Birth Defects Foundation
1275 Mamaroneck Avenue
White Plains, NY 10605　　　　914-997-4488
　　　　　　　　　　　　888-663-4637
　　　　　　　　　　　　Fax: 914-997-4763
　　　　　e-mail: answers@marchofdimes.com
　　　　　　　　www.marchofdimes.com

Partnership of volunteers and professionals dedicates to improving the health of babies by preventing birth defects and infant mortality. Over 100 chapters are located across the country and can be located through the National Office.

Jennifer L Howse, President

4351 Thyroid Foundation of America
Ste 300
Boston, MA 02210　　　　　617-534-1500
　　　　　　　　　　　　800-832-8321
　　　　　　　　　　　　Fax: 617-534-1515
　　　　　　　　e-mail: info@allthyroid.org
　　　　　　　　　　www.allthyroid.org

TFA's mission is to become the best at providing credible, unbiased information on thyroid topics using electronic, print, and voice technology for benefit of patients with thyroid disorders, their families and the general public. It is also to ensure timely diagnosis, appropriate treatment, and ongoing support for all individuals with thyroid disease.

4352 Thyroid Society for Education and Research
7515 S Main Street, Suite 545
Houston, TX 77030　　　　　713-799-9909
　　　　　　　　　　　　800-849-7643
　　　　　　　　　　　　Fax: 713-799-9919
　　　　　e-mail: help@the-thyroid-society.org
　　　　　　　www.the-thyroid-society.org

A nonprofit organization whose mission is to pursue the prevention, treatment and cure of thyroid disease.

Libraries & Resource Centers

4353 National Digestive Diseases Information Clearinghouse
Bldg 31, Rm 9A06, 31 Center Drive
Bethesda, MD 20892　　　　　301-496-3583
　　　　　　　　　　　　800-891-5389
　　　　　　　　　　　　Fax: 301-907-8906
　　　　　e-mail: nddic@info.niddk.nih.gov
　　　　　　　　www2.niddk.nih.gov

The National Institute of Diabetes and Digestive and Kidney Diseases conducts and supports research on many of the most serious diseases affecting public health. The Institute supports much of the clinical research on the diseases of internal medicine and related subspecialty fields as well as many basic science disciplines.

Griffin P. Rodgers, M.D, CHAIRPERSON
Brent B. Stanfield, EXECUTIVE SECRETARY
Camille M. Hoover, M.S.W, Executive Officer

Web Sites

4354 American Association of Clinical Endocrinologists
245 Riverside Avenue Suite 200
Jacksonville,, FL 32202　　　　904-353-7878
　　　　　　　　　　　　Fax: 904-353-8185
　　　　　　　　　　　　www.aace.com

The American Association of Clinical Endocrinologists is a professional medical organization devoted to the enhancement of the practice of clinical endocrinology.

R. Mack Harrell, President
George Grunberger, President Elect
Pauline M. Camacho, Vice President

4355 Online Mendelian Inheritance in Man
8600 Rockville Pike
Bethesda, MD 20894　　　　　301-594-5983
　　　　　　　　　　　　888-346-3656
　　　　　　　　　　　　Fax: 301-402-1384
　　　　　　　　　　　　TDD: 800-735-2258
　　　　　e-mail: custserv@nlm.nih.gov
　　　　　　www.ncbi.nlm.nih.gov/omim

Is an online database catalog of human genes and genetic disorders. The database contains textual information and references. It also contains copious links to MEDLINE and sequence records in the Entrenz System, and links to additional related resources at NCBI and elsewhere.

Christine E Seidman M.D, Chairman
David J Lipman M.D, Executive Secretary
Scott Edwards, Member

4356 Thyroid Federation International
P.O. Box 471
Bath, ON K0H 1　　e-mail: webmaster@thyroid-fed.org
　　　　　　　　　　www.thyroid-fed.org/

The Thyroid Federation International aims to work for the benefit of those affected by thyroid disorders throughout the world. Its objectives are to encourage and assist the formation of patient oriented thyroid organizations, to work closely with the medical professions to promote awareness and understanding of thyroid disorders and their complications, to provide through member organizations, information and moral support to those affected by thyroid disorders and to promote education.

Ashok Bhaseen, President
Beate BartSs, Secretary
Asta Tirronen, Treasurer

Book Publishers

4357 Endocrine & Metabolic Disorders Sourcebook
Omnigraphics
PO Box 8002
Aston, PA 19014　　　　　800-234-1340
　　　　　　　　　　　　Fax: 800-875-1340
　　　　　e-mail: info@omnigraphics.com
　　　　　　　　omnigraphics.com

Basic information for the lay person about pancreatic and insulin-related disorders such as pancreatitis, diabetes and hypoglycemia; adrenal gland disorders such as Cushing's syndrome, Addison's disease and congenital adrenal hyperplasia; pituitary gland disorders such as growth hormone deficiency, acromegaly and pituitary tumors; and thyroid disorders such as hypothyroidism, Grave's disease, Hashimoto's disease and goiter.

574 pages
ISBN: 0-780802-07-1

Journals

4358 Journal of Clinical Endocrinology
245 Riverside Avenue Suite 200
Jacksonville, FL 32204　　　　904-353-7878
　　　　　　　　　　　　Fax: 904-353-8185
　　　　　　　　　　　　www.aace.com

Hypothyroidism / Pamphlets

Original research and articles, visual vignettes and other clinical information spanning the science of endocrinology.

R. Mack Harrell, President
George Grunberger, President Elect
Pauline M. Camacho, Vice President

Pamphlets

4359 Congenital & Acquired Hypothyroidism
Human Growth Foundation
P.O. Box 872
Pine, CO 80470

303-400-9040
888-999-9428
Fax: 303-838-0753
e-mail: jmoore@erols.com
www.genetic.org/hgf

Myra Byrd, Chair
Gary Glissman, Vice Chair
Shiela Clark, Secretary

498

Description

4360 ICHTHYOSIS

Covers these related disorders: Collodion baby, Congenital ichthyosiform erythroderma, Epidermolytic hyperkeratosis, Harlequin fetus, Ichthyosis vulgaris, X-linked ichthyosis

Involves the following Biologic System(s):

Dermatologic Disorders

Ichthyosis, literally meaning "fish skin," is a group of disorders characterized by abnormal thickening, dryness, and scaling of the skin due to abnormalities in the production of keratin, a protein that is the primary component of the skin, hair, and nails. Most forms of ichthyosis are genetic disorders that are usually apparent at birth (congenital) or during the first months of life. The genes that cause some congenital forms of ichthyosis have been mapped to particular chromosomes. Ichthyosis may also be due to other underlying genetic syndromes or may be an acquired condition due to certain nutritional deficiencies, the administration of particular drugs, or certain conditions, such as abnormally decreased activity of the thyroid gland (hypothyroidism) or Hodgkin's disease, a malignancy of the lymphatic system.

One congenital form of ichthyosis is known as harlequin fetus and may result from several different genetic abnormalities, most of which are thought to be transmitted as an autosomal recessive trait. Affected newborns may be covered with thickened, ridged, armor-like plates that confine the fingers and toes, restrict movements of the joints, and flatten the nose and ears. Additional features may include eyelids that are turned outward (ectropion), causing eyes to be indistinct; gaping lips; and absent hair and nails. Newborns with the condition may experience difficulties breathing, be susceptible to repeated skin infections, and develop life-threatening complications during the first days or weeks of life.

Another congenital form of ichthyosis, known as collodion baby, may also result from many different genetic abnormalities. Affected newborns are covered by a thick membrane that resembles an oiled parchment (collodion membrane), causing flattening of the nose and ears, abnormalities of the eyelids (ectropion), gaping of the lips, or other abnormalities. The membrane begins to crack as patients breathe and is gradually shed in large sheets. This condition is usually an early manifestation of specific genetic forms of ichthyosis (e.g., lamellar ichthyosis or congenital ichthyosiform erythroderma). Patients may develop potentially life-threatening symptoms due to skin infection, inflammation of the lungs (pneumonia), excessive loss of bodily fluids (dehydration), or other abnormalities.

Congenital ichthyosiform erythroderma is an autosomal recessive disorder that typically becomes apparent shortly after birth and may often present as collodion baby, the name given to a baby who is born encased in a skin that resembles a yellow, tight and shiny film or dried collodion (sausage skin) This form of ichthyosis is characterized by abnormal redness of the skin (erythroderma); generalized, fine, white scaling of the skin; and potentially severe itching (pruritus). Many children also have abnormally thickened skin (hyperkeratosis) on the palms of the hands and soles of the feet as well as around the knees, ankles, and elbo. Additional

findings may include unusually sparse hair and abnormalities of the nails. Another form of the disorder, known as lamellar ichthyosis or nonbullous congenital ichthyosiform erythroderma, is usually inherited as an autosomal recessive trait. This form of ichthyosis becomes apparent shortly after birth and may also present as a collodion baby. After the collodion membrane is shed, the skin becomes covered with relatively large, coarse scales. Scaling often affects all surfaces of the body and may be associated with pruritus. Patients may also have thickened skin on the palms and soles, usually small ears, ectropion, and abnormally sparse, fine hair.

Another form of the disorder, known as X-linked ichthyosis, is often apparent at birth or during early infancy. Although males are primarily affected, some females who carry a single copy of the disease gene may also experience some symptoms. Patients develop prominent darkened scales on the scalp, ears, neck, arms and legs, torso, or other areas. Scaling may gradually worsen in severity and progress to affect other areas of the skin. By late childhood or adolescence, many patients develop clouding of the corneas (corneal opacities) that does not interfere with vision.

The most common form of the disorder is ichthyosis vulgaris, also known as ichthyosis simplex, an autosomal dominant disorder that affects about one in 250 to 300 children. Symptoms, which typically become apparent by the age of six months, may include slight roughness and scaling of the skin, particularly of the back and the legs. Scaling may worsen upon exposure to cold temperatures and may subside during warm months of the year. There may also be overgrowth of hair follicles (keratosis pilaris), particularly those of the thighs and upper arms, as well as abnormal thickening of the skin of the palms and soles. The condition may gradually improve or subside with age.

Another form of ichthyosis, known as epidermolytic hyperkeratosis or bullous congenital ichthyosiform erythroderma, may occur randomly for unknown reasons or be inherited as an autosomal dominant trait. This form of ichthyosis typically becomes apparent shortly after birth and is characterized by erythroderma, hyperkeratosis in certain areas, and small, rough, wart-like scales over body surfaces. Skin overgrowth may be most apparent on the neck and hips, under the arms, or at the elbows or knees and may affect the skin of the palms and soles. Recurrent blistering (bullae) may also develop, particularly on the lower legs, knees, or elbows.

The methods used to treat ichthyosis depend upon the specific disorder type as well as the severity and extent of associated symptoms. In severe neonatal forms, such as collodion baby and harlequin fetus, supportive measures may include administration of fluids to prevent dehydration; use of specialized support equipment such as an incubator that provides a heated, appropriately moisturized (hum idified) environment; and use of measures to help prevent or aggressively treat infections. Treatment may also include the administration of certain vitamin A derivatives (retinoids) or emulsifying ointments or lubricants. Bathing with oils may help to moisten the skin, and the application of certain emulsifying ointments and lubricants that soften the skin may alleviate dryness and scaling. In addition, applying topical agents that promote skin softening and peeling (keratolytic agents) may facilitate the removal of scales. In some patients, the use of air conditioning in warmer months and exposure to a high-humidity environment during the colder months may also be beneficial. Additional treatment is symptomatic and supportive.

Government Agencies

4361 NIH/National Institute of Allergy and Infectious Diseases
6610 Rockledge Drive, Room 4017, MSC 6606. PO Box
Bethesda, MD 20817
301-496-2644
866-284-4107
Fax: 301-402-7123
TDD: 800-877-8339
e-mail: niaidnews@niaid.nih.gov
www.niaid.nih.gov

Conducts and supports basic and applied research to better understand, treat, and ultimately prevent infectious, immunologic, and allergic diseases.

Anthony S Fauci MD, Director

4362 NIH/National Institute of Arthritis and Mu sculoskeletal and Skin Diseases
1AMS Circle. PO Box 3675
Bethesda, MD 20892
301-495-4484
877-226-4267
Fax: 301-718-6366
TTY: 301-565-2966
TDD: 301-565-2966
e-mail: niamsinfo@mail.nih.gov
www.niams.nih.gov

The mission of the NIAMS, a part of the NIH, is to support research into the causes, treatment, and prevention of arthritis and musculoskeletal and skin diseases, the training of basic and clinical scientists to carry out this research, and the dissemination of information on research progress in these diseases.

Stephen I Katz MD PhD, Director
Robert H Carter MD, Deputy Director

4363 NIH/National Institute of Child Health and Human Development
31 Center Drive, Building 31, Room 2A32
Bethesda, MD 20892
301-496-1333
800-370-2943
Fax: 866-760-5947
TTY: 888-320-6942
e-mail: NICHDInformationResourceCenter@mail.nih.
www.nichd.nih.gov

Established in 1962 by congress, today the institute conducts and supports research on topics related to the health of children, adults, families and populations. Some of these topics include: developmental disabilities, growth and development, infant death, reproductive health and birth defects.

Jay H Hoofnagle, Director
Lisa Kaeser, Program & Public Liaison

National Associations & Support Groups

4364 American Academy of Pediatrics
141 Northwest Point Boulevard
Elk Grove Village, IL 60007
847-434-4000
800-433-9016
Fax: 847-434-8000
www.aap.org

The American Academy of Pediatrics and its member pediatricians are committed to the attainment of optimal physical, mental and social health and well-being for all infants, children, adolescents, and young adults.

Sandra Hassink, MD, FAAP, President

4365 FIRST: Foundation for Ichthyosis and Related Skin Types
2616 North Broad Street
Colmar, PA 18915
215-997-9400
800-545-3286
Fax: 215-997-9403
e-mail: info@firstskinfoundation.org
www.firstskinfoundation.org

Dedicated to helping individuals and families affected by the inherited skin diseases collectively called the Ichthyoses. Provides support, information, education, and advocacy for individuals and families affected by ichthyosis.

Mike Briggs, President
Larry Silverman, CFO

4366 Genetic Alliance
4301 Connecticut Avenue NW
Washington, DC 20008
202-966-7955
800-336-4363
Fax: 202-966-8553
e-mail: info@geneticalliance.org
www.geneticalliance.org

A coalition of voluntary genetic support groups, consumers and professionals addressing the needs of individuals and families affected by genetic disorders from a national perspective.

Joan Oppenheimer Weiss, Founder
Sharon Terry, President

4367 March of Dimes Birth Defects Foundation
1275 Mamaroneck Avenue
White Plains, NY 10605
914-997-4488
888-663-4637
Fax: 914-997-4763
e-mail: answers@marchofdimes.com
www.marchofdimes.com

Partnership of volunteers and professionals dedicates to improving the health of babies by preventing birth defects and infant mortality. Over 100 chapters are located across the country and can be located through the National Office.

Jennifer L Howse, President

4368 National Registry for Ichthyosis and Related Disorders
University of Washington, Dermatology Department
Box 356524, Rm.BB1353, 1959 NE Pacific St.
Seattle, WA 98195
800-595-1265
Fax: 206-543-2489
e-mail: info@skinregistry.org
www.skinregistry.org

Identifies individuals in the USA who have an inherited disorder of keratinization; confirms the diagnosis by strict clinical, histiopathic and biological criteria, and by using molecular resources to assist in diagnosis, assistance with research, and a means of empowerment for affected individuals and their families.

Philip Fleckman, MD, Principal Investigator

4369 Society for Pediatric Dermatology
8365 Keystone Crossing, Suite 107
Indianapolis, IN 46240
317-202-0224
Fax: 317-205-9481
e-mail: spd@hp-assoc.com
www.pedsderm.net

National organization dedicated to promote, develop and advance education, research and care of skin disease in all pediatric age groups.

Kent Lindeman, Executive Director
Carol Caldwell, Office Secretary

Web Sites

4370 Family Village
www.familyvillage.wisc.edu

A global community that integrates information, resources and communication opportunities on the Internet for persons with cognitive and other disabilities, for their families and for those that provide them services and support.

4371 Ichthyosis Information
www.ichthyosis.com/

e-mail: chris@ichthyosis.com
www.ichthyosis.com/

This website is to furnish users with general information.

Pamphlets

4372 Ichthyosis: An Overview
FIRST: Foundation for Ichthyosis and Related Skin
2616 N. Broad Street
Colmar, PA 18915

215-997-9400
800-545-3286
Fax: 215-619-0780
e-mail: info@firstskinfoundation.org
www.firstskinfoundation.org

An overview of ichthyosis; descriptions of the primary types of ichthyosis and frequently asked questions. Available in Spanish.

18 pages

Jeff Hoerle, President
Moise Levy, Vice President
Larry Silverman, CFO

4373 Ichthyosis: The Genetics of Its Inheritance
FIRST: Foundation for Ichthyosis and Related Skin
2616 N. Broad Street
Colmar, PA 18915

215-997-9400
800-545-3286
Fax: 215-619-0780
e-mail: info@firstskinfoundation.org
www.firstskinfoundation.org

A description of the genetic inheritance patterns for the different forms of ichthyosis: autosomal dominant, autosomal recessive and X-linked recessive. With illustrations. Also available in Spanish.

23 pages

Jeff Hoerle, President
Moise Levy, Vice President
Larry Silverman, CFO

Description

4374 INTRAVENTRICULAR HEMORRHAGE

Synonyms: IVH, germinal matrix hemorrhage, GMH,
Periventricular hemorrhage, PVH

Involves the following Biologic System(s):
Neonatal and Infant Disorders, Neurologic Disorders

Intraventricular Hemorrhage (IVH) is a disease of premature
infants in which there is bleeding inside or around the ventricles, the spaces in the brain that contain the cerebrospinal
fluid (CSF). Bleeding in the brain can put pressure on the
nerve cells and damage them. Severe damage to cells can lead
to brain injury. Intraventricular hemorrhage is most common
in premature babies, especially very low birthweight babies.
The younger the gestational age, the higher the incidence of
IVH. It is not clear why IVH occurs. Bleeding can occur because blood vessels in a premature baby's brain are very fragile and immature and easily rupture. The risk of rupture is
greatest in the first 4-5 days after birth. Abrupt changes in cerebral blood flow are thought to be one of the causes of IVH.
Symptoms of IVH include apnea (stopped breathing),
bradycardia (slow heart rate), pale or blue coloring
(cyanosis), weak suck, high-pitched cry, and seizures.

IVH is diagnosed by cranial ultrasound and graded I through
IV (IV being most severe). Infants with IVH are at higher risk
for neurological disease including seizures, developmental
delay, and hydrocephalus. Infants with IVH also have a
higher incidence of death. With higher grades of IVH, the
risk of future morbidity and mortality increases.

The treatment of IVH is supportive care. The best prevention
of IVH is to prevent premature birth. When this is unavoid-
able, the use of anti-inflammatory medication (indomethacin)
in the first 48 hours of life has been shown to decrease the
incidence of IVH.

National Associations & Support Groups

4375 American Academy of Pediatrics
141 Northwest Point Boulevard
Elk Grove Village, IL 60007
847-434-4000
800-433-9016
Fax: 847-434-8000
www.aap.org

The American Academy of Pediatrics and its member pediatricians are committed to the attainment of optimal physical, mental
and social health and well-being for all infants, children, adolescents, and young adults.

Sandra Hassink, MD, FAAP, President

4376 Children's Hospital at Montefiore
3415 Bainbridge Avenue. PO Box 2940
Bronx, NY 10467
718-741-2426
Fax: 718-741-2460
e-mail: montekids@montefiore.org
www.montekids.org

The Children's Hospital at Montefiore is one of the most technologically advanced hospitals for children in the world. Staffed by
the nationally renowned faclty of the Albert Einstein College of
Medicine, our pediatric specialists and caregivers are ranked
amoung the best in the nation.

Steven M. Safyer, President/CEO
Philip O. Ozuah, Executive VP
Alfredo Cabrera, Sr. VP

4377 Children's Hospital of New York Presbyterian
3959 Broadway (165th Street and Broadway)
New York, NY 10032
212-305-5437
www.childrensnyp.org

Provides a comprehensive continuum of accessible, high-quality,
family-centered children's services. Improves the health status of
children in our community and maintain a world class academic
center for children's health care services, teaching and research.

Taisha Benjamin, Executive Director

4378 IVH Parents
PO Box 56-1111
Miami, FL 33256
305-232-0381
Fax: 305-232-9890
e-mail: mailto:72167.633@compuserve.com
www.familyvillage.wisc.edu

Support group for parents of children suffering from
intaventricular hemorrhage.

4379 Lucile Packard Children's Hospital
725 Welch Road
Palo Alto, CA 94304
650-497-8000
800-690-2282
Fax: 650-497-8612
www.lpch.org/index.html

Devoted entirely to the care of babies, children, adolescents and
expectant mothers. To best serve our communitites we advocate
on behalf of the children and expectant mothers, advance family
centered care, foster innovation, and educate health care
providers and leaders.

Christopher Dawes, Ceo

Web Sites

4380 Children's Hospital at Montefiore
3415 Bainbridge Avenue
Bronx, NY 10467
718-741-2426
TTY: 718-920-5027
e-mail: lbank@montefiore.org
www.montekids.org

Web site of one of the most technologically advanced hospitals
with highly ranked pediatric specialists and caregivers.

Steven M Safyer, President & CEO
Philip O Ozuah, Executive Vice President
Joel A Perlman, Executive Vice President

4381 Children's Hospital of New York Presbyterian
nyp.org/kids/index.html

Provides comprehensive information for children with serious
disearse, associated with Children's Hospital of New York
Presbyterian.

4382 IVH Parents
www.familyvillage.wisc.edu

Provides support for parents of children with intaventricular hemorrhage.

4383 Yale University School of Medicine
330 Cedar St, Boardman 110, P.O. Box 208056
New Haven, CT 06520
medicine.yale.edu/intmed/cardio/

Information on heart conditions, including Intraventricular Hemorrhage — symptoms, treatments and support.

Henry Scott Cabin, Professor of Medicine
Joseph Akar, Associate Professor of Medicine
Henry Cabin, Acting Section Chief

Description

4384 JUVENILE RHEUMATOID ARTHRITIS

Synonym: JRA

Covers these related disorders: Pauciarticular juvenile arthritis, Systemic-onset juvenile arthritis (Still's disease), Type I polyarticular juvenile arthritis, Type II polyarticular juvenile arthritis

Involves the following Biologic System(s):

Immunologic and Rheumatologic Disorders

Juvenile rheumatoid arthritis (JRA) is a group of disorders of childhood characterized by inflammation (arthritis), tenderness, pain, and swelling of one or more joints, potentially causing impaired development, limited movements, and permanent bending or extension of affected joints in various fixed postures (contractures). The symptoms and findings associated with JRA occur as the result of inflammation of the synovial membrane of affected joints (synovitis). Synovial membranes are connective tissue membranes that line the spaces between joints and bones and secrete a thick fluid to lubricate the joints. Although the cause of JRA is unknown, researchers speculate that the disorder may be the result of infection by an unidentified microorganism, an excessive immune response to a substance that the body perceives as foreign (hypersensitivity response), or abnormal immune responses against the body's own cells or tissues (autoimmune response). Certain antibodies often present in the blood of adults with rheumatoid arthritis (e.g., rheumatoid factors) are only rarely present in children with JRA. In such cases, researchers indicate that affected children may have some genetic predisposition for certain forms of JRA. Approximately 250,000 children are thought to be affected by JRA in the United States. Females are more commonly affected than males.

There are three major categories of JRA: polyarticular (30 percent), pauciarticular (50 percent), and systemic-onset juvenile arthritis (20 percent). Polyarticular juvenile arthritis typically involves several joints. Associated symptoms and findings include inflammation, swelling, abnormal warmth, tenderness, and pain of affected joints. This form of JRA often affects joints of the elbows, wrists, fingers, knees, feet, and ankles. In addition, patients may have involvement of joints of the jaw (temporomandibular joints), causing limited opening of the mouth; the neck (cervical spine), resulting in neck pain and stiffness; and the hips, causing pain, stiffness, and limited movements. Normal growth may be delayed during periods of active disease, causing such abnormalities as unusually short fingers, small feet, or underdevelopment of the jaw (micrognathia). Some children with polyarticular juvenile arthritis may also experience more generalized symptoms, such as low-grade fever, lack of appetite (anorexia), increased irritability, a mild decrease in the level of circulating red blood cells (anemia), swelling of certain lymph nodes (lymphadenopathy), or mild enlargement of the liver and spleen (hepatosplenomegaly).

Pauciarticular juvenile arthritis is characterized by involvement of larger joints, usually four or fewer for six consecutive weeks. Type I pauciarticular juvenile arthritis primarily affects females and has an early onset. Affected joints typically include the elbows, knees, and ankles. In addition, other joints may sometimes be affected, such as those of a single finger or toe, the wrists, the neck, or the jaw. Patients are also at risk (girls more than boys) for chronic inflammation of the colored region of the eye (iris) and its muscle (iridocyclitis). One or both eyes may be affected. Some patients may experience associated redness, sensitivity to light (photophobia), pain, or decreased clearness of vision (visual acuity). Without appropriate treatment, visual impairment or, in severe cases, blindness may result. Boys are at higher risk of arthritis of the spine. Symptoms may include a general feeling of ill health (malaise), low-grade fever, mild hepatosplenomegaly, and mild anemia. Type II pauciarticular juvenile arthritis is most common in males older than age eight. Affected joints usually include those of the hips, knees, toes, and heels. In some patients, joints of the elbows, fingers, wrists, or jaw may also be affected. In patients with this form of JRA, associated foot and hip pain may sometimes be disabling. In addition, chronic, progressive, inflammatory disease of joints of the spine (spondyloarthropathy) may develop. Symptoms may include pain, stiffness, and loss of mobility of joints of the upper and lower back (ankylosing spondylitis). In addition, some affected children may experience sudden (acute) episodes of iridocyclitis.

Systemic-onset juvenile arthritis appears to affect females and males equally. This form of JRA usually begins with generalized symptoms, such as a high, intermittent fever that rapidly returns to normal; a characteristic rash; anemia; hepatosplenomegaly; lymphadenopathy; mild liver dysfunction (hepatitis); and, in about one third of patients, inflammation of the membranous sac surrounding the heart (pericarditis) or the membrane lining the lungs and chest cavity (pleuritis). The fever associated with systemic JRA tends to rise in the evenings, although it may also be elevated in the mornings, and is often associated with shaking chills. During fever episodes, a temporary, salmon-colored rash often appears on the trunk or arms or legs (extremities), although it may appear anywhere on the body. Such a rash may also temporarily appear in association with heat exposure or stress. In patients with systemic disease, joint inflammation, swelling, stiffness, and pain may occur at disease onset or months later. Joint involvement is usually similar to that seen in patients with polyarticular juvenile arthritis. Systemic symptoms and findings typically have a self-limited course that lasts for several months. However, such findings may recur in some patients.

In approximately 75 percent of affected children, symptoms associated with JRA completely disappear with little loss of function or deformity. However, other patients, particularly those with multiple joint involvement or rheumatoid factor, may experience repeated or chronic joint inflammation and permanent stiffness, limited movement, and deformity of certain affected joints. In addition, some patients with pauciarticular juvenile arthritis may later experience additional joint involvement (polyarthritis) or ongoing symptoms due to progressive, inflammatory disease of joints of the spine (spondyloarthropathy).

Children with JRA should receive regular eye (e.g., slit-lamp) examinations to ensure early detection and treatment of iridocyclitis. Treatment of iridocyclitis includes the use of corticosteroid eyedrops and drugs that widen (dilate) the pupil. Joint inflammation, pain, and stiffness may be alleviated with aspirin, nonsteroidal anti-inflammatory drugs (NSAIDs), medications such as methotrexate or hydroxychloroquine, or, in extremely severe cases, corticosteroids administered by mouth (orally). Due to the potential association of aspirin and the occurrence of Reye's syndrome, NSAIDs (e.g., tolmetin, naproxen, etc.) are currently being prescribed more frequently than aspirin as a treatment for JRA. Children with JRA who do not respond to NSAIDs therapy may be treated with low-dose methotrexate. If JRA is severe and systemic or, in patients in whom iridocyclitis is uncontrolled by corticosteroid eyedrops, oral corticosteroid therapy may be prescribed. However, oral corticosteroid therapy is usually avoided in children, if possible, since such therapy may slow the growth rate and is associated with other negative side effects. Children who don't respond well to methotrexate can be offered similar medications, sometimes referred to as disease-modifying antirheumatic drugs (DMARDs). Agents being tried in therapy of JRA include sulfasalazine, intravenous immunoglobulin, and cyclosporine. Splints may be used during the day to help rest inflamed joints and at night to minimize the risk of contracture development and associated deformity. Special exercises may also be recommended to help reduce possible muscle wasting and contractures. In some patients, surgery may be required to help correct contractures. Children should also be monitored for growth abnormalities, nutritional deficiencies, and school/social impairment.

Government Agencies

4385 NIH/National Institute of Arthritis & Musculoskeletal & Skin Diseases
National Institutes of Health
1AMS Circle. PO Box 3675
Bethesda, MD 20892

301-495-4484
877-226-4267
Fax: 301-718-6366
TTY: 301-565-2966
TDD: 301-565-2966
e-mail: niamsinfo@mail.nih.gov
www.niams.nih.gov

The mission of the NIAMS, a part of the NIH, is to support research into the causes, treatment, and prevention of arthritis and musculoskeletal and skin diseases, the training of basic and clinical scientists to carry out this research, and the dissemination of information on research progress in these diseases.

Stephen I Katz MD PhD, Director
Robert H Carter MD, Deputy Director

4386 NIH/National Institute of Arthritis and Mu sculoskeletal and Skin Diseases
1AMS Circle. PO Box 3675
Bethesda, MD 20892

301-495-4484
877-226-4267
Fax: 301-718-6366
TTY: 301-565-2966
TDD: 301-565-2966
e-mail: niamsinfo@mail.nih.gov
www.niams.nih.gov

The mission of the NIAMS, a part of the NIH, is to support research into the causes, treatment, and prevention of arthritis and musculoskeletal and skin diseases, the training of basic and clinical scientists to carry out this research, and the dissemination of information on research progress in these diseases.

Stephen I Katz MD PhD, Director
Robert H Carter MD, Deputy Director

National Associations & Support Groups

4387 American Academy of Pediatrics
141 Northwest Point Boulevard
Elk Grove Village, IL 60007

847-434-4000
800-433-9016
Fax: 847-434-8000
www.aap.org

The American Academy of Pediatrics and its member pediatricians are committed to the attainment of optimal physical, mental and social health and well-being for all infants, children, adolescents, and young adults.

Sandra Hassink, MD, FAAP, President

4388 American Juvenile Arthritis Organization
1330 West Peachtree Street Suite 100
Atlanta, GA 30309

404-872-7100
800-283-7800
Fax: 404-872-9559
e-mail: info.ga@arthritis.org
www.arthritis.org

Devoted to serving the special needs of children, teens, and young adults with childhood rheumatic diseases and their families. Offers both support and information through national and local programs that serve the needs of families, friends and health professionals. Serves as a clearinghouse of information, sponsors an annual national conference, monitors and promotes legislation, sponsors research, and offers training to both parents and health professionals.

Sage Rhodes, President
Sharon Davenport

4389 Arthritis Foundation
1330 W. Peachtree Street., Suite 100
Atlanta, GA 30309

404-872-7100
800-283-7800
Fax: 404-872-0457
www.arthritis.org

The only nonprofit organization that supports the more than 100 types of arthritis and related conditions with advocacy, programs, services and research.

Daniel T. McGowan, Chair
John H. Klippel, M.D., President/CEO
Patricia Novak Nelson, Vice Chair

4390 Genetic Alliance
4301 Connecticut Avenue NW
Washington, DC 20008

202-966-7955
800-336-4363
Fax: 202-966-8553
e-mail: info@geneticalliance.org
www.geneticalliance.org

A coalition of voluntary genetic support groups, consumers and professionals addressing the needs of individuals and families affected by genetic disorders from a national perspective.

Joan Oppenheimer Weiss, Founder
Sharon Terry, President

4391 Kids on the Block Arthritis Programs
Arthritis Foundation
9385-C Gerwig Lane
Columbia, MD 21046

410-290-9095
800-368-5437
Fax: 410-290-9358
e-mail: kob@kotb.com
www.kotb.com

State and local programs that use puppetry to help children understand what it is like for children and adults who have arthritis.

Aric Darroe, President

Research Centers

4392 Pediatric Rheumatoid Clinic
Duke Medical Center
Box 3212
Durham, NC 27710   919-684-6575

Clinical and laboratory pediatric rheumatoid studies.

Dr. Deborah Kredich, Chairman
Stacy Ardman

Web Sites

4393 Online Mendelian Inheritance in Man
8600 Rockville Pike
Bethesda, MD 20894   301-594-5983
                                           888-346-3656
                                      Fax: 301-402-1384
                                      TDD: 800-735-2258
                             e-mail: custserv@nlm.nih.gov
                                       www.ncbi.nlm.nih.gov

This database is a catalog of human genes and genetic disorders.

Christine E Seidman M.D, Chairman
David J Lipman M.D, Executive Secretary
Scott Edwards, Member

Book Publishers

4394 Arthritis
Franklin Watts
90 Old Sherman Turnpike
Danbury, CT 06816   203-797-3500
                                           800-724-6527
                                      Fax: 203-797-3197
                                       www.scholastic.com

This book offers a clear explanation of the various forms and effects of the disease of arthritis and what treatments are available.

96 pages Grades 7-12
ISBN: 0-531108-01-5

Dick Robinson, President & CEO

4395 Arthritis Sourcebook
Omnigraphics
PO Box 8002
Aston, PA 19014   800-234-1340
                                      Fax: 800-875-1340
                             e-mail: info@omnigraphics.com
                                       omnigraphics.com

Basic consumer health information on specific forms of arthritis
and related disorders.

550 pages Hardcover
ISBN: 0-780802-01-2

**4396 Educational Rights for Children With Arthritis: Parents
Manual**
AJAO
1330 W. Peachtree Street, Suite 100
Atlanta, GA 30309   404-872-7100
                                      Fax: 404-872-9559
                               e-mail: help@arthritis.org
                                         www.arthritis.org

A self-instructional manual helping parents to identify and obtain
school services needed by their child with arthritis. Covers laws
and special services, explores strategies for working with school
personnel and stresses good communication and advocacy
techniques.

Daniel T. McGowan, Chairman
John H. Klippel, President & CEO
Michael V. Ortman, Secretary

4397 JRA and Me
American Juvenile Arthritis Organization
PO Box 19000
Atlanta, GA 30326   800-283-7800

A workbook for school-aged children who have juvenile arthritis.
This book offers a variety of educational games, puzzles and
worksheets to teach children about their illness and how to take
care of themselves.

57 pages

4398 Living with Arthritis
Franklin Watts
90 Old Sherman Turnpike
Danbury, CT 06816   203-797-3500
                                           800-621-1115
                                      Fax: 203-797-3197
                                       www.scholastic.com

Shows how people with arthritis can overcome their pain and lead
productive, full lives.

32 pages Grades 5-7

Dick Robinson, President & CEO

4399 Understanding Juvenile Rheumatoid Arthritis
American Juvenile Arthritis Organization
1330 W. Peachtree Street, Suite 100
Atlanta, GA 30309   404-872-7100
                                           800-568-4045
                               e-mail: help@arthritis.org
                                         www.arthritis.org

A manual for health professionals to use in teaching children
with JRA and their families about disease management and
self-care.

372 pages

Daniel T. McGowan, Chairman
John H. Klippel, President & CEO
Michael V. Ortman, Secretary

4400 We Can: Guide for Parents of Children with Arthritis
American Juvinile Arthritis Association
1330 W. Peachtree Street, Suite 100
Atlanta, GA 30309   404-872-7100
                                           800-568-4045
                                      Fax: 404-872-9559
                               e-mail: help@arthritis.org
                                         www.arthritis.org

Offers parents tips for daily living and practical points for helping their child toward independent adulthood.

Daniel T. McGowan, Chairman
John H. Klippel, President & CEO
Michael V. Ortman, Secretary

4401 Yard Sale Coloring Book
American Juvenile Arthritis Organization
PO Box 19000
Atlanta, GA 30326   800-283-7800

A coloring/activity book based on a Kids on the Block script,
written for third and fourth grade students. It can be used with
Kids on the Block performances, as a stand-alone piece or with a
free lesson plan packet.

Newsletters

4402 AJAO Newsletter
American Juvenile Arthritis Organization
1330 W. Peachtree Street, Suite 100
Atlanta, GA 30309   404-872-7100
                                           800-283-7800
                                      Fax: 404-872-0457
                            e-mail: kgatmail@arthritis.org
                                         www.arthritis.org

This reliable and comprehensive newsletter for families coping with childhood arthritis and related conditions contains the latest research findings, responsible advice from pediatric specialists, practical methods to help improve quality of life, and informative updates about medications and how they affect children. Articles are written in clear understandable language. Timely medical insights and life enhancing information that provides solutions to everyday problems.

Quarterly

Michael V. Ortman, Chair
Ann M. Palmer, President & CEO
Meagan Fulmer, Chief Development Officer

Pamphlets

4403   Arthritis Information: Children
Arthritis Foundation
1330 W. Peachtree Street, Suite 100
Atlanta, GA 30309

404-872-7100
800-283-7800
Fax: 404-872-0457
www.arthritis.org

Michael V. Ortman, Chair
Ann M. Palmer, President & CEO
Meagan Fulmer, Chief Development Officer

4404   Arthritis in Children and La Artritis Infantojuvenil
American Juvenile Arthritis Organization
PO Box 7669
Atlanta, GA 30357

404-872-7100
800-568-4045

A medical information booklet about juvenile rheumatoid arthritis. This booklet is written for parents or other adults and includes details about different forms of JRA, medications, therapies and coping issues.

4405   Arthritis in Children: Resources for Children, Parents and Teachers
National Arthritis and Skin Diseases Clearinghouse
9000 Rockville Pike
Bethesda, MD 20892

301-495-4484
www.niams.nih.gov/health_info

A resource offering information on juvenile arthritis, causes, treatments and prevention.

38 pages

4406   Rheumatoid Arthritis
NAMSIC, National Institutes of Health
1 AMS Circle
Bethesda, MD 20892

301-495-4484
877-226-4267
Fax: 301-718-6366
TTY: 301-565-2966
e-mail: NIAMSinfo@mail.nih.gov
www.nih.gov/niams/

Offers an introduction and definition of rheumatoid arthritis, treatments, causes, objectives, daily living, resources and medical information.

Stephen I. Katz, M.D., Ph.D., Director

4407   When Your Student Has Arthritis: Guide for Teachers
Arthritis Foundation
1330 W. Peachtree Street, Suite 100
Atlanta, GA 30309

404-872-7100
800-283-7800
Fax: 404-872-0457
www.arthritis.org

A medical information booklet written for teachers or other adults who have arthritis. The booklet describes different forms of juvenile arthritis, how arthritis might affect the child at school, and how to help the child work around these problems.

Michael V. Ortman, Chair
Ann M. Palmer, President & CEO
Meagan Fulmer, Chief Development Officer

Description

4408 KAWASAKI DISEASE

Synonyms: MLNS, Mucocutaneous lymph node syndrome

Involves the following Biologic System(s):

Cardiovascular Disorders, Immunologic and Rheumatologic Disorders

Kawasaki disease is a syndrome of unknown origin that primarily affects infants and young children. The disease was initially observed in Japanese children after World War II. Kawasaki disease is becoming increasingly frequent in the United States, has been reported worldwide, and is currently considered the leading cause of acquired heart disease in children in the U.S. Although Kawasaki disease has been reported in people in all racial groups, individuals of Japanese descent appear to be most commonly affected. The disease may occur commonly in a random or an isolated manner (sporadic form) or, rarely, may suddenly affect large numbers of individuals (epidemic form). Although the cause of Kawasaki disease is unknown, researchers suspect that toxic substances produced by certain bacteria (e.g., staphylococcal toxins) may play some role. There is no evidence of transmission of the disease from one affected individual to another (person-to-person transmission).

Kawasaki disease most commonly affects children who are five years of age or younger. Affected children typically develop a sudden, sustained, high fever that is often greater than 104 degrees and unresponsive to therapy with fever-reducing (antipyretic) medications. Most patients also have inflammation of the whites of both eyes and the lining inside the eyelids (bilateral conjunctivitis), causing redness but no associated discharge; dry, red (erythematous), cracked (fissured) lips; a strawberry-red tongue; and swelling of one or several lymph nodes, particularly those of the neck (cervical lymphadenopathy). Patients also typically develop a reddish skin rash that may consist of flat, discolored spots and small, raised areas (maculopapular) or appear similar to that seen in measles (morbilliform). The trunk, the hands and feet, and the face may be affected. Patients usually experience subsequent swelling and associated pain of the hands and feet. By approximately the second to third week, affected skin may begin to peel (desquamate) from the palms of the hands, the soles of the feet, and the tips of the fingers and toes. Such peeling may also involve other affected areas, such as the trunk. In addition, children with Kawasaki disease are usually irritable and may develop joint swelling and pain (arthritis), abdominal pain, diarrhea, vomiting, coughing, inflammation of the gall bladder, or enlargement of the liver and spleen (hepatosplenomegaly). Additional symptoms and findings may include inflammation of certain muscles (myositis), nasal discharge of a thin fluid (rhinorrhea), episodes of increased electrical activity in the brain (seizures), mild inflammation of the protective membrane surrounding the brain (aseptic meningitis), or other abnormalities.

The most serious complication potentially associated with Kawasaki disease is involvement of the heart. Within the first few weeks after disease onset, approximately 25 percent of untreated patients develop inflammation of arteries that carry blood to the heart muscle (coronary arteritis) and associated widening or bulging (aneurysms) of the walls of these arteries. In rare cases, affected children, particularly those under the age of one year, may experience few early symptoms associated with the disease, yet later develop coronary arteritis. Patients with cardiac involvement may develop inflammation of heart muscle (myocarditis); deficient blood supply to heart muscle (myocardial ischemia), resulting in localized loss of tissue (infarction); and inflammation of the membranous sac surrounding the heart (pericarditis). Additional findings may include inflammation of the membrane lining the internal surfaces of the cavities of the heart (endocarditis), an inability of the heart to sufficiently pump blood to the lungs and the rest of the body (heart failure), or abnormalities of the rhythm or rate of the heartbeat (arrythmias). In some cases, without appropriate treatment, patients with severe cardiac involvement may experience potentially life-threatening complications.

All patients with diagnosed or suspected Kawasaki disease should undergo specialized diagnostic tests, such as chest x-rays, electrocardiograms, and echocardiograms. Additional testing (e.g., two-dimensional echocardiogram) may also be conducted during the first two weeks of disease. The treatment of children with Kawasaki disease should include intravenous (IV) infusion with a preparation of antibodies (immunoglobulins) obtained from plasma, the liquid portion of the blood (intravenous gammaglobulin), and therapy with high-dose aspirin (salicylate therapy). Early (within 10 days of fever onset) intravenous gammaglobulin therapy helps to alleviate fever and other associated symptoms; in addition, controlled studies have demonstrated that such therapy decreases heart involvement to some patients. Once the fever has subsided, patients may receive therapy with lower doses of aspirin. Such therapy typically continues until coronary arteritis resolves. In the rare patient with large or multiple coronary artery aneurysms, treatment may include therapy with anticlotting medications, such as warfarin or heparin. Other treatment is symptomatic and supportive. All children diagnosed with Kawasaki disease receive outpatient follow-up with a pediatric cardiologist.

Government Agencies

4409 NIH/National Heart, Lung and Blood Institu te
National Institute of Health
Building 31, Room 5A52, 31 Center Drive MSC 2486
Bethesda, MD 20892   301-592-8573
                                                     Fax: 301-592-8563
                                                     TTY: 240-629-3255
                                           e-mail: NHLBIinfo@nhlbi.nih.gov
                                                     www.nhlbi.nih.gov

Primary responsibility of this organization is the scientific investigation of heart, blood vessel, lung and blood disorders. Oversees research, demonstration, prevention, education, control and training activities in these fields and emphasizes the prevention and control of heart diseases.

Elizabeth G Nabel, MD, Director
Susan Shurin, MD, Deputy Director
Sheila Pohl, Chief of Staff

4410 NIH/National Institute of Allergy and Infectious Diseases
6610 Rockledge Drive, Room 4017, MSC 6606. PO Box
Bethesda, MD 20817   301-496-2644
                                                          866-284-4107
                                                     Fax: 301-402-7123
                                                     TDD: 800-877-8339
                                          e-mail: niaidnews@niaid.nih.gov
                                                     www.niaid.nih.gov

Conducts and supports basic and applied research to better understand, treat, and ultimately prevent infectious, immunologic, and allergic diseases.

Anthony S Fauci MD, Director

507

4411 NIH/National Institute of Child Health and Human Development
31 Center Drive, Building 31, Room 2A32
Bethesda, MD 20892
301-496-1333
800-370-2943
Fax: 866-760-5947
TTY: 888-320-6942
e-mail: NICHDInformationResourceCenter@mail.nih.
www.nichd.nih.gov

Established in 1962 by congress, today the institute conducts and supports research on topics related to the health of children, adults, families and populations. Some of these topics include: developmental disabilities, growth and development, infant death, reproductive health and birth defects.

Jay H Hoofnagle, Director
Lisa Kaeser, Program & Public Liaison

National Associations & Support Groups

4412 American Academy of Pediatrics
141 Northwest Point Boulevard
Elk Grove Village, IL 60007
847-434-4000
800-433-9016
Fax: 847-434-8000
www.aap.org

The American Academy of Pediatrics and its member pediatricians are committed to the attainment of optimal physical, mental and social health and well-being for all infants, children, adolescents, and young adults.

Sandra Hassink, MD, FAAP, President

4413 Kawasaki Disease Foundation
PO Box 45
Boxford, MA 01921
978-356-2070
Fax: 978-356-2079
e-mail: info@kdfoundation.org

Raising awareness among the medical community, childcare providers, and the general public is critical to early diagnosis and treatment. Facilitating support among families is essential to helping families cope with this uncommon illness and the potentially devastating effects of heart damage. Increasing funding for research is necessary to advance diagnostic guidelines, enhance the existing treatment, improve short-term and long-term follow-up care and find a cause.

Gregory Chin, President
Anthony Olaes, VP

4414 Kawasaki Families' Network
46-111 Nahewai Place
Kaneohe, HI 96744
808-525-8053
Fax: 808-525-8055
e-mail: kawasaki@compuserve.com
ourworld.compuserve.com/homepage/kawasaki

A network that works to share information on research, to share information and support through occasional mailings, and to provide links to medical literature.

Description

National Associations & Support Groups

4415 KELOIDS

Synonym: Cheloids

Involves the following Biologic System(s):

Dermatologic Disorders

Keloids are firm, nodule-like overgrowths of scar tissue that occur at the sites of surgery, injury, or trauma to the skin. These overgrowths result from the formation, during the healing process, of excessive amounts of the fibrous protein collagen, which is a major structural component of connective tissue. Doctors do not understand exactly why keloids form in certain people or situations and not in others. Changes in the signals sent out by cells that control growth and proliferation may be related to the process of keloid formation, but these changes have not yet been scientifically proven. Keloids may be itchy and are usually pink in color, shiny, smooth, irregularly shaped, firm, and rubbery. Some keloids may be tender or painful. Although keloids may appear on the face, neck, earlobes, legs, or other areas, they most often occur over the breastbone (sternum) and the shoulders.

Keloid development may sometimes result following surgery, body piercing, and other types of trauma to the skin such as burns or scalds. In addition, keloids may develop in association with severe acne and occasionally with certain connective tissue disorders such as Ehlers-Danlos syndrome or skin disorders such as Touraine-Solente-Gole syndrome. In some cases, keloid development may be inherited as an autosomal recessive or autosomal dominant trait. In addition, keloids are more common in black individuals.

Without treatment, keloids tend to flatten out and become less obvious within a period of months or years. However, monthly injections of certain corticosteroid drugs directly into the lesions (intralesional) may successfully decrease their size and reduce itching, but treatment should be initiated early in their development. Treatment of large keloids may include surgical removal followed by corticosteroid injections into the lesions. Surgery alone most often results in a recurrence of the keloid. Other treatment may include laser therapy that reduces the redness of the keloid; freezing keloids (cryotherapy) may also flatten them. The direct application of silicone patches or sheeting may promote shrinkage.

Government Agencies

4416 NIH/National Institute of Arthritis and Mu sculoskeletal and Skin Diseases

1AMS Circle. PO Box 3675
Bethesda, MD 20892

301-495-4484
877-226-4267
Fax: 301-718-6366
TTY: 301-565-2966
TDD: 301-565-2966
e-mail: niamsinfo@mail.nih.gov
www.niams.nih.gov

The mission of the NIAMS, a part of the NIH, is to support research into the causes, treatment, and prevention of arthritis and musculoskeletal and skin diseases, the training of basic and clinical scientists to carry out this research, and the dissemination of information on research progress in these diseases.

Stephen I Katz MD PhD, Director
Robert H Carter MD, Deputy Director

4417 American Academy of Dermatology (AAD)

PO Box 4014
Schaumburg, IL 60168

847-240-1280
866-503-7546
Fax: 847-240-1859
e-mail: MRC@aad.org
www.aad.org

Committed to the highest quality standards in continuing medical education. Developed a platform to promote and advance the science and art of medicine and surgery related to the skin; promotes the highest possible standards in clinical practice, education and research in dermatology and related disciplines; and supports and enhances patient care and promotes the public interest relating to dermatology.

Stephen P Stone MD, President
William P Coleman III, MD, VP
David M Pariser MD, Secretary/Treasurer

4418 American Academy of Pediatrics

141 Northwest Point Boulevard
Elk Grove Village, IL 60007

847-434-4000
800-433-9016
Fax: 847-434-8000
www.aap.org

The American Academy of Pediatrics and its member pediatricians are committed to the attainment of optimal physical, mental and social health and well-being for all infants, children, adolescents, and young adults.

Sandra Hassink, MD, FAAP, President

4419 American Osteopathic College of Dermatology

1501 E Illinois Street, PO Box 7525
Kirksville, MO 63501

660-665-2184
800-449-2623
Fax: 660-627-2623
e-mail: info@aocd.org
www.aocd.org

Strives to improve the standards of the practice of dermatology, to stimulate the study and extend knowledge in the field of dermatology, and to promote a more general understanding of the nature and scope of services rendered by osteopathic dermatologists to other divisions of practice, hospitals, clinics and the public.

David Grice, President
Suzanne Rozenberg, President-Elect
Rick Lin, First VP

4420 American Skin Association

6 East 43rd Street, 28th Floor
New York, NY 10017

212-889-4858, 800-499-7546
Fax: 212-889-4959
e-mail: info@americanskin.org; www.americanskin.org

The American Skin Association is the only volunteer led health organization dedicated through research, education and advocacy to saving lives and alleviating human suffering caused by the full spectrum of skin disorders.

Howard P. Milstein, Chairman
George W. Hambrick, President/Founder
Nora M. Jordan, Vice Chair

4421 Society for Pediatric Dermatology

8365 Keystone Crossing, Suite 107
Indianapolis, IN 46240

317-202-0224; Fax: 317-205-9841
e-mail: spd@hp-assoc.com
www.pedsderm.net

A national organization specifically dedicated to the field of pediatric dermatology, with the objective of promoting, developing, and advancing education, research and care of skin disease in all pediatric age groups. The organization holds meetings twice a year to educate physicians about advances in pediatric dermatology, help them support children with dermatological diseases and improve the care of these children.

Sheila Friedlander, President
Richard Antaya, President-Elect
Anthony Mancini, Secretary/Treasurer

Description

4422 KERNICTERUS

Synonym: Bilirubin encephalopathy

Involves the following Biologic System(s):

Neonatal and Infant Disorders

Kernicterus refers to a rare neurologic condition in which excessive amounts of bilirubin accumulate in the brain of affected newborns, resulting in damage to the central nervous system. Bilirubin, a reddish-yellow pigment present in bile, is derived from the breakdown of the protein in red blood cells that carries oxygen (hemoglobin). Premature infants and newborns with certain congenital disorders (e.g., erythroblastosis fetalis and Crigler-Najjar syndrome) are at risk for this life-threatening condition. In premature infants, the processes needed for bilirubin excretion may not be fully developed. Factors that put extra strain on this immature metabolic process may result in increased levels of bilirubin in the blood (hyperbilirubinemia). If these levels become excessive and are left untreated, bilirubin may be deposited in the brain. For example, in infants with erythroblastosis fetalis, antibodies from the mother's blood cross the placental barrier and destroy red blood cells of the fetus, resulting in release of excessive amounts of bilirubin. In some cases, bilirubin builds up faster than the liver is able to eliminate it, resulting in hyperbilirubinemia. Signs of this condition include a yellowing of the eyes, skin, and mucous membranes (jaundice).

Crigler-Najjar syndrome results from the deficiency of an enzyme that is required to convert bilirubin to a form that may be excreted from the body, thus causing hyperbilirubinemia. Other conditions or disorders that cause hyperbilirubinemia place the newborn, especially those who are born prematurely, at risk for kernicterus.

Symptoms of kernicterus usually become apparent within the first week of life. However, hyperbilirubinemia that occurs anytime within the first month of life may result in kernicterus. Symptoms and characteristic findings may include difficulty in feeding; vomiting; lethargy; and lack of a normal response to sudden, loud noises (Moro or startle reflex). Further signs of this condition may include breathing difficulties; severe muscle spasms resulting in a backward arching of the back and neck (opisthotonos); twitching of the arms, legs, and face; a high-pitched cry; and convulsions. In some affected infants, severe involvement of the central nervous system may cause life-threatening complications. In others, findings associated with permanent disability may be observed periodically until the third year of life when the complete neurologic picture emerges. Symptoms may include involuntary spasms of the muscles, hearing loss, eye movement irregularities, deficiencies in motor development, difficulties in speech, seizures, and mental retardation. Some infants who experience only slight kernicterus may experience mild irregularities in neuromuscular coordination, moderate deafness, and slight retardation.

Treatment of kernicterus is directed toward prevention involving the correction of hyperbilirubinemia and jaundice before kernicterus can develop. Treatment may include phototherapy in which, under careful monitoring, the infant's skin is exposed to high-intensity fluorescent light. Although phototherapy is often effective in reducing levels of bilirubin, the underlying cause of hyperbilirubinemia and jaundice must be identified and treated as well. Some infants, especially those at higher risk for kernicterus, may be effectively treated with exchange blood transfusions in which small amounts of the infant's circulating blood are repeatedly withdrawn and replaced with equal amounts of whole blood from a donor until about 80 percent of the newborn's blood has been replaced. Other treatment is symptomatic and supportive.

Government Agencies

4423 NIH/National Institute of Child Health and Human Development

31 Center Drive, Building 31, Room 2A32
Bethesda, MD 20892

301-496-1333
800-370-2943
Fax: 866-760-5947
TTY: 888-320-6942
e-mail: NICHDInformationResourceCenter@mail.nih.
www.nichd.nih.gov

Established in 1962 by congress, today the institute conducts and supports research on topics related to the health of children, adults, families and populations. Some of these topics include: developmental disabilities, growth and development, infant death, reproductive health and birth defects.

Jay H Hoofnagle, Director
Lisa Kaeser, Program & Public Liaison

National Associations & Support Groups

4424 American Academy of Pediatrics

141 Northwest Point Boulevard
Elk Grove Village, IL 60007

847-434-4000
800-433-9016
Fax: 847-434-8000
www.aap.org

The American Academy of Pediatrics and its member pediatricians are committed to the attainment of optimal physical, mental and social health and well-being for all infants, children, adolescents, and young adults.

Sandra Hassink, MD, FAAP, President

4425 American Liver Foundation

39 Broadway, Suite 2700
New York, NY 10006

212-668-1000
800-465-4837
Fax: 212-483-8179
e-mail: info@liverfoundation.org
www.liverfoundation.org

Nonprofit, national voluntary organization dedicated to the prevention, treatment, and cure of hepatitis and other liver diseases through research, education and advocacy on behalf of those affected by or at risk of liver disease.

Thomas F. Nealon, Chairman
Daniel E. Weil, Treasurer
Carlo Frappolli, Secretary

4426 Genetic Alliance

4301 Connecticut Avenue NW, Suite 404
Washington, DC 20008

202-966-7955
800-336-4363
Fax: 202-966-8553
e-mail: info@geneticalliance.org
www.geneticalliance.org

A coalition of voluntary genetic support groups, consumers and professionals addressing the needs of individuals and families affected by genetic disorders from a national perspective.

Joan Oppenheimer Weiss, Founder
Sharon Terry, MA, President/CEO
Kemp Battle, Treasurer

4427 March of Dimes Birth Defects Foundation
1275 Mamaroneck Avenue
White Plains, NY 10605   914-997-4488
                                          888-663-4637
                                          Fax: 914-997-4763
                          e-mail: answers@marchofdimes.com
                                     www.marchofdimes.com

Partnership of volunteers and professionals dedicates to improving the health of babies by preventing birth defects and infant mortality. Over 100 chapters are located across the country and can be located through the National Office.

Jennifer L Howse, President

4428 United Liver Foundation
5777 W Century Boulevard
Los Angeles, CA 90045   310-670-4624
                                          Fax: 310-670-4672
                              e-mail: pbrady@liver411.com
                                          www.liver411.com

A national organization that promotes research and cures for hepatitis and other liver diseases.

Pam Brady, Contact Person
Donna Gracon, Chapter Director

Libraries & Resource Centers

4429 National Digestive Diseases Information Clearinghouse
Bldg 31, Rm 9A06, 31 Center Drive
Bethesda, MD 20892   301-496-3583
                                          800-891-5389
                                          Fax: 301-907-8906
                          e-mail: nddic@info.niddk.nih.gov
                                        www2.niddk.nih.gov

The National Institute of Diabetes and Digestive and Kidney Diseases conducts and supports research on many of the most serious diseases affecting public health. The Institute supports much of the clinical research on the diseases of internal medicine and related subspecialty fields as well as many basic science disciplines.

Griffin P. Rodgers, M.D, Chairman, Executive Board
Brent B. Stanfield, EXECUTIVE SECRETARY
Camille M. Hoover, M.S.W, Executive Officer

Web Sites

4430 Online Mendelian Inheritance in Man
8600 Rockville Pike
Bethesda, MD 20894   301-594-5983
                                          888-346-3656
                                          Fax: 301-402-1384
                                          TDD: 800-735-2258
                             e-mail: custserv@nlm.nih.gov
                                     www.ncbi.nlm.nih.gov

This database is a catalog of human genes and genetic disorders.

Christine E Seidman M.D, Chairman
David J Lipman M.D, Executive Secretary
Scott Edwards, Member

4431 Parents of Infants and Children with Kernicterus
www.pickonline.org

Provides information and support to families of children with kernicterus.

4432 Rare Genetic Diseases in Children (NYU)
550 First Avenue
New York, NY 10016   212-263-7300
                                          www.med.nyu.edu

We target issues arising from rare genetic diseases affecting children. Also, to assist in the endeavor to bring knowledge and hope to those for whom there is, at present, so little.

Robert I. Grossman, MD, Dean & CEO
Steven B Abramson, Senior Vice President
Andrew W Brotman, SVP & Chief Clinical Officer

4433 Save Babies Through Screening Foundation
P. O. Box 42197
Cincinnati, OH 45242   888-454-3383
                                 e-mail: email@savebabies.org
                                          www.savebabies.org

Is a national nonprofit public charity run by volunteers. Its mission is to improve the lives of babies by working to prevent disabilities and early death resulting from disorders detectable through newborn screening.

Jill Levy-Fisch, President
Micki Gartzke, Vice President
Laura Larks, Secretary

Description

4434 KLINEFELTER SYNDROME

Synonyms: Chromosome XXY, XXY syndrome

Covers these related disorders: 45, X/46, XY/47, XXY mosaicism, 46, XY/47, XXY mosaicism, 46, XY/48, XXYY mosaicism, 46, XX/47, XXY mosaicism, 48, XXXY, 49, XXXYY

Involves the following Biologic System(s):

Genetic/Chromosomal/Syndrome/Metabolic Disorders

Klinefelter syndrome is a chromosomal disorder that appears to affect approximately one in 1,000 males. Males usually have one X and one Y chromosome; however, those with Klinefelter syndrome have an extra X chromosome in cells of the body. In some patients, only a certain percentage of cells contain the XXY chromosomal abnormality. This finding is known as chromosomal mosaicism. Other cells may have the normal XY chromosomal pair or other sex chromosome abnormalities (e.g., XX, XXYY, etc.). Some males may have Klinefelter variants in which some or all cells contain more than two X chromosomes.

Because only a few or subtle symptoms may be associated with Klinefelter syndrome, the disorder is rarely diagnosed before puberty. Males with the disorder may have extremely variable I.Q.s (intelligence quotients), ranging from well above to far below average; however, most affected males have an I.Q. within average limits (mean of 85 to 90). Some children with Klinefelter syndrome may have learning problems, such as difficulties with verbal expression, reading, and spelling, potentially requiring special assistance or full-time special education classes. Children with the disorder also tend to have behavioral problems, such as immaturity, excessive shyness, anxiety, poor judgment, aggressive activity, and poor social skills. Such behavioral difficulties tend to begin when affected children begin school.

Many children with Klinefelter syndrome have slim, tall stature; long legs; and small testes and a relatively small penis (hypogenitalism). As affected males enter puberty, they may experience partial, inadequate development of secondary sexual characteristics (impaired virilization). For example, facial hair tends to be unusually sparse, the testes remain unusually small, and, in many cases, there is abnormal enlargement of the breasts (gynecomastia). In addition, many affected males experience inadequate production of the male hormone testosterone and deficient production of male reproductive cells (azoospermia), resulting in infertility. In males with deficient testosterone production, treatment may include testosterone replacement therapy beginning at approximately 11 to 12 years of age. In most cases, Klinefelter syndrome results from errors during the division of a parent's reproductive cells (meiosis). In rare cases, the disorder may result from errors during cellular division after fertilization (mitosis).

In males with XY/XXY mosaicism (i.e., a percentage of cells containing the normal XY chromosomal pair), the range and severity of associated symptoms and findings may be less severe, and there may be an increased likelihood of fertility and improved psychosocial adjustment. Affected males with Klinefelter variants (i.e., in which cells contain more than two X chromosomes) may have more severe symptoms and findings, such as a greater risk of mental retardation and impaired virilization and fertility as well as additional physical abnormalities, including malformations of the head and facial (craniofacial) areas and other skeletal abnormalities.

Government Agencies

4435 NIH/National Institute of Child Health and Human Development
31 Center Drive, Building 31, Room 2A32
Bethesda, MD 20892 301-496-1333
800-370-2943
Fax: 866-760-5947
TTY: 888-320-6942
e-mail: NICHDInformationResourceCenter@mail.nih.
www.nichd.nih.gov

Established in 1962 by congress, today the institute conducts and supports research on topics related to the health of children, adults, families and populations. Some of these topics include: developmental disabilities, growth and development, infant death, reproductive health and birth defects.

Jay H Hoofnagle, Director
Lisa Kaeser, Program & Public Liaison

National Associations & Support Groups

4436 49 XXY Syndrome Association
10001 NE 74th Street
Vancouver, WA 98662 360-892-7547
e-mail: kimbj@juno.com

4437 A&K Associates
7 Independence Avenue
Derry, NH 03038 603-432-5755
888-999-9428
e-mail: info@akassociates911.com
www.akassociates911.com

Nonprofit organization that provides information about Klinefelter syndrome, common characteristics, and treatment. Information on current research projects and other resources.

Melissa Aylstock, Executive Director

4438 American Academy of Pediatrics
141 Northwest Point Boulevard
Elk Grove Village, IL 60007 847-434-4000
800-433-9016
Fax: 847-434-8000
www.aap.org

The American Academy of Pediatrics and its member pediatricians are committed to the attainment of optimal physical, mental and social health and well-being for all infants, children, adolescents, and young adults.

Sandra Hassink, MD, FAAP, President

4439 Genetic Alliance
4301 Connecticut Avenue NW
Washington, DC 20008 202-966-7955
800-336-4363
Fax: 202-966-8553
e-mail: info@geneticalliance.org
www.geneticalliance.org

A coalition of voluntary genetic support groups, consumers and professionals addressing the needs of individuals and families affected by genetic disorders from a national perspective.

Joan Oppenheimer Weiss, Founder
Sharon Terry, President

4440 Klinefelter Syndrome and Associates
PO Box 872
Pine, CO 80470 916-773-2999
888-999-9428
Fax: 303-838-0753
e-mail: info@genetic.org
genetic.org

Nonprofit organization.

Myra Byrd, Chair
Gary Glissman, Vive Chair
Sheila Clark, Secretary/Treasurer

4441 Klinefelter's Syndrome Association
N5879 30th Street
Pine River, WI 54965   920-987-5782

4442 Support and Educational Exchange for Klinefelter Syndrome
1417 25th Avenue, Drive W
Bradenton, FL 34205   813-750-8044

Web Sites

4443 Klinefelter Syndrome Support Group
www.klinefeltersyndrome.org/

An online support group which offers information about the group, organizations, online pharmacies, other web sites, and current research studies.

4444 NIH/National Institute of Mental Health
6001 Executive Boulevard, Room 6200
Bethesda, MD 20892   301-443-8431
                            866-615-6464
                            TTY: 866-415-8051
                            e-mail: nimhinfo@nih.gov
                            www.nimh.nih.gov

The mission is to reduce the burden of mental illness and behavioral disorders through research on mind, brain, and behavior. This public health mandate demands that we harness powerful scientific tools to achieve better understanding, treatment, and eventually prevention of these disabling conditions that affect millions of Americans.

Thomas Insel, Director
Philip Sung Wang, Deputy Director
Tracy Holt, Program Analyst

Newsletters

4445 Even Exchange Newsletter
KS&A
P.O. Box 872
Pine, CO 80470   303-400-9040
                        888-999-9428
                        Fax: 303-838-0753
                        e-mail: info@genetic.org
                        www.genetic.org

Information on support groups, meetings, research being conducted, book and product reviews, and ask the doctor column.

3 times a year

Myra Byrd, Chair
Gary Glissman, Vice Chair
Shiela Clark, Secretary/ Treasurer

4446 Klinefelter Syndrome Newsletter
P.O. Box 872
Pine, CO 80470   303-400-9040
                        888-999-9428
                        Fax: 303-838-0753
                        e-mail: jmoore@erols.com
                        www.genetic.org

News on Klinefelter syndrome, education and support. You'll find a wealth of information on this very common, but underdiagnosed condition.

Myra Byrd, Chair
Gary Glissman, Vice Chair
Shiela Clark, Secretary

Description

4447 KLIPPEL-FEIL SYNDROME

Synonym: KFS

Covers these related disorders: Klippel-Feil syndrome Type I, Klippel-Feil syndrome Type II, Klippel-Feil syndrome Type III

Involves the following Biologic System(s):

Genetic/Chromosomal/Syndrome/Metabolic Disorders

Klippel-Feil syndrome (KFS) is a congenital malformation characterized by the fusion of two or more vertebrae, especially in the neck or cervical region (congenital synostosis) or by the absence of one or more cervical vertebrae. Klippel-Feil syndrome Type I involves extensive fusion of several cervical vertebrae and thoracic vertebrae located in the upper back. Type II involves fusion of a limited number of incompletely developed vertebrae (hemivertebrae) and vertebrae, fusion of the uppermost cervical vertebra with the bone at the back of the skull (occipital bone), and other irregularities. Klippel-Feil syndrome Type III is characterized by fusion of the cervical, lower thoracic, or lumbar vertebrae. Physical findings associated with Klippel-Feil syndrome may include a short neck with limited range of motion, a low hairline, and irregularities of the urinary tract and reproductive, cardiovascular, pulmonary, and nervous systems. Additional abnormalities may include curvatures of the spine (scoliosis or kyphosis), an inclination of the neck to one side (torticollis), webbing of the neck (pterygium colli) and fingers (syndactyly), and other irregularities of the bones and muscles.

Treatment of Klippel-Feil syndrome may be directed toward the particular physical findings and symptoms associated with this disorder. Such treatment may include measures to correct or halt the progression of various spinal irregularities and to correct other abnormalities as warranted. Other treatment is supportive.

In some children, Klippel-Feil syndrome is transmitted as an autosomal dominant trait, while transmission by autosomal recessive inheritance is possible in others. In addition, some affected children have no recognizable pattern of genetic transmission.

Government Agencies

4448 NIH/National Institute of Arthritis & Musculoskeletal & Skin Diseases

National Institutes of Health
1AMS Circle, PO Box 3675
Bethesda, MD 20892

301-495-4484
877-226-4267
Fax: 301-718-6366
TTY: 301-565-2966
TDD: 301-565-2966
e-mail: niamsinfo@mail.nih.gov
www.niams.nih.gov

The mission of the NIAMS, a part of the NIH, is to support research into the causes, treatment, and prevention of arthritis and musculoskeletal and skin diseases, the training of basic and clinical scientists to carry out this research, and the dissemination of information on research progress in these diseases.

Stephen I Katz MD PhD, Director
Robert H Carter MD, Deputy Director

4449 NIH/National Institute of Child Health and Human Development

31 Center Drive, Building 31, Room 2A32
Bethesda, MD 20892

301-496-1333
800-370-2943
Fax: 866-760-5947
TTY: 888-320-6942
e-mail: NICHDInformationResourceCenter@mail.nih.
www.nichd.nih.gov

Established in 1962. The institute conducts and supports research on topics related to the health of children.

Jay H Hoofnagle, Director
Lisa Kaeser, Program & Public Liaison

4450 NIH/Osteoporosis and Related Bone Diseases National Resource Center

2 AMS Circle, PO Box 3676
Bethesda, MD 20892

202-223-0344
800-624-2663
Fax: 202-293-2356
TTY: 202-466-4315
e-mail: NIHBoneInfo@mail.nih.gov
www.bones.nih.gov

The National Resource Center is an information service that provides general information on metabolic bone conditions.

Stephen I Katz MD, PhD, Director

National Associations & Support Groups

4451 American Academy of Pediatrics

141 Northwest Point Boulevard
Elk Grove Village, IL 60007

847-434-4000
800-433-9016
Fax: 847-434-8000
www.aap.org

The American Academy of Pediatrics and its member pediatricians are committed to the attainment of optimal physical, mental and social health and well-being for all infants, children, adolescents, and young adults.

Sandra Hassink, MD, FAAP, President

4452 Klippel-Feil Syndrome Support Group

311 Bracken Avenue
Pittsburgh, PA 15227

412-884-2969

Describes congenital fusion of at least two of the seven vertebrae in the cervical-spine. In addition there may be fusion or anomalies of vertebrae in the thoracic or lumbar-spine.

4453 March of Dimes Birth Defects Foundation

1275 Mamaroneck Avenue
White Plains, NY 10605

914-997-4488
888-663-4637
Fax: 914-997-4763
e-mail: answers@marchofdimes.com
www.marchofdimes.com

Partnership of volunteers and professionals dedicates to improving the health of babies by preventing birth defects and infant mortality. Over 100 chapters are located across the country and can be located through the National Office.

Jennifer L Howse, President

Web Sites

4454 Online Mendelian Inheritance in Man

8600 Rockville Pike
Bethesda, MD 20894

301-594-5983
888-346-3656
Fax: 301-402-1384
TDD: 800-735-2258
e-mail: custserv@nlm.nih.gov
www.ncbi.nlm.nih.gov

This database is a catalog of human genes and genetic disorders.

Christine E Seidman M.D, Chairman
David J Lipman M.D, Executive Secretary
Scott Edwards, Member

4455 Rare Genetic Diseases in Children (NYU)
550 First Avenue
New York, NY 10016

212-263-7300
www.med.nyu.edu

We target issues arising from rare genetic diseases affecting children. Also, to assist in the endeavor to bring knowledge and hope to those for whom there is, at present, so little.

Robert I. Grossman, MD, Dean & CEO
Steven B Abramson, Senior Vice President
Andrew W Brotman, SVP & Chief Clinical Officer

4456 Wheeless' Textbook of Orthopaedics
www.wheelessonline.com

410-494-4994
www.wheelessonline.com

Derives from a variety of sources, including journals, articles, national meetings lectures and other textbooks.

Clifford R. Wheeless, Editor in chief
James A Nunley, Managing Editor
James R. Urbaniak, Managing Editor

Description

4457 LAZY EYE

Synonym: Amblyopia

Covers these related disorders: Anisometropic Amblyopia

Involves the following Biologic System(s):

Ophthalmologic Disorders

Lazy eye, also known as amblyopia, is a condition in which the vision in one eye is impaired because the images of objects seen by the affected eye are not clearly transmitted to the brain. This visual impairment results from interference with the vision in the affected eye, such as from a cataract, or from an eye-muscle weakness. This impairment prevents the affected eye from turning normally and focusing clearly on objects.

Typically, lazy eye affects only one eye, and develops in 1 to 5% of children, usually before the age of 6 years. Its existence is not always apparent, but its symptoms may include favoring the use of one eye over another, or a tendency to miss objects in the periphery of vision, causing patients to bump into objects on the side of the affected eye. However, symptoms of this condition are not always obvious either to the patient or to others, since it neither reduces the amount of light entering the affected eye nor interferes with the vision in the unaffected eye. Thus, any adjustments made by patients seem normal to them. In many cases, persons with lazy eye discover it only through an eye examination.

If not corrected early in life, lazy eye may prevent the affected eye from ever developing clear and effective vision. Because of this, it is recommended that infants have an eye examination at the age of 6 months, and that examinations are repeated regularly and at frequent intervals, up until 6 years of age. (R)(R)Treatment of lazy eye may in volve forcing the use of the amblyopic eye by applying a patch over its neighboring (good) eye, for periods ranging from weeks to months. This has been shown to strengthen the vision in the weakened eye. Eyeglasses may be prescribed to improve the visual acuity in the affected eye. In some cases surgery can repair muscles of the affected eye, thus improving its coordination with the non-affected eye in looking at and focusing on objects. Eye exercises, to strengthen the affected eye, are often used by themselves or in conjunction with surgery.

Government Agencies

4458 National Eye Institute
31 Center Drive MSC 2510, PO Box 2510
Bethesda, MD 20892
301-496-5248
e-mail: 2020@nei.nih.gov
www.nei.nih.gov

As part of the federal government's National Institutes of Health (NIH), the institute conducts and supports training, research, and disseminates information regarding blinding eye diseases, visual disorders, preservation of sight and mechanisms of visual function.

Paul A. Seiving MD, PhD, Director

National Associations & Support Groups

4459 American Academy of Pediatrics
141 Northwest Point Boulevard
Elk Grove Village, IL 60007
847-434-4000
800-433-9016
Fax: 847-434-8000
www.aap.org

The American Academy of Pediatrics and its member pediatricians are committed to the attainment of optimal physical, mental and social health and well-being for all infants, children, adolescents, and young adults.

Sandra Hassink, MD, FAAP, President

4460 American Foundation for the Blind
2 Penn Plaza, Suite 1102
New York, NY 10121
212-502-7600
800-232-5463
Fax: 888-545-8331
e-mail: afbinfo@afb.net
www.afb.org

The foundation is a national nonprofit that has been eliminating barriers that prevent people with vision loss from reaching their potential. Their priorities include broadening access to technology; elevating the quality of information and tools for professionals; and promoting healthy independent living for those with vision loss.

Carl Augusto, President/CEO

4461 Autism, Strabismus & Amblyopia (Lazy Eye)
www.mdjunction.com
800-273-8255
www.mdjunction.com

Online support group and forum.

4462 Eye Patch Club
Prevent Blindness America
211 West Wacker Drive, Suite 1700
Chicago, IL 60606
800-331-2020
www.preventblindness.org/children/EyePatchClub.html

A supportive and fun program for families going through their children's Amblyopia patching treatment. The club kit contains a newsletter, calendar and stickers for each day of wearing the patch, member-only online content, and a pen pal form.

James E. Anderson, Chair
Marge Axelrad, Sr. VP/Editorial Director
Gary Davis, Commercial VP

4463 EyeCare America
Foundation of American Academy of Ophthalmology
PO Box 429098
San Francisco, CA 94142
877-887-6327
Fax: 415-561-8567
e-mail: comm@aao.org
www.eyecareamerica.org/eyecare/conditions/amblyopia/

EyeCare America is a public service foundation of the American Academy of Ophthalmology. It is a partner in the EyeSmart campaign, offering multiple programs to help with free or reduced cost eye examinations. In addition, online educational materials are available.

Betty Lucas, Director
Gail Nyman-York, Program Manager
Allison Neves, Director, Communications

4464 Lighthouse International
Goldman Bldg, 111 E 59th Street, PO Box 1202
New York, NY 10022
212-821-9200
800-829-0500
Fax: 212-821-9707
TTY: 212-821-9713
e-mail: info@lighthouse.org
www.lighthouse.org

Provides services, information, resource contacts, education and research related to the needs of children who are visually impaired and their families. Resources include an Early Intervention Program and the Child Development Center.

Joseph A. Ripp, Chairman
Sarah E. Smith, Vice Chair/Treasurer
Jonathan M. Wainwright, Vice Chair/Secretary

4465 Lions Club International
300 W 22nd Street, PO Box 8842
Oak Brook, IL 60523   630-571-5466
                                           800-747-4448
               www.lionsclubs.org/EN/our-work/sight-programs/

Provides support for sight programs and services, including vision screenings, eye banks and eyeglass recycling. Also provides financial assistancefor eye care to individuals through local clubs.

4466 National Association for Parents of Children with Visual Impairments
Jewish Guild Healthcare, 1 North Lexington Avenue,
White Plains, NY 10601   617-972-7441
                                           800-562-6265
                                      Fax: 617-972-7444
                           e-mail: napvi@guildhealth.org
                                   www.spedex.com/napvi/

Enables parents to find resources and information for their children who are visually impaired, blind or have additional disabilities. NAPVI provides support, leadership, and training.

Julie Urban, President
Venetia Hayden, VP
Randi Sher, Secretary

4467 Sight for Students - Vision Service Plan
www.vspglobal.com/cms

                                           888-867-8867
                                      Fax: 916-858-5388
                          e-mail: vspglobal@vspglobal.com
                                   www.vspglobal.com/cms

Provides free vision exams and glasses to low-income uninsured children. It operates on a national level through a network of community partners who identify children in need and VSP (Vision Service Plan) network doctors who provide the eyecare services.

Rob Lynch, President/CEO

4468 Vision USA-American Optometric Association
243 North Lindbergh Blvd. Floor 1
St Louis, MO 63141   314-983-4200
                                           800-365-2219
                                      Fax: 314-991-4101
                            e-mail: foundation@aoa.org
                                 www.aoa.org/visionusa.xml

The Vision USA program offers free eye exams to low income working families and their children. It was established by AOA (American Optometric Association) doctors of optometry who donate their services.

Dennis Holter, Chief Advancement Officer
Rebecca Hildebrand, Development Officer
Emily Stenberg, Heritage Services Specialist

Libraries & Resource Centers

4469 Talking Books - National Library Service
NLS for the Blind & Physically Handicapped
Library of Congress
Washington, DC 20542   202-707-5100
                                           888-657-7323
                                      Fax: 202-707-0712
                                      TDD: 202-707-0744
                                 e-mail: nls@loc.gov
                                        www.loc.gov/nls

Administers a free library program of audio materials through a network of cooperating libraries to eligible borrowers in the U.S.

Karen Keninger, Director
Jane Caulton, Head, Publications & Media
Marsha Jackson, Head, Administrative Section

Research Centers

4470 Visual Systems Research Group
Cincinnati Children's Research Foundation
3333 Burnet Avenue, PO Box 3026
Cincinnati, OH 45229   513-636-4200
                                           800-344-2462
                                      Fax: 513-636-4317
                                      TTY: 513-636-4900
                          e-mail: richard.lang@chmcc.org
                www.cincinnatichildrens.org/research/project/vsg/

A collaboration between the Developmental Biology and Pediatric Ophthalmology divisions, the program is designed to bring basic research to Ophthalmology and to foster research efforts of the clinical faculty.

Richard Lang, PhD, Principal Investigator

Web Sites

4471 3D Vision
www.vision3d.org

Learn about binocular or stereoscopic vision in a fun way.

4472 All About Amblyopia (Lazy Eye)
58 Mohonk Road
High Falls, NY 12440   www.lazyeye.org

Research and information from the National Eye Institute (part of the National Institutes of Health, NIH).

4473 All About Vision
1010 Turquoise Street, Suite 275
San Diego, CA 92109   858-454-2145
                                      www.allaboutvision.org

Lists humanitarian eye care organizations that serve the needs of those with vision challenges.

Joseph T. Barr, Advisory Board
Brian S. Boxer Wachler, Advisory Board
Michael DePaolis, Advisory Board

4474 All About Vision.Com
1010 Turquoise Street, Suite 275
San Diego, CA 92109   858-454-2145
                                      www.allaboutvision.com

Provides consumers with information resources on eye health and vision correction options.

Joseph T. Barr, Advisory Board
Brian S. Boxer Wachler, Advisory Board
Michael DePaolis, Advisory Board

4475 Attention Disorders and Eyesight
58 Mohonk Road
High Falls, NY 12440   212-923-0496
                                      www.optometrists.org

Provides information on the link between vision problems and ADD/ADHD. Articles by third-party professionals are added/updated each year.

4476 Children Special Needs-Pediatric Eye Care
58 Mohonk Road
High Falls, NY 12440   212-923-0496
                                      www.optometrists.org

Provides information on visual health including: pediatric eye doctor search; tools for parents (glossary, checklists, book list); and descriptions of vision impairments.

4477 Convergence Insufficiency
58 Mohonk Road
High Falls, NY 12440   212-923-0496
                                      www.optometrists.org

Contains an in-depth review of Convergence Insufficiency (CI) including what it is; the symptoms; how common it is; detection and diagnosis; and treatment.

4478 FamilyConnect
www.familyconnect.org

e-mail: familyconnect@afb.net
www.familyconnect.org

An online, multimedia community resource for parents and guardians of children with visual impairments. 24-hour support and access to message boards, real life videos, parent blogs, and parenting articles.

4479 Lazy Eye Discussion Group
health.groups.yahoo.com/group/LazyEye/

An email list (955 members) for parents of children with amblyopia, strabismus or other conditions associated with the disorder.

4480 Optometrists Network
58 Mohonk Road
High Falls, NY 12440   212-923-0496
www.optometrists.org

Twelve education websites for patients that are free of advertisements and require no registraion. There is also a free eye doctor referral directory.

4481 Prevent Blindness America Affiliates & Divisions
211 West Wacker Drive, Suite 1700
Chicago, IL 60606   800-331-2020
www.preventblindness.org

Users will be able to find Prevent Blindness programs, services, chapters and branches by state.

Paul G. Howes, Chairman
Andy Alcorn, President
Kevin Bakewell, Senior Vice President

4482 Strabismus
58 Mohonk Road
High Falls, NY 12440   212-923-0496
www.strabismus.org

All about strabismus: what is it? who does it affect? what types exist? and how can it be treated?

4483 Vision Therapy
58 Mohonk Road
High Falls, NY 12440   212-923-0496
www.visiontherapy.org

The site provides an interview of frequently asked questions with an eye doctor who is an expert in the field of vision therapy. The effectiveness of therapy and what it involves is addressed.

4484 Vision Therapy Success Stories
58 Mohonk Road
High Falls, NY 12440   212-923-0496
www.visiontherapystories.org

Children and adult vision therapy patients express their own success stories. There are over 525 stories covering many topics.

Book Publishers

4485 All Children Have Different Eyes
Edie Glaser / Dr. Maria Burgio, author

Vidi Press
11721 Whittier Blvd, #203
Whittier, CA 90601   800-409-7170
e-mail: service@vidipress.com
www.lowvisionkids.com

An illustrated book for children that models for children with visual impairment how to play and make friends competently and with confidence.

48 pages

4486 Blueberry Eyes
Monica Driscoll Beatty, author

Health Press
2920 Carlisle Blvd, NE
Albuquerque, NM 87110   505-888-1394
877-411-0707
www.healthpress.com

Children's book that addresses the different aspects of eye treatment including eye patches, eye muscle surgery, and wearing glasses. Reading level: ages 4 thru 8.
32 pages
ISBN: 0-929173-24-4

4487 My Travelin' Eye
Jenny Sue Kostecki-Shaw, author

Henry Holt & Company, Inc.
175 Fifth Avenue
New York, NY 10010   646-307-5151
Fax: 212-633-0748
e-mail: customerservice@mpsvirginia.com
us.macmillan.com

Audience: pre-school- grade 3. Jenny has an eye that wanders sometimes. Although this makes her different, she is also able to see the world in a special way.
40 pages Hardcover
ISBN: 0-805081-69-0

Stefan von Holtzbrinck, Chairman, Executive Board
Klaus-Dieter Lehmann, Chairman, Supervisory Board
Sandra Dittert, Senior Vice President

4488 The Patch
Justina Chen Headley, author

Charlesbridge Publishing
85 Main Street
Watertown, MA 02472   617-926-0329
800-225-3214
Fax: 800-926-5775
e-mail: books@charlesbridge.com
www.charlesbridge.com

Becca wears glasses and an eye patch. She leads the kids in her class on an imaginative adventure to explain her new fashion accessories.
32 pages
ISBN: 1-580890-49-0

Brian Walker, VP Production
Mary Ann Sabia, VP Marketing and Sales and Associat
Bob Sammartino, Sammartino

Magazines

4489 Eye on NEI
31 Center Dr, MSC 2510
Bethesda, MD 20892   301-496-5248
e-mail: 2020@nei.nih.gov
www.nei.nih.gov

The National Eye Institute's online news magazine is published two times a month. It features articles on vision research projects, answers to eye questions, interviews with scientists, and provides a general look into the vision research process.

Dr. Paul A. Sieving, Director
Dr. Belinda Seto, Deputy Director
Allyson T. Collins, Editor

4490 EyeWorld
American Society Cataract/Refractive Surgery-ASCRS
4000 Legato Road, Suite 700
Fairfax, VA 22033   703-591-2220
Fax: 703-591-0614
e-mail: dlong@eyeworld.org
www.eyeworld.org

The monthly news magazine for the American Society of Cataract & Refractive Surgery (ASCRS).

David F. Chang, Chief Medical Editor
John A. Vukich, International Editor
Bonnie An Henderson, Cataract Editor

Journals

4491 Journal of Pediatric Health Care
Natl Assoc. of Ped. Nurse Practitioners (NAPNAP)
5 Hanover Square, Suite 1401
New York, NY 10004

917-746-8300
877-662-7627
Fax: 212-785-1713
e-mail: info@napnap.org
www.napnap.org

Bi-monthly pediatric journal that contains articles about research and current developments in pediatric care.

5 pages Pub # EY-145

Felicia Taylor, MBA, BA, Director, Communications

Newsletters

4492 Awareness
NAPVI
PO Box 317
Watertown, MA 2471

800-562-6265
e-mail: jobs@spedex.com
www.spedex.com

Quarterly newsletter of the National Association for Parents of Children with Visual Impairments. It contains regional news and announcements, notices of events and conferences, legislative updates and articles.

32 pages

Pamphlets

4493 Amblyopia
National Eye Institute (NIH)
Information Office, 31 Center Dr, MSC 2510
Bethesda, MD 20892

301-496-5248
catalog.nei.nih.gov/productcart/pc/

Provides a description of the causes, symptoms, diagnosis and treatment for the disorder. The information is also available in Spanish.

5 pages Pub # EY-145

Description

4494 LEAD POISONING

Involves the following Biologic System(s):

Developmental/Behavioral/Psychiatric Disorders, Neurologic Disorders

Children and adults exposed to lead chronically over time can develop toxic levels in their blood. Traditionally, the lead level that raises concern is 10mcg/dl or above. Lead is much more harmful to children than adults because it can affect children's developing nerves and brains. The younger the child, the more harmful lead can be. Unborn children are the most vulnerable. However, many children with these levels may be asymptomatic. There are a number of sources for lead exposure. Although paint is a common source of lead, other products that may contain lead include ceramics, crystal, gasoline, batteries, and cosmetics. In the United States, the primary sources for lead exposure include household plumbing, paint made prior to 1977, and gasoline with tetraethyl lead as an additive. Although there has been a growing movement in the US to restrict the use of lead in these products, its prior use in many products continues to pose a hazard to the general population, especially young children. Lead may be inadvertently ingested, inhaled, or absorbed through the skin. One of the most common ways small children become exposed to lead is through the ingestion of fine dust from lead based paints, by licking their hands that are coated with lead dust, or by inhaling lead dust that is then swallowed. Lead makes things taste sweet, so children are attracted to the taste of lead paint chips and especially to lead dust. Lead that enters the body gets absorbed into the blood stream. It is then deposited in soft tissue and organs, or excreted through the kidney. Most of the lead that remains in the body, though, is deposited in bones. Lead toxicity primarily involves the central nervous system and the gastrointestinal system. Although many children with lead ingestion will have asymptomatic disease, they may show increased behavioral problems, poor school performance, decreased height, and decreased cognitive function. Children with more severe lead exposure may complain of anorexia, nausea, vomiting, abdominal pain and constipation. These symptons have been reported at lead levels as low as 20 mcg/dl but more commonly seen at lead levels greater than 50 mcg/dl. Neurological symptoms may include ataxia (staggering gait), seizures, coma, and encephalopathy. Screening for lead exposure should be performed in all children under 5. A thorough history should be taken, focusing on age of the patient's home, behavioral changes, exposure to battery factories or ceramics, recent home renovations (in homes pre-1978), and history of lead poisoning in a sibling. The frequency of the blood test screening will increase based on the patient's environmental exposure. A lead level of 10 mcg/dl or greater is considered a significant exposure and warrants further evaluation. An assessment of the home should be undertaken and the patient should have repeat blood lead levels tested no later than 3 months of age. The American Academy of Pediatrics recommends repeating a lead level by 3 months. Lead exposure may in some cases also be confirmed by x-ray, studies in the abdomen and in bones (lead lines). Therapy for lead exposure/toxicity generally focuses on removing the lead from the patient's environment, diminishing hand to mouth behaviors, improving nutrition in exposed patients and removing the lead from the patient's body. Homes may be cleaned properly by professionals and old paint must be removed from environment or sealed in a fashion that will eliminate the family's exposure to paint dust and chips. Some children will need to be moved to a lead-free safehouse while this is occurring. Frequent washing of hands and toys will cut down on exposure from hand to mouth behavior exhibited by young children. Lead levels greater than 44mcg/dl are considered significant enough to warrant chelation therapy and levels greater than 70 mcg/dl should prompt referral for chelation and hospitalization. Chelation therapy involves giving patients chelating, or binding, agents which bind to the lead and make it easier to excrete from the body. This type of therapy should begin only after the source of lead in the environment has been eliminated.

National Associations & Support Groups

4495 American Academy of Pediatrics
141 Northwest Point Boulevard
Elk Grove Village, IL 60007

847-434-4000
800-433-9016
Fax: 847-434-8000
www.aap.org

The American Academy of Pediatrics and its member pediatricians are committed to the attainment of optimal physical, mental and social health and well-being for all infants, children, adolescents, and young adults.

Sandra Hassink, MD, FAAP, President

4496 National Lead Information Center
8601 Georgia Avenue Suite 503
Silver Spring, MD 20910

800-424-5323
Fax: 301-585-7976
e-mail: hotline.lead@epa.gov

Offers support and referrals for patients and their families. Provides testing kits, evaluation techniques, and resource materials, including publications and tapes.

State Agencies & Support Groups

4497 Connecticut Lead Poisoning Prevention Program
410 Capitol Avenue, Ms#51LED P.O. Box 340308
Hartford, CT 06134

860-509-7299
Fax: 860-509-7295

Workshops and literature on how to diagnose and prevent lead poisoning.

Web Sites

4498 Consumer Product Safety Commission Hotline
4330 East West Highway
Bethesda, MD 20814

301-504-7923
Fax: 301-504-0124
www.cpsc.gov

CPSC is an Independent Federal Regulatory Agency that works to save lives and keep families safe by reducing the risk of injuries and deaths associated with consumer products.

Elliot F. Kaye, Chairman

4499 National Conference of State Legislatures
444 North Capitol Street, N.W., Suite 515
Washington, D. 20001

202-624-5400
Fax: 202-737-1069
e-mail: ncslnet-admin@ncsl.org.
www.ncsl.org

The National Conference of State Legislatures is a bipartisan organization that serves the legislators and staffs of the nation's 50 states, its commonwealths and territories. NCSL provides research, technical assistance and opportunities for policymakers to exchange ideas on the most pressing state issues. NCSL is an effective and respected advocate for the interests of state governments before Congress and federal agencies.

Senator Pamela, President
Jean Cantrel, Vice President
Tom Wright, Secretary/Treasurer

4500 Safe Drinking Water Hotline
www.epa.org/safewater/

Together with the states, tribes, and its many partners, protects public health by ensuring safe drinking water and protecting ground water. Along with EPS's ten regional drinking water programs, oversees implementation of the SAFE DRINKING WATER ACT, which is the national law safeguarding tap water in America.

Description

4501 LEARNING DISABILITY/READING DYSLEXIA

Synonyms: Learning Disorders, LDD

Covers these related disorders: Dyscalculia, Dyslexia, Dysgraphia

Involves the following Biologic System(s):
Developmental/Behavioral/Psychiatric Disorders

Learning Disability (LD) is a general term that refers to a group of disorders characterized by problems with learning, processing, or expressing information. When LD involves speech and language, it can affect how a person hears words (receptive language disorder), how they put thoughts into words (expressive language disorder), or how words are put together when spoken (articulation disorder).

LD can also affect academic skills. Dyscalculia is a learning disability characterized by difficulty in using mathematical symbols and understanding mathematical concepts. Dysgraphia is the difficulty in the physical process of writing letters and words. A person with dyspraxia can understand sentences in a normal way, but has difficulty putting words together into a coherent sentence. Dyslexia is characterized by the impairment in the ability to process written symbols.

Young children with dyslexia may have difficulty remembering the correct names of letters and numbers. Some school aged children may reverse letters and words when writing. For example, affected children may substitute the letter P for Q, reverse the word WAS to become SAW, or transpose letters so that BETS becomes BEST. Children with dyslexia may also have difficulty reading due to an impaired ability to determine the sequence of letters within words and to distinguish right from left. The hallmark of this learning disability is the fact that despite their difficulties, affected children are of average or above average intelligence by IQ testing and scholastic achievement.

Although learning disabilities occur in very young children, the disorders are usually not recognized until the child reaches school age. Early diagnosis of LD is an important factor in treatment. Children nearing the end of first grade who exhibit difficulties with word skills, or any children whose reading, writing, or mathematical skills are not commensurate with that of their other scholastic abilities should be tested for LD. Although LD is not related to eye defects, an ophthalmologic evaluation is beneficial in eliminating vision problems as a cause for symptoms. Treatment for LD is geared towards remedial teaching techniques specific to the disability.

LD is thought to be a familial disorder and may be inherited in an autosomal dominant fashion.

National Associations & Support Groups

4502 AVKO Dyslexia Research Foundation
3084 W Willard Road Suite W. PO Box 9404
Birch Run, MI 48415

810-686-9283
866-285-6612
Fax: 810-686-1101
e-mail: webmaster@avko.org
www.avko.org

Nonprofit organization founded to help determine what dyslexia is, why traditional methods of teaching and writing fail and help most dyslexics learn to read and write.
1974

Barry Chute, President
Julie Guyette, VP
Clifford Schroeder, Treasurer

4503 American Academy of Pediatrics
141 Northwest Point Boulevard
Elk Grove Village, IL 60007

847-434-4000
800-433-9016
Fax: 847-434-8000
www.aap.org

The American Academy of Pediatrics and its member pediatricians are committed to the attainment of optimal physical, mental and social health and well-being for all infants, children, adolescents, and young adults.

Sandra Hassink, MD, FAAP, President

4504 American School Counselor Association
1101 King Street, Suite 310
Alexandria, VA 22314

703-683-2722
800-306-4722
Fax: 703-997-7572
e-mail: asca@schoolcounselor.org
www.schoolcounselor.org

The mission of ASCA is to represent professional school counselors and to promote professionalism and ethical practices.

Richard Wong, Executive Director
Jeff Broderson, Information Technology Admin.
Kathleen M Rakestraw, Director of Communications

4505 American Speech Language Hearing Associati on (ASHA)
2200 Research Boulevard, PO Box 3289
Rockville, MD 20850

301-296-5700
800-638-8255
Fax: 301-296-8580
TTY: 301-296-5650
e-mail: nsslha@asha.org
www.asha.org

A certifying body of 123,000 professionals providing speech, language and hearing services to the public. It is an accrediting agency for college and university graduate school programs in speech-language pathology and audiology.

Patricia A. Prelock, President
Elizabeth S. McCrea, President-Elect
Donna Fisher Smiley, VP for Audiology Practice

4506 Council for Learning Disabilities
11184 Antioch Road Box 405
Overland Park, KS 66210

913-491-1011
Fax: 913-491-1012
e-mail: CLDInfo@cldinternational.org
www.cldinternational.org

An international organization that promotes effective teaching and research. CDL is composed of professionals who represent diverse disciplines and who are committed to enhancing the education and life span development of individuals with learning disabilities.

Caroline Kethley, President
Silvana Watson, President-Elect
Steve Chamberlain, VP

4507 Division for Learning Disabilities
1110 N Glebe Road Suite 300
Arlington, VA 22201

703-524-0099
888-232-7733
Fax: 703-264-9494
TTY: 703-264-9446
www.teachingld.org

The Division for Learning Disabilities is a national professional organization consisting of teacher, higher education professionals, administrators, and parents. The major purpose of DLD is to promote the education and general welfare of persons with learning disabilities, provide a forum for discussion of issues facing the field of learning disabilities, and to encourage interaction amoung the many groups whose research and service efforts impact persons with learning disabilities.

Jenette Klingner, President
Erica Lembke, President-Elect
David Chard, VP

4508 Dyslexia Research Institute
5746 Centerville Road
Tallahassee, FL 32309   850-893-2216
                                Fax: 850-893-2440
                        e-mail: dri@dyslexia-add.org
                                www.dyslexia-add.org

Addresses academic, social and self-concept issues for dyslexic and ADD children and adults. College prep courses, study skills, advocacy, diagnostic testing, seminars, teachers training, day school, tutoring and adult literacy and life skills programs are available using an accredited MSLE approach.

Patricia K. Hardman, Executive Director
Robyn A Rennick MS, Assistant Director

4509 Federation for Children with Special Needs
529 Main Street, Suite 1102
Boston, MA 02129   617-236-7210
                                   800-331-0688
                                Fax: 617-241-0330
                        e-mail: fcsninfo@fcsn.org
                                www.fcsn.org

The mission of the Federation for Children with Special Needs provides information, support, and assistance to parents of children with disabilities, and encouraging full participation in community life by all people, especially those with isabilities.

Sonya Andrade, Executive Assistant
Robin Foley, Director

4510 International Dyslexia Association
40 York Road, Suite 400, 4th Floor
Baltimore, MD 21204   410-296-0232
                                   800-223-3123
                                Fax: 410-321-5069
                        e-mail: info@interdys.org
                                www.interdys.org

Our mission is to pursue and provide the most comprehensive range of information and services that address the full scope of dyslexia and related difficulties in learning to read and write.

Steve Peregoy, Executive Director
Gerri Morris, Corrdinator Information/Referral
Robert Hott, Director of Development

4511 Learning Disabilities Association of Ameri ca
4156 Library Road
Pittsburgh, PA 15234   412-341-1515
                                   888-300-6710
                                Fax: 412-344-0224
                        e-mail: info@LDAAmerica.org
                                www.ldaamerica.org

Helps families of the affected individual through information and referral to professionals in their area. A membership organization with affiliates across the country.

Sheila Buckley, Executive Director

4512 National Center For Learning Disabilities With Disabilities
381 Park Avenue S Suite 1401
New York, NY 10016   212-545-7510
                                   888-575-7373
                                Fax: 212-545-9665
                                www.ncld.org

The mission is to increase opportunities for all individuals with learning disabilities to achieve their potential.NCLD accomplishes this mission by increasing public awareness and understanding of learning disabilities, conducting educational programs and services leat promote research-based knowledge, and providing national leadership in shaping public policy.

Frederic M. Poses, Chairman of the Board
Anne Ford, Chairman
John R. Langeler, Treasurer

4513 National Dissemination Center for Children with Disabilities
PO Box 1492
Washington, DC 20013   202-884-8200
                                   800-695-0285
                                Fax: 202-884-8441
                        e-mail: nichcy@aed.org
                                www.nichcy.org

Provides parents with information about special education and the rights children and youth with disabilities have under the law. NICHY can also provide parents and others with a State Resource Sheet, useful for identifying resources within their state. This sheet includes, names, addresses and phone numbers of state agencies disability organizations, and parent groups serving individuals with disabilities and their families. A variety of other publications are available upon request.

Suzanne Ripley, Executive Director

4514 New England Center for Children
33 Turnpike Road, PO Box 2108
Southborough, MA 01772   508-481-1015
                                Fax: 508-485-3421
                        e-mail: info@necc.org
                                www.necc.org

Serving students between the ages of 3 and 22 diagnosed with autism, learning disabilities, language delays, mental retardation, behavior disorders and related disabilities; educational curriculum encompasses both the teaching of functional life skills and traditional academics; communication skills are taught throughout all activities in the school, residence, and community. Tuition and fees are set by the state. Consulting services also available.

Lisel Macenka, Chairman of the Board
James C. Burling, Vice Chair of the Board
L. Vincent Strully, President

4515 Parents Helping Parents: Family Resources for Children with Special Needs
1400 Parkmoor Avenue, Suite 100
San Jose, CA 95126   408-727-5775
                                   855-727-5775
                                Fax: 408-286-1116
                        e-mail: info@php.com
                                www.php.com

Helping children with special needs receive the resources, love, hope, respect, health care, education and other services they need to achive their full potential by providing them with strong families and dedicated professional to serve them.

Suzanne Cistulli, Board Chair
Robert Badagliacco, Board Treasurer
Lisa Caywood, Board Member

Libraries & Resource Centers

4516 Berkshire Center
18 Park Street #160
Lee, MA 01238   413-243-2576

A postsecondary program for young adults with learning disabilities ages eighteen-twenty-six. Half the students attend Berkshire Community College part-time while others go directly into the working world. Services include vocational/adacademic preparation, tutoring, college liason, life skills instruction, driver's education, money management, psychotherapy, and more. The program is year-round with an average stay of two years.

4517 Carroll Center for the Blind
770 Centre Street
Newton, MA 02458   617-969-6200
                                   800-852-3131
                                Fax: 617-969-6204
                                www.carroll.org

Assists blind and visually impaired adults and adolescents to adjust to loss of vision. The goal of this dynamic program is to help the person become more independent, to restore self-confidence, prepare for employment and improve the quality of life. Programs of individual counseling are offered as part of the program.

4637 MSUD:(Maple Syrup Urine Disease) Family Support Group
82 Ravine Road
Powell, OH 43065   614-389-2739
                                         e-mail: dbulcehr@aol.com
                                              www.msud-support.org

MSUD is a nonprofit (501)(c)(3) organization for parents of children with MSUD, adults with MSUD, health-care professionals and others interested in MSUD. Dedicated to providing opportunities for support and personal contact for those with MSUD and their families, distributing information and raising public awareness of MSUD, strengthening the liaison between families and professionals and encouraging newborn screening programs and research for MSUD.

Sandy Bulcher, Director
Marcia Hubbard, Secretary
Dave Bulcher, Treasurer

4638 March of Dimes Birth Defects Foundation
1275 Mamaroneck Avenue
White Plains, NY 10605   914-997-4488
                                                    888-663-4637
                                              Fax: 914-428-8203
                                  e-mail: answers@marchofdimes.com
                                              www.marchofdimes.com

Partnership of volunteers and professionals dedicates to improving the health of babies by preventing birth defects and infant mortality. Over 100 chapters are located across the country and can be located through the National Office.

Jennifer L Howse, President

Libraries & Resource Centers

4639 National Digestive Diseases Information Clearinghouse
2 Information Way
Bethesda, MD 20892   301-496-3583
                                                    800-891-5389
                                              Fax: 301-907-8906
                                   e-mail: nddic@info.niddk.nih.gov
                                              www2.niddk.nih.gov

The National Institute of Diabetes and Digestive and Kidney Diseases conducts and supports research on many of the most serious diseases affecting public health. The Institute supports much of the clinical research on the diseases of internal medicine and related subspecialty fields as well as many basic science disciplines.

Griffin P. Rodgers, M.D, Chairman, Executive Board
Brent B. Stanfield, Executive Secretary
Camille M. Hoover, M.S.W, Executive Officer

Web Sites

4640 Family Village
www.familyvillage.wisc.edu

A global community that integrates information, resources and communication opportunities on the Internet for persons with cognitive and other disabilities, for their families and for those that provide them services and support.

Book Publishers

4641 Let's Talk About Going to the Hospital
Rosen Publishing Group's PowerKids Press
29 E 21st Street
New York, NY 10010   212-777-3017
                                                    800-237-9932
                                              Fax: 888-436-4643
                                   e-mail: rosenpub@tribeca.ios.com
                                              www.rosenpublishing.com

If a child has to check into the hospital, chances are he or she is already upset about being ill. Knowing how a hospital functions and what the procedures are, such as when family members can visit, will help in what is already a stressful situation. Grades K-5.

24 pages
ISBN: 0-823950-36-0
Roger Rosen, President

Newsletters

4642 MSUD Newsletter
MSUD Family Support Group
82 Ravine Road
Powell, OH 43065   740-548-4475
                                              www.msud-support.org

Provides the latest information on the treatment of the disorder, reports on the latest research, current diet information, family news and related topics.

16 pages
Sandy Bulcher, Director
Dave Bulcher, Treasurer
K R Dollins, Editor

Description

4643 MARFAN SYNDROME
Synonym: MFS
Covers these related disorders: Neonatal or infantile Marfan syndrome
Involves the following Biologic System(s):
Cardiovascular Disorders,
Genetic/Chromosomal/Syndrome/Metabolic Disorders, Orthopedic and Muscle Disorders

Marfan syndrome is a connective tissue disorder that may result in heart (cardiac), blood vessel, skeletal, and eye (ocular) abnormalities. Children with Marfan syndrome tend to be unusually tall and slim; in some cases, this may be apparent at birth. Many affected infants also have deficiency of the layer of fat under the skin and abnormally diminished muscle tone (hypotonia) that may contribute to motor delays. In addition, in some infants with Marfan syndrome, several additional characteristic symptoms and findings may be apparent during later childhood. Neonatal or infantile Marfan syndrome is characterized by abnormal flexions (contractures), dislocations, and limited ranges of movement; an abnormally long head and face (dolichocephaly); a highly arched roof of the mouth (palate); unusually large corneas of the eyes (megalocornea); abnormal quivering movements of the colored portions of the eyes (irides); and heart defects (e.g., aortic root dilatation, mitral valve prolapse).

Older children with Marfan syndrome also tend to have an unusually long, narrow face as well as a narrow, highly arched palate and abnormal crowding of the teeth. Affected children and adults also have unusually long, thin arms and legs; a wide arm span; and long, thin fingers (arachnodactyly) with abnormally increased extension (hyperflexibility). Additional skeletal abnormalities are often present, such as unusually thin, fragile ribs; abnormal protrusion or depression of the breastbone (pectus carinatum or excavatum); and, in older children and adolescents, progressive abnormal sideways curvature (scoliosis) or front-to-back curvature (kyphosis) of the spine.

In many cases, affected children also have additional ocular abnormalities, such as dislocation (subluxation) of the lenses of the eyes (ectopia lentis); abnormal bluish coloration of the tough, outer membrane of the eyes; and severe nearsightedness (myopia). In addition, in some cases, the nerve-rich membrane at the back of the eyes (retina) may become detached.

Most individuals with Marfan syndrome also experience abnormalities of the heart and certain blood vessels (cardiovascular defects) that may be life-threatening. These may include progressive widening of the major artery of the body (aorta), causing leakage of blood through the valve between the left ventricle and the aorta (aortic regurgitation). In addition, the valve between the left ventricle and the left upper chamber (atrium) of the heart may bulge backward (prolapse) into the atrium, causing leakage of blood into the atrium.

The treatment of Marfan syndrome is directed toward preventing potential complications associated with progression of the disease. Affected children should receive regular evaluations to detect ocular defects, abnormal spinal curvatures, or cardiovascular defects. Treatment includes symptomatic and supportive measures, such as orthopedic techniques to help prevent or treat scoliosis or kyphosis; therapy with certain medications (beta-adrenergic blocking agents, e.g., propranolol) that may help to prevent or reduce the progression of certain cardiovascular abnormalities (e.g., aortic dilatation and associated complications); or surgical correction of cardiovascular defects as required. At one time, affected individuals were provided with antibiotic medications before dental visits and surgical procedures to reduce the incidence of endocarditis (an infection of the heart wall or heart valvle when bacteria enter the bloodstream). The American Heart Association no longer recommends taking routine antibiotics before certain dental procedures except for people at highest risk for bad outcomes if they develop endocarditis. Individuals with Marfan syndrome do not fall into this high-risk category.

Marfan syndrome results from abnormal changes (mutations) in a gene (fibrillin gene) located on the long arm of chromosome 15 (15q21.1). Such mutations may occur spontaneously (sporadically) for unknown reasons or may be inherited as an autosomal dominant trait. In individuals with the disease gene, the range and severity of associated symptoms and findings may vary from case to case (variable expressivity). Marfan syndrome is thought to affect about one in 10,000 individuals.

Government Agencies

4644 NIH/National Institute of Arthritis and Mu sculoskeletal and Skin Diseases
1AMS Circle, PO Box 3675
Bethesda, MD 20892
301-495-4484
877-226-4267
Fax: 301-718-6366
TTY: 301-565-2966
TDD: 301-565-2966
e-mail: niamsinfo@mail.nih.gov
www.niams.nih.gov

The mission of the NIAMS, a part of the NIH, is to support research into the causes, treatment, and prevention of arthritis and musculoskeletal and skin diseases, the training of basic and clinical scientists to carry out this research, and the dissemination of information on research progress in these diseases.

Stephen I Katz MD PhD, Director
Robert H Carter MD, Deputy Director

National Associations & Support Groups

4645 American Academy of Pediatrics
141 Northwest Point Boulevard
Elk Grove Village, IL 60007
847-434-4000
800-433-9016
Fax: 847-434-8000
www.aap.org

The American Academy of Pediatrics and its member pediatricians are committed to the attainment of optimal physical, mental and social health and well-being for all infants, children, adolescents, and young adults.

Sandra Hassink, MD, FAAP, President

4646 Genetic Alliance
4301 Connecticut Avenue NW
Washington, DC 20008
202-966-5557
800-336-4363
Fax: 202-966-8553
e-mail: info@geneticalliance.org
www.geneticalliance.org

A coalition of voluntary genetic support groups, consumers and professionals addressing the needs of individuals and families affected by genetic disorders from a national perspective.

Joan Oppenheimer Weiss, Founder
Sharon Terry, President

4647 March of Dimes Birth Defects Foundation
1275 Mamaroneck Avenue
White Plains, NY 10605
914-997-4488
888-663-4637
Fax: 914-428-8203
e-mail: answers@marchofdimes.com
www.marchofdimes.com

Partnership of volunteers and professionals dedicates to improving the health of babies by preventing birth defects and infant mortality. Over 100 chapters are located across the country and can be located through the National Office.

Jennifer L Howse, President

4648 National Marfan Foundation
22 Manhasset Avenue
Port Washington, NY 11050
516-883-8712
800-862-7326
Fax: 516-883-8040
e-mail: staff@marfan.org
www.marfan.org

A nonprofit voluntary health organization dedicated to saving lives and improving the quality of life for individuals and families affected by the Marfan Syndrome and related disorders.

Ray Chevallier, Chair
Mary J. Roman, Vice Chairman
Teri Dean, Treasurer

Web Sites

4649 National Marfan Foundation
22 Manhasset Avenue
Port Washington, NY 11050
516-883-8712
Fax: 516-883-8040
e-mail: staff@marfan.org
www.marfan.org

A nonprofit voluntary health organization dedicated to saving lives and improving the quality of life for individuals and families affected by the Marfan Syndrome and related disorders.

Raymond Chevallier, Chair
Mary J. Roman, Vice Chair
Cory Eaves, Secretary

4650 Wheeless' Textbook of Orthopaedics
www.wheelessonline.com
410-494-4994
www.wheelessonline.com

Derives from a variety of sources, including journals, articles, national meetings lectures and other textbooks.

Clifford R. Wheeless, Editor in chief
James A Nunley, Managing Editor
James R. Urbaniak, Managing Editor

Book Publishers

4651 Let's Talk About Going to the Hospital
Rosen Publishing Group's PowerKids Press
29 E 21st Street
New York, NY 10010
212-777-3017
800-237-9932
Fax: 888-436-4643
e-mail: rosenpub@tribeca.ios.com
www.rosenpublishing.com

If a child has to check into the hospital, chances are he or she is already upset about being ill. Knowing how a hospital functions and what the procedures are, such as when family members can visit, will help in what is already a stressful situation. Grades K-5.

24 pages
ISBN: 0-823950-36-0
Roger Rosen, President

Pamphlets

4652 Marfan Syndrome
March of Dimes Pregnancy & Newborn Health Edu Ctr
1275 Mamaroneck Avenue
White Plains, NY 10605
914-977-4488
888-663-4637
Fax: 914-997-4763
e-mail: answers@marchofdimes.com
www.marchofdimes.org

A series of fact sheets each discussing an aspect of Marfan, inlcuding prevention, research, causes, treamtents, diagnosis, affects, eye problems, heart problems, and skeletal problems.

Description

4653 MCCUNE-ALBRIGHT SYNDROME

Synonyms: Albright syndrome, MAS, PFD, POFD, Polyostotic fibrous dysplasia, Precocious puberty with polyostotic

Involves the following Biologic System(s):

Endocrinologic Disorders,

Genetic/Chromosomal/Syndrome/Metabolic Disorders

McCune-Albright syndrome is a genetic disorder characterized by multiple areas of abnormal, fiber-like tissue growths (bone lesions) that replace normal bone tissue (polyostotic fibrous dysplasia); irregular, patchy areas of light brown pigmentation on the skin (cafe-au-lait spots); and abnormalities of certain hormone-producing glands that assist in regulating the body's growth, controlling the rate of metabolism, and promoting the development of secondary sexual characteristics. Although bone lesions are most common in the pelvis and the long bones of the arms and legs, other bones may be affected, including the ribs, skull and facial bones, and bones of the spinal column (vertebrae). These bone lesions may cause abnormal thickness and deformity of affected bones, susceptibility to fractures, and bone pain. In addition, lesions may cause corresponding bones to develop unevenly. For example, one leg may appear unusually short, or one side of the face may appear different from the other (facial asymmetry). Bone lesions of the skull and face may eventually result in hearing loss and visual impairment.

Many girls with McCune-Albright syndrome undergo early development of secondary sexual characteristics (precocious puberty), including early breast development and onset of menstrual cycles (menstruation). Some boys with the disorder may also experience precocious puberty, including genital development and unusually accelerated growth. In many patients, additionalendocrine abnormalities may be present. For example, some affected children may produce excessive amounts of the hormone cortisol, resulting in Cushing's syndrome. This disorder is characterized by excessive weight gain in the chest and abdominal area; a moon-shaped, rounded face; abnormal pads of fat in certain areas of the body; high blood pressure (hypertension); weakening of bones, causing increased susceptibility to fractures; thin, and fragile skin.

Some children with McCune-Albright syndrome may also produce excessive amounts of thyroid hormones (hyperthyroidism), potentially leading to heart palpitations, anxiety, heat intolerance, excessive sweating, muscle weakness, or weight loss. In addition, some affected children may be prone to developing tumors of the pituitary gland, resulting in increased secretion of growth hormone, which stimulates body growth and development. Affected children may experience enlargement of bones and soft tissues of the hands, feet, and face (acromegaly); lengthening and coarsening of the face; and enlargement of certain organs (e.g., heart). In some patients, excessive growth during childhood (gigantism) and tall stature may occur.

McCune-Albright syndrome may be obvious at birth because of unusual skin pigmentation. Alternatively, it may not be apparent until late infancy or early childhood when precocious puberty or bone lesions become apparent. The disorder is caused by spontaneous (sporadic) changes (mutations) of a gene known as the GNAS1 gene. The disease gene is located on the long arm (q) of chromosome 20 (20q13.2). Because the gene mutation is present in only some cells of the body (mosaicism), symptoms and findings may vary among affected individuals, depending upon the specific body cells affected. Treatment of McCune-Albright syndrome includes symptomatic and supportive measures. These may include drug therapy to help prevent or treat precocious puberty, surgical removal of pituitary tumors or the thyroid gland, and appropriate treatment of bone lesions and associated abnormalities.

Government Agencies

4654 NIH/National Institute of Arthritis and Mu sculoskeletal and Skin Diseases
1AMS Circle, PO Box 3675
Bethesda, MD 20892

301-495-4484
877-226-4267
Fax: 301-718-6366
TTY: 301-565-2966
TDD: 301-565-2966
e-mail: niamsinfo@mail.nih.gov
www.niams.nih.gov

The mission of the NIAMS, a part of the NIH, is to support research into the causes, treatment, and prevention of arthritis and musculoskeletal and skin diseases, the training of basic and clinical scientists to carry out this research, and the dissemination of information on research progress in these diseases.

Stephen I Katz MD PhD, Director
Robert H Carter MD, Deputy Director

4655 NIH/National Institute of Child Health and Human Development
31 Center Drive, Building 31, Room 2A32
Bethesda, MD 20892

301-496-1333
800-370-2943
Fax: 866-760-5947
TTY: 888-320-6942
e-mail: NICHDInformationResourceCenter@mail.nih.
www.nichd.nih.gov

Established in 1962 by congress, today the institute conducts and supports research on topics related to the health of children, adults, families and populations. Some of these topics include: developmental disabilities, growth and development, infant death, reproductive health and birth defects.

Jay H Hoofnagle, Director
Lisa Kaeser, Program & Public Liaison

National Associations & Support Groups

4656 American Academy of Pediatrics
141 Northwest Point Boulevard
Elk Grove Village, IL 60007

847-434-4000
800-433-9016
Fax: 847-434-8000
www.aap.org

The American Academy of Pediatrics and its member pediatricians are committed to the attainment of optimal physical, mental and social health and well-being for all infants, children, adolescents, and young adults.

Sandra Hassink, MD, FAAP, President

4657 Genetic Alliance
4301 Connecticut Avenue NW
Washington, DC 20008

202-966-5557
800-336-4363
Fax: 202-966-8553
e-mail: info@geneticalliance.org
www.geneticalliance.org

A coalition of voluntary genetic support groups, consumers and professionals addressing the needs of individuals and families affected by genetic disorders from a national perspective.

Joan Oppenheimer Weiss, Founder
Sharon Terry, President

4658 International Skeletal Dysplasia Registry
Medical Genetics Institute
8700 Beverly Blvd
Los Angeles, CA 90048

310-423-9915
800-233-2771
Fax: 310-423-1528
e-mail: maryann.priore@cshs.org
www.cedars-sinai.edu

The International Skeletal Dysplasia Registry at Cedars-Sinai Medical Center is a referral center for research into the diagnosis; management and etiology of the skeletal dysplasias.

Lawrence B. Platt, Chair
Thomas M. Prislac, President/CEO
Vera Guerin, Vice Chair

4659 MAGIC Foundation: Major Aspects of Growth in Children
6645 W North Avenue
Oak Park, IL 60302

708-383-0808
800-362-4423
Fax: 708-383-0899
e-mail: ContactUs@magicfoundation.org
www.magicfoundation.org

A national nonprofit organization providing support and education regarding growth disorders in children and related adult disorders. Provides educational information, networking, a national conference, a kids' program and an extensive medical library.

10,000 members

Rich Buckley, Chairman
Ken Dickard, Vice Chairman
Courtney Lance, Secretary

4660 March of Dimes Birth Defects Foundation
1275 Mamaroneck Avenue
White Plains, NY 10605

914-997-4488
888-663-4637
Fax: 914-428-8203
e-mail: answers@marchofdimes.com
www.marchofdimes.com

Partnership of volunteers and professionals dedicates to improving the health of babies by preventing birth defects and infant mortality. Over 100 chapters are located across the country and can be located through the National Office.

Jennifer L Howse, President

Web Sites

4661 Human Growth Foundation
997 Glen Cove Ave, Suite 5
Glen Head, NY 11545

800-451-6434
Fax: 516-671-4055
e-mail: hgf1@hgfound.org
www.hgfound.org

Helps children and adults with growth or growth hormone related disorders through research, education, support and advocacy.

Pisit Pitukcheewanont, President
Emily German - Lee, Vice President
Patricia Costa, Executive Director

4662 University Alabama Birmingham
1720 2nd Ave South
Birmingham, AL 35294

205-934-4011
TDD: 205-934-4642
www.uab.edu/home

Dr. Margaret A. Purcell, Executive Director
Michael A Bownes, Secretary
Linda Beasley, Assistant to Secretary

Book Publishers

4663 Let's Talk About Going to the Hospital
Rosen Publishing Group's PowerKids Press
29 E 21st Street
New York, NY 10010

212-777-3017
800-237-9932
Fax: 888-436-4643
e-mail: rosenpub@tribeca.ios.com
www.rosenpublishing.com

If a child has to check into the hospital, chances are he or she is already upset about being ill. Knowing how a hospital functions and what the procedures are, such as when family members can visit, will help in what is already a stressful situation. Grades K-5.

24 pages
ISBN: 0-823950-36-0

Roger Rosen, President

Description

4664 MENINGITIS

Covers these related disorders: Bacterial meningitis, Chronic meningitis, Neonatal meningitis, Viral meningitis

Involves the following Biologic System(s):

Infectious Disorders, Neurologic Disorders

Meningitis is an inflammation of the protective membranes that cover the brain and spinal cord (meninges). It most often occurs from infancy to young adulthood, but can develop in persons of any age, and is most commonly caused by a viral (viral meningitis) or bacterial infection (bacterial meningitis) that reaches the meninges by way of the blood and through the cerebrospinal fluid (CSF) that surrounds the brain and spinal cord. Meningitis may also be caused by fungi and other kinds of microorganisms, by noninfectious disease, head injury, medications, and exposure to chemical substances. Cases of meningitis in which no causative infecting organism can be identified are sometimes called aseptic meningitis. However, specialized testing often reveals specific kinds of bacteria or viruses as the cause of such disease.

All types of meningitis are serious and require prompt medical attention to prevent injury to the brain, and death, but bacterial meningitis is typically more serious than viral meningitis. Bacterial meningitis most commonly affects children from 1 month to 5 years old. In children aged approximately 2 months to 12 years, bacterial meningitis is most commonly caused by two species of bacteria: *Neisseria meningitidis* (meningococcus), and *Streptococcus pneumoniae*. These bacteria are spread by the inhalation of airborne cough or sneeze droplets from infected persons, or through contact with feces or other infected body products. Viral meningitis is more common and typically less severe than bacterial meningitis, but is spread in the same way, through saliva, mucus, fecal matter, and other infected body materials.

Symptoms of meningitis include headache and stiff neck, nausea and vomiting, fever, sensitivity to light (photophobia), unnatural sleepiness, confusion, and seizures. Symptoms of meningitis in infants and young children may include irritability and loss of appetite. Meningitis that occurs within the first month of life, known as neonatal meningitis, may produce a different pattern of symptoms than that seen in older infants and children. Such meningitis affects approximately 0.2 to 0.4 in every 1,000 newborns, and is more frequent among infants born prematurely (before 37 weeks). As a result of increased fluid pressure, meningitis in newborns may cause bulging of the skull in the fontanels at the forward sides of the head, where bones of the skull have not fully fused, and enlargement of the head (hydrocephalus). Other symptoms of meningitis in children include coughing and difficulty in breathing. Without prompt treatment, these effects of meningitis can progress to coma and death.

The diagnosis of meningitis, and the type microorganism causing a particular case of infectious meningitis, is made by testing a sample of CSF from the lower back. As the treatment of meningitis proceeds, lumbar puncture and analysis of the CSF are repeated to assess the patient's response to treatment..

Prompt diagnosis and immediate treatment of bacterial meningitis are essential to help prevent brain damage and potentially life-threatening complications. Treatment requires immediate hospitalization and the intravenous administration of antibiotics, as well as careful, close monitoring and measures for reducing the increased pressure on the brain caused by fluid that passes through the inflamed meninges. Antibiotic treatment for bacterial meningitis usually lasts for a couple of weeks, but may continue after a patient is discharged from the hospital. Additional treatment of bacterial meningitis is symptomatic and supportive. Preventive antibiotic therapy may be recommended for persons who have had close contact with children or other persons who have bacterial meningitis. Currently, routine childhood immunization plays an essential role in preventing meningitis caused by the species of bacteria known as Haemophilus influenzae type b (Hib), which used to be one of the most common causes of childhood bacterial meningitis. Vaccines that can protect against some other types of meningitis are also available, such as that caused by *Streptococcus pneumoniae*.

Like bacterial meningitis, viral meningitis requires prompt medical attention, but usually disappears gradually of its own accord within a period of 2 weeks. Because they do not affect viruses, antibiotic drugs are not useful for treating this type of meningitis. Instead, treatment of viral meningitis is usually focused on relieving fever and its other symptoms, and on supporting the patient's respiration, nutrition, and movement. In more severe cases, however medications specifically directed at viruses, known as antiviral drugs, may be given to patients with viral meningitis.

Some patients with meningitis may develop fever, headache, a stiff neck, back pain, vomiting, and other symptoms that last for a month or longer. This condition, known as chronic meningitis, may result from certain bacterial, viral, or other infections, or may be due to noninfectious disorders that can affect the brain, such as sarcoidosis or multiple sclerosis; certain medications, such as some anticancer drugs; or other factors. Individuals whose immune systems have been impaired by disease or by surgical or medical treatment for disease may also be more susceptible to chronic meningitis. The treatment of chronic meningitis is based on the underlying cause of the condition.

For more information on a meningitis vaccine, see chapter on Preventable Childhood Infections.

Government Agencies

4665 NIH/National Institute of Allergy and Infectious Diseases
6610 Rockledge Drive, Room 4017, MSC 6606, PO Box
Bethesda, MD 20817
301-496-2644
866-284-4107
Fax: 301-402-7123
TDD: 800-877-8339
e-mail: niaidnews@niaid.nih.gov
www.niaid.nih.gov

Conducts and supports basic and applied research to better understand, treat, and ultimately prevent infectious, immunologic, and allergic diseases.

Anthony S Fauci MD, Director

National Associations & Support Groups

4666 American Academy of Pediatrics
141 Northwest Point Boulevard
Elk Grove Village, IL 60007

847-434-4000
800-433-9016
Fax: 847-434-8000
www.aap.org

The American Academy of Pediatrics and its member pediatricians are committed to the attainment of optimal physical, mental and social health and well-being for all infants, children, adolescents, and young adults.

Sandra Hassink, MD, FAAP, President

4667 March of Dimes Birth Defects Foundation
1275 Mamaroneck Avenue
White Plains, NY 10605

914-997-4488
888-663-4637
Fax: 914-428-8203
e-mail: answers@marchofdimes.com
www.marchofdimes.com

Partnership of volunteers and professionals dedicates to improving the health of babies by preventing birth defects and infant mortality. Over 100 chapters are located across the country and can be located through the National Office.

Jennifer L Howse, President

4668 Meningitis Foundation of America
PO Box 1818
El Mirage, AZ 85335

480-270-2652
800-668-1129
Fax: 317-595-6370
e-mail: support@musa.org
www.musa.org

Goals and objectives are: help support sufferers of Spinal Meningitis and their families; provide information to educate the public and medical professionals about meningitis so that its early diagnosis and treatment will save lives; and support development of vaccines and other preventions.

Daisi Pollard Sepulveda, National President
Courtney Martin, National VP
Caroline L. Petrie, National Secretary

Web Sites

4669 MGH Neurology Web Forums
www.mgh.harvard.edu/forum

4670 Maryland Department of Health
www.dhml.state.md.us

4671 Meningitis Foundation of America
P. O. Box 1818
El Mirage, AZ 85335

480-270-2652
www.musa.org

Help support sufferers of meningitis and their families and the development of vaccines and other means of treating and/or preventing meningitis.

Caroline Petrie, National Secretary
Alexander James Flatley, Board Member

4672 World Health Organization
1211 Geneva 27
Switzerland,

122-791-2111
Fax: 122-791-3111
e-mail: who_reform@who.int
www.who.int/topics/meningitis/en

WHO's objective, as set out in its Constitution, is the attainment by all peoples of the highest possible level of health.

Book Publishers

4673 Let's Talk About Going to the Hospital
Rosen Publishing Group's PowerKids Press
29 E 21st Street
New York, NY 10010

212-777-3017
800-237-9932
Fax: 888-436-4643
e-mail: rosenpub@tribeca.ios.com
www.rosenpublishing.com

If a child has to check into the hospital, chances are he or she is already upset about being ill. Knowing how a hospital functions and what the procedures are, such as when family members can visit, will help in what is already a stressful situation. Grades K-5.

24 pages
ISBN: 0-823950-36-0

Roger Rosen, President

Description

4674 MENTAL RETARDATION

Synonym: Mental deficiency

Involves the following Biologic System(s):

Developmental/Behavioral/Psychiatric Disorders, Neurologic Disorders

Mental retardation is characterized by impaired or below average intellectual functioning that results in deficits in learning ability and adaptive behaviors. The disorder is thought to affect approximately three percent of the general population. About 80 to 90 percent of patients have mild mental retardation, whereas 10 to 20 percent are affected by moderate to profound degrees of impairment.

The causes of mental retardation may be biological as well as psychosocial or sociocultural in nature. In other words, the disorder may be due to a combination of several factors and influenced both by biological abnormalities of the brain as well as the nature of a child's life experiences, such as those resulting from parent-child interactions and overall family dynamics. Biological causes of mental retardation may include fetal exposure to certain drugs, maternal infections, or radiation therapy; premature birth; or certain underlying disorders, such as inborn errors of metabolism, chromosomal abnormalities including Down syndrome and fragile X syndrome, or other genetic disorders. Mental retardation may also result from head injuries or low levels of oxygen to the brain during delivery, childhood exposure to lead, or certain infections during infancy or early childhood, such as inflammation of the protective membranes surround|ing the brain and spinal cord (meningitis). Some underlying causes may be correctable before mental retardation occurs, such as phenylketonuria (PKU), which is a metabolic disorder, or hypothyroidism, a condition characterized by decreased activity of the thyroid gland. Additional contributing factors may include malnutrition; dysfunctional interactions between caregivers and infants; or other psychosocial or sociocultural factors. In many children with mental retardation, the specific causes remain unknown. The condition may occur as the result of the interactions of several genes (polygenic inheritance), possibly in association with certain environmental influences (multifactorial).

During normal development, infants and children acquire mental, physical, and behavioral skills in certain stages known as developmental milestones. Although the particular rate of development is variable, most children acquire such skills at certain ages. However, infants and children with mental retardation typically experience delays in achieving certain developmental milestones. For example, with severe levels of mental retardation, patients may initially have delays in the acquisition of certain motor skills. With more moderate levels of retardation, children may achieve early motor milestones yet be delayed in acquiring certain skills that require the coordination of physical and mental abilities (psychomotor delays), such as delayed speech and language skills. In children with mild or borderline impairment, below average intellectual functioning may not be suspected until the early school years. Varying degrees of mental retardation are based upon the different levels of support that may be required for daily functioning as well as intelligence quotient (I.Q.), which is a standardized, age-related measure of intelligence. Mental retardation may be defined as having an I.Q. below 70 and is often subdivided into mild, moderate, severe, and profound mental retardation. Most individuals in the general population have an I.Q. between 80 and 120.

Children with what is known as borderline intellectual functioning have very mild intellectual deficits (e.g., I.Q. between 70 to 85) and minor impairments in adaptive behaviors. These behaviors include certain adaptive skills, such as social, self-care, communication, and vocational skills. Patients with mild retardation (I.Q. between 50 and 70) may develop academic skills up to the sixth grade level. In addition, with appropriate support, they may achieve social skills that enable them to function relatively independently during adulthood. Patients with moderate impairment (I.Q. between 35 and 50) may learn to communicate and tend to have only fair motor development. Although these patients rarely develop academic skills up to the second grade level, they may benefit from vocational training and achieve limited independence with appropriate supervision. Children with severe mental retardation (I.Q. between 20 and 35) typically have poor motor development and little speech or communication skills. With appropriate education and support, they may develop speech by late adolescence. In addition, with close supervision, they may learn basic hygienic skills and simple tasks by adulthood. Although children with profound impairment (I.Q. under 20) may learn some basic hygienic skills, they typically have limited psychomotor development and require close, ongoing supervision.

In infants with suspected mental retardation, a number of specialized laboratory tests may be conducted to rule out certain underlying disorders, such as fragile X syndrome or other chromosomal or genetic syndromes. The management of mental retardation is individualized for each child and may include therapeutic and special educational services as well as special social support and counseling services. Early diagnosis and the prompt development of an individualized, comprehensive intervention program is essential in helping affected children reach their potential. Prenatal screening for genetic defects, and genetic counseling for families at risk for known heritable disorders can decrease the incidence of genetically caused mental retardation. Primary care pediatricians lay an important role in consulting with specialists and other health care providers as required and developing an appropriate intervention program. As patients with mild to moderate impairment reach adolescence, specialized services may include a focus on vocational training and community living.

National Associations & Support Groups

4675 ARC of the United States
1825 K Street MW, Suite 1200
Washington, DC 20006

202-534-3700
800-433-5255
Fax: 202-534-3731
e-mail: info@thearc.org
www.thearc.org

The ARC is the national organization of and for people with mental retardation and related developmental disabilities and their families. Devoted to promoting and improving supports and services for people with mental retardation and their families. The association also fosters research and education regarding the prevention of mental retardation in infants and young children. The ARC was founded in 1950 by a small group of parents and other concerned individuals.

Nancy Webster, President
Ronald Brown, VP
Elise McMillan, Secretary

4676 American Academy of Pediatrics
141 Northwest Point Boulevard
Elk Grove Village, IL 60007   847-434-4000
                                     800-433-9016
                                     Fax: 847-434-8000
                                     www.aap.org

The American Academy of Pediatrics and its member pediatricians are committed to the attainment of optimal physical, mental and social health and well-being for all infants, children, adolescents, and young adults.

Sandra Hassink, MD, FAAP, President

4677 American Association of People with Disabilities
2013 H Street, NW, 5th Floor
Washington, DC 20006   800-840-8844
                              Fax: 866-536-4461
                              TTY: 202-457-0046
                              www.aapd.com

It is the nation's largest disability rights organization. We promote equal opportunity, economic power, independent living, and political participation for people with disabilities.

Mark Perriello, President and CEO
Henry Claypool, Executive Vice President
TaKeisha Bobbitt, Managing Director

4678 American Association on Health and Disabilities
110 N. Washington Street, Suite 328-J
Rockville, MD 20850   301-545-6140
                             Fax: 301- 54- 614
                             www.aahd.us

It is dedicated to improve overall health and reduce health disparities for people with disabilities through health promotion and wellness.

Ronald G. Blankenbaker, MD, President
Roberta Carlin, MS, JD, Executive Director
E. Clarke Ross, DPA, Public Policy Director

4679 American Mental Health Foundation (AMHF)
PO Box 3
Riverdale, NY 10471
USA   212-737-9027
e-mail: elomke@americanmentalhealthfoundation.or
www.americanmentalhealthfoundation.org

Dedicated to the extensive and intensive research in the theories and techniques of treatment of emotional illness and to the implementation of reforms in the mental health system. Efforts have resulted in development of better and less expensive treatment methods. Findings are disseminated in English and other major languages.

Sister Joan Curtin, Director
John P. Fowler, Treasurer
Eugene Gollogly, VP

4680 American Network of Community Options & Resources
1101 King Street, Suite 380,
Alexandria, VA 22314   703-535-7850
                              e-mail: ancor@ancor.org
                              www.ancor.org

It is the advocate and resource for private community providers of services to people with disabilities.

Barbara Merrill, Chief Executive Officer
Gabrielle Sedor, Chief Operations Officer

4681 American Occupational Therapy Association
4720 Montgomery Ln Ste 200
Bethesda,, MD 20814   800-729-2682
                             Fax: 240-762-5150
                             www.aota.org

4682 American Public Health Association
800 I Street, NW
Washington, DC 20001   202-777-2742
                              Fax: 202-777-2534
                              TTY: 202-777-2500
                              www.apha.org

APHA champions the health of all people and all communities. They aim to strengthen the public health profession and speak out for public health issues and policies backed by science.

Georges C. Benjamin, MD, Executive Director
Kemi Oluwafemi, MBA, CPA, Chief Financial Officer
Susan Polan, PhD, Associate Executive Director

4683 Arc (The)
1825 K Street, NW, Suite 1200
Washington, DC 20006   202-534-3700
                              800-433-5255
                              Fax: 202-534-3731
                              e-mail: tnguyen@thearc.org.
                              www.thearc.org

An organization advocating for and serving people with intellectual and developmental disabilities and their families. They encompass all ages and all spectrums from autism, Down syndrome, Fragile X and various other developmental disabilities.

Ronald Brown, President
Elise McMillan, Vice President
M.J. Bartelmay, Jr., Secretary

4684 Association of Developmental Disabilities
1671 Worcester Road (Rt. 9W), Suite 201
Framingham, MA 1701   508-405-8000
                             Fax: 508-405-8001
                             www.addp.org

The mission is to promote and ensure the strength of the community-based provider community and its members so that our members can be successful in improving the quality, access and value of community based services.

Jean Phelps,, Chair
Chris White, Vice-Chair
Michael Andrade, Clerk

4685 Association of Professional Developmental Disabilities Administrators
www.apdda.org

The mission is to supports the continuous improvement of a comprehensive array of individual and accessible services designed to enhance the quality of life for persons with intellectual disabilities and other developmental disabilities.

David J. Thomas, President
Julene Hollenbach, President Elect

4686 Association of University Centers on Disabilities
1100 Wayne Ave., Suite 1000
Silver Spring, MD 20910   301-588-8252
                                 Fax: 301-588-2842
                                 e-mail: aucdinfo@aucd.org
                                 www.aucd.org

The Association of University Centers on Disabilities (AUCD) is a membership organization that supports and promotes a national network of university-based interdisciplinary programs.

Andrew J. Imparato, JD, Executive Director
Abigail (Abbey) Alberico, MPH, Project Manager
Leon Barnett, MSEd, Program Specialist

4687 Bethpage Mission
4980 W 118th Street, Suite A
Omaha, NE 68137   402-896-3884
                         800-628-7070
                         Fax: 402-896-1511
                         e-mail: psanchez@bethpage.org
                         www.bethpage.org

4688 Bethphage
2245 Midway Road, #300
Carrolton, TX 75006
972-866-9989
800-628-7070
Fax: 972-991-0834
e-mail: hbranicki@bethphage.org
www.bethphage.org

Bethphage is an affiliate of the Evangelical Lutheran Church in America, serves and advocates for people with disabilities so that they may achieve their full potential. Bethphage provides living and vocational services to individuals with developmental disabilities, including group homes, supervised apartment living and job skills training.

4689 Center for Disabilities and Development
University of Iowa Hospitals and Clinics
451 Newton Road, 200 Medicine Administration Build
Iowa City, IA 52242
319-353-6900
877-686-0031
Fax: 319-356-8284
e-mail: cdd-webmaster@uiowa.edu
www.medicine.uiowa.edu

A trusted resource for healthcare, training, research and information for people with disabilities that include: behavior disorders, brain injury, cerebral palsy, diabetes, down syndrome, learning disabilities, mental retardation, sleep disorders and spina bifida.

Debra A. Schwinn, Dean
Donna L. Hammond, Interim Executive Associate Dean
Christopher Cooper, Associate Dean for Student Affairs

4690 Council for Exception Children - Division on Autism and Development Disabilities
daddcec.org

It is an organization composed of persons committed to enhancing the quality of life of individuals, especially children and youth, with autism, intellectual disability, and other developmental disabilities.

Dianne Zager, President
Gardner Umbarger, Treasurer

4691 Council on Quality and Leadership (The)
100 West Road, Suite 300
Towson, MD 21204
410-583-0060
e-mail: info@thecouncil.org
www.c-q-l.org

CQL offers training, accreditation, consultation and certification services to organizations and systems that share our vision of dignity, opportunity and community for all people.

Cathy Ficker Terrill, President/ CEO
Kerri Melda, VP, Research and Special Projects
Tammi Watkins, VP, Operations

4692 Developmental Disabilities Nurses Association
1501 South Loop 288, Suite 104 - PMB 381
Denton, TX 76205
800-888-6733
Fax: 844-336-2329
ddna.org

Developmental Disabilities Nurses Association (DDNA) is a 501(c)(3) not-for-profit nursing specialty organization that is committed to advocacy, education, and support for nurses who provide services to persons with intellectual and developmental disabilities (IDD).

Karen Green McGowan, RN, CDDN, President
Deb Maloy, RN, CDDN, President-Elect
Wendy Herbers, RN, CDDN, QDDP, Vice-President

4693 Judge David L. Bazelon Center for Mental Health
1101 15th Street, NW, Suite 1212
Washington, DC 20005
202-467-5730
Fax: 202-223-0409
TDD: 202-467-4232
e-mail: communications@bazelon.org
www.bazelon.org

The mission of the Judge David L. Bazelon Center for Mental Health Law is to protect and advance the rights of adults and children who have mental disabilities.

Robert Bernstein, President/ CEO
Ira Burnim, Director
Jennifer Mathis, Deputy Director

4694 Mosaic
4980 S. 118th St.
Omaha, NE 68137
877-3MO-SAIC
Fax: 402-896-1511
e-mail: info@mosaicinfo.org
www.mosaicinfo.org

Mosaic is a faith-based organization serving people with intellectual disabilities.

Linda Timmons, President/ CEO
Raul Saldivar, Chief Operating Officer
Cindy Schroeder, Chief Financial Officer

4695 NADD: National Association for the Dually Diagnosed
132 Fair Street
Kingston, NY 12401
845-331-4336
800-331-5362
Fax: 845-331-4569
e-mail: info@thenadd.org
www.thenadd.org

Nonprofit organization designed to promote the interests of professional and parent development with resources for individuals who have the coexistence of mental illness and mental retardation. Provides conferences, educational services and training materials to professionals, parents, concerned citizens and service organizations. Formerly known as the National Association for the Dually Diagnosed.

Donna McNelis, President
Dan Baker, VP
Julia Pearce, Secretary

4696 NYSARC
393 Delaware Ave.
Delmar, NY 12054
518-439-8311
Fax: 518-439-1893
e-mail: info@nysarc.org
www.nysarc.org

NYSARC's mission is to advocate for persons with intellectual and other developmental disabilities in every manner possible. In its advocacy role, NYSARC is committed to a full quality of life for every person, as it recognizes the challenges of the present and has a clear vision for the future.

Laura J. Kennedy, President
Steven Kroll, Executive Director
Tania F. Seaburg, Esq., Chief Policy and Operations Officer

4697 National Alliance on Mental Illness
3803 N. Fairfax Drive, Suite 100
Arlington, VA 22203
703-524-7600
800-950-6264
Fax: 703-524-9094
e-mail: info@nami.org
www.nami.org

Grassroots mental health organization dedicated to building better lives for the millions of Americans affected by mental illness. - See more at:
http://www.nami.org/About-NAMI#sthash.1Ytjmu5h.dpuf

Jim Payne, J.D., President
David Levy, Chief Financial Officer
Mary Giliberti, J.D., Executive Director

4698 National Association for Dually Diagnosed
132 Fair Street
Kingston, NY 12401
845-331-4336
800-331-5362
Fax: 845-331-4569
e-mail: rfletcher@thenadd.org
thenadd.org

NADD is a not-for-profit membership association established for professionals, care providers and families to promote understanding of and services for individuals who have developmental disabilities and mental health needs.

Robert J. Fletcher DSW, Chief Executive Officer
Donna McNelis, Ph.D., President
Michelle Jordan, Office Manager

4699 National Association of Councils on Developmental Disabilities
1825 K. Street, N.W. Suite 600
Washington, DC 20006   202-506-5813
e-mail: mjones@nacdd.org
www.nacdd.org

The National Association of Councils on Developmental Disabilities (NACDD) is a national membership organization representing the 56 State and Territorial Councils on Developmental Disabilities.

Claire Mantonya, President
Donna A Meltzer, Chief Executive Officer
Sheryl Matney, Director

4700 National Association of QDDPs
301 Veterans Parkway
New Lenox, IL 60451   815-320-7301
Fax: 815-320-7357
e-mail: hjanczak@qddp.org
www.qddp.org

The National Association of Qualified Developmental Disability Professionals was formed in 1996 by Trinity Services staff as the result of a recognized need by QDDPs - Qualified Developmental Disability Professionals/QMRPs - Qualified Mental Retardation Professionals (also known as Case Managers) to establish a strong resource for research, networking, and addressing issues that concern QDDPs today.

Holly Janczak, Executive Director
Kevin Schaefer, Associate Director
Lori Elgas, Conference/Membership Coordinator

4701 National Association of State Directors of Developmental Disabilities Services
301 N Fairfax Street, Suite 101
Alexandria, VA 22314   703-683-4202
e-mail: nthaler@nasddds.org
www.nasddds.org

The NASDDDS mission is to assist member state agencies in building person-centered systems of services and supports for people with intellectual and developmental disabilities and their families.

Laura L. Nuss, President
Bernard Simons, Vice President/President Elect
Nancy Thaler, Executive Director

4702 National Association of State Mental Health Program Directors
66 Canal Center Plaza, Suite 302
Alexandria, VA 22314   703-739-9333
Fax: 703-548-9517
e-mail: webmaster@nasmhpd.org
www.nasmhpd.org

Founded in 1959 and based in Alexandria, VA, the National Association of State Mental Health Program Directors (NASMHPD) represents the $37.6 billion public mental health service delivery system serving 7.1 million people annually in all 50 states, 4 territories, and the District of Columbia.

Jay Meek, CPA, MBA, Chief Financial Officer
Robert W. Glover, PhD, Executive Director
David Miller, MPAff, Project Director

4703 National Disability Rights Network
820 1st Street NE, Suite 740
Washington, DC 20002   202-408-9514
Fax: 202-408-9520
TTY: 220-408-9521
www.ndrn.org

The National Disability Rights Network (NDRN) works to improve the lives of people with disabilities by guarding against abuse; advocating for basic rights; and ensuring accountability in health care, education, employment, housing, transportation, and within the juvenile and criminal justice systems.

Curtis L. Decker, JD, Executive Director
Janice K. Johnson Hunter, Deputy Executive Director
Eric Buehlmann, Deputy Executive Director

4704 People First International
PO Box 12642
Salem, OR 97309   503-362-0336
Fax: 503-585-0287
e-mail: people1@people1.org
www.people1.org

Developmentally disabled people joining together to learn how to speak for themselves. Offers support, information, assistance and advocacy.

Dennis L Heath, Manager

4705 Rehabilitation Research Training Center on Developmental Disabilities and Health
1640 West Roosevelt Road, M/C 626
Chicago, IL 60608   312-413-1520
800-996-8845
Fax: 312-996-6942
TTY: 312-413-0453
www.rrtcadd.org

The Rehabilitation Research and Training Center on Developmental Disabilities and Health (RRTCDD) has the following goals for people with I/DD: increase understanding of health status, health access, and health behaviors; improve health and function through health promotion interventions; and, improve health care access through integrated care practices.

Tamar Heller, PhD, Center Director
Jasmina Sisirak, PhD, MPH, Associate Director
Erika Magallanes, M.Ed., Business Manager

4706 Research and Training Center on Community Living
204 Pattee Hall, 150 Pillsbury Drive S.E.
Minneapolis, MN 55455   612-624-6328
Fax: 612-625-6619
e-mail: rtc@umn.edu
rtc.umn.edu

The Research and Training Center on Community Living provides research, evaluation, training, technical assistance and dissemination to support the aspirations of persons with developmental disabilities to live full, productive and integrated lives in their communities.

Amy Hewitt, Director

4707 VOR
836 S. Arlington Heights Rd., #351
Elk Grove Village, IL 60007   877-399-4867
Fax: 847-253-0675
e-mail: info@vor.net
www.vor.net

VOR's mission is to advocate for high quality care and human rights for all people with intellectual and developmental disabilities (I/DD).

Ann Knighton, President
Geoffrey Dubrowsky, First Vice President
Julie Huso, Executive Director

4708 Voice of the Retarded
836 S Arlington Heights Road #351
Elk Grove Village, IL 60007   847-399-4VOR
Fax: 605-399-1631
e-mail: info@vor.net
www.vor.net

Voice of the Retarded supports a full range of choices for individuals with mental retardation and their families and guardians. VOR is a national, nonprofit organization that advocates for a full continuum of quality care for persons with mental retardation.

Ann Knighton, President
Geoffrey Dubrowsky, First Vice President
Barbara Cukierski, Treasurer

State Agencies & Support Groups

4709 Center for Family Support
333 7th Avenue, 9th Floor
New York, NY 10001
212-629-7939
Fax: 212-239-2211
www.cfsny.org

The Center for Family Support (CFS) is a not-for-profit human service agency providing support and assistance to individuals with developmental disabilities and traumatic brain injuries throughout New York City, Long Island, the lower Hudson Valley region and New Jersey.

Steven Vernikoff, Executive Director
Barbara Greenwald, Associate Executive Director
Mike Mazzocco, Associate Executive Director

4710 KenCrest Services
502 W Germantown Pike Suite 200
Plymouth Meeting, PA 19462
610-825-9360
Fax: 610-825-4127
www.kencrest.org

Multi-service organization with programs specifically designed for children and youth with developmental disabilities and autism, throughout Pennsylvania, Delaware, & Connecticut.

Bill Nolan, Executive Director
Jim McFalls, Executive Director
Toni McNeal, CFO

Web Sites

4711 American Association on Intellectual and D evelopmental Disabilities
501 3rd Street, NW Suite 200
Washington, DC 20001
202-387-1968
Fax: 202-387-2193
www.aamr.org

AAMR promotes progressive policies, sound research, effective practices, and universal human rights for people with intellectual disabilites.

Hank Bersani PhD, President
Doreen Croser, Executive Director
Danielle Webber, Manager

4712 NADD: National Association for the Dually Diagnosed
132 Fair Street
Kingston, NY 12401
845-331-4336
e-mail: info@thenadd.org
www.thenadd.org

Nonprofit organization designed to promote the interests of professional and care providers for individuals who have the coexistence of mental illness and mental retardation. NADD provides conferences, educational services and training materials to professionals, parents, concerned citizens and service organizations.

Donna McNelis, President
Don Baker, Vice President
Julia Pearce, Secretary

Book Publishers

4713 Art Projects for the Mentally Retarded Child
Ellen J Sussman, author

Charles C Thomas Publishing
2600 South First Street
Springfield, IL 62704
217-789-8980
800-258-8980
Fax: 217-789-9130
e-mail: books@ccthomas.com
www.ccthomas.com

108 pages Softcover
ISBN: 0-398035-35-8

Charles Thomas, Publisher

4714 Children with Mental Retardation
Woodbine House
6510 Bells Mill Road
Bethesda, MD 20817
301-468-8800
800-843-7323
Fax: 301-897-5838
e-mail: info@woodbinehouse.com
www.woodbinehouse.com

A book for parents of children with mild to moderate mental retardation, whether or not they have a diagnosed syndrome or condition. It provides a complete and compassionate introduction to their child's medical, therapeutic, and educational needs, and discusses the emotional impact on the family. New parents can rely on Children with Mental Retardation to provide the solid foundation and confidence they need to help their child reach his or her highest potential.

437 pages Softcover
ISBN: 0-933149-39-5

4715 Music Curriculum Guidelines for Moderately Retarded Adolescents
Charles C Thomas Publishing
2600 S 1st Street
Springfield, IL 62704
217-789-8980
800-258-8980
Fax: 217-789-9130
e-mail: books@ccthomas.com
www.ccthomas.com

122 pages Spiral-Paper
ISBN: 0-398047-57-X

Charles Thomas, Publisher

4716 Retarded Isn't Stupid, Mom!
Sandra Z Kaufman, author

Brookes Publishing
PO Box 10624
Baltimore, MD 21285
410-337-9580
800-638-3775
Fax: 410-337-8539
e-mail: webmaster@brookespublishing.com
www.brookespublishing.com

This book goes through the triumphs and sorrows of one young woman and her family and the emotions and events encountered as her daughter moves toward adulthood.

272 pages Softcover
ISBN: 1-557663-78-5

Paul Brookes, President
Jeff Brookes, President
Melissa A. Behm, Executive Vice President

Magazines

4717 American Journal on Mental Retardation
AAMR
501 3rd Street, NW Suite 200
Washington, DC 20001
202-387-1968
800-424-3688
Fax: 202-387-2193
e-mail: maclean@uwyo.edu
aaidd.org

AAMR promotes progressive policies, sound research, effective practices, and universal human rights for people with intellectual and developmental disabilities.

Margaret A. Nygren, EdD, Executive Director/ CEO
Paul D. Aitken, CPA, Director, Finance & Administration
Kathleen McLane, Director, Publications Program

4718 Mental Retardation
AAMR
501 3rd Street, NW Suite 200
Washington, DC 20001
202-387-1968
Fax: 202-387-2193
e-mail: staylo01@mailbox.syr.edu
www.aamr.org

Provides information on the latest program advances, current research, and information on products and services in the developmental disabilities field.

Bimonthly

Steven J Taylor, Editor

Newsletters

4719 Association for the Help of Retarded Children
83 Maiden Lane
New York, NY 10038 212-780-2500
Fax: 212-777-5893
TTY: 800-662-1220
e-mail: ahrcnyc@dti.net
www.ahrcnyc.org

Developmentally disabled children and adults, their families, and interested individuals. Provides support services, training programs, clinics, schools and residential facilities to the developmentally disabled. Publications: The Chronicle, quarterly newsletter.

Biannually

Laura J Kennedy, President
Gary Lind, Executive Director
Amy West, Chief Financial Officer

4720 NADD Bulletin
132 Fair Street
Kingston, NY 12401 845-331-4336
800-331-5362
Fax: 845-331-4569
e-mail: info@thenadd.org
www.thenadd.org

Official publication of the National Association for the Dually Diagnosed. It features articles that address clinical, programmatic, research or family oriented issues concerning mental health aspects in persons with disabilities.

20 pages Bimonthly

Donna McNelis, President
Don Baker, Vice President
Julia Pearce, Secretary

Camps

4721 Camp Huntington
56 Bruceville Road
High Falls, NY 12440 845-687-7840
855-707-2267
Fax: 845-687-7211
e-mail: camohtgtn@aol.com
www.camphuntington.com

Summer activities include recreational, academic and vocational programs for the learning disabled, neurologically impaired and mildly ADA to mild/moderately retarded. An Olympic pool, horse riding and a special work training program are featured. Programs are tailored to meet individual needs, ages 6-21, and campers may enroll for 4 to 8 weeks.

Dr. Bruria Falik, Director
Michael Bednarz, Executive Director
Alex Mellor, Program Director

4722 Council for Extended Care of Mentally Retarded Citizens
1600 S Hanley Road
Saint Louis, MO 314-781-4950
Fax: 314-781-3850
e-mail: cecmrc@aol.com

Services are provided to adults and children with developmental disabilities. Supported living arrangements are located in St. Louis city and St. Charles County. Group home and camp services are located in Dittmer, MO. Travel program also available.

Cynthia Compton, Executive Director
Marge Lindhorst, Supported Living Director
Angela Jackson, Development Director Camp

4723 Crotched Mountain School & Rehabilitation Center
1 Verney Drive
Greenfield, NH 3047 603-547-3311
800-800-966
Fax: 603-547-3232
e-mail: info@crotchedmountain.org
www.cmf.org

Currently serves children ages 6-22 with multiple-handicaps including: Cerebral Palsy, Spina Bifida, visual and hearing impairments and neurological disabilities, developmental disorders, mental retardation, autism, behavioral and emotional disorders, seizure disorders, spinal cord and head injuries. Member of the National Association of Independent Schools and accredited with the NE Association of Schools and Colleges, Independent Schools of Northern NE.

Donald L Shumway, President & CEO
Tom Zubricki, Chief Financial Officer
Michael Redmond, Senior Vice President

4724 Easter Seal Kysoc
2050 Versailles Road
Lexington, KY 40504 859-254-5701
800-233-3260
Fax: 502-732-0783
e-mail: ek1@cardinalhill.org
www.cardinalhill.org

Designed for the fullest camping experience for children or adults with physical disabilities, blind, deaf, behavior disorders, mental retardation, diabetes and multiple handicaps, ages 7 and up.

Gary Payne, President & CEO
Heide Miller, CCD, CTRS, Director

4725 New Jersey Camp Jaycee
985 Livingston Avenue
North Brunswick, NJ 8902 732-246-2525
Fax: 732-214-1834
e-mail: infor@campjaycee.org
www.campjaycee.org

This camp is for children and adults with mental retardation and is sponsored jointly by the New Jersey Jaycees and the ARC of New Jersey. Activities at the 185-acre Pocono Mountain camp include arts and crafts, games and sports, music, nature, swimming, boating, horseback riding and self-help skills.

Frank Pirrello, President
John O'Brien, Vice President
Patricia Rhein, Secretary

4726 Raven Rock Lutheran Camp
17912 Harbaugh Valley Road
Sabillasville, MD 717-794-2667

Christ-centered program for youth and mentally retarded adults.

Lee Sodowsky

4727 Thorpe Camp
680 Capen Hill Road
Goshen, VT 5733 802-247-6611
e-mail: info@campthorpe.org
www.campthorpe.com

Summer camp for children and adults with special needs.

Description

4728   MICROCEPHALY

Synonyms: Microcephalia, Microcephalism, Microencephaly

Involves the following Biologic System(s):

Neurologic Disorders

Microcephaly is a developmental abnormality in which an infant's or child's head circumference is smaller than would be expected for his or her age and sex (i.e., two or three standard deviations below the mean). In most affected infants and children, underdevelopment of the brain (microencephaly) may result in varying degrees of mental retardation. Microcephaly is considered a relatively common condition, particularly among individuals affected by mental retardation.

In some affected infants and children, microcephaly occurs as an isolated genetic condition. Familial cases of isolated microcephaly have been reported that appear to have autosomal recessive or dominant inheritance. Autosomal recessive microcephaly is characterized by a narrow, sloping forehead; a flat back portion of the head (occiput); varying levels of mental retardation (although severe retardation is most common); and, in some cases, episodes of uncontrolled electrical disturbances in the brain (seizures). Autosomal dominant microcephaly may be characterized by mild slanting of the forehead, upslanting eyelid folds (palpebral fissures), prominent ears, short stature, and borderline or mild mental retardation. In others, the condition occurs in association with certain underlying genetic disorders, such as Cornelia de Lange syndrome. It may also be part of chromosomal malformation syndromes, such as trisomy 13 and trisomy 18 syndromes.

Microcephaly may also occur secondary to particular environmental factors, such as exposure before birth to radiation, certain chemical agents (e.g., alcohol), or certain maternal infections (e.g., rubella). In addition, the condition may result from particular conditions (e.g., meningitis, hyperthermia, etc.) during periods of rapid brain development after birth, particularly during the first two years of life.

When infants and children have a very small head circumference, the underlying abnormality may have begun during early embryonic or fetal development. Although the exact cause is not understood, the condition is thought to result from abnormal development of the outer region of the brain (cerebral cortex).

When infants or children are diagnosed with microcephaly, physicians typically take thorough family histories to determine whether other family members are affected or other disorders or syndromes may be present that are associated with microcephaly. The head circumference is measured periodically for a direct comparison to measurements at birth. Head circumference measurements may also be taken of both parents and any siblings. Additional testing may be undertaken to rule out potential underlying disorders or associated conditions. These tests may include advanced imaging techniques (e.g., CT scanning, MRI) of the brain, chromosomal testing (karyotyping), or certain laboratory tests to detect antibodies against certain infectious agents (e.g., rubella titers) in the child's and mother's bloodstream. Treatment of infants and children with microcephaly includes symptomatic and supportive measures, such as the prescription of certain medications to help treat or control seizures (e.g., anticonvulsants) and special education and other multidisciplinary measures to help ensure that affected children with mental retardation reach their potential. Prenatal screening for genetic defects, and genetic counseling for families at risk for known heritable disorders can decrease the incidence of genetically caused mental retardation. Primary care pediatricians lay an important role in consulting with specialists.

Government Agencies

4729   ARC of the United States
1825 K Street MW, Suite 1200
Washington, DC 20006
                                    202-534-3700
                                    800-433-5255
                              Fax: 202-534-3731
                           e-mail: info@thearc.org
                                   www.thearc.org

The ARC is the national organization of and for people with mental retardation and related developmental disabilities and their families. Devoted to promoting and improving supports and services for people with mental retardation and their families. The association also fosters research and education regarding the prevention of mental retardation in infants and young children. The ARC was founded in 1950 by a small group of parents and other concerned individuals.

Nancy Webster, President
Ronald Brown, VP
Elise McMillan, Secretary

4730   NIH/National Institute of Child Health and Human Development
National Institues of Health
31 Center Drive, Building 31, Room 2A32
Bethesda, MD 20892
                                    301-496-1333
                                    800-370-2943
                              Fax: 866-760-5947
                              TTY: 888-320-6942
      e-mail: NICHDInformationResourceCenter@mail.nih.
                                   www.nichd.nih.gov

Established in 1962 by congress, today the institute conducts and supports research on topics related to the health of children, adults, families and populations. These topics include: developmental disabilities, mental retardation, growth and development, infant death, reproductive health, and rehabilitation.

Jay H Hoofnagle, Director
Lisa Kaeser, Program & Public Liaison

National Associations & Support Groups

4731   American Academy of Pediatrics
141 Northwest Point Boulevard
Elk Grove Village, IL 60007
                                    847-434-4000
                                    800-433-9016
                              Fax: 847-434-8000
                                      www.aap.org

The American Academy of Pediatrics and its member pediatricians are committed to the attainment of optimal physical, mental and social health and well-being for all infants, children, adolescents, and young adults.

Sandra Hassink, MD, FAAP, President

4732   Birth Defect Research for Children
976 Lake Baldwin Lane, Suite 104
Orlando, FL 32814
                                    407-895-0802
                              Fax: 407-895-0824
                        e-mail: staff@birthdefects.org
                                  www.birthdefects.org

Organization that helps families with free birth defect information, parent matching that links families of children with similar defects and research through the National Birth Defect Registry to discover the causes of birth defects. Support group information and newsletter on Internet.

James Murphy, Associate Professor
JD Sherman, Adjunct Professor

4733 Genetic Alliance
4301 Connecticut Avenue NW
Washington, DC 20008   202-966-5557
                                        800-336-4363
                                   Fax: 202-966-8553
                    e-mail: info@geneticalliance.org
                          www.geneticalliance.org

A coalition of voluntary genetic support groups, consumers and
professionals addressing the needs of individuals and families affected by genetic disorders from a national perspective.

Joan Oppenheimer Weiss, Founder
Sharon Terry, President

4734 March of Dimes Birth Defects Foundation
1275 Mamaroneck Avenue
White Plains, NY 10605   914-997-4488
                                        888-663-4637
                                   Fax: 914-428-8203
                  e-mail: answers@marchofdimes.com
                          www.marchofdimes.com

Partnership of volunteers and professionals dedicates to improving the health of babies by preventing birth defects and infant
mortality. Over 100 chapters are located across the country and
can be located through the National Office.

Jennifer L Howse, President

4735 National Dissemination Center for Children with Disabilities
1825 Connecticut Avenue NW, Suite 700
Washington, DC 20009   202-884-8200
                                        800-695-0285
                                   Fax: 202-884-8441
                       e-mail: nichcy@fhi360.org
                          www.nichcy.org

A national information and referral center that provides information on disabilities and disability-related issues for families, educators and other professionals.

Suzanne Ripley, Executive Director

Web Sites

4736 Online Mendelian Inheritance in Man
8600 Rockville Pike
Bethesda, MD 20894   301-594-5983
                                        888-346-3656
                                   Fax: 301-402-1384
                                   TDD: 800-735-2258
                    e-mail: custserv@nlm.nih.gov
                          www.ncbi.nlm.nih.gov

This database is a catalog of human genes and genetic disorders.

Christine E Seidman M.D, Chairman
David J Lipman M.D, Executive Secretary
Scott Edwards, Member

Description

4737 **MICRODONTIA**

Synonym: Microdontism

Involves the following Biologic System(s):

Dental Disorders

Microdontia is a term that refers to a developmental dental ir-regularity in which one or more teeth are abnormally small. This tooth abnormality often occurs in association with cer-tain disorders, conditions, and syndromes and usually affects a single tooth or specific groups of teeth, namely the second or lateral incisors and the molars of the upper jaw. However, in rare instances, microdontia occurs in association with cer-tain other disorders and may affect all or most of the teeth. These other disorders may include pituitary dwarfism, Down's syndrome, and certain forms of congenital heart dis-ease.

Children with certain abnormalities of the face or skull (craniofacial defects) may often exhibit some form of microdontia. These disorders include Turner syndrome, a chromosomal disorder affecting females and characterized by various symptoms including a narrow palate and a small jaw (micrognathia); Crouzon's disease, an autosomal dominant disorder characterized by underdevelopment of the upper jaw and protrusion of the lower jaw (prognathism), a beaked nose, and other symptoms; and cleft lip, a congenital defect in which there is a split or fissure (cleft) in the upper lip. Microdontia is also manifested in several other disorders (e.g., focal dermal hypoplasia, progeria, oculomandibulodyscephaly, oculo-auriculo-vertebral anom-aly, and others). Small teeth with a characteristic cone shape are often present in conjunction with missing teeth (anodontia) in certain syndromes known as ectodermal dysplasias, in which there is abnormal development of embry-onic tissues that give rise to tooth enamel, hair, nails, skin glands, the outermost layer of the skin (epidermis), the ner-vous system, the ears and eyes, and mucous membranes of the anus and mouth. Other syndromes that involve microdontia include Williams syndrome, in which the second primary mo-lar of the upper jaw is abnormally small. Aglossia-adactylia syndrome is characterized by partial or total absence of the tongue and missing or abnormally small incisors in the lower jaw.

Microdontia is thought to be genetically transmitted and re-sults from an unknown factor or factors that affect the normal development of the main component of teeth (dentin) and their outermost covering (enamel). This condition is slightly more prevalent in females than males. Treatment may include oral surgery, orthodontic procedures, tooth restoration, and the use of implants or other dental appliances.

Government Agencies

4738 **NIH/National Institute of Child Health and Human Development**
31 Center Drive, Building 31, Room 2A32
Bethesda, MD 20892

301-496-1333
800-370-2943
Fax: 866-760-5947
TTY: 888-320-6942
e-mail: NICHDInformationResourceCenter@mail.nih.
www.nichd.nih.gov

Established in 1962 by congress, today the institute conducts and supports research on topics related to the health of children, adults, families and populations. Some of these topics include: developmental disabilities, growth and development, infant death, reproductive health and birth defects.

Jay H Hoofnagle, Director
Lisa Kaeser, Program & Public Liaison

4739 **NIH/National Institute of Dental and Crani ofacial Research**
National Institutes of Health
31 Center Drive, MSC 2290, Building 31
Bethesda, MD 20892

301-496-3571
866-232-4528
Fax: 301-480-4098
e-mail: nidcrinfo@mail.nih.gov
www.nidcr.nih.gov

Provides leadership for a national research program designed to understand, treat and prevent the infectious and inherited craniofacial-oral-dental diseases and disorders.

Dr Lawrence A Tabak, Director
Thomas G Murphy, Acting Executive Director

National Associations & Support Groups

4740 **American Academy of Pediatrics**
141 Northwest Point Boulevard
Elk Grove Village, IL 60007

847-434-4000
800-433-9016
Fax: 847-434-8000
www.aap.org

The American Academy of Pediatrics and its member pediatri-cians are committed to the attainment of optimal physical, mental and social health and well-being for all infants, children, adoles-cents, and young adults.

Sandra Hassink, MD, FAAP, President

4741 **American Dental Association**
211 E Chicago Avenue
Chicago, IL 60611

312-440-2500
Fax: 312-440-7494
www.ada.org

Professional association of dentists committed to the public's oral health, ethics, science and professional advancement; leading a unified profession through initiatives in advocacy, education, research and the development of standards.

Kathleen O'Loughlin, Executive Director

Web Sites

4742 **American Dental Association**
211 East Chicago Ave
Chicago, IL 60611

312-440-2500
e-mail: affiliates@ada.org
www.ada.org

Professional association of dentists committed to the public's oral health, ethics, science and professional advancement; leading a unified profession through initiatives in advocacy, education, research and the development of standards.

Dr. Maxine Feinberg, President
Dr. Carol Gomez Summerhays, President-Elect:
Dr. Kathleen T O'Loughlin, Executive Director

4743 **Dental Consumer Advisory**
toothinfo.com/

Purpose is to provide useful and practical information for the public concerning issues of dental care.

4744 **Dental Resources on the Web**
dental-resources.com/

Dental sites for education, practices, laboratories, office supplies, dental care and associations.

Description

4745 MIGRAINE HEADACHES

Covers these related disorders: Common migraine (Migraine without aura), Classic migraine (Migraine with aura)

Involves the following Biologic System(s):
Developmental/Behavioral/Psychiatric Disorders

The term migraine refers to a headache that is recurring and accompanied by three or more symptoms or findings that include the presence of certain visual, motor, or other sensations (aura or prodrome) preceding onset; head throbbing; pain on one side of the head (unilateral); nausea; vomiting; and abdominal pain. Additional associated findings include cessation of pain following sleep and a history of migraines in other family members. Migraines are the most common type of recurrent headaches that occur among children. In children younger than 10 years of age, boys are slightly more apt to develop migraines, while adolescent girls and adult females are more prone to migraines than are adolescent boys or adult men. Migraines may be caused by several different factors, alone or in combination. Such factors include genetic influences; stress-related factors; certain foods such as chocolate, citrus fruit, cheese, monosodium glutamate, etc.; red wine; stimuli such as bright lights, loud noises, etc.; medications such as birth control pills; menstruation; and other factors. Pain associated with migraines results from the narrowing and subsequent widening of the arteries that lead to the brain. This action triggers the pain receptors in that region, thus producing the characteristic pain of migraine headaches. More recent theories relate to the role played by the nervous system in the development of migraine headaches. It has been found that nerve cells in blood vessels of the migraine patient release a compound called "substance P." Substance P triggers pain and its release into the arteries is associated with the dilation of blood vessels and the release of histamine and other allergic compounds.

Migraine without aura (formerly called common migraine), is the type of migraine most likely to occur in children. Common migraine is characterized by a pounding or throbbing pain in the front or side(s) of the head. This headache may or may not be one-sided, may persist from one to 24 hours, and is usually accompanied by nausea, vomiting, and abdominal pain. Other associated symptoms may include fever, an unusual sensitivity to light (photophobia), numbness or tingling of the hands and feet, and dizziness or lightheadedness.

Migraine with aura (formerly called classic migraine), is characterized by similar symptoms and findings to those associated with common migraine; however, classic migraine is always preceded by an aura that occurs from 10 to 30 minutes before onset of the headache. This phenomenon may be characterized by visual, motor, or other sensations such as the appearance of shimmering or flashing lights (photopsia) as well as distorted images, loss of vision in part of the visual field (blind spot or scotoma), dizziness, tingling or weakness in an arm or leg, prickling or burning sensation around the mouth, and other irregularities.

In addition to the two primary types of migraine headaches, some children may develop unusual migraine headaches, called migraine variants, that may be characterized by vomiting that recurs at irregular intervals, sudden attacks of dizzi-

ness, and confusion. Children with this type of migraine, especially infants, may experience monthly episodes of severe vomiting resulting in excessive fluid loss (dehydration); the loss of essential compounds, known as electrolytes, in the fluid portion of the blood (i.e., sodium, calcium, and potassium); and associated fever, abdominal pain, and diarrhea. Children with migraine variants may at times appear disoriented, hyperactive, and nonresponsive. Other types of migraine include complicated migraine and cluster headaches. Complicated migraines refer to migraine headaches accompanied by neurologic findings that persist beyond the headache and may be further categorized as basilar migraine, ophthalmoplegic migraine, and hemiplegic migraine. These types of headaches may sometimes indicate the presence of an underlying lesion. Basilar migraine is characterized by problems with equilibrium, double or blurred vision, loss of vision in part of the visual field, lack of muscular coordination (ataxia), seizures, or other irregularities. Ophthalmoplegic migraine, which is characterized by paralysis of the eye muscles on the same side as the migraine, does not commonly occur in children. Amaurosis fugax, a variant of complicated migraine, is characterized by reversible blindness or partial blindness in one eye. Hemiplegic migraine is characterized by numbness and muscular weakness or paralysis affecting only one side of the body. It is rare for children to experience more than one hemiplegic migraine episode. Cluster headaches do not commonly occur in children.

Treatment for migraine headaches may first be directed toward prevention by identifying and removing or avoiding stimulating influences such as certain foods, medications, or underlying stress factors. Many children may benefit from simply resting in a quiet, darkened room. Treatment for pain and vomiting associated with migraine headaches may include administration of pain relievers such as acetaminophen or ibuprofen along with drugs to reduce vomiting (antiemetics). These drugs are often administered rectally in suppository form. In more severe episodes, older children and adolescents may require the administration of a preparation called ergotamine, which is most effective if taken during the early stages of the migraine episode. Ergotamine should not be administered to children with hemiplegic migraines. Some children and adolescents may benefit from behavior management therapy. Other treatment is symptomatic and supportive.

Government Agencies

4746 NIH/National Eye Institute
31 Center Drive MSC 2510
Bethesda, MD 20892
                                             301-496-5248
                                   e-mail: 2020@nei.nih.gov
                                              www.nei.nih.gov

Conducts and supports research that helps prevent and treat eye diseases and other disorders of vision. This research leads to sight-saving treatments, reduces visual impairment and blindness, and improves the quality of life for people of all ages. NEI-supported research has advanced our knowledge of how the eye functions in health and disease.

Paul A Sieving M.D., Ph.D., Director

National Associations & Support Groups

4747 American Academy of Neurology
1080 Montreal Avenue Ste 100
Saint Paul, MN 55116
651-695-1940
800-879-1960
Fax: 651-695-2791
e-mail: memberservices@aan.com
www.aan.com

Medical society established to advance the art and science of neurology, and thereby promote the best possible care for patients with neurological disorders by: ensuring appropriate access to neurological care, supporting and advocating for an environment which ensures ethical, high quality neurological care and supporting clinical and basic research in the neurosciences and related fields.

19,000 members

Catherine Rydell, CEO
Timonthy A. Pedley, President
Stephen Sergay, President Elect

4748 American Academy of Pediatrics
141 Northwest Point Boulevard
Elk Grove Village, IL 60007
847-434-4000
800-433-9016
Fax: 847-434-8000
www.aap.org

The American Academy of Pediatrics and its member pediatricians are committed to the attainment of optimal physical, mental and social health and well-being for all infants, children, adolescents, and young adults.

Sandra Hassink, MD, FAAP, President

4749 American Headache Society
19 Mantua Road
Mount Royal, NJ 8061
856-423-0043
Fax: 856-423-0082
e-mail: ahshg@talley.com
www.americanheadachesociety.org

A professional society of health care providers dedicated to the study and treatment of headache and face pain. It was founded in 1959 and sponsors the American Council for Headache Education (ACHE), which will soon become a committee of the AHS.

Paul Winner, Chair
Linda McGillicuddy, Executive Director
Fred Sheftell, MD, President

4750 Migraine Awareness Group: National Understanding for Migraineurs (MAGNUM)
100 N Union Street, Suite B
Alexandria, VA 22314
703-349-1929
Fax: 703-739-2432
e-mail: comments@migraines.org
www.migraines.org

Works to bring public awareness, utilizing the electronic, print, and artistic mediums, to the fact that Migraine is a true, biologic disease. Advocates on behalf of Migraine head pain sufferers worldwide.

Michael John Coleman, Founder/Executive Director
Terri Miller-Burchfield, Executive VP
Doug Johnson, Webmaster

4751 National Headache Foundation
820 N Orleans, Ste 217
Chicago, IL 60610
312-274-2650
888-643-5552
Fax: 312-640-9049
e-mail: info@headaches.org
www.headaches.org

Nonprofit organization dedicated to the education of headache sufferers and health care professionals about the causes and treatment of headaches.

Seymour Diamond, Chairman/Founder
Roger K. Cady MD, Vice President
Edmond J. Bergeron, Treasurer

Research Centers

4752 Kennedy Krieger Institute
Pediatric Headache Program
707 N Broadway
Baltimore, MD 21205
443-923-9200
800-873-3377
e-mail: webmaster@kennedykrieger.org
www.kennedykrieger.org

The Pediatric Headache Program was started in 2005 in order to facilitate the diagnosis, treatment and management of children and adolescents who suffer from persistent headaches, including migraine, tension and chronic daily.

John J Laterra, Program Clinical Coordinator
Terri Holbrook, Neurology/Nursing Staff Coordinator

Web Sites

4753 American Academy of Neurology
201 Chicago Avenue
Minneapolis, MN 55415
800-879-1960
Fax: 612-454-2746
e-mail: memberservices@aan.com
www.aan.com

Medical society established to advance the art and science of neurology, and therby promote the best possible care for patients with neurological disordes by: ensuring appropriate access to neurological care, supporting and advocating for an environment which ensures ethical, high quality neurological care and supporting clinical and basic research in the neurosciences and reltated fields.

4754 Migraine Awareness Group: A National Understanding for Migraineurs
100 North Union Street, Suite B
Alexandria, VI 22314
e-mail: comments@migraines.org
www.migraines.org

Brings public awareness to the fact that Migraine is a true, biological neurological disease using the electronic, print and artistic mediums of expression.

Michael John Coleman, President
Terri Miller Burchfield, Executive VP
P. Elizabeth Pirsch, General Council

4755 National Headache Foundation
820 N Orleans, Suite 411
Chicago, IL 60610
312-274-3650
888-643-5552
e-mail: info@headches.com
www.headches.org

A nonprofit organization dedicated to educating headache sufferers and healthcare professionals about headache causes and treatments.

Seymour Diamond, Executive Chairman
Arthur H. Elkind MD, President
Vincent Martin MD, Vice President

Book Publishers

4756 Freedom From Headaches
Joel Saper, author

Simon & Schuster
100 Front Street
Riverside, NJ 8075
856-461-6500
800-223-2336
Fax: 212-698-7099
www.simonandschuster.com

236 pages paperback
ISBN: 0-671254-04-9

Carolyn Reidy, President and Chief Executive Offic
Liz Perl, Senior Vice President, Marketing
Dennis Eulau, Executive Vice President, Operation

4757 Handbook of Headache
Lippincott Williams & Wilkins
351 W Camden Street
Baltimore, MD 21201   410-528-4000
                                   800-638-3030
                                   www.lww.com

2004 400 pages softbound
ISBN: 0-781752-23-0

Edward B. Hutton Jr., Chief Executive Officer, President
E. Passano Jr., Vice Chairman of the Board and Secr

4758 Headache Book: Prevention & Treatment for All Types of Headaches
Frank B. Minirth, author

Thomas Nelson Publishers
1 Gateway Plaza
Port Chester, NY 10573   914-937-2320
                                   Fax: 914-937-3183
                                   www.fsw.org

1994
ISBN: 0-785282-56-4

Susan B. Wayne, President/CEO
Geoffrey Barsky, CFO
Polly Kerrigan, Senior Vice President Program Opera

4759 Management of Headache & Headache Medications
Lawrence D. Robbins, author

Spring-Verlag
175 5th Avenue
New York, NY 10010   646-307-5151
                                   Fax: 212-633-0748
                                   www.us.macmillan.com

1994 294 pages
ISBN: 0-387989-44-7

Stefan von Holtzbrinck, Chairman, Executive Board
Klaus-Dieter Lehmann, Chairman, Supervisory Board
Sandra Dittert, Senior Vice President

4760 Migraine and Other Headaches: Vascular Mechanisms
Raven Press
19710 Ventura Blvd., Ste 108
Woodland Hills, CA 91364   818-888-3388
                                   Fax: 818-888-1881
                                   www.raven.com

Leading international experts present new concepts on the mechanisms of migraine and other vascular headaches and detail the latest strategies for diagnosis and treatment of migraine with and without aura, tension-type headaches, cluster headaches and other vascular disorders.

368 pages
ISBN: 0-881677-95-7

4761 Overcoming Headaches & Migraines
Longmeadow Press
PO Box 10218
Stamford, CT 06904   203-352-2110

1993 128 pages Paperback
ISBN: 0-681417-92-7

4762 Treating the Headache Patient
Roger K. Cady, author

Marcell Dekker, Inc.
270 Madison Avenue
New York, NY 10016   212-696-9000
                                   Fax: 800-228-1160

1994 366 pages
ISBN: 0-824791-09-6

4763 Wolff's Headaches & Other Head Pain
Stephen D. Silberstein, author

Oxford University Press
198 Madison Avenue
New York, NY 10016   212-726-6000
                                   800-445-9714
                                   Fax: 919-677-1303
                                   e-mail: custserv.us@oup.com
                                   www.us.oup.com/us

1993
ISBN: 0-195082-50-8

Newsletters

4764 Headache
American Council for Headache Education
19 Mantua Road
Mount Royal, NJ 8061   856-423-0043
                                   Fax: 856-423-0082
                                   e-mail: achehq@talley.com
                                   www.achenet.org

Provides valuable and current information on new treatments, as well as time-proven headache management strategies. All articles are written or reviewed by headache experts from the American Headache Society (AHS). Recent issues have included articles by headache experts on drug and nondrug treatment options and information on new treatments and research is regularly included.

12 pages Quarterly

Paul Winner, Chair
Arthur H. Elkind MD, President
Vincent Martin MD, Vice President

4765 NHF Head Lines
National Headache Foundation
820 N Orleans, Suite 411
Chicago, IL 60610   312-274-3650
                                   888-643-5552
                                   e-mail: info@headches.org
                                   www.headaches.org

Offers the latest information on headaches, causes and treatments. Contains news on drugs and medical forums, in-depth discussions of headaches and preventions and a question and answer section in which physicians respond to reader inquiries and support group information.

Bimonthly

Seymour Diamond, Executive Chairman
Arthur H. Elkind MD, President
Vincent Martin MD, Vice President

Pamphlets

4766 52 Proven Stress Reducers
National Headache Foundation
820 N Orleans, Suite 411
Chicago, IL 60610   312-274-3650
                                   888-643-5552
                                   Fax: 773-525-7357
                                   e-mail: info@headches.com
                                   www.headaches.org

Seymour Diamond, Executive Chairman
Arthur H. Elkind MD, President
Vincent Martin MD, Vice President

4767 About Headaches
National Headache Foundation
820 N Orleans, Suite 411
Chicago, IL 60610   312-274-3650
                                   888-643-5552
                                   Fax: 312-640-9049
                                   e-mail: info@headches.com
                                   www.headaches.org

Contains an in-depth look at headaches, tips on when to seek medical advice, methods of treatment and more.

16 pages

Seymour Diamond, Executive Chairman
Arthur H. Elkind MD, President
Vincent Martin MD, Vice President

4768 Analgesic Rebound Headaches-Fact Sheet
National Headache Foundation
820 N Orleans, Suite 411
Chicago, IL 60610
312-274-3650
888-643-5552
Fax: 312-640-9049
e-mail: info@headaches.org
www.headaches.org

Offers information on analgesic agents or drugs used to control pain including migraine and other types of headaches.

Seymour Diamond, Executive Chairman
Arthur H. Elkind MD, President
Vincent Martin MD, Vice President

4769 Cluster Headache-Fact Sheet
National Headache Foundation
820 N Orleans, Suite 411
Chicago, IL 60610
312-274-3650
888-643-5552
Fax: 312-640-9049
e-mail: info@headaches.org
www.headaches.org

Offers information on cluster headaches and the treatment available for them.

Seymour Diamond, Executive Chairman
Arthur H. Elkind MD, President
Vincent Martin MD, Vice President

4770 Diet and Headache-Fact Sheet
National Headache Foundation
820 N Orleans, Suite 411
Chicago, IL 60610
312-274-3650
888-643-5552
Fax: 312-640-9049
e-mail: info@headaches.org
www.headaches.org

Offers information on what foods should be avoided, and what foods trigger headaches in all migraine sufferers.

Seymour Diamond, Executive Chairman
Arthur H. Elkind MD, President
Vincent Martin MD, Vice President

4771 Headache Facts-What Everyone Should Know
American Council for Headache Education
19 Mantua Road
Mount Royal, NJ 8061
856-423-0043
Fax: 856-423-0082
e-mail: achehq@talley.com
www.achenet.org

Paul Winner, DO, Chair
Barry Baumel, Chair Of Funding Committee
John Rothrock, Journal Editor

4772 Headache Handbook
National Headache Foundation
820 N Orleans, Suite 411
Chicago, IL 60610
312-274-2650
888-643-5552
Fax: 312-640-9049
e-mail: info@headaches.org
www.headaches.org

Gives information and coauses on five common types of headaches as well as treatments available.

8 pages

Arthur H. Elkind MD, President
Vincent Marin, M.D., Vice President
Chad Beste, Treasurer

4773 Headache Q & A
National Headache Foundation
820 N Orleans, Suite 411
Chicago, IL 60610
312-274-2650
888-643-5552
Fax: 312-640-9049
e-mail: info@headaches.org
www.headaches.org

Handy, fact-filled card contains the most frequently asked questions and answers concerning headache triggers and treatments.

Arthur H. Elkind MD, President
Vincent Marin, M.D., Vice President
Chad Beste, Treasurer

4774 Headache in Children-Fact Sheet
National Headache Foundation
820 N Orleans, Suite 411
Chicago, IL 60610
312-274-2650
888-643-5552
Fax: 312-640-9049
e-mail: info@headaches.org
www.headaches.org

Offers information on vascular headaches, tension-type headaches, traction and inflammatory headaches and treatment.

Arthur H. Elkind MD, President
Vincent Marin, M.D., Vice President
Chad Beste, Treasurer

4775 How to Talk to Your Doctor About Headaches
National Headache Foundation
820 N Orleans, Suite 411
Chicago, IL 60610
312-274-2650
888-643-5552
Fax: 312-640-9049
e-mail: info@headaches.com
www.headaches.org

Learn how to keep a headache diary to pinpoint symptoms and effective diagnosis.

Arthur H. Elkind MD, President
Vincent Marin, M.D., Vice President
Chad Beste, Treasurer

4776 Impact of Migraine-A Disabling and Costly Condition
American Council for Headache Education
19 Mantua Road
Mount Royal, NJ 8061
856-423-0043
Fax: 856-423-0082
e-mail: achehq@talley.com
www.achenet.org

Paul Winner, DO, Chair
Barry Baumel, Chair Of Funding Committee
John Rothrock, Journal Editor

4777 Migraine and Coexisting Conditions-Other Illnesses That May Affect Migraine
American Council for Headache Education
19 Mantua Road
Mount Royal, NJ 8061
856-423-0043
Fax: 856-423-0082
e-mail: achehq@talley.com
www.achenet.org

Paul Winner, DO, Chair
Barry Baumel, Chair Of Funding Committee
John Rothrock, Journal Editor

4778 Migraine-Fact Sheet
National Headache Foundation
820 N Orleans, Suite 411
Chicago, IL 60610
312-274-2650
888-643-5552
Fax: 312-640-9049
e-mail: info@headaches.com
www.headaches.org

Offers information on migraines and treatments.

Arthur H. Elkind MD, President
Vincent Marin, M.D., Vice President
Chad Beste, Treasurer

4779 Tap the Best Resource
National Headache Foundation
820 N Orleans, Suite 411
Chicago, IL 60610

312-274-2650
888-643-5552
Fax: 312-640-9049
e-mail: info@headaches.org
www.headaches.org

Informational brochure offering facts and statistics on headaches.
Everything from muscle contraction, vascular headaches, sinus
headaches, TMJ, and much more.

Arthur H. Elkind MD, President
Vincent Marin, M.D., Vice President
Chad Beste, Treasurer

4780 What's the Best Medicine for My Headaches?
American Council for Headache Education
19 Mantua Road
Mount Royal, NJ 8061

856-423-0043
Fax: 856-423-0082
e-mail: achehq@talley.com
www.achenet.org

Paul Winner, DO, Chair
Barry Baumel, Chair Of Funding Committee
John Rothrock, Journal Editor

**4781 When Are Opioid (Narcotic) Drugs Appropriate for
Headache?**
American Council for Headache Education
19 Mantua Road
Mount Royal, NJ 8061

856-423-0043
Fax: 856-423-0082
e-mail: achehq@talley.com
www.achenet.org

Paul Winner, DO, Chair

4782 Women and Headache
American Council for Headache Education
19 Mantua Road
Mount Royal, NJ 8061

856-423-0043
Fax: 856-423-0082
e-mail: achehq@talley.com
www.achenet.org

Paul Winner, DO, Chair

Description

4783 MILK PROTEIN ALLERGY/LACTOSE INTOLERANCE

Involves the following Biologic System(s):

Gastrointestinal Disorders

Milk protein allergy is an allergic reaction to the proteins found in cow's milk and is the most common food allergy in children. Cow's milk is a large source of nutrition for infants and children. Infant formulas are primarily composed of cow's milk proteins, and milk products are often a major source of calories, protein, vitamins, and minerals in a child's diet. Cow's milk contains proteins, sugars (carbohydrates), as well as fats. Breastmilk can also contain these proteins from the mother's diet. There are several distinct diseases entities that would fall under the category of milk allergy or intolerance.

Most infants show symptoms of cow's milk protein allergy within the first three to six months of exposure. The immune system of the infant recognizes the milk protein as foreign and reacts by making immune proteins (antibodies also known as immunoglobulins) to defend the body against the foreign protein. Milk protein allergy can be either an immediate-onset or delayed-onset allergic reaction. Immediate-onset reactions can manifest acutely with gastrointestinal (diarrhea, vomiting, abdominal pain), respiratory (asthma, wheezing), or dermatologic (eczema, hives) symptoms. Delayed-onset reactions usually manifest with chronic diarrhea that may be bloody (hematochezia). More severe disease leads to small bowel damage and poor weight gain (failure to thrive).

The diagnosis of milk protein allergy can be made by history and physical exam. Stool, blood, skin and/or milk challenge tests may also be used to aid in diagnosis. Milk protein allergy is reported in up to 4% of infants, and usually resolves by age three. Until that time, infants on formula are fed special formulas (hydrolysate formula) and breastfeeding mothers should avoid milk and milk products. Infants with cow's milk protein allergy have a higher chance of having soy milk protein allergy and therefore soy formulas are not recommended. As children get older, milk is slowly reintroduced. Fortunately, most babies outgrow their milk allergies by their second or third year.

Lactose intolerance is not an allergic reaction, but an inability to digest the primary sugar found in milk (lactose). In the small intestine there is an enzyme (lactase) that breaks lactose down into smaller sugars to be used by the body. Symptoms of lactose intolerance include abdominal cramping, bloating, diarrhea, and flatulence. There are large racial differences in the incidence of lactose intolerance; persons of Asian and African descent have a higher incidence in comparison to Caucasians.

Symptoms of lactose intolerance can occur any time after age 5 because lactase enzyme activity peaks in infancy and early childhood. One exception is congenital lactase deficiency. In this genetic disorder, infants are born without the enzyme lactase and symptoms, such as abdominal bloating and diarrhea, occur in the first week of life.

The treatment for lactose intolerance is avoidance of milk or lactase enzyme supplementation (available in pill form or added to milk products).

National Associations & Support Groups

4784 American Academy of Pediatrics
141 Northwest Point Boulevard
Elk Grove Village, IL 60007
847-434-4000
800-433-9016
Fax: 847-434-8000
www.aap.org

The American Academy of Pediatrics and its member pediatricians are committed to the attainment of optimal physical, mental and social health and well-being for all infants, children, adolescents, and young adults.

Sandra Hassink, MD, FAAP, President

4785 International Foundation for Functional Gastrointestinal Disorders (IFFGD)
700 W. Virginia St., #201
Milwaukee, WI 53217
414-964-1799
888-964-2001
Fax: 414-964-7176
e-mail: iffgd@iffgd.org
www.iffgd.org

A nonprofit education and research organization founded in 1991. IFFGD addresses the issues surrounding life with gastrointestinal functional and motility disorders and increases the awareness about these disorders among the general public, researchers, and the clinical care community.

Nancy J Norton, Founder
William Norton, VP
Michael Cohen, Director

4786 North American Society for Pediatric Gastroenterology/Hepatology/Nutrition
PO Box 6
Flourtown, PA 19031
215-233-0808
Fax: 215-233-3918
e-mail: naspghan@naspghan.org
www.naspghan.org

Strives to improve the care of infants, children and adolescents with digestive disorders by promoting advances in clinical care of children with chronic abdominal pain, diarrhea, constipation, vomiting, bleeding from the GI tract, inflammatory bowel disease, liver diseases, diseases of the pancreas, poor weight gain and nutritional problems.

Margaret K Stallings, Executive Director
Kate Ho, Associate Director
Kim Rose, Membership Coordinator

4787 Parents of Galactosemic Children
P.O. Box 2401
Mandeville, LA 70470
228-497-5886
866-900-7421
e-mail: president@galactosemia.org
www.galactosemia.org

A nonprofit national organization founded in 1985 by a small group of mothers in New York. It offers support and educational information to galactosemic families and facilitates communication between them and professionals.

Michelle Fowler, President
Diane Flynn, Secretary
Paul Fowler, Treasurer

Web Sites

4788 Galactosemia Resources and Information
P.O. Box 1512
Deerfield Beach, FL 33443
215-233-0808
866-900-7421
Fax: 215-233-3939
e-mail: scott.shepard@galactosemia.org
galactosemia.org

A repository for information about galactosemia and a jumping-off point to other places on the web.

Scott Shepard, President
Scott Saylor, Vice-President
Paul Fowler, Treasurer

4789 International Foundation for Functional Gastrointestinal Disorders (IFFGD)
700 W. Virginia St., #201
Milwaukee, WI 53204
414-964-1799
888-964-2001
Fax: 414-964-7176
e-mail: iffgd@iffgd.org
www.iffgd.org

Nancy J. Norton, President
William Norton, Vice President
Eleanor Cautley, Vice President

4790 NASPGHAN
PO Box 6
Flourtown, PA 19031
215-233-0808
Fax: 215-233-3918
e-mail: naspghan@naspghan.org
www.naspghan.org

Offering information on pediatric gastroenterology, hepatology and nutrition.

Carlo Di Lorenzo, MD, President
James Heubi, MD, President-Elect
Michael Narkewicz, MD, Secretary-Treasurer

4791 Parents of Galactosemic Children
P.O. Box 1512
Deerfield Beach, FL 33443
866-900-7421
e-mail: scott.shepard@galactosemia.org
galactosemia.org

Offering support and educational information to galactosemic families and interested professionals.

Scott Shepard, President
Scott Saylor, Vice-President
Paul Fowler, Treasurer

Book Publishers

4792 Raising Your Child Without Milk: Reassuring Advice and Recipes For Parent
Simon & Simon
100 Front Street
Riverside, NJ 08075
856-461-6500
800-488-4308
Fax: 800-943-9831
e-mail: info@simonsays.com
www.simonandschuster.com

This book offers parents of milk-allergic or lactose intolerant children and the most up-to-date medical and nutritional information. It contains 125 dairy free recipes, and answers questions sent in from parents across the country.

384 pages Paperback

Carolyn Reidy, President/CEO
Liz Perl, Senior Vice President, Marketing
Dennis Eulau, Executive Vice President, Operation

4793 Why Does Milk Bother Me?
NDDIC
2 Information Way
Bethesda, MD 20892
800-891-5389
Fax: 703-738-4929
e-mail: nddic@info.niddk.nih.gov
www2.niddk.nih.gov

Defines lactose intolerance and provides information on symptoms, diagnosis and treatment.

16 pages

Griffin P. Rodgers, M.D, Chairman, Executive Board
Brent B. Stanfield, Executive Secretary
Camille M. Hoover, M.S.W, Executive Officer

Journals

4794 Managing Food Allergy and Intolerance
Janice Vickerstaff Joneja, PhD, author

J A Hall Publications
2401-9304 Salish Court
Burnaby, BC
Canada
604-738-9688
888-993-6133
Fax: 604-738-9425
e-mail: info@hallpublications.com
www.hallpublications.com

This is a fully-referenced, extensively researched and indexed manual for health care professionals counseling those with food allergy or intolerance.

581 pages
ISBN: 0-968209-80-7

Newsletters

4795 NASPGHAN News
PO Box 6
Flourtown, PA 19031
215-233-0808
Fax: 215-233-3918
e-mail: naspghan@naspghan.org
www.naspghan.org

Publication of the North American Society for Pediatric Gastroenterolgy, Hepatology and Nutrition, which strives to improve the care of infants, children and adolescents with digestive disorders by promoting advances in clinical care of children with chronic abdominal pain, diarrhea, constipation, vomiting, bleeding from the GI tract, inflammatory bowel disease, liver diseases, diseases of the pancreas, poor weight gain and nutritional problems.

Carlo Di Lorenzo, MD, President
James Heubi, MD, President-Elect
Michael Narkewicz, MD, Secretary-Treasurer

Pamphlets

4796 Lactose Intolerance
NDDIC
2 Information Way
Bethesda, MD 20892
301-496-3583
800-891-5389
Fax: 703-738-4929
e-mail: nddic@info.niddk.nih.gov
www.niddk.nih.gov

8 pages

Griffin P. Rodgers, M.D., Director
Dr. Gregory Germino, Deputy Director
Kevin Abbott, Program Director

Description

4797 MUCOLIPIDOSES

Synonym: ML

Involves the following Biologic System(s):

Genetic/Chromosomal/Syndrome/Metabolic Disorders

The mucolipidoses (ML) are inborn errors of metabolism that belong to a group of diseases known as lysosomal storage disorders. Lysosomes are the major digestive structures within cells. Certain proteins known as enzymes break down or digest nutrients, such as particular fats or carbohydrates. The mucolipidoses are characterized by a deficiency or the abnormal functioning of certain lysosomal enzymes, causing the abnormal accumulation of complex carbohydrates (glycosaminoglycans) and fats (lipids) in cells within particular tissues. Such tissues may include those of the brain and spinal cord (central nervous system), skeleton, joints, heart, liver, spleen, or eyes. The mucolipidoses are thought to be inherited as an autosomal recessive trait.

Specific names as well as Roman numerals are used to classify the different forms of ML. Different types of mucolipidosis include I-Cell disease (ML II), pseudo-Hurler polydystrophy (ML III), and Berman syndrome (ML IV). Some forms of ML are further divided into different subtypes, such as sialidosis (ML I) types I and II, based on age of onset, associated symptoms, or other factors.

In children with mucolipidosis, associated symptoms and findings may be variable, depending upon the specific form of ML that is present. However, certain abnormalities occur in association with most forms of ML. Such findings include mild to severe coarsening of facial features, characteristic skeletal abnormalities (known as dysostosismultiplex), changes of the joints, and varying levels of mental retardation. In children with ML, skeletal malformations may include short stature; abnormal front-to-back or sideways curvature of the spine (kyphosis or scoliosis) or both; improper development of the hips (hip dysplasia); abnormally short neck; or premature fusion of the fibrous joints (sutures) between certain bones of the skull. Many affected children may develop joint stiffness and abnormal bending of certain joints in a fixed position (contractures). In addition, in some patients, neuromuscular abnormalities may be present, such as unusually decreased muscle tone (hypotonia) followed by abnormally exaggerated reflexes (hyperreflexia); shock-like contractions of certain muscles or muscle groups (myoclonus); or involuntary, rapid or writhing movements of the arms and legs (choreoathetoid movements).

Some forms of ML may also be associated with distinctive eye abnormalities, such as clouding of the corneas (corneal opacities), the development of abnormal red circular areas of the middle layer of the eyes (cherry-red spots), or other defects, causing visual impairment. Additional physical abnormalities associated with ML may include bulging of part of the intestine through a weak area in the abdominal wall (hernias), enlargement of the liver or spleen, enlargement of the heart or other heart defects, or increased susceptibility to repeated respiratory infections. Some children with these disorders may also experience delays in the acquisition of skills that require the coordination of physical and mental activities (psychomotor retardation) and may develop progressively se-

vere mental retardation. Other patients may experience mild, nonprogressive mental retardation. Some of the mucolipidoses may result in potentially life-threatening complications during childhood, adolescence, or young adulthood.

The treatment of children with mucolipidosis is symptomatic and supportive. Such measures may include therapies to help prevent or aggressively treat respiratory infections; surgical correction of joint contractures, heart abnormalities, hernias, or other defects; physical therapy; special education; or other measures as required.

National Associations & Support Groups

4798 American Academy of Pediatrics
141 Northwest Point Boulevard
Elk Grove Village, IL 60007

847-434-4000
800-433-9016
Fax: 847-434-8000
www.aap.org

The American Academy of Pediatrics and its member pediatricians are committed to the attainment of optimal physical, mental and social health and well-being for all infants, children, adolescents, and young adults.

Sandra Hassink, MD, FAAP, President

4799 March of Dimes Birth Defects Foundation
1275 Mamaroneck Avenue
White Plains, NY 10605

914-997-4488
888-663-4637
Fax: 914-428-8203
e-mail: answers@marchofdimes.com
www.marchofdimes.com

Partnership of volunteers and professionals dedicates to improving the health of babies by preventing birth defects and infant mortality. Over 100 chapters are located across the country and can be located through the National Office.

Jennifer L Howse, President

4800 Mucolipidosis IV Foundation
719 E 17th Street
Brooklyn, NY 11230

718-434-5064
877-654-5459
www.ml4.org

Funds three major institutions comprised of the best genetic scientists recognized worldwide.

Paul Tanenholz, President
Randy Gold, VP
Paula Kutner, Secretary and Treasurer

4801 National MPS Society
PO Box 14686
Durham, NC 27709

919-806-0101
877-MPS-1001
Fax: 919-806-2055
e-mail: info@mpssociety.org
www.mpssociety.org

Organization that serves as a support group for those affected by mucopolysaccharidoses and related disorders. Raises funds to promote research and increases awareness of the disorder.

Stephanie Bozarth, President
Kim Whitecotton, Vice President
Lisa Todd, Treasurer

Web Sites

4802 Healthfinder
1101 Wootton Parkway
Rockville, MD 20852

e-mail: healthfinder@hhs.gov
www.healthfinder.gov

Links to carefully selected information and Web sites from over 1,500 health-related organizations.

4803 Mucolipidosis IV Foundation
3500 Piedmont Road Suite 500
Atlanta, GA 30305   877-654-5459
                                               www.ml4.org

Funds three major institutions comprised of the best genetic scientists recognized worldwide.

Paul Tanenholz, Past President

4804 National MPS Society
PO Box 14686
Durham, NC 27709   919-806-0101
                                               www.mpssociety.org

Shares information on the care and management of the children with Mucopolysaccharide diseases. The conference also brings in Medical Researchers reporting on advances in research related to these diseases.

Stephanie Bozarth, President
Kim Whitecotton, Vice President
Lisa Todd, Treasurer

4805 Online Mendelian Inheritance in Man
National Library of Medicine Building 38A
Bethesda, MD 20894   888-346-3656
                              e-mail: info@ncbi.nlm.nih.gov
                                            www.ncbi.nlm.nih.gov

This database is a catalog of human genes and genetic disorders.

Book Publishers

4806 Let's Talk About Going to the Hospital
Rosen Publishing Group's PowerKids Press
29 E 21st Street
New York, NY 10010   212-777-3017
                                               800-237-9932
                                          Fax: 888-436-4643
                          e-mail: rosenpub@tribeca.ios.com
                                         www.rosenpublishing.com

If a child has to check into the hospital, chances are he or she is already upset about being ill. Knowing how a hospital functions and what the procedures are, such as when family members can visit, will help in what is already a stressful situation. Grades K-5.

24 pages
ISBN: 0-823950-36-0

Roger Rosen, President

Description

4807 MUCOPOLYSACCHARIDOSES

Synonym: MPS

Involves the following Biologic System(s):

Genetic/Chromosomal/Syndrome/Metabolic Disorders

The mucopolysaccharidoses (MPS) are hereditary metabolic disorders that belong to a group of diseases known as lysosomal storage disorders. Lysosomes are the major digestive units within cells. Enzymes within lysosomes break down nutrients, such as certain fats and carbohydrates. The mucopolysaccharidoses are characterized by deficiency of certain lysosomal enzymes, causing the abnormal accumulation of complex carbohydrates in cells within particular tissues of the body. Affected tissues and organs typically include the skeleton, joints, brain and spinal cord (central nervous system), heart, liver, spleen, and eyes. The genes that encode most of these enzymes have been mapped to particular chromosomes. All of the mucopolysaccharidoses are inherited as an autosomal recessive trait, with the exception of Hunter syndrome, which has X-linked recessive inheritance. Collectively, these disorders are thought to affect approximately one in 10,000 newborns.

The various forms of MPS are typically designated by a Roman numeral and a specific name, such as Hunter syndrome (MPS II) or Sanfilippo syndrome (MPS III). In addition, some forms of MPS are divided into different subtypes, such as Hurler syndrome (MPS I H) and Hurler-Scheie syndrome (MPS I H/S), based on different changes (mutations) of the disease gene, age of onset, clinical course, or other factors. The range and severity of associated symptoms and findings may vary, depending upon the specific form of MPS that is present. However, certain findings are common to most forms of MPS, such as characteristic skeletal abnormalities (known as dysostosis multiplex), changes of the joints, growth delays, a characteristic facial appearance, and progressive mental retardation. For example, beginning in the first year of life or during later childhood, many patients develop progressively coarse facial features. Many children with MPS also experience delays in the acquisition of skills requiring the coordination of physical and mental activities (psychomotor retardation), a gradual loss of previously acquired skills (developmental regression), and progressively severe mental retardation. However, in a few forms of MPS, children may have average intelligence.

Many children with MPS also have short stature; sideways or front-to-back curvature of the spine (scoliosis or kyphosis) or both; other bone abnormalities; joint stiffness; and abnormal bending of certain joints in a fixed position (contractures). Other common findings include clouding of the corneas of the eyes and associated visual impairment, abnormal bulging of part of the intestine through a weak area in the abdominal wall (hernias), and enlargement of the liver and spleen (hepatosplenomegaly). Some patients also have associated abnormalities of the heart and its major blood vessels (cardiovascular defects), such as narrowing of the arteries supplying the heart; improper closure of one of the heart valves, allowing blood to leak back into the left upper chamber of the heart (mitral insufficiency); or other cardiac defects. Many of these disorders may result in potentially life-threatening complications during childhood or adolescence.

The treatment of children with MPS includes symptomatic and supportive measures, such as surgical correction of hernias, cardiovascular defects, joint contractures, or other abnormalities as required; physical therapy; or special education. In patients with some forms of MPS, enzyme replacement therapy has been shown to provide some temporary benefit. In addition, bone marrow transplantation may be effective in some patients with certain forms of mucopolysaccharidosis (e.g., Hurler syndrome).

National Associations & Support Groups

4808 American Academy of Pediatrics
141 Northwest Point Boulevard
Elk Grove Village, IL 60007
847-434-4000
800-433-9016
Fax: 847-434-8000
www.aap.org

The American Academy of Pediatrics and its member pediatricians are committed to the attainment of optimal physical, mental and social health and well-being for all infants, children, adolescents, and young adults.

Sandra Hassink, MD, FAAP, President

4809 Association for Neuro-Metabolic Disorders
5223 Brookfield Lane
Sylvania, OH 43560
419-885-1809
e-mail: volk4olks@aol.com

Nonprofit organization that serves as an advocate organization for families of patients with the following neuro-metabolic disorders: phenylketonuria, maple syrup urine disease, galactosemia, and biotinidase deficiency. Provides educational information for parents and children; provides networking information on support groups for new parents; supports scientific research into the treatments of these four neuro-metabolic disorders.

Cheryl Volk, Contact Person

4810 March of Dimes Birth Defects Foundation
1275 Mamaroneck Avenue
White Plains, NY 10605
914-997-4488
888-663-4637
Fax: 914-428-8203
e-mail: answers@marchofdimes.com
www.marchofdimes.com

Partnership of volunteers and professionals dedicates to improving the health of babies by preventing birth defects and infant mortality. Over 100 chapters are located across the country and can be located through the National Office.

Jennifer L Howse, President

4811 National MPS Society
PO Box 14686
Durham, NC 27709
919-806-0101
Fax: 919-806-2055
e-mail: info@mpssociety.org
www.mpssociety.org

Organization that serves as a support group for those affected by mucopolysaccharidoses and related disorders. Raises funds to promote research and increases awareness of the disorder.

Stephan Holland, President
Stephanie Bozarth, VP
Tom Gniazdowski, Treasurer

Web Sites

4812 Canadian Society for Mucopolysaccharide & Related Diseases
Po Box 30034 RPO Parkgate
North Vancouver, BC v7h2y
canada
604-924-5130
800-667-1846
Fax: 604-924-5131
www.mpssociety.ca

Provides information and support to affected individuals and their families.

Bernie Geiss, Chair
Judy Byrne, Secretary
Brent Nichols, Treasurer

4813 Healthfinder
1101 Wootton Parkway
Rockville, MD 20852
e-mail: healthfinder@hhs.gov
www.healthfinder.gov

Links to carefully selected information and Web sites from over 1,500 health-related organizations.

4814 Mucopolysaccharidoes & Related Diseases
Po Box 30034 RPO Parkgate
North Vancouver, BC v7h2y
604-924-5130
800-667-1846
Fax: 604-924-5131
www.mpssociety.ca/

Provides information and support to affected individuals and their families.

Bernie Geiss, Chair
Judy Byrne, Secretary
Brent Nichols, Treasurer

4815 National MPS Society
PO Box 14686
Durham, NC 27709
919-806-0101
www.mpssociety.org

Shares information on the care and management of the children with Mucopolysaccharide diseases. The conference also brings in Medical Researchers reporting on advances in research related to these diseases.

Stephanie Bozarth, President
Kim Whitecotton, Vice President
Lisa Todd, Treasurer

4816 Online Mendelian Inheritance in Man
National Library of Medicine Building 38A
Bethesda, MD 20894
888-346-3656
e-mail: info@ncbi.nlm.nih.gov
www.ncbi.nlm.nih.gov

This database is a catalog of human genes and genetic disorders.

4817 Society for Mucopolysaccharide Diseases
MPS House, Repton Place, White Lion Road
Amersham, Bu HP7 9
345-389-9901
Fax: 345-389-9902
e-mail: mps@mpssociety.org.uk
www.mpssociety.co.uk

A voluntary support group that represents from throughout the UK over 1200 children and adults suffering from mucopolysaccharide and related diseases, their families, care-givers and professionals. It is a registered charity entirely supported by voluntary donations and fundraising. It is managed by the members themselves.

Book Publishers

4818 Let's Talk About Going to the Hospital
Rosen Publishing Group's PowerKids Press
29 E 21st Street
New York, NY 10010
212-777-3017
800-237-9932
Fax: 888-436-4643
e-mail: rosenpub@tribeca.ios.com
www.rosenpublishing.com

If a child has to check into the hospital, chances are he or she is already upset about being ill. Knowing how a hospital functions and what the procedures are, such as when family members can visit, will help in what is already a stressful situation. Grades K-5.

24 pages
ISBN: 0-823950-36-0

Roger Rosen, President

Description

4819 MUSCULAR DYSTROPHIES

Synonyms: Duchenne muscular dystrophy, Becker muscular dystrophy, Landouzy-Dejerine disease

Involves the following Biologic System(s):

Neurologic Disorders, Orthopedic and Muscle Disorders

Muscular dystrophies are a group of inherited neuromuscular disorders characterized by the progressive weakness and degeneration of muscles without accompanying nerve tissue involvement. Each of these disorders is different from the others with respect to its age of onset, clinical manifestations, severity, course, and underlying genetic defect.

Duchenne muscular dystrophy, the most common of these disorders, is transmitted as an X-linked recessive trait and, as such, is fully expressed in boys; however, on rare occasions, girls who are carriers of the disease gene may exhibit mild symptoms. The incidence rate for this disorder is about one out of every 3,600 newborn boys. Although some affected infants may exhibit signs of diminished muscle tone such as poor head control, most boys do not develop symptoms until three to seven years of age. Early symptoms may include weakness in the pelvic girdle area that may be manifested by an unusual method of moving from the supine position to the standing position (Gowers' sign). In addition, boys with this disorder may develop a waddling manner of walking (Trendelenburg gait), be prone to stumbling and falling, or having difficulty climbing stairs and standing up from a sitting position. As the disease progresses, muscles around the joints may contract resulting in the inability to fully extend the knees and elbows. In addition, the spine may develop a side-to-side curve (scoliosis) and muscles, especially of the calves, become bulky due to the enlargement (hypertrophy) of the muscle fibers, the infiltration of fat into the muscles, and the increase of connective tissue protein (collagen) in the muscles. Other findings include involvement of the heart muscle (cardiomyopathy) and intellectual impairment ranging from learning disabilities to mental retardation. Most boys with Duchenne muscular dystrophy are able to walk until the age of 10 or 12 years, at which time they may be confined to a wheelchair. Life-threatening complications such as pneumonia, respiratory failure, and congestive heart failure often occur during late adolescence or early adulthood. This disorder is believed to result from the deficiency of the essential muscle protein dystrophin. The gene for Duchenne muscular dystrophy is located on the short arm of the X chromosome (Xp21).

Duchenne muscular dystrophy is initially diagnosed through evaluation of physical findings and through tests that show increased blood levels of the enzyme creatinine kinase. Additional diagnostic screening may include the use of an electrical muscle function test called electromyography or EMG. Confirmation, however, must be determined through microscopic examination of a muscle tissue sample (biopsy). Treatment is symptomatic and supportive. For example, nutritional vigilance and immunizations against flu and other childhood diseases may help to avoid or postpone complications. The administration of digitalis medications may help to alleviate certain heart-related complications. Some children may benefit from physical therapy, exercise, or surgical intervention to aid in walking.

Becker muscular dystrophy results in symptoms similar to those of Duchenne muscular dystrophy; however, these symptoms are usually less severe, do not appear until about the age of 10 years, and follow a long course. Patients usually remain ambulatory, and most survive into their 30s and 40s. The gene for Becker muscular dystrophy is also located on the short arm of the X chromosome (Xp21); however, the essential muscle protein dystrophin is defective and dysfunctional rather than deficient.

Less common forms of muscular dystrophy include facioscapulohumeral muscular dystrophy (Landouzy-Dejerine disease), limb-girdle muscular dystrophy, and others. Facioscapulohumeral muscular dystrophy, which is an autosomal dominant disorder occurring in both males and females, is characterized by facial and shoulder muscle weakness and sometimes weakness in the lower legs. This is a relatively mild disease that usually occurs between seven years of age and early or mid-adulthood. The gene for this disorder is located on the long arm of chromosome 4 (4q35). Limb-girdle muscular dystrophy is usually transmitted as an autosomal recessive trait, although autosomal dominant inheritance has also been documented. This disorder usually occurs in late childhood or early adulthood and is characterized by the progressive weakness and degeneration of the muscles of the hips and shoulders. Treatment for these types of muscular dystrophy is symptomatic and supportive.

National Associations & Support Groups

4820 American Academy of Pediatrics

141 Northwest Point Boulevard
Elk Grove Village, IL 60007

847-434-4000
800-433-9016
Fax: 847-434-8000
www.aap.org

The American Academy of Pediatrics and its member pediatricians are committed to the attainment of optimal physical, mental and social health and well-being for all infants, children, adolescents, and young adults.

Sandra Hassink, MD, FAAP, President

4821 Duchenne Parent Project Muscular Dystrophy

401 Hackensack Avenue, 9th Floor
Hackensack, NJ 07601

201-250-8440
800-714-5437
Fax: 201-250-8435
e-mail: info@parentprojectmd.org
www.parentprojectmd.org

Parent Project Muscular Dystrophy is a not-for-profit organization founded in 1994 by parents of children with Duchenne and Becker muscular dystrophy. Today, the focus is on areas such as; seeking to ensure that all families, caregivers, health care professionals and others have access to state-of-the-art information about treatment and care options for children with Duchenne and Becker MD, and to ensure that the voices of people with and affected by Duchenne and Becker are heard.

Pat Furlong, Founding President/CEO
Kimberly Galberaith, Executive VP
Ryan Fischer, Office Manager

4822 Facioscapulohumeral Dystrophy Society

450 Bedford Street
Lexington, MA 02420

781-301-6060
Fax: 781-862-1116
e-mail: info@fshsociety.org
www.fshsociety.org

Daniel Paul Perez, President/CEO
Nancy Van Zant, Executive Director

4823 Muscular Dystrophy Association
3300 E Sunrise Drive
Tucson, AZ 85718
520-529-2000
800-572-1717
Fax: 520-529-5300
e-mail: mda@mdausa.org
www.mda.org

Voluntary health agency aimed at conquering neuromuscular diseases that affect more than 1,000,000 Americans. The diseases in MDA's program include nine forms of muscular dystrophy, amyotrophic lateral sclerosis (Lou Gehrig's disease), spinal muscular atrophy, Charcot-Marie-Tooth disease, and other neuromuscular conditions. With over 200 offices across the country, MDA conducts research, medical and community services, clinics, support groups, summer camps for youngsters and much more.

Jennifer Lopez, Assoc. Director of Health Care Svcs

4824 Muscular Dystrophy Family Foundation
1033 Third Avenue SW, Suite 108
Indianapolis, IN 46032
317-249-8488
800-544-1213
Fax: 317-853-6743
e-mail: mdff@mdff.org
www.mdff.org

Provides adaptive equipment and emotional support to individuals and families affected by one of the over forty neuromuscular diseases. Established in 1958, some of the equipment provided includes: hospital beds, wheelchairs, ramps, communication devices, and lifts.

Paula McDonald, Executive Director
Hazel M Walker, Vice President

4825 Reflex Sympathetic Dystrophy Syndrome Association
PO Box 502
Milford, CT 06460
203-877-3790
877-662-7737
Fax: 203-882-8362
e-mail: info@rsds.org
www.rsds.org

The Reflex Sympathetic Dystrophy Syndrome Association was founded in 1984 to promote public and professional awareness of Reflex Sympathetic Dystrophy Syndrome, also known as Complex Regional Pain Syndrome. Educates those afflicted with this syndrome, their family, friends, insurance and healthcare providers, on the disabling pain the syndrome causes. Publishes quarterly newsletter, clinical practice guidelines, and has a very helpful website.

James E Tyrrell Jr. Esquire, Chairman of the Board
Paul R. Charlesworth, President
Donald F. McKee, Vice President, Treasurer

Research Centers

4826 Rusk Institute of Rehabilitation Medicine
NYU Langone Medical Center
400 E 34th Street
New York, NY 10016
212-263-6034
Fax: 212-263-8510
e-mail: gwen.treharne@nyumc.org
www.rusk.med.nyu.edu

The world's first university-affiliated facility devoted entirely to rehabilitation medicine, Rusk is among the most renowned center of its kind for the treatment of adults and children with disabilities-home to innovations and advances that have set the standard in rehabilitation care for every stage of life and for every stage of recovery.

Dr. Steven Flanagan, Professor & Chairman
Marilyn Shoo, Pediatrics Director

Minnesota

4827 Mayo Clinic and Foundation
200 First Street S.W.
Rochester, MN 55905
507-284-2511
800-660-4582
Fax: 507-284-0161
www.mayo.edu

Neuromuscular clinical research center with a primary research interest in neuropathies.

Julie E Hammack, CEO

New York

4828 Columbia Presbyterian Medical Center
Neurology Institute of NY/Research Center
630 W 168th Street
New York, NY 10032
212-305-3880
e-mail: alscenter@columbia.edu
www.nyp.org

Neuromuscular clinical research center.

Steven J. Corwin, CEO
Robert E. Kelly, President

4829 NYU Rusk Institute
301 East 17th Street, Second Avenue
New York, NY 10003
212-263-6034
Fax: 212-263-8510
www.rusk.med.nyu.edu

Focuses on Muscular Dystrophy and related bone disorders.

Jeffrey Cohen MD, Director
Marilyn Shoo, Pediatrics Director

Ohio

4830 Parent Project for Muscular Dystrophy Research
401 Hackensack Avenue, 9th Floor
Hackensack, NJ 07601
201-250-8440
800-714-5437
Fax: 201-250-8435
e-mail: info@parentprojectmd.org
www.parentprojectmd.org

Organization of families around the world who have children diagnosed with DMD/BMD. The goal is to invest significant amounts of money raised into medical research with clinical application.

Robert J McDonald, Chairman
John Killian, Treasurer
Daniel Garofalo, Secretary

Pennsylvania

4831 Penn Neurological Institute
Hospital of the University of Pennsylvania
3417 Spruce Street
Philadelphia, PA 19104
215-662-3396
800-789-7366
www.pennmedicine.org

Research program centering its efforts on finding better ways to prevent and treat neuromuscular disorders.

Michael E Selzer, Director Neuromuscular Diseases

Texas

4832 Baylor College of Medicine
Neuromuscular Disease Research
1 Baylor Plaza
Houston, TX 77030
713-798-4951
e-mail: neurons@bcm.tmc.edu
www.bcm.edu

Offers research into biochemistry, molecular genetics and neuromuscular disorders.

Laura J Morrison, Professor And Chair
Michael Vincent Abene M.D., Assistant Professor
Farah F. Atassi, Instructor

Utah

4833 University of Utah
Eccles Institute of Human Genetics
15 N 2030 E, Room 2100
Salt Lake City, UT 84112

801-581-4422
Fax: 801-581-7796
e-mail: efry@genetics.utah.edu
www.genetics.utah.edu

John F Atkins PhD, Research Professor
Mario R. Capecchi Ph.D, Distinguished Professor & Co-Chair
Richard M. Cawthon, M.D. Ph.D., Research Associate Professor

Audio Video

4834 Muscular Dystrophy
Films for Humanities/Films Media Group
132 West 31st Street, 17th Floor
New York, NY 10001

800-322-8755
Fax: 609-671-0266
e-mail: custserv@filsmediagroup.comm
www.films.com

Muscular Dystrophy attacks muscles, so that people lose the ability to walk, talk, and in some cases, to breath. About two thirds of those affected are children, but symptoms can appear any time between birth and adolescence. This video looks at how people deal with a disease that has no cure. A young boy, a six year old girl, and a young mother are managing their disease and show us the medical interventions used to help them live more fully.

1990 VHS/DVD
ISBN: 1-421336-46-4

Web Sites

4835 Muscular Dystrophy Association
222 S. Riverside Plaza, Suite 1500
Chicago, IL 60606

800-572-1717
www.mda.org

Information regarding muscular dystrophy.
Steven M. Derks, President and CEO
Valerie A. Cwik, M.D., EVP, Chief Medical & Scientific
Julie Faber, EVP, CFO

4836 Muscular Dystrophy Family Foundation
P.O. Box 776
Carmel, IN 46082

317-615-9140
www.mdff.org

Provides adaptive equipment and emotional support to individuals and families affected by one of the over forty neuromuscular diseases. Established in 1958, some of the equipment provided includes: hospital beds, wheelchairs, ramps, communication devices, and lifts.

Tim Doyle, President/Chair
Emily Munson, Vice President/Vice Chair
Matthew D. Haab, Treasurer

4837 Parent Project Muscular Dystrophy
401 Hackensack Avenue, 9th Floor
Hackensack, NJ 7601

201-250-8440
800-714-5437
Fax: 201-250-8435
e-mail: info@parentprojectmd.org
www.parentprojectmd.org

The Parent Project Muscular Dystrophy moblizes people in the United States and worldwide in collaborative effort to enable people with Duchenne and becker muscular dystrophy to survive, thrive and fully participate within their families and communities into adulthood and beyond.

Anessa Gaydou-Fehsenfeld, Board Chairman
Lance Hester, Board Treasurer
Daniel P. Garofalo, Board Secretary

Book Publishers

4838 Journey of Love: Parent's Guide to Duchenne Muscular Dystrophy
Muscular Dystrophy Association
3300 E Sunrise Drive
Tucson, AZ 85718

520-529-2000
800-572-1717
Fax: 520-529-5300
e-mail: mda@mdausa.org
www.mda.org/publications/journey/misc.html

Complete guide for parents with children diagnosed with DMD. Information includes explanation of the disease, treatments, research, services provided by MDA, guides to finding assistance and more. Available in paperback and online; free from a local MDA office to families with a member affected by DMD or BMD who is registered with the MDA.

1988 170 pages

R. Rodney Howell, M.D, Chairman
Steven M Derks, Chief Executive Officer
Roxan Olivas, Vice President - Public Relations

4839 Let's Talk About Going to the Hospital
Rosen Publishing Group's PowerKids Press
29 E 21st Street
New York, NY 10010

212-777-3017
800-237-9932
Fax: 888-436-4643
e-mail: rosenpub@tribeca.ios.com
www.rosenpublishing.com

If a child has to check into the hospital, chances are he or she is already upset about being ill. Knowing how a hospital functions and what the procedures are, such as when family members can visit, will help in what is already a stressful situation. Grades K-5.

24 pages
ISBN: 0-823950-36-0

Roger Rosen, President

4840 Medifocus Guidebook On Reflex Sympathetic Dystrophy
Medifocus.Com
11529 Daffodil Lane, Suite 200
Silver Spring, MD 20902

301-649-9300
800-965-3002
e-mail: info@medifocus.com
www.medifocus.com

A patient's comprehensive guide to treatment options and the latest medical advances for RSD. The book provides information about the signs and symptoms of RSD, the treatment options including drug therapy, sympathetic nerve blocks, chemical and surgical sympathectomy, physical therapy, and other methods used for controlling pain and improving quality of life. Updated regularly, purchase includes free updates for 1 year. Available online or in print; see website for details of print vs. online.

April 2009 130 pages Print

4841 Muscular Dystrophy and Allied Diseases: Im pacts on Patients, Family, and Staff

Leon I Charash, author

Center for Thanatology Research & Education
391 Atlantic Avenue
Brooklyn, NY 11217

718-858-3026
Fax: 718-852-1846
e-mail: thanatology@pipeline.com
www.thanatology.org

An Internet best-seller, it covers Duchenne Muscular Dystrophy, psychosocial aspects, anticipatory grief of parents, education issues, etc.

1988 90 pages Paper
ISBN: 0-930194-38-1

Roberta Halporn, Director

4842 Muscular Dystrophy and Other Neuromuscular Diseases
Haworth Press
711 Third Avenue
New York, NY 10017   212-216-7800
                                          800-429-6784
                                    Fax: 212-244-1563
                      e-mail: getinfo@haworthpress.com
                                      www.tandf.co.uk

A thoughtful book from professionals who assist persons afflicted
with neuromuscular disorders to help them and their families
adapt to lifestyle changes accompanying the onset of these
disorders.

1991 250 pages Hardcover
ISBN: 1-560240-77-6

4843 My Life-Melinda's Story

Melinda Lawrence, author

Children's Hospice International
1101 King Street, Suite 360
Alexandria, VA 22314   703-684-0330
                                          800-242-4453
                                    Fax: 703-684-0226
                          e-mail: info@chionline.org
                           www.chionline.org/publications

Written by Melinda, a child with Muscular Dystrophy. This heartwarming story teaches children and their families how to cope
with the illness.

ISBN: 0-317618-38-5

Ann Armstrong-Dailey, Founding Director/CEO
Richard Larkin, Secretary/Treasurer
Rebecca Brant, Director

4844 Realities in Coping with Progressive Neuromuscular Diseases
Charles C. Thomas
2037 Chestnut Street, PO Box 15715
Philadelphia, PA 19103   215-561-2786
                                    Fax: 215-600-1248
                     e-mail: mailbox@charlespresspub.com
                             www.charlespresspub.com

248 pages Hardcover
ISBN: 0-914783-20-3

**4845 Travis:I Got Lots of Neat Stuff Children Living with Muscular
Dystrophy**

Kathy L Gordon, author

Muscular Dystrophy Association
3300 E Sunrise Drive
Tucson, AZ 85718   800-572-1717
                        e-mail: publications@mdausa.org
                         www.mda.org/publications/travis/

Travis' mother shares his story with other children, helping them
to accept their muscular dystrophy and see the world of possibilities before them.

Online

R. Rodney Howell, M.D, Chairman
Steven M Derks, Chief Executive Officer
Roxan Olivas, Vice President - Public Relations

Magazines

4846 MDA/ALS Newsmagazine
Muscular Dystrophy Association
222 S. Riverside Plaza, Suite 1500
Chicago, IL 60606   520-529-2000
                                          800-322-8755
                                    Fax: 520-529-5300
                        e-mail: publications@mdausa.org
                                        www.mda.org

A national magazine that goes out to everyone registered with
MDA, MDA clinics, reseacgers and subscribers. It presents news
related to ALS including research, personal profiles, fund raising
activities, patient services, and lifestyle information including
products and trends.

125,000 circ Bimonthly

Steven M. Derks, President and CEO
Valerie A. Cwik, M.D., EVP, Chief Medical & Scientific
Julie Faber, EVP, CFO

4847 Quest Magazine
MDA Publications
222 S. Riverside Plaza, Suite 1500
Chicago, IL 60606   520-529-2000
                                          800-322-8755
                                    Fax: 520-529-5300
                        e-mail: publications@mdausa.org
                                        www.mda.org

A national magazine that goes out to everyone registered with
MDA, MDA clinics, researchers and subscribers. It presents news
related to muscular dystrophy and other neuromuscular diseases
including research, personal profiles, fund raising activities, patient services, and lifestyle information including products and
trends.

Bimonthly

Steven M. Derks, President and CEO
Valerie A. Cwik, M.D., EVP, Chief Medical & Scientific
Julie Faber, EVP, CFO

Newsletters

4848 Helping Children & Youth with RSD/CRPS Succeed in School
RSDSA
PO Box 502
Milford, CT 6460   203-877-3790
                                          877-662-7737
                                    Fax: 203-882-8362
                             e-mail: info@rsds.org
                                        www.rsds.org

This brochure is designed to help schools accoommadate the special needs of children with CRPS. Available online.

Peter Moskovitz, MD, Chairman of the Board
Francis Ludington, III, Co-President
Guy M. Tufo, Treasurer

4849 Pediatrics CRPS Tri-Fold Brochure
RSDSA
PO Box 502
Milford, CT 6460   203-877-3790
                                          877-662-7737
                                    Fax: 203-882-8362
                             e-mail: info@rsds.org
                                        www.rsds.org

This brochure offers information and resources for the family and
friends of youth with CRPS, and those who want to help.

Peter Moskovitz, MD, Chairman of the Board
Francis Ludington, III, Co-President
Guy M. Tufo, Treasurer

4850 RSDA Review
Reflex Sympathetic Dystrophy Syndrome Association
PO Box 502
Milford, CT 6460   203-877-3790
                                          877-662-7737
                                    Fax: 203-882-8362
                             e-mail: info@rsds.org
                                        www.rsds.org

Quarterly newsletter of the Reflex Sympathetic Dystrophy Syndrome Association

Peter Moskovitz, MD, Chairman of the Board
Francis Ludington, III, Co-President
Guy M. Tufo, Treasurer

Pamphlets

4851 101 Hints to "Help with Ease" for Patients with Neuromuscular Disease

Irwin M Siegel MD, author

Muscular Dystrophy Association
3300 E Sunrise Drive
Tucson, AZ 85718

520-529-2000
800-572-1717
Fax: 520-529-5300
e-mail: publications@mdausa.org
www.mda.org/publications/101hints/

A do-it-yourself guide to everyday living with NMD's. Chapters include Housekeeping, Exercising & Managing Contractures, Eating, Sleeping, Grooming, Dressing, Toileting, Sitting, Transferring & Mobility, Recreating, and Communicating. Also in Spanish and online.

2007 30 pages Paperback

Carol Sowell, Director Publications

4852 101 Hints to Help with Ease"" for Patients with Neuromuscular Disease

222 S. Riverside Plaza, Suite 1500
Chicago, IL 60606

520-529-2000
800-572-1717
Fax: 520-529-5300
e-mail: publications@mdausa.org
www.mda.org/publications/101hints/

A do-it-yourself guide to everyday living with NMD's. Chapters include Housekeeping, Exercising & Managing Contractures, Eating, Sleeping, Grooming, Dressing, Toileting, Sitting, Transferring & Mobility, Recreating, and Communicating. Also in Spanish and online.

Steven M. Derks, President and CEO
Valerie A. Cwik, M.D., EVP, Chief Medical & Scientific
Julie Faber, EVP, CFO

4853 Breathe Easy: Respiratory Care in Neuromus cular Disorders

Muscular Dystrophy Association
222 S. Riverside Plaza, Suite 1500
Chicago, IL 60606

520-529-2000
800-322-8755
Fax: 520-529-5300
e-mail: publications@mdausa.org
www.mda.org/publications/breathe/

Respiratory health is a vital issue for children and adults with NMDs, which progressively weaken muscles, sometimes including those we need to breathe. A guide to respiratory care for children with muscular dystrophy. This guide is the result of efforts by a number of highly respected experts in the fileds of NMDs and children's medicine. Also available in Spanish and online.

2006

Steven M. Derks, President and CEO
Valerie A. Cwik, M.D., EVP, Chief Medical & Scientific
Julie Faber, EVP, CFO

4854 Conference on the Cause and Treatment of Facioscapulohumeral Muscular Dystrophy

National Inst. of Neurological Disorders/Stroke
P.O. Box 5801
Bethesda, MD 20824

301-496-5751
800-352-9424
www.ninds.nih.gov

4855 Congressional Testimony on Muscular Dystrophy

National Inst. of Neurological Disorders/Stroke
P.O. Box 5801
Bethesda, MD 20824

301-496-5751
800-352-9424
www.ninds.nih.gov

Testimony by Dr. Audrey Penn, Acting Director, NINDS, from February, 2001.

4856 Everybody's Different, Nobody's Perfect

Muscular Dystrophy Association
222 S. Riverside Plaza, Suite 1500
Chicago, IL 60606

520-529-2000
800-572-1717
Fax: 520-529-5300
e-mail: mda@mdausa.org
www.mda.org/publications/nobody/

Explains how muscular dystrophy affects children and describes how people are different from each other in many ways. Emphasizing fun, friendship, and caring, this booklet is ideal for heightening awareness and encouraging understanding of persons with disabilities. Pre-school edition also available; and in Spanish and online.

1999 11 pages

Steven M. Derks, President and CEO
Valerie A. Cwik, M.D., EVP/ CMO/ CSO
Julie Faber, EVP, CFO

4857 Facts About Duchenne and Becker Muscular Dystrophies

Muscular Dystrophy Association
222 S. Riverside Plaza, Suite 1500
Chicago, IL 60606

520-529-2000
800-322-8755
Fax: 520-529-5300
e-mail: publications@mdausa.org
www.mda.org/publications/

Describes in layman's terms Duchenne and Becker Muscular Dystrophies and addresses the most currently asked questions about these diseases, research, inheritance and treatments. Also available in Spanish or online.

2009

Steven M. Derks, President and CEO
Valerie A. Cwik, M.D., EVP, Chief Medical & Scientific
Julie Faber, EVP, CFO

4858 Facts About Facioscapulohumeral Muscular Dystrophy

Muscular Dystrophy Association
222 S. Riverside Plaza, Suite 1500
Chicago, IL 60606

520-529-2000
800-322-8755
Fax: 520-529-5300
e-mail: publications@mdausa.org
www.mda.org/publications/

Explains facioscapulohumeral muscular dystrophy (FHSD) in layman's terms and answers commonly asked questions. Also available in Spanish.

2009 20 pages Paperback

Steven M. Derks, President and CEO
Valerie A. Cwik, M.D., EVP, Chief Medical & Scientific
Julie Faber, EVP, CFO

4859 Facts About Inflammatory Myopathies-DM, PM and IBM

Muscular Dystrophy Association
222 S. Riverside Plaza, Suite 1500
Chicago, IL 60606

520-529-2000
800-322-8755
Fax: 520-529-5300
e-mail: publications@mdausa.org
www.mda.org/publications/fa-myosi.html

Outlines these forms of inflammatory myopathy. Current approaches to treatment and MDA's efforts in continued research are described. Also available in Spanish and online.

Steven M. Derks, President and CEO
Valerie A. Cwik, M.D., EVP, Chief Medical & Scientific
Julie Faber, EVP, CFO

4860 Facts About Limb-Girdle Muscular Dystrophy

Muscular Dystrophy Association
222 S. Riverside Plaza, Suite 1500
Chicago, IL 60606

520-529-2000
800-322-8755
Fax: 520-529-5300
e-mail: publications@mdausa.org
www.mda.org/publications/fa-lgmd.html

Overview of the various forms of LGMD encompassed by MDA's program. Addresses commonly asked questions and highlights MDA's research efforts aimed at finding the causes of and effective treatments for these disorders. Also available in Spanish and online.

2007 19 pages

Steven M. Derks, President and CEO
Valerie A. Cwik, M.D., EVP, Chief Medical & Scientific
Julie Faber, EVP, CFO

4861   Facts About Metabolic Diseases of Muscle
Muscular Dystrophy Association
222 S. Riverside Plaza, Suite 1500
Chicago, IL 60606   520-529-2000
                                       800-322-8755
                                 Fax: 520-529-5300
             www.mda.org/publications/fa-metab.html

Provides an overview of the 10 heritable metabolic diseases of muscle encompassed by MDA's program. Addresses commonly asked questions and highlights MDA's research efforts aimed at finding the causes of and effective treatments for these disorders. Also online and in Spanish.

Steven M. Derks, President and CEO
Valerie A. Cwik, M.D., EVP, Chief Medical & Scientific
Julie Faber, EVP, CFO

4862   Facts About Mitochondrial Myopathies
Muscular Dystrophy Association
222 S. Riverside Plaza, Suite 1500
Chicago, IL 60606   520-529-2000
                                       800-572-1717
                                 Fax: 520-529-5300
             e-mail: publications@mdausa.org
   www.mda.org/publications/mitchondrial_myopathies.htm

Explains Mitochondrial myopathies in layman's terms and answers the most frequently asked questions about this disease. Also available in Spanish and online.

2008 24 pages

Steven M. Derks, President and CEO
Valerie A. Cwik, M.D., EVP, Chief Medical & Scientific
Julie Faber, EVP, CFO

4863   Facts About Muscular Dystrophy
Muscular Dystrophy Association
222 S. Riverside Plaza, Suite 1500
Chicago, IL 60606   520-529-2000
                                       800-322-8755
                                 Fax: 520-529-5300
             www.mda.org/publications/fa-md-help.html

Answers many questions commonly asked about the forty-plus forms of the disease encompassed by MDA's program.

Steven M. Derks, President and CEO
Valerie A. Cwik, M.D., EVP, Chief Medical & Scientific
Julie Faber, EVP, CFO

4864   Facts About Myasthenia Gravis (MG, LEMS, & CMS)
Muscular Dystrophy Association
222 S. Riverside Plaza, Suite 1500
Chicago, IL 60606   520-529-2000
                                       800-322-8755
                                 Fax: 520-529-5300
             e-mail: publications@mdausa.org
             www.mda.org/publications/fa-mg.html

Explains myasthenia gravis and Lambert-Eaton syndrome in layman's terms and answers the most frequently asked questions about these diseases. Also available in Spanish and online.

2001 19 pages

Steven M. Derks, President and CEO
Valerie A. Cwik, M.D., EVP, Chief Medical & Scientific
Julie Faber, EVP, CFO

4865   Facts About Myopathies
Muscular Dystrophy Association
222 S. Riverside Plaza, Suite 1500
Chicago, IL 60606   520-529-2000
                                       800-322-8755
                                 Fax: 520-529-5300
             www.mda.org/publications/fa-myop.html

Describes the six inheritable myopathies encompassed by MDA's program, as well as current methods for diagnosing and managing these disorders. Also online and in Spanish.

2003

Steven M. Derks, President and CEO
Valerie A. Cwik, M.D., EVP, Chief Medical & Scientific
Julie Faber, EVP, CFO

4866   Facts About Myotonic Muscular Dystrophy
Muscular Dystrophy Association
222 S. Riverside Plaza, Suite 1500
Chicago, IL 60606   520-529-2000
                                       800-322-8755
                                 Fax: 520-529-5300
             e-mail: publications@mdausa.org
             www.mda.org/publications/fa-mmd.html

Basic knowledge about Myotonic Muscular Dystrophy, precautions, treatments, research and answers to most commonly asked questions. Also available in Spanish and online.

2009 23 pages

Steven M. Derks, President and CEO
Valerie A. Cwik, M.D., EVP, Chief Medical & Scientific
Julie Faber, EVP, CFO

4867   Facts About Plasmapheresis
Muscular Dystrophy Association
222 S. Riverside Plaza, Suite 1500
Chicago, IL 60606   520-529-2000
                                       800-322-8755
                                 Fax: 520-529-5300
             e-mail: publications@mdausa.org
             www.mda.org/publications/fa-plasmaph.html

Describes plasmapheresis, a plasma exchange procedure often utilized as a treatment for autoimmune diseases such as myasthenia gravis and Lambert-Eaton syndrome. Available in paperback or online.

2005

Steven M. Derks, President and CEO
Valerie A. Cwik, M.D., EVP, Chief Medical & Scientific
Julie Faber, EVP, CFO

4868   Facts About Rare Muscular Dystrophies
Muscular Dystrophy Association
222 S. Riverside Plaza, Suite 1500
Chicago, IL 60606   520-529-2000
                                       800-322-8755
                                 Fax: 520-529-5300
             e-mail: publications@mdausa.org
                                 www.mda.org

This brochure gives basic facts about four forms of muscular dystrophy (congenital, distal, Emery-Dreifuss and oculopharyngeal) and addresses commonly asked questions. Also available in Spanish.

28 pages

Steven M. Derks, President and CEO
Valerie A. Cwik, M.D., EVP, Chief Medical & Scientific
Julie Faber, EVP, CFO

4869   Genetics and Neuromuscular Diseases
Muscular Dystrophy Association
222 S. Riverside Plaza, Suite 1500
Chicago, IL 60606   520-529-2000
                                       800-322-8755
                                 Fax: 520-529-5300
             e-mail: publications@mdausa.org
                                 www.mda.org

An up-to-date review of genetics information relating to neuromatic diseases, specifically describing what a genetic disorder is, genetic testing and counseling and inheritance patterns. Also available in Spanish and online.

19 pages

Steven M. Derks, President and CEO
Valerie A. Cwik, M.D., EVP, Chief Medical & Scientific
Julie Faber, EVP, CFO

4870 Hey! I'm Here, Too!
Irwin M Siegel, MD, author

Muscular Dystrophy Association
222 S. Riverside Plaza, Suite 1500
Chicago, IL 60606   520-529-2000
                                           800-322-8755
                                      Fax: 520-529-5300
                      e-mail: publications@mdausa.org
                       www.mda.org/publications/hey/

Help for siblings of boys with Duchenne muscular dystrophy. Explores how they feel about themselves, their brothers, and their families. Also provides specific answers to some questions that siblings may wonder about. Has the option for an introduction for parents or for children. Available online and in Spanish.

1989

Steven M. Derks, President and CEO
Valerie A. Cwik, M.D., EVP, Chief Medical & Scientific
Julie Faber, EVP, CFO

4871 Learning to Live with Neuromuscular Disease: A Message for Parents
Muscular Dystrophy Association
222 S. Riverside Plaza, Suite 1500
Chicago, IL 60606   520-529-2000
                                           800-322-8755
                                      Fax: 520-529-5300
                      e-mail: publications@mdausa.org
                     www.mda.org/publications/learning/

Intended to help parents and families cope with the knowledge that their child has a neuromuscular disease and with the impact the disease will have on everyday life. Online and in Spanish.

2006

Steven M. Derks, President and CEO
Valerie A. Cwik, M.D., EVP, Chief Medical & Scientific
Julie Faber, EVP, CFO

4872 MDA Fact Sheet
Muscular Dystrophy Association
222 S. Riverside Plaza, Suite 1500
Chicago, IL 60606   520-529-2000
                                           800-572-1717
                                      Fax: 520-529-5300
                      e-mail: publications@mdausa.org
                          www.mda.org/publications/

Outlines the history of MDA, the diseases included in MDA's program, and the services available through the Association.

Steven M. Derks, President and CEO
Valerie A. Cwik, M.D., EVP, Chief Medical & Scientific
Julie Faber, EVP, CFO

4873 MDA Services for the Individual, Family and Community
Muscular Dystrophy Association
222 S. Riverside Plaza, Suite 1500
Chicago, IL 60606   520-529-2000
                                           800-322-8755
                                      Fax: 520-529-5300
                      e-mail: publications@mdausa.org
                     www.mda.org/publications/mdasvcs/

Contains a list of the diseases covered by MDA as well as eligibility criteria for MDA's services program, a list of MDA-sponsored clinics nationwide, and the services available through these clinics. Also in Spanish and online.

2009

Steven M. Derks, President and CEO
Valerie A. Cwik, M.D., EVP, Chief Medical & Scientific
Julie Faber, EVP, CFO

4874 MDA Summer Camp Brochure
Muscular Dystrophy Association
222 S. Riverside Plaza, Suite 1500
Chicago, IL 60606   520-529-2000
                                           800-322-8755
                                      Fax: 520-529-5300
                          www.mda.org/clinics/camp

Highlights the activities of MDA summer camps for youngsters diagnosed with one of the more than 40 diseases in MDA's program. Shares camper and volunteer reactions. Also available in Spanish and online.

Steven M. Derks, President and CEO
Valerie A. Cwik, M.D., EVP, Chief Medical & Scientific
Julie Faber, EVP, CFO

4875 Teacher's Guide to Neuromuscular Disease
Muscular Dystrophy Association
222 S. Riverside Plaza, Suite 1500
Chicago, IL 60606   520-529-2000
                                           800-322-8755
                                      Fax: 520-529-5300
                      e-mail: publications@mdausa.org
                     www.mda.org/publications/tchrdmd/

A source of guidance and information to educators detailing neuromuscular disease, how it affects school participation, and ways that teachers can help meet the academic and social needs of students affected by the disorder. Online and in Spanish.

2005

Steven M. Derks, President and CEO
Valerie A. Cwik, M.D., EVP, Chief Medical & Scientific
Julie Faber, EVP, CFO

4876 Workshop on Therapeutic Approaches for Duchenne Muscular Dystrophy
National Inst. of Neurological Disorders/Stroke
PO Box 5801
Bethesda, MD 20824   301-496-5751
                                           800-352-9424
             www.ninds.nih.gov/news_and_events/proceedings/

Camps

4877 MDA Summer Camp
Muscular Dystrophy Association
222 S. Riverside Plaza, Suite 1500
Chicago, IL 60606   520-529-2000
                                           800-322-8755
                                      Fax: 520-529-5300
                            e-mail: mda@mdausa.org
                          www.mda.org/clinics/camp

With over 90 camps across the country MDA camp is a magical place where year-round skills are developed and where a child with a disability can just be a kid. In addition to camp and medical staff, most campers have their own 1-on-1 volunteer to help with fun and personal care. Activites are designed for young people with limited mobility or wheelchairs, and include swimming, boating, baseball, football, horseback riding, arts, crafts and talent shows. Free for famlies registered with MDA.

Steven M. Derks, President and CEO
Valerie A. Cwik, M.D., EVP, Chief Medical & Scientific
Julie Faber, EVP, CFO

Description

4878 NARCOLEPSY

Synonyms: Gelineau's syndrome, Hypnolepsy, Paroxysmal sleep

Involves the following Biologic System(s):

Neurologic Disorders

Narcolepsy refers to a sleep disorder characterized by profound drowsiness during the day and sudden daytime attacks of sleep that may last from a few seconds to one or more hours. These episodes are sometimes accompanied by sudden loss of muscle tone (hypotonia) in response to emotional stimuli such as anger, fear, joy, or surprise (cataplexy). During a cataplectic episode, the patient remains conscious but is not able to speak or move. Some patients experience sleep paralysis and are unable to move at the onset of sleep or immediately upon waking. Hypnagogic hallucinations are disquieting occurrences that take place at onset of sleep or, less commonly, upon awakening. During these hallucinations, patients may see or hear things that are not grounded in reality. In most cases, narcolepsy begins during adolescence or early adulthood and persists throughout the life of the affected individual. Sleep attacks associated with narcolepsy may occur at any time and may take place many times during the day; however, most individuals may be easily awakened.

Very few people with narcolepsy exhibit all the symptoms associated with this disorder and, occasionally, children and adults who do not have this disorder may experience similar signs and symptoms. For this reason, diagnosis of narcolepsy may necessitate confirmation by a sleep study which uses a procedure called electroencephalography (EEG), during which electrical brain-wave activity is recorded. An EEG may demonstrate an abnormal sleep pattern in which rapid eye movement or REM-type sleep occurs at the onset of sleep. There are no pathologic changes that occur in the brain. In individuals who do not have narcolepsy, REM sleep or periods of deep sleep normally follow nonrapid eye movement sleep (NREM). The cause of narcolepsy is unknown, but researchers think that, in some cases, it may be related to genetic influences as evidenced by the tendency of this disorder to occur within families. Approximately 200,000 people in the United States are affected by narcolepsy.

Treatment for narcolepsy may include regular napping and the administration of stimulant medications to control attacks of drowsiness and sleep, while antidepressant medications may help control episodes of cataplexy. Because this disorder may increase the risk of accidents, appropriate care and caution is advised in the performance of certain tasks or jobs. Other treatment is symptomatic and supportive.

Government Agencies

4879 NIH/National Institute of Neurological Dis orders and Stroke (NINDS)
PO Box 5801
Bethesda, MD 20824

301-496-5751
800-352-9424
Fax: 301-496-0296
TTY: 301-468-5981
www.ninds.nih.gov

Works to reduce the burden of neurological disease by conducting, fostering, coordinating and guiding research on the causes, prevention, diagnosis and treatment of neurological disorders and stroke, while supporting basic research in related scientific areas.

Story C Landis Ph.D., Director
Audrey S Penn M.D., Deputy Director
Audrey S. Penn, Special Advisor To Director

National Associations & Support Groups

4880 American Academy of Pediatrics
141 Northwest Point Boulevard
Elk Grove Village, IL 60007

847-434-4000
800-433-9016
Fax: 847-434-8000
www.aap.org

The American Academy of Pediatrics and its member pediatricians are committed to the attainment of optimal physical, mental and social health and well-being for all infants, children, adolescents, and young adults.

Sandra Hassink, MD, FAAP, President

4881 American Academy of Sleep Medicine
2510 N Frontage Road
Darien, IL 60561

630-737-9700
Fax: 630-737-9790
e-mail: inquiries@aasmnet.org
www.aasmnet.org

Provides full diagnostic and treatment services to improve the quality of care for patients with all types of sleep disorders.

Jerome A. Barrett, Executive Director
Nancy Collop, President-Elect
Timothy I. Morgenthaler, Secretary/Treasurer

4882 Association of Professional Sleep Societies
2510 N Frontage Road
Darien, IL 60561

630-737-9700
Fax: 630-737-9790
e-mail: jmarkkanen@aasmnet.org
www.apss.org

A joint venture of the AASM and the Sleep Research Society. It works to facilitate the research and development of sleep disorders medically by encouraging exchange of information among members.

Jennifer Markkanen, Assistant Executive Director

4883 Florida Narcolepsy Association
2631 59th Street, PO Box 15352
Sarasota, FL 34232

941-355-5359
e-mail: sleepymc@yahoo.com
www.flnarcolepsy.org

The Association is a collective of people that helps or comforts others afflicted with Narcolepsy; as well as their families, doctors and friends.

Marion L Cikovic, Vice President

4884 Genetic Alliance
4301 Connecticut Avenue NW
Washington, DC 20008

202-966-5557
800-336-4363
Fax: 202-966-8553
e-mail: info@geneticalliance.org
www.geneticalliance.org

A coalition of voluntary genetic support groups, consumers and professionals addressing the needs of individuals and families affected by genetic disorders from a national perspective.

Joan Oppenheimer Weiss, Founder
Sharon Terry, President

4885 NIH/National Institute of Neurological Dis orders and Stroke (NINDS)
PO Box 5801
Bethesda, MD 20824

301-496-5751
800-352-9424
Fax: 301-496-0296
TTY: 301-468-5981
www.ninds.nih.gov

Information and advocacy resources for families and professionals. Includes listings of organizations providing general tips and organizations focusing on more specific areas of concern to families and young adults who have disabilities.

Story C Landis Ph.D., Director
Walter J Koroshetz, Deputy Director
Audrey S. Penn, Special Advisor To Director

4886 Narcolepsy Institute
Montefiore Medical Center
111 E 210th Street
Bronx, NY 10467

718-920-6799
Fax: 718-654-9580
e-mail: mgoswami@narcolepsyinstitute.org
www.NarcolepsyInstitute.org

The Narcolepsy Institute, at Montefiore Medical Center, provides support services to individuals who have narcolepsy and their families in New York City. Free services are provided for people who narcolepsy qualifies as a developmental disability. The Institute provides screening, counseling, case management, crisis intervention, and advocacy for affected individuals and their families.

Dr Meeta Goswami, Phd, Director

4887 Narcolepsy Network
129 Waterwheel Lane
North Kingstown, RI 02852

401-667-2523
888-292-6522
Fax: 401-633-6567
e-mail: narnet@narcolepsynetwork.org
www.narcolepsynetwork.org

Nonprofit organization that serves as a resource center, to assist support groups, to educate the public, to facilitate early diagnosis, to protect the rights of those with narcolepsy, and to encourage on-going scientific research in sleep medicine.

Sara Kowalczyk, President
Sarah DiDavide, Co VP
Heidi Shilensky, Co-VP

4888 National Sleep Foundation
1010 N Glebe Road
Arlington, VA 22201

703-243-1697
Fax: 202-347-3472
e-mail: nsf@sleepfoundation.org
www.narap.org

Works to improve the quality of life for millions of Americans who suffer from sleep disorders, and to prevent the catastrophic accidents that are related to poor or disordered sleep through research, education and the dissemination of information towards the cause of the Narcolepsy Project. Seeks patients to aid new research project targeting the cause of the disorder.

Richard Gelula, CEO
Inne Barber, Board of Directors
Robin Choi, Board of Directors

State Agencies & Support Groups

Arizona

4889 Arizona Sleep Disorders Center
University of Arizona, College of Medicine
1501 N Campbell Avenue, PO Box 245017
Tucson, AZ 85724

520-626-4555
Fax: 520-626-6623
www.medicine.arizona.edu/centers/index.cfm

The newest addition to the University of Arizona's College of Medicine. Program and website under development at time of publication.

Steven Goldschmid, Dean
Judith DiMarco, Associate Dean

California

4890 Loma Linda University Sleep Disorders Cent er
11139 Anderson St.
Loma Linda, CA 92350

909-558-6344
Fax: 909-558-6343
www.llu.edu

Richard H Hart, CEO
Philip M. Gold, Medical Director
Richard E. Chinnock, MD, Medical Director

4891 Stanford University Center for Narcolepsy
450 Broadway Street, Pav B, 2nd Floor
Redwood City, CA 94063

650-721-7550
Fax: 650-721-3466
e-mail: einen@stanford.edu
www.med.stanford.edu/school/psychiatry/narcolepsy/
Theodore Chen, Director

Connecticut

4892 Gaylord Hospital Sleep Medicine
Gaylord Farm Road, PO Box 400
Wallingford, CT 06492

203-284-2800
866-429-5673
TTY: 203-284-2700
TDD: 203-284-2700
e-mail: lcrispino@gaylord.org
www.gaylord.org

Nadine Cartwright

District of Columbia

4893 Georgetown University Sleep Disorders Center
3800 Reservoir Road NW
Washington, DC 20007

202-444-2000
Fax: 202-444-2336
e-mail: pme2@gunet.georgetown.edu
www.georgetownuniversityhospital.org

Anne O'Donnel, Chair
Raoul L Wientzen, President

Indiana

4894 Methodist Hospital Sleep Disorders Center
Rehab Centers
8701 Broadway
Merrillville, IN 46410

219-738-5500
800-909-3627
Fax: 219-738-6624
www.methodisthospitals.org

Ian E. McFadden, President/CEO
Robin Logsdon, Manager

4895 MidWest Medical Center - Sleep Disorders Center
3232 N Meridian Street
Indianapolis, IN 46208
Kenneth Wiesert, MD

317-927-2100

4896 Sleep Disorder Center, St Elizabeth Medica l Center
1501 Hartford Street, PO Box 7501
Lafayette, IN 47903

766-423-6518
800-371-6011
Fax: 765-423-6525
www.glhsi.org

Dr Shahid M Ahsan, Medical Director

4897 Sleep Disorders Center-Good Samaritan Hospital
520 S 7th Street
Vincenne, IN 47591

812-885-3988
812-882-5220
e-mail: gsh@gshvin.org
www.gshvin.org/goodsamaritan/

4898 Sleep/Wake Disorders Center-Community Heal th Network
1500 N Ritter Avenue, Suite 451
Indianapolis, IN 46219
317-355-1411
Fax: 317-351-2785
e-mail: sleepcenter@ecommunity.com
www.ecommunity.com/sleep/
Marvin E Vollmer, MD, Co-Director

Maryland

4899 Johns Hopkins University Sleep Disorders Center
Francis Scott Key Medical Center
301 Bayview Boulevard
Baltimore, MD 21224
410-550-0571
Fax: 410-550-3374
e-mail: nschube1@jhmi.edu
Alan Schwartz, MD, Medical Director

Massachusetts

4900 Sleep Disorders Unit, Beth Israel Hospital
330 Brookline Avenue
Boston, MA 02215
617-667-7000
800-439-0183
Fax: 617-975-5506
e-mail: patsite@bidmc.harvard.edu
www.bidmc.org
Stephan B. Kay, Chair
Daniel Jick, First Vice Chair
Carol Anderson, Vice Chairperson

Michigan

4901 Center for Sleep Science at University of Michigan
University of Michigan Health System
2799 West Grand Boulevard Cfp3
Detroit, MI 48202
313-916-5176
Fax: 313-916-5150
e-mail: dhudgel1@hfhs.org
www.med.umich.edu/umsleepscience/

The center's main goal is to advance knowledge and understanding in these three areas: the physiology of normal sleep; the diagnosis of sleep disorders; and the treatment of sleep problems.

Ronald D Chervin MD, Director
Barbara T Felts MD, Pediatrics

Minnesota

4902 Center for Sleep Diagnostics
1455 St. Frances Ave.
Shakopee, MN 55379
952-428-3000
e-mail: askstfrancis@allina.com
www.stfrancis-shakopee.com

Is dedicated to providing information, education, and support for all your sleep needs. Our goal is to be the center of sleep information and discussion on the internet.

David Zelinsky, Chair
Kelly J. DiGrado, Vice Chairman
Lee Shimek, Secretary

New Hampshire

4903 Dartmouth-Hitchcock Sleep Disorders Center Dartmouth Medical Center
One Medical Center Drive
Lebanon, NH 03756
603-650-7534
Fax: 603-650-7820
www.dartmouth-hitchcock.org
Rocco R Addante, Director
Glen Greenough MD, Fellowship Director
Joanne MacQuarrie, BS,RPSGT,RRT, Administrator

4904 Sleep/Wake Disorders Center, Hampstead Hospital
218 East Road
Hampstead, NH 03841
603-329-5311
Fax: 603-329-4746
www.hampsteadhospital.com
Philip Kubaik, CEO
Cynthia Gove, COO
Scott Ranks, Director support Services

New Jersey

4905 Newark Sleep Disorders Center
Newark Beth Israel Medical Center
201 Lyons Avenue
Newark, NJ 07112
973-926-7163
Fax: 973-926-6672
e-mail: mkaretzky@sbhcs.com
www.njsleephelp.com
Dr Monroe S Karetzky, Director

New York

4906 Capital Regional Sleep-Wake Disorders Center
Saint Peter's Hospital & Albany Medical Center
1220 New Scotland Road
Slingerlands, NY 12159
518-439-4326
Fax: 518-439-6143
e-mail: bwenzel@stpetershealthcare.org
www.capitalregionspecialsurgery.com/sleep-wake/
William Wenzel, Manager

4907 Center for Sleep Medicine of the Mount Sinai Medical Center
Box 1232, One Gustave L Levy Place
New York, NY 10029
212-241-6500
800-637-4624
Fax: 212-987-5584
www.mountsinai.org
Kenneth L. Davis, President/CEO
Dennis S. Charney, Executive VP
Douglas Jabs, CEO

4908 Columbia Presbyterian Medical Center Sleep Disorders Center
630 West 168th St
New York, NY 10032
212-305-5371
Fax: 212-305-5496
www.nyp.org
Ronald E Drusin

4909 Saint Joseph's Hospital Health Center Sleep Laboratory
301 Prospect Ave.
Syracuse, NY 13203
315-448-5111
888-785-6371
www.sjhsyr.org
George Deptula, Chairperson
Kathryn H. Ruscitto, President
Sister Mary Obrist, Secretary

4910 Sleep Center, Community General Hospital
4900 Broad Road
Syracuse, NY 13215
315-492-5877
www.chg.org
Robert Westlake, MD

4911 Sleep Disorders Center of Western New York Millard Fillmore Hospital
3 Gates Circle
Buffalo, NY 14209
716-887-5337
Fax: 716-887-5332
e-mail: drifkin@kaleidahealth.org
www.sleepcenterwny.com
Daniel Rifkin MD, Medical Director

4912 Sleep Disorders Center, University Hospital
101 Nicolls Road
Stony Brook, NY 11794   631-444-4000
                                    Fax: 631-444-8821
                  e-mail: craig.lehmann@stonybrook.edu
                  www.healthtechnology.stonybrookmedicine.edu
Craig A. Lehmann, Dean
Richard W. Johnson, Associate Dean
Carol Vidal, Associate Dean for community Engage

**4913 Sleep-Wake Disorders Center, Montefiore Sleep Disorders
       Center**
111 E 210th Street
Bronx, NY 10467   718-920-4841
                                    Fax: 718-798-4352
                        e-mail: thorpy@aecom.yu.edu
                        www.cloud9.net/~thorpy/mmc

Center that provides diagnostic and treatment services for children with sleep disorders, such as sleep apnea, narcolepsy, insomnia, daytime sleepiness, sleepwalking, or night terrors.

Michael J Thorpy, MD, Medical Director
Karen Balaban-Gil, MD

**4914 Sleep-Wake Disorders Center, New York Presbyterian
       Hospital**
Cornell Medical Center
21 Bloomingdale Road
White Plains, NY 10605   914-997-5751
                                         800-694-7533
                                    Fax: 914-682-6911
                     e-mail: mmoline@med.cornell.edu
                  www.cornellphysicians.com/sleepWake/

Provides outpatient diagnostic evaluation and treatment for adults
and children with problems associated with sleeping and waking.
More common pediatric sleep problems include complaints of difficulty falling asleep and staying asleep, snoring, sleep apnea,
sleepwalking, sleep terrors, nightmares, excessive difficulty waking up, bedwetting, and narcolepsy. Many can be successfully
treated in one or several visits although some may require an
overnight or daytime sleep study.

Margaret Moline, PHD, Director

4915 Unity Sleep Disorders Clinic Unity Health System
89 Genesee Street
Rochester, NY 14611   585-723-7000
                                    Fax: 585-442-6259
                        e-mail: Oncall@unityhealth.org
                                www.unityhealth.org
Warren Hern, President/CEO
Annette Leahy, President
Tom Crilly, Executive VP/CFO

4916 Winthrop-University Hospital Sleep Disorders Center
1300 Franklin Avenue, Suite UL-5
Garden City, NY 11530   516-663-3907
                                    Fax: 516-663-4788
                        e-mail: mweinstein@winthrop
            www.winthrop.org/departments/specialtycenters/?id=31
Charles M. Strain, Chairman
John F. Collins, President/CEO
Michael Weinstein, Medical Director

Ohio

4917 Bethesda Oak Hospital, Sleep Disorders Center
619 Oak St.
Cincinnati, OH 45206   513-569-5400
                                    Fax: 513-745-1691
                  e-mail: michael_fletcher@trihealth.com
                                www.trihealth.com
Anthony P Borzotta

4918 Center for Sleep & Wake Disorders, Miami Valley Hospital
One Wyoming Street
Dayton, OH 45409   937-208-8000
                                    Fax: 937-208-2006
                        e-mail: khuban@wor.rr.com
                        www.miamivalleyhospital.com

M Dallal, Manager

4919 Cleveland Clinic Foundation, Sleep Disorders Center
9500 Euclid Avenue FA20
Cleveland, OH 44195   216-444-4508
                                         800-223-2273
                                    Fax: 216-445-6205
                        e-mail: foldvan@ccf.org
                            my.clevelandclinic.org

Petra Podmore, Manager

4920 Kettering Medical Center, Sleep Disorders Center
3095 Dayton-Xenia Rd
Beavercreek, OH 45439   937-458-4010
                                www.ketteringhealth.org
George G. Burton MD, Medical Director

4921 NW Ohio Sleep Disorders Center
Toledo Hospital
2121 Hughes Drive Harris-McIntosh Tower 2nd Floor
Toledo, OH 43606   419-291-5629
                                    Fax: 419-479-6954
                     e-mail: pam.lang@promedica.org
                            www.nwosemsleep.org
Navin K. Jain, President
Michael Neeb, VP
James Kusina, Secretary

4922 Ohio Sleep Medicine Institute
4975 Bradenton Avenue
Dublin, OH 43017   614-766-0773
                                    Fax: 614-766-2599
                     e-mail: info@sleepmedicine.com
                            www.sleepmedicine.com
Dr. Markus Schmidt, MD, President
Dr. Asim Roy, Clinic Associate

4923 Ohio State University Hospitals, Sleep Disorders Center
410 W 10th Avenue
Columbus, OH 43210   614-293-8652
                                    Fax: 614-257-2551
                            www.medicalcenter.osu.edu
Larry Anstine, CEO

4924 Saint Vincent Medical Center, Sleep Disorders Center
3829 Woodley Road Suite 1
Toledo, OH 43606   419-250-5702
                                    Fax: 419-251-0574
                                www.stvincent.org
Joseph Schaffer, PhD, Director
Gary Fammartino, Site Admin

Pennsylvania

4925 Community Medical Center, Sleep Disorders Clinic
1800 Mulberry Street
Scranton, PA 18510   570-969-8000
                                www.cmchealthsys.org
Michael Aronica, Director

4926 Crozer-Chester Medical Center
Sleep Disorders Center
Department of Neurology
Upland-Chester, PA 19013   610-447-2689
                                         800-254-3258
                        e-mail: CKHSInfo@crozer.org
                            www.crozerkeystone.org
Joan Richards, President/CEO
Calvin Stafford, MD, Director

**4927 Geisinger Wyoming Valley Medical Center, Sleep Disorders
       Center**
1000 E. Mountain Blvd.
Wilkes-Barre, PA 18711   570-808-7300
                                         800-275-6401
                                    Fax: 570-826-7650
                        e-mail: lvender@geisinger.edu
                            www.geisinger.org
John W. McBurney, MD, Medical Director

4928 Lankenau Hospital, Sleep Disorders Center
100 Lancaster Avenue
Wynnewood, PA 19096   484-476-2000
                                                                  866-CAL- MLH
                                                             Fax: 610-645-2291
                                                   e-mail: pressmanm@mlhs.org
                                                       www.mainlinehealth.org

Sandra V Abramson, Director

4929 Medical College of Pennsylvania, Sleep Disorders Center
3300 Henry Avenue
Philadelphia, PA 19129   215-842-6000
Farhana Bashar, Director

4930 Mercy Hospital of Johnstown, Sleep Disorders Center
1086 Franklin Street
Johnstown, PA 15905   814-534-9000
William F Pruchnic, Director

4931 Penn Center for Sleep Disorders, Hospital of the University of Pennsylvania
3624 Market Street, Suite 201
Philadelphia, PA 19104   215-590-3703
                                                             800-789-PENN
                                                             Fax: 215-590-2632

Indira Gurubhagavatula, MD, Director

4932 Presbyterian-University Hospital, Pulmonary Sleep Evaluation Center
200 Lothrop Street
Pittsburgh, PA 15213   412-647-2345
                                                               www.upmc.com

Mark Sanders, MD, Director

4933 Thomas Jefferson University Sleep Disorders Center
Jefferson Medical College
Suite 500, 211 S 9th St
Philadelphia, PA 19107   215-955-6175
                                                             Fax: 215-923-8219
                                                     www.jeffersonhospital.org

Karl Doghramji, MD, Director

4934 Western Psychiatric Institute & Clinic, Sleep Evaluation Center
3811 O'Hara Street
Pittsburgh, PA 15213   412-624-3934
                                                             Fax: 412-246-5300

David Alan Lewis, Director

Rhode Island

4935 Sleep Disorders Center of Lifespan Hospita ls
Rhode Island Hospital
167 Point Street
Providence, RI 02903   401-444-3500
                                                             Fax: 404-431-5429
                                                 e-mail: millman@lifespan.org
                                                            www.lifespan.org

Timonthy J. Babineau, President/CEO
Kenneth E. Arnold, Senior Vice-President
August Cordeiro, President

Texas

4936 Sleep Disorders Center for Children
Children's Medical Center of Dallas
1935 Medical District Dr
Dallas, TX 75235   214-456-7000
                                                             Fax: 214-456-8740
                                           e-mail: larry.brewer@childrens.com
                                                          www.childrens.com

Dr S K Naqvi, Medical Director
Dr John Herman PhD, Contact for Children

4937 Sleep Medicine Associates of Texas
5477 Glen Lakes Drive, Suite 100
Dallas, TX 75231   214-750-7776
                                                             Fax: 214-750-4621
                                                            www.sleepmed.com

Philip M Becker, President

4938 University of Texas Sleep/Wake Disorders Center
Southwestern Medical Center
5323 Harry Hines Boulevard
Dallas, TX 75235   214-648-3111
                                                             Fax: 214-648-3112

Studies sleep/wake disorders including insomnia, apnea and narcolepsy.

Howard Roffwrag, MD, Director

Research Centers

Illinois

4939 Center for Narcolepsy Research at the University of Illinois at Chicago
College of Nursing M/C 802
845 S Damen Avenue
Chicago, IL 60612   312-996-5176
                                                             Fax: 312-996-7008
                                              e-mail: CNSHR@listserv.uic.edu
                                                                  www.uic.edu

David W. Carley, PhD, Director
Mary Kapella, Associate Director
Julie Law, Center Administration

Iowa

4940 Mercy Sleep Laboratory
Mercy Medical Center
1111 6th Avenue
Des Moines, IA 50314   515-358-9600
                                                             Fax: 515-643-8905
                                         e-mail: cmann@mercydesmoines.org
                                                      www.mercydesmoines.org

Sleep is an integral part of life, but it's not always a welcome or peaceful close to a busy day. Some people suffer almost unbearable torture as they toss and turn. Others find sleepiness an uncontrollable intruder. It's been estimated that 30 to 40 percent of the population suffers from a sleeping problem at some time in their lives. Mercy's Sleep Center helps patients with sleep problems.

Donald L. Burrows, MD, Medical Director

Maine

4941 Sleep Laboratory, Maine Medical Center
930 Congress Street
Portland, ME 04102   207-662-4535
                                                             Fax: 207-662-6005
                                                                  www.mmc.org

Christopher W. Emmons, Chairman
Frank H. Frye, Vice-Chairman
Richard W. Peterson, President

Maryland

4942 University of Maryland Medical Center
Pediatric Sleep Disorders Center
22 S Greene Street
Baltimore, MD 21201   866-408-6885
                                                             800-492-5538
                                                           TDD: 800-735-2258
                                                                  www.umm.edu

Carol J Blaisdell MD, Director

Ohio

4943 Tri-State Sleep Disorders Center Center for Research in Sleep Disorders
1275 E Kemper Road
Cincinnati, OH 45246
513-671-3101
800-838-4322
Fax: 513-671-4159
e-mail: web@tristatesleep.com
www.tristatesleep.com

Provides diagnostics and treatment services to thousands of people in Cincinnati and throughout the country at our state-of-the-art sleep clinic through cutting edge research efforts.

Martin B Scharf, Executive Director
Dr. David Berkowitz
Cara Zurmehly PA-C

Texas

4944 Baylor Sleep Wellness Center
Baylor Clinic
6620 Main Street
Houston, TX 77030
713-798-1000
800-229-5671
www.baylorclinic.com

A comprehensive program with a multidisciplinary approach to sleep disorders.

Sr Shyam Subramanian, Director, Sigworth
VP Rose, Clinical Psychologist

4945 University of Texas Medical Branch at Galveston, Clinical Research Center
301 University Boulevard
Galveston, TX 77555
409-772-2222
800-917-8906
Fax: 409-772-6216
e-mail: public.affairs@utmb.edu
www.utmb.edu

Research focusing on sleep disorders including apnea and narcolepsy.

David L. Callender, President
Cary W. Cooper, VP/Dean
William R. Elger, Executive VP

Audio Video

4946 Narcolepsy
Fanlight Productions
32 Court Street
Brooklyn, NY 11201
718-488-8900
800-876-1710
Fax: 718-488-8642
e-mail: info@fanlight.com
www.fanlight.com

Presents the experiences of three individuals whose lives and relationships have been disrupted by narcolepsy, while offering solid, comprehensive scientific information about the disorder.
ISBN: DVD: 1-57295-974-6; VHS: 1-572953-23-2

25 minutes DVD or VHS

Ben Achtenberg, President
Anthony Sweeney, Marketing Director
Nicole Johnson, Publicity Coordinator

4947 Narcolepsy: A Guide for Understanding, Dia gnosing & Treating Narcolepsy
National Sleep Foundation
1010 N. Glebe Road, Suite 310
Arlington, VA 22201
703-243-1697
e-mail: nsf@sleepfoundation.org
www.sleepfoundation.org

A comprehensive PowerPoint™, 114 slide presentation to educate health care providers about narcolepsy.

Charles A. Czeisler, PhD, MD, Chairman
Max Hirshkowitz, PhD, Vice Chairman
Joseph Ojile, MD, Secretary

4948 Narcolepsy: Evaluation and Treatment
American Academy of Sleep Medicine
2510 North Frontage Road
Darien, IL 60561
630-737-9700
Fax: 630-737-9790
www.aasmnet.org

A 97 slide presentation designed as a foundation for a teaching curriculum on the recognition and traetment of narcolepsy.

Timothy I. Morgenthaker, MD, President
Nathaniel F. Watson, MD, President-Elect
Ronald D. Chervin, MD, MS, Secretary/Treasurer

Web Sites

4949 Narcolepsy
129 Waterwheel Lane
North Kingstown, RI 2852
401-667-2523
888-292-6522
Fax: 401-633-6567
e-mail: NarNet@narcolepsynetwork.org
narcolepsynetwork.org

Narcolepsy Internet jumpstation.

4950 Online Mendelian Inheritance in Man
National Library of Medicine Building 38A
Bethesda, MD 20894
888-346-3656
e-mail: info@ncbi.nlm.nih.gov
www.ncbi.nlm.nih.gov

This database is a catalog of human genes and genetic disorders.

Christine E. Seidman, M.D., Chair
David J. Lipman, Executive Secretary

4951 Sleep Disorders
http://talhost.net/sleep/narcolepsy.htm

Descriptions of certain sleep disorders and useful links.

4952 Talk About Sleep
www.talkaboutsleep.com

Sleep disorder information and resources.

Book Publishers

4953 Narcolepsy Primer
Montefiore Medical Center
111 E 210th Street
Bronx, NY 10467
718-920-4321
e-mail: info@Montefiore.org
www.montefiore.org

A guide for physicians, patients and their families on the affects, causes and prevention of narcolepsy.

Steven M. Safyer, MD, President/CEO
Philip O. Ozuah, Chief Operating Officer
Joel A. Perlman, Chief Financial Officer

4954 Psychosocial Aspects of Narcolepsy

Meeta Goswami, author

Haworth Press
PO BOX 8002
Aston, PA 19014
800-234-1340
Fax: 800-875-1340
e-mail: info@omnigraphics.com
www.omnigraphics.com

Addresses the diagnosis, treatment and management of narcolepsy with particular emphasis on psychological and social aspects of care.

567 pages Hardcover
ISBN: 1-560242-22-1

Peter Ruffner, Publisher

4955 Sleep Disorders Sourcebook
Omnigraphics
PO Box 8002
Aston, PA 19014
800-234-1340
Fax: 800-875-1340
e-mail: info@omnigraphics.com
www.omnigraphics.com

Basic consumer health information about sleep and its disorders, including narcolepsy, insomnia, sleepwalking, sleep apnea, and restless leg syndrome.

567 pages 2nd edition
ISBN: 0-780807-43-0

Peter Ruffner, Publisher

4956 Sleep Disorders and Psychiatry

Daniel J Buysse MD, author

American Psychiatric Publishing
1000 Wilson Boulevard, Ste 1825
Arlington, VA 22209
703-907-7322
800-368-5777
Fax: 703-907-1091
e-mail: appi@psych.org
www.appi.org

Summarizes the major categories of sleep disorders including parasomnias and narcolepsy.

2005 256 pages Paperback
ISBN: 1-585622-29-0

Robert E. Hales, M.D., Editor-in-Chief
Rebecca D. Rinehart, Publisher
John McDuffie, Editorial Director

Pamphlets

4957 Living with Narcolepsy
National Sleep Foundation
1010 N. Glebe Road, Suite 310
Arlington, VA 22201
703-243-1697
Fax: 202-347-3472
e-mail: nsf@sleepfoundation.org
www.sleepfoundation.org

For people with narcolepsy and their families; defines and describes narcolepsy, as well as the effects on education, social and family life.

packet of 25

Charles A. Czeisler, PhD, MD, Chairman
Max Hirshkowitz, PhD, Vice Chairman
Joseph Ojile, MD, Secretary

4958 Narcolepsy
American Academy of Sleep Medicine
2510 North Frontage Road
Darien, IL 60561
630-737-9700
Fax: 630-737-9790
www.aasmnet.org

Describes the causes, symptoms and treatments of a disorder characterized by excessive sleepiness.

Lot of 50

Timothy I. Morgenthaker, MD, President
Nathaniel F. Watson, MD, President-Elect
Ronald D. Chervin, MD, MS, Secretary/Treasurer

Description

4959 NEONATAL HERPES SIMPLEX

Synonym: Congenital herpes

Involves the following Biologic System(s):

Infectious Disorders, Neonatal and Infant Disorders

Neonatal herpes simplex refers to an infection of the newborn caused by the herpes simplex virus (HSV) that is transmitted before birth from mother to fetus through the placenta, or more commonly, during birth as the baby passes through the birth canal. There are two strains of herpes simplex virus known as HSV-1 and HSV-2. Herpes simplex virus type 1 commonly causes infections of the skin and mucous membranes of the lips, mouth, and eyes, while type 2 typically causes genital herpes as well as approximately 75 percent of all neonatal herpes simplex infections.

Herpes simplex may be categorized as an initial (primary) infection or a recurrent infection. After an initial infection, the virus becomes inactive or latent; however, the virus may be reactivated by many different factors including stress, sun exposure, suppression of the immune system, and certain foods or drugs. Mothers with a primary genital herpes simplex virus infection have an approximately 45 percent chance of transmitting HSV-2 to their infants, while risk of transmission from a recurrent infection is less than five percent. In addition, newborns are at risk for HSV-1 transmission through such direct contact as kissing near the eyes or mouth by someone with a cold sore.

Symptoms of HSV infection transmitted through contact with infectious secretions during the birthing process may occur anywhere from one to four weeks after birth and may sometimes commence with the appearance of small, fluid-filled blisters (vesicles) on the skin or inflammation of the front part of the eyeball (cornea) and the delicate mucous membranes (conjunctiva) that line the inside of the eyelids and the whites of the eyes (keratoconjunctivitis). Other findings may include fever, drowsiness, loss of muscle tone, irritability, seizures, and inflammation of the liver (hepatitis) and brain (encephalitis), as well as other severe irregularities. If left untreated, HSV infection may cause potentially life-threatening complications. Some infants may have no skin involvement but manifest such symptoms as fluctuating temperature, listlessness, poor sucking, chills, shaking, nausea, vomiting, and diarrhea.

Transmission of the herpes simplex virus through the placenta is a rare but potentially life-threatening occurrence. This type of infection usually affects the skin, eyes, and central nervous system and is characterized by blister-type rashes and scarring, abnormally small eyes (microphthalmia) and other eye abnormalities, an abnormally small head (microcephaly), and brain and spinal cord irregularities. Some infants may also have hepatitis or lung involvement.

Prevention of neonatal herpes simplex infection may include delivery by Cesarean section, especially if the mother has a primary genital herpes infection. Treatment is directed toward early diagnosis and intervention. Such therapy may include the intravenous administration of antiviral drugs such as acyclovir in conjunction with regular testing to preclude possible associated toxic side effects related to kidney dysfunction. Eye involvement may indicate the application of antiviral ointments or drops directly into the eyes. Other treatment is symptomatic and supportive.

Government Agencies

4960 NIH/National Institute of Allergy and Infectious Diseases
6610 Rockledge Drive, Room 4017, MSC 6606. PO Box
Bethesda, MD 20817
301-496-2644
866-284-4107
Fax: 301-402-7123
TDD: 800-877-8339
e-mail: niaidnews@niaid.nih.gov
www.niaid.nih.gov

Conducts and supports basic and applied research to better understand, treat, and ultimately prevent infectious, immunologic, and allergic diseases.

Anthony S Fauci MD, Director

National Associations & Support Groups

4961 American Academy of Pediatrics
141 Northwest Point Boulevard
Elk Grove Village, IL 60007
847-434-4000
800-433-9016
Fax: 847-434-8000
www.aap.org

The American Academy of Pediatrics and its member pediatricians are committed to the attainment of optimal physical, mental and social health and well-being for all infants, children, adolescents, and young adults.

Sandra Hassink, MD, FAAP, President

4962 American Social Health Association
PO Box 13827
Research Triangle Park, NC 27709
919-361-8400
919-361-8488
Fax: 919-361-8425
e-mail: info@ashastd.org
www.ashastd.org

The American Social Health Association is dedicated to improving the health of individuals, families, and communities, with a focus on preventing sexually transmitted diseases and their harmful consequences.

Lynn Barclay, President/CEO

4963 National Health Information Center: Office of Disease Preventive/Health Promotion
US Dept of Health and Human Services
PO Box 1133
Washington, DC 20013
240-453-8280
800-336-4797
Fax: 240-453-8282
e-mail: info@nhif.org
www.nhic.org

The National Health Information Center is a health information referral service that links consumers and health professionals who have health questions to organizations best able to provide reliable health information.

Libraries & Resource Centers

4964 Herpes Resource Center
American Social Health Association
PO Box 13827
Research Triangle Park, NC 27709
919-361-8400
Fax: 919-361-8425
e-mail: customerservice@ashastd.org
www.ashastd.org

Tom Beall, Chairman
Lynn Barclay, President and Chief Executive Offic
Deborah Arrindell, Vice President, Health Policy

Web Sites

4965 American Social Health Association
www.ashastd.org

Dedicated to improving the health of individuals, families, and communities, with a focus on preventing sexually transmitted diseases and their harmful consequences.

4966 Health Research Project (HaRP)
www.harpnet.org

e-mail: harp@aimglobalhealth.org
www.harpnet.org

A program by USAID, the project strives to improve the health status of infants, children, mothers and families through the development and research of new tools, technologies, policies and approaches.

4967 HerpeSite
www.herpesite.org

800-273-8255
TTY: 800-799-4889
www.herpesite.org

Provides online personal empowerment and support; a compedium of information outlining aspects and issues relating to Herpes Simplex Virus.

4968 Herpes.com
www.herpes.com

Purpose of this website is to fill the desperate need for herpes education, make it easier to manage herpes, inform people of ways to limit herpes reoccurrences, to inform people of the beneficial products for herpes sufferers, to show the relationship between good health and herpes, to provide an opportunity for herpes sufferers to share their personal experiences and to provide communication via our live chat.

4969 Infectious Diseases in Children
6900 Grove Road
Thorofare, NJ 8086   856-848-1000
e-mail: editor@healio.com
http://idinchildren.com

A leading provider of healthcare information, educational programs, and meeting and exhibit management services worldwide.

4970 International Herpes Alliance
www.herpesalliance.org

4971 Virtual Pediatric Hospital
www.virtualpediatrichospital.org

A digital library of pediatric informaion dedicated to helping patients find the highest quality medical information in the world today. Offers patients the tools necessary to make informed treatment decisions within the short time lines dictated by their illness or disease.

Book Publishers

4972 Understanding Herpes
Dr Lawrence R Stanberg, author

University Press of Mississippi
3825 Ridgewood Road
Jackson, MS 39211   601-432-6205
800-737-7788
Fax: 601-432-6217
e-mail: press@ihl.state.ms.us
www.upress.state.ms.us

A most informative overview of herpes written for the general reader.

120 pages Cloth
ISBN: 1-578060-40-0

Leila W. Salisbury, Director
Cynthia Foster, Administrative Assistant
Tracey Curtis, Assistant For Development

Description

4973 NEONATAL JAUNDICE

Synonym: Icterus neonatorum

Involves the following Biologic System(s):

Neonatal and Infant Disorders

Neonatal jaundice refers to a condition of the newborn in which high blood levels of the reddish-orange bile pigment bilirubin cause a yellowing of the skin, eyes, and mucous membranes. Bilirubin is derived from the breakdown of the protein, hemoglobin, in red blood cells. Neonatal jaundice may be the result of many different factors including metabolic disturbances or deficiencies; certain genetic disorders; conditions associated with an increased rate of red blood cell destruction (hemolysis); conditions that affect liver function; and certain types of infections.

Blood levels of bilirubin may be somewhat elevated after the first day of life, usually peak by the fourth day, and fall to normal levels by the end of the first week. This temporary rise, frequently accompanied by jaundice, results from the increased destruction of fetal red blood cells and the inability of a still-developing metabolic mechanism to efficiently eliminate bile from the body. In addition, an enzyme present in the intestines of newborns may convert bilirubin to a form that allows it to be reabsorbed into the blood, resulting in even higher bilirubin blood levels. Premature infants are particularly at risk for jaundice. If no other underlying cause is responsible, jaundice typically resolves spontaneously along with bilirubin level stabilization.

The appearance of jaundice in a newborn is carefully evaluated for underlying causes. Factors that may indicate the presence of an underlying disorder may include jaundice within the first 24 hours of life; a higher and faster-than-expected rise in bilirubin levels; birth defects, especially those that affect the liver such as biliary atresia; a family history of diseases that cause the early destruction of red blood cells such as hemolytic disease of the newborn; or rare disorders associated with hyperbilirubinemia (e.g., Crigler-Najjar syndrome, transient familial neonatal hyperbilirubinemia, etc.). Other suspect findings may include an enlarged liver (hepatomegaly), enlarged spleen (splenomegaly), lethargy, unusual paleness, difficulty in feeding, vomiting, or excessive weight loss.

Treatment of neonatal jaundice depends upon the underlying cause. Some infants with jaundice associated with breast-feeding may benefit from phototherapy. During this treatment, which is carefully monitored, the infant's bare skin is exposed to high intensity fluorescent lights that speed up the excretion and elimination of bilirubin in the skin. Other treatment is symptomatic and supportive.

Government Agencies

4974 NIH/National Institute of Child Health and Human Development

31 Center Drive, Building 31, Room 2A32
Bethesda, MD 20892

301-496-1333
800-370-2943
Fax: 866-760-5947
TTY: 888-320-6942
e-mail: NICHDInformationResourceCenter@mail.nih.
www.nichd.nih.gov

Established in 1962 by congress, today the institute conducts and supports research on topics related to the health of children, adults, families and populations. Some of these topics include: developmental disabilities, growth and development, infant death, reproductive health and birth defects.

Jay H Hoofnagle, Director
Lisa Kaeser, Program & Public Liaison

National Associations & Support Groups

4975 American Academy of Pediatrics

141 Northwest Point Boulevard
Elk Grove Village, IL 60007

847-434-4000
800-433-9016
Fax: 847-434-8000
www.aap.org

The American Academy of Pediatrics and its member pediatricians are committed to the attainment of optimal physical, mental and social health and well-being for all infants, children, adolescents, and young adults.

Sandra Hassink, MD, FAAP, President

4976 American College of Gastroenterology

6400 Goldsboro Rd, Ste 200
Bethesda, MD 20817

301-263-9000
Fax: 301-263-9025
www.acg.gi.org

Founded to advance the scientific study and medical practice of diseases of the gastrointestinal (GI) tract.

Ronald J. Vender, President
Harry E. Sarles, Jr., President Elect
Stephen B. Hanauer, VP

4977 American Liver Foundation

39 Broadway, Suite 2700
New York, NY 10006

212-668-1000
800-465-4837
Fax: 212-483-8179
e-mail: info@liverfoundation.org
www.liverfoundation.org

Nonprofit, national, voluntary health organization dedicated to the prevention, treatment and cure of hepatitis and other liver diseases through research, education, and advocacy on behalf of those affected by or at risk of liver disease.

Thomas F. Nealon III, Chairman
Daniel E. Weil, Treasurer
Carlo Frappolli, Secretary

4978 Digestive Disease National Coalition

507 Capitol Court NE, Suite 200
Washington, DC 20002

202-544-7497
Fax: 202-546-7105
e-mail: ddnc@hmcw.org
www.ddnc.org

Advocacy organization comprised of 22 voluntary and professional societies concerned with the many diseases of the digestive tract and liver.

Diane Paley, Chairperson
James DeGerome, MD, President
Andrew Spiegel, Vice-Chairman

4979 Greater Los Angeles Chapter
American Liver Foundation
130 N. Brand Blvd., Suite 305
Glendale, CA 91203

818-500-8636
Fax: 818-500-8638
e-mail: cshort@liverfoundation.org
www.cai-glac.org/

A national organization that promotes research and cures for hepatitis and other liver diseases.

Matt D. Ober, Partner
Katy Krupp, VP
Gregg Lotane, Treasurer

4980 International Foundation for Functional Gastrointestinal Disorders
700 W. Virginia St., #201
Milwaukee, WI 53204

414-964-1799
888-964-2001
Fax: 414-964-7176
e-mail: iffgd@iffgd.org
www.iffgd.org

Nonprofit education and research organization founded in 1991. IFFGD addresses the issues surrounding life with gastrointestinal (GI) functional and mobility disorders and increases the awareness about these disorders among the general public, researchers and the clinical care community.

Nancy J Norton, Founder
William Norton, VP/Director
Eleanor Cautley, VP/Director

4981 March of Dimes Birth Defects Foundation
1275 Mamaroneck Avenue
White Plains, NY 10605

914-997-4488
888-663-4637
Fax: 914-428-8203
e-mail: answers@marchofdimes.com
www.marchofdimes.com

Partnership of volunteers and professionals dedicates to improving the health of babies by preventing birth defects and infant mortality. Over 100 chapters are located across the country and can be located through the National Office.

Jennifer L Howse, President

4982 North American Society for Pediatric Gastroenterology/Hepatology/Nutrition
PO Box 6
Flourtown, PA 19031

215-233-0808
Fax: 215-233-3918
e-mail: naspghan@naspghan.org
www.naspghan.org

Strives to improve the care of infants, children and adolescents with digestive disorders by promoting advances in clinical care of children with chronic abdominal pain, diarrhea, constipation, vomiting, bleeding from the GI tract, inflammatory bowel disease, liver diseases, diseases of the pancreas, poor weight gain and nutritional problems.

Philip Sherman, President
Margaret K Stallings, Executive Director

Libraries & Resource Centers

4983 National Digestive Diseases Information Clearinghouse
2 Information Way
Bethesda, MD 20892

301-654-3810; 800-891-5389
Fax: 301-907-8906
e-mail: nddic@info.niddk.nih.gov
www2.niddk.nih.gov

The National Institute of Diabetes and Digestive and Kidney Diseases conducts and supports research on many of the most serious diseases affecting public health. The Institute supports much of the clinical research on the diseases of internal medicine and related subspecialty fields as well as many basic science disciplines.

Griffin P. Rodgers, M.D, Chairman, Executive Board
Brent B. Stanfield, Executive Secretary
Camille M. Hoover, M.S.W, Executive Officer

Web Sites

4984 American Liver Foundation
39 Broadway, Suite 2700
New York, NY 10006

212-668-1000; Fax: 212-483-8179
www.liverfoundation.org

Nonprofit, national, voluntary health organization dedicated to the prevention, treatment and cure of hepatitis and other liver diseases through research, education, and advocacy on behalf of those affected by or at risk of liver disease.

Thomas F. Nealon III, Chairman
Daniel E. Weil, Treasurer
Carlo Frappolli, Secretary

4985 Liver 411
www.liver411.com

4986 National Digestive Diseases Information Clearinghouse
www.digestive.niddk.nih.gov

301-496-3583
www.digestive.niddk.nih.gov

The National Institute of Diabetes and Digestive and Kidney Diseases conducts and supports research on many of the most serious diseases affecting public health. The Institute supports much of the clinical research on the diseases of internal medicine and related subspecialty fields as well as many basic science disciplines.

4987 Online Mendelian Inheritance in Man
National Library of Medicine Building 38A
Bethesda, MD 20894

888-346-3656
e-mail: info@ncbi.nlm.nih.gov
www.ncbi.nlm.nih.gov

This database is a catalog of human genes and genetic disorders.

Journals

4988 Journal of Pediatric Gastroenterology and Nutrition
NASPGHAN, author

Lippincott Williams & Wilkins
2001 Market Street
Philadelphia, PA 19103

215-521-8300; Fax: 215-521-8902
www.lww.com

Publication of the North American Society for Pediatric Gastroenterolgy, Hepatology and Nutrition, which strives to improve the care of infants, children and adolescents with digestive disorders by promoting advances in clinical care of children with chronic abdominal pain, diarrhea, constipation, vomiting, bleeding from the GI tract, inflammatory bowel disease, liver diseases, diseases of the pancreas, poor weight gain and nutritional problems.

Newsletters

4989 NASPGHAN News
PO Box 6
Flourtown, PA 19031

215-233-0808; Fax: 215-233-3939
e-mail: naspghan@naspghan.org
www.naspghan.org

Publication of the North American Society for Pediatric Gastroenterolgy, Hepatology and Nutrition, which strives to improve the care of infants, children and adolescents with digestive disorders by promoting advances in clinical care of children with chronic abdominal pain, diarrhea, constipation, vomiting, bleeding from the GI tract, inflammatory bowel disease, liver diseases, diseases of the pancreas, poor weight gain and nutritional problems.

Carlo Di Lorenzo, MD, President
James Heubi, MD, President-Elect
Michael Narkewicz, MD, Secretary-Treasurer

Description

4990 NEPHROTIC SYNDROME

Synonyms: Minimal change nephrotic syndrome, MCNS

Covers these related disorders: Infantile nephrotic syndrome, Primary nephrotic syndrome, Secondary nephrotic syndrome

Involves the following Biologic System(s):
Renal and Urologic Disorders

Nephrotic syndrome is characterized by an abnormality of the kidney that allows proteins to leak out of the blood and into the urine. The loss of these proteins leads to proteinuria (protein in the urine), edema (swelling) of the body, hypoproteinemia (low blood levels of protein), hyperlipidemia (high fat levels in the blood) and lipiduria (fat in the urine). Clinical examination of a patient with nephrotic syndrome will reveal swelling of the eyelids and skin around the eyes (periorbital edema), swelling of the extremities, especially feet and lower legs, and fluid in the abdomen (ascites). Laboratory examination will show large amounts of urinary protein, low serum albumin and high cholesterol.

There are three categories of nephrotic syndrome: infantile; primary; and secondary:

Infantile nephrotic syndrome is usually the result of an inherited form and symptoms occur in the first few months of life. Secondary nephrotic syndrome is nephrotic syndrome associated with another disease process. These can include infection, connective tissue disorders such as lupus erythematosus, allergen exposure and medications.

Primary nephrotic syndrome results from disease in the kidney alone. The most common form is minimal change nephrotic syndrome (MCNS), or minimal change disease. It is called minimal change because little change is seen in the kidneys when a biopsy of the kidney is examined. Minimal change nephrotic syndrome almost always responds to steroids. Although relapses are not uncommon the long-term prognosis is excellent. Other causes of primary nephrotic syndrome, such as focal segmental glomerulosclerosis, mesangial proliferative glomeruloephritis, and membranous nephropathy, may or may not improve with the steroids and generally have a worse prognosis than MCNS. These patients can be treated with immunosuppressive therapy but may progress to end-stage renal disease requiring dialysis or kidney transplant.

Children with nephrotic syndrome are at risk for several complications. These include increased risk of infection, blood clots and cardiovascular disease. Dietary management includes restriction of sodium and fluid intake. Excessive sunlight should be avoided, because sensitivity to light (photosensitivity) is common.

National Associations & Support Groups

4991 American Academy of Pediatrics
141 Northwest Point Boulevard
Elk Grove Village, IL 60007

847-434-4000
800-433-9016
Fax: 847-434-8000
www.aap.org

The American Academy of Pediatrics and its member pediatricians are committed to the attainment of optimal physical, mental and social health and well-being for all infants, children, adolescents, and young adults.

Sandra Hassink, MD, FAAP, President

4992 American Kidney Fund
11921 Rockville Pike, Suite 300
Rockville, MD 20852

301-881-3052
800-638-8299
Fax: 301-881-0898
e-mail: helpline@kidneyfund.org
www.akfinc.org

The American Kidney Fund is the nation's leading voluntary health organization serving people with and at risk for kidney disease through direct financial assistance, comprehensive education, clinical research and community service programs.

Timothy G. Morgan, Chair
John P. Butler, Chair-Elect
Myra A. Kleinpeter, Chair Medical Affairs

4993 National Kidney Foundation
30 E 33rd Street
New York, NY 10016

212-889-2210
855-653-2273
Fax: 212-689-9261
e-mail: info@kidney.org
www.kidney.org

A major voluntary health organization, seeking to prevent kidney and urinary tract diseases, improve the health and well-being of individuals and families affected by these diseases, and increases the availability of all organs for transplant.

James Carlson, CEO
Joseph A Vassalotti MD, Chief Medical Officer

4994 NephCure Foundation
15 Waterloo Avenue
Berwyn, PA 19312

610-540-0186
866-637-4287
Fax: 610-540-0190
e-mail: info@nephcure.org
www.nephcure.org

The only organization committed exclusively to support research seeking the cuses of the potentially debilitating kidney diseases, Nephrotic Syndrome and Focal Segmental Glomerulosclerosis (FSGS), improve treatment and find a cure.

Irvine Smokler, President
Ron Cohen, VP
Michael Levine, VP

Web Sites

4995 American Kidney Fund
11921 Rockville Pike, Suite 300
Rockville, MD 20852

www.akfinc.org

Providing information for people with and at risk for kidney disease such as Nephrotic Syndrome.

John P. Butler, Chair
LaVarnee A. Burton, President & Chief Executive Officer
Donald J. Roy, Jr, EVP, CFO, COO

4996 National Kidney Foundation
30 East 33rd Street
New York, NY 10016

800-622-9010
Fax: 212-689-9261
e-mail: info@kidney.org
www.kidney.org

A site that offers information to prevent kidney and urinary tract diseases, improve the health and well-being of individuals and families affected by these diseases, and increases the availability of all organs for transplant.

Bruce Skyer, CEO
Joseph Vassalotti, MD, Chief Medical Officer
Petros Gregoriou, CPA, Senior Vice President & CFO

4997 NephCure Foundation
150 S. Warner Road Suite 402
King of Prussia, PA 19406
e-mail: info@nephcure.org
nephcure.org

The only organization committed exclusively to support research seeking the cuses of the potentially debilitating kidney diseases, Nephrotic Syndrome and Focal Segmental Glomerulosclerosis (FSGS), improve treatment and find a cure.

Irving Smokler, Ph.D. , President
Ron Cohen , Vice President
Andrew Silverman , Treasurer

Book Publishers

4998 The Official Parent's Sourcebook on Childhood Nephrotic Syndrome

James N. Parker, author

Icon Group International
9606 Tierra Grande St., Suite 205
San Diego, CA 92126
Fax: 858-635-9414
e-mail: orders@icongroupbooks.com
www.icongrouponline.com

A comprehensive manual for anyone interested in self-directed research on childhood Nephrotic Syndrome. Fully referenced with ample internet listings and glossary.

2002 136 pages Paperback
ISBN: 0-597832-16-1

Newsletters

4999 NephCure Now
NephCure Foundation
150 S. Warner Road, Suite 402
King of Prussia, PA 19406
610-540-0186
Fax: 610-540-0190
e-mail: info@nephcure.org
www.nephcure.org

The NephCure Foundation's newsletter that contains news and information on a variety of topics including the latest research updates, NephCure events and fundraisers and much more.

Irving Smokler, Ph.D., President
Ron Cohen , Vice President
Andrew Silverman, Treasurer

5000 Renalink
National Kidney Foundation
30 E 33rd Street
New York, NY 10016
212-889-2210
800-622-9010
Fax: 212-689-9261
e-mail: info@kidney.org
www.kidney.org/professionals/journals/login.cfm

Renalink is the joint newsletter of the Council of Nephrology Nurses and Technicians, the Council of Nephrology Social Work and the Council of Renal Nutrition of the National Kidney Foundation. Renalink includes news for each Council, information vital to the renal care team and ideas that should lead to further collaboration among allied health professionals in the renal field.

Quarterly

Bruce Skyer, CEO
Joseph Vassalotti, MD, Chief Medical Officer
Petros Gregoriou, CPA, Senior Vice President & CFO

Pamphlets

5001 Childhood Nephrotic Syndrome
Information Clearinghouse
2 Information Way
Bethesda, MD 20892
301-496-3583
Fax: 301-907-8906
e-mail: nddic@info.niddk.nih.gov
www.niddk.nih.gov

5002 Children and Kidney Disease
American Kidney Fund
30 East 33rd Street
New York, NY 10016
301-881-3052
800-622-9010
Fax: 212-689-9261
e-mail: info@kidney.org
www.kidney.org

Bruce Skyer, CEO
Joseph Vassalotti, MD, Chief Medical Officer
Petros Gregoriou, CPA, Senior Vice President & CFO

5003 Financial Assistance and Insurance for People with Kidney Disease
Information Clearinghouse
2 Information Way
Bethesda, MD 20892
301-496-3583
Fax: 301-907-8906
e-mail: nddic@info.niddk.nih.gov
www.niddk.nih.gov

5004 Kidney Disease of Diabetes
Information Clearinghouse
1 Information Way
Bethesda, MD 20892
301-496-3583
Fax: 301-907-8906
e-mail: ndoc@info.niddk.nih.gov
www.niddk.nih.gov

Description

5005 NEUROFIBROMATOSIS

Synonym: NF

Covers these related disorders: Neurofibromatosis type I (von Recklinghausen disease) (NF1), Neurofibromatosis type II (NF2)

Involves the following Biologic System(s):
Dermatologic Disorders, Orthopedic and Muscle Disorders

The term neurofibromatosis is often used to refer to neurofibromatosis type I (NF1), an autosomal dominant disorder that affects approximately one in 3,500 to 4,000 individuals. Neurofibromatosis type I, also known as von Recklinghausen disease, is characterized by the appearance of pale tan or light brown discolorations (macules) on the skin (cafe-au-lait spots) and multiple benign, fibrous tumors of nerves and skin (neurofibromas). A second, distinctive form of neurofibromatosis (NF), known as neurofibromatosis type II (NF2), accounts for about 10 percent of all cases of NF. Neurofibromatosis type II, also an autosomal dominant disorder, is characterized by the development of benign tumors on both acoustic nerves (bilateral acoustic neuromas), resulting in progressive hearing impairment.

In most children with neurofibromatosis type I, skin discoloration may develop by the age of one year. Such skin lesions typically increase in number and size over time, and most affected individuals have six or more spots measuring 1.5 centimeters or more in diameter after the onset of puberty. Although these cafe-au-lait spots are often distributed in various areas of the body, they are most commonly present on the trunk. In addition, after three years of age, areas of freckling, particularly under the arms (axillary) and in the groin (inguinal) area, may also be present.

In approximately 95 percent of children with NF1 over six years of age, two or more benign, tumor-like nodules, known as Lisch nodules, are present on the pigmented areas of the eyes. Benign, fibrous tumors of the skin (cutaneous neurofibromas) tend to develop during the second decade of life, typically appearing as small, soft, raised, and slightly purplish discolorations of the overlying skin. These tumors, which rarely develop before six years of age, may increase in number and size during puberty. In addition, large benign tumors composed of bundles of nerves (plexiform neurofibromas) may be apparent at birth or during early childhood. Approximately two to four percent of individuals with NF1 may develop malignant tumors (e.g., neurofibrosarcomas). Physical findings that may be associated with malignant transformation include increasing tumor size, associated pain, or various neurologic symptoms due to tumor growth. Approximately 15 percent of affected individuals may also develop tumors of the optic nerve (optic glioma), which is the cranial nerve that carries visual impulses from the back of the eye (retina) to the brain. These tumors are usually considered relatively benign and may cause no associated symptoms (asymptomatic). However, in some cases, depending upon their specific location, growth, and nature, such tumors may affect vision. In these patients, associated findings may include visual impairment; degeneration (atrophy) of the optic nerve; abnormal deviation of the eye (strabismus); or involuntary, rhythmic eye movements (nystagmus). In addition, some affected individuals may have an increased risk of developing tumors of the brain and spinal cord (e.g., astrocytomas, meningiomas, neurilemmomas, etc.).

Some individuals with NF1 may also experience associated skeletal abnormalities, such as bowing of the lower legs; improper development of a bone at the base of the skull (sphenoid wing dysplasia), potentially causing pronounced bulging of the eyes (exophthalmos); and progressive sideways curvature of the spine (scoliosis). Additional abnormalities may be present, such as mild short stature, abnormal largeness of the head (macrocephaly), and episodes of uncontrolled electrical activity in the brain (seizures). In addition, many affected children may have learning disabilities and speech abnormalities. Neurofibromatosis type I is caused by abnormal changes (mutations) of a gene located on the long arm of chromosome 17 (17q11.2). In approximately 50 percent of patients, the disease gene is inherited an an autosomal dominant trait; the remaining cases result from new (sporadic) mutations of the gene that occur for unknown reasons.

Neurofibromatosis type II (NF2) is also characterized by bilateral acoustic neuromas that are responsible for carrying sound impulses from the inner ear to the brain. Symptoms may become apparent during childhood or the second or third decades of life. These may include a facial numbness or weakness, headache, dizziness, unsteadiness, and progressive hearing loss. Individuals with NF2 may also develop clouding of the lenses of the eyes (i.e., posterior subcapsular opacities), have an increased risk of developing tumors of the brain and spinal cord (e.g., gliomas, meningiomas, schwannomas, etc.), or experience progressive visual impairment. NF2 is caused by a disease gene located on the long arm of chromosome 22 (22q12.2).

The treatment of neurofibromatosis is directed toward ensuring early detection and prompt, appropriate management of potentially associated findings or complications. Affected individuals are typically regularly monitored with complete neurologic evaluations (e.g., including visual and auditory screening) and thorough examinations to detect potential complications associated with NF. In most cases, symptoms of NF1 are mild, and patients live normal and productive lives. In some cases, however, NF1 can be severely debilitating. In some cases of NF2, the damage to nearby vital structures, such as other cranial nerves, can be life-threatening. Some tumors may be surgically removed or treated using other appropriate methods (e.g., radiation or chemotherapy for certain malignancies). Other treatment is symptomatic and supportive.

National Associations & Support Groups

5006 American Academy of Pediatrics
141 Northwest Point Boulevard
Elk Grove Village, IL 60007

847-434-4000
800-433-9016
Fax: 847-434-8000
www.aap.org

The American Academy of Pediatrics and its member pediatricians are committed to the attainment of optimal physical, mental and social health and well-being for all infants, children, adolescents, and young adults.

Sandra Hassink, MD, FAAP, President

5007 Children's Tumor Foundation
95 Pine Street, 16th Floor
New York, NY 10005

212-344-6633
800-323-7938
Fax: 212-747-0004
e-mail: info@ctf.org
www.ctf.org

The Children's Tumor Foundation funds research, patient support, and public awareness of the neurofibromatoses (NF1, NF2 & Schwannomatosis) genetic disorders that cause random tumor growth throughout the body.

Stuart Match Suna, Chairperson
John W Risner, President
Linda Halliday Martin, Vice Chairperson

5008 Genetic Alliance
4301 Connecticut Avenue NW
Washington, DC 20008

202-966-5557
800-336-4363
Fax: 202-966-8553
e-mail: info@geneticalliance.org
www.geneticalliance.org

A coalition of voluntary genetic support groups, consumers and professionals addressing the needs of individuals and families affected by genetic disorders from a national perspective.

Joan Oppenheimer Weiss, Founder
Sharon Terry, President

5009 March of Dimes Birth Defects Foundation
1275 Mamaroneck Avenue
White Plains, NY 10605

914-997-4488
888-663-4637
Fax: 914-428-8203
e-mail: answers@marchofdimes.com
www.marchofdimes.com

Partnership of volunteers and professionals dedicates to improving the health of babies by preventing birth defects and infant mortality. Over 100 chapters are located across the country and can be located through the National Office.

Jennifer L Howse, President

5010 National Brain Tumor Foundation
55 Chapel Street, Suite 200
Newton, MA 02458

617-924-9997
800-934-2873
Fax: 617-924-9998
e-mail: info@braintumor.org
www.braintumor.org

NBTF is a national nonprofit health organization dedicated to providing information and support for brain tumor patients, family members, and healthcare professionals, while supporting innovative research into better treatment options and a cure for brain tumors.

Jeffrey Kolodin, Chair
Michael Nathanson, Vice-Chair
Michael Corkin, Treasurer

5011 Neurofibromatosis Support & Information Group
Parents Helping Parents
3041 Olcott Street
Santa Clarka, CA 95054

408-727-5775
Fax: 408-727-0182
e-mail: info@php.com
www.php.com

Helping children with special needs receive the resources, love, hope, respect, health care, education and other services they need to achieve their full potential by providing them with strong families and dedicated professionals to serve them.

Alexandra Cramer, Receptionist/Admin. Assistant
Carlos A. Gallegos, Kids on the Block Coordinator
Cathie Silverberg

5012 Neurofibromatosis, Inc
213 S. Wheaton Ave.
Wheaton, IL 60187

630-510-1115
800-942-6825
Fax: 630-510-8508
e-mail: admin@nfnetwork.org
www.nfnetwork.org

An organization of independent state and regional chapters that provides support and services to families coping with neurofibromatosis. Works closely with clinical and research professionals who specialize in the treatment of NF. Has a newsletter and other printed materials.

Cheri Stewart, President
Rosemary Anderson, VP
Nicole Hicks, Secretary

State Agencies & Support Groups

Arizona

5013 Neurofibromatosis, Inc - Arizona Chapter
PO Box 2718
Chandler, AZ 85244

480-945-9650
e-mail: info@nfarizona.org
www.nfarizona.org

Arkansas

5014 Children's Tumor Foundation-Arkansas Chapter
1 Children's Way
Little Rock, AR 72202

501-364-1850
e-mail: paws4me@cox.net
www.ctf.org/Chapters-Affiliates/Arkansas/

Julie Jarrett, Contact
Rolla Shbarou, Clinic Director
Shaneika Lewis-Williams, Clinic Coordinators

5015 Children's Tumor Foundation-Arkansas Infor www.php.com
PO Box 7262
Little Rock, AR 72217

501-920-5588
e-mail: loslica@gmail.com
www.ctfarkansas.com

Lesley Oslica, Contact

California

5016 Neurofibromatosis, Inc - California Chapter
PO Box 1234
Vacaville, CA 95696

707-469-0467
Fax: 866-571-2366
e-mail: info@nfcalifornia.org
www.nfcalifornia.org

Debbie Bell, President
Dana Inigues, VP
Katie Sperring, Secretary

Colorado

5017 Children's Tumor Foundation - Colorado Chapter
13121 E. 17th Ave.
Aurora, CO 80045

303-724-2370
e-mail: ilaskey@peakpeak.com
www.ctf.org/Chapters-Affiliates/Colorado/

Mark Ebel, Chapter President
Gary Bellus, Clinic Director
Katherine Howard, Clinic Coordinators

Florida

5018 Children's Tumor Foundation - Florida Chap ter
3100 SW 62nd Avenue, Suite 301
Miami, FL 33155   305-663-8595
                                               800-540-5721
                              e-mail: hehrli@aol.com
                              www.ctf.org/Chapters-Affiliates/florida/
Hannah Erli, Chapter President
Sue Bresnahan, Office Contact
Mislen Bauer, Clinic Director

Georgia

5019 Children's Tumor Foundation - Georgia
5 Ardmore Circle
Cartersville, GA 30120   678-428-9711
                              e-mail: ctfgeorgia@bellsouth.net
                              www.ctf.org/Chapters-Affiliates/Georgia/
Beth O'Brien-Burke, President
Melissa Lee, VP
Julie Santana, Patient Outreach Committee Chair

Illinois

5020 Children's Tumor Foundation - Illinois
2300 Children's Plaza
Chicago, IL 60614   773-880-4462
                              Fax: 217-732-8568
                              e-mail: mmoscatello@ctf.org
                              www.ctf.org/Chapters-Affiliates/Illinois/

2500 members

Paul Beach, Chapter President
Joel Charrow, Clinic Co-Director
Michelle Gilats, Clinic Coordinators

5021 Children's Tumor Foundation - Illinois Cha pter
2300 Children's Plaza
Chicago, IL 60614   773-880-4462
                              Fax: 217-732-8568
                              e-mail: mmoscatello@ctf.org
                              www.ctf.org/Chapters-Affiliates/Illinois/
Paul Beach, Chapter President
Joel Charrow, Clinic Co-Director
Michelle Gilats, Clinic Coordinators

5022 Neurofibromatosis, Inc - Illinois
213 S. Wheaton Ave
Wheaton, IL 60187   630-510-1115
                                               800-942-6825
                              Fax: 630-510-8508
                              e-mail: admin@nfnetwork.org
                              www.nfnetwork.org

A leading national organization advocating for the development
of local NF organizations and for federal funding for NF research

Cheri Stewart, President
Rosemary Anderson, Vice President
Mike Montgomery, Treasurer

5023 Neurofibromatosis, Inc - Illinois/Midwest
473 Dunham Rd, Suite 3
St. Charles, IL 60174   630-945-3562
                                               800-322-6363
                              Fax: 630-932-8119
                              e-mail: Diana@nfmidwest.org
                              www.nfmidwest.org
Diana Haberkamp, Executive Director
Jenny Perkins, Development Director
Liz Campana, Administrative Assistant

Indiana

5024 Children's Tumor Foundation - Indiana Affi liate
Suite 4700, 355 W, 16th Street
Indiannapolis, IN 46202   317-948-5450
                              Fax: 317-963-7533
                              e-mail: kym1577@sbcglobal.net
                              www.indiananf.com
Kim Bebley, Affiliate Representative

Iowa

5025 Children's Tumor Foundation - Iowa Chapter
200 Hawkins Drive
Iowa City, IA 52242   319-356-2229
                              Fax: 515-277-1526
                              e-mail: Drev@aol.com
                              www.ctf.org/Chapters-Affiliates/Iowa/
Sheila Drevyanko, Chapter President
Pamela Trapane, Director
Catherine Evers, Clinic Co-Coordinators

Kansas

5026 Neurofibromatosis, Inc - Kansas & Central Plains
9218 Metcalf, Ste. 335
Overland Park, KS 66212   316-669-8453
                                               800-942-6825
                              e-mail: nprieb@southwind.net
                              www.nfcentralplains.org

Nichole Servos, President
Mike Montgomery, VP
Sharon Loftspring, Secretary

Maryland

5027 Neurofibromatosis, Inc - MidAtlantic
2 Village Square., Suite #213, 5100 Falls Road
Baltimore, MD 21210   443-423-0535
                              Fax: 410-889-0400
                              e-mail: info@nfmidatlantic.org
                              www.nfmidatlantic.org
Diana Bark, President
Lee Herman, Board of Directors
Aaron Jumani, VP

Massachusetts

5028 Children's Tumor Foundation - Northern New England
300 Longwood Ave
Boston, MA 02115   617-355-4699
                                               888-585-5316
                              Fax: 617-663-4801
                              e-mail: seburne@ctf.org
                              www.ctf.org/Northern-New-England
Samantha Eburne, VP, NE Development

5029 Neurofibromatosis, Inc - New England/North east
213 S. Wheaton Ave.
Wheaton, IL 60187   630-510-1115
                                               800-942-6825
                              Fax: 630-510-8508
                              e-mail: admin@nfnetwork.org
                              www.nfnetwork.org
Cheri Stewart, President
Rosemary Anderson, VP
Nicole Hicks, Secretary

Michigan

5030 Children's Tumor Foundation - Michigan Cha pter
6069 Brynthrop
Shelby Township, MI 48316   586-731-7811
e-mail: hawkeyenf@wideopenwest.com
www.ctf.org/Chapters-Affiliates/michigan/
Peter Dingeman, Chapter President
Wendy Schaffer, Treasurer
Xia Wang, Director

Missouri

5031 Children's Tumor Foundation - Missouri Cha pter
Thompson Coburn LLP
1046 Grand Blvd.
St Louis, MO 63104   314-552-6139
Fax: 314-552-7139
e-mail: dcox@thompsoncoburn.com
www.ctf.org/Chapters-Affiliates/missouri/
Thomas Geller, Director
Julie Engel, Clinic Coordinator
Annette Novak

Nevada

5032 Children's Tumor Foundation - Nevada
8351 Mountain Destiny Ave
Las Vegas, NV 89131   702-457-0745
Fax: 775-972-1885
e-mail: twnsmommy@msn.com
www.ctf.org/Chapters-Affiliates/Nevada/
Jennifer Halbert, Chapter Representative
Lori Bjorkquist, Chapter Representative

Ohio

5033 Children's Tumor Foundation - Ohio
3333 Burnet Avenue
Cincinnati, OH 45229   513-636-8826
e-mail: mmoscatello@ctf.org
www.ctf.org/Chapters-Affiliates/Ohio/
Elizabeth Schorry, Director
Anne Lovell, Coordinator

Oregon

5034 Children's Tumor Foundation - Oregon Suppo rt Group
Oaks Park, 7805 SE Oaks Park Way
Portland, OR 97202   503-333-6797
Fax: 503-674-9256
e-mail: kellerko@ohsu.edu
www.ctf.org/Chapters-Affiliates/Oregon/
Kory Keller, Genetic Counselor

5035 Legacy Good Samaritan Hospital & Medical C enter
Neurofibromatosis Support Group
1015 NW 22nd Avenue, N-300
Portland, OR 97210   503-413-7711
800-733-9959
e-mail: mflorian@lhs.org
www.legacyhealth.org
Amy Marr, Coordinator

South Carolina

5036 Children's Tumor Foundation - South Caroli na Chapter
111 Oakview Drive
Darlington, SC 29532   843-393-9672
Fax: 843-393-9673
e-mail: pmchrisley@aol.com
www.ctf.org/Chapters-Affiliates/South-Carolina/
Susan Luttrell, President

Tennessee

5037 Children's Tumor Foundation - Tennessee Af filiate
3501 Central Ave.
Nashville, TN 37924   865-633-5858
Fax: 865-633-5859
www.ctf.org/Chapters-Affiliates/Tennessee/
Cynthia Hester, President

Utah

5038 Children's Tumor Foundation - Utah Chapter
Sugarhouse Park, 1500 East 2100 South
Salt Lake City, UT 84115   801-485-2801
Fax: 801-277-4042
e-mail: uteNFmom@gmail.com
www.ctf.org/Chapters-Affiliates/Utah/
Kelly Carpenter, President
Andrea Davis, VP
Kelsey Richards, Secretary

Virginia

5039 Children's Tumor Foundation - MidAtlantic Region Chapter
42010 Village Center Plz Ste 180
Aldie, VA 22066   703-444-1624
e-mail: bentleyaw@aol.com
www.ctf.org/Home/Chapters-Affiliates/Mid-Atlantic/
Anne Bentley

Washington

5040 Children's Tumor Foundation - Washington C hapter
12722 166th St Ct E
Puyallup, WA 98374   253-370-9509
e-mail: kkaralus74@yahoo.com
www.ctf.org/Chapters-Affiliates/washington/

Provides information, support services and referrals for patients
and families affected by neurofibromatosis, while supporting
medical research toward effective treatments and a cure.

Stuart Match Suna, Chairperson
John Risner, President
Linda Halliday Martin, Vice-Chairperson

Wisconsin

5041 Children's Tumor Foundation - Wisconsin Ch apter
6562 W Glenbrook Road
Brown Deer, WI 53223   414-716-5001
Fax: 414-362-0212
e-mail: epankownf@aol.com
www.ctf.org/Chapters-Affiliates/Wisconsin/
Elaine Pankow, President

Research Centers

5042 NF Clinic - University of Pittsburgh Children's Hospital
5501 Old York Road
Philadelphia, PA 19141   215-456-8722
Fax: 215-456-2356
e-mail: scheida@einstein.edu
www.nfmidatlantic.org

Jennifer Berkowitz, Contact

5043 Neurofibromatosis Center at North Broward Medical Center
303 SE 17th Street
Fort Lauderdale, FL 33316   954-784-1521
www.browardhealth.org

Frank Nask, President

5044 Neuroscience Institute at Mercy Hospital
4120 W Memorial Road
Oklahoma City, OK 73120
405-302-2661
Fax: 405-302-2670
www.mercy..net

Gary Brown PhD, Contact

Web Sites

5045 Children's Tumor Foundation
120 Wall Street, 16th Floor
New York, NY 10005
212-344-6633
e-mail: info@ctf.org
www.ctf.org

A nonprofit medical foundation dedicated to improving the health and well being of individuals and families affected by NF.

Linda Halliday Martin, Chairperson
Annette Bakker, PhD, President
Colin Bryar, Vice Chairperson

5046 Neurofibromatosis, Inc
213 S. Wheaton Ave.
Wheaton, IL 60187
630-510-1115
800-942-6825
Fax: 630-510-8508
e-mail: admin@nfnetwork.org
www.nfinc.org

An organization made up of independent state and regional chapters, providing support and services to NF families. In addition to assisting individuals and families, NF, Inc. works closely with clinical and research professionals who specialize in the treatment of NF.

Cheri Stewart, President
Nicole Hicks, Secretary
Mike Montgomery, Treasurer

5047 Online Mendelian Inheritance in Man
National Library of Medicine Building 38A
Bethesda, MD 20894
888-346-3656
e-mail: info@ncbi.nlm.nih.gov
www.ncbi.nlm.nih.gov

This database is a catalog of human genes and genetic disorders.

Book Publishers

5048 Let's Talk About Going to the Hospital
Rosen Publishing Group's PowerKids Press
29 E 21st Street
New York, NY 10010
212-777-3017
800-237-9932
Fax: 888-436-4643
e-mail: rosenpub@tribeca.ios.com
www.rosenpublishing.com

If a child has to check into the hospital, chances are he or she is already upset about being ill. Knowing how a hospital functions and what the procedures are, such as when family members can visit, will help in what is already a stressful situation. Grades K-5.

24 pages
ISBN: 0-823950-36-0

Roger Rosen, President

5049 Neurofibromatosis: A Handbook for Patients , Families and Health Care Professionals

Dr Bruce R Korf; Dr Allan E Rubenstein, author

Children's Tumor Foundation
95 Pine Street, 16th Floor
New York, NY 10005
212-344-6633
800-323-7938
Fax: 212-747-0004
e-mail: info@ctf.org
www.ctf.org/patientinfo/

2005-2nd Ed 264 pages Hardbound
Stuart Match Suna, Chairperson
John Risner, President
John McCarthy, Treasurer

5050 Who Says It Has to Be Fair
Theda Schott, author

PublishAmerica
213 S. Wheaton Ave.
Wheaton, IL 60187
630-510-1115
800-942-6825
Fax: 630-510-8508
e-mail: admin@nfnetwork.org
www.nfnetwork.org; www.publishamerica.com

A mother's story about raising a child with neurofibromatosis.
2006 184 pages Paperback
ISBN: 1-424118-09-3

Cheri Stewart, President
Rosemary Anderson, Vice President
Nicole Hicks, Secretary

Newsletters

5051 Neurofibromatosis Ink
Neurofibromatosis, Inc
213 S. Wheaton Ave.
Wheaton, IL 60187
630-510-1115
800-942-6825
Fax: 630-510-8508
e-mail: admin@nfnetwork.org
www.nfinc.org

Cheri Stewart, President
Nicole Hicks, Secretary
Mike Montgomery, Treasurer

5052 Neurofibromatosis News
Children's Tumor Foundation
120 Wall Street, 16th Floor
New York, NY 10005
212-344-6633
800-323-7938
Fax: 212-747-0004
e-mail: info@cft.org
www.ctf.org

Offers information on the newest advances in neurofibromatosis, related events and foundation activities.

Quarterly

Linda Halliday Martin, Chairperson
Annette Bakker, PhD, President
Colin Bryar, Vice Chairperson

Pamphlets

5053 About Neurofibromatosis 1
Children's Tumor Foundation
120 Wall Street, 16th Floor
New York, NY 10005
212-344-6633
800-323-7938
Fax: 212-747-0004
e-mail: info@ctf.org
www.ctf.org/patientinfo/

A pamphlet providing an introductory overview of NF1 for patients, families, and healthcare providers with the hope that readers will seek additional information about the disorder according to their own needs.

2007 36 pages

Linda Halliday Martin, Chairperson
Annette Bakker, PhD, President
Colin Bryar, Vice Chairperson

5054 Achieving in Spite of...A Booklet on Learn ing Disabilities
Children's Tumor Foundation
120 Wall Street, 16th Floor
New York, NY 10005

212-344-6633
800-323-7938
Fax: 212-747-0004
www.ctf.org

Designed for use by parents, teachers and health professionals-information on learning disabilities and what to do about them.

34 pages

Linda Halliday Martin, Chairperson
Annette Bakker, PhD, President
Colin Bryar, Vice Chairperson

5055 Facing Neurofibromatosis: A Guide for Teen s
Children's Tumor Foundation
120 Wall Street, 16th Floor
New York, NY 10005

212-344-6633
800-323-7938
Fax: 212-747-0004
e-mail: info@ctf.org
www.ctf.org

Offers information for teenagers on how to face neurofibromatosis on a daily basis.

Linda Halliday Martin, Chairperson
Annette Bakker, PhD, President/ Chief Scientific Officer
Colin Bryar, Vice Chairperson

5056 Neurofibromatosis Type 1: A Guide for Educ ators
Children's Tumor Foundation
120 Wall Street, 16th Floor
New York, NY 10005

212-344-6633
800-323-7938
Fax: 212-747-0004
e-mail: info@ctf.org
www.ctf.org/patientinfo/

Offers concise and practical information as well as recommendations about the cognitive, physical and behavioral manifestations of the disorder. Free online PDF; English or Spanish.

12 pages

Linda Halliday Martin, Chairperson
Annette Bakker, PhD, President
Colin Bryar, Vice Chairperson

5057 Neurofibromatosis Type 2: Information for Patients and Families
Children's Tumor Foundation
120 Wall Street, 16th Floor
New York, NY 10005

212-344-6633
800-323-7938
Fax: 212-747-0004
e-mail: info@ctf.org
www.ctf.org/patientinfo/

Offers extensive information on what NF2 is and answers the most asked about questions regarding the illness. Free online PDF; English or Spanish.

2007 13 pages

Linda Halliday Martin, Chairperson
Annette Bakker, PhD, President
Colin Bryar, Vice Chairperson

5058 Neurofibromatosis: Questions and Answers
Children's Tumor Foundation
120 Wall Street, 16th Floor
New York, NY 10005

212-344-6633
803-237-938
Fax: 212-747-0004
www.ctf.org

Information about neurofibromatosis.

Linda Halliday Martin, Chairperson
Annette Bakker, PhD, President
Colin Bryar, Vice Chairperson

5059 The Child with NF1
Children's Tumor Foundation
120 Wall Street, 16th Floor
New York, NY 10005

212-344-6633
800-323-7938
Fax: 212-747-0004
e-mail: info@cft.org
www.ctf.org

This brochure is dedicated to the families who live with neurofibromatosis and the friends who provide support and en-couragements. It's the purpose of this brochure to attempt to place mild or early NF in perspective. To some extent, NF is an unpredictable condition and uncertainty is inevitable. It is hoped, however, that access to accurate medical information will make this uncertainty easier to live with and to understand. Free online PDF.

2008 9 pages

Linda Halliday Martin, Chairperson
Annette Bakker, PhD, President
Colin Bryar, Vice Chairperson

Camps

5060 Camp New Friends
Neurofibromatosis, Inc
213 S. Wheaton Ave.
Wheaton, IL 60187

630-510-1115
800-942-6825
Fax: 630-510-8508
e-mail: admin@nfnetwork.org
www.nfinc.org

A summer camp for those affected with NF1 or NF2, between the ages of 7 and 15. Those aged 18 and over may apply as counsel-ors or counselors-in-training. The camp is held in collaboration with Children's National Medical Center.

Cheri Stewart, President
Nicole Hicks, Secretary
Mike Montgomery, Treasurer

5061 International NF Summer Camp
Children's Tumor Foundation
120 Wall Street, 16th Floor
New York, NY 10005

212-344-6633
800-323-7938
Fax: 212-747-0004
e-mail: ppanza@ctf.org
www.ctf.org

Campers have the chance to connect with other children who un-derstand what it's like to live with NF. Held at Camp Kotsopoulos, in Emigration Canyon, Utah for the 13th year, there will be swimming, horse-back riding, fishing, canoeing, climbing wall, movie night, a day at the water park, and, of course, camp-fires. Campers can register for either of the two, one-week ses-sions. Thanks to donations, scholarships are available, and in some cases, travel assistance.

Linda Halliday Martin, Chairperson
Annette Bakker, PhD, President
Colin Bryar, Vice Chairperson

Description

5062 NEUROBLASTOMA

Synonym: NB

Involves the following Biologic System(s):

Hematologic and Oncologic Disorders

Neuroblastomas are malignant tumors that account for approximately eight to 10 percent of childhood cancers. They are the most common solid tumors that develop outside the skull in children. About 500 to 600 new cases are reported each year in the United States, with males affected slightly more frequently than females. In approximately 90 percent of affected infants and children, neuroblastoma is diagnosed before age five. Neuroblastoma sometimes occurs in members of certain families (kindreds), although the specific underlying cause is unknown.

Neuroblastomas may originate in any part of the sympathetic nervous system but most commonly develop in the inner region of the adrenal gland (adrenal medulla). In other patients, neuroblastomas may arise in the chest. The sympathetic nervous system controls certain involuntary activities during times of stress, such as raising blood pressure and increasing the heart rate. The adrenal glands, two relatively small organs that curve over the top of each kidney, secrete certain hormones directly into the bloodstream.

A neuroblastoma often invades surrounding tissues and spreads to small, node-like structures located along the course of the lymphatic vessels (lymph nodes). The tumor may then spread to other parts of the body (metastasize), particularly the liver, skeleton, and bone marrow. Rarely, neuroblastomas spread to the lungs or the brain. Associated symptoms and findings are highly variable and depend upon the specific location of the tumor and the extent to which it may have spread. Many infants and children may have a hard, solid, painless lump or mass in the neck or a large mass that may be felt in the abdomen or on the back. Patients often have a general feeling of ill health (malaise) and appear pale (pallor). Those with skeletal involvement typically experience tumor-associated bone pain. In addition, because the bone marrow is a blood-producing tissue, tumor infiltration of the bone marrow may result in abnormally decreased levels of the different blood cells, including circulating red blood cells (anemia), platelets (thrombocytopenia), and certain white blood cells, (neutropenia). Due to low levels of platelets, patients may experience abnormal bleeding and easy bruising. Decreased levels of white blood cells may cause an increased susceptibility to certain infections.

Depending upon the location and potential spread of the tumor, additional symptoms and findings may occur. If a neuroblastoma spreads to the bony cavities surrounding the eyes, associated symptoms may include abnormal protrusion of the eyes (proptosis) and the appearance of bluish-purple patches (ecchymosis) around the eyes. Tumor development near the spinal cord may result in weakness or paralysis of the legs (paresis). In addition, involvement of the liver typically causes abnormal liver enlargement (hepatomegaly). Tumor growth within the adrenal glands may cause excessive secretion of the hormones epinephrine and norepinephrine, resulting in increased irritability, high blood pressure (hypertension), increased heart rate (tachycardia), flushing of the skin, severe diarrhea, and other symptoms.

Some patients may also develop Horner's syndrome, which is characterized by ptosis, absence of sweating (anhidrosis), and narrowing of the pupil of the eye (miosis). Skin abnormalities may also be present, including firm, bluish nodules under the skin or skin lesions on the scalp. Approximately four percent of patients experience a sudden onset of neuromuscular symptoms due to abnormal functioning of the cerebellum (acute cerebellar encephalopathy). The cerebellum is a region of the brain that plays an essential role in maintaining normal postures, sustaining balance, and producing coordinated movements. Neuroblastoma symptoms may include an impaired ability to coordinate voluntary movements (cerebellar ataxia); random, rapid, uncontrolled eye movements (opsoclonus); and shock-like contractions of certain muscles or muscle groups (myoclonic jerks).

In infants and children with neuroblastoma, treatment may depend upon the location of the tumor, whether it has spread, the patient's age, or other factors. If the tumor is contained and has not spread, treatment may consist of surgical removal of the tumor. When the tumor may not be removed surgically or has spread to other parts of the body, treatment measures may include the use of certain drugs (chemotherapy) or radiation therapy. Additional treatments for advanced disease may be considered.

Government Agencies

5063 NIH/National Cancer Institute

6116 Executive Boulevard, Room 3036A
Bethesda, MD 20892   800-422-6237
                                      www.cancer.gov

The National Cancer Institute coordinates the National Cancer Program, which conducts and supports research, training, health information dissemination, and other programs with respect to the cause, diagnosis, prevention, and treatment of cancer, rehabilitation from cancer, and the continuing care of cancer patients and the families of cancer patients.

John E Niederhuber MD, Director

National Associations & Support Groups

5064 American Academy of Pediatrics

141 Northwest Point Boulevard
Elk Grove Village, IL 60007   847-434-4000
                                      800-433-9016
                                      Fax: 847-434-8000
                                      www.aap.org

The American Academy of Pediatrics and its member pediatricians are committed to the attainment of optimal physical, mental and social health and well-being for all infants, children, adolescents, and young adults.

Sandra Hassink, MD, FAAP, President

5065 CancerCare

275 7th Avenue, Floor 22
New York, NY 10001   212-712-8400
                                      800-813-4673
                                      Fax: 212-712-8495
                                      e-mail: info@cancercare.org
                                      www.cancercare.org

CancerCare is a national nonprofit, 501(c)(3) organization that provides free, professional support services to anyone affected by cancer: people with cancer, caregivers, children, loved ones, and the bereaved. CancerCare programs - including counseling and support groups, education, financial assistance and practical help - are provided by professional oncology social workers and are completely free of charge.

Helen Miller, LCSW, Chief Executive Officer
John Rutigliano, Chief Operating Officer
Rosalie Canosa, Program Division Director

5066 Candlelighters Childhood Cancer Foundation
PO Box 498
Kensington, MD 20895

301-962-3520
800-366-2223
Fax: 310-962-3521
e-mail: staff@candlelighters.org
www.candlelighters.org

The Candlelighters Childhood Cancer Foundation National Office was founded in 1970 by concerned parents of children with cancer. Today our membership of over 50,000 members of the national office and more than 100,000 members across the across the country, including Candlelighters affiliate groups, includes, parents of children who are being treated or have been treated for cancer.

Ruth Hoffman, Executive Director
Naomi Bartley, President
Janine Lynne, Vice President

5067 Children's Wish Foundation International
8615 Roswell Road
Atlanta, GA 30350

770-393-9474
800-323-9474
Fax: 770-393-0683
e-mail: wish@childrenswish.org
www.childrenswish.org

Children's Wish Foundation International is dedicated to bringing joy and hope to seeiously ill children and their families world wide by involving the public in putting children first with opportunities to experience the enhanced value and quality of life through the magic of a fulfilled wish.

Arthur Stein, President
Linda Dozoretz, Founder/Executive Director

5068 Genetic Alliance
4301 Connecticut Avenue NW
Washington, DC 20008

202-966-5557
800-336-4363
Fax: 202-966-8553
e-mail: info@geneticalliance.org
www.geneticalliance.org

A coalition of voluntary genetic support groups, consumers and professionals addressing the needs of individuals and families affected by genetic disorders from a national perspective.

Joan Oppenheimer Weiss, Founder
Sharon Terry, President

5069 Neuroblastoma Children's Cancer Society
PO Box 957672
Hoffman Estates, IL 60195

847-605-1245
800-532-5162
Fax: 847-605-0705
e-mail: info@neuroblastomacancer.org
www.neuroblastomacancer.org

The Neuroblastoma Children's Cancer Society is a group made up of volunteers, many of whom have children or relatives who are victims or survivors of this disease. The organization is an advocate for the children who suffer from neuroblastoma and is dedicated to serving as a support center for their families.

Research Centers

5070 Children's Cancer Research Institute
University of Texas Health Science Ctr
8403 Floyd Curl Drive
San Antonio, TX 78229

210-562-9000
Fax: 210-562-9014
e-mail: chessher@uthscsa.edu
ccri.uthscsa.edu

It is the mission of the institute to advance scientific knowledge relevant to childhood cancer and to accelerate the translation of knowledge into therapies.

Sharon Murphy MD, Director
Bill Chessher, Administrator

Web Sites

5071 CancerCare
275 Seventh Avenue 22nd Floor
New York, NY 10001

212-712-8400
800-813-4673
Fax: 212-712-8495
www.cancercare.org

CancerCare is a national nonprofit, 501(c)(3) organization that provides free, professional support services to anyone affected by cancer: people with cancer, caregivers, children, loved ones, and the bereaved. CancerCare programs - including counseling and support groups, education, financial assistance and practical help - are provided by professional oncology social workers and are completely free of charge.

Patricia J. Goldsmith, CEO
John Rutigliano, COO
Sue Lee, Senior Director of Development

5072 Children's Cancer Web
www.cancerindex.org/ccw

An independent nonprofit site, established to provide a directory of childhood cancer resources.

5073 Online Mendelian Inheritance in Man
National Library of Medicine Building 38A
Bethesda, MD 20894

888-346-3656
e-mail: info@ncbi.nlm.nih.gov
www.ncbi.nlm.nih.gov

This database is a catalog of human genes and genetic disorders.

Book Publishers

5074 Let's Talk About Going to the Hospital
Rosen Publishing Group's PowerKids Press
29 E 21st Street
New York, NY 10010

212-777-3017
800-237-9932
Fax: 888-436-4643
e-mail: rosenpub@tribeca.ios.com
www.rosenpublishing.com

If a child has to check into the hospital, chances are he or she is already upset about being ill. Knowing how a hospital functions and what the procedures are, such as when family members can visit, will help in what is already a stressful situation. Grades K-5.

24 pages
ISBN: 0-823950-36-0

Roger Rosen, President

5075 Let's Talk About When Kids Have Cancer

Melanie Apel Gordon, author

Rosen Publishing Group's PowerKids Press
29 E 21st Street
New York, NY 10010

212-777-3017
800-237-9932
Fax: 888-436-4643
e-mail: customerservice@rosenpub.com
www.rosenpublishing.com

In a straightforward yet comforting way, this book explains what cancer is, what kinds of treatments surround the disease and how to cope if a child or the friend of a child has cancer.

24 pages Papperback
ISBN: 0-823951-95-2

Roger Rosen, President

5076 Pediatric Cancer Sourcebook

Edward J. Prucha, author

Omnigraphics
PO Box 8002
Aston, PA 19014

800-234-1340
Fax: 800-875-1340
e-mail: info@omnigraphics.com
www.omnigraphics.com

Basic consumer health information about leukemias, brain tumors, sarcomas, lymphomas and other cancers in infants, children and adolescents.

1999 587 pages
ISBN: 0-780802-45-4

Peter Ruffner, Publisher

5077 Resource Survival Handbook

Neuroblastoma Children's Cancer Society
PO Box 957672
Hoffman Estates, IL 60195

847-605-0705
800-532-5162
Fax: 847-605-0705
www.neuroblastomacancer.org

An accumulation of resource information of facts about neuroblastoma and related treatments, national and local resources for families and patients, health claim forms, pamphlets, and other relevant forms.

Online

Jim Sexton, Chairman

5078 Surviving Childhood Cancer: A Guide for Families

Margot Joan Fromer, author

New Harbinger Publications
5674 Shattuck Avenue
Oakland, CA 94609

510-652-0215
800-748-6273
Fax: 800-652-1613
e-mail: customerservice@newharbinger.com
www.newharbinger.com

Cancer in a child is an overwhelming experience for a family. This book explains common medical procedures and offers readers practical advice about how to cope with emotions and stress during this time.

232 pages Paperback
ISBN: 1-572241-02-0

Journals

5079 Candlelighters Childhood Cancer Foundation
PO Box 498
Kensington, MD 20895

301-962-3520
855-858-2226
Fax: 310-962-3521
e-mail: staff@candlelighters.org
www.candlelighters.org

Provides the latest information on CCCF programs and childhood cancer.

Quarterly

Ruth Hoffman, Executive Director
Naomi Bartley, President
Janine Lynne, Vice President

Description

5080 NEUTROPENIA

Covers these related disorders: Chronic neutropenia, Transient neutropenia

Involves the following Biologic System(s):
Hematologic and Oncologic Disorders

Neutropenia is a blood condition characterized by decreased numbers of circulating white blood cells known as neutrophils. These white blood cells play an essential role in fighting bacterial infections by detecting, engulfing, and digesting invading bacteria (phagocytosis). Neutrophils mature in the bone marrow and are then released into the bloodstream, where they may circulate for approximately six to eight hours. When responding to invading microorganisms or inflammation, neutrophils may leave the blood circulation, move into affected tissues, and digest microbes or other invaders as required.

Neutropenia is specifically defined as the presence of fewer than 1,500 neutrophils per microliter of blood. The condition may result from deficient production of neutrophils by the bone marrow or abnormally increased loss of neutrophils from the blood circulation. Depending upon the nature of the condition, its underlying cause, and other factors, neutropenia may occur for only days or weeks (transient neutropenia) or be present for months or a patient's lifetime (chronic neutropenia). In addition, the findings potentially associated with neutropenia are extremely variable and may include no apparent symptoms (asymptomatic), mild infections of the mucous membranes and the skin, or, in severe cases, potentially life-threatening complications.

In children, transient neutropenia may be caused by certain viral or bacterial infections; a deficiency of folic acid or vitamin B12; or the administration of certain medications, such as a class of antipsychotic drugs (phenothiazines), penicillin preparations, nonsteroidal anti-inflammatory agents, or anticancer drugs that may suppress bone marrow production. Chronic neutropenia also has several different causes and occurs in many different forms. Benign chronic neutropenia is a condition of childhood in which patients have chronically low levels of circulating neutrophils in the blood. This may result in increased susceptibility to recurrent infections of the skin, the mouth, or other areas. The condition typically resolves on its own by age four. Patients with immune deficiency disorders that are present at birth (primary inherited immunodeficiencies) or acquired (such as acquired immune deficiency syndrome, AIDS) often develop chronic neutropenia during infancy or early childhood. These children often fail to grow and gain weight at the expected rate (failure to thrive) and may experience recurrent bacterial infections, enlargement of the liver and spleen (hepatosplenomegaly), and potentially life-threatening complications.

Other uncommon forms of childhood neutropenia include cyclic neutropenia and Kostmann's disease. In patients with cyclic neutropenia, neutropenia recurs in regular cycles (e.g., every 18 to 21 days). When circulating neutrophils are abnormally decreased, these patients may experience fever, a general feeling of ill health (malaise), and susceptibility to mouth ulcers and infections of the skin, mucous membranes, and tissues that surround and support the teeth. Cyclic neutropenia typically becomes apparent during childhood and often runs in certain families. Kostmann's disease, also known as genetic infantile agranulocytosis, is a rare, autosomal recessive disorder characterized by persistent, extremely low levels of circulating neutrophils (fewer than 200 per microliter), frequent bacterial infections, and potentially life-threatening complications by approximately age three.

Neutropenia may also occur as a component of certain genetic, multisystemic diseases, such as Shwachman syndrome and metaphyseal chondrodysplasia, or in association with certain cancers, including leukemia and lymphoma.

The treatment of children with neutropenia depends upon the condition's severity and its underlying cause. In those with mild neutropenia, treatment may not be required. If a particular medication is responsible for the condition, such drug therapy is discontinued if possible. In patients with chronic neutropenia, physicians may recommend steps to help prevent bacterial infection and institute immediate antibiotic therapy should infections occur. In severe cases of bacterial infection, hospitalization may be required. In addition, in some patients with severe neutropenia, therapies may be administered to help stimulate the bone marrow's production of neutrophils (granulocyte colony-stimulating factor [G-CSF]). In some cases, bone marrow transplantation is an option, a procedure in which healthy bone marrow is given to replace defective bone marrow.

Government Agencies

5081 NIH/National Heart, Lung and Blood Institute
National Institute of Health
PO Box 30105
Bethesda, MD 20824
301-592-8573
Fax: 301-592-8563
TTY: 240-629-3255
e-mail: NHLBIinfo@nhlbi.nih.gov
www.nhlbi.nih.gov

Primary responsibility of this organization is the scientific investigation of heart, blood vessel, lung and blood disorders. Oversees research, demonstration, prevention, education, control and training activities in these fields and emphasizes the prevention and control of heart diseases.

Gary H. Gibbons, Director
Susan Shurin, MD, Deputy Director
Nakela Cook, Chief of Staff

5082 NIH/National Institute of Child Health and Human Development
31 Center Drive, Building 31, Room 2A32
Bethesda, MD 20892
301-496-1333
800-370-2943
Fax: 866-760-5947
TTY: 888-320-6942
e-mail: NICHDInformationResourceCenter@mail.nih.
www.nichd.nih.gov

Established in 1962 by congress, today the institute conducts and supports research on topics related to the health of children, adults, families and populations. Some of these topics include: developmental disabilities, growth and development, infant death, reproductive health and birth defects.

Jay H Hoofnagle, Director
Lisa Kaeser, Program & Public Liaison

National Associations & Support Groups

5083 American Academy of Pediatrics
141 Northwest Point Boulevard
Elk Grove Village, IL 60007
847-434-4000
800-433-9016
Fax: 847-434-8000
www.aap.org

The American Academy of Pediatrics and its member pediatricians are committed to the attainment of optimal physical, mental and social health and well-being for all infants, children, adolescents, and young adults.

Sandra Hassink, MD, FAAP, President

5084 American Autoimmune Related Diseases Association
22100 Gratiot Avenue
East Detroit, MI 48021
586-776-3900
800-598-4668
Fax: 586-776-3903
e-mail: aarda@aarda.org
www.aarda.org

Dedicated to the eradiction of autoimmune diseases and the alleviation of suffering and the socio-economic impact of autoimmunity through fostering and facilitating collaboration in the areas of education, public awareness, research and patient services in an effective, ethical and efficient manner.

Betty Diamond, Chair
Noel R. Rose, Chairman Emeritus
Stanley M. Finger, Chairman of Board of Director

5085 Genetic Alliance
4301 Connecticut Avenue NW, Suite 404
Washington, DC 20008
202-966-5557
800-336-4363
Fax: 202-966-8553
e-mail: info@geneticalliance.org
www.geneticalliance.org

A coalition of voluntary genetic support groups, consumers and professionals addressing the needs of individuals and families affected by genetic disorders from a national perspective.

Sharon Terry, President & CEO

5086 March of Dimes Birth Defects Foundation
1275 Mamaroneck Avenue
White Plains, NY 10605
914-997-4488
888-663-4637
Fax: 914-428-8203
e-mail: answers@marchofdimes.com
www.marchofdimes.com

Partnership of volunteers and professionals dedicates to improving the health of babies by preventing birth defects and infant mortality. Over 100 chapters are located across the country and can be located through the National Office.

Jennifer L Howse, President

5087 Severe Chronic Neutropenia International Registry (SCNIR)
1107 NE 45th Street, Suite 345
Seattle, WA 98105
206-543-9749
800-726-4463
Fax: 206-543-3668
e-mail: bolyard@u.washington.edu
www.depts.washington.edu/registry

The SCNIR was established in the United States, Australia, Canada, and the European Community. The SCNIR is directed by a scientific advisory board of physicians from around the world who care for SCN patients. Our mission is to established a world-wide database of treatment and disease-related outcomes for persons diagnosed with SCN. Collection of this information will lead to improved medical care and is used for research to determine the causes of neutropenia.

Audrey Anna Bolyard, Clinical Manager

Web Sites

5088 American Autoimmune Related Diseases Association
22100 Gratiot Ave.
Eastpointe, MI 48021
586-776-3900
Fax: 586-776-3903
www.aarda.org

Dedicated to the eradiction of autoimmune diseases and the alleviation of suffering and the socio-economic impact of autoimmunity through fostering and facilitating collaboration in the areas of education, public awareness, research and patient services in an effective, ethical and efficient manner.

Herbert G. Ford, D. Min., Chairperson
Stanley M. Finger, Ph.D., Vice Chairperson
Virginia T. Ladd, R.T., President

5089 National Neutropenia Network
www.neutropenianet.org

Supports general and clinical research and provides information to the families, the medical community and the general public. Also committed to helping affected families and individuals work with hospitals, physicians, nurses, and other health care professionals.

5090 Online Mendelian Inheritance in Man
National Library of Medicine Building 38A
Bethesda, MD 20894
888-346-3656
e-mail: info@ncbi.nlm.nih.gov
www.ncbi.nlm.nih.gov

This database is a catalog of human genes and genetic disorders.

Book Publishers

5091 Let's Talk About Going to the Hospital
Rosen Publishing Group's PowerKids Press
29 E 21st Street
New York, NY 10010
212-777-3017
800-237-9932
Fax: 888-436-4643
e-mail: rosenpub@tribeca.ios.com
www.rosenpublishing.com

If a child has to check into the hospital, chances are he or she is already upset about being ill. Knowing how a hospital functions and what the procedures are, such as when family members can visit, will help in what is already a stressful situation. Grades K-5.

24 pages
ISBN: 0-823950-36-0

Roger Rosen, President

Description

5092 NIGHTMARES

Involves the following Biologic System(s):

Developmental/Behavioral/Psychiatric Disorders

Nightmares are a type of sleep disturbance that occurs during the rapid eye movement (REM) phase of sleep, or deep sleep stage. Vivid, disturbing dreams often evoke feelings of extreme and inescapable fear, terror, anxiety, and distress. Nightmares are often so intense that they awaken the sleeping individual, who is then usually able to recall all or most details of the dream.

Nightmares are quite common in children, particularly in the eight to 10 year old age group. Girls are more prone to this type of sleep disturbance than boys. Precipitating factors vary and may include breathing irregularities caused by the common cold or other illnesses; violent movies or television programs, especially in younger children; separation anxiety; and other traumatic experiences or events. In addition, children with certain types of psychological disturbances (e.g., affective, mood, or anxiety disorders) may experience repeated episodes of nightmares.

It is common for most children to experience occasional nightmares and, until the anxiety or fear of the experience passes, understanding and comfort by parents or caregivers is usually helpful. However, children who experience frequent nightmares may require a careful evaluation to determine if these episodes are a manifestation of an underlying psychologic disorder or other irregularity. If this is the case, treatment may be directed toward the underlying condition. Other treatment is supportive. For example, parents and caregivers are encouraged to be reassuring, understanding, and firm but nonthreatening. Reading or other quiet or soothing activities or rituals before bedtime may also be beneficial. In addition, night lights or other reasonable accommodations may be provided to reassure or comfort affected children.

Government Agencies

5093 Center for Mental Health Services Knowledge Exchange Program
US Department of Health and Human Services
PO Box 42557
Washington, DC 20015   800-789-2647
                                        Fax: 240-221-4295
                                        TDD: 866-889-2647
                                        http://mentalhealth.samhsa.gov

Supplies the public with responses to their commonly asked questions about mental health issues and services.

Kathryn Power, M.Ed., Director
Edward B. Searle M.B.A., Deputy Director
Jeffrey A. Buck, Ph.D, Associate Director

5094 NIH/National Institute of Mental Health
6001 Executive Boulevard, Room 8184, MSC 9663
Rockville, MD 20852   301-443-4513
                                        866-615-6464
                                        Fax: 301-443-4279
                                        TTY: 301-443-8431
                                        e-mail: NIMHinfo@mail.nih.gov
                                        www.nimh.nih.gov

Conducts strategic planning for specific research areas as well as for the Institute as a whole.

Dr Thomas R Insel, Director

National Associations & Support Groups

5095 American Academy of Pediatrics
141 Northwest Point Boulevard
Elk Grove Village, IL 60007   847-434-4000
                                        800-433-9016
                                        Fax: 847-434-8000
                                        www.aap.org

The American Academy of Pediatrics and its member pediatricians are committed to the attainment of optimal physical, mental and social health and well-being for all infants, children, adolescents, and young adults.

Sandra Hassink, MD, FAAP, President

5096 American Academy of Sleep Medicine
2510 North Frontage Road
Darien, IL 60561   630-737-9700
                                        Fax: 630-737-9790
                                        www.aasmnet.org

National not-for-profit professional membership organization dedicated to the advancement of sleep medicine. The Academy's mission is to assure quality care for patients with sleep disorders, promote the advancement of sleep research and provide public and professional education. The AASM delivers programs, information and services to and through its members and advocates sleep medicine supportive policies in the medical community and the public sector.

Timothy I. Morgenthaler, MD, President
Nathaniel F. Watson, MD, President-Elect
Ronald D. Chervin, MD,, Secretary/Treasurer

5097 American Association of Sleep Technologists
2510 North Frontage Road
Darien, IL 60561   630-737-9704
                                        Fax: 630-737-9788
                                        e-mail: coordinator@aastweb.org
                                        www.aastweb.org

The American Association of Sleep Technologists is the leading advocate for the sleep technologist profession. Our mission is to promote and advance the profession through the continued development of educational, technical and clinical excellence in sleep disorders.

Rita Brooks, President
Laura A. Linley, President-Elect
David Gregory, Secretary

5098 American Board of Sleep Medicine
2510 North Frontage Road
Darien, IL 60561   630-737-9700
                                        Fax: 630-737-9790
                                        e-mail: absm@absm.org
                                        www.absm.org

The American Board of Sleep Medicine (ABSM) is an independent, nonprofit organization whose certificates are recognized throughout the world as a credential signifying a high level of competence for sleep medicine physicians, PhDs, behavioral sleep medicine specialists and sleep technologists.

Kelly Carden, MD, President
Nathaniel Watson, MD, MS, Past President
Ron Chervin, MD, Secretary-Treasurer

5099 American Mental Health Foundation (AMHF)
P.O. Box 3
Riverdale, NY 10471
USA   212-737-9027
          e-mail: elomke@americanmentalhealthfoundation.or
                   www.americanmentalhealthfoundation.org

Dedicated to the extensive and intensive research in the theories and techniques of treatment of emotional illness and to the implementation of reforms in the mental health system. Efforts have resulted in development of better and less expensive treatment methods. Findings are disseminated in English and other major languages.

Sister Joan Curtin, Director
John P. Fowler, Treasurer
Eugene Gollogly, VP

5100 American Sleep Association
1002 Lititz Pike #229
Lititz, PA 17543   www.sleepassociation.org

The American Sleep Association (ASA) is an organization dedicated to improving public awareness about sleep disorders and sleep health, promoting sleep medicine research, and providing a portal for communication between patients, physicians, healthcare professionals, corporations, and scientists.

5101 American Sleep Medicine Foundation
2510 North Frontage Road
Darien, IL 60561   630-737-9700
                                    Fax: 630-737-9790
                        e-mail: asmfinfo@aasmnet.org
                                    www.discoversleep.org

The American Sleep Medicine Foundation (ASMF) promotes sleep research and education.

Merrill Wise, MD, President
Ronald D. Chervin, MD, MS, Secretary/Treasurer
Jerome A. Barrett, Executive Director

5102 Christian Horizons
PO Box 6646
Saginaw, MI 48608   616-956-7063
                                    Fax: 616-956-7064
                    e-mail: info@christianhorizonsinc.org
                        www.christianhorizonsinc.org

To share Christ's love as we equip and support Adults with developmental disabilities.

5103 Federation of Families for Children's Mental Health
9605 Medical Center Drive, Suite 280
Rockville, MD 20850   240-403-1901
                                    Fax: 240-403-1909
                            e-mail: ffcmh@ffcmh.org
                                    www.ffcmh.org

The National family run organization is dedicated exclusively to helping children with mental health needs and their families achieve a better quality of life.

Teka Dempson, President
Sherri Luthe, Vice President
Josh Ross, Secretary

5104 NADD: National Association for the Dually Diagnosed
132 Fair Street
Kingston, NY 12401   845-331-4336
                                    800-331-5362
                                    Fax: 845-331-4569
                            e-mail: info@thenadd.org
                                    www.thenadd.org

Nonprofit organization designed to promote the interests of professional and parent development with resources for individuals who have the coexistence of mental illness and mental retardation. Provides conferences, educational services and training materials to professionals, parents, concerned citizens and service organizations.

Donna McNelis, President
Dan Baker, VP
Julia Pearce, Secretary

5105 National Alliance for the Mentally Ill
3803 N Fairfax Drive, Suite 100
Arlington, VA 22203   703-524-7600
                                    888-999-6264
                                    Fax: 703-524-9094
                                    TDD: 703-516-7227
                            e-mail: info@nami.org
                                    www.nami.org

NAMI is a nonprofit, grassroots, self-help, support and advocacy organization of consumers, families and friends of people with severe mental illness, such as schizophrenia, bipolar disorder, major depressive disorder, obsessive compulsive disorder, anxiety disorders, autism and other severe and persistent mental illnesses that affect the brain.

Keris J.,n Myrick, President
Kevin B. Sullivan, First Vice President
Jim Payne, Second VP

5106 National Mental Health Association
2000 N Beauregard Street, 6th Floor
Alexandria, VA 22311   703-684-7722
                                    800-969-6642
                                    Fax: 703-684-5968
                                    TTY: 800-433-5959
                        www.mentalhealthamerica.net

Addresses all aspects of mental health and mental illness. NMHA with over 340 affiliates works to improve the mental health of all Americans.

David Shern, CEO

5107 National Mental Health Consumers' Self-Help Clearinghouse
1211 Chestnut Street, Suite 1207
Philadelphia, PA 19107   267-507-3810
                                    800-553-4539
                                    Fax: 215-636-6312
                        e-mail: info@mhselfhelp.org
                                    www.mhselfhelp.org

Offers information, support and appropriate referrals; and promotes public and professional education. Provides networking for those with special interests related to albinism. Promotes and supports research and funding that will improve diagnosis and management of albinism and hypopigmentation.

Joseph Rogers, Executive Director & Founder
Susan Rogers, Director
Christa Burkett, Technical Assistance Coordinator

5108 National Sleep Foundation
1522 K Street NW, Suite 500
Washington, DC 20005   202-464-1308
                                    Fax: 202-347-3472
                        e-mail: nsf@sleepfoundation.org
                                    www.narap.org

An independent, nonprofit organization dedicated to improving public health and safety by achieving public understanding of sleep and sleep disorders, and by supporting public education, sleep-related research, and advocacy. Actively collaborates with sleep centers, support groups for patients with sleep disorders and safety organizations.

Richard Gelula, CEO

5109 Sleep Research Society
2510 North Frontage Road
Darien, IL 60561   630-737-9702
                                    Fax: 630-737-9790
                        e-mail: coordinator@srsnet.org
                                    www.sleepresearchsociety.org

The Sleep Research Society (SRS) is organization for scientific investigators who educate and research sleep and sleep disorders. The SRS serves its members and the field of sleep research through training and education, and by providing forums for the collaboration and the exchange of ideas.

Allan I. Pack, PhD, MBChB, President
Sean P.A. Drummond, PhD, President-Elect
Jerome A. Barrett, Executive Director

5110 Society of Behavioral Sleep Medicine
2510 North Frontage Road
Darien, IL 60561   630-737-9706
                                    Fax: 630-737-9790
                        e-mail: membership@behavioralsleep.org
                                    www.behavioralsleep.org

Behavioral Sleep Medicine is the field of clinical practice and scientific inquiry that encompasses: the study of behavioral, psychological, and physiological factors underlying normal and disordered sleep across the life span; and, the development and application of evidence-based behavioral and psychological approaches to the prevention and treatment of sleep disorders and co-existing conditions.

Ryan G. Wetzler, PsyD, CBSM, President
Michael Scherer, PhD, CBSM, President-Elect
Valerie M. Crabtree, PhD, CBSM, Secretary/Treasurer

State Agencies & Support Groups

5111 Center for Family Support
333 7th Avenue, #901
New York, NY 10001

212-629-7939
Fax: 212-239-2211
www.cfsny.org

The Center for Family (CFS) is a not-for-profit human service agency providing support and assistance to individuals with developmental disabilities and traumatic brain injuries throughout New York City, Long Island, the lower Hudson Valley region and New Jersey.

Steven Vernikoff, Executive Director
Barbara Greenwald, Associate Executive Director
Mike Mazzocco, Associate Executive Director

Libraries & Resource Centers

5112 American Academy of Somnology
PO Box 27077
Las Vegas, NV 89126

702-371-0947
e-mail: somnology@aol.com
www.hopperinstitute.com/aas_intro.html

Covers about 75 physicians, dentists, nurses, psychologists, technicians, and students and sponsoring organizations, including associations, institutions, and corporations, with a special interest in sleep.

David Hopper, Director

Web Sites

5113 CyberPsych
www.cyberpsych.org

CyberPsych presents information about psychoanalysis, psychotherapy, and special topics such as anxiety disorder, the problematic use of alcohol, homophobia, and the traumatic effects of racism. CyberPsych is a nonprofit network which offers free web hosting and technical support for internet communication, to non profit groups and individuals.

5114 NADD: National Association for the Dually Diagnosed
132 Fair Street
Kingston, NY 12401

845-331-4336
800-331-5362
Fax: 845-331-4569
www.thenadd.org

Nonprofit organization designed to promote the interests of professional and care providers for individuals who have the coexistence of mental illness and mental retardation. NADD provides conferences, educational services and training materials to professionals, parents, concerned citizens and service organizations.

Donna McNelis, PhD, President
Dan Baker, PhD., Vice President
Julia Pearce, Secretary

5115 Planetpsych
www.planetpsych.com

Planetpsych is an online resource for mental health information.

5116 Psych Central
55 Pleasant St., Suite 207
Newburyport, MA 1950

www.psychcentral.com

Offers free informational and educational articles and resources on psychology, support and mental health online.

John M. Grohol, CEO
Rick Nauert, Ph.D., Senior News Editor
Bailey Apple, Associate Editor

5117 Sleep Disorders
http://talhost.net/sleep/parasomnia.htm

For those who have sleep disorders and have a problem sleeping.

5118 Sleepdisorders.com
www.sleepdisorders.com

Updated monthly and organized by sleep disorders with quality links.

Book Publishers

5119 Concise Guide to Evaluation and Management of Sleep Disorders
American Psychiatric Publishing
1000 Wilson Boulevard, Suite 1825
Arlington, VA 22209

703-907-7322
800-368-5777
Fax: 703-907-1091
e-mail: appi@psych.org
www.appi.org

Overview of sleep disorders medicine, sleep physiology and pathology, insomnia complaints, excessive sleepiness disorders, parasomnias, medical and psychiatric disorders and sleep, medications with sedative-hypnotic properties, special problems and populations.

2002 296 pages Paper 3rd Ed
ISBN: 1-585620-45-6

Robert E. Hales, M.D., Editor-in-Chief
Rebecca D. Rinehart, Publisher
John McDuffie, Editorial Director

5120 Sleep Disorders and Psychiatry

Daniel J Buysse MD, author

American Psychiatric Publishing
1000 Wilson Boulevard, Ste 1825
Arlington, VA 22209

703-907-7322
800-368-5777
Fax: 703-907-1091
e-mail: appi@psych.org
www.appi.org

Summarizes the major categories of sleep disorders including parasomnias and narcolepsy.

2005 256 pages Paperback
ISBN: 1-585622-29-0

Robert E. Hales, M.D., Editor-in-Chief
Rebecca D. Rinehart, Publisher
John McDuffie, Editorial Director

5121 Snoring From A to Zzzz
Spencer Press
2525 NW Lovejoy Street, Suite 402
Portland, OR 97210

503-223-4959
Fax: 503-223-1608
e-mail: dereklipman@aol.com

Covers organizations, associations, support groups, and manufacturers of sleep-related medical products relevant to sleep disorders. Discussess every aspect of snoring abd sleep apnea from causes to cures.

256 pages Paperback
ISBN: 0-965070-81-6

Derek Lipman MD, Author/Editor

Description

5122 NIGHT TERRORS

Synonyms: Pavor nocturnus, Sleep-terror disorder

Involves the following Biologic System(s):

Developmental/Behavioral/Psychiatric Disorders

Night terrors is a sleep disorder characterized by episodes of sudden awakening from sleep in an extremely anxious or terrified state. This sleep disturbance occurs in from two to five children out of every hundred, and, in most cases, begins during the fourth to seventh year of life. Sleep-terror disorder more commonly affects boys than girls and often disappears before the onset of adolescence.

Episodes of night terrors usually take place during the third or fourth stage of the nonrapid eye movement or NREM phase of sleep. Each stage of NREM sleep is a successively deeper sleep leading up to rapid eye movement sleep or a deep REM during which dreams may occur. Typically, affected children awaken abruptly and may be screaming and extremely frightened. They may be in a semiconscious state and unaware of or unable to recognize people or surroundings. These children are generally inconsolable and may exhibit such physical symptoms as sweating; widening (dilation) of the pupils; elevated heart rate (tachycardia); abnormally deep, rapid breathing (hyperventilation); and violent thrashing. In about a third of patients, sleepwalking (somnambulism) may also occur. Children are usually able to fall back to sleep within minutes of these short-lived episodes and have no memory of the event when they awaken.

Night terrors are most often confused with nightmares, but unlike night terrors, a child having a nightmare is usually easily woken up and comforted. Sleep disorders such as night terrors often result from childhood fears or anxieties. For example, some young children may be apprehensive about going to bed because this actually represents a temporary separation from their parents (separation anxiety). In addition, any issues affecting the family or child (e.g., separation, divorce, death, school performance, social interactions, etc.) may translate into disturbances in normal sleep patterns. Other contributing factors may include the presence of a fever, depression, or other emotional disorders.

Although the administration of certain antianxiety and antidepressant drugs may, in some cases, be of benefit, treatment of night terrors is mainly supportive. If the precipitating cause can be determined, steps may then be taken to alleviate the fear or anxiety. In any case, parents or caregivers are encouraged to be supportive and firm, but nonjudgmental. Excitement before bedtime is discouraged; however, reading or other quiet, pleasurable activities may be beneficial.

Government Agencies

5123 Center for Mental Health Services Knowledge Exchange Program
US Department of Health and Human Services
4301 Connecticut Avenue, NW, Suite 100
Washington, DC 20008
877-871-0744
Fax: 240-747-5470
TTY: 877-871-0665
TDD: 866-889-2647
www.ncwd-youth.info/node/245

Supplies the public with responses to their commonly asked questions about mental health issues and services.

5124 NIH/National Institute of Mental Health
6001 Executive Boulevard, Room 8184, MSC 9663
Rockville, MD 20852
301-443-4513
866-615-6464
Fax: 301-443-4279
TTY: 301-443-8431
e-mail: NIMHinfo@mail.nih.gov
www.nimh.nih.gov

Conducts strategic planning for specific research areas as well as for the Institute as a whole.

Dr Thomas R Insel, Director

National Associations & Support Groups

5125 American Academy of Pediatrics
141 Northwest Point Boulevard
Elk Grove Village, IL 60007
847-434-4000
800-433-9016
Fax: 847-434-8000
www.aap.org

The American Academy of Pediatrics and its member pediatricians are committed to the attainment of optimal physical, mental and social health and well-being for all infants, children, adolescents, and young adults.

Sandra Hassink, MD, FAAP, President

5126 American Academy of Sleep Medicine
2510 North Frontage Road
Darien, IL 60561
630-737-9700
Fax: 630-737-9790
www.aasmnet.org

National not-for-profit professional membership organization dedicated to the advancement of sleep medicine. The Academy's mission is to assure quality care for patients with sleep disorders, promote the advancement of sleep research and provide public and professional education. The AASM delivers programs, information and services to and through its members and advocates sleep medicine supportive policies in the medical community and the public sector.

Sam Fleishman, President
M. Safran Badr, President-Elect
Timothy I. Morgenthaler, Secretary

5127 American Mental Health Foundation (AMHF)
P.O. Box 3
Riverdale, NY 10471
USA
212-737-9027
e-mail: elomke@americanmentalhealthfoundation.or
www.americanmentalhealthfoundation.org

Dedicated to the extensive and intensive research in the theories and techniques of treatment of emotional illness and to the implementation of reforms in the mental health system. Efforts have resulted in development of better and less expensive treatment methods. Findings are disseminated in English and other major languages.

Sister Joan Curtin, Director
John P. Fowler, Treasurer
Eugene Gollogly, VP

5128 Center for Disabilities and Development
University of Iowa Hospitals and Clinics
451 Newton Road, 200 Medicine Administration Build
Iowa City, IA 52242
319-353-6900
877-686-0031
Fax: 319-356-8284
e-mail: cdd-webmaster@uiowa.edu
www.medicine.uiowa.edu

A trusted resource for healthcare, training, research and information for people with disabilities that include: behavior disorders, brain injury, cerebral palsy, diabetes, down syndrome, learning disabilities, mental retardation, sleep disorders and spina bifida.

Debra A. Schwinn, Dean
Donna L. Hammond, Interim Executive Associate Dean
Christopher Cooper, Associate Dean for Student Affairs

5129 Christian Horizons
PO Box 6646
Saginaw, MI 48608
616-956-7063
Fax: 616-956-7064
e-mail: info@christianhorizonsinc.org
www.christianhorizonsinc.org

To share Christ's love as we equip and support Adults with developmental disabilities.

5130 Federation of Families for Children's Mental Health
9605 Medical Center Drive, Suite 280
Rockville, MD 20850
240-403-1901
Fax: 240-403-1909
e-mail: ffcmh@ffcmh.org
www.ffcmh.org

The National family run organization is dedicated exclusively to helping children with mental health needs and their families achieve a better quality of life.

Teka Dempson, President
Sherri Luthe, Vice President
Josh Ross, Secretary

5131 NADD: National Association for the Dually Diagnosed
132 Fair Street
Kingston, NY 12401
845-331-4336
800-331-5362
Fax: 845-331-4569
e-mail: info@thenadd.org
www.thenadd.org

Nonprofit organization designed to promote the interests of professional and parent development with resources for individuals who have the coexistence of mental illness and mental retardation. Provides conferences, educational services and training materials to professionals, parents, concerned citizens and service organizations.

Donna McNelis, President
Dan Baker, VP
Julia Pearce, Secretary

5132 National Mental Health Consumers' Self-Help Clearinghouse
1211 Chestnut Street, Suite 1207
Philadelphia, PA 19107
267-507-3810
800-553-4539
Fax: 215-636-6312
e-mail: info@mhselfhelp.org
www.mhselfhelp.org

Offers information, support and appropriate referrals; and promotes public and professional education. Provides networking for those with special interests related to albinism. Promotes and supports research and funding that will improve diagnosis and management of albinism and hypopigmentation.

Joseph Rogers, Executive Director & Founder
Susan Rogers, Director
Christa Burkett, Technical Assistance Coordinator

5133 National Sleep Foundation
1522 K Street NW, Suite 500
Washington, DC 20005
202-464-1308
Fax: 202-347-3472
e-mail: nsf@sleepfoundation.org
www.narap.org

An independent, nonprofit organization dedicated to improving public health and safety by achieving public understanding of sleep and sleep disorders, and by supporting public education, sleep-related research, and advocacy. Actively collaborates with sleep centers, support groups for patients with sleep disorders and safety organizations.

Richard Gelula, CEO

State Agencies & Support Groups

5134 Center for Family Support
333 7th Avenue, #901
New York, NY 10001
212-629-7939
Fax: 212-239-2211
www.cfsny.org

The Center for Family (CFS) is a not-for-profit human service agency providing support and assistance to individuals with developmental disabilities and traumatic brain injuries throughout New York City, Long Island, the lower Hudson Valley region and New Jersey.

Steven Vernikoff, Executive Director
Barbara Greenwald, Associate Executive Director
Mike Mazzocco, Associate Executive Director

Libraries & Resource Centers

5135 American Academy of Somnology
PO Box 27077
Las Vegas, NV 89126
702-371-0947
e-mail: somnology@aol.com
www.hopperinstitute.com/aas_intro.html

Covers about 75 physicians, dentists, nurses, psychologists, technicians, and students and sponsoring organizations, including associations, institutions, and corporations, with a special interest in sleep.

David Hopper, Director

Research Centers

5136 UC Berkeley School of Social Welfare
Mental Health & Social Welfare Research Group
120 Haviland Hall #7400
Berkeley, CA 94720
510-642-4341
Fax: 510-643-6126
e-mail: spsegal@berkeley.edu
www.socialwelfare.berkeley.edu

Steven P Segal, Director

Web Sites

5137 About.com on Sleep Disorders
www.sleepdisorders.about.com

Well-organized information including new developments and a chat room.

5138 CyberPsych
www.cyberpsych.org

Presents information about psychoanalysis, psychtherapy and special topics such as anxiety disorder, the problamatic use of alcohol, homophobia, and the traumatic effects of racism.

5139 NADD: National Association for the Dually Diagnosed
132 Fair Street
Kingston, NY 12401
845-331-4336
800-331-5362
Fax: 845-331-4569
www.thenadd.org

Nonprofit organization designed to promote the interests of professional and care providers for individuals who have the coexistence of mental illness and mental retardation. NADD provides conferences, educational services and training materials to professionals, parents, concerned citizens and service organizations.

Donna McNelis, PhD, President
Dan Baker, PhD., Vice President
Julia Pearce, Secretary

5140 Planetpsych
www.planetpsych.com

Online resource for mental health information.

5141 Psych Central
55 Pleasant St., Suite 207
Newburyport, MA 1950
www.psychcentral.com

Offers free informational and educational articles and resources on psychology, support and mental health online.

John M. Grohol, CEO
Rick Nauert, Ph.D., Senior News Editor
Bailey Apple, Associate Editor

5142 Sleep Disorders
http://talhost.net/sleep/parasomnia.htm

For those who have sleep disorders and have a problem sleeping.

5143 Sleepdisorders.com
www.sleepdisorders.com

Updated monthly and organized by sleep disorders with quality links.

Book Publishers

5144 Concise Guide to Evaluation and Management of Sleep Disorders
American Psychiatric Publishing
1000 Wilson Boulevard, Suite 1825
Arlington, VA 22209   703-907-7322
                                                 800-368-5777
                                           Fax: 703-907-1091
                                         e-mail: appi@psych.org
                                               www.appi.org

Overview of sleep disorders medicine, sleep physiology and pathology, insomnia complaints, excessive sleepiness disorders, parasomnias, medical and psychiatric disorders and sleep, medications with sedative-hypnotic properties, special problems and populations.

2002 296 pages Paper 3rd Ed
ISBN: 1-585620-45-6

Robert E. Hales, M.D., Editor-in-Chief
Rebecca D. Rinehart, Publisher
John McDuffie, Editorial Director

5145 Principles and Practice of Sleep Medicine
Elsevier Health Sciences Division
1600 John F Kennedy Blvd, Suite 1800
Philadelphia, PA 19103   215-239-3900
                                                 800-523-1649
                                           Fax: 215-239-3990
                                      www.us.elsevierhealth.com

Covers the recent advances in basic sciences as well as sleep pathology in adults. Encompasses developments in this rapidly advancing field and also includes topics related to psychiatry, circadian rhythms, cardiovascualr diseases and sleep apnea diagnosis and treatment. Hardcover.

2005 1552 pages 4th Edition
ISBN: 0-721607-97-7

5146 Sleep Disorders and Psychiatry

Daniel J Buysse MD, author

American Psychiatric Publishing
1000 Wilson Boulevard, Ste 1825
Arlington, VA 22209   703-907-7322
                                                 800-368-5777
                                           Fax: 703-907-1091
                                         e-mail: appi@psych.org
                                               www.appi.org

Summarizes the major categories of sleep disorders including parasomnias and narcolepsy.

2005 256 pages Paperback
ISBN: 1-585622-29-0

Robert E. Hales, M.D., Editor-in-Chief
Rebecca D. Rinehart, Publisher
John McDuffie, Editorial Director

5147 Snoring From A to Zzzz
Spencer Press
2525 NW Lovejoy Street, Suite 402
Portland, OR 97210   503-223-4959
                                           Fax: 503-223-1608
                                    e-mail: dereklipman@aol.com

Covers organizations, associations, support groups, and manufacturers of sleep-related medical products relevant to sleep disorders. Discussess every aspect of snoring abd sleep apnea from causes to cures.

256 pages Paperback
ISBN: 0-965070-81-6

Derek S Lipman, MD, Author/Editor

Description

5148 NOCTURNAL ENURESIS

Synonym: Bed-wetting

Involves the following Biologic System(s):

Developmental/Behavioral/Psychiatric Disorders, Renal and Urologic Disorders

Nocturnal enuresis or bed-wetting refers to the discharge of urine during the night by children who have achieved urinary control during other periods of the day. It affects an estimated 5 to 7 million children in the United States. This type of bed-wetting is considered primary enuresis if nightly urinary incontinence has persisted since birth. Nocturnal enuresis that occurs in children who were previously continent during the night for a period of one year or more is considered secondary enuresis, a regressive form of this abnormality. Bed-wetting is a very common problem that occurs more often in boys than in girls and tends to run in families. In most cases, enuresis resolves spontaneously. The causes of nocturnal enuresis are varied and may include delayed maturation of certain functions of the nervous system that regulate bladder control, psychological influences, spinal abnormalities (e.g., spina bifida), structural abnormalities or defects, underlying disease (e.g., diabetes mellitus), urinary tract infection, or other physical causes. Secondary enuresis may be precipitated by stressful or traumatic events such as the birth of another child, death, divorce, or other situations that impact on the normal day-to-day routine.

Children with enuresis may undergo evaluation in order to determine if the condition is caused by neurological or physical problems. If this is the case, treatment is geared toward the underlying problem. Other treatment may include such supportive measures as establishing a reward system to give the child incentive to cooperate, charting the child's progress in order to offer positive reinforcement, limiting liquid intake before bedtime, having the child urinate directly before going to bed, and having affected older children take part in laundering soiled clothing and remaking the bed. Parents and caregivers are typically counseled to remain supportive and nonjudgmental. Additional treatment may include behavioral therapy and other counseling that involves both the parents or caregivers and the affected child. Bed-wetting alarms that detect small amounts of urine and certain types of medication (e.g., imipramine and desmopressin acetate nasal spray) may also be used to control enuresis. Imipramine is an antidepressant drug that is usually effective within two weeks; however, relapses are common after the drug is gradually stopped and, therefore, a longer course of administration may become necessary. Desmopressin acetate nasal spray reduces urine output in approximately 70 percent of affected children; however, its beneficial effect is temporary. Other treatment is supportive.

Government Agencies

5149 NIH/National Institute of Mental Health
6001 Executive Boulevard, Room 8184, MSC 9663
Rockville, MD 20892

301-443-4513
866-615-6464
Fax: 301-443-4279
TTY: 301-443-8431
e-mail: nimhinfo@nih.gov
www.nimh.nih.gov

Conducts strategic planning for specific research areas as well as for the Institute as a whole.

Dr Thomas R Insel, Director

5150 National Kidney and Urologic Diseases Information Clearinghouse
Bldg 31, Rm 9A06, 31 Center Drive, MSC 2560
Bethesda, MD 20892

301-496-3583
800-891-5390
Fax: 703-738-4929
e-mail: nkudic@info.niddk.nih.gov
www2.niddk.nih.gov

To increase knowledge and understanding about diseases of the kidneys and urologic system among people with these conditions and their families, health care professionals and the general public.

Griffin P. Rogers, Director

National Associations & Support Groups

5151 American Academy of Pediatrics
141 Northwest Point Boulevard
Elk Grove Village, IL 60007

847-434-4000
800-433-9016
Fax: 847-434-8000
www.aap.org

The American Academy of Pediatrics and its member pediatricians are committed to the attainment of optimal physical, mental and social health and well-being for all infants, children, adolescents, and young adults.

Sandra Hassink, MD, FAAP, President

5152 American Urological Association Foundation
1000 Corporate Boulevard, Suite 410
Linthicum, MD 21090

410-689-3700
866-746-4282
Fax: 410-689-3800
e-mail: auafoundation@auafoundation.org
www.auanet.org

Partners with physicians, researchers, healthcare professionals, patients, families, caregivers and the public to support, promote research, and patient/public education and advocacy in improving the prevention, detection, treatment and cure of urologic diseases.

Veronica Gilliard, Manager
Robert C. Flannigan MD, Secretary
William F. Gee MD, Treasurer

5153 Association for the Bladder Exstrophy Community
6737 West Washington Street, Ste 3265
West Allis, WI 53214

414-918-9002
866-300-2222
Fax: 414-918-9001
e-mail: admin@bladderexstrophy.com
www.bladderexstrophy.com

The ABC is an international support network of individuals with bladder exstrophy (includes classic exstrophy, cloacal exstrophy, and epispadias), local parent-exstrophy support groups, and health care providers working with patients and families living with bladder exstrophy.

Dr. Jeffrey Niezgoda, President/Founder
Pamela Block, President
Tom Exler, Vice-President

5154 Federation of Families for Children's Mental Health
9605 Medical Center Drive, Suite 280
Rockville, MD 20850

240-403-1901
Fax: 240-403-1909
e-mail: ffcmh@ffcmh.org
www.ffcmh.org

The National family run organization is dedicated exclusively to helping children with mental health needs and their families achieve a better quality of life.

Teka Dempson, President
Sherri Luthe, Vice President
Josh Ross, Secretary

5155 National Mental Health Association
2000 N Beauregard Street, 6th Floor
Alexandria, VA 22311   703-684-7722
                                    800-969-6642
                                    Fax: 703-684-5968
                                    TTY: 800-433-5959
                                    www.mentalhealthamerica.net

Addresses all aspects of mental health and mental illness. NMHA with over 340 affiliates works to improve the mental health of all Americans.

David Shern, CEO

5156 National Mental Health Consumers' Self-Help Clearinghouse
1211 Chestnut Street, Suite 1207
Philadelphia, PA 19107   215-751-1810
                                    800-553-4539
                                    Fax: 215-636-6312
                                    e-mail: info@mhselfhelp.org
                                    www.mhselfhelp.org

Offers information, support and appropriate referrals; and promotes public and professional education. Provides networking for those with special interests related to albinism. Promotes and supports research and funding that will improve diagnosis and management of albinism and hypopigmentation.

Joseph Rogers, Executive Director & Founder
Susan Rogers, Director
Christa Burkett, Technical Assistance Coordinator

5157 National Sleep Foundation
1522 K Street NW, Suite 500
Washington, DC 20005   202-464-1308
                                    Fax: 202-347-3472
                                    e-mail: nsf@sleepfoundation.org
                                    www.narap.org

An independent, nonprofit organization dedicated to improving public health and safety by achieving public understanding of sleep and sleep disorders, and by supporting public education, sleep-related research, and advocacy. Actively collaborates with sleep centers, support groups for patients with sleep disorders and safety organizations.

Richard Gelula, CEO

Web Sites

5158 American Urological Association Foundation
1000 Corporate Boulevard
Linthicum, MD 21090   410-689-3700
                                    800-828-7866
                                    Fax: 410-689-3998
                                    e-mail: info@urologycarefoundation.org
                                    www.urologyhealth.org

Provides information on enuresis as well as other pediatric disorders related to the kidneys and bladder.

Richard A. Memo, MD, Chair
Steven Schlossberg, MD, MBA, Secretary/Treasurer
Martin Dineen, Member-at-Large

5159 Bedwetting Online
www.bedwetting.ferring.ca

Helps parents and children deal with Nocturnal Enuresis.

5160 Child Development Institute
500 State College, Suite 1100
Orange, CA 92868childdevelopmentinfo.com/disorders/bedwetting.shtml

Child development and parent information for learning, health and safety, as well as child disorders.

5161 Dr. Koop
750 Third Avenue, 6th Floor
New York, NY 10017   212-695-2223
                                    Fax: 212-695-2936
                                    www.healthcentral.com

Information on the condition, causes, symptoms, tests and treatment.

Michael Cunnion, Chief Executive Officer
Jim Curtis, Chief Revenue Officer
Rebecca Farwell, Chief Content Officer

5162 National Kidney Foundation
30 East 33rd Street
New York, NY 10016   800-622-9010
                                    Fax: 212-689-9261
                                    e-mail: info@kidney.org
                                    www.kidney.org/patients/bw/index.cfm

Information for parents, kids and teens, and medical professionals on bed-wetting.

Bruce Skyer, CEO
Joseph Vassalotti, MD, Chief Medical Officer
Petros Gregoriou, SVP, CFO

Description

5163 NON-HODGKIN'S LYMPHOMA

Synonym: NHL

Covers these related disorders: Non-Hodgkin's lymphoma, large cell type, Non-Hodgkin's lymphoma, lymphoblastic type, Non-Hodgkin's lymphoma, small noncleaved cell(SNC)

Involves the following Biologic System(s):
Hematologic and Oncologic Disorders

Non-Hodgkin's lymphoma (NHL) consists of a group of cancers of the body's lymphatic system. This specialized system consists of the spleen, thymus gland, adenoids and tonsils, lymph nodes, and lymph ducts. Together these structures carry the clear fluid known as lymph and the white blood cells known as lymphocytes, and drain fluid and waste products from the body's organs and tissues. The lymph nodes act as tiny sieves that filter invading organisms and cancerous cells from the lymph that passes through the nodes, while lymphocytes in the nodes and elsewhere in the lymphatic system attack and destroy these hostile organisms and malignant cells. Besides its presence in these lymphatic structures, lymphatic tissue is present in the skin, stomach, and small intestine.

Non-Hodgkin lymphoma (NHL) is characterized by the proliferation of either T- or B-lymphocytes (white blood cells).T-lymphocytes act directly against infecting microorganisms and body cells that have turned cancerous by coming into contact with these hostile organisms or cells and secreting substances that either kill them directly or mark them for killing by other blood cells. B-cells combat infection by secreting antibodies that target alien microorganisms for killing by other cells. Types of NHL that occur among T-cells include the diseases known as mycosis fungoides, anaplastic large cell lymphoma, and precursor T-lymphoblastic lymphoma. Most NHLs occurring in the United States are B-cell lymphomas, whichinclude chronic lymphocytic leukemia/small lymphocytic lymphoma (CLL/SLL), diffuse large B-cell lymphoma, follicular lymphoma, Burkitt's lymphoma, immunoblastic large cell lymphoma, precursor B-lymphoblastic lymphoma, and mantle cell lymphoma, as well as the condition named hairy-cell leukemia because of the hair-like projections that extend from the abnormal B-lymphocytes in this disease.

Most types of NHL arise from lymph nodes in the head and neck, the chest cavity, or the abdomen. Some types may develop in lymph nodes at other sites in the body or affect other structures of the lymphoid system or other tissues, and a close association exists between specific types of NHL and the sites at which these diseases initially occur. For example, lymphoblastic NHL, which affects the immature cells that become lymphocytes, tends to arise in the head and neck or in the front of the chest cavity (anterior mediastinum).

Besides consisting of these different diseases, NHL is classified as being either aggressive, where lymphocytes multiply rapidly, or indolent, where cells proliferate slowly. Every individual case is further classified into one of four stages, based on the degree of progression. NHL symbolized by "E" indicates that the disease exists in lymphatic structures or tissues besides or beyond the lymph nodes; "S" indicates that it exists in the spleen.

Although lymphomas can occur at any age, they are the third most common kinds of childhood cancers in the United States, affecting about 13 of every 1 million children annually. While all lymphomas originate with a genetic defect in white cells or their immature precursor cells, other factors may instigate these lymphoid cancers or increase susceptibility to them. Thus, NHL particularly affects children with impaired immune systems. These include patients with acquired immune deficiency syndrome (AIDS) or certain genetic immunodeficiency disorders that are present at birth (primary immunodeficiencies), such as Wiskott-Aldrich syndrome, a condition marked by deficiencies in the numbers of platelet cells in the blood and in the body's immune system; X-linked lymphoproliferative syndrome; or ataxia-telangiectasia. Other sources of increased risk of developing NHL include infection with Epstein-Barr virus, which causes infectious mononucleosis; a high dietary meat or fat intake; and exposure to various pesticides and other toxic substances.

The diagnosis of NHL is based on physical examination, which may reveal swelling of the lymph nodes and other telltale signs of the disease; a complete blood count (CBC) that reveals increased numbers of either T- or B-lymphocytes and possibly decreased numbers of other kinds of blood cells; a decreased content of the oxygen-carrying substance known as hemoglobin in the body's red blood cells; abnormalities in tissue specimens taken from lymph nodes or other structures of the lymphatic system or in the bone marrow where lymphocyte progenitor cells originate. Procedures used to determine the stage of NHL in a particular patient include chest X-rays, computed tomography (CT), positron emission tomography (PET), magnetic resonance imaging (MRI), and the technique known as gallium scanning, in which a minuscule quantity of the element known as gallium is injected into the body and accumulates at sites where cancerous cells are proliferating, providing images of such disease activity.

In children with NHL, initial symptoms and findings vary and depend upon the specific type of the disease, its location, and its stage, or level of involvement. Findings often include painless swelling of lymph nodes in the neck, groin, or deep within the abdominal or chest region. Tumor growth in the chest cavity area may result in abnormal accumulations of fluid (pleural effusion) between layers of the lung lining (pleura), as well as difficulty in breathing and abnormal swelling of tissues of the face, neck, and arms, causing difficulty in swallowing. Other symptoms can include nausea, vomiting, lack of appetite (anorexia), abdominal pain and swelling (distension), severe constipation, or other digestive symptoms. Some cases of NHL affect the skin, resulting in dark, thickened, itchy patches. Tumors in the bone marrow may result in decreased numbers of red blood cells (anemia) or platelets (thrombocytopenia). In advanced cases of NHL, involvement of the brain may cause increased fluid pressure around the brain, severe headache, and p aralysis of certain nerves. As it progresses, NHL may also increasingly cripple the body's immune system and impair its infection-fighting ability, leading to potentially severe or life-threatening infections.

NHL is classified into different stages, based upon the number and location of tumors, the degree that the disease has spread, and other factors. Both the prognosis or outlook for patients with NHL and their treatment depend on the stage and type of their disease.

Treatment typically involves the use of drugs that kill cancerous cells known as cytotoxic drugs; radiation therapy, in which X-rays are directed at lymph nodes and other body sites affected by disease; immunotherapy, in which substances that bolster the immune system are given to help restore its infection-fighting and other capabilities; and biotherapy, in which a drug named rituximab, belonging to a highly cell- and tissue-specific group of newer drugs known as monoclonal antibodies, is used to hone in on cancerous cells and assist the immune system in destroying them. Treatment may also include the use of bone marrow transplantation to help restore the ability of the bone marrow to generate new lymphocytes and other blood cells to replace those affected by NHL or destroyed by the drugs or radiation used to treat it. In many cases, two or more of these treatment methods are combined with one another to combat NHL. In the recent technique known as radioimmunotherapy, monoclonal antibodies that specifically hone in on cancerous cells are linked to radioactive substances that carry these substances directly to such cells and kill them.

Both chemotherapy and radiation therapy for NHL can have side effects, including nausea and vomiting, diarrhea, weight loss, hair loss, and fatigue. Some children also experience psychological depression. Most of these effects are transitory, and gradually disappear after treatment is completed. More potentially serious side effects are declines in the numbers of infection-fighting cells. Severe neutrophil deficiency, or neutropenia, can open the way to infection, and may require treatment with granulocyte colony-stimulating factor (G-CSF), which promotes the proliferation of neutrophils and thus reduces the risk of infection. In some cases, antibiotics are used to prevent and treat infection occurring in patients with NHL. Serious but infrequent complications of treatment for NHL include sterility, from radiation therapy; osteoporosis, from treatment-related damage to bone cells; and damage to the heart by some drugs used in chemotherapy for NHL.

Government Agencies

5164 NIH/National Cancer Institute
9609 Medical Center Drive, 7th Floor, West Tower,
Bethesda, MD 20892
240-276-6340
800-422-6237
www.cancer.gov

The National Cancer Institute coordinates the National Cancer Program, which conducts and supports research, training, health information dissemination, and other programs with respect to the cause, diagnosis, prevention, and treatment of cancer, rehabilitation from cancer, and the continuing care of cancer patients and the families of cancer patients.

John E Niederhuber MD, Director

National Associations & Support Groups

5165 American Academy of Pediatrics
141 Northwest Point Boulevard
Elk Grove Village, IL 60007
847-434-4000
800-433-9016
Fax: 847-434-8000
www.aap.org

The American Academy of Pediatrics and its member pediatricians are committed to the attainment of optimal physical, mental and social health and well-being for all infants, children, adolescents, and young adults.

Sandra Hassink, MD, FAAP, President

5166 CancerCare
275 7th Avenue, Floor 22
New York, NY 10001
212-712-8400
800-813-4673
Fax: 212-712-8495
e-mail: info@cancercare.org
www.cancercare.org

CancerCare is a national nonprofit, 501(c)(3) organization that provides free, professional support services to anyone affected by cancer: people with cancer, caregivers, children, loved ones, and the bereaved. CancerCare programs - including counseling and support groups, education, financial assistance and practical help - are provided by professional oncology social workers and are completely free of charge.

Helen Miller, LCSW, Chief Executive Officer
John Rutigliano, Chief Operating Officer
Rosalie Canosa, Program Division Director

5167 Candlelighters Childhood Cancer Foundation
PO Box 498
Kensington, MD 20895
301-962-3520
855-858-2226
Fax: 310-962-3521
e-mail: staff@candlelighters.org
www.acco.org

The Candlelighters Childhood Cancer Foundation National Office was founded in 1970 by concerned parents of children with cancer. Today our membership of over 50,000 members of the national office and more than 100,000 members across the across the country, including Candlelighters affiliate groups, includes, parents of children who are being treated or have been treated for cancer.

Ruth Hoffman, Executive Director
Amber Masso, Program Director
Liz Dicus, Administrative Co-ordinator

5168 Leukemia & Lymphoma Society
1311 Mamaroneck Avenue, Suite 310
White Plains, NY 10605
914-949-5213
Fax: 914-949-6691
www.lls.org

Large voluntary health organization dedicated to funding blood cancer research, education and patient services.

Timothy S. Durst, Chairman
James H. Davis, Vice-Chair
Kenneth Schwartz, Secretary

5169 Lymphoma Research Foundation
115 Broadway, Suite 1301
New York, NY 10006
212-349-2910
800-235-6848
Fax: 212-349-2886
e-mail: LRF@lymphoma.org
www.lymphoma.org

Voluntary lymphoma-focused voluntary health organization devoted to funding lymphoma research and providing critical information on the disease.

Diane Blum, CEO
Kathleen Brown, Director of Research
Jen Davis, Director of Special Events

5170 National Childhood Cancer Foundation
4600 East West Highway, Suite 600
Bethesda, MD 20814
301-718-0042
800-458-6223
Fax: 301-718-0047
e-mail: info@curesearch.org
www.curesearch.org

CureSearch unites the world's largest childhood cancer research organization, the Children's Oncology Group, and the National Childhood Cancer Foundation through our mission to cure childhood cancer. Research is the key to the cure.

Stuart Siegal, Chairman
Timothy Harmon, Vice-Chair
Mary Payne, Treasurer

5171 Wellness Community
1990 S. Bundy Dr., Suite 100
Los Angeles, CA 90025

310-314-2555
Fax: 310-314-7586
e-mail: info@twc-wla.org
www.cancersupportcommunitybenjamincenter.org

Helps people with cancer and their loved ones enhance their health and well-being by providing a professional program of emotional support, education and hope.

Horald H. Benjamin, Co-Founder
Bonnie Schuman, Communications & Media Relations

Web Sites

5172 CancerCare
275 Seventh Avenue 22nd Floor
New York, NY 10001

212-712-8400
800-813-4673
Fax: 212-712-8495
www.cancercare.org

CancerCare is a national nonprofit, 501(c)(3) organization that provides free, professional support services to anyone affected by cancer: people with cancer, caregivers, children, loved ones, and the bereaved. CancerCare programs - including counseling and support groups, education, financial assistance and practical help - are provided by professional oncology social workers and are completely free of charge.

Patricia J. Goldsmith, CEO
John Rutigliano, COO
Sue Lee, Senior Director of Development

5173 Children's Cancer Web
www.cancerindex.org/ccw

An independent nonprofit site, established to provide a directory of childhood cancer resources.

5174 Leukemia and Lymphoma Society of America
1311 Mamaroneck Avenue, Suite 310
White Plains, NY 10605

914-949-5213
Fax: 914-949-6691
www.leukemia.org

Is the largest voluntary health organization dedicated to funding blood cancer research, education and patient services. The mission is to cure leukemia, lymphoma, Hodgkin's disease and myeloma, and to improve the quality of life of patients and their families.

James H. Davis, Chair
Elizabeth J. Clark, Vice Chair
Kenneth Schwartz, Secretary/Treasurer

5175 Lymphoma Innovations
www.lymphomainnovations.com

Targeted information for people with Non Hodgkins Lymphoma.

Book Publishers

5176 Let's Talk About Going to the Hospital
Rosen Publishing Group's PowerKids Press
29 E 21st Street
New York, NY 10010

212-777-3017
800-237-9932
Fax: 888-436-4643
e-mail: rosenpub@tribeca.ios.com
www.rosenpublishing.com

If a child has to check into the hospital, chances are he or she is already upset about being ill. Knowing how a hospital functions and what the procedures are, such as when family members can visit, will help in what is already a stressful situation. Grades K-5.

24 pages
ISBN: 0-823950-36-0

Roger Rosen, Predident

5177 Let's Talk About When Kids Have Cancer

Melanie Apel Gordon, author

Rosen Publishing Group's PowerKids Press
29 E 21st Street
New York, NY 10010

212-777-3017
800-237-9932
Fax: 888-436-4643
e-mail: customerservice@rosenpub.com
www.rosenpublishing.com

In a straightforward yet comforting way, this book explains what cancer is, what kinds of treatments surround the disease and how to cope if a child or the friend of a child has cancer.

24 pages Paperback
ISBN: 0-823951-95-2

Roger Rosen, President

5178 Pediatric Cancer Sourcebook
Omnigraphics
PO Box 8002
Aston, PA 19014

800-234-1340
Fax: 800-875-1340
e-mail: info@omnigraphics.com
www.omnigraphics.com

Basic consumer health information about leukemias, brain tumors, sarcomas, lymphomas and other cancers in infants, children and adolescents.

1999 587 pages
ISBN: 0-780802-45-4

Peter Ruffner, Publisher

5179 Surviving Childhood Cancer: A Guide for Families
New Harbinger Publications
5674 Shattuck Avenue
Oakland, CA 94609

510-652-0215
800-748-6273
Fax: 800-652-1613
e-mail: customerservice@newharbinger.com
www.newharbinger.com

Cancer in a child is an overwhelming experience for a family. This book explains common medical procedures and offers readers practical advice about how to cope with emotions and stress during this time.

232 pages Paperback
ISBN: 1-572241-02-0

Camps

5180 Arizona Camp Sunrise
PO Box 27872
Tempe, AZ 85285

602-952-7550
Fax: 602-404-1118
e-mail: melissa@azcampsunrise.org
www.azcampsunrise.org

The camp is dedicated to provide an exciting, medically safe camp program for children who have or have had cancer and their siblings.

Melissa Lee, Camp Director

5181 Camp Catch-A-Rainbow
American Cancer Society
One Children's Plaza
Dayton, OH 45404

937-641-3000
800-228-4055
www.childrensdayton.org

Open to any child who has, or has had, cancer.

5182 Camp Sunshine Dreams
PO Box 28232
Fresno, CA 93729

e-mail: contact@campsunshinedreams.com
www.campsunshinedreams.com

Summer camp for children with cancer.

5183 Okizu Foundation Camps
16 Digital Drive, Suite 130
Novato, CA 94949

415-382-9083
Fax: 415-382-8384
e-mail: info@okizu.org
www.okizu.org

This foundation runs family camp programs for children who have cancer and their families, and for children who have or had a parent with cancer.

John H. Bell, Chairman
Michael D. Amylon, M.D., Vice Chairman
Suzanne B. Randall, Secretary

Description

5184 NOONAN SYNDROME

Synonyms: Female Pseudo-Turner syndrome, Male Turner syndrome, NS

Involves the following Biologic System(s):
Cardiovascular Disorders,
Genetic/Chromosomal/Syndrome/Metabolic Disorders

Noonan syndrome is a genetic disorder that is usually apparent at birth (congenital) and interferes with the normal development of various body structures and organs. The symptoms and findings associated with the disorder may be extremely variable, differing in range and severity from case to case. However, children with Noonan syndrome often have short stature, webbing of the neck (pterygium colli), and characteristic abnormalities of the head and facial (craniofacial) area, such as downwardly slanting eyelid folds (palpebral fissures), drooping of the upper eyelids (ptosis), a small jaw (micrognathia), and prominent, low-set ears that are rotated toward the back of the head. In addition, in many males with Noonan syndrome, the testes fail to descend into the scrotum (cryptorchidism) before birth or during the first year of life. Therefore, in some cases, the male reproductive cells (sperm) may fail to develop appropriately within the testes, potentially causing infertility.

The genetic mutations responsible for Noonan syndrome chiefly affect four genes, which may be inherited from a parent, or result spontaneously from mutations occurring in the embryo. Most estimates indicate that this syndrome affects one in 1,000 to 2,500 newborns, but it may be difficult to determine the true frequency of Noonan syndrome because of the wide variation in its effects.

Many children with Noonan syndrome have distinctive skeletal malformations, such as abnormal depression of the lower portion of the breastbone (pectus excavatum) and protrusion of the upper portion of the breastbone (pectus carinatum); outward deviation of the elbows upon extension (cubitus valgus); sideways curvature of the spine (scoliosis); or front-to-back curvature of the spine (kyphosis). Affected children may also have structural abnormalities of the heart that are present at birth (congenital heart defects). These include obstruction of normal blood flow from the lower right pumping chamber (ventricle) of the heart to the lungs (pulmonary valvular stenosis). During infancy, there may also be an abnormal accumulation of lymph fluid in body tissues and a consequent swelling of these tissues (lymphedema) as the result of malformations in the body's lymphatic system. Additional symptoms and findings in Noonan syndrome may include deficient functioning of the blood cells known as platelets, which play an essential role in preventing or stopping bleeding; abnormally small numbers of platelets in circulating blood (thrombocytopenia); or defects in blood clotting (coagulation factor), potentially causing abnormal bleeding and susceptibility to bruising. In some cases, children with Noonan syndrome may have mental retardation or experience delays in acquiring certain skills that require the coordination of physical and mental activities (psychomotor retardation).

The diagnosis of Noonan syndrome is based on its physical effects, such as distortions in the chest, neck, ears, or eyelids, together with ultrasound or computed tomographic (CT) scans that reveal congenital heart, or other internal organ, defects, and tests that reveal disorders in blood clotting. The severity of Noonan syndrome in an infant or child is assessed through physical, neurological, and optical examinations; studies of heart function and body development; studies of the brain, spine, and rib cage done with X-ray images and the technique known as magnetic resonance imaging (MRI); ultrasound examination of the kidneys and urinalyses to assess kidney function; hearing tests; and blood and genetic testing.

The treatment of children with Noonan syndrome depends upon its severity and may include drugs, surgery to manage or correct congenital heart defects or to move undescended testes into the scrotum (orchiopexy) in males with cryptorchidism; hormone therapy (i.e., human growth hormone therapy); administration of platelets, blood-clotting factors, and other appropriate measures for treating thrombocytopenia, platelet dysfunction, and abnormalities in blood clotting, special education; and other treatment measures as required. Genetic counseling is recommended if there is a family history of Noonan syndrome.

National Associations & Support Groups

5185 American Academy of Pediatrics
141 Northwest Point Boulevard
Elk Grove Village, IL 60007

847-434-4000
800-433-9016
Fax: 847-434-8000
www.aap.org

The American Academy of Pediatrics and its member pediatricians are committed to the attainment of optimal physical, mental and social health and well-being for all infants, children, adolescents, and young adults.

Sandra Hassink, MD, FAAP, President

5186 Genetic Alliance
4301 Connecticut Avenue NW
Washington, DC 20008

202-966-5557
800-336-4363
Fax: 202-966-8553
e-mail: info@geneticalliance.org
www.geneticalliance.org

A coalition of voluntary genetic support groups, consumers and professionals addressing the needs of individuals and families affected by genetic disorders from a national perspective.

Joan Oppenheimer Weiss, Founder
Sharon Terry, President

5187 Human Growth Foundation
997 Glen Cove Avenue, Suite 5
Glen Head, NY 11545

516-671-4041
800-451-6434
Fax: 516-671-4055
e-mail: hgfl@hgfound.org
www.hgfound.org

Nonprofit organization devoted to research and advocacy regarding people with growth and growth hormone disorders.

Pisit Pitukcheewanont, President
Emily Germain-Lee, VP
Patricia D Costa, Executive Director

5188 MAGIC Foundation: Major Aspects of Growth in Children
6645 W North Avenue
Oak Park, IL 60302

708-383-0808
800-362-4423
Fax: 708-383-0899
e-mail: mary@magicfoundation.org
www.magicfoundation.org

The National family run organization is dedicated exclusively to helping children with mental health needs and their families achieve a better quality of life.

Teka Dempson, President
Sherri Luthe, VP
Sheila Pires, Treasurer

5363   Genetic Alliance
4301 Connecticut Avenue NW
Washington, DC 20008   202-966-5557
                                        800-336-4363
                                        Fax: 202-966-8553
                                        e-mail: info@geneticalliance.org
                                        www.geneticalliance.org

A coalition of voluntary genetic support groups, consumers and professionals addressing the needs of individuals and families affected by genetic disorders from a national perspective.

Joan Oppenheimer Weiss, Founder
Sharon Terry, President

5364   NADD: National Association for the Dually Diagnosed
132 Fair Street
Kingston, NY 12401   845-331-4336
                                        800-331-5362
                                        Fax: 845-331-4569
                                        e-mail: info@thenadd.org
                                        www.thenadd.org

Nonprofit organization designed to promote the interests of professional and parent development with resources for individuals who have the coexistence of mental illness and mental retardation. Provides conferences, educational services and training materials to professionals, parents, concerned citizens and service organizations.

Donna McNelis, President
Dan Baker, VP
Julia Pearce, Secretary

5365   National Alliance for the Mentally Ill
3803 N Fairfax Drive, Suite 100
Arlington, VA 22203   703-524-7600
                                        888-999-6264
                                        Fax: 703-524-9094
                                        TDD: 703-516-7227
                                        e-mail: info@nami.org
                                        www.nami.org

NAMI is a nonprofit, grassroots, self-help, support and advocacy organization of consumers, families and friends of people with severe mental illness, such as schizophrenia, bipolar disorder, major depressive disorder, obsessive compulsive disorder, anxiety disorders, autism and other severe and persistent mental illnesses that affect the brain.

Keris J,,n Myrick, President
Kevin B. Sullivan, First Vice President
Jim Payne, Second VP

5366   National Anxiety Foundation
3135 Custer Drive
Lexington, KY 40517   859-281-0003
                                        www.lexington-on-line.com/naf.html

A volunteer nonprofit organization. Its goal is to educate the public and health professionals about anxiety and anxiety disorders (such as panic disorder and obsessive-compulsive disorder) through printed materials and electronic media.

Stephen Cox MD, President & Medical Director
Linda Vernon Blair, Vice President
C. Todd Strecker, Treasurer

5367   National Mental Health Association
2000 N Beauregard Street, 6th Floor
Alexandria, VA 22311   703-684-7722
                                        800-969-6642
                                        Fax: 703-684-5968
                                        TTY: 800-433-5959
                                        www.mentalhealthamerica.net

Addresses all aspects of mental health and mental illness. NMHA with over 340 affiliates works to improve the mental health of all Americans.

Ann Boughtin, Chairman
Eric Ashton, Vice-Chair
David Theobald, President

5368   National Mental Health Consumers' Self-Help Clearinghouse
1211 Chestnut Street, Suite 1207
Philadelphia, PA 19107   267-507-3810
                                        800-553-4539
                                        Fax: 215-636-6312
                                        e-mail: info@mhselfhelp.org
                                        www.mhselfhelp.org

Offers information, support and appropriate referrals; and promotes public and professional education. Provides networking for those with special interests related to albinism. Promotes and supports research and funding that will improve diagnosis and management of albinism and hypopigmentation.

Joseph Rogers, Executive Director & Founder
Susan Rogers, Director
Britani Nestel, Program Specialist

5369   Obsessive Compulsive Anonymous
PO Box 215
New Hyde Park, NY 11040   516-739-0662
                                        e-mail: howardsedlitz@gmail.com
                                        www.obsessivecompulsiveanonymous.org

A fellowship of individuals dedicated to sharing their experience, strength and hope with one another to enable them to solve their common problems and help others recover from OCD. The Twelve Steps are adapted for OCA, to help obtain relief from obsessions and compulsions. Consisting of approximately 1,000 members and 50 chapters, OCA is not allied with any sect, denomination or organization.

5370   Obsessive Compulsive Foundation
PO Box 961029
Boston, MA 02196   617-973-5801
                                        Fax: 617-973-5803
                                        e-mail: info@ocfoundation.org
                                        www.ocfoundation.org

Provides vital support to educate the public and professional communities about OCD and related disorders, provides assistance to individuals with OCD and related disorders, their families and friends. The foundation also funds research into the causes and effective treatments of OCD and related disorders.

Denise Egan Stack, President
Susan B. Dailey, VP
Michael J. Stack, Treasurer

5371   Suncoast Residential Training Center/Developmental Services Program
Goodwill Industries-Suncoast
10596 Gandy Boulevard
Saint Petersburg, FL 33702   727-523-1512
                                        888-279-1988
                                        Fax: 727-563-9300
                                        TTY: 727-579-1068
                                        www.goodwill-suncoast.org

A large group home which serves individuals diagnosed as mentally retarded with a secondary diagnosis of psychiatric difficulties as evidenced by problem behavior. Providing residential, behavioral and instructional support and services that will promote the development of adaptive, socially appropriate behavior, each individual is assessed to determine socialization, basic academics and recreation. The primary intervention strategy is applied behavior analysis.

Oscar J. Horton, Chairman
Martin W. Gladysz, Sr. Vice Chair
Steven M. Erickson, Vice Chair

State Agencies & Support Groups

5372   Center for Family Support
333 7th Avenue #901
New York, NY 10001   212-629-7939
                                        Fax: 212-239-2211
                                        www.cfsny.org

The Center for Family (CFS) is a not-for-profit human service agency providing support and assistance to individuals with developmental disabilities and traumatic brain injuries throughout New York City, Long Island, the lower Hudson Valley region and New Jersey.

Steven Vernikoff, Executive Director
Barbara Greenwald, Associate Executive Director
Mike Mazzocco, Associate Executive Director

5373 Obsessive Compulsive Foundation of Metropo litan Chicago
2300 Lincoln Park West
Chicago, IL 60614

773-661-9530
Fax: 773-661-9535
e-mail: info@ocfchicago.org
www.ocdchicago.org

Serves adults and children with OCD, their families, and the mental health professionals who treat them. The only Chicago area organization dedicated to OCD.

Ellen Sawyer, Executive Director

Research Centers

5374 National Alliance for Research on Schizophrenia and Depression
60 Cutter Mill Road, Suite 404
Great Neck, NY 11021

516-829-0091
800-829-8289
Fax: 516-487-6930
e-mail: info@bbrfoundation.org
www.bbrfoundation.org

NARSAD raises and distributes funds for scientific research into the causes, cures, treatments, and prevention of severe mental illnesses, primarily schizophrenia.

Steve Lieber, Chairman
Suzzane Golden, VP
John B. Hollister, Secretary

Audio Video

5375 Hope and Solutions for OCD
ADD WareHouse
300 NW 70th Avenue, Suite 102
Plantation, FL 33317

954-792-8100
800-233-9273
Fax: 954-792-8545
e-mail: sales@addwarehouse.com
www.addwarehouse.com

A video series about obsessive compulsive disorder with some straight forward solutions and advice for individuals with OCD, their families, doctors, and school personnel. Viewers will learn what OCD is and how to treat it. Discusses how OCD can affect students in school and the impact on the family life.

85 Minutes
ISBN: 1-886941-37-8

5376 It's Not Me...It's My OCD: A Look at Behav ioral Therapy
Aquarius Health Care Videos
3435 Main Street, Bldg. 28
Buffalo, NY 14214

716-829-5744
888-440-2963
Fax: 508-650-1665
emro.lib.buffalo.edu

1997 28 Minutes
ISBN: 1-581403-38-0

Lori Widzinski, Editor
Oksana Dykyj, Associate Editor
Angela Davis, Social Network Coordinator

5377 Touching Tree
Awareness Films, author

Pyramid Media
3200 Airport Ave, Ste 19
Santa Monica, CA 90405

310-398-6149
800-421-2304
Fax: 310-398-7869
e-mail: info@pyramidmedia.com
www.pyramidmedia.com

Chronicles of a young boy trapped in the pain of OCD; how he faces his fears and begins the slow recovery with professional help. A film ideal for teaching the need for sensitivity when dealing with special children and their differences.

38 Minutes

Web Sites

5378 Anxiety Disorders Association of America

Offers resources and information for persons with anxiety and stress-related disorders.

5379 CyberPsych
www.cyberpsych.org

CyberPsych presents information about psychoanalysis, psychotherapy, and special topics such as anxiety disorder, the problematic use of alcohol, homophobia, and the traumatic effects of racism. CyberPsych is a nonprofit network which offers free web hosting and technical support for internet communication, to nonprofit groups and individuals.

5380 Guidelines for Families Coping with OCD
4901 NW 17th Way, Suite 101
Fort Lauderdale, FL 33309

954-962-6662
Fax: 954-962-6164
www.ocdhope.com/gdlines.htm

Offers 19 guidelines for families coping with OCD.

Dr. Bruce Hyman, Founder & Director
Dr. Stacy Sanders Shaup, Associate
Dr. Jennifer Hochman, Associate

5381 NADD: National Association for the Dually Diagnosed
132 Fair Street
Kingston, NY 12401

845-331-4336
800-331-5362
Fax: 845-331-4569
www.thenadd.org

Nonprofit organization designed to promote the interests of professional and care providers for individuals who have the coexistence of mental illness and mental retardation. NADD provides conferences, educational services and training materials to professionals, parents, concerned citizens and service organizations.

Donna McNelis, PhD, President
Dan Baker, PhD., Vice President
Julia Pearce, Secretary

5382 National Anxiety Foundation
www.lexington-on-line.com/naf.html

Nonprofit organization that provides education to the public and professionals about anxiety through printed and electronic media.

Stephen Cox, MD, President
Linda Vernon Blair, Vice-President
C. Todd Strecker, Secretary-Treasurer

5383 National Mental Health Consumers' Self-Help Clearinghouse
www.mhselfhelp.org

A consumer run national technical assistance center serving the mental health consumer movement. We help connect individuals to self-help and advocacy resources, and we offer expertise to self-help groups, and other peer-run services for mental health consumers.

Joseph Rogers, Executive Director
Susan Rogers, Director
Christa Burkett, Technical Assistance Coordinator

5384 Obsessive Compulsive Disorder (OCD)
6001 Executive Boulevard
Rockville, MD 20852   e-mail: NIMHinfo@mail.nih.gov
www.nimh.nih.gov/healthinformation/ocdmenu.cfm

Discusses the diagnosis of obsessive-compulsive disorder, its prevalence among both children and adults. Descibes types of treatment including pharmacotherapy. Gives sources of information for both the individual who has OCD and the family.

5385 Obsessive Compulsive Foundation
P.O. Box 961029
Boston, MA 2196   617-973-5801
                                Fax: 617-973-5803
                              e-mail: info@iocdf.org
                                       iocdf.org

An international nonprofit organization composed of people with obsessive compulsive disorder and related disorders, their families, friends, professionals, and other concerned individuals.

Denise Egan Stack, LMHC, President
Susan B. Dailey, Vice President
Michael J Stack, CFA, Treasurer

5386 Planetpsych
www.planetpsych.com

Planetpsych is an online resource for mental health information.

5387 Psych Central
55 Pleasant St., Suite 207
Newburyport, MA 1950   www.psychcentral.com

Offers free informational and educational articles and resources on psychology, support and mental health online.

John M. Grohol, CEO
Rick Nauert, Senior News Editor
Bailey Apple, Associate Editor

Book Publishers

5388 Boy Who Couldn't Stop Washing: The Experience and Treatment of OCD

Judith L Rapoport, author

Penguin Group
375 Hudson Street
New York, NY 10014   212-366-2372
                                Fax: 212-366-2933
                       e-mail: online@us.penguingroup.com
                                us.penguingroup.com

A comprehensive treatment of obsessive-compulsive disorder that summarizes evidence that the disorder is neurobiological. It also describes the effect of medication combined with behavioral therapy.

1991 304 pages Paperback
ISBN: 0-451172-02-0

John Makinson, CHAIRMAN
Coram Williams, CFO
David Shanks, CEO

5389 Brain Lock: Free Yourself from Obsessive Compulsive Behavior

Jeffrey M Schwartz, author

Harper Collins
10 E 53rd Street
New York, NY 10022   212-207-7000
                                     800-242-7737
                                Fax: 212-207-7901
                    e-mail: feedback2@harpercollins.com
                                www.harpercollins.com

A simple four-step method for overcoming OCD that is so effective, it's now used in academic treatment centers throughout the world. Proven by brain-imaging tests to actually alter the brain's chemistry, this method doesn't rely on psychopharmaceuticals but cognitive self-therapy and behavior modification to develop new patterns of response. Offers real-life stories of actual patients.

1997 256 pages Paperback
ISBN: 0-060987-11-1

5390 Brief Strategic Solution-Oriented Therapy of Phobic and Obsessive Disorders

Giorgio Nardone, author

Jason Aronson Publishers
4501 Forbes Boulevard, Suite 200
Lanham, MD 20706   301-459-3366
                                     800-462-6420
                                Fax: 301-429-5748
                                     www.aronson.com

1996 188 pages Cloth
ISBN: 1-568218-04-4

5391 Childhood Obsessive Compulsive Disorder

Greta Francis, author

Sage Publications
2455 Teller Road
Thousand Oaks, CA 91320   800-818-7243
                                     800-818-7243
                                Fax: 800-583-2665
                     e-mail: supplements@sagepub.com.
                                     www.sagepub.com

1996 120 pages
ISBN: 0-803959-22-2

Sara Miller McCune, Chairman
Blaise R. Simqu, President & CEO
Chris Hickok, Senior Vice President & Chief Finan

5392 Freeing Your Child from Obsessive-Compulsi ve Disorder

Tamar E Chansky PhD, author

Crown Publishing Group/Random House
280 Park Avenue
New York, NY 10017   212-940-7381
                                     800-733-3000
                                www.crownpublishing.com

ISBN: 0-812931-17-4

5393 It's Nobody's Fault-New Hope and Help for Difficult Children and Their Parents
ADD WareHouse
300 NW 70th Avenue, Suite 102
Plantation, FL 33317   954-792-8100
                                     800-233-9273
                                Fax: 954-792-8545
                                www.addwarehouse.com

This book explains that neither the parents nor children are causes of mental disorders and related problems.

1997 320 pages Paperback
ISBN: 0-812929-21-7

5394 Obsessive Compulsive Disorder: Helping Children and Adolescents

Mitzi Waltz, author

O'Reilly Media
1005 Gravenstein Highway N
Sebastopol, CA 95472   707-827-7019
                                     800-889-8969
                                Fax: 707-829-0104
                                     www.oreilly.com

This book helps parents secure an accurate and complete diagnosis, and live with OCD children using effective parenting techniques. Offers support systems, medical interventions and explores therapeutic and other interventions, such as cognitive therapy; helps to secure care with an existing health plan even with no coverage of mental disorders, navigate the special education system and find resources.

2000 404 pages
ISBN: 1-565927-58-3

Tim O'Reilly, Founder & CEO

5395 Obsessive-Compulsive Disorder in Children and Adolescents
American Psychiatric Publishing
1000 Wilson Boulevard, Suite 1825
Arlington, VA 22209

703-907-7322
800-368-5777
Fax: 703-907-1091
e-mail: appi@psych.org
www.appi.org

Examines the early development of obsessive-compulsive disorder and describes effective treatments.

1989 368 pages Hardcover
ISBN: 0-880482-82-0

Robert E. Hales, M.D, Editor-in-Chief
Rebecca D. Rinehart, Publisher
John McDuffie, Editorial Director

5396 School Personnel: A Critical Link in the Identification and Management of OCD

Gail B Adams, author

Obsessive Compulsive Foundation
18 Tremont Street, Suite 903
Boston, MA 02108

617-973-5801
Fax: 617-973-5803
e-mail: info@ocfoundation.org
www.ocfoundation.org

Recognizing OCD in the school setting, current treatments, the role of school personnel in identification, assessment, and educational interventions are thoroughly covered in this brief, but informative booklet especially targeted to educators and guidance counselors.

2003 32 pages Booklet

Denise Egan Stack, President
Susan B. Dailey, Vice President
Diane Davey, Secretary

5397 Talking Back to OCD: The Program That Help Kids & Teens Say No Way

John March W/ Christine Benton, author

Guilford Publications
72 Spring Street
New York, NY 10012

212-431-9800
800-365-7006
Fax: 212-966-6708
e-mail: info@guilford.com
www.guilford.com

Dr March's 8-step program to empower young people overcome OCD. Each chapter begins with a section that helps young readers zero in on specific problems and develop skills they can use to tune out the obsessions and resist compulsions. Filled with tips for parents to seperate the disorder from the child and to encourage their child in recovery. Hard- or paperback.

2007 276 pages Paperback
ISBN: 1-593853-55-6

Bob Matloff, President
Seymour Weingarten, Editor-in-Chief

5398 Teaching the Tiger
Hope Press
PO Box 188
Duarte, CA 91009

800-321-4039
Fax: 626-358-3520
e-mail: dcomings@earthlink.net
www.hopepress.com

A handbook for individuals involved in the education of students with Attention Deficit Disorder, Tourette Syndrome, or Obsessive Compulsive Disorder.

ISBN: 1-878267-34-5

David E Comings MD, Presenter

5399 Key Update
National Mental Health Consumer's Self-Help Clrhs.
1211 Chestnut Street, Suite 1207
Philadelphia, PA 19107

215-751-1810
800-553-4539
Fax: 215-636-6312
e-mail: info@mhselfhelp.org
www.mhselfhelp.org

A monthly e-newsletter that provides timely news and notes on important mental health issues, details on upcoming events, and recent publications on policy issues. Topics addressed in the newsletter include self-advocacy, self-care, community integration, human rights and mental health treatments and services.

Monthly

Joseph Rogers, Executive Director
Susan Rogers, Director
Christa Burkett, Technical Assistance Coordinator

5400 OCD Newsletter
Obsessive Compulsive Foundation
P.O. Box 961029
Boston, MA 2196

617-973-5801
Fax: 617-973-5803
e-mail: info@iocdf.org
iocdf.org

For sufferers of obsessive-compulsive disorder and their families and friends.

16-20 pages 6 times/yr

Denise Egan Stack, LMHC, President
Susan B. Dailey, Vice President
Michael J Stack, CFA, Treasurer

5401 Children and Adolescents
Madison Institute of Medicine
7617 Mineral Point Road, Suite 300
Madison, WI 53717

608-827-2470
Fax: 608-827-2479
e-mail: mim@miminc.org
www.miminc.org

Literature packet: diagnosis, treatment and other information on OCD in young children and adolescents.

5402 Obsessive Compulsive Disorder General Pack et
Madison Institute of Medicine
7617 Mineral Point Road, Suite 300
Madison, WI 53717

608-827-2470
Fax: 608-827-2479
e-mail: mim@miminc.org
www.miminc.org

Literature packet: overview of OCD, including information on prevalence, diagnosis and treatment.

5403 Obsessive-Compulsive Disorder, A Real Illn ess
National Institute of Mental Health
Public Info, 6001 Executive Blvd, Rm 8184
Rockville, MD 20852

301-443-4513
866-615-6464
Fax: 301-443-4279
TTY: 301-443-8431
e-mail: NIMHinfo@mail.nih.gov
www.nimh.nih.gov

Easy-to read booklet on OCD, explaining what it is, when it starts, how long it lasts and how to get help. The booklet also includes a self-test.

Camps

5404 Tourette Syndrome Camp Organization
6933 N Kedzie, #816
Chicago, IL 60640
                                      773-465-7536
                        e-mail: info@tourettecamp.com
                        www.tourettecamp.com

Dedicated to promoting camping opportunities for children with
Tourette Syndrome and its assocaited disorders, Obsessive Compulsive Disorder (OCD) and Attention Deficit/Hyperactivity
Disorder (ADD/ADHD).

Monica Newman, Camp Director
Marleen Martinez, Assistant Director
Sarah Matchen, Director

Description

5405 OMPHALOCELE

Involves the following Biologic System(s):

Gastrointestinal Disorders, Neonatal and Infant Disorders

An omphalocele is a birth defect characterized by bulging or protrusion of a portion of the intestines through an abnormal opening in the abdominal wall near the navel, the region where the umbilical cord meets the abdomen during fetal growth and development. The bulging area of the intestines is covered by a thin, membrane-like sac consisting of part of the amnion and peritoneum. The amnion is the inner layer of membrane that forms the amniotic sac, the fluid-filled sac within which a fetus grows and develops. The peritoneum is the thin membrane that lines the abdominal cavity and covers the internal abdominal organs.

Depending upon the size of the abdominal wall defect in an affected newborn, varying amounts of intestine or, in severe cases, other abdominal organs, may protrude through the navel. Associated complications may include rupture of the protruding, membranous sac, damage to body tissues due to drying, or onset of infection. Because these complications may be life-threatening, an omphalocele is usually surgically repaired immediately after birth.

An omphalocele is thought to affect approximately one in 4,000 newborns. Prenatal ultrasounds often identify infants with an omphalocele before birth. Otherwise, physical examination of the infant is sufficient to diagnose this condition. In many infants, omphaloceles occur in association with other birth defects, such as abnormalities of the urinary and reproductive systems, central nervous system, or cardiovascular system. This condition may also occur in association with certain rare malformation syndromes that are apparent at birth. These include Beckwith-Wiedemann syndrome, also known as exomphalos-macroglossia-gigantism, and Shprintzen omphalocele syndrome, also called pharynx and larynx hypoplasia with omphalocele.

In other cases, omphaloceles may occur as isolated findings for unknown reasons. Omphaloceles are repaired with surgery, although not always immediately; complete recovery is expected. There have been reports of multiple cases of isolated omphaloceles within certain families (kindreds). In these families, the condition may be caused by abnormal changes (mutations) in a gene or genes that may be inherited as an autosomal recessive or X-linked trait. It is also possible that the interaction of several different genes in association with certain environmental factors (multifactorial inheritance) may play a role in the development of some omphaloceles.

Government Agencies

5406 Division of Birth Defects & Developmental Disabilities
1600 Clifton Road
Atlanta, GA 30333
404-639-3311
800-232-4636
Fax: 404-639-3534
TTY: 888-232-6348
www.cdc.gov

Information and advocacy resources for families and professionals dealing with children with birth defects and developmental disabilities.

National Associations & Support Groups

5407 American Academy of Pediatrics
141 Northwest Point Boulevard
Elk Grove Village, IL 60007
847-434-4000
800-433-9016
Fax: 847-434-8000
www.aap.org

The American Academy of Pediatrics and its member pediatricians are committed to the attainment of optimal physical, mental and social health and well-being for all infants, children, adolescents, and young adults.

Sandra Hassink, MD, FAAP, President

5408 American College of Gastroenterology
6400 Goldsboro Rd., Ste 200
Bethesda, MD 20817
301-263-9000
www.acg.gi.org

Founded to advance the scientific study and medical practice of diseases of the gastrointestinal (GI) tract.

Jack A DiPalma, President
Amy E Foxx-Orenstein, VP

5409 March of Dimes Birth Defects Foundation
1275 Mamaroneck Avenue
White Plains, NY 10605
914-997-4488
888-663-4637
Fax: 914-428-8203
e-mail: answers@marchofdimes.com
www.marchofdimes.com

Partnership of volunteers and professionals dedicates to improving the health of babies by preventing birth defects and infant mortality. Over 100 chapters are located across the country and can be located through the National Office.

Jennifer L Howse, President

5410 North American Society for Pediatric Gastroenterology/Hepatology/Nutrition
PO Box 6
Flourtown, PA 19031
215-233-0808
Fax: 215-233-3918
e-mail: naspghan@naspghan.org
www.naspghan.org

Strives to improve the care of infants, children and adolescents with digestive disorders by promoting advances in clinical care of children with chronic abdominal pain, diarrhea, constipation, vomiting, bleeding from the GI tract, inflammatory bowel disease, liver diseases, diseases of the pancreas, poor weight gain and nutritional problems.

Philip Sherman, President
Margaret K Stallings, Executive Director

Libraries & Resource Centers

5411 National Digestive Diseases Information Clearinghouse
2 Information Way
Bethesda, MD 20892
301-654-3810
800-891-5389
Fax: 703-738-4929
e-mail: nddic@info.niddk.nih.gov
www2.niddk.nih.gov

The National Institute of Diabetes and Digestive and Kidney Diseases conducts and supports research on many of the most serious diseases affecting public health. The Institute supports much of the clinical research on the diseases of internal medicine and related subspecialty fields as well as many basic science disciplines.

Griffin P. Rodgers, M.D, Chairman, Executive Board
Brent B. Stanfield, Executive Secretary
Camille M. Hoover, M.S.W, Executive Officer

Web Sites

5412 Mothers of Omphaloceles
www.omphalocele.com

Support and Webring.

5413 National Digestive Diseases Information Clearinghouse
www.digestive.niddk.nih.gov

The National Institute of Diabetes and Digestive and Kidney Diseases conducts and supports research on many of the most serious diseases affecting public health. The Institute supports much of the clinical research on the diseases of internal medicine and related subspecialty fields as well as many basic science disciplines.

5414 Online Mendelian Inheritance in Man
National Library of Medicine Building 38A
Bethesda, MD 20894   888-346-3656
                            e-mail: info@ncbi.nlm.nih.gov
                                       www.ncbi.nlm.nih.gov

This database is a catalog of human genes and genetic disorders.

5415 Pediatric Surgery Update
P.O. Box 10426
San Juan, PR 922   home.coqui.net/titolugo/PSU11.htm#1152

An online handbook about many differnt diseases and disablilies.

Journals

5416 Journal of Pediatric Gastroenterology and Nutrition
NASPGHAN, author

Lippincott Williams & Wilkins
2700 Lake Cook Road
Riverwoods, IL 60015   847-580-5000
                                         Fax: 215-521-8902
                                              www.lww.com

Publication of the North American Society for Pediatric Gastroenterolgy, Hepatology and Nutrition, which strives to improve the care of infants, children and adolescents with digestive disorders by promoting advances in clinical care of children with chronic abdominal pain, diarrhea, constipation, vomiting, bleeding from the GI tract, inflammatory bowel disease, liver diseases, diseases of the pancreas, poor weight gain and nutritional problems.

Newsletters

5417 NASPGHAN News
PO Box 6
Flourtown, PA 19031   215-233-0808
                                         Fax: 215-233-3939
                          e-mail: naspghan@naspghan.org
                                        www.naspghan.org

Publication of the North American Society for Pediatric Gastroenterolgy, Hepatology and Nutrition, which strives to improve the care of infants, children and adolescents with digestive disorders by promoting advances in clinical care of children with chronic abdominal pain, diarrhea, constipation, vomiting, bleeding from the GI tract, inflammatory bowel disease, liver diseases, diseases of the pancreas, poor weight gain and nutritional problems.

Carlo Di Lorenzo, MD, President
James Heubi, MD, President-Elect
Michael Narkewicz, MD, Secretary-Treasurer

Description

5418 OPPOSITIONAL DEFIANT DISORDER

Synonym: ODD

Involves the following Biologic System(s):

Developmental/Behavioral/Psychiatric Disorders

Oppositional Defiant Disorder (ODD) is a disruptive behavioral disorder along with conduct disorder. It is marked by an ongoing pattern of negativistic, argumentative, and hostile behaviors when interacting with some or all authority figures. The symptoms are usually seen in multiple settings, but may be more noticeable at home or at school. Five to fifteen percent of all school-age children have ODD. This disorder is usually apparent before age eight. Although it is more common in boys in the pre-pubertal years, the sex ratio evens out post puberty. The causes of ODD are unknown, but many parents report that their child with ODD was more rigid and demanding than the child's siblings from an early age. Biological and environmental factors may have a role. ODD can also be a precursor to conduct disorder later in life. Children with ODD also have a higher risk of other conditions, including ADHD (attention deficit hyperactivity disorder), anxiety and depression.

ODD is diagnosed by the presence of at least six months of hostile, negative and defiant behavior that is more frequent and intense than expected for a child's age. The behavior must cause significant functional impairment, either socially, academically or occupationally. ODD can not be diagnosed in patients who are actively psychotic or who meet criteria for conduct disorder or antisocial personality disorder.

Treatment for ODD centers upon evaluating the child's physical and psychosocial environment, ruling out or treating co-morbid conditions and assisting parents in anticipating and modifying behavior. Problems in the family or environment that may be driving the behaviors also need to be addressed. Many children with ODD will respond to the positive parenting techniques. A child with ODD can be very difficult for parents who need support and understanding. Older school age children and adolescents with ODD are more likely to benefit from an intensive intervention program.

National Associations & Support Groups

5419 American Academy of Child and Adolescent Psychiatry
3615 Wisconsin Avenue NW
Washington, DC 20016
202-966-7300
Fax: 202-966-2891
e-mail: clinical@aacap.org
www.aacap.org

The AACAP (American Academy of Child and Adolescent Psychiatry) is the leading national professional medical association dedicated to treating and improving the quality of life for children, adolescents, and families affected by these disorders. The AACAP is a 501 (c)(3) nonprofit organization established in 1953.

Elizabeth Hughes, Asst. Director of Education & Recer
Quentin Bernhard III, CME Coordinator
Alan Ezagui, Deputy Director of Development

5420 American Academy of Pediatrics
141 Northwest Point Boulevard
Elk Grove Village, IL 60007
847-434-4000
800-433-9016
Fax: 847-434-8000
www.aap.org

The American Academy of Pediatrics and its member pediatricians are committed to the attainment of optimal physical, mental and social health and well-being for all infants, children, adolescents, and young adults.

Sandra Hassink, MD, FAAP, President

Audio Video

5421 Explosive Child

Ross W Greene PhD, author

HarperCollins Publishers
1350 Avenue of the Americas
New York, NY 10019
212-261-6500
800-242-7737
www.harpercollins.com

A new approach for understanding and parenting easily frustrated, cronically inflexible children. Dr Greene offers help for you and your child. Now updated with new practical information, The Explosive Child lays out a sensitive, practical approach to helping your child at home and school.

1999 Audio Cassette
ISBN: 0-694521-90-6

Brian Murray, President and CEO
Chantal Restivo-Alessi, Chief Digital Officer
Janet Gervasio, SVP & CFO

Web Sites

5422 American Academy of Child and Adolescent Psychiatry
3615 Wisconsin Avenue, N.W.
Washington, DC 20016
202-966-7300
Fax: 202-966-2891
www.aacap.org

Information on treating and improving the quality of life for children, adolescents, and families affected by such disorders as Oppositional Defiant.

Book Publishers

5423 Disruptive Behavior Disorders in Children and Adolescents

Robert L Hendren, DO, author

American Psychiatric Publishing
1000 Wilson Boulevard, Suite 1825
Arlington, VA 22209
703-907-7322
800-368-5777
Fax: 703-907-1091
e-mail: appi@psych.org
www.appi.org

Comprehensively reviews current research and clinical observations on this timely topic. The authors look at three subtypes of attention-deficit/hyperactivity disorder (ADHD), conduct disorder, and oppositional defiant disorder, all of which are common among youths and often share similar symptoms of impulse control problems.

1999 216 pages Paperback
ISBN: 0-880489-60-7

Robert E. Hales, M.D, Editor-in-Chief
Rebecca D. Rinehart, Publisher
John McDuffie, Editorial Director

Quarterly

Journals

5424 Explosive Child

Ross W Greene PhD, author

HarperCollins Publishers
10 East 53rd Street
New York, NY 10022

212-207-7000
800-242-7737
Fax: 212-207-7901
e-mail: feedback2@harpercollins.com
www.harpercollins.com

A new approach for understanding and parenting easily frustrated, cronically inflexible children. Dr Greene offers help for you and your child. Now updated with new practical information, The Explosive Child lays out a sensitive, practical approach to helping your child at home and school.

2005 334 pages Paperbcak
ISBN: 0-060931-02-7

5425 Helping the Noncompliant Child

Robert McMahon, Rex Forehand, author

Guilford Press
72 Spring Street
New York, NY 10012

212-431-9800
800-365-7006
Fax: 212-966-6708
e-mail: info@guilford.com
www.guilford.com

An empirically proven program for teaching parents to manage non-compliance in 3- to 8- year olds. Practitioners are provided step-by-step guidelines for child and family assessment, detailed descriptions of parent training procedures, effective adjunctive treatment strategies, and complete protocols for conducting the program. Hard- or soft-cover.

2005 264 pages Paperback
ISBN: 1-593852-41-2

Bob Matloff, President
Seymour Weingarten, Editor-in-Chief

5426 New Strong-Willed Child

James C Dobson, author

Tyndale House Publishers
351 Executive Drive
Carol Stream, IL 60188

800-323-9400
Fax: 800-684-0247
www.tyndale.com

A complete update of The Strong-Willed Child for a new generation of parents and teachers. It offers practical advice on raising difficult-to-handle children and incorporates the latest research.

2004 270 pages Hardcover
ISBN: 0-842336-22-2

Magazines

5427 EHealth

UAB Health System
1802 6th Avenue South
Birmingham, AL 35233

205-934-4011
800-822-8816
Fax: 205-934-9991
www.uabmedicine.org

A health and fitness publication packed with all the latest news and health tips from the UAB Health System.

Journals

5428 Official Journal of the American Academy of Child and Adolescent Psychiatry

Lippincott Williams & Wilkins
351 West Camden Street
Baltimore, MD 21201

410-528-4200
800-638-3030
Fax: 410-528-8557
www.jaacap.com

The journal is recognized as THE major journal focusing exclusively on today's psychiatric research and treatment of the child and adolescent.

12x a year

Mina K Dulcan MD, Editor
Sara Tiner, Editorial Coordinator

Newsletters

5429 AACAP News

American Academy of Child & Adolescent Psychiatry
3615 Wisconsin Avenue NW
Washington, DC 20016

202-966-7300
Fax: 202-966-2891
www.aacap.org

Official membership publication; provides the latest information on issues that directly affect child and adolescent psychiatrists.

6400 48 pages Bi-monthly

Paramjit T. Joshi, M.D., President
Gregory K. Fritz, M.D., President-Elect
Aradhana Sood, M.D., Secretary

5430 DevelopMentor

American Academy of Child & Adolescent Psychiatry
3615 Wisconsin Avenue NW
Washington, DC 20016

202-966-7300
Fax: 202-966-2891
www.aacap.org

Introduces medical students and residens to the clinical, academic, and research opportunities in child and adolescent psychiatry. Ideal for training directors.

Semi-annual

Paramjit T. Joshi, M.D., President
Gregory K. Fritz, M.D., President-Elect
Aradhana Sood, M.D., Secretary

Description

5431 OSTEOGENESIS IMPERFECTA

Synonyms: Brittle bone disease, OI

Covers these related disorders: Osteogenesis imperfecta Type I (OI Type I), Osteogenesis imperfecta Type II (OI Type II), Osteogenesis imperfecta Type III (OI Type III), Osteogenesis imperfecta Type IV (OI Type IV)

Involves the following Biologic System(s):
Genetic/Chromosomal/Syndrome/Metabolic Disorders, Orthopedic and Muscle Disorders

Osteogenesis imperfecta (OI) is an inherited genetic disorder characterized by abnormally brittle, fragile bones that are prone to fracture. The genetic abnormality responsible for OI produces defects in collagen, a protein that forms connective tissue such as bone, and is essential to normal bone growth and development.

Eight types of OI have been recognized, with each type having specific characteristics. The most common forms of OI are Types I through VI. Types VII and VIII of OI are recently recognized forms of the disease, of which only a few cases have so far been identified. Symptoms of OI, and how the disease is acquired, vary according to Type.

Of the eight types of OI, Type I is the least severe and most frequent. It occurs in approximately one in every 30,000 live births, and is inherited in an autosomal dominant manner, meaning that the defective gene that causes it can be inherited from only one parent, who will also have OI because of its dominant nature. Although the bones of infants and children with Type I are fragile and easily broken, and their teeth may be predisposed to cavities and breakage, there is little deformity of the bones. Other characteristics associated with Type I include flat feet, short stature, and a blue, purple, or gray coloration of the whites of the eyes. As children with this type of OI reach adolescence, they may experience bone fractures much less often than when they were younger.

OI Type II is the most severe form of the disease. Infants with Type II typically have a low birth weight, skeletal abnormalities of the limbs, ribs, and face, and frequent breakage of bones in prenatal fetuses. As many as half of births with OI of Type II are stillbirths, and many infants born with Type II die soon after birth from defects in the rib cage, resulting respiratory problems. Approximately one in 60,000 infants is affected with OI Type II. Both Types I and II are inherited as an autosomal dominant trait, or an recessive trait. The disease can also be caused by a genetic mutation, occurring only in the individual in whom the disease develops.

OI Type III is inherited as an autosomal recessive trait or as the result of a new mutation in affected offspring. It is a progressive form of the condition, characterized by multiple fractures and severely fragile bones in newborns, followed by deformity of the skeleton and skull. Other features of children with this type of OI include a triangular-shaped face, curvature of the spine, a barrel-shaped rib cage, diminished muscle development in the arms and legs, and short stature. Although many children with this type of OI reach adolescence, most do not reach adulthood.

OI Type IV, inherited as an autosomal dominant trait, is characterized by a reduced density of bones (osteoporosis) that causes them to be easily broken, and by shortness of stature. Bone fractures may be present at birth or at any time up to adulthood. As in Type I, curvature of thespine is likely to occur in Type IV, as is a barrel-shaped rib cage and triangular shape of the face, as well as brittleness of the teeth.

Type V is inherited in an autosomal dominant manner, and resembles Type IV, with the added symptom of calluses that develop at sites of bone fractures or surgical procedures. In many cases, the characteristics and symptoms of Type VI resemble those of Type IV, but it is not yet known whether this type of OI is inherited in a dominant or recessive manner. Type VII has so far been identified in only a small number of cases, some similar to Type IV, while others resembling the severe Type II, with surviving infants having short arm and leg bones, a short stature, a round face, and a small head. Type VIII OI resembles Type II or Type III, but surviving infants have seriously deficient growth and bones with a deficient mineral content.

OI is often detected as the result of a bone fracture, which then prompts further studies of an infant or child. Because of its effects on bone structure, OI can often be detected before birth by ultrasound examination, in which high-frequency sound waves are reflected by the bones and organs of a fetus in such a way as to permit a detailed examination of their structure. In some cases, laboratory tests can reveal the specific genetic defects responsible for OI.

OI cannot be completely cured or corrected. Treatment for most types and cases of the disease is medical and orthopedic, involving the use of drugs that reduce bone loss and others that promote growth of the body; casts and splints to repair fractures; and either braces or spinal fusion, in which bones of the spine are joined or fused to one another, to ease curvature of the spine and improve its supportive strength. Depending on the type and severity of OI, surgery may be done to treat fractures or to insert metal rods into the long bones of the arms and legs to strengthen and straighten them during growth. Physical therapy and exercise, including swimming, are used to build muscle, aid bone development, and strengthen the body.

Government Agencies

5432 NIH/National Institute of Child Health and Human Development
National Institutes of Health
Building 31, Room 2A32
Bethesda, MD 20892

301-496-5133
Fax: 301-496-7107
www.nichd.nih.gov

Supports several basic and clinical research projects on osteogenesis imperfecta.
Nancy D Wirth, Director
Lisa Kaeser, Program & Public Liaison

5433 NIH/Osteoporosis and Related Bone Diseases National Resource Center
2 AMS Circle
Bethesda, MD 20892

202-223-0344
800-624-2663
Fax: 202-293-2356
TTY: 202-466-4315
e-mail: NIAMSBoneinfo@mail.nih.gov
www.bones.nih.gov

The National Resource Center is an information service that provides general information on metabolic bone conditions including osteoporosis, osteogenesis imperfecta, and Paget's disease of bone.

Stephen I Katz MD, PhD, Director

National Associations & Support Groups

5434 American Academy of Pediatrics
141 Northwest Point Boulevard
Elk Grove Village, IL 60007   847-434-4000
                                                800-433-9016
                                           Fax: 847-434-8000
                                                www.aap.org

The American Academy of Pediatrics and its member pediatricians are committed to the attainment of optimal physical, mental and social health and well-being for all infants, children, adolescents, and young adults.

Sandra Hassink, MD, FAAP, President

5435 Genetic Alliance
4301 Connecticut Avenue NW
Washington, DC 20008   202-966-5557
                                                800-336-4363
                                           Fax: 202-966-8553
                                   e-mail: info@geneticalliance.org
                                          www.geneticalliance.org

A coalition of voluntary genetic support groups, consumers and professionals addressing the needs of individuals and families affected by genetic disorders from a national perspective.

Sharon Terry, President
Natasha Bonhomme, Vice President of Strategic Develop
Vaughn ÿEdelson, Assistant Director of Health Commun

5436 Little People of America
250 El Camino Real, Suite 201
Tustin, CA 92780   714-368-3689
                                                888-572-2001
                                           Fax: 714-368-3367
                                     e-mail: info@lpaonline.org
                                            www.lpaonline.org

A nonprofit organization that provides support and information to people of short stature and their families.

Lois Gerage-Lamb, President
Bill Bradford, Senior Vice President
Jon North, Vice President, Finance

5437 March of Dimes Birth Defects Foundation
1275 Mamaroneck Avenue
White Plains, NY 10605   914-997-4488
                                                888-663-4637
                                           Fax: 914-428-8203
                                  e-mail: answers@marchofdimes.com
                                           www.marchofdimes.com

Partnership of volunteers and professionals dedicates to improving the health of babies by preventing birth defects and infant mortality. Over 100 chapters are located across the country and can be located through the National Office.

Jennifer L Howse, President

5438 National Dissemination Center for Children with Disabilities
1825 Connecticut Avenue NW, Suite 700
Washington, DC 20009   202-884-8200
                                                800-695-0285
                                           Fax: 202-884-8441
                                       e-mail: nichcy@aed.org
                                             www.nichcy.org

A national information and referral center for families, educators and other professionals on: disabilities in children and youth; programs and services; IDEA, the nation's special education law; and research-based information on effective practices.

Suzanne Ripley, Executive Director

5439 Osteogenesis Imperfecta Foundation
804 W Diamond Avenue
Gaithersburg, MD 20878   301-947-0083
                                                800-981-2663
                                           Fax: 301-947-0456
                                     e-mail: bonelink@oif.org
                                                www.oif.org

This foundation serves the needs of people affected by osteogenesis imperfecta, a brittle bone disorder. Offers information, resources, support and a biannual conference.

Tracy Hart, Ceo
Mary Beth Huber, Information/Resource Director

State Agencies & Support Groups

Arkansas

5440 Little People of America - District 7
250 El Camino Real, Suite 201
Tustin, CA 92780   714-368-3689
                                                888-572-2001
                                           Fax: 714-368-3367
                                     e-mail: info@lpaonline.org
                                            www.lpaonline.org

District 7 of the Little People of America represents short stature individuals from the states of Arkansas, Kansas, Missouri and Oklahoma.

Karen Shelby, Director
Jack Dohr, Vice Director
Cyndy Dohr, Treasurer

California

5441 Little People of America - San Francisco Bay Area Chapter
National Headquarters
250 El Camino Real, Suite 201
Tustin, CA 92780   714-368-3689
                                                888-572-2001
                                           Fax: 714-368-3367
                                     e-mail: info@lpaonline.org
                                           www.lpabayarea.org

A nonprofit organization that provides support and information to people of short stature and their families.

Lee Uniacke, President
Keren Stronach, Co-Vice President
Caroline Jones, Co-Vice President

Colorado

5442 Little People of America - Front Range Chapter
7117 E Euclid Drive
Englewood, CO 80111   303-740-8555
                                 e-mail: ebennettebennett@netscape.net
                                        http://frontrangelpa26.org

Little People of America, Inc. (LPA), will assist dwarfs with their physical and developmental concerns resulting from short stature. By providing medical, environmental, educational, vocational, and parental guidance, short-stature individuals and their families may enhance their lives and lifestyles with minimal limitations. Through peer support and personal example, members will be supportive of all those who reach out to LPA.

Chris & Bob Kotzian, President
Souda Bell, Vice President
Brandi VanAnne, Treasurer

Kansas

5443 Little People of America - District 7
250 El Camino Real, Suite 201
Tustin, CA 92780   714-368-3689
                                          888-572-2001
                                          Fax: 714-368-3367
                                          e-mail: info@lpaonline.org
                                          www.lpaonline.org

District 7 of the Little People of America represents short stature
individuals from the states of Arkansas, Kansas, Missouri and
Oklahoma.

Karen Shelby, Director
Jack Dohr, Vice Director
Cyndy Dohr, Treasurer

Missouri

5444 Little People of America - District 7
250 El Camino Real, Suite 201
Tustin, CA 92780   714-368-3689
                                          888-572-2001
                                          Fax: 714-368-3367
                                          e-mail: info@lpaonline.org
                                          www.lpaonline.org

District 7 of the Little People of America represents short stature
individuals from the states of Arkansas, Kansas, Missouri and
Oklahoma.

Karen Shelby, Director
Jack Dohr, Vice Director
Cyndy Dohr, Treasurer

New Jersey

5445 Little People of America - District 2
National Headquarters
250 El Camino Real, Suite 201
Tustin, CA 92780   714-368-3689
                                          888-572-2001
                                          Fax: 714-368-3367
                                          e-mail: info@lpaonline.org
                                          www.lpaonline.org

A nonprofit organization that provides support and information to
people of short stature and their families.

Joe Zrinski, District Director
Patty Ott, Assistant District Director
Jim Davis, District Treasurer

New York

5446 Little People of America - District 2
National Headquarters
250 El Camino Real, Suite 201
Tustin, CA 92780   714-368-3689
                                          888-572-2001
                                          Fax: 714-368-3367
                                          e-mail: info@lpaonline.org
                                          www.lpaonline.org

A nonprofit organization that provides support and information to
people of short stature and their families.

Joe Zrinski, District Director
Patty Ott, Assistant District Director
Jim Davis, District Treasurer

Oklahoma

5447 Little People of America - District 7
250 El Camino Real, Suite 201
Tustin, CA 92780   714-368-3689
                                          888-572-2001
                                          Fax: 714-368-3367
                                          e-mail: info@lpaonline.org
                                          www.lpaonline.org

District 7 of the Little People of America represents short stature
individuals from the states of Arkansas, Kansas, Missouri and
Oklahoma.

Karen Shelby, Director
Jack Dohr, Vice Director
Cyndy Dohr, Treasurer

Pennsylvania

5448 Little People of America - District 2
National Headquarters
250 El Camino Real, Suite 201
Tustin, CA 92780   714-368-3689
                                          888-572-2001
                                          Fax: 714-368-3367
                                          e-mail: info@lpaonline.org
                                          www.lpaonline.org

A nonprofit organization that provides support and information to
people of short stature and their families.

Joe Zrinski, District Director
Patty Ott, Assistant District Director
Jim Davis, District Treasurer

Utah

5449 Little People of America - Utah Seagulls
250 El Camino Real, Suite 201
Tustin, CA 92780   714-368-3689
                                          888-572-2001
                                          Fax: 714-368-3367
                                          e-mail: info@lpaonline.org
                                          www.utahlittlepeople.org

A nonprofit organization that provides support and information to
people of short stature and their families.

Steve Hatch, President

Libraries & Resource Centers

**5450 NIH/Osteoporosis and Related Bone Diseases National
Resource Center**
2 AMS Circle
Bethesda, MD 20892   202-223-0344
                                          800-624-2663
                                          Fax: 202-293-2356
                                          TTY: 202-466-4315
                                          e-mail: NIHBoneInfo@mail.nih.gov
                                          www.niams.nih.gov/bone/

Devoted to the dissemination of knowledge regarding the disease
along with several helpful medias to explore.

Stephen I Katz MD, PhD, Director

Conferences

5451 LPA National Conference
Little People of America
250 El Camino Real, Suite 201
Tustin, CA 92780   714-368-3689
                                          888-572-2001
                                          Fax: 714-368-3367
                                          e-mail: info@lpaonline.org
                                          www.lpaonline.org

July
Joanna Campbell, Executive Director
Gary Arnold, President
Bill Bradford, Senior Vice President

5452 National Conference on OI
Osteogenesis Imperfecta Foundation
804 W Diamond Avenue, Suite 210
Gaithersburg, MD 20878   301-947-0083
800-981-2663
Fax: 301-947-0456
e-mail: bonelink@oif.org
www.oif.org

Annual conference that allows the Foundation to build on important advocacy efforts while providing an exciting conference.

Sharon Trahan, President
Mark Birdwhistell, Vice President
Tracy Smith Hart, Chief Executive Officer

Audio Video

5453 Plan for Success: Educator's Guide to Students with Osteogenesis Imperfecta
Osteogenesis Imperfecta Foundation
804 W Diamond Avenue, Suite 210
Gaithersburg, MD 20878   301-947-0083
844-889-7579
Fax: 301-947-0456
e-mail: bonelink@oif.org
www.oif.org

Information for parents and educators on planning steps that will help children with osteogenesis imperfecta to fully particapate in school activities.

15 minutes

Heller An Shapiro, Executive Director
Mary Beth Huber, Information/Resource Director

Web Sites

5454 Little People of America
250 El Camino Real, Suite 211
Tustin, CA 92780   714-368-3689
888-LPA-2001
Fax: 714-368-3367
www.lpaonline.org

Offers resources pertaining to dwarfism and Little People of America, medical data, instructions on how to join an e-mail discussion group, and links to numerous other dwarfism-related sites.

Gary Arnold, President
April Brazier, Senior Vice President
Clinton Brown, Finance Director

5455 Online Mendelian Inheritance in Man
National Library of Medicine Building 38A
Bethesda, MD 20894   888-346-3656
e-mail: info@ncbi.nlm.nih.gov
www.ncbi.nlm.nih.gov

This database is a catalog of human genes and genetic disorders.

5456 Osteogenesis Imperfecta Foundation
804 W Diamond Avenue, Suite 210
Gaithersburg, MD 20878   301-947-0083
844-889-7579
Fax: 301-947-0456
www.oif.org

Is the only voluntary national health organization dedicated to helping people cope with the problems associated with osteogenesis imperfecta. The foundations mission is to improve the quality of life for individuals affected by OI through research to find treatments and a cure, education, awareness, and mutual support.

5457 Osteoporosis and Related Bone Diseases - National Resource Center
2 AMS Circle
Bethesda, DC   202-223-0344
800-624-2663
Fax: 202-293-2356
TTY: 202-466-4315
e-mail: NIHBoneInfo@mail.nih.gov
www.niams.nih.gov/bone/

The National Resource Center is dedicated to increasing the awareness, knowledge and understanding of physicians, health professionals, patients, underserves and at-risk populations and the general public about the prevention, early detection and treatment of osteoperosis and related bone diseases.

5458 Shriner's Hospital Research Study Report
www.shrinershq.org

Provides patients, health professionals, and the public with an important link to resources and information on metabolic bone disease, including osteoporosis, Paget's disease of the bone, osteogenesis imperfecta, and hyperparathyroidism. It is dedicated to increasing the underserved and at-risk populations and the general public about the prevention, early detection and treatment of osteoporosis and related bone disease.

5459 Wheeless' Textbook of Orthopaedics
www.wheelessonline.com

Derives from a variety of sources, including journals, articles, national meetings lectures and other textbooks.

Clifford R. Wheeless III, MD, Editor-in-Chief
James A. Nunley, II, MD, Managing Editor
James R. Urbaniak, MD, Managing Editor

Book Publishers

5460 Children with Osteogenesis Imperfecta: Str ategies to Enhance Performance
Osteogenesis Imperfecta Foundation
804 W Diamond Avenue
Gaithersburg, MD 20878   301-947-0083
Fax: 301-947-0456
e-mail: BoneLink@oif.org
www.oif.org

A guide to fitness and exercise for children and teens who have OI. It focuses on practical strategies designed to maximize mobility and function, and prevent some of the complications related to immobility.

2005 270 pages Paperback
ISBN: 0-964218-95-0

Sharon Trahan, President
Mark Birdwhistell, Vice President
Tracy Smith Hart, Chief Executive Officer

5461 Growing Up with OI: Guide for Children
Osteogenesis Imperfecta Foundation
804 W Diamond Avenue, Suite 210
Gaithersburg, MD 20878   301-947-0083
800-981-2663
Fax: 301-947-0456
e-mail: bonelink@oif.org
www.oif.org

Tips and experiences from families of people who have osteogenesis imperfecta.

2001 122 pages Paperback
ISBN: 0-964218-92-5

Sharon Trahan, President
Mark Birdwhistell, Vice President
Tracy Smith Hart, Chief Executive Officer

5462 Growing Up with OI: Guide for Families and Caregivers
Osteogenesis Imperfecta Foundation
804 W Diamond Avenue, Suite 210
Gaithersburg, MD 20878   301-947-0083
800-981-2663
Fax: 301-947-0456
e-mail: bonelink@oif.org
www.oif.org

Tips and experiences from families of people who have
Osteogenesis Imperfecta.

2001 295 pages Paperback
ISBN: 0-964218-91-7

Sharon Trahan, President
Mark Birdwhistell, Vice President
Tracy Smith Hart, Chief Executive Officer

5463 Jason's First Day!
Osteogenesis Imperfecta Foundation
804 W Diamond Avenue
Gaithersburg, MD 20878   301-947-0083
Fax: 301-947-0456
e-mail: BoneLink@oif.org
www.oif.org

This picture book tells the story of the first day of school for a
child with OI. It can be read to preschool, kindergarten and first
grade children. The book includes a teacher's guide and resources
for educators to make the transition to school easier for children
with OI or other mobility impairing disabilities.

2004 43 pages Paperback
ISBN: 0-964218-94-1

Sharon Trahan, President
Mark Birdwhistell, Vice President
Tracy Smith Hart, Chief Executive Officer

5464 Let's Talk About Going to the Hospital
Rosen Publishing Group's PowerKids Press
29 E 21st Street
New York, NY 10010   212-777-3017
800-237-9932
Fax: 888-436-4643
e-mail: rosenpub@tribeca.ios.com
www.rosenpublishing.com

If a child has to check into the hospital, chances are he or she is
already upset about being ill. Knowing how a hospital functions
and what the procedures are, such as when family members can
visit, will help in what is already a stressful situation. Grades
K-5.

24 pages
ISBN: 0-823950-36-0

Roger Rosen, President

5465 Managing Osteogenesis Imperfecta: a Medical Manual
Osteogenesis Imperfecta Foundation
804 W Diamond Avenue, Suite 210
Gaithersburg, MD 20878   301-947-0083
800-981-2663
Fax: 301-947-0456
e-mail: bonelink@oif.org
www.oif.org

The manual is designed for physicians, physical and occupational
therapists, orthopedic technologists, early intervention providers
and others who come in contact with persons with OI. It covers a
broad range of topics including genetics, diagnosis, pregnancy,
arthritis, and osteoperosis.

1997

Sharon Trahan, President
Mark Birdwhistell, Vice President
Tracy Smith Hart, Chief Executive Officer

5466 Osteogenesis Imperfecta: A Guide for Nurse s
Osteogenesis Imperfecta Foundation
804 W Diamond Avenue
Gaithersburg, MD 20878   301-947-0083
Fax: 301-947-0456
e-mail: BoneLink@oif.org
www.oif.org

A comprehensive guide to assist nursing professionals as they
come into contact with people who have OI of all ages. Topics include diagnosis, family education, standard treatments, emergencies and medical procedures. It is intended for nursing
professionals, nursing students and familes.

2003 64 pages Paperback

Sharon Trahan, President
Mark Birdwhistell, Vice President
Tracy Smith Hart, Chief Executive Officer

Newsletters

5467 Breakthrough
Osteogenesis Imperfecta Foundation
804 W Diamond Avenue
Gaithersburg, MD 20878   301-947-0083
844-889-7579
Fax: 301-947-0456
e-mail: bonelink@oif.org
www.oif.org

Newsletter of the Osteogenesis Imperfecta Foundation that provides information on current research and OIF fundraising activities as well as support features. Free within the United States.

24 pages Quarterly

Heller An Shapiro, Executive Director
Mary Beth Huber, Information/Resource Director

Pamphlets

5468 Caring for Infants and Children with Osteogenesis Imperfecta
Osteogenesis Imperfecta Foundation
804 W Diamond Avenue
Gaithersburg, MD 20878   301-947-0083
844-889-7579
Fax: 301-947-0456
e-mail: BoneLink@oif.org
www.oif.org

Presents information on caring for a babies and toddlers with OI.
Available in Spanish.

17 pages

5469 Osteogenesis Imperfecta: A Guide for Medical Professionals, Ind. & Families
Osteogenesis Imperfecta Foundation
804 W Diamond Avenue
Gaithersburg, MD 20878   301-947-0083
844-889-7579
Fax: 301-947-0456
e-mail: BoneLink@oif.org
www.oif.org

Briefly describes osteogenesis imperfecta, its diagnosis and treatment.

10 pages Paperback

5470 Therapeutic Strategies for OI: A Guide for Physical and Occupational Therapists
Osteogenesis Imperfecta Foundation
804 W Diamond Avenue
Gaithersburg, MD 20878   301-947-0083
844-889-7579
Fax: 301-947-0456
e-mail: BoneLink@oif.org
www.oif.org

It covers the role of physical and occupational therapy in managing OI. Topics include safe handling of children and adults with
OI and strategies for safe, successful therapy.

14 pages Paperback

Heller An Shapiro, Executive Director
Mary Beth Huber, Information/Resource Director

Description

5471 OTITIS MEDIA

Synonym: Tympanitis

Covers these related disorders: Acute otitis media, Chronic otitis media, Secretory otitis media

Involves the following Biologic System(s):

Infectious Disorders

Otitis media refers to an infection or inflammation of the middle ear, the irregularly-shaped cavity that lies in the temporal bone on each side of the skull, and contains structures essential to hearing. Otitis media is one of the most common disorders of childhood, especially in children from the ages of 6 months to 3 years.

Acute otitis media usually occurs in conjunction with or as a complication of upper respiratory tract infections such as the common cold. Infections of the respiratory tract can extend to the middle ear and cause otitis media by way of the eustachian tube, a narrow canal that extends from the rear of the nasal area to the middle ear and helps to maintain normal air pressure in the middle ear. Infants and young children are especially vulnerable to otitis media because they have a short and narrow eustachian tube that is positioned somewhat horizontally, making them more susceptible to the backward flow of infectious secretions from the nasal area and into the middle ear. Further increasing the risk of otitis media during colds and other respiratory infections in infants and young children is swelling of the lymph nodes known as the adenoids, which are located at the back of the throat, near the opening of the eustachian tube that extends to each ear, and which can block these tubes and limit their ability to drain infected secretions out of the middle ear.

Symptoms of acute otitis media often develop soon after the onset of a respiratory tract infection, and include sudden and severe ear pain (otalgia), ringing in the ears (tinnitus), fever, temporary hearing loss, and discomfort. Infants and young children with otitis media may exhibit the following symptoms: irritability; pulling at the infected ear; fluid draining from the infected ear; nausea; vomiting; and diarrhea. The eardrum (tympanic membrane) of the infected ear may rupture, thus releasing fluid, which usually relieves the pain in an infected ear. The eardrum may then heal within a short period, but if healing does not occur, this rupture can result in a permanent impairment of hearing, leading to difficulties in speech. Symptoms such as dizziness, headache, sudden and significant hearing loss or deafness, chills, and fever may suggest complications that may result from otitis media or which may occur in conjunction with it, including inflammation of the membranes surrounding the brain and spinal cord (meningitis), infection of the inner ear canals (labyrinthitis), or infection in the mastoid bone behind the ear (mastoiditis).

Otitis media can be detected with an otoscope, an instrument that allows examination of the eardrum to see whether it is inflamed or swollen, thus reflecting an infection of the middle ear, located behind the eardrum. A pneumatic otoscope is used to deliver a puff of air onto the eardrum to check for flexibility or swelling. A microphone can also be used to hear the sound that the air makes.

Treatment of acute otitis media depends upon its cause. If the infection causing an episode of otitis media is bacterial, antibiotics may be given. Some children may require a surgical procedure known as myringotomy, in which an incision is made in the eardrum to relieve pressure and allow the release of pus and other secretions, or through tympanocentesis, a procedure in which the eardrum is surgically punctured to release fluid. Other treatment of otitis media is symptomatic and supportive, with pain relievers, antihistamines, nasal decongestants, and other medications.

Some children with otitis media develop secretory otitis media, which sometimes follows blockage of the eustachian tube, or the successful treatment of acute otitis media. This is characterized by the escape of thin (serous), thick (mucoid), or pus-like fluid from the ear. Symptoms associated with secretory otitis media may include dizziness and tinnitus. Although this condition may resolve spontaneously, its treatment is often indicated to prevent possible hearing loss and subsequent difficulties in the acquisition of speech and language. This may be accomplished through surgical incision and the insertion of tubes into the eardrum to allow the drainage of fluid. Children who do not respond to such treatment may benefit by having their adenoids removed surgically (adenoidectomy) to drain fluids from the eustachian tubes and allow a normal flow of air through them.

An infection of the middle ear that persists beyond the usually course of acute otitis media is known as chronic otitis media Such infection is much less common than acute otitis media, but its symptoms, being less severe, may persist for varying periods without being noticed. This can impair hearing, learning, and speech. Chronic otitis media may, for example, result in small growths (polyps) in the ear and damage to the small bones (ossicles) of the middle ear, impairing the ability of the ear to conduct sound. Chronic otitis media may be treated by the continued administration of antibiotics for a longer period than for the acute condition, as well as by drainage of the ear and the other procedures used in acute otitis media, and by the surgical repair of a ruptured eardrum (tympanoplasty). Tympanoplasty may also be used to restore the mechanism by which the middle ear transmits sound, which involves three small bones known as the malleus, incus, and stapes. The incus transmits vibrations it receives from the malleus to the stapes, which in turn sends the vibrations through a membrane and into the fluid-filled canal of the inner ear, where the vibrations are transformed into nerve signals that travel to the hearing centers of the brain for sensing and comprehension.

Government Agencies

5472 NIH/National Institute of Allergy and Infectious Diseases
6610 Rockledge Drive, MSC 6612
Bethesda, MD 20892

301-496-5717
866-284-4107
Fax: 301-402-3573
TDD: 800-877-8339
e-mail: ocposfoffice@niaid.nih.gov
www.niaid.nih.gov

Conducts and supports basic and applied research to better understand, treat, and ultimately prevent infectious, immunologic, and allergic diseases.

Anthony S Fauci MD, Director

National Associations & Support Groups

5473 American Academy of Audiology
11480 Commerce Park Drive, Ste 220
Reston, VA 20191
703-790-8466
800-222-2336
Fax: 703-790-8631
e-mail: info@audiology.org
www.audiology.org

A professional organization dedicated to providing high quality and balanced hearing care to the public. Provides professional development, education and research and provides increased public awareness of hearing disorders and audiologic services.
ISSN: 1050-0545

Allison Grimes, President
Sydney Hawthorne Davis, Director Communications

5474 American Academy of Pediatrics
141 Northwest Point Boulevard
Elk Grove Village, IL 60007
847-434-4000
800-433-9016
Fax: 847-434-8000
www.aap.org

The American Academy of Pediatrics and its member pediatricians are committed to the attainment of optimal physical, mental and social health and well-being for all infants, children, adolescents, and young adults.

Sandra Hassink, MD, FAAP, President

5475 American Hearing Research Foundation
8 S Michigan Avenue, Suite 1205
Chicago, IL 60603
312-726-9670
Fax: 312-726-9695
e-mail: ahrf@american-hearing.org
www.american-hearing.org

Funds medical research and education into the causes, prevention, and cures of hearing losses, and balance disorders. Also keeps physicians and the public informed of the latest developments in hearing research and education.

Richard G. Muench, Chairman
Alan G. Micco, President
Mark R. Muench, Vice President

5476 March of Dimes Birth Defects Foundation
1275 Mamaroneck Avenue
White Plains, NY 10605
914-997-4488
888-663-4637
Fax: 914-428-8203
e-mail: answers@marchofdimes.com
www.marchofdimes.com

Partnership of volunteers and professionals dedicates to improving the health of babies by preventing birth defects and infant mortality. Over 100 chapters are located across the country and can be located through the National Office.

Jennifer L Howse, President

5477 World Health Organization
Avenue Appia 20
CH-1211 Geneva 27, SL
Switzerland
122-791-2111
Fax: 122-791-3111
www.who.int

WHO is the directing and coordinating authority for health within the United Nations system.

Dr Margaret Chan, Director General

Web Sites

5478 Baylor College of Medicine-Pathology & Pathogenesis of Otitis Media
One Baylor Plaza
Houston, TX 77030
713-798-4951
www.bcm.edu

Paul Klotman, M.D., President/ CEO & Executive Dean
William T. Butler, M.D., Chancellor Emeritus
Alicia Monroe, M.D., Provost/ SVP

5479 Indiana State University School of Medicin e
340 West 10th Street, Suite 6200
Indianapolis, IN 46202
317-274-8157
medicine.iu.edu

Provides a presentation of the disease including signs, symptoms and illustrations.

Jay L. Hess, M.D., Vice President
Stephen P. Bogdewic, PhD, Executive Vice Dean
Diane Iseminger, Chief of Staff

5480 PDR.net
5 Paragon Drive
Montvale, NJ 7645
888-227-6469
e-mail: PDRnet@pdr.net
www.pdr.net

Offers integrated medical information and education tools. Updated frequently, this site contains the drug information resources needed daily by its prescriber user base arranged together in one site for convenience and ease-of-use.

5481 University of Texas Medical Branch
301 University Boulevard
Galveston, TX 77555
www.utmb.edu/oto/
David L. Callender, President
Danny O. Jacobs, MD, Executive Vice President
Carolee King, JD, Senior Vice President

Book Publishers

5482 Let's Talk About Going to the Hospital
Rosen Publishing Group's PowerKids Press
29 E 21st Street
New York, NY 10010
212-777-3017
800-237-9932
Fax: 888-436-4643
e-mail: rosenpub@tribeca.ios.com
www.rosenpublishing.com

If a child has to check into the hospital, chances are he or she is already upset about being ill. Knowing how a hospital functions and what the procedures are, such as when family members can visit, will help in what is already a stressful situation. Grades K-5.

24 pages
ISBN: 0-823950-36-0

Roger Rosen, President

5483 Living with Hearing Loss

Marcia B Dugan, author

Gallaudet University Press
800 Florida Avenue NE
Washington, DC 20002
202-651-5488
Fax: 202-651-5489
TTY: 888-630-9347
e-mail: gupress@gallaudet.edu
gupress.gallaudet.edu

192 pages
ISBN: 1-563681-34-0

5484 Screening for Hearing Loss and Other Otiti s Media

Jackson Roush PhD, author

AGB Association for the Deaf and Hard of Hearing
3417 Volta Place NW
Washington, DC 20007
202-337-5220; 800-432-7543
Fax: 202-337-8314; TTY: 202-337-5221
e-mail: info@agbell.org
www.listeningandspokenlanguage.org

2001 245 pages Softcover
ISBN: 0-769300-00-6

Donald M. Goldberg, President
Alexander T. Graham, Executive Director/CEO
Ted A. Meyer, MD, Ph.D. (SC), Secretary-Treasurer

Description

5485 PASSIVE-AGGRESSIVE BEHAVIOR

Involves the following Biologic System(s):

Developmental/Behavioral/Psychiatric Disorders

Passive-aggressive behavior refers to a type of disruptive conduct that is apparent in approximately 20 percent of children and adolescents. Although seemingly compliant, affected individuals usually harbor negative, aggressive, or hostile feelings, but are unable to directly express them. These negative, hostile feelings are typically manifested indirectly and nonviolently through procrastination, forgetfulness, inefficiency, pouting or sullenness, stubbornness, obstructionism, and resistance to requests or demands. When infants and toddlers, passive-aggressive children and adolescents may have manifested their negativistic personalities through difficulties with feeding and toilet training.

Passive-aggressive individuals may be unaware that they are using their behavior to counteract or offset certain frustrations (e.g., feelings of inadequacy). They may persist in these behaviors in an attempt to regain control of a situation or to punish and retaliate. These stubbornly compliant behaviors are apparent in other situations that typically provoke direct displays of assertiveness, hostility, or other forms of aggression. Parents may be overly, but inconsistently, demanding and critical; conversely, affected individuals may, in some cases, be reared by parents or caregivers who are overly permissive and tolerant.

Treatment for passive-aggressive behavior includes the cooperation of parents or caregivers who are often in the best position to provide motivation for children to learn to appropriately express their assertiveness. Such motivation may be further supported by the establishment of firm rules and guidelines, the setting of realistic goals, and the prioritizing of responsibilities. Some parents or caregivers may benefit from direct management training that teaches the necessary skills to facilitate proper behavior and other social skills. Individual, group, and family psychotherapy may also be indicated. Other treatment is supportive.

Government Agencies

5486 NIH/National Institute of Mental Health
6001 Executive Boulevard, Room 8184, MSC 9663
Bethesda, MD 20892
301-443-4513
866-615-6464
Fax: 301-443-4279
TTY: 301-443-8431
e-mail: nimhinfo@nih.gov
www.nimh.nih.gov

Conducts strategic planning for specific research areas as well as for the Institute as a whole.

Dr Thomas R Insel, Director

National Associations & Support Groups

5487 American Academy of Pediatrics
141 Northwest Point Boulevard
Elk Grove Village, IL 60007
847-434-4000
800-433-9016
Fax: 847-434-8000
www.aap.org

The American Academy of Pediatrics and its member pediatricians are committed to the attainment of optimal physical, mental and social health and well-being for all infants, children, adolescents, and young adults.

Sandra Hassink, MD, FAAP, President

5488 American Mental Health Foundation (AMHF)
PO Box 3
Riverdale, NY 10471
USA
212-737-9027
e-mail: elomke@americanmentalhealthfoundation.or
americanmentalhealthfoudnation.org

Dedicated to the extensive and intensive research in the theories and techniques of treatment of emotional illness and to the implementation of reforms in the mental health system. Efforts have resulted in development of better and less expensive treatment methods. Findings are disseminated in English and other major languages.

Evander Lomke, President/Executive Director

5489 Christian Horizons
25 Sportsworld Crossing Road
Kitchener, MI N2P 0
519-650-0966
866-362-6810
Fax: 519-650-8984
e-mail: info@christian-horizons.org
www.christian-horizons.org

To share Christ's love as we equip and support Adults with developmental disabilities.

5490 Federation of Families for Children's Mental Health
9605 Medical Center Drive, Suite 280
Rockville, MD 20850
240-403-1901
Fax: 240-403-1909
e-mail: ffcmh@ffcmh.org
www.ffcmh.org

The National family run organization is dedicated exclusively to helping children with mental health needs and their families achieve a better quality of life.

Sandra Spencer, Executive Director

5491 NADD: National Association for the Dually Diagnosed
132 Fair Street
Kingston, NY 12401
845-331-4336
800-331-5362
Fax: 845-331-4569
e-mail: info@thenadd.org
www.thenadd.org

Nonprofit organization designed to promote the interests of professional and parent development with resources for individuals who have the coexistence of mental illness and mental retardation. Provides conferences, educational services and training materials to professionals, parents, concerned citizens and service organizations.

Dr Robert Fletcher, CEO
Michelle Jordan, Office Manager
Lisa Christie, Conference Planner

5492 National Alliance for the Mentally Ill
3803 N Fairfax Drive, Suite 100
Arlington, VA 22203
703-524-7600
888-999-6264
Fax: 703-524-9094
TDD: 703-516-7227
e-mail: info@nami.org
www.nami.org

NAMI is a nonprofit, grassroots, self-help, support and advocacy organization of consumers, families and friends of people with severe mental illness, such as schizophrenia, bipolar disorder, major depressive disorder, obsessive compulsive disorder, anxiety disorders, autism and other severe and persistent mental illnesses that affect the brain.

Suzanne Vogel-Scibilia MD, President

5493 National Mental Health Association
2000 N Beauregard Street, 6th Floor
Alexandria, VA 22311

703-684-7722
800-969-6642
Fax: 703-684-5968
TTY: 800-433-5959
www.mentalhealthamerica.net

Addresses all aspects of mental health and mental illness. NMHA with over 340 affiliates works to improve the mental health of all Americans.

David Shern, CEO

5494 National Mental Health Consumers' Self-Help Clearinghouse
1211 Chestnut Street, Suite 1207
Philadelphia, PA 19107

215-751-1810
800-553-4539
Fax: 215-636-6312
e-mail: info@mhselfhelp.org
www.mhselfhelp.org

Offers information, support and appropriate referrals; and promotes public and professional education. Provides networking for those with special interests related to albinism. Promotes and supports research and funding that will improve diagnosis and management of albinism and hypopigmentation.

Joseph Rogers, Executive Director & Founder

State Agencies & Support Groups

5495 Center for Family Support
2811 Zuletteÿ Avenue
Bronx, NY 10461

718-518-1500
Fax: ÿ71- 51- 820
e-mail: svernikoff@cfsny.org
www.cfsny.org

The Center for Family (CFS) is a not-for-profit human service agency providing support and assistance to individuals with developmental disabilities and traumatic brain injuries throughout New York City, Long Island, the lower Hudson Valley region and New Jersey.

Steven Vernikoff, Executive Director
Barbara Greenwald, Associate Executive Director

Web Sites

5496 Borderline Personality Disorder Sanctuary
borderlinepersonality.ca/bpdlinks.htm

Offers a bookstore, resources, articles, hotlines and answers questions about mental health.

5497 CyberPsych
www.cyberpsych.org

CyberPsych presents information about psychoanalysis, psychotherapy, and special topics such as anxiety disorder, the problematic use of alcohol, homophobia, and the traumatic effects of racism. CyberPsych is a nonprofit network which offers free web hosting and technical support for internet communicatios, to nonprofit groups and individuals.

5498 Dual Diagnosis
1050 Hull Street
Baltimore, MD 21230

410-209-6799
877-438-8623
Fax: 410-244-5042
www.toad.net/~arcturus/dd/papd.htm

Review of personality disorders including PAPD.

5499 El Rolphe Center
members.aol.com/elrolphe/PassiveAggressive.html

Description and overview of the Passive/Aggressive Personality by Dr Sidney Langston.

5500 I.D. Weeks Library
414 E. Clark St.
Vermillion, SD 57069

www.usd.edu/library/

5501 NADD: National Association for the Dually Diagnosed
132 Fair Street
Kingston, NY 12401

845-331-4336
800-331-5362
Fax: 845-331-4569
www.thenadd.org

Nonprofit organization designed to promote the interests of professional and care providers for individuals who have the coexistence of mental illness and mental retardation. NADD provides conferences, educational services and training materials to professionals, parents, concerned citizens and service organizations.

Donna McNelis, PhD, President
Dan Baker, PhD., Vice President
Julia Pearce, Secretary

5502 National Anxiety Foundation
www.lexington-on-line.com/naf.html

Offers information and help to persons with panic disorders, manic and depressive disorders and mental illness.

Stephen Cox, MD, President
Linda Vernon Blair, Vice-President
C. Todd Strecker, Secretary

5503 New York Online Access to Health
National Library of Medicine Building 38A
Bethesda, MD 20894

888-346-3656
e-mail: info@ncbi.nlm.nih.gov
www.ncbi.nlm.nih.gov

Provides access to high quality full-text consumer health information that is accurate, timely, relevant and unbiased.

5504 Planetpsych
www.planetpsych.com

e-mail: webmaster@planetpsych.com
www.planetpsych.com

Planetpsych is an online resource for mental health information.

5505 Psych Central
55 Pleasant St., Suite 207
Newburyport, MA 1950

e-mail: talkback@psychcentral.com
www.psychcentral.com

Offers free informational and educational articles and resources on psychology, support and mental health online.

John M. Grohol, Psy.D., CEO & Founder
Holly R. Counts, Psy.d., Clinical Psychologist
Marie Hartwell-Walker, Ed.D., Psychologist/ Therapist

Book Publishers

5506 Challenging Behaviour

Eric Emerson, author

Cambridge University Press
32 Avenue of the Americas
New York, NY 10013

212-924-3900
800-872-7423
Fax: 212-691-3239
e-mail: information@cup.org
www.cup.org

Analysis and intervention in people with severe intellectual disabilities

2nd Edition 232 pages Paperback
ISBN: 0-521794-44-7

5507 Clinical Assessment and Management of Severe Personality Disorders
American Psychiatric Press
1000 Wilson Boulevard, Suite 1825
Arlington, VA 22209

703-907-7322
800-368-5777
Fax: 703-907-1091
e-mail: appi@psych.org
www.appi.org

Focuses on issues relevant to the clinician in private practice, including the diagnosis of a wide range of personality disorders and alternative management approaches.

1996 250 pages Hardcover
ISBN: 0-880484-88-6

Robert E. Hales, M.D, Editor-in-Chief
Rebecca D. Rinehart, Publisher
John McDuffie, Editorial Director

5508 Personality and Psychopathology
American Psychiatric Press
1000 Wilson Boulevard, Suite 1825
Arlington, VA 22209

703-907-7322
800-368-5777
Fax: 703-907-1091
e-mail: appi@psych.org
www.appi.org

Compiles the most recent findings from more than 30 internationally recognized experts. Analyzes the association between personality and psychopathology from several interlocking perspectives: descriptive, developmental, etiological, and theraputic.

1999 544 pages Hardcover
ISBN: 0-880489-23-2

Robert E. Hales, M.D, Editor-in-Chief
Rebecca D. Rinehart, Publisher
John McDuffie, Editorial Director

Description

5509 PATENT DUCTUS ARTERIOSUS

Synonym: PDA

Involves the following Biologic System(s):

Cardiovascular Disorders

Patent ductus arteriosus is characterized by the persistence of a fetal vessel that maintains a passageway between the major artery that carries oxygen-rich blood to the tissues of the body (descending aorta) and the artery that carries deoxygenated blood to the lungs (pulmonary artery). Before birth, fetal blood receives oxygen from the mother's blood rather than from its own lungs, making it unnecessary for fetal blood to pass from the right side of the heart to the lungs to be oxygenated. To accommodate this fetal blood flow, blood passes through an opening (foramen ovale) in the wall (septum) between the two upper chambers of the heart (atria). Fetal blood is diverted away from the lungs through a vessel known as the ductus arteriosus that connects the pulmonary artery and the aorta. Normally, both the foramen ovale and ductus arteriosus close soon after birth. The persistence of the opening (patency) of the ductus arteriosus causes some blood from the aorta to flow into the pulmonary artery to the lungs instead of moving away from the heart to nourish the tissues of the body.

Symptoms and physical findings associated with patent ductus arteriosus depend upon the size of the opening and the volume of the diverted blood. A small defect may result in no symptoms while a larger opening may result in difficulty in breathing (dyspnea), rapid heartbeat (tachycardia), failure to gain weight, inflammation of the lining of the heart (bacterial endocarditis), and inefficient pumping by the heart (heart failure). Physical findings may include enlargement of the heart (cardiomegaly); characteristic heart sounds; a machinery-like heart murmur; and, if left untreated, abnormally high pressure in the lung's circulatory system (pulmonary hypertension).

Premature infants may require early intervention through restriction of fluid intake, certain drug therapy, or surgery to prevent malfunctioning of the heart or lungs. However, if no immediate surgical or medicinal intervention is required or administered, this defect may spontaneously close in many premature newborns.

In full-term infants and children, a patent ductus arteriosus may require intervention (surgical or catheter closure). Such treatment may be helpful in preventing or alleviating associated complications. The exact cause of patent ductus arteriosus in the full-term infant is unknown. It is thought to result from different genetic and environmental factors (multifactorial). For example, this irregularity may be associated with maternal German measles (rubella) infection. In addition, patent ductus arteriosus is often accompanied by other congenital heart defects. This defect appears in approximately 60 of 100,000 births and is more prevalent in females than males by a ratio of about two to one. The patent ductus arteriosus is non routinely closed in a non-surgical, outpatient catheter procedure in otherwise healthy children.

Government Agencies

5510 NIH/National Heart, Lung and Blood Institu te
National Institute of Health
31 Center Dr MSC 2486, Bldg 31, Room 5A48
Bethesda, MD 20892
      301-592-8573
      Fax: 240-629-3246
      TTY: 240-629-3255
    e-mail: NHLBIinfo@nhlbi.nih.gov
      www.nhlbi.nih.gov

Primary responsibility of this organization is the scientific investigation of heart, blood vessel, lung and blood disorders. Oversees research, demonstration, prevention, education, control and training activities in these fields and emphasizes the prevention and control of heart diseases.

Elizabeth G Nabel, MD, Director
Susan Shurin, MD, Deputy Director
Sheila Pohl, Chief of Staff

5511 NIH/National Institute of Child Health and Human Development
31 Center Drive, Building 31
Bethesda, MD 20892
      301-496-1333
      Fax: 301-496-1104
      www.nichd.nih.gov

Established in 1962 by congress, today the institute conducts and supports research on topics related to the health of children, adults, families and populations. Some of these topics include: developmental disabilities, growth and development, infant death, reproductive health and birth defects.

Jay H Hoofnagle, Director
Lisa Kaeser, Program & Public Liaison

National Associations & Support Groups

5512 American Academy of Pediatrics
141 Northwest Point Boulevard
Elk Grove Village, IL 60007
      847-434-4000
      800-433-9016
      Fax: 847-434-8000
      www.aap.org

The American Academy of Pediatrics and its member pediatricians are committed to the attainment of optimal physical, mental and social health and well-being for all infants, children, adolescents, and young adults.

Sandra Hassink, MD, FAAP, President

5513 American Heart Association
7272 Greenville Avenue
Dallas, TX 75231
      214-373-6300
      800-242-8721
      Fax: 214-706-1341
   e-mail: review.personal.info@heart.org
      www.americanheart.org

Supports research, education and community service programs with the objective of reducing premature death and disability from cardiovascular diseases and stroke; coordinates the efforts of health professionals, and others engaged in the fight against heart and circulatory disease.

M Cass Wheeler, CEO

5514 Genetic Alliance
4301 Connecticut Avenue NW
Washington, DC 20008
      202-966-5557
      800-336-4363
      Fax: 202-966-8553
   e-mail: info@geneticalliance.org
      www.geneticalliance.org

A coalition of voluntary genetic support groups, consumers and professionals addressing the needs of individuals and families affected by genetic disorders from a national perspective.

Sharon Terry, President
Natasha Bonhomme, Vice President of Strategic Develop
Vaughn ÿEdelson, Assistant Director of Health Commun

650

5515 March of Dimes Birth Defects Foundation
1275 Mamaroneck Avenue
White Plains, NY 10605   914-997-4488
                                           888-663-4637
                                      Fax: 914-428-8203
                    e-mail: answers@marchofdimes.com
                              www.marchofdimes.com

Partnership of volunteers and professionals dedicates to improving the health of babies by preventing birth defects and infant mortality. Over 100 chapters are located across the country and can be located through the National Office.

Jennifer L Howse, President

Web Sites

5516 Congenital Heart Information Network
www.tchin.org

An international organization that provides reliable information, support services and resources to families of children with congenital heart defects and acquired heart disease, adults with congenital heart defects, and the professionals who work with them.

5517 Southern Illinois University School of Medicine
P.O.Box 19658
Springfield, IL 62794   217-545-8000
                       www.siumed.edu/peds/index.htm

Mission is to assist the people of central and southern Illinois in meeting their present and future health care needs through education, clinical service and research.

5518 Yale University School of Medicine
333 Cedar Street
New Haven, CT 6510   203-737-1770
                                       medicine.yale.edu

A helpful site that explains the causes, symptoms and treatments for Patent Ductus Arteriosus.

Peter Salovey, President
Richard Belitsky, Deputy Dean
Benjamin Polak, Provost

Book Publishers

5519 Congenital Disorders Sourcebook
Omnigraphics
PO Box 625
Holmes, PA 19043   800-234-1340
                                      Fax: 800-875-1340
                      e-mail: info@omnigraphics.com
                              www.omnigraphics.com

Basic consumer health information on disorders aquired during gestation, including spina bifida, hydrocephalus, cerebral palsy, heart defects, craniofacial abnormalities and fetal alcohol syndrome.

650 pages
ISBN: 0-780809-45-9

Peter Ruffner, Publisher

Description

5520 PEMPHIGUS

Involves the following Biologic System(s):

Dermatologic Disorders

Pemphigus refers to a group of chronic skin disorders that are characterized by the appearance of blisters on the skin and delicate mucous membranes that line the mouth, for example. Pemphigus most often occurs amoung the adult population, but may appear at any age. Associated findings include a phenomenon known as Nikolsky's sign, characterized by the tendency of the upper layer of the skin to separate or slough off from the lower layer upon rubbing or other minor trauma. Pemphigus is thought to result from an autoimmune reaction during which the body mistakenly attacks healthy cells. In this case, antibodies attack the cells that glue skin together, resulting in disruptions in contact between the cells.

Benign familial pemphigus is a relatively mild form of this disorder that is inherited as an autosomal dominant trait and is characterized by the persistent and recurrent formation of blisters mainly in the groin area, the armpit (axillary) region, the sides of the neck, and on the bending surfaces of the arms and legs. These localized or widespread lesions rupture, erode, and then crust over and heal. This form of pemphigus is also known as Hailey-Hailey disease.

Pemphigus foliaceus is a rare, usually mild form of the disorder that is characterized by small blisters that are usually localized and rupture easily, erode, and then heal by crusting over or scaling. These lesions most commonly appear on the scalp, neck, face, and trunk. The blisters may cause itching, pain, or burning in the affected areas. Affected individuals may also experience the sloughing off of the upper skin layer (Nikolsky's sign). Some affected individuals may develop a more generalized pattern of eruptions characterized by excessive shedding or peeling of the skin. Treatment for pemphigus foliaceus may include therapy with corticosteriod drugs. In some cases, topical application of corticosteroid ointments, salves, or creams proves beneficial.

Pemphigus vulgaris is a very severe form of disease that is manifested by eruptions of painful, ulcerative lesions in the delicate mucous membranes that line the mouth. Later findings include the appearance of large blisters on previously unaffected areas of the face, chest, abdomen, armpit region, groin area, and the various pressure points of the body. These lesions enlarge and rupture, leaving raw areas that may partially crust over, but have little or no tendency to heal. These raw or denuded areas sometimes give rise to wart-like granulations that emit a strong, offensive odor. This stage of pemphigus vulgaris is sometimes referred to as pemphigus vegetans. The folds of the skin are particularly susceptible to the development of these wart-like lesions. Individuals with pemphigus vulgaris also exhibit Nikolsky's sign. Life-threatening complications associated with pemphigus vulgaris may include secondary bacterial infections such as sepsis or debilitating conditions such as malnutrition and the loss of essential elements, known as electrolytes, in the fluid portion of the blood (e.g., sodium, potassium, and calcium). For this reason, early diagnosis and treatment of pemphigus vulgaris is essential to its successful management. Positive diagnosis may be determined through microscopic examination of a skin sample, obtained through biopsy, that indicates the presence of certain antibody deposits. Initial treatment may include high-dose corticosteroid therapy, followed by long-term administration of corticosteroid or other immunosuppressive drugs to control the disease. Antibiotic therapy may be indicated for treatment of skin or secondary bacterial infections.

Neonatal pemphigus vulgaris develops in the unborn fetus of an affected mother by transmission of the mother's antibodies through the placenta. In most cases, the severity of disease in the fetus is related to the severity of the mother's disease. If the mother is severely affected, the placental transmission of antibodies may potentially threaten the life of the unborn child.

Government Agencies

5521 NIH/National Institute of Arthritis and Musculoskeletal and Skin Diseases

1AMS Circle
Bethesda, MD 20892

301-402-4484
877-226-4267
Fax: 301-718-6366
TDD: 301-565-2966
e-mail: niamsinfo@mail.nih.gov
www.niams.nih.gov

The mission of the NIAMS, a part of the NIH, is to support research into the causes, treatment, and prevention of arthritis and musculoskeletal and skin diseases, the training of basic and clinical scientists to carry out this research, and the dissemination of information on research progress in these diseases.

Stephen I Katz MD PhD, Director
Robert H Carter MD, Deputy Director

5522 NIH/National Institute of Child Health and Human Development

31 Center Drive, Building 31
Bethesda, MD 20892

301-496-1333
Fax: 301-496-1104
www.nichd.nih.gov

Established in 1962 by congress, today the institute conducts and supports research on topics related to the health of children, adults, families and populations. Some of these topics include: developmental disabilities, growth and development, infant death, reproductive health and birth defects.

Jay H Hoofnagle, Director
Lisa Kaeser, Program & Public Liaison

National Associations & Support Groups

5523 American Academy of Pediatrics

141 Northwest Point Boulevard
Elk Grove Village, IL 60007

847-434-4000
800-433-9016
Fax: 847-434-8000
www.aap.org

The American Academy of Pediatrics and its member pediatricians are committed to the attainment of optimal physical, mental and social health and well-being for all infants, children, adolescents, and young adults.

Sandra Hassink, MD, FAAP, President

5524 American Autoimmune Related Diseases Association

22100 Gratiot Avenue
Eastpointe, MI 48021

586-776-3900
800-598-4668
Fax: 586-776-3903
e-mail: aarda@aarda.org
www.aarda.org

Dedicated to the eradiction of autoimmune diseases and the alleviation of suffering and the socio-economic impact of autoimmunity through fostering and facilitating collaboration in the areas of education, public awareness, research and patient services in an effective, ethical and efficient manner.

Virginia Ladd, Executive Director

5525 Genetic Alliance
4301 Connecticut Avenue NW
Washington, DC 20008
202-966-5557
800-336-4363
Fax: 202-966-8553
e-mail: info@geneticalliance.org
www.geneticalliance.org

A coalition of voluntary genetic support groups, consumers and professionals addressing the needs of individuals and families affected by genetic disorders from a national perspective.

Sharon Terry, President

5526 International Pemphigus Foundation
1331 Garden Highway, Ste 100
Sacramento, CA 95833
916-922-1298
Fax: 916-922-1458
e-mail: pemphigus@pemphigus.org
www.pemphigus.org

A nonprofit organization with these goals: to increase awareness of pemphigus and pemphigold among the public and the medical community; to provide information and emotional support to pemphigus and pemphigold patients and caregivers; to provide referrals to specialists and to support research into advanced treatments and a cure.

Molly Stuart, CEO
David A Sirois PhD, President
Will Zrnchik, Director Development/Communications

5527 March of Dimes Birth Defects Foundation
1275 Mamaroneck Avenue
White Plains, NY 10605
914-997-4488
888-663-4637
Fax: 914-428-8203
e-mail: answers@marchofdimes.com
www.marchofdimes.com

Partnership of volunteers and professionals dedicates to improving the health of babies by preventing birth defects and infant mortality. Over 100 chapters are located across the country and can be located through the National Office.

Jennifer L Howse, President

5528 Society for Pediatric Dermatology
8365 Keystone Crossing, Suite 107
Indianapolis, IN 46240
317-202-0224
Fax: 317-205-9481
e-mail: spd@hp-assoc.com
www.pedsderm.net

Objective is to promote, develop and advance education, research and care of skin disease in all pediatric age groups.

Kent Lindeman, Executive Director

State Agencies & Support Groups

California

5529 International Pemphigus Foundation: Southe rn California Support Group
310-559-5462
e-mail: lynntg@prodigy.net

Lynn Glick

Maryland

5530 International Pemphigus Foundation: Baltim ore Support Group
410-750-1618
e-mail: byrnete@comcast.net

Erica Byrne

Massachusetts

5531 International Pemphigus Foundation: Massac husetts Support Group
978-463-0965
e-mail: alppy@comcast.net

Alan Papert

New York

5532 International Pemphigus Foundation: New Yo rk Support Group
Valley Stream, NY
516-825-4594
e-mail: mayykoe@aol.com

Matt Koenig

South Carolina

5533 International Pemphigus Foundation: South Carolina Support Group
Gray Court, SC 29645
864-386-1620
e-mail: bubba2coggins@juno.com

Cheryl Jordan

Texas

5534 International Pemphigus Foundation
2701 Cottage Way #16
Sacramento, CA 95825
916-922-1298
Fax: 916-922-1458
e-mail: pemphigus@pemphigus.org
www.pemphigus.org

A nonprofit organization with these goals: to increase awareness of pemphigus and pemphigold among the public and the medical community; to provide information and emotional support to pemphigus and pemphigold patients and caregivers; to provide referrals to specialists and to support research into advanced treatments and a cure.

Molly Stuart, CEO
David A Sirois PhD, President
Will Zrnchik, Director Development/Communications

5535 International Pemphigus Foundation Dallas Support Group
817-557-9642
e-mail: angela.bob@netzero.net

Angela Vickers

5536 International Pemphigus Foundation: Housto n Support Group
5231 Kinglet Street
Houston, TX 77035
713-723-5647
Fax: 713-726-0286
e-mail: richardm@hal-pc.org

Richard M Schwartz

Audio Video

5537 International Pemphigus Foundation Promoti onal Video
International Pemphigus Foundation
1331 Garden Highway, Ste 100
Sacramento, CA 95833   916-922-1298
                    e-mail: info@pemphigus.org
                    www.pemphigus.org

Promotional video available ($5.00 S/H).

Free 15 Minutes

Victoria Werth, M.D., Chair
Sergei Grando, M.D., Ph.D., Vice Chair
Badri Rengarajan, M.D., President

Web Sites

5538 American Autoimmune Related Diseases Association
22100 Gratiot Ave.
Eastpointe, MI 48021   586-776-3900
                    Fax: 586-776-3903
                    www.aarda.org

Dedicated to the eradiction of autoimmune diseases and the alleviation of suffering and the socio-economic impact of
autoimmunity through fostering and facilitating collaboration in
the areas of education, public awareness, research and patient services in an effective, ethical and efficient manner.

Betty Diamond, M.D., Chair
Stanley M. Finger, Ph.D. , Vice Chairperson
Virginia Ladd, President/ Executive Director

5539 Pemphigus FAQ
www.pemphigus.org.uk

Offers information about pemphigus.

Newsletters

5540 IPF Quarterly
1331 Garden Highway, Ste 100
Sacramento, CA 95833   916-922-1298
                    e-mail: pemphigus@pemphigus.org
                    www.pemphigus.org

The International Pemphigus Foundation's newsletter. Dedicated
exclusively to the subject of pemphigus and pemphigoid, providing the latest medical research news and reports on treatment,
drugs and events.

12 pages Quarterly

Victoria Werth, M.D., Chair
Sergei Grando, M.D., Ph.D., Vice Chair
Badri Rengarajan, M.D., President

Pamphlets

5541 An Introduction to Pemphigus
1331 Garden Highway, Ste 100
Sacramento, CA 95833   916-922-1298
                    Fax: 916-922-1458
                    e-mail: pemphigus@pemphigus.org
                    www.pemphigus.org/pubs.html

An overview of pemphigus

14 pages Handbook

Victoria Werth, M.D., Chair
Sergei Grando, M.D., Ph.D., Vice Chair
Badri Rengarajan, M.D., President

5542 Pemphigus and Pemphigoid At a Glance
1331 Garden Highway, Ste 100
Sacramento, CA 95833   916-922-1298
                    Fax: 916-922-1458
                    e-mail: pemphigus@pemphigus.org
                    www.pemphigus.org/pubs.html

An introductory brochure designed for the doctors office. It provides a helpful overview of each disease.

2 pages Brochure

Victoria Werth, M.D., Chair
Sergei Grando, M.D., Ph.D., Vice Chair
Badri Rengarajan, M.D., President

Description

5543 PHENYLKETONURIA (PKU)

Synonyms: Classic phenylketonuria, PKU

Involves the following Biologic System(s):

Genetic/Chromosomal/Syndrome/Metabolic Disorders

Phenylketonuria (PKU) is an inherited metabolic disorder characterized by the absence or deficiency of phenylalanine hydroxylase (PAH), an enzyme that assists in processing or metabolizing the amino acid known as phenylalanine — which is present in almost all foods — so that cells can use it for various purposes. The role of PAH is to convert phenylalanine into another amino acid named tyrosine. An absence or deficiency of PAH results in the accumulation of excessive phenylalanine in the blood. This may lead to severe mental retardation that is frequently accompanied by seizures and other neurologic problems.

Phenylketonuria gets its name from the appearance in the urine of abnormally large quantities of byproducts of phenylalanine known as phenylketones, which give an unpleasant odor to the sweat and urine of infants and children with PKU.

Phenylketonuria is transmitted as an autosomal recessive trait, meaning that both parents must carry and transmit the mutated genes for their child develop PKU. The mutations that cause the disease occur in the genes that carry instructions for making PAH. In the United States, approximately one in 16,000 infants is affected by PKU. All infants born in hospitals in the United States are now routinely screened for PKU. This procedure, known as the Guthrie or PKU test, takes a small sample of blood from an infant's heel and examining it for phenylalanine.

Initially, most newborns with PKU have no symptoms.Early symptoms may include severe vomiting and poor eating. As they increase in age, children with untreated PKU may have an abnormally small head, irregularities of the teeth and upper jaw (maxilla), abnormalities in the structure and function of the heart, and mental retardation that develops slowly but progressively and may become apparent within the first few months of life. Other effects of untreated PKU include unusual paleness of the skin, accompanied by skin disorders such as eczema, behavioral abnormalities, and neuromuscular irregularities such as involuntary, continuous, slow movements of the arms and legs (athetosis). Other findings may include seizures and hyperactivity, sometimes accompanied by rhythmic behaviors such as rocking; light-colored skin, blonde hair, and blue eyesand an eczema-type rash that disappears with age.

Treatment for PKU is aimed toward reducing dietary intake of phenylalanine in order to prevent or reduce damage to the brain. The most effective treatment consists of a special diet of foods that help control the amount of PAH consumed (some PAH is needed for normal growth and development). The diet is begun as soon after birth as PKU is identified, and is monitored under close supervision. It consists of fruits and vegetables, breads, pastas, and cereals with a low protein content, since proteins contain relatively large quantities of phenylalanine. The diet does not contain high-protein foods such as eggs, cheeses, meat, milk, or nuts. People with PKU who are on this diet from birth or shortly thereafter develop normally and often have no symptoms of PKU. It is recommended that pregnant women with PKU or affected women who are planning to become pregnant maintain a low phenylalanine diet to avoid the risk of miscarriage. Infants born to women with PKU and are not on a special diet are at high risk of experiencing serious effects of the disease.

National Associations & Support Groups

5544 American Academy of Pediatrics
141 Northwest Point Boulevard
Elk Grove Village, IL 60007

847-434-4000
800-433-9016
Fax: 847-434-8000
www.aap.org

The American Academy of Pediatrics and its member pediatricians are committed to the attainment of optimal physical, mental and social health and well-being for all infants, children, adolescents, and young adults.

Sandra Hassink, MD, FAAP, President

5545 Children's PKU Network
3306 Bumann Rd
Encinitas, CA 92024

858-509-0767
800-377-6677
Fax: 858-509-0768
e-mail: pkunetwork@aol.com
www.pkunetwork.org

Provides support services and treatment products to families affected by phenylketonuria (PKU). Services include referral, newborn express packages, digital scale sales and crises intervention aid.

Cindy Neptune, Executive Director

5546 March of Dimes Birth Defects Foundation
1275 Mamaroneck Avenue
White Plains, NY 10605

914-997-4488
888-663-4637
Fax: 914-428-8203
e-mail: answers@marchofdimes.com
www.marchofdimes.com

Partnership of volunteers and professionals dedicates to improving the health of babies by preventing birth defects and infant mortality. Over 100 chapters are located across the country and can be located through the National Office.

Jennifer L Howse, President

State Agencies & Support Groups

5547 PKU Organization of Illinois
PO Box 102
Palatine, IL 60078

630-415-2219
Fax: 208-978-8963
e-mail: info@pkuil.org
www.pkuil.org

Resource for families in Illinois and around the world dealing with phenylketonuria. Founded in 1969 for the benefit of patients and families.

Joseph Annunzio, President
Lisa Irgang, VP
Christine Davis, Treasurer

Web Sites

5548 National Human Genome Research Institute
biotech.law.lsu.edu/research/fed/tfgt/appendix5.htm

Report on the history of phenylketonuria screening in newborns in the U.S.

Diane B. Paul, Author

5549 National Society for Phenylketonuria (UK)
PO Box 3143
Purley, CR 89DD
303-040-1090
Fax: 845-004-8341
e-mail: info@nspku.org
www.nspku.org

Helps and supports people with PKU, their families and caregivers. The NSPKU actively promotes the care and treatment of PKU and works closely with medical professionals in the UK.

Eric Lange, Chair
Iain Williamson, Secretary
Lisa Lee, Treasurer

5550 Online Mendelian Inheritance in Man
National Library of Medicine,Building 38A
Bethesda, MD 20894
888-346-3656
e-mail: info@ncbi.nlm.nih.gov
www.ncbi.nlm.nih.gov

This database is a catalog of human genes and genetic disorders.

5551 PKU Kid Zone
www.pkuil.org/kidzone.htm

Provides activities for chidren to have fun online.

5552 PKU Mailing List
PO Box 3143
Purley, CR 89DD
303-040-1090
Fax: 845-004-8341
e-mail: info@nspku.org
www.nspku.org/listserve

Worldwide mailing list making communication between families dealing with PKU easier.

Eric Lange, Chair
Iain Williamson, Secretary
Lisa Lee, Treasurer

5553 PKU Organization of Illinois
PO Box 102
Palatine, IL 60078
630-344-9758
e-mail: pkuillinois@gmail.com
www.pkuil.org

Committed to the support of appropriate research initiatives to better understand PKU and eventually find a cure. Support services include: get togethers for kids and parents to express their concerns and share ways of coping with the disease, annual picnics throughout the state and family camp to get to know other PKU families, and activities on both state and national levels in protecting the interests of PKU families.

5554 Star-G: Screening, Technology and Research in Genetics
741 Sunset Avenue
Honolulu, HI 96816
808-733-9039
Fax: 808-733-9068
e-mail: lianne@hawaiigenetics.org
www.newbornscreening.info

General and newborn screening information for amino acid disorders including PKU.

Newsletters

5555 National PKU News
6869 Woodland Avenue NE, Suite 116
Seattle, WA 98115
206-525-8140
Fax: 206-525-5023
e-mail: schuett@pkunews.org
www.pkunews.org

Nonprofit organization dedicated to providing up-to-date, accurate news and information to families and professionals dealing with phenylketonuria through this newsletter.

2000+ 3 issues/year

Virginia Schuett, Director/Editor

5556 PKU Press
PKU Organization of Illinois
PO Box 102
Palatine, IL 60078
630-344-9758
Fax: 208-978-8963
e-mail: pkuillinois@gmail.com
www.pkuil.org

Provides information, support, and highlights achievements for the benefit of the PKU community.

20 pages 3x/year

Joseph Annunzio, President
Lisa Irgang, VP
Christine Davis, Treasurer

Pamphlets

5557 Phenylketonuria (PKU) Information Sheet
March of Dimes Pregnancy & Newborn Health Edu Ctr
1275 Mamaroneck Avenue
White Plains, NY 10605
914-997-4488
Fax: 914-997-4763
e-mail: answers@marchofdimes.com
www.marchofdimes.org/pregnancy.aspx

Defines and discusses the implications and causes of PKU, as well as testing, treatment, prevention and research.

Description

5558 PHOBIAS

Involves the following Biologic System(s):

Developmental/Behavioral/Psychiatric Disorders

A phobia is a persistent, exaggerated, unreasonable fear or dread of certain activities, situations, objects, or events. Exposure to the activity, situation, or object that arouses fear typically elicits signs of anxiety or panic reaction. Such symptoms may include nausea, abdominal pain, irregular pulsation or racing of the heart (palpitations), sweating, and dizziness. In contrast to adults, children, especially younger one, don't see their fear as excessive or unreasonable. Most children are fearful of particular things as they reach certain age plateaus. For example, young children are often afraid of monsters or of being alone in the dark. Older children may be fearful of death or other distressing situations. Children may become fearful of events or situations that they view on television. Others may have fear or dread related to conflicts in the home. These fears are not unusual and may often be alleviated by reassurances and comforting by parents and caregivers. However, a fear or phobia that interferes with normal, day-to-day functioning is considered pathologic.

Simple or specific phobias include fear of certain animals and insects or particular situations (e.g., fear of flying, etc.). Social phobias, often appearing in late childhood or adolescence, include fear and avoidance of certain social situations such as using public bathroom facilities or eating, speaking, performing, or writing in public. Researchers believe that some simple phobias may result from an associated, traumatic childhood experience or from the existence of a similar fear in a parent or caregiver. More complicated specific phobias (e.g., fear of attending school, etc.) may be associated with such conflicts as a hostile-dependent relationship between the parent or caregiver and the child.

Treatment for phobias is dependent upon the specific fear, the extent of the fear, and the effect of the phobias on day-to-day living. Parents or caregivers are counseled to remain calm and patient when confronted with a phobic episode. Behavioral therapy, including relaxation therapy for older children, may be indicated and may include the training of parents or caregivers in the use of supportive measures and techniques. Slow and orderly exposure to the activity, situation, or object of fear (desensitization) may help to alleviate the fear. Older children and adolescents with social phobias may learn to overcome their particular fear through social skills training. Other treatment is symptomatic and supportive.

Government Agencies

5559 Center for Mental Health Services Knowledge Exchange Program
US Department of Health and Human Services
PO Box 42557
Washington, DC 20015
800-789-2647
Fax: 240-747-5470
TDD: 866-889-2647
http://mentalhealth.samhsa.gov

Supplies the public with expert responses to commonly asked questions about various mental health disorders, and directs the caller to appropriate resources.

5560 NIH/National Institute of Mental Health
6001 Executive Boulevard, Room 8184, MSC 9663
Bethesda, MD 20892
301-443-4513
866-615-6464
Fax: 301-443-4279
TTY: 301-443-8431
e-mail: nimhinfo@nih.gov
www.nimh.nih.gov

Conducts strategic planning for specific research areas as well as for the Institute as a whole.

Dr Thomas R Insel, Director

National Associations & Support Groups

5561 Agoraphobics in Motion
P.O. Box 725363
Berkley, MI 48072
248-547-0400
e-mail: anny@ameritech.net
www.aimforrecovery.com

A.I.M. has been helping people with anxiety disorders since 1983.

James Fortune, President
Robert Diedrich, Vice President
Mary Ann Gogoleski, SWT, Director

5562 American Academy of Pediatrics
141 Northwest Point Boulevard
Elk Grove Village, IL 60007
847-434-4000
800-433-9016
Fax: 847-434-8000
www.aap.org

The American Academy of Pediatrics and its member pediatricians are committed to the attainment of optimal physical, mental and social health and well-being for all infants, children, adolescents, and young adults.

Sandra Hassink, MD, FAAP, President

5563 American Counseling Association
6101 Stevenson Ave
Alexandria, VA 22304
703-823-9800
800-347-6647
Fax: 703-823-0252
e-mail: webmaster@counseling.org
www.counseling.org

Represents professional counselors in various practice settings, and stands ready to serve more than 55,000 members with the resources they need to make a difference. From webinars, publications, and journals to Conference education sessions and legislative action alerts, ACA is where counseling professionals turn for powerful, credible content and support.

Robert L. Smith, President

5564 American Mental Health Foundation (AMHF)
PO Box 3
Riverdale, NY 10028
212-737-9027
e-mail: elomke@americanmentalhealthfoundation.or
americanmentalhealthfoudnation.org

Dedicated to the extensive and intensive research in the theories and techniques of treatment of emotional illness and to the implementation of reforms in the mental health system. Efforts have resulted in development of better and less expensive treatment methods. Findings are disseminated in English and other major languages.

Monroe W Spero, MD
Evander Lomke, Executive Director

5565 American Psychiatric Association
1000 Wilson Boulevard, Suite 1825
Arlington, VA 22209
703-907-7300
888-35 -7924
e-mail: apa@psych.org
www.psychiatry.org

It is a medical specialty society representing growing membership of more than 36,000 psychiatrists.

5566 American Psychological Association
750 First St. NE
Washington, DC 20002
202-336-5500
800-374-2721
TTY: 202-336-6123
www.apa.org

The mission is to advance the creation, communication and application of psychological knowledge to benefit society and improve people's lives.

Norman B. Anderson, PhD, CEO/ EVP
L. Michael Honaker, PhD, Deputy Chief Executive Officer
Ellen G. Garrison, PhD, Senior Policy Advisor

5567 American School Counselor Association
1101 King Street, Suite 310
Alexandria, VA 22314
703-683-2722
800-306-4722
Fax: 703-997-7572
e-mail: asca@schoolcounselor.org
www.schoolcounselor.org

The mission of ASCA is to represent professional school counselors and to promote professionalism and ethical practices.

Richard Wong, Executive Director
Jeff Broderson, Information Technology Admin.
Kathleen M Rakestraw, Director of Communications

5568 Anxiety Disorders Association of America
8730 Georgia Avenue, Suite 600
Silver Spring, MD 20910
240-485-1001
Fax: 240-485-1035
e-mail: information@adaa.org
www.adaa.org

Offers resources and information for persons with anxiety and stress-related disorders.

Alies Muskin, Executive Director

5569 Anxiety Disorders Institute
1 Dunwoody Park Suite 112
Atlanta, GA 30338
770-395-6845

Provides support, training, and services for those suffering from anxiety disorders, and their families.

5570 Anxiety and Depression Association of America
8701 Georgia Ave., Suite #412
Silver Spring, MD 20910
240-485-1001
Fax: 240-485-1035
www.adaa.org

ADAA is a national nonprofit organization dedicated to the prevention, treatment, and cure of anxiety, depression, OCD, PTSD, and related disorders and to improving the lives of all people who suffer from them through education, practice, and research.

Mark H. Pollack, MD, President
Alies Muskin, Executive Director
Jean Kaplan Teichroew

5571 Anxiety and Phobia Treatment Center
Whire Plains Hospital Center
Davis Avenue & East Post Road
White Plains, NY 10601
914-681-1038
Fax: 914-681-2284
e-mail: jchessa@wphospital.org
phobia-anxiety.com

Treatment groups for individuals suffering from phobias. Deals with fears through contextual therapy, a treatment and study of the phobia in the actual setting in which the phobic reactions occur. Conducts Intensive Courses, Phobia Self-Help Groups, 8-week Phobia Clinics and individual treatment. Publications: PM Newsletter, bimonthly. Articles and papers. Annual conference.

Fredrick J Neumen, MD, Director

5572 Federation of Families for Children's Mental Health
9605 Medical Center Drive, Suite 280
Rockville, MD 20850
240-403-1901
Fax: 240-403-1909
e-mail: ffcmh@ffcmh.org
www.ffcmh.org

The National family run organization is dedicated exclusively to helping children with mental health needs and their families achieve a better quality of life.

Sandra Spencer, Executive Director

5573 Freedom From Fear
308 Seaview Avenue
Staten Island, NY 10305
718-351-1717
Fax: 718-667-8893
e-mail: help@freedomfromfear.org
www.freedomfromfear.org

The mission of Freedom From Fear is to aid and counsel individuals and their families who suffer from anxiety and depressive illness.

Mary Guardino, Founder

5574 National Alliance for the Mentally Ill
3803 N Fairfax Drive, Suite 100
Arlington, VA 22203
703-524-7600
888-999-6264
Fax: 703-524-9094
TDD: 703-516-7227
e-mail: info@nami.org
www.nami.org

NAMI is a nonprofit, grassroots, self-help, support and advocacy organization of consumers, families and friends of people with severe mental illness, such as schizophrenia, bipolar disorder, major depressive disorder, obsessive compulsive disorder, anxiety disorders, autism and other severe and persistent mental illnesses that affect the brain.

Suzanne Vogel-Scibilia MD, President

5575 National Alliance on Mental Illness
3803 N. Fairfax Drive, Suite 100
Arlington, VA 22203
703-524-7600
800-950-6264
Fax: 703-524-9094
e-mail: info@nami.org
www.nami.org

Grassroots mental health organization dedicated to building better lives for the millions of Americans affected by mental illness. - See more at:
http://www.nami.org/About-NAMI#sthash.lYtjmu5h.dpuf

Jim Payne, J.D., President
David Levy, Chief Financial Officer
Mary Giliberti, J.D., Executive Director

5576 National Anxiety Foundation
3135 Custer Drive
Lexington, KY 40517
859-281-0003
www.lexington-on-line.com/naf.html

Nonprofit organization that provides education to the public and professionals about anxiety through printed and electronic media.

Stephen Cox MD, President & Medical Director

5577 National Mental Health Association
2000 N Beauregard Street, 6th Floor
Alexandria, VA 22311
703-684-7722
800-969-6642
Fax: 703-684-5968
TTY: 800-433-5959
www.mentalhealthamerica.net

Addresses all aspects of mental health and mental illness. NMHA with over 340 affiliates works to improve the mental health of all Americans.

David Shern, CEO

5578 National Mental Health Consumers' Self-Help Clearinghouse
1211 Chestnut Street, Suite 1207
Philadelphia, PA 19107
215-751-1810
800-553-4539
Fax: 215-636-6312
e-mail: info@mhselfhelp.org
www.mhselfhelp.org

Offers information, support and appropriate referrals; and promotes public and professional education. Provides networking for those with special interests related to albinism. Promotes and supports research and funding that will improve diagnosis and management of albinism and hypopigmentation.

Joseph Rogers, Executive Director & Founder

5579 Phobia Society of America
133 Rollins Avenue, Suite 4B
Rockville, MD 20852

301-231-9350
Fax: 301-231-7392
www.adaa.org

Offers support for those suffering from phobia and panic attacks.

5580 Phobics Anonymous
PO Box 1180
Palm Springs, CA 92263

706-327-2148

Twelve-step program for panic disorders and anxiety. Publications available.

Marily Gellis PhD, Contact

5581 Selective Mutism Foundation
PO Box 25972
Tamarac, FL 33320

305-748-7714
Fax: 305-748-7714
www.selectivemutismfoundation.org

Promotes awareness and understanding for individuals and families affected by selective mutism, an inherited anxiety disorder in which children with normal or deficient language skills are unable to speak in school or social situations. SM is often mistaken for normal shyness and may go undetected for as long as two years. Encourages research and treatment. Maintains speakers' bureau. Publications: Let's Talk, annual newsletter. Selective Mutism, A Silent Cry for Help, brochure.

Sue Newman, Co-Founder & Director

5582 Social Anxiety Association
socialphobia.org

The Social Anxiety Association is a non-profit organization founded in 1997 to meet the growing needs of people with social anxiety.

Thomas A. Richards, Ph.D., President

5583 Special Interest Group on Phobias and Related Anxiety Disorders (SIGPRAD)
245 E 87th Street
New York, NY 10128

212-860-5560
Fax: 212-744-5751
e-mail: lindy@interport.net
www.cyberpsych.org

For psychologists, psychiatrists, social workers and other individuals interested in treatment of anxiety disorders. Objectives are to increase knowledge, facilitate communication, and support research and treatment of phobias and related anxiety disorders. Conducts programs at professional meetings. Affiliated with the Association for Advancement of Behavior Therapy. Periodic symposiums and workshops.

Carol Lindemann, PhD, CEO

5584 Territorial Apprehensiveness (TERRAP) Programs
932 Evelyn Street
Menlo Park, CA 94025

800-274-6242

To disseminate information concerning the recognition, causes, and treatment of anxieties, fears and phobias especially agoraphobia. Provides information and counseling for those with phobias. Sponsors service centers and training for psychotherapists and counselors. Publications: TERRAP Manual, audiotapes, booklets, monographs, and videos.

Crucita V Hardy, Director

State Agencies & Support Groups

5585 Center for Family Support
333 7th Avenue #901
New York, NY 10001

212-629-7939
Fax: 212-239-2211
www.cfsny.org

The Center for Family (CFS) is a not-for-profit human service agency providing support and assistance to individuals with developmental disabilities and traumatic brain injuries throughout New York City, Long Island, the lower Hudson Valley region and New Jersey.

Steven Vernikoff, Executive Director

Research Centers

5586 UC Berkeley School of Social Welfare
Mental Health & Social Welfare Research Group
120 Haviland Hall #7400
Berkeley, CA 94720

510-642-4341
e-mail: spsegal@berkeley.edu
socialwelfare.berkeley.edu/mhswrg/mhswrg.html
Steven P Segal, Director

Audio Video

5587 Acquiring Courage: Audio Cassette Program for the Rapid Treatment of Phobias
New Harbinger Publications
5674 Shattuck Avenue
Oakland, CA 94609

510-652-2002
800-748-6273
Fax: 510-652-5472
e-mail: customerservice@newharbinger.com
newharbinger.com

ISBN: 1-879237-03-2

5588 Anxiety Disorders
American Counseling Association
6101 Stevenson Ave.
Alexandria, VA 22304

703-823-9800
800-347-6647
Fax: 703-823-0252
e-mail: webmaster@counseling.org
counseling.org

Increase your awareness of anxiety disorders, their symptoms, and effective treatments. Learn the effect these disorders can have on life and how treatment can change the quality of life for people presently suffering from these disorders. Includes 6 audiotapes and a study guide.

Robert L. Smith, Ph.D., NCC, FPPR, President
Brain Canfield, Treasurer
Richard Yep, Chief Executive Officer

5589 Fear of Illness
New Harbinger Publications
5674 Shattuck Avenue
Oakland, CA 94609

510-652-2002
800-748-6273
Fax: 510-652-5472
e-mail: customerservice@newharbinger.com
newharbinger.com

120 minute videotape that reduces fears arising from unexplained pain or symptoms; learn to relax while you desensitize to strange body sensations.

ISBN: 1-572240-15-6

5590 Flying
New Harbinger Publications
5674 Shattuck Avenue
Oakland, CA 94609

510-652-2002
800-748-6273
Fax: 510-652-5472
e-mail: customerservice@newharbinger.com
newharbinger.com

120 minute videotape that reduces fear to the point where you can take longer and longer flights; desensitize to the sensations of flying.

ISBN: 1-879237-90-3

5591 Heights
New Harbinger Publications
5674 Shattuck Avenue
Oakland, CA 94609

510-652-2002
800-748-6273
Fax: 510-652-5472
e-mail: customerservice@newharbinger.com
newharbinger.com

120 minute videotape that makes you feel more comfortable in high - rise buildings, on bridges, and on mountain roads.

ISBN: 1-879237-91-1

Web Sites

5592 Answers to Your Questions about Panic Disorder
750 First St. NE
Washington, DC 20002

202-336-5500
800-374-2721
www.apa.org/pubinfo/panic.html

The objects of the APA shall be to advance psychology as a science and profession and as a means of promoting health, education, and human welfare by: encouragement of psychology in all its branches in the broadest and most liberal manner, the promotion of research in psychology and the improvement fo research methods and conditions, and the improvement of the qualifications and usefulness of psychologists through high standards of ethics, conduct, education, and achievement.

Barry S. Anton, PhD, President
Bonnie Markham, Treasurer
Norman B. Anderson, CEO & VP

5593 Anxiety Disorders Association of America

Offers resources and information for persons with anxiety and stress-related disorders.

5594 Anxiety Panic Internet Resource
www.algy.com/anxiety/

It is the web's first and still best self-help resource for those with anxiety disorders, Panic attacks, phobias, extreme shyness, obsessive-compulsive behaviors, and generalized anxiety disrupt the lives of an estimated 15% of the population. It is a free grass-root website dedicated to providing information, relief, and support for those recovering from debilitating anxiety.

5595 Basic Guided Relaxation: Advanced Technique
1258 Eagle Crest Dr.
Oak Harbor, WA 98277

360-593-3833
e-mail: wellness@dstress.com
www.dstress.com/guided.htm

A guide to relaxation.
L. John Mason, Founder

5596 Causes of Anxiety and Panic Attacks
www.algy.com/anxiety/files/barlow.html

Provides information concerning phobias, what they are, the symptoms, and the effects of phobias.

5597 CyberPsych
www.cyberpsych.org

CyberPsych presents information about psychoanalysis, psychotherapy, and special topics such as anxiety disorder, the problematic use of alcohol, homophobia, and the traumatic effects of racism. CyberPsych is a nonprofit network which offers free web hosting and technical support for internet communication, to nonprofit groups and individuals.

5598 National Anxiety Foundation
3135 Custer Dr.
Lexington, KY 40517   www.lexington-on-line.com/naf.html

Endeavours to educate the public and professionals about anxiety through printed and electronic media. A volunteer, nonprofit entity.

Stephen Cox, President
Linda Vermon Blair, Vice-President
C. Todd Strecker, Secretary-Treasurer

5599 National Panic/Anxiety Disorder Newsletter
www.npadnews.com

e-mail: editor@npadnews.com
www.npadnews.com

We provide the most up to date material which is gathered from many resourced and contributors form all corners of the globe.

5600 Panic Disorder, Separation, Anxiety Disorder
www.klis.com/chandler/pamphlet/panic

Provides information about panic attacks and more, about what can be done and what medican treatments there are.

5601 Planetpsych
www.planetpsych.com

e-mail: webmaster@planetpsych.com
www.planetpsych.com

Planetpsych is an online resource for mental health information.

5602 Recovery Panic Anxiety
www.alt.recovery.panic.anxiety.self-help

An online support group t talk about anxiety recovery.

Book Publishers

5603 An End to Panic: Breakthrough Techniques for Overcoming Panic Disorder

Elke Zuercher-White, author

New Harbinger Publications
5674 Shattuck Avenue
Oakland, CA 94609

510-652-2002
800-748-6273
Fax: 510-652-5472
TTY: 800-652-1613
e-mail: customerservice@newharbinger.com
www.newharbinger.com

A state of the art treatment program covers breathing retraining, taking charge of fear-fueling thoughts, overcoming the fear of physical symptoms, coping with phobic situations, avoiding relapse, and living in the here and now.

232 pages Paperback
ISBN: 1-572241-13-6

5604 Anxiety & Phobia Workbook

Edmund J Bourne, author

New Harbinger Publications
5674 Shattuck Avenue
Oakland, CA 94609

510-652-2002
800-748-6273
Fax: 510-652-5472
TTY: 800-652-1613
e-mail: customerservice@newharbinger.com
www.newharbinger.com

This comprehensive guide is recommended to those struggling with anxiety disorders. Includes step-by-step instructions for the crucial cognitive-behavioral techniques that have given real help to hundreds of thousands of readers struggling with anxiety disorders.

448 pages 4th Edition
ISBN: 1-572244-13-5

5605 Anxiety Cure: An Eight-Step Program for Ge tting Well
John Wiley & Sons
10475 Crosspoint Boulevard
Indianapolis, IN 46256   877-762-2974
                                               Fax: 800-597-3299
                                                 www.wiley.com

A practical guide, written by a father and his two daughters, featuring a step-by-step program for curing the six main kinds of anxiety.

272 pages 2nd Edition
ISBN: 0-471464-87-2

Peter B. Wiley, Chairman
Stephen M. Smith, President & CEO
Ellis E. Cousens, Executive Vice President, Chief Fin

5606 Anxiety Disorders
Cambridge University Press
40 W 20th Street
New York, NY 10011   212-924-3900
                                                  800-872-7423
                                               Fax: 914-937-4712
                                        e-mail: marketing@cup.org
                                                        cup.org

This comprehensive text covers all the anxiety disorders found in the latest DSM and ICD classifications. Provides detailed information about seven principal disorders, including anxiety in the medically ill. For each disorder, the book covers diagnosis criteria, epidemiology, etiology and pathogenesis, clinical features, natural history and different diagnoses. Describes treatment approaches, both psychological and pharmacological.

354 pages

5607 Anxiety Disorders: Practioner's Guide
John Wiley & Sons
605 3rd Avenue
New York, NY 10058   212-850-6000
                                               Fax: 212-850-6008
                                          e-mail: info@wiley.com
                                                     wiley.com

210 pages
ISBN: 0-471931-12-8

Peter B. Wiley, Chairman
Stephen M. Smith, President & CEO
Ellis E. Cousens, Executive Vice President, Chief Fin

5608 Encyclopedia of Phobias, Fears, and Anxieties
Facts on File
11 Penn Plaza, Room M274
New York, NY 10001   212-290-8090
                                                  800-322-8755

500 pages

5609 Helping Your Anxious Child
New Harbinger Publications
5674 Shattuck Avenue
Oakland, CA 94609   510-652-2002
                                                  800-748-6273
                                               Fax: 510-652-5472
                                                TTY: 800-652-1613
                              e-mail: customerservice@newharbinger.com
                                              www.newharbinger.com

Step-by-step guide for parents of anxious children to help them overcome their fears and anxieties. Detailed strategies and techniques.

168 pages Paperback
ISBN: 1-572241-91-8

5610 It's Nobody's Fault: New Hope and Help for Difficult Children and Their Parents
ADD WareHouse
300 NW 70th Avenue
Plantation, FL 33317   954-792-8944
                                                  800-233-9273
                                               Fax: 954-792-8545
                                                 addwarehouse.com

This book explains that neither the parents nor children are causes of mental disorders and related problems.

184 pages

5611 Perfectionism: What's Bad About Being Too Good
Free Spirit Pub

With help for superkids, workaholics, type A's. straight A's, procrastinators, overacheivers, and caring adults, this book explains the differance between healthy ambition and unhealthy perfectionism and gives straight strategies for getting out of the perfectionist trap- from recognizing the symptoms to rewarding yourself for who you are, not what you do. It explains why some people become perfectionists, what it does to the body, and why girls are more prone to it, and more.

1999 144 pages

Miriam Adderholt, PhD, Author
Miriam Elliot, Author
Judy Galbraith, Author

5612 Psychological Trauma
American Psychiatric Press
1400 K Street, NW
Washington, DC 20005   202-682-6262
                                                  800-368-5777
                                               Fax: 202-789-2648
                                          e-mail: order@appi.org
                                                   www.appi.org

Epidemiology of trauma and post-tramatic stress disorder. Evaluation, neuroimaging, neuroendocrinology and pharmacology.

1998 206 pages

Robert E. Hales M.D, Editor-in-Chief
Rebecca D. Rinehart, Publisher
John McDuffie, Editorial Director

5613 Shy Children, Phobic Adults: Nature and Treatment of Social Phobia
American Psychological Press
1400 K Street, NW
Washington, DC 20005   202-682-6262
                                                  800-368-5777
                                               Fax: 202-789-2648
                                         e-mail: orders@appi.org
                                                   www.appi.org

Describes the similiarities and differences in the syndrome across all ages. Draws from the clinical, social and developmental literatures, as well as from extensive clinical experience. Illustrates the impact of developmental stage on phenomenology, diagnosis and assessment and treatment of social phobia.

1998 321 pages

Robert E. Hales M.D, Editor-in-Chief
Rebecca D. Rinehart, Publisher
John McDuffie, Editorial Director

Pamphlets

5614 5 Smart Steps to Less Stress
ETR Associates
PO Box 1830
Santa Cruz, CA 95061   831-438-4060
                                                  800-321-4407
                                               Fax: 800-435-8433

Steps to managing stress include: know what stresses you, manage your stress, take care of your body, take care of your feelings, ask for help.

5615 Anxiety Disorders
National Institute of Mental Health
6001 Executive Boulevard, Room 6200
Bethesda, MD 20892   301-443-4513
                                                      866-615-6464
                                                  Fax: 301-443-4279
                                                  TTY: 301-443-8431
                                         e-mail: nimhinfo@nih.gov
                                                  www.nimh.nih.gov

This brochure helps to identify the symptoms of anxiety disorders, explains the role of research in understanding the causes of
these conditions, describes effective treatments, helps you learn
how to obtain treatment and work with a doctor or therapist, and
suggests ways to make treatment more effective.

Francis Collins, M.D., Director
Tom Insel, Director

5616 Anxiety Disorders Fact Sheet
Center for Mental Health Services
PO Box 42490
Washington, DC 20015   800-789-2647
                                                  Fax: 301-984-8796
                                       e-mail: ken@mentalhealth.org
                                                  mentalhealth.org

This fact sheet presents basic information on the symptoms, formal diagnosis, and treatment for generalized anxiety disorder,
panic disorders, phobias, and post traumatic stress disorder.

3 pages

5617 Anxiety Disorders in Children and Adolescents
Center for Mental Health Services
PO Box 42490
Washington, DC 20015   800-789-2647
                                                  Fax: 301-984-8796
                                       e-mail: ken@mentalhealth.org
                                                  mentalhealth.org

This fact sheet defines anxiety disorders, identifies warning signs,
discusses risk factors, describes types of help available, and suggests what parents or other caregivers can do.

3 pages

5618 Families Can Help Children Cope with Fear, Anxiety
Center for Mental Health Services
PO Box 42490
Washington, DC 20015   800-789-2647
                                                  Fax: 301-984-8796
                                       e-mail: ken@mentalhealth.org
                                                  mentalhealth.org

This fact sheet defines conduct disorder, identifies risk factors,
discusses types of help available, and suggests what parents or
other caregivers responses should be to common signs of fear and
anxiety.

5619 Panic Attacks
ETR Associates
PO Box 1830
Santa Cruz, CA 95061   831-438-4060
                                                      800-321-4407
                                                  Fax: 800-435-8433

Describes causes of panic attacks, including genetics, stress, and
drug use; prevention and treatment, and how to stop a panic attack in its tracks.

Description

5620 PHOTOSENSITIVITY

Covers these related disorders: Photoallergic reaction, Phototoxic reaction

Involves the following Biologic System(s):
Dermatologic Disorders

Photosensitivity, sometimes referred to as sun allergy, is an abnormal reaction of the skin to sunlight or artificial light that is usually characterized by the rapid development of redness, swelling, tenderness, peeling, blistering, hives, or other skin irregularities. The skin reactions associated with photosensitivity are often induced by the interaction of light and certain substances known as photosensitizers that are ingested or applied directly to the skin. Such photosensitizers may include antibiotics, antifungal agents, and other drugs as well as some perfumes, soaps, dyes, and plants (e.g., buttercups, parsley, parsnips, mustard, etc.).

Particular wavelengths of light interact with photosensitizers to produce skin inflammations (dermatitis) that may be considered photoallergic or phototoxic. A photoallergic reaction is a delayed immune or allergic response of the skin that results from having been previously exposed to a photosensitizer and light. Such photosensitizers may include barbiturates, certain antibiotics such as tetracycline, and other medications as well as certain topical agents such as coal tar derivatives, perfume oils such as bergamot, etc. A phototoxic reaction is a nonimmune response to the accumulation of certain chemicals in the skin. This type of skin reaction may be similar in appearance to a severe sunburn; some individuals may develop hives or blisters. The initial inflammation is usually followed by abnormally increased skin pigmentation (hyperpigmentation). Phototoxic reactions result from high doses of certain photosensitizers that may cause photoallergic reactions in lower doses, as well as from additional chemical substances. Treatment includes the withdrawal of offending medications and other photosensitizers and sunlight avoidance. In addition, administration of antihistamines and topical corticosteroids may be effective in eliminating associated itching (pruritus).

Photosensitivity is also associated with certain disorders in children. Such disorders may include congenital erythropoietic porphyria (EPP), an autosomal recessive disorder that results from a deficiency of an enzyme. This particular enzyme is necessary for the synthesis of heme, which is the oxygen-carrying component of a certain protein (hemoprotein) found in the tissues of the body. Congenital erythropoietic porphyria develops within a few months of birth and is characterized by a severe sensitivity to light that may cause blistering eruptions on the skin, leading to severe scarring, abnormally increased skin pigmentation, and other skin irregularities. Children with this disorder may also have numerous other abnormalities. Erythropoietic protoporphyria is an autosomal dominant disorder that results from a deficiency of an enzyme that is also essential to the proper synthesis of heme. This disorder appears during early childhood and is characterized by pain, tingling, and a burning feeling upon exposure to sunlight. The skin may redden, swell, and form blisters or hives. In addition to having nail irregularities, children may develop fever and chills. Repeated exposure to sunlight may result in skin thickening and other

chronic associated irregularities; however, some children experience improvement during their preadolescent years. Treatment for these types of disorders includes the avoidance of direct sunlight and the use of protective clothing and appropriate sunscreens. In addition, the administration of sufficient quantities of beta-carotene to cause a light yellowing of the skin may be effective in reducing sensitivity to sunlight. Photosensitivity is a feature of many other disorders that may include Cockayne syndrome, xeroderma pigmentosum, hydroa vacciniforme, Rothmund-Thomson syndrome, and other diseases.

Occasionally, some individuals experience an unusual photosensitive reaction to sunlight in the absence of any apparent photosensitizer or associated disease. This type of photosensitivity is called polymorphous light eruption and is one of the most common sun-related skin problems. It is characterized by the appearance of hives or other itchy, rash-type reactions on exposed areas. Polymorphous light eruption usually occurs after a prolonged initial sun exposure in the spring or summer. The eruption may occur within hours or days of the exposure and may remain for hours, days, or weeks. Treatment may include oral or topical corticosteroid therapy. In addition, susceptible people are counseled to avoid the sun, wear protective clothing, and use sunscreen.

Individuals with certain types of photosensitivity may benefit from the cautious administration of photosensitizing drugs that enhance pigmentation of the skin (psoralens). In addition, certain types of phototherapy may be effective. Other treatment is symptomatic and supportive.

Government Agencies

5621 NIH/National Eye Institute
31 Center Drive MSC 2510
Bethesda, MD 20892
301-496-5248
e-mail: 2020@nei.nih.gov
www.nei.nih.gov

Conducts and supports research that helps prevent and treat eye diseases and other disorders of vision. This research leads to sight-saving treatments, reduces visual impairment and blindness, and improves the quality of life for people of all ages. NEI-supported research has advanced our knowledge of how the eye functions in health and disease.

Paul A Sieving M.D., Ph.D., Director

5622 NIH/National Institute of Arthritis and Mu sculoskeletal and Skin Diseases
1AMS Circle
Bethesda, MD 20892
301-402-4484
877-226-4267
Fax: 301-718-6366
TDD: 301-565-2966
e-mail: niamsinfo@mail.nih.gov
www.niams.nih.gov

The mission of the NIAMS, a part of the NIH, is to support research into the causes, treatment, and prevention of arthritis and musculoskeletal and skin diseases, the training of basic and clinical scientists to carry out this research, and the dissemination of information on research progress in these diseases.

Stephen I Katz MD PhD, Director
Robert H Carter MD, Deputy Director

5623 NIH/National Institute of Child Health and Human Development
31 Center Drive, Building 31
Bethesda, MD 20892
301-496-1333
Fax: 301-496-1104
www.nichd.nih.gov

Established in 1962 by congress, today the institute conducts and supports research on topics related to the health of children, adults, families and populations. Some of these topics include: developmental disabilities, growth and development, infant death, reproductive health and birth defects.

Jay H Hoofnagle, Director
Lisa Kaeser, Program & Public Liaison

National Associations & Support Groups

5624 American Academy of Pediatrics
141 Northwest Point Boulevard
Elk Grove Village, IL 60007

847-434-4000
800-433-9016
Fax: 847-434-8000
www.aap.org

The American Academy of Pediatrics and its member pediatricians are committed to the attainment of optimal physical, mental and social health and well-being for all infants, children, adolescents, and young adults.

Sandra Hassink, MD, FAAP, President

5625 Genetic Alliance
4301 Connecticut Avenue NW
Washington, DC 20008

202-966-5557
800-336-4363
Fax: 202-966-8553
e-mail: info@geneticalliance.org
www.geneticalliance.org

A coalition of voluntary genetic support groups, consumers and professionals addressing the needs of individuals and families affected by genetic disorders from a national perspective.

Sharon Terry, President
Natasha Bonhomme, Vice President of Strategic Develop
Vaughn ÿEdelson, Assistant Director of Health Commun

5626 March of Dimes Birth Defects Foundation
1275 Mamaroneck Avenue
White Plains, NY 10605

914-997-4488
888-663-4637
Fax: 914-428-8203
e-mail: answers@marchofdimes.com
www.marchofdimes.com

Partnership of volunteers and professionals dedicates to improving the health of babies by preventing birth defects and infant mortality. Over 100 chapters are located across the country and can be located through the National Office.

Jennifer L Howse, President

5627 Society for Pediatric Dermatology
8365 Keystone Crossing, Suite 107
Indianapolis, IN 46240

317-202-0224
Fax: 317-205-9481
e-mail: spd@hp-assoc.com
www.pedsderm.net

Objective is to promote, develop and advance education, research and care of skin disease in all pediatric age groups.

Kent Lindeman, Executive Director

Libraries & Resource Centers

California

5628 University of California, San Francisco Dermatology Drug Research
515 Spruce Street
San Francisco, CA 94115

415-476-4701
Fax: 415-502-4126
cc.ucsf.edu/people

Conducts clinical testing of new or existing pharmalogic agents used in the treatment of skin disorders.

John Koo, MD, Director

Delaware

5629 Delaware Division of Libraries for the Blind and Physically Handicapped
121 Duke of York Street
Dover, DE 19901

302-736-4748
800-282-8676
Fax: 302-736-6787
TDD: 302-739-4748
e-mail: bedpg@lib.de.us

Braille readers receive service from Philadelphia and Pennsylvania, summer reading program, Braille writer and cassettes.

Beth Landon, Librarian

Illinois

5630 Dermatology Information Network (DERMINFONET)
American Academy of Dermatology
PO Box 4014
Schaumburg, IL 60168

847-330-0230
Fax: 847-330-0050

Consists of a collection of dermatologic databases that are available to members on a subscription and/or purchase basis. These databases are designed to run on a wide variety of personal computers.

5631 National Library of Dermatologic Teaching Slides
American Academy of Dermatology
930 E. Woodfield Road
Shaumburg, IL 60173

847-240-1280
866-503-7546
Fax: 847-240-1859
www.aad.org

A collection of dermatologic teaching slides offering the most comprehensive series ever assembled. Each set offers a realistic presentation of classic clinical skin conditions encountered by the dermatologist.

New York

5632 Laboratory of Dermatology Research
Memorial Sloan-Kettering Cancer Center
1275 York Avenue
New York, NY 10065

212-639-2000
Fax: 212-639-3576
www.mskcc.org

Specific studies on the identification of skin disorders and dermatology.

Biijan Safai, MD, Head

5633 Rockefeller University Laboratory for Investigative Dermatology
1230 York Avenue
New York, NY 10065

212-327-8000
Fax: 212-327-7974

Research into skin disorders and the whole specialty of dermatology in general.

Barry Coller, Head

Research Centers

5634 University of California, San Francisco Dermatology Drug Research
515 Spruce Street
San Francisco, CA 94115

415-476-4701
Fax: 415-502-4126
cc.ucsf.edu/people

Conducts clinical testing of new or existing pharmalogic agents used in the treatment of skin disorders.

John Koo, MD, Director

Magazines

5635 International Journal of Dermatology
International Society of Dermatology
2323 North State Street #30
Bunnell, FL 32110
386-437-4405
Fax: 386-437-4427
e-mail: info@intsocderm.org
www.intsocderm.org

Focuses on information for dermatologists and the whole specialty of dermatology research and education.

10 times a year

Evangeline Handog, MD, President
Luca Borradori, Vice President
Paulo Rowilson Cunha, Vice President

5636 Journal of Dermatologic Surgery and Oncology
International Society for Dermatologic Surgery
930 N Meachan Road
Schaumburg, IL 60173
847-330-9830
Fax: 847-330-1135

Focuses on medical updates and information on dermatology.

Monthly

Newsletters

5637 Awareness
NAPVI
PO Box 317
Watertown, MA 2471
617-972-7441
800-562-6265
Fax: 617-972-7444
www.spedex.com/napvi

Newsletter offering regional news, sports and activities, conferences, camps, legislative updates, book reviews, audio reviews, professional question and answer column and more for the visually impaired and their families.

Quarterly

5638 DVH Quarterly
University of Arkansas at Little Rock
2801 S University Avenue
Little Rock, AR 72204
Fax: 501-663-3536

Offers information on upcoming events, conferences and workshops on and for visual disabilities. Book reviews, information on the newest resources and technology, educational programs, want ads and more.

Quarterly

Bob Brasher, Editor

5639 Dermatology Focus
Dermatology Foundation
1560 Sherman Avenue, Suite 870
Evanston, IL 60201
847-328-2256
Fax: 847-328-0509
e-mail: dfgen@dermatologyfoundation.org
dermatologyfoundation.org

Includes membership activities, research articles and lists recipients of foundation awards.

Quarterly

Bruce U. Wintroub, Chairman
Michael D. Tharp, M.D., President
Staurt R. Lessin, M.D., Vice President

5640 Dermatology World
American Academy of Dermatology
930 E. Woodfield Road
Schaumburg, IL 60173
847-240-1280
866-503-7546
Fax: 847-240-1859
www.aad.org/dw

Offers Academy members information outside the clinical realm. It carries news of government actions, reports of socioeconomic issues, societal trends and other events which impinge on the practice of dermatology.

Monthly

Brett M. Coldiron, MD, President
Elise A. Olsen, MD, Vice President
Suzanne M. Olbricht, MD, Secretary-Treasurer

5641 Progress in Dermatology
Dermatology Foundation
1560 Sherman Avenue, Suite 870
Evanston, IL 60201
847-328-2256
Fax: 847-328-0509
e-mail: dfgen@dermatologyfoundation.org
dermatologyfoundation.org

Bulletin offering information on research reports and clinical trials.

Quarterly

Bruce U. Wintroub, Chairman
Michael D. Tharp, M.D., President
Staurt R. Lessin, M.D., Vice President

Camps

5642 Camp Discovery
American Academy of Dermatology
930 E Woodfield Road
Schaumburg, IL 60173
847-240-1280
866-503-7546
Fax: 847-240-1859
e-mail: jmueller@aad.org
www.aad.org/dermatology-a-to-z/for-kids/camp-discove

A camp for young people with chronic skin conditions. There is no fee and transportation is provided. Three locations: Camp Horizon in Millville, PA, Camp Knutson in Crosslake, MN, and Camp Dermadillo in Burton, TX.

Brett M. Coldiron, MD, President
Elise A. Olsen, MD, Vice President
Suzanne M. Olbricht, MD, Secretary-Treasurer

Description

5643 PHYSICAL & SEXUAL ABUSE

Involves the following Biologic System(s):

Developmental/Behavioral/Psychiatric Disorders

Child abuse is a pervasive societal disease that has been gaining increasing recognition in the last 40 years. Maltreatment of children includes neglect, physical abuse and sexual abuse. In 1996, one million children were confirmed by protective US agencies as having been abused. Reporting figures since that time have been on the rise.

Neglect is the most common form of abuse, and covers a wide range of irresponsible behaviors that negatively impact the growth and well being of a child. Inadequate supervision may result in injury from falling, usage of a dangerous object such as a knife, scissors or other tools, or ingestion of toxic products and medications. Neglect may also include providing insufficient food, clothing and shelter for a child, which carries a high risk of malnutrition, illness, and poor emotional development. Parents or guardians who do not ensure proper medical care for their children are also negligent, particularly for children with chronic serious medical illnesses.

Physical abuse encompasses a wide range of symptoms but always involves purposeful injury inflicted on a child. Physical abuse can be difficult to identify, especially in toddlers, because children are prone to accidents and receive bruises and cuts as routine events. One key element in the diagnosis is ascertaining whether the injury could have happened the way it was reported. Another important clue is whether the child at a given developmental stage, could have performed the reported event. For example, a report of a six-month old who "fell" and broke his femur (thigh bone) should raise suspicion as a six-month old infant is too young to walk. Common abusive injuries include bruises from belts, hands or cords, burns from cigarettes or hot water immersion, fractures or brain injury from vigorous shaking and internal abdominal injuries from trauma to the back and abdomen. It is important for health care providers, or friends and family members, to record all injuries as a pattern may develop that will help diagnose the situation.

Sexual abuse occurs when a child is involved in sexual activities that he/she cannot fully comprehend, he/she cannot give consent to, or that violate societal norms. Common ages of abuse are between 9 and 12 years. Approximately 25 percent of women and 12 percent of men report histories of being sexually abused as children. Normal sexual play between children of similar age and developmental level can be distinguished from abuse by assessing disparity of age/development and the level of coercion involved. Abusive acts include fondling, intercourse, oral-genital and anal-genital contact, as well as voyeurism, exhibitionism and pornography. Perpetrators are more commonly male adults and adolescents, although women have been known to commit these crimes as well. This type of abuse is often very difficult to recognize because there are frequently no physical signs or symptoms and victims are reluctant and embarrassed to disclose the information. There is often a trusting and/or fearful relationship between the perpetrator and victim that binds the victim to secrecy. Certain telltale signs include inappropriate sexualized behaviors and language, and sexually transmitted diseases such as gonorrhea and chlamydia or symptoms such as discharge or bleeding. Physical evidence may include abrasions, hymenal tears, bruising, foul discharge or even pregnancy.

Professionals working with children, including teachers, social workers and health care providers are all mandated reporters, which means that if abuse is suspected they must report the family to the local protective service agency. It is critical to note that the burden of proof does not lie with the reporter, so even if there is a degree of uncertainty, one is required to act upon his or her concern.

Government Agencies

5644 Administration for Children & Families-Child Abuse and Neglect Prevention
Department of Health & Human Services
330 C Street SW, Room 2422
Washington, DC 20201
202-205-8618
Fax: 202-205-8221
www.acf.hhs.gov/programs/cb
Wade F Horn PhD, Assistant Secretary

National Associations & Support Groups

5645 AMT Children of Hope Foundation
c/o Nassau County Police Department
1490 Franklin Avenue
Mineola, NY 11501
516-781-3511
877-796-4673
Fax: 516-781-0691
www.amtchildrenofhope.com

Safe infant abandonment, nationwide, 24-hour crisis line. Confidential referrals to 'safe havens' and professional services.

Timothy Jaccard, Founder & President

5646 American Academy of Pediatrics
141 Northwest Point Boulevard
Elk Grove Village, IL 60007
847-434-4000
800-433-9016
Fax: 847-434-8000
www.aap.org

The American Academy of Pediatrics and its member pediatricians are committed to the attainment of optimal physical, mental and social health and well-being for all infants, children, adolescents, and young adults.

Sandra Hassink, MD, FAAP, President

5647 American Professional Society on the Abuse of Children
350 Poplar Avenue, PO Box 30669
Elmhurst,, IL 60126
843-764-2905
877-402-7722
Fax: 803-753-9823
e-mail: apsac@comcast.net
www.apsac.org

Dedicated to providing professional education which promotes effective, culturally sensitive and interdisciplinary approaches to the identification, intervention, treatment and prevention of child abuse and neglect.

Daphne Wright, National Operations Manager

5648 Child Abuse Prevention Association
503 E 23rd Street
Independence, MO 64055
816-252-8388
Fax: 816-252-1337
e-mail: capa@childabuseprevention.org
www.childabuseprevention.org

Mission is to prevent and treat all forms of child abuse by creating changes in individuals, families and society which strengthen relationships and promote healing.

Jenatta Issa, CEO
Tamara Tucker, Program Director
Diana Castillo, Resource/Communications Dierctor

5649 Child Welfare League of America
1726 M Street NW, Suite 500
Washington, DC 20036   202-688-4200
                                   Fax: 202-833-1689
                                        www.cwla.org

National nonprofit organization dedicated to developing and promoting policies and programs to protect America's children from
harm and strengthen America's families.

Shay Bilchik, President/CEO
Joyce Johnson, Public Relations

5650 Childhelp
Childhelp National Headquarters
15757 N 78th Street
Scottsdale, AZ 85260   480-922-8212
                                   Fax: 480-922-7061
                                  TDD: 800-2AC-HILD
                                      www.childhelp.org

Dedicated to meeting the physical, emotional and spiritual needs
of abused and neglected children through focusing its efforts and
resources upon treatment, prevention and research.

Sara O'Mara, CEO
Yvonne Federson, Co-Founder/President
John Rteid, Executive Director

5651 Childhelp National Child Abuse Hotline
15757 N. 78th Street, Ste B
Scottsdale,, AZ 85260   480-922-8212
                                       800-4AC-HILD
                                   Fax: 480-922-7061
                                  TDD: 800-2AC-HILD
                                e-mail: www.childhelp.org
                                      www.childhelp.org

Abuse crisis counseling and referral services available 24/7 with
assistance in over 140 languages.

5652 Children's Defense Fund
25 E Street NW
Washington, DC 20001   202-628-8787
                                       800-233-1200
                                   Fax: 202-662-3510
                          e-mail: cdfinfo@childrensdefense.org
                                  www.childrensdefense.org

Mission is to ensure every child a healthy start, a head start, a fair
start, a safe start and a moral start in life.

Mariane Wright-Edelman, President
DD Eisenberg, Child Advocate/Commissioner

5653 IVAT: Institute on Violence, Abuse and Tra uma
10065 Old Grove Road
San Diego, CA 92131   858-527-1860
                                   Fax: 858-527-1743
                                    www.ivatcenters.org

Formerly the Family Violence & Sexual Assault Institute. Shares
and disseminates vital information, improves networking among
professionals, and assists with program evaluation, consultation
and training that promotes violence-free living.

Robert Geffner PhD, President
Dawn Alley PhD, Community Relations & Outreach
Sandi C Morrison, Executive President

5654 KidsPeace National Centers/Hospital
5300 KidsPeace Drive
Orefield, PA 18069   610-799-8471
                                       800-854-3123
                           e-mail: admissions@kidspeace.org
                                      www.kidspeace.org

Counseling, info and referral services for children and youth in
crisis.

Richard Zelko, Executive Director

5655 KlaasKids Foundation for Children
PO Box 925
Sausalito, CA 94966   415-331-6867
                                   Fax: 415-331-5633
                              e-mail: info@klaaskids.org
                                      www.klaaskids.org

Established in 1994 to give meaning to the death of
twelve-year-old kidnap and murder victim Polly Hannah Klaas
and to create a legacy in her name that would be protective of
children for generations to come. The Foundation's mission is to
stop crimes against children.

Marc Klaas, President

5656 National Center for Missing & Exploited Children
Charles B Wang International Children's Building
699 Prince Street
Alexandria, VA 22314   703-224-2150
                                       800-843-5678
                                   Fax: 703-224-2122
                                     www.missingkids.com

Private, nonprofit organization, co-founded in 1984 by John
Walsh, whose son Adam was abducted and murdered. NCMEC
serves as a focal point in providing assistance to parents, children, law enforcement, schools and the community in recovering
missing children and raising public awareness about ways to help
prevent child abduction, molestation and sexual exploitation.
NCMEC spends 94 cents of every dollar directly on programs and
services.

Ernie Allen, CEO

**5657 National Center for Missing and Exploited Children: 24-hour
Hotline**

                                       800-843-5678
                                       800-THE-LOST

The primary means by which NCMEC serves as an information
clearinghouse and delivers technical assistance.

5658 National Child Pornography Tipline and Cyber Tipline
www.cybertipline.com

                                       703-224-2150
                                       800-843-5678
                                   Fax: 703-224-2122
                                     www.cybertipline.com

The National Center for Missing and Exploited Children, in conjunction with the US Postal Inspection Service, US Customs Service and the Federal Bureau of Investigation, serves as the
tipline, handling calls from individuals reporting the sexual exploitation of children through the production and distribution of
pornography. For online reporting visit the website.

5659 National Children's Advocacy Center
210 Pratt Avenue
Huntsville, AL 35801   256-533-5437
                                   Fax: 256-534-6883
                        e-mail: prevention@nationalcac.org
                                      www.nationalcac.org

A non profit organization that provides training, prevention, intervention and treatment services to fight child abuse and neglect.

Deborah Callins, Executive Director
JoAnn Jaco Plucker, Federal Programs Director

5660 National Children's Alliance
516 C Street NE
Washington, DC 20002   202-548-0090
                                       800-239-9950
                                   Fax: 202-548-0099
                              e-mail: info@nca-online.org
                                      www.nca-online.org

Nationwide nonprofit membership organization which promotes
and supports communities in providing a coordinated investigation and response to victims of severe child abuse.

Janet Fine, Executive Director
Julie Pape, Director Programs
Benjamin Murray, Director Member Services

5661 National Exchange Club Foundation
3050 Central Avenue
Toledo, OH 43606   419-535-3232
                                       800-924-2643
                                   Fax: 419-535-1989
                  e-mail: ÿÿÿinfo@nationalexchangeclub.org
                              www.nationalexchangeclub.org

667

Committed to making a difference in the lives of children, families and communities through its national project, the prevention of child abuse.

Dave Nershi, VP

5662 Prevent Child Abuse America
228 S Wabash Avenue
Chicago, IL 60604
312-663-3520
Fax: 312-939-8962
e-mail: mailbox@preventchildabuse.org
www.preventchildabuse.org

Mission is to prevent the abuse and neglect of the nation's children. Supports education and research.

Jim Hmurovich, President

5663 Project Cuddle
2973 Harbor Boulevard, # 326
Costa Mesa, CA 92626
714-432-9681
888-628-3353
Fax: 714-433-6815
e-mail: info@projectcuddle.org
www.projectcuddle.org

Safe infant abandonment, nationwide, 24-hour crisis line. All calls are confidential. Help in finding a safe, legal alternative to abandonment.

Debbe Magnusen, Owner

5664 Rape, Abuse and Incest National Network (RAINN)
1220 L Street, NW, Ste 505
Washington, DC 20036
202-544-3064
800-656-HOPE
Fax: 202-544-3556
e-mail: info@rainn.org
www.rainn.org

Operates a 24 hour national sexual assault hotline and carries out programs to prevent sexual assault, help victims and ensure that rapists are brought to justice.

Darcey West, Communications Manager
Chelsea Bowers, Membership Information

5665 Safe Place for Newborns
120 S 6th Street, Suite 1150
Minneapolis, MN 55402
414-447-3030
877-440-2229
Fax: 612-317-2899
e-mail: safeplace@safeplacefornewborns.com
www.safeplacefornewborns.com

Crisis line. Will provide a list of hospitals in Minnesota and Wisconsin which accept healthy babies up to three days old with no questions asked. Will provide information on other states with 'safe place' programs.

Laure Krupp, Executive Director

5666 Stop It Now! (DBA Child Sex Abuse Preventi on & Protection
351 Pleasant Street, Suite B-319
Northampton, MA 01060
413-587-3500
888-773-8368
Fax: 413-587-3505
e-mail: info@stopitnow.org
www.stopitnow.org

Deborah Donoran Rice, Executive Director

5667 The Kempe Center: For the Prevention & Tre atment of Child Abuse and Neglect
13123 E 16th Avenue B390
Aurora, CO 80045
303-864-5300
Fax: 303-837-2599
e-mail: questions@kempe.org
http://kempecenter.org

Provides education, clinical services and research on child abuse and neglect. Can provide referrals to local agencies.

Rob Clyman, Executive Director
Gene Liffick, Operations Director
Lindsey Zimmerman, Communications Director

5668 Youth Crisis Hotline
Youth Development International
PO Box 178408
San Diego, CA 92177
800-843-5200
http://hometown.aol.com/garnierlaw/hithome.html

Services for runaway/homeless youth, referrals to resources for abuse and crisis counseling.

State Agencies & Support Groups

Alaska

5669 Rid Alaska of Child Abuse
PO Box 35595
Juneau, AK 99803
800-478-4444
e-mail: Help@RIDAlaskaOfChildAbuse
www.ridalaskaofchildabuse.org

Nonprofit organization dedicated to providing resources and information, raising public awareness of the occurrence of child abuse, lessening the stigma placed on child sexual abuse victims/survivors, promoting child safety and abuse prevention programs, researching and posting safety tips and maintaining a website.

Debra Gerrish, President/State Coordinator
Tia M Holley, VP
Patti Fay Hickox, Treasurer/Secretary

Arizona

5670 Crisis Nursery
2334 East Polk Street
Phoenix, AZ 85006
602-273-7363
Fax: 602-244-1316
e-mail: cninfo1@crisisnurseryphx.com
www.crisisnurseryphx.org

Offers hope and support, through prevention and protection, to children in our community threatened with abuse and neglect. Since 1977, over 13,000 children have found a safe refuge at Crisis Nursery. Its mission is to provide a last resort for parents and families who are simply overwhelmed, a safe and healthy place for children who can no longer remain with their families, a temporary home for children who haven't one to call their own and a transitional placement with follow up for services.

Marsha Porter, Executive Director

California

5671 Child Sexual Abuse Treatment Program (Giar retto)
EMQ Children & Family Services
232 E Gish Road
San Jose, CA 95112
408-453-7616
e-mail: csc@emq.org
www.emq.org

Sexual abuse treatment center

F Jerome Doyle, CEO
Kristine Austin, Director Public Relations

Georgia

5672 Prevent Child Abuse Georgia
PO Box 3995
Atlanta, GA 30302
404-413-1281
800-244-5373
Fax: 404-413-1299
e-mail: feedback@pcageorgia.org
www.preventchildabusega.org

Private, statewide, community-based nonprofit organization with the sole mission of preventing child abuse and neglect.

Doug Middleton, Executive Director
Sonda Abernathy, College Facilities Manager
Frances Marine, Director of Communications

Rosie Allen, CEO

Illinois

5673 Prevent Child Abuse Illinois
528 S 5th Street, Suite 211
Springfield, IL 62701
217-522-1129
Fax: 217-522-0655
e-mail: rharley@preventchildabuseillinois.org
www.preventchildabuseillinois.org
Roy Harley, Executive Director

Indiana

5674 Prevent Child Abuse Indiana
3833 N Meridian Suite 101
Indianapolis, IN 46208
317-775-6439
888-542-7064
Fax: 317-775-6420
e-mail: Generalinfo.pcain@villages.org
www.pcain.org

Sandy Runkle, Manager

Iowa

5675 Prevent Child Abuse Iowa
505 Fifth Avenue, Suite 900
Des Moines, IA 50309
515-244-2200
Fax: 515-280-7835
e-mail: sscott@pcaiowa.org
www.pcaiowa.org
Stephen Scott, Executive Director

New York

5676 Child Abuse Prevention Project: Be'ad HaYeled (For the Sake of the Child)
Board of Jewish Education of Greater New York
135 West 50th Street
New York, NY 10020
212-582-9100
Fax: 646-472-5421
e-mail: admin@jbfcs.org
www.bjeny.org

Be'ad HaYeled was created in 1995 specifically for the Jewish community by the Board of Jewish Education of Greater New York and the Jewish Board of Family and Children's Services. Training workshops give educators, parents and communal workers the skills needed to recognize signs of abuse and to intervene in an effective and appropriate manner Halachically, clinically and legally. Additional programs deal with parenting methods, communication skills and other relevant family issues.

Martin Haber, President

5677 Prevent Child Abuse New York
33 Elk Street Suite 201
Albany, NY 12207
518-445-1273
Fax: 518-436-5889
e-mail: cdeyss@preventchildabuseny.org
www.preventchildabuseny.org

Not-for-profit agency whose singular mission is to prevent child abuse in all its forms. Prevent Child Abuse New York is a chartered state chapter of Prevent Child Abuse America.

Christine Deyss, Executive Director
Jennifer Matrazzo, Associate Executive Director

North Carolina

5678 Prevent Child Abuse North Carolina
3701 National Drive, Suite 211
Raleigh, NC 27612
919-829-8009
Fax: 919-832-0308
e-mail: info@preventchildabusenc.org
www.prventchildabusenc.org

Statewide not-for-profit organization with the mission of ending child abuse in the state of North Carolina.

Virginia

5679 Childhelp Children's Center of Virginia
11230 Waples Mill Road #105
Fairfax, VA 22030
703-208-1500
Fax: 703-208-1540
e-mail: mail@childhelpva.org
www.childhelpusa.org/regional/virginia2

Dedicated to meeting the physical, emotional and spiritual needs of abused and neglected children through focusing its efforts and resources upon treatment, prevention and research.

Stanley D Beder

Libraries & Resource Centers

5680 Child Welfare Information Gateway
Children's Burea/ACYF
1250 Maryland Avenue SW, 8th Floor
Washington, DC 20024
703-385-7565
800-394-3366
Fax: 703-385-3206
e-mail: info@childwelfare.gov
www.childwelfare.gov

The National Clearinghouse on Child Abuse and Neglect Information and the National Adoption Information Clearinghouse have consolidated and expanded to create the Child Welfare Information Gateway. It is a service of the US DHHS and provides access to information and resources to help protect children and strengthen families.

Research Centers

5681 National Center on Child Abuse Prevention Research
228 S Wabash Avenue
Chicago, IL 60604
312-663-3520
Fax: 312-939-8962
e-mail: ÿmailbox@preventchildabuse.org
www.preventchildabuse.org

Established with the support of the Skillman Foundation to increase understanding of the complex causes of child maltreatment, to evaluate the effectiveness of prevention programs, and to disseminate this information out into the field and public.

Gregory Hilton, Owner

Conferences

5682 Annual New York State Child Abuse Prevention Conference
33 Elk Street, Suite 201
Albany, NY 12207
518-445-1273
800-244-5373
Fax: 518-436-5889
e-mail: rreyes@preventchildabuseny.org
www.preventchildabuseny.org/conf06/

Presented by Prevent Child Abuse New York, a not-for-profit agency whose singular mission is to prevent child abuse in all its forms. PCANY is a chartered state chapter of Prevent Child Abuse America. Conference attendees include those who work in home-based and center-based family support programs, child abuse prevention and child protective services, intervention and treatment, health care and mental health, schools, religious and civic organizations, and parents, themselves.

Christine Deyss, Executive Director
Robin Christenson, President
Dean Geesler, Vice President

Audio Video

5683 Break the Silence: Kids Against Child Abuse
The Health Connection
55 W Oak Ridge Drive
Hagerstown, MD 21740
301-393-3270
800-765-6955
Fax: 888-294-8405
www.adventistbookcenter.com/resources/health-connect

Jane Seymore explains physical abuse, sexual abuse and neglect. Animation illustrates each story. All the stories end happily, and the main point is that children should tell a trusted adult. 28 minutes. Grades 1-5.
1994

5684 I Am the Boss of My Body: Preventing Child Sexual Abuse
The Health Connection
55 W Oak Ridge Drive
Hagerstown, MD 21740
301-393-3270
800-765-6955
Fax: 888-294-8405
www.adventistbookcenter.com/resources/health-connect

Children feel empowered when they see this video and learn that they have the authority and the right to say no to any touch that makes them feel strange. Grades 1-4.
1999 18 Minutes

Web Sites

5685 American Professional Society on the Abuse of Children
1706 E. Broad Street
Columbus, OH 43203
614-827-1321
877-402-7722
Fax: 614-251-6005
e-mail: apsac@apsac.org
www.apsac.org

Dedicated to providing professional education which promotes effective, culturally sensitive and interdisciplinary approaches to the identification, intervention, treatment and prevention of child abuse and neglect.

Frank E. Vandevort, President
Tricia Gardner, Vice President
Michael L. Haney, Ph.D., Executive Director

5686 Bikers Against Child Abuse
www.bacausa.com

Has the intent to create a safer environment for abused children. An established, united body of bikers in a stand to empower children to not feel afraid of the world in which they live. They work in conjunction with local officials who are already in place to protect children.

Scootr , President
Pipes , Vice President

5687 Child Abuse Legislation
www.childabuse.com/legislat.htm

Prevention through education and awareness.

5688 Child Abuse Prevention Network
child-abuse.com

For professionals in the field of child abuse and neglect. Child maltreatment, physical abuse, psychological maltreatment, neglect, sexual abuse and emotional abuse and neglect are the key areas of concern. Provides unique and powerful tools for all workers to support the identification, investigation, treatment, adjudication and prevention of child abuse and neglect.

5689 Child Abuse Quilts: Revealing and Healing the Pain of Child Abuse
mbgoodman.tripod.com/caq/caq1.html

Site shows 28 quilts made dealing with the subject of child abuse, child abuse prevention and violence against children. Some of the quiltmakers knew the pain of abuse first hand, others knew it through the eyes of others, often close family members. Quilts are displayed in the hope that each person who sees them will leave re-awakened to the tragedy of child abuse and resolved to prevent it.

5690 Child Abuse.com
1231 W. Northern Lights Blvd, STE 458
Anchorage, AL 99503
www.childabuse.com

Comprehensive resource bringing awareness and education in preventing child abuse and related issues. The site was created to inform, support and encourage those dealing with any aspect of child abuse, in a positive non-threatening environment.

5691 Child Trauma Academy
www.childtraumaacademy.com

Provides information on free online courses that offer creative and practical approaches to understanding and working with maltreated children.

5692 Children's Bureau
1250 Maryland Avenue, SW Eighth Floor
Wasington, DC 20024
www.acf.hhs.gov/programs/cb

Is responsible for programs that promote the economic and social well-being of families, chidren, individuals, and communities. Programs aim to achieve the following: families and individuals empowered to increase their own economic independence and productivity, and strong healthy, supportive commuities that have a positive impact on the quality of life and the development of children.

Joe Bock, Director/Commissioner

5693 Children's House
child-abuse.com/childhouse/

An interactive resource center and meeting place for the exchange of information that serves the well-being of children.

5694 Connect for Kids
Benton Foundation
P.O. Box 45372
Westlake, OH 44145
440-250-5563
e-mail: info@connectingforkids.org
www.connectforkids.org

Family-friendly politics and information on how to connect with hundreds of groups working on behalf of children.

Kathy Nash, President
Andrea Campesino, Secretary
Rebecca Baker, Treasurer

5695 Intrafamilial (Incest) Abuse Resources
www.vachss.com/help_text/incest.html

Many resources on the subject of child abuse, both physical and sexual.

5696 KidsPeace
4085 Independence Drive
Schnecksville, PA 18078
800-257-3223
e-mail: kpinfo@KidsPeace.org
www.kidspeace.org

Counseling, info and referral services for children and youth in crisis.

L. Richard Plunkett, Chairman
Larry Bell, Vice Chairman
William R. Isemann, President/ CEO

5697 Making Daughters Safe Again
mdsa-online.org

Is the only organization in the world specializing in mother-daughter sexual abuse. We are also distinguished by the innovative online group experience we provide for survivors.

5698 National Council on Child Abuse & Family Violence
1025 Connecticut Avenue NW, Suite 1000
Washington, DC 20036   202-429-6695
Fax: 202-521-3479
e-mail: info@nccafv.org
www.nccafv.org

Providing intergenerational violence prevention services since 1984.

5699 Pandora's Box
www.prevent-abuse-now.com

Offers more than 270 pages of resource information on child abuse prevention and child protection.

5700 Prevent Child Abuse America
228 South Wabash Avenue, 10th Floor
Chicago, IL 60604   312-663-3520
800-244-5373
Fax: 312-939-8962
e-mail: mailbox@preventchildabuse.org
www.preventchildabuse.org

Providing and inspiring hope to everyone involved in the effort to prevent the abuse and neglect of our nations children. Working with 40 statewide chapters to provide leadership in promoting and implementing prevention efforts at both the national and local levels.

Fred M. Riley, Chair
David Rudd, Vice Chair
James Hmurovich, President/ CEO

5701 Prevent Child Abuse California
P.O. Box 6400
Columbia, MD 21045   410-381-0911
Fax: 410-381-0924
www.pca.org

Mission is to prevent child abuse in all its forms by maximizing resources throughout the state of California.

Caren Cooper, President
Thomas Gorsuch, Vice President
Cindy Jacisin, Secretary

5702 Rape, Abuse and Incest National Network (RAINN)
1220 L Street, NW, Suite 505
Washington, DC 20005   202-544-3064
Fax: 202-544-3556
e-mail: info@rainn.org
www.rainn.org

Operates a 24 hour national sexual assault hotline and carries out programs to prevent sexual assault, help victims and ensure that rapists are brought to justice.

Regan Burke, Chairperson
Scott Berkowitz, President and Founder
Cybele Daley, Treasurer

5703 Sibling Abuse Survivors' Information & Adv ocacy Network
www.sasian.org

Provides information about problems associated with domestic sibling incest abuse.

5704 Stop Child Abuse Now
www.efn.org/~scan/scan.html

Is a nonprofit organization dedicated to stopping child abuse of all forms, and improving the lives of survivors of all types of abuse and loss. By speaking out about abuse, we increase the public's awareness of the prevalence of abuse. Our goal is to join with other organizations and individuals who wish to ultimately put a stop to child abuse.

Book Publishers

5705 A Child Called It: One Child's Courage to Survive
Dave Pelzer, author

Health Communications, Inc (HCI)
3201 SW 15th Street
Deerfield Beach, FL 33442   954-360-0909
800-441-5569
Fax: 954-360-0034
www.hci-online.com

The author's true story of abuse he suffered as a child.
ISBN: 1-558743-66-9

5706 Body Language of the Abused Child
Jacqueline A Rankin, author

Rankin File/Signature Book Printing
8041 Cessna Avenue
Gaithersburg, MD 20879   301-258-8353
Fax: 301-670-4147
e-mail: book@sbpbooks.com
www.signaturebook.com/Books/rankin.htm

Uses body language to identify a suspected victim.
1999 271 pages Paperback
ISBN: 1-887711-06-6

5707 It's My Body
Lory Freeman, author

Parenting Press
PO Box 75267
Seattle, WA 98175   206-364-2900
800-992-6657
Fax: 206-364-0702
www.parentingpress.com

Helps adults and preschool children talk about sexual abuse together. Introduces touching codes children can use for their protection. Ages 3-8.
32 pages Paperback
ISBN: 1-403408-96-3

5708 My Body is Mine, My Feelings are Mine
Susan Hoke, author

YouthLight
714 Cove Trail, PO Box 115
Chapin, SC 29036   800-209-9774
Fax: 803-345-0888
e-mail: yl@sc.rr.com
www.youthlightbooks.com

For K-5th grade. First part to be read to children, the second part teaches adults how to educate children about body safety. Sexual victimization can be prevented through explanation of how to identify inappropriate touching and what to do about it.
77 pages Paperback

5709 Out of Harm's Way: A Parent's Guide to Pro tecting Young Children from Sexual Abuse
Janie Hart-Rossi, author

Parenting Press
PO Box 75267
Seattle, WA 98175   206-364-2900
800-992-6657
Fax: 206-364-0702
e-mail: office@parentingpress.com
www.parentingpress.com

An authoritative and objective look at child sexual abuse, which can be used at home and in school, or as a complement to existing school safety curricula. It describes how community members or extended family members might groom a child for abuse, as well as how to watch for such grooming and how to discuss it with children.

32 pages Paperback
Homer J Henderson, Operations Manager

5710 Something Happened and I'm Scared to Tell

Patricia Kehoe PhD, author

Parenting Press
PO Box 75267
Seattle, WA 98175   206-364-2900
800-992-6657
Fax: 206-364-0702
www.parentingpress.com

With the help of a friendly lion, a young sexual abuse victim is able to talk about sexual abuse and recover self-esteem. A gentle and positive approach to reassure children. Ages 3-7.

32 pages Paperback
ISBN: 0-943990-28-9

5711 Soul Murder Revisited

Leonard Shengold, author

Yale University Press
PO Box 209040
New Haven, CT 06520   203-432-0960
800-405-1619
Fax: 203-432-0948
e-mail: marketing@yale.edu.
yalepress.yale.edu/yupbooks

Further reflections on how abuse occurs and its consequences. Discusses the psychopathology of soul murder and appropriate therapy for victims.

2000 336 pages Paperback
ISBN: 0-300086-99-7

John Donatich, Director

5712 Treating Abused and Traumatized Children

Eliana Gil, author

Guilford Press
72 Spring Street
New York, NY 10012   800-365-7006
Fax: 212-966-6708
e-mail: info@guilford.com
www.guilford.com

The author presents a program combining play, art, and expressive therapies, with strategies from cognitave-behvior therapy and family therapy, as she demonstrates how to tailor the treatment to the needs of each child. Paperback or e-book.

2006 254 pages Paperback
ISBN: 1-593853-34-1

Bob Matloff, President
Seymour Weingarten, Editor-in-Chief

5713 Trouble with Secrets

Karen Johnson, author

Parenting Press
PO Box 75267
Seattle, WA 98175   206-364-2900
800-992-6657
Fax: 206-364-0702
www.parentingpress.com

Helps children distinguish between secrets that should be kept and those that shouldn't.

32 pages Paperback
ISBN: 0-943990-22-X

Newsletters

5714 APSAC Advisor
American Profess. Society on the Abuse of Children
1706 E. Broad Street
Columbus, OH 43203   614-827-1321
877-402-7722
Fax: 614-251-6005
e-mail: apsac@apsac.org
www.apsac.org

News journal for professionals in the field of child abuse and neglect. It provides succint, data-based articles that keep professionals informed of the latest developments in policy and practice in the field of child maltreatment.

Frank E. Vandevort, President
Tricia Gardner, Vice President
Michael L. Haney, Ph.D., Executive Director

5715 Lookin' Up
Prevent Child Abuse America
228 South Wabash Avenue, 10th Floor
Chicago, IL 60604   312-663-3520
800-244-5373
Fax: 312-939-8962
e-mail: mailbox@preventchildabuse.org
www.preventchildabuse.org

Newsletter of Prevent Child Abuse America.

Quarterly
Fred M. Riley, Chair
David Rudd, Vice Chair
James Hmurovich, President/ CEO

Pamphlets

5716 Understanding SBS/Shaken Impact Syndrome B rochure
National Center on Shaken Baby Syndrome
1433 N 1075 W Ste 110
Farmington, UT 84025   801-447-9360
888-273-0071
Fax: 801-447-9364
e-mail: mail@dontshake.com
www.dontshake.com

Information brochure on shaken baby syndrome.
Jill Moore, Chairperson
Lori Frasier, Vice Chairperson
Ryan Steinbeigle, Executive Director

Description

5717 PICA

Involves the following Biologic System(s):

Developmental/Behavioral/Psychiatric Disorders

Pica is a type of eating disorder characterized by the recurrent or chronic ingestion of nonfood or nonnutritive substances such as dirt, flaking paint or plaster, clay, charcoal, ashes, wool, and other nonfoods. Although this psychological disorder usually commences during the first or second year of life, some children are affected during infancy. The pattern should last at least one month to fit the diagnosis of pica. Pica is often self-limiting with resolution occurring during the childhood years; however, sometimes it may persist into adolescence or adulthood. If the symptoms associated with pica occur initially in older children or adults (e.g., pregnant women), this is usually indicative of a nutritional deficiency, such as iron or zinc, rather than a psychological disorder.

Children who are mentally retarded are particularly susceptible to development of this unusual disorder. Other factors that may influence the evolution of pica include environmental influences such as family discord, lack of or ineffective nurturing, and nutritional and emotional neglect. In addition, pica is sometimes associated with certain psychiatric disorders.

Children who eat nonfood or nonnutritive substances may be at risk of developing certain types of parasitic infections. For example, the ingestion of dirt (geophagia) may result in toxocariasis, an infection resulting from the spread of the larvae of the common roundworm (Toxocara canis) throughout the body. Symptoms of toxocariasis are often mild and may include fever, weakness, and discomfort. Other children may develop a cough, wheezing, enlarged liver (hepatomegaly), and eye lesions. In addition, another parasitic infection known as toxoplasmosis may develop from dirt ingestion. This common parasitic infection is caused by Toxoplasma gondii and may produce no symptoms or may sometimes be characterized by rash, fever, and other mononucleosis-type symptoms. In individuals with compromised immune systems, toxoplasmosis may result in more serious, widespread disease. Children who eat paint, paint dust, or paint flakes are at risk of developing lead poisoning that may damage the central nervous system, red blood cells, and digestive system.

Any nutritional deficiencies and other medical problems, such as lead toxicity, should be addressed. Treatment emphasizes psychosocial, environmental, and family education approaches. Nutritional supplements may be considered.

National Associations & Support Groups

5718 American Academy of Pediatrics
141 Northwest Point Boulevard
Elk Grove Village, IL 60007

847-434-4000
800-433-9016
Fax: 847-434-8000
www.aap.org

The American Academy of Pediatrics and its member pediatricians are committed to the attainment of optimal physical, mental and social health and well-being for all infants, children, adolescents, and young adults.

Sandra Hassink, MD, FAAP, President

5719 International Association of Eating Disorders Professionals Foundation
PO Box 1295
Pekin, IL 61555

309-346-3341
800-800-8126
Fax: 775-239-1597
e-mail: iaedpmembers@earthlink.net
www.iaedp.com

Well-known for providing first-quality education and high-level training standards to an international multidisciplinary group of healthcare treatment providers who treat the full spectrum of eating disorder problems.

Emmett R Bishop MD, President
Bonnie Harken, Managing Director

5720 NIH/National Institute of Mental Health Eating Disorders Program
6001 Executive Boulevard, Room 8184
Bethesda, MD 20892

301-443-4513
Fax: 301-443-4279

5721 National Alliance for the Mentally Ill
3803 N Fairfax Drive, Suite 100
Arlington, VA 22203

703-524-7600
888-999-6264
Fax: 703-524-9094
TDD: 703-516-7227
e-mail: info@nami.org
www.nami.org

NAMI is a nonprofit, grassroots, self-help, support and advocacy organization of consumers, families and friends of people with severe mental illness, such as schizophrenia, bipolar disorder, major depressive disorder, obsessive compulsive disorder, anxiety disorders, autism and other severe and persistent mental illnesses that affect the brain.

Suzanne Vogel-Scibilia MD, President

5722 National Eating Disorders Association (NED A)
603 Stewart Street, Suite 803
Seattle, WA 98101

206-382-3587
800-931-2237
Fax: 206-829-8501
e-mail: info@NationalEatingDisroders.org
www.nationaleatingdisorders.org

Dedicated to the elimination of eating disorders through prevention efforts, education, referral and support services, advocacy, training and research. Offers free information and referrals as well as educational curriculum and materials for sale. A toll free information & referral helpline is also available, linking more than 1,200 callers per month to vital information and life-saving treatment.

Lynn S Grefe, CEO
Lynn S Grefe, Chief Executive Officer
Tracy Kahlo, Chief Operating Officer

5723 National Mental Health Association
2000 N Beauregard Street, 6th Floor
Alexandria, VA 22311

703-684-7722
800-969-6642
Fax: 703-684-5968
TTY: 800-433-5959
www.mentalhealthamerica.net

Addresses all aspects of mental health and mental illness. NMHA with over 340 affiliates works to improve the mental health of all Americans.

David Shern, CEO

5724 National Mental Health Consumers' Self-Help Clearinghouse
1211 Chestnut Street, Suite 1207
Philadelphia, PA 19107

215-751-1810
800-553-4539
Fax: 215-636-6312
e-mail: info@mhselfhelp.org
www.mhselfhelp.org

Offers information, support and appropriate referrals; and promotes public and professional education. Provides networking for those with special interests related to albinism. Promotes and supports research and funding that will improve diagnosis and management of albinism and hypopigmentation.

Joseph Rogers, Executive Director & Founder

Web Sites

5725 Eating Disorder Referrals
www.eating-disorder-referral.com/pica.php

866-690-7238
www.eating-disorder-referral.com/pica.php

A free referral resource with listings across the nation. Can also access by phone, toll free at 866-323-5608

5726 KidsHealth for Parents
kidshealth.org/parent/emotions/behavior/pica.html

General overview of pica.

Neil Izenberg, MD, Editor-in-Chief & Founder

5727 Pica Information Page
archive.tobacco.org/resources/health/pica

A small group of citizens that seeks to alert the public about a new category of hazardous waste.

Description

5728 PINWORM (ENTEROBIUS VERMICULARIS)

Synonyms: Enterobiasis, Oxyuriasis, Threadworm

Involves the following Biologic System(s):

Infectious Disorders

Pinworm infection (enterobiasis) refers to a common condition in which small, white, parasitic worms (Enterobius vermicularis) infect the human intestinal tract. Such infection results from ingestion of parasitic eggs. The eggs hatch in the stomach, and the larvae then typically migrate to and grow within the upper part of the large intestine (cecum). On rare occasions, pinworms may migrate to the vagina of affected girls, potentially causing such symptoms as vaginal irritation or itching. Pinworms can also cause appendicitis, cystitis (infection of the urinary tract), and diverticulitis (inflammation from out-pouchings in the colon (large intestinal tract).

At night, pinworms migrate from the intestines to the anal region where they deposit their eggs, potentially causing itching (pruritus), irritation, and sleeplessness. Scratching often results in reinfestation from ingestion of eggs that become imbedded under the fingernails and are inadvertently deposited in the mouth. Parasitic eggs are also often deposited from the anal area onto clothing, bedding, furniture, or toys, where they may then be transferred from the fingers to the mouth, causing reinfection or infection of others. In addition, in some cases, eggs may be inhaled from the air and swallowed. Parasitic eggs may remain viable for up to three weeks at regular room temperature.

The diagnosis of enterobiasis is made by detecting parasitic eggs or pinworms. The eggs or worms may be obtained by pressing sticky tape against the perianal region of affected children during early morning hours before the children awaken. The tape is then examined under a microscope to verify the presence of pinworms or eggs. In addition, pinworms may sometimes be detected by the naked eye. Treatment may include the administration of drugs that destroy pinworms (anthelmintic drugs), such as pyrantel pamoate or mebendazole, and, in some patients, topical anti-itch ointments that help relieve itching and irritation. Anthelmintic medications should also be given to all other members of the household. Handwashing after going to the bathroom and before meals is critical. Linens should be washed thoroughly.

Enterobiasis is a very common infection that may occur in individuals of all ages. However, children between the ages of five to 14 years are most commonly affected.

Government Agencies

5729 NIH/National Institute of Allergy and Infectious Diseases
6610 Rockledge Drive, MSC 6612
Bethesda, MD 20892
301-496-5717
866-284-4107
Fax: 301-402-3573
TDD: 800-877-8339
e-mail: ocposfoffice@niaid.nih.gov
www.niaid.nih.gov

Conducts and supports basic and applied research to better understand, treat, and ultimately prevent infectious, immunologic, and allergic diseases.

Anthony S Fauci MD, Director

5730 NIH/National Institute of Child Health and Human Development
31 Center Drive, Building 31
Bethesda, MD 20892
301-496-1333
Fax: 301-496-1104
www.nichd.nih.gov

Established in 1962 by congress, today the institute conducts and supports research on topics related to the health of children, adults, families and populations. Some of these topics include: developmental disabilities, growth and development, infant death, reproductive health and birth defects.

Jay H Hoofnagle, Director
Lisa Kaeser, Program & Public Liaison

National Associations & Support Groups

5731 American Academy of Pediatrics
141 Northwest Point Boulevard
Elk Grove Village, IL 60007
847-434-4000
800-433-9016
Fax: 847-434-8000
www.aap.org

The American Academy of Pediatrics and its member pediatricians are committed to the attainment of optimal physical, mental and social health and well-being for all infants, children, adolescents, and young adults.

Sandra Hassink, MD, FAAP, President

5732 World Health Organization
Avenue Appia 20
CH-1211 Geneva 27,
Switzerland
www.who.int

WHO is the directing and coordinating authority for health within the United Nations system.

Dr Margaret Chan, Director General

Web Sites

5733 KidsHealth for Parents
www.kidshealth.org

Signs, symptoms, doagnosis, and treatment of pinworms.

Neil Izenberg, MD, Editor-in-Chief & Founder

5734 MayoClinic.com
www.mayoclinic.com/health/pinworm/DS00687

Introduction, risk factors, prevention and treatment of pinworms.

Pamphlets

5735 Pinworm Infection
CDC
13400 E. Shea Blvd.
Scottsdale, AZ 85259
480-301-8000
800-446-2279
www.mayoclinic.org/about-mayo-clinic

Pinworm infection factsheet provided by the CDC.

Description

5736   PITYRIASIS ROSEA

Involves the following Biologic System(s):

Dermatologic Disorders, Infectious Disorders

Pityriasis rosea is an inflammatory skin condition that may develop at any age but mostly commonly affects children and young adults. In some cases, the onset of the condition may be preceded by certain generalized symptoms, such as fever, inflammation of the throat (pharyngitis), and muscle and joint pain (myalgia and arthralgia). Pityriasis rosea typically begins with the development of a single oval or round patch known as a herald patch. This patch is usually red, pink, or light brown with a raised border and is covered with fine scales. A herald patch varies in diameter from one to 10 centimeters and may occur anywhere on the body. About five to 10 days after the appearance of the herald patch, there is a widespread eruption of similar, smaller patches (lesions), particularly on the torso and upper arms and thighs. These lesions, which are less than one centimeter in diameter, are usually slightly raised, oval or round, and red, pink, or light brown. In addition, they may be scaly and tend to peel. Lesions may continue to appear over several days and develop on other areas of the body, such as the forearms and calves, face, and scalp. The lesions are typically distributed along the subtle lines in the skin that indicate the direction of skin fibers (Langer's or cleavage lines). Some individuals with the condition may experience no associated symptoms (asymptomatic). Others may experience mild to severe itching (pruritus). Pityriasis rosea is a self-limited condition that has a duration of approximately two to 12 weeks, with an average of approximately four to five weeks. As skin lesions heal, affected areas may have abnormally increased or diminished pigmentation (postinflammatory hyperpigmentation or hypopigmentation) that gradually resolves after several weeks or months.

If individuals with pityriasis rosea experience no associated symptoms, treatment may not be necessary. Those with widespread lesions and scaling may benefit from using a cream that softens the skin (emollient). Associated itching may be relieved by lubricating lotions that contain the natural compounds camphor or menthol or medicated skin creams, such as a nonfluorinated topical corticosteroid. Certain medications taken by mouth such as oral antihistamines may help those who experience bothersome itching while attempting to sleep. Antihistamines, which are medications that often induce drowsiness, reduce the effects of histamine, a chemical that is released during allergic inflammatory reactions.

The cause of pityriasis rosea is unknown. However, many researchers speculate that the condition results from infection with a viral agent.

Government Agencies

5737   NIH/National Institute of Arthritis and Musculoskeletal and Skin Diseases
1AMS Circle
Bethesda, MD 20892

301-402-4484
877-226-4267
Fax: 301-718-6366
TDD: 301-565-2966
e-mail: niamsinfo@mail.nih.gov
www.niams.nih.gov

The mission of the NIAMS, a part of the NIH, is to support research into the causes, treatment, and prevention of arthritis and musculoskeletal and skin diseases, the training of basic and clinical scientists to carry out this research, and the dissemination of information on research progress in these diseases.

Stephen I Katz MD PhD, Director
Robert H Carter MD, Deputy Director

National Associations & Support Groups

5738   American Academy of Dermatology (AAD)
930 E. Woodfield Roa, PO Box 4014
Schaumburg, IL 60173

847-240-1280
866-503-7546
Fax: 847-240-1859
e-mail: mrc@aad.org
www.aad.org

Dedicated to achieving high quality dermatologic care for everyone which encompasses: responsiveness, unification and representation of the specialty, and excellence in patient care, education and research.

Ronald Moy MD, President
Suzanne Connolly, VP
Robert Greenberg, Secretary/Treasurer

5739   American Academy of Pediatrics
141 Northwest Point Boulevard
Elk Grove Village, IL 60007

847-434-4000
800-433-9016
Fax: 847-434-8000
www.aap.org

The American Academy of Pediatrics and its member pediatricians are committed to the attainment of optimal physical, mental and social health and well-being for all infants, children, adolescents, and young adults.

Sandra Hassink, MD, FAAP, President

5740   Society for Pediatric Dermatology
8365 Keystone Crossing, Suite 107
Indianapolis, IN 46240

317-202-0224
Fax: 317-205-9481
e-mail: spd@hp-assoc.com
www.pedsderm.net

Objective is to promote, develop and advance education, research and care of skin disease in all pediatric age groups.

Kent Lindeman, Executive Director

Web Sites

5741   DermNet NZ: The Dermatology Resource
www.dermnetnz.org

Information about the skin from the New Zealand Dermatological Society.

Marius Rademaker, Chairperson
Anthony Young, Secretary
Sandra Winhoven, Treasurer

Pamphlets

5742 Pityriasis Rosea
American Academy of Dermatology
PO Box 4014
Schaumburg, IL 60168

847-240-1280
866-503-7546
Fax: 847-240-1859
e-mail: mrc@aad.org
www.aad.org

Discusses the appearance, symptoms, and causes of this common rash. Diagnosis and treatment are also explained.

Pkgs of 50

Brett M. Coldiron, President
Elise A. Olsen, MD, Vice President
Suzanne M. Olbricht, Secretary-Treasurer

Description

5743 PNEUMONIA

Involves the following Biologic System(s):

Infectious Disorders, Respiratory Disorders

Pneumonia refers to a group of disorders characterized by an acute inflammation of the lungs. The causes of pneumonia are many and may include infection by certain bacteria, viruses, bacteria-like organisms, fungi, yeasts, and protozoa. In addition, noninfectious causes include the inhalation (aspiration) of food or other substances into the airway and lungs, an abnormal response of the immune system to certain substances (hypersensitivity reaction), and an inflammatory response to radiation or certain drugs. Pneumonia may also result as a complication of surgery or injury, due to the impaired ability to cough, breathe deeply, or expel mucus.

Pneumonia in very young children is most commonly caused by certain respiratory viruses, such as RSV, or respiratory syncytial virus; influenza; parainfluenza (the virus that causes croup); and adenoviruses. Symptoms and findings associated with this type of pneumonia in infants and young children may include cough, nasal discharge, fever, rapid breathing (tachypnea), or a bluish color to the skin and mucous membranes (cyanosis). Antibiotics do not treat viral infections, though some viruses are susceptible to new antiviral therapies. Most infants and children recover from viral pneumonia with no complications. However, some may develop subsequent lung irregularities.

Although bacterial pneumonia is not common among children, certain conditions (e.g., viral respiratory illnesses, immune deficiency disorders, certain congenitaldefects, blood irregularities, etc.) may put them at increased risk for developing this type of pneumonia. The most common types of bacteria that cause pneumonia in children include Streptococcus pneumoniae (pneumococcus), Streptococcus pyogenes, Staphylococcus aureus, and Haemophilus influenzae type b. Symptoms associated with bacterial pneumonia vary according to age, type of bacteria involved, and other factors. Infants and young children may develop a stuffy nose and other signs of upper respiratory infection, loss of appetite, sudden onset of fever, restlessness, respiratory distress, and cyanosis. In addition, infants with Staphylococcus aureus infection, a more serious type of disease, may develop lethargy, increased irritability, difficulty breathing (dyspnea), vomiting, or diarrhea. Abscesses may form in the lungs and may lead to the development of air-containing cysts (pneumatoceles). Accumulation of pus, or empyema, may occur in the space surrounding the lungs. Older children and adolescents with bacterial pneumonia may develop symptoms commonly associated with mild upper respiratory tract infection followed by chills, shaking, fever, drowsiness, rapid breathing, coughing, or chest pain. Treatment for bacterial pneumonia includes the use of appropriate antibiotics. In the case of Staphylococcus aureus infection, drainage of pus accumulations may be indicated. Other treatment is symptomatic and supportive. Vaccination is important for preventing pneumonia in children. Vaccinations against Haemophilus influenzae and Streptococcus pneumoniae in the first year of life have greatly reduced their role in pneumonia in children.

Atypical pneumonias include those resulting from infection by bacteria-like microorganisms such as Mycoplasma pneumoniae and Chlamydia pneumoniae. Symptoms associated with these types of infections include fatigue, sore throat, cough, joint pain, or rash. Treatment may include the use of certain antibiotics.

Children with compromised immune systems are at risk for developing certain types of pneumonia infections caused by fungi (e.g., histoplasmosis, coccidioidomycosis, cryptococcosis, etc.) and other common organisms such as Pneumocystis carinii. Pneumocystis pneumonia is particularly prevalent among individuals with AIDS. Choice of drug therapy relates to the appropriate identification of the causative organism. Other treatment is symptomatic and supportive.

Government Agencies

5744 NIH/National Institute of Allergy and Infectious Diseases
6610 Rockledge Drive, MSC 6612
Bethesda, MD 20892

301-496-5717
866-284-4107
Fax: 301-402-3573
TDD: 800-877-8339
e-mail: ocpsfoffice@niaid.nih.gov
www.niaid.nih.gov

Conducts and supports basic and applied research to better understand, treat, and ultimately prevent infectious, immunologic, and allergic diseases.

Anthony S Fauci MD, Director

National Associations & Support Groups

5745 American Academy of Pediatrics
141 Northwest Point Boulevard
Elk Grove Village, IL 60007

847-434-4000
800-433-9016
Fax: 847-434-8000
www.aap.org

The American Academy of Pediatrics and its member pediatricians are committed to the attainment of optimal physical, mental and social health and well-being for all infants, children, adolescents, and young adults.

Sandra Hassink, MD, FAAP, President

5746 March of Dimes Birth Defects Foundation
1275 Mamaroneck Avenue
White Plains, NY 10605

914-997-4488
888-663-4637
Fax: 914-428-8203
e-mail: answers@marchofdimes.com
www.marchofdimes.com

Partnership of volunteers and professionals dedicates to improving the health of babies by preventing birth defects and infant mortality. Over 100 chapters are located across the country and can be located through the National Office.

Jennifer L Howse, President

5747 World Health Organization
Avenue Appia 20
CH-1211 Geneva 27,
Switzerland

www.who.int

WHO is the directing and coordinating authority for health within the United Nations system.

Dr Margaret Chan, Director General

Research Centers

5748 National Jewish Medical & Research Center
1400 Jackson Street
Denver, CO 80206
303-388-4461
877-225-5654
www.njc.org

National Jewish is a nonsectarian, nonprofit independent clinical research, medical center that focuses on respiratory, immunologic, allergic, and infectious diseases.

Russell P Bowler, President/CEO
J Verne Singleton, COO
Gary Cott MD, Medical & Clinical Services

Web Sites

5749 American Lung Association
55 W. Wacker Drive, Suite 1150
Chicago, IL 60601
Fax: 202-452-1805
www.lung.org

Information regarding lung disease in all its forms, with special emphasis on asthma, tobacco control and environmental health. Includes information and a fact sheet on pneumonia.

Kathryn A. Forbes, Chair
John F. Emanuel, Vice Chair
Harold Wimmer, President/ CEO

5750 Department of Health and Human Services
540 Gaither Road
Rockville, MD 20850
301-427-1364
www.ahrq.gov

Pneumonia research findings for consumers.

5751 Kid's Health
kidshealth.org/parent/infections/

Kids health is the largest and most visited site on the web providing doctor-approved health information about children from before birth through adolescense. Kids health provides families with accurate, up to date and jargon free health information they can use.

Neil Izenberg, MD, Editor-in-Chief & Founder

5752 Mayo Clinic
13400 E. Shea Blvd.
Scottsdale, AZ 85259
480-301-8000
800-446-2279
www.mayoclinic.com/health/pneumonia/DS00135

5753 National Jewish Medical & Research Center
1400 Jackson St.
Denver, CO 80206
877-225-5654
www.nationaljewish.org

National Jewish is a nonsectarian, nonprofit independent clinical research, medical center. Focusing on respiratory, immunologic, allergic, and infectious diseases. The Center's mission is to develop and provide innovative clinical programs for treating and rehabilitating patients of all ages and for preventing disease, discovering knowledge to enhance prevention, treatment and cures through an integrated program of basic and clinical research, and educating professionals and the public.

Michael Salem, MD, FACS, President & CEO

Book Publishers

5754 Let's Talk About Going to the Hospital
Rosen Publishing Group's PowerKids Press
29 E 21st Street
New York, NY 10010
212-777-3017
800-237-9932
Fax: 888-436-4643
e-mail: rosenpub@tribeca.ios.com
www.rosenpublishing.com

If a child has to check into the hospital, chances are he or she is already upset about being ill. Knowing how a hospital functions and what the procedures are, such as when family members can visit, will help in what is already a stressful situation. Grades K-5.

24 pages
ISBN: 0-823950-36-0

Roger Rosen, President

Description

5755 POLYDACTYLY

Synonyms: Polydactylia, Polydactylism

Involves the following Biologic System(s):

Genetic/Chromosomal/Syndrome/Metabolic Disorders, Orthopedic and Muscle Disorders

Poldactyly refers to an abnormality that is present at birth (congenital) in which an infant has more than the usual number of fingers or toes. Defects associated with this abnormality may range from simple skin tags or stumps of flesh to extra fingers or toes that are completely developed. In some families polydactyly is passed from generation to generation.

Polydactyly involving the toes occurs in approximately two out of every 1,000 births. Although the fifth toe is the digit most often duplicated, polydactyly sometimes affects the great or big toe. Careful evaluation is indicated so that treatment of possible associated abnormalities may be appropriately coordinated. However, if the extra digit is small or rudimentary, it may be tied off (ligated) at birth or soon thereafter. This method allows for the digit to spontaneously detach itself after a period of time. In those cases where the digit is jointed, treatment usually involves surgical amputation of the extra digit and repair of other associated structures and tissues. Surgical intervention of this type is usually performed at approximately one year of age.

Duplication of a finger usually appears near the small finger (pinky) or thumb. As in polydactyly of the toes, small, rudimentary digits may be tied off, while more complex deformities typically require surgical intervention at about one year of age.

Polydactyly may also occur in association with several genetic disorders. These disordersinclude acrocephalopolysyndactyly type II (Carpenter's syndrome), characterized by mental retardation and irregularities involving the head, hand, and genitalia; trisomy 13 syndrome (Patau's syndrome), characterized by cleft lip and palate, polydactyly, mental retardation, and irregularities of the central nervous system, heart, genitalia, and internal organs; chondroectodermal dysplasia (Ellis-van Creveld syndrome), a bone growth disorder characterized by short stature, cardiac defects, polydactyly, and developmental defects of the teeth, and nails (hypoplastic). The efficacy of treating polydactyly associated with these and other disorders depends upon the exact nature of the disorder in question.

Government Agencies

5756 NIH/National Institute of Arthritis and Mu sculoskeletal and Skin Diseases

1AMS Circle
Bethesda, MD 20892

301-402-4484
877-226-4267
Fax: 301-718-6366
TDD: 301-565-2966
e-mail: niamsinfo@mail.nih.gov
www.niams.nih.gov

The mission of the NIAMS, a part of the NIH, is to support research into the causes, treatment, and prevention of arthritis and musculoskeletal and skin diseases, the training of basic and clinical scientists to carry out this research, and the dissemination of information on research progress in these diseases.

Stephen I Katz MD PhD, Director
Robert H Carter MD, Deputy Director

5757 NIH/National Institute of Child Health and Human Development

31 Center Drive, Building 31
Bethesda, MD 20892

301-496-1333
Fax: 301-496-1104
www.nichd.nih.gov

Established in 1962 by congress, today the institute conducts and supports research on topics related to the health of children, adults, families and populations. Some of these topics include: developmental disabilities, growth and development, infant death, reproductive health and birth defects.

Jay H Hoofnagle, Director
Lisa Kaeser, Program & Public Liaison

National Associations & Support Groups

5758 American Academy of Pediatrics

141 Northwest Point Boulevard
Elk Grove Village, IL 60007

847-434-4000
800-433-9016
Fax: 847-434-8000
www.aap.org

The American Academy of Pediatrics and its member pediatricians are committed to the attainment of optimal physical, mental and social health and well-being for all infants, children, adolescents, and young adults.

Sandra Hassink, MD, FAAP, President

5759 CHERUB-Association of Families and Friends of Children with Limb Disorders

Children's Hospital of Buffalo
936 Delaware Avenue
Buffalo, NY 14209

716-762-9997
888-881-0805
e-mail: pffdvsg@ohio.net
www.ohio.net

Offers support to families of juveniles diagnosed with a limb disorder.

Sandra Richenberg
Kathy Gura

5760 Genetic Alliance

4301 Connecticut Avenue NW
Washington, DC 20008

202-966-5557
800-336-4363
Fax: 202-966-8553
e-mail: info@geneticalliance.org
www.geneticalliance.org

A coalition of voluntary genetic support groups, consumers and professionals addressing the needs of individuals and families affected by genetic disorders from a national perspective.

Sharon Terry, President
Natasha Bonhomme, Vice President of Strategic Develop
Vaughn ÿEdelson, Assistant Director of Health Commun

5761 March of Dimes Birth Defects Foundation

1275 Mamaroneck Avenue
White Plains, NY 10605

914-997-4488
888-663-4637
Fax: 914-428-8203
e-mail: answers@marchofdimes.com
www.marchofdimes.com

Partnership of volunteers and professionals dedicates to improving the health of babies by preventing birth defects and infant mortality. Over 100 chapters are located across the country and can be located through the National Office.

Jennifer L Howse, President

5762 Shriners Hospitals for Children
Headquarters
12502 USF Pine Drive
Tampa, FL 33607 813-972-2250
800-237-5055
Fax: 813-975-7125
e-mail: aargiz-lyons@shrinenet.org
www.shrinershospitalsforchildren.org

Network of 22 hospitals that provide expert, no-cost orthopedic
and burn care to children under 18.

Peter F Armstrong, VP

Web Sites

5763 On The Other Hand
www.ontheotherhand.org

Provides information, support, and suggestions for parents, relatives. and friends of children with hand anomalies.

5764 Polydactyly
www.eatonhand.com/hw/hw024.htm

Explanation and general overview of the disorder.

Description

5765 PORPHYRIA

Synonyms: EPP, Erythrohepatic protoporphyria, Ferrochelatase deficiency, Protoporphyria

Involves the following Biologic System(s):

Hematologic and Oncologic Disorders

Porphyria is a rare group of hereditary metabolic disorders characterized by enzyme deficiencies that result in the abnormal accumulation of chemicals known as porphyrins in certain tissues of the body. Porphyrins are formed during the manufacture of heme, the pigmented, iron-containing component of hemoglobin, which is the oxygen-carrying protein in red blood cells. The porphyrias may be classified as erythropoietic or hepatic porphyrias. The erythropoietic porphyrias are characterized by overproduction of porphyrins in the blood-forming tissue of the bone marrow. In individuals with hepatic porphyrias, there is abnormally increased production of porphyrins in the liver. The range and severity of associated symptoms and the age at onset are variable and depend on the underlying enzyme deficiency and the form of porphyria present. Erythropoietic protoporphyria is the most common form of porphyria and is thought to affect approximately one in 5,000 to 10,000 individuals.

In patients with erythropoietic protoporphyria, also known as EPP, deficiency of the enzyme ferrochelatase results in excessive accumulation of protoporphyrin in red blood cells and the fluid portion of the blood (plasma). Excessive protoporphyrin is also concentrated in a liquid secreted by the liver (bile) and is eliminated in the feces. In some patients, abnormal accumulations of protoporphyrin also become deposited within the liver itself.

Symptoms associated with EPP usually begin in childhood before age 10. The most common symptom is an abnormal sensitivity of the skin to sunlight and certain forms of artificial light (photosensitivity). Affected children typically experience pain, burning, and itching of the skin within an hour of exposure to sunlight. Such symptoms are often followed hours later by redness and inflammation of the skin and abnormal accumulation of fluid (edema) beneath the skin in affected areas. However, abnormal burning sensations of the skin may occur in the absence of associated redness or fluid accumulation. Rarely, if sun exposure is prolonged, fluid-filled blisters (vesicles) may develop or there may be bleeding in the skin or mucous membranes, appearing as pinpoint purplish spots (petechiae) or small bluish-purple patches (purpura). Such blistering or bruising may persist for several days after exposure to the sun. In addition, prolonged, repeated sun exposure may cause mild scarring, abnormal thickening of the skin in certain areas, or an abnormality of the nails in which the nails become separated from the nail beds (onycholysis). Although symptoms associated with photosensitivity typically become apparent during infancy or early childhood, the condition sometimes does not occur until adolescence or adulthood.

Many patients with EPP may also develop lumps of solid matter in the gall bladder (gallstones or cholelithiasis) at an unusually early age. The gall bladder is a small, muscular sac under the liver that stores and concentrates bile from the liver. In addition, uncommonly, there may be mildly decreased levels of circulating red blood cells (anemia). Rarely, patients may develop progressive liver damage that may lead to liver failure.

EPP is caused by changes (mutations) in the gene that regulates the production of the enzyme ferrochelatase. This gene is located on the long arm of chromosome 18 (18q21.3). Several different mutations of the gene have been identified in individuals with the disorder. In most cases, EPP has autosomal dominant inheritance. However, there have been reports in which patients inherited two different mutations of the gene, one from each parent. In addition, some individuals who inherit one copy of the disease gene may have slightly elevated levels of protoporphyrin, yet do not experience symptoms associated with the disease.

Patients with EPP benefit from avoiding sunlight, using topical sunscreens, and wearing protective clothing, such as sunglasses, hats, long sleeves, and double layers. Administration of beta-carotene by mouth may help improve tolerance to sunlight. Therapy with cholestyramine, a medication that acts upon the liver's bile acids, may help to alleviate skin symptoms and liver disease. Additional treatment is symptomatic and supportive.

Government Agencies

5766 NIH/National Institute of Child Health and Human Development

31 Center Drive, Building 31

Bethesda, MD 20892

301-496-1333

Fax: 301-496-1104

www.nichd.nih.gov

Established in 1962 by congress, today the institute conducts and supports research on topics related to the health of children, adults, families and populations. Some of these topics include: developmental disabilities, growth and development, infant death, reproductive health and birth defects.

Jay H Hoofnagle, Director

Lisa Kaeser, Program & Public Liaison

National Associations & Support Groups

5767 American Academy of Pediatrics

141 Northwest Point Boulevard

Elk Grove Village, IL 60007

847-434-4000

800-433-9016

Fax: 847-434-8000

www.aap.org

The American Academy of Pediatrics and its member pediatricians are committed to the attainment of optimal physical, mental and social health and well-being for all infants, children, adolescents, and young adults.

Sandra Hassink, MD, FAAP, President

5768 American Porphyria Foundation

4900 Woodway, Suite 780, PO Box 22712

Houston, TX 77056

713-266-9617

866-273-3635

Fax: 713-840-9552

e-mail: porphyrus@aol.com

www.porphyriafoundation.com

Dedicated to improving the health and wellness of individuals and families affected by porphyria through enhanced public awareness; support of research; and development of educational programs and educational material.

Desiree Lyon Howe, Executive Director

5769 Erythropoietic Protoporphyria Research & Education Fund
Brigham & Women's Hospital
Channing Laboratory, 181 Longwood Avenue
Boston, MA 02115   617-525-8249
                                            Fax: 617-731-1541
                    e-mail: mmmathroth@rics.bwh.harvard.edu
                          www.brighamandwomens.org/eppref

A support group for patients with Erythropoietic Protoporphyria
and their families and their physicians, providing information on
this disease and publishing a bi-annual newsletter available online on the website.

Micheline Mathews Roth, MD, Medical Director

5770 Genetic Alliance
4301 Connecticut Avenue NW
Washington, DC 20008   202-966-5557
                                                800-336-4363
                                            Fax: 202-966-8553
                          e-mail: info@geneticalliance.org
                               www.geneticalliance.org

A coalition of voluntary genetic support groups, consumers and
professionals addressing the needs of individuals and families affected by genetic disorders from a national perspective.

Sharon Terry, President
Natasha Bonhomme, Vice President of Strategic Develop
Vaughn ÿEdelson, Assistant Director of Health Commun

5771 March of Dimes Birth Defects Foundation
1275 Mamaroneck Avenue
White Plains, NY 10605   914-997-4488
                                                888-663-4637
                                            Fax: 914-428-8203
                     e-mail: answers@marchofdimes.com
                            www.marchofdimes.com

Partnership of volunteers and professionals dedicates to improving the health of babies by preventing birth defects and infant
mortality. Over 100 chapters are located across the country and
can be located through the National Office.

Jennifer L Howse, President

Libraries & Resource Centers

5772 National Digestive Diseases Information Clearinghouse
2 Information Way
Bethesda, MD 20892   301-654-3810
                                                800-891-5389
                                            Fax: 703-738-4929
                          e-mail: nddic@info.niddk.nih.gov
                               www2.niddk.nih.gov

The National Institute of Diabetes and Digestive and Kidney Diseases conducts and supports research on many of the most serious
diseases affecting public health. The Institute supports much of
the clinical research on the diseases of internal medicine and related subspecialty fields as well as many basic science
disciplines.

Griffin P. Rodgers, M.D, Chairman, Executive Board
Brent B. Stanfield, Executive Secretary
Camille M. Hoover, M.S.W, Executive Officer

Newsletters

5773 APF Newsletter
American Porphyria Foundation
4900 Woodway, Suite 780
Houston, TX 77056   713-266-9617
                                                866-APF-3635
                                            Fax: 713-840-9552
                          e-mail: porphyrus@aol.com
                            www.porphyriafoundation.com

The newsletter provides updates on treatment and reserach, as
well as informative articles on patients and specialists who treat
porphyria.

Quarterly
James V. Young, Chairman
Desiree H. Lyon, Executive Director
Dr. William McCutchen, Board Member

Pamphlets

5774 Porphyria Fact Sheet
Nat'l Digestive Diseases Information Clearinghouse
2 Information Way
Bethesda, MD 20892   301-496-3583
                                                800-891-5389
                                            Fax: 703-738-4929
                          e-mail: nddic@info.niddk.nih.gov
                               www.niddk.nih.gov

Griffin P. Rodgers, M.D., Director

Description

5775 POST-TRAUMATIC STRESS DISORDER
Synonym: PTSD
Involves the following Biologic System(s):
Developmental/Behavioral/Psychiatric Disorders

Traumatic events can stay with children for a long time. Such events can range from the rare and horrific, such as severe torture, to more common events such as an automobile accident or a violent crime. With immediate media coverage of violence in our world, children are often exposed to the violent acts of war and terror through the television. Moreover, children may be directly or indirectly affected by events of terror and violence that now pervade our society. Effects of some childhood experiences can last well into adulthood. When the after-effects of a traumatic event are so severe and so persistent that they impair normal childhood functioning, behavior or development, professional help should be considered.

Post-Traumatic Stress Disorder, or PTSD, is a diagnosis made to describe the psychological and physiological symptoms that arise from experiencing, witnessing or participating in a traumatic event. PTSD in a child may result from exposure to a traumatic event which the child experienced or witnessed. It may occur if the child was confronted by death or serious injury, or a threat to the physical integrity of self or others. Studies indicate that 15 to 43% of girls and 14 to 43% of boys have experienced at least one traumatic event in their lifetime. Of those children and adolescents who have experienced a trauma, 3 to 15% of girls and 1 to 6% of boys meet criteria for PTSD. Researchers and clinicians are beginning to recognize that PTSD may not present itself in children in the same way as it does in adults. The classical triad of symptoms includes re-experiencing, numbing of responsiveness, and hyperarousal. Other symptoms include regression, bedwetting, separation anxiety and new fears previously not expressed. Children are also more likely to exhibit their 're-experience' in play. Very young children may present with few PTSD symptoms. Instead, young children may report more generalized fears such as stranger or separation anxiety, avoidance of situations that may or may not be related to the trauma, sleep disturbances, and a preoccupation with words or symbols that may or may not be related to the trauma. Elementary school-aged children may be unable to recall the sequence of the events related to the trauma or believe that there were warning signs that predicted the trauma. PTSD in adolescents may begin to more closely resemble PTSD in adults. Adolescents are more likely to engage in traumatic reenactment in which they incorporate aspects of the trauma into their daily lives. In addition, adolescents are more likely than younger children or adults to exhibit impulsive and aggressive behaviors. Response to traumatic events can also vary from child to child. Some characteristics, however, are common among all children with PTSD. If a child has survived a life-threatening event, there may be a profound sense of guilt, particularly if others did not survive the event. These guilt feelings may be exacerbated if the child had to do extraordinary things to survive. In other cases, a child with PTSD may complain of physical symptoms that have no discernible anatomic or physiological explanation, but which are manifestations of psychic distress; these are known as somatic complaints. The child with PTSD is also liable to experience a range of feelings that make it difficult or impossible for him or her to carry on with life in a normal fashion. They may feel that the trauma they experienced damaged them permanently and irreparably. Children who suffer from PTSD may also experience depression, Obsessive-Compulsive Disorder, social phobia or in the adolescent population, substance abuse.

Therapies include medication and/or psychotherapy. Behavior therapy focuses on helping the child recognize the thought processes that result in traumatic stress reactions. Behavior therapy may involve exposing the patient in a safe and controlled environment to stimuli that prompt a stress reaction; through repeated exposures, the child slowly is desensitized and in time will be able to experience the stimuli without having a stress reaction. As with many psychiatric disorders, treatment often involves some combination of therapy and medication.

Early intervention with skilled providers is vital for successful treatment of children with PTSD.

Government Agencies

5776 National Center for PTSD
www.ptsd.va.gov

802-296-6300
e-mail: ncptsd@va.gov
www.ptsd.va.gov

A special center within the US Department of Veterans Affairs, which advances clinical care and social welfare through research, education, training and diagnosis.

National Associations & Support Groups

5777 American Academy of Pediatrics
141 Northwest Point Boulevard
Elk Grove Village, IL 60007

847-434-4000
800-433-9016
Fax: 847-434-8000
www.aap.org

The American Academy of Pediatrics and its member pediatricians are committed to the attainment of optimal physical, mental and social health and well-being for all infants, children, adolescents, and young adults.

Sandra Hassink, MD, FAAP, President

5778 American Counseling Association
6101 Stevenson Ave
Alexandria, VA 22304

703-823-9800
800-347-6647
Fax: 703-823-0252
e-mail: webmaster@counseling.org
www.counseling.org

Represents professional counselors in various practice settings, and stands ready to serve more than 55,000 members with the resources they need to make a difference. From webinars, publications, and journals to Conference education sessions and legislative action alerts, ACA is where counseling professionals turn for powerful, credible content and support.

Robert L. Smith, President

5779 American Psychological Association
750 First St. NE
Washington, DC 20002

202-336-5500
800-374-2721
TTY: 202-336-6123
www.apa.org

The mission is to advance the creation, communication and application of psychological knowledge to benefit society and improve people's lives.

Norman B. Anderson, PhD, CEO/ EVP
L. Michael Honaker, PhD, Deputy Chief Executive Officer
Ellen G. Garrison, PhD, Senior Policy Advisor

5780 Anxiety Disorders Association of America
8730 Georgia Avenue, Suite 600
Silver Spring, MD 20910
240-485-1001
Fax: 240-485-1035
e-mail: information@adaa.org
www.adaa.org

Offers resources and information for persons with anxiety and
stress-related disorders.

Alies Muskin, Executive Director

5781 Association of Traumatic Stress Specialists
88 Pompton Avenue
Verona, NJ 07044
973-559-9200
800-991-2877
Fax: 973-227-7169
e-mail: admin@atss.info
www.atss.info

An international membership organization which develops standards of service and education for qualified individuals who provide services, intervention and treatment in the field of traumatic
stress.

Mike Garone, CEO
Barbara Maurer, Vice President

5782 CEDAR Associates
39 Smith Ave.
Mount Kisco, NY 10549
914-224-1904
e-mail: info@cedarassociates.com
www.cedarassociates.com

CEDAR Associates is a multi-disciplinary private group practice
for the treatment of a full range of mental health issues for individuals and their family. CEDAR Associates specializes in the
prevention and treatment of eating disorders and the problems
that often accompany them including depression, self-harm, anxiety, relational issuel, sexual and physical trauma and body image
issues.

Judy Scheel, Ph.D., LCSW, Executive Director

5783 International Critical Incident Stress Foundation
3290 Pine Orchard Lane, Suite 106
Ellicott City, MD 21042
410-750-9600
410-750-9601
Fax: 410-750-9601
e-mail: info@icisf.org
www.icisf.org

Nonprofit, open membership foundation dedicated to the prevention and mitigation of disabling stress by education, training and
support services for all emergency service professionals; Continuing education and training in emergency mental health services
for psychologists, psychiatrists, social workers and licensed
professional counselors.

Donald Howell, Executive Director
Stephanie Beam, General Information

**5784 National Child Traumatic Stress Network NCCTS - University
of California, LA**
11150 W Olympic Blvd., Suite 650
Los Angeles, CA 90064
310-235-2633
Fax: 310-235-2612
www.nctsnet.org

The mission is to raise the standard of care and improve access to
services for traumatized children, their families and communities
throughout the United States.

Robert S Pynoos, Co-Director
Alan Steinberg, Associate Director
Jenifer Maze, Co-Managing Director

5785 Traumatic Incident Reduction Association
5145 Pontiac Trail
Ann Arbor, MI 48105
734-761-6268
800-499-2751
Fax: 734-663-6861
e-mail: info@tir.org
www.tir.org

Devoted to reducing the effects of traumatic incidents and providing education on how to deal with traumatic events.

Marian Volkman, President
Ragnhild Malnati, VP

Research Centers

5786 International Society for Traumatic Stress Studies
111 Deer Lake Road Suite 100
Deerfield, IL 60015
847-480-9028
Fax: 847-480-9282
e-mail: istss@istss.org
www.istss.org

Provides a forum for sharing research, clinical strategies, public
policy concerns and theoretical formulation on trauma in the US
and worldwide. Dedicated to discovery and dissemination of
knowledge and to the stimulation of policy, program and service
initiatives that seek to reduce traumatic stressors and their permanent and long-term consequences. Members include psychiatrists,
psychologists, social workers, nurses, counselors, researchers,
administrators, advocates, and others.

Marylene Cloitre PhD, President
Karestan C Koenen PhD, Vice President
Dean G Kilpatrick PhD, Treasurer

Audio Video

5787 Complex PTSD in Children
Sidran Institute
PO Box 436
Brooklandville, MD 21022
410-825-8888
888-825-8249
Fax: 410-560-0134
e-mail: help@sidran.org
www.sidran.org

Tape I: Etiology, Assessment, Advocacy; Tape II: Therapeutic Interventions

VHS 41 Minutes

Esther Giller, President and Director
Sheila Giller, Secretary/Treasurer
Tracy Howard, Book Sales/ Office Manager

5788 PTSD in Children: Move in the Rhythm of th e Child
Sidran Institute
PO Box 436
Brooklandville, MD 21022
410-825-8888
888-825-8249
Fax: 410-560-0134
e-mail: help@sidran.org
www.sidran.org

Trauma experts explain the circumstances, symptoms and therapy
techniques for PTSD in children and the effect on our communities. Primarily for use by mental health professionals, it is an excellent resource for any who work with children.

VHS 58 Minutes

Esther Giller, President and Director
Sheila Giller, Secretary/Treasurer
Tracy Howard, Book Sales/ Office Manager

5789 Significant Event Childhood Trauma
Sidran Institute
PO Box 436
Brooklandville, MD 21022
410-825-8888
888-825-8249
Fax: 410-560-0134
e-mail: help@sidran.org
www.sidran.org

Topics discussed inlude: effects; targeting resources; in the classroom; single parents; divorce; violence; addiction; and intervention.

DVD

Esther Giller, President and Director
Sheila Giller, Secretary/Treasurer
Tracy Howard, Book Sales/ Office Manager

Web Sites

5790 Association of Traumatic Stress Specialists
5000 Old Buncombe Road, Suite 27-11
Greenville, SC 29617   864-294-4337
www.atss.info

An international membership organization which develops standards of service and education for qualified individuals who provide services, intervention and treatment in the field of traumatic stress.

Chrys Harris, President
Bill Mc Dermott, Vice President
Linda Hood, Secretary

5791 David Baldwin's Trauma Information Pages
www.trauma-pages.com

Brief summary of what is known about traumatic symptoms and responses including PTSD and coping strategies. Pages include additional links to more detailed references, online articles and web resources.

5792 Facts for Health: PTSD
ptsd.factsforhealth.org

5793 Helping Kids Cope With a New Threat
750 First St. NE
Washington, DC 20002   202-336-5500
                                          800-374-2721
www.apa.org/monitor/apr02/helpingkids.html

An online article about the issues of traumatic stress in children in particular after the September 11 attacks.

Barry S. Anton, PhD, President
Bonnie Markham, Treasurer
Linda Frye Campbell, Member

5794 International Critical Incident Stress Foundation
3290 Pine Orchard Lane, Suite 106
Ellicott City, MD 21042   410-750-9600
www.icisf.org

Nonprofit, open membership foundation dedicated to the prevention and mitigation of disabling stress by education, training and support services for all emergency service professionals; Continuing education and training in emergency mental health services for psychologists, psychiatrists, social workers and licensed professional counselors.

Becky Stoll, Chair
Lisa Joubert, Secretary
Richard Bloch, Counsel

5795 Madison Institute of Medicine
www.miminc.org

Disseminates innovative approaches to the education of professionals and the general public on many mental health topics such as PTSD, OCD, depression, SAD and others.

5796 PTSD Alliance
www.ptsdalliance.org

A group of professional and advocacy organizaions that have joined forces to provide educational resources to individuals diagnosed with PTSD and their loves ones; those at risk for developing PTSD; and medical, healthcare and other frontline professionals.

5797 Sidran Institute - Traumatic Stress Educat ion & Advocacy
PO Box 436
Brooklandville, MD 21022   410-825-8888
                                          888-825-8249
                                     Fax: 410-560-0134
                                 e-mail: help@sidran.org
                                          www.sidran.org

Provides education, resources, information and advocacy, publications, training and consulting on traumatic stress.

Esther Giller, President and Director
Sheila Giller, Secretary/Treasurer
Tracy Howard, Book Sales/ Office Manager

Book Publishers

5798 Coping with Post-Traumatic Stress Disorder
Rosen Publishing Group
29 E 21st Street
New York, NY 10010   800-237-9932
                                     Fax: 888-436-4643
                                 www.rosenpublishing.com

Revised 2002 192 pages
Roger Rosen, President

5799 Effective Treatments for PTSD, 2nd Ed
Foa, Keane, Friedman, & Cohen, author

Guilford Press
72 Spring Street
New York, NY 10012   800-365-7006
                                     Fax: 212-966-6708
                                e-mail: info@guilford.com
                                          www.guilford.com

Represents the collaborative work of experts across a range of theoretical orientations and professional backgrounds. Addresses general treatment considerations and methodological issues, reviews and evaluates literature on treatment approaches for children, adolescents and adults.

2008 604 pages Paperback
ISBN: 1-606230-01-5

Bob Matloff, President
Seymour Weingarten, Editor-in-Chief

5800 Helping Kids Heal - 75 Activities to Help Children Recover from Trauma & Loss
Rebecca Carman CSW, author

Sidran Institute
PO Box 436
Brooklandville, MD 21022   410-825-8888
                                          888-825-8249
                                     Fax: 410-560-0134
                                 e-mail: info@sidran.org
                                          www.sidran.org

75 activities to use with school-aged children after traumatic events. Broken down into 13 sections that follow the natural sequence of recovery.

117 pages Paperback

Esther Giller, President & Director
Sheila Giller, Secretary/Treasurer
Ruta Mazelis, Editor

5801 PTSD Workbook
Courage to Change
PO Box 486
Wilkes-Barre, PA 18703   800-440-4003
                                     Fax: 800-772-6499
                                 www.couragetochange.com

Outlines simple and effective techniques employed by PTSD experts for trauma survivors in order to conquer their most distressing symptoms. Readers learn to evaluate their type of trauma and then learn the most effective strategies to overcome them.

5802 Post Traumatic Stress Disorder Sourcebook
Glenn R Schiraldi, author

McGraw Hill Publishers
860 Taylor Station Road
Blacklick, 43004   877-833-5524
                                          877-833-5524
                                     Fax: 614-759-3823
                   e-mail: pbg.ecommerce_custserv@mcgraw-hill.com
                                          www.mhprofessional.com

Offers help and hope for lasting recovery. A guide for sufferers and theor loved ones.

446 pages Paperback
ISBN: 0-737302-65-8

Lloyd G. Waterhouse, President & CEO
Patrick Milano, CFO
David Stafford, Senior Vice President

5803 Posttraumatic Stress Disorder in Children and Adolescents

Raul R Silva MD, author

Sidran Institute
PO Box 436
Brooklandville, MD 21022   410-825-8888
                                          888-825-8249
                                          Fax: 410-560-0134
                                          e-mail: info@sidran.org
                                          www.sidran.org

An expert guide to the most importatnt issues pertaining to PTSD, trauma, stress and concurrent conditions. Includes 15 chapters that address different aspects of childhood and adolescent trauma.

384 pages Paperback

Esther Giller, President & Director
Sheila Giller, Secretary/Treasurer
Ruta Mazelis, Editor

5804 Treating Psychological Trauma and PTSD

John Wilson et al, author

Sidran Institute
PO Box 436
Brooklandville, MD 21022   410-825-8888
                                          888-825-8249
                                          Fax: 410-560-0134
                                          e-mail: info@sidran.org
                                          www.sidran.org

Identifies 65 PTSD symptoms contained within five symptom clusters, and then addresses 80 target objectives for treatment, which can be treated by 11 different psychotherapeutic approaches.

443 pages Paperback

Esther Giller, President & Director
Sheila Giller, Secretary/Treasurer
Ruta Mazelis, Editor

5805 Treating Trauma & Traumatic Grief in Child ren and Adolescents

J Cohen, A Mannarino, E Deblinger, author

Guilford Press
72 Spring Street
New York, NY 10012   800-365-7006
                                          Fax: 212-966-6708
                                          e-mail: info@guilford.com
                                          www.guilford.com

The book presents a systematic treatment approach, grounded in CBT, for traumatized children and their families. Provides a comprehensive frameworkl for assessing PTSD, depression, anxiety, and other symptoms; assists in developing a flxible, patient-specific treatment plan to work with the children and parents in building core skills. Includes age and culture specific treatment components. Print or e-book.

2006 256 pages
ISBN: 1-593853-08-2

Bob Matloff, President
Seymour Weingarten, Editor-in-Chief

Pamphlets

5806 Helping Children and Adolescents Cope with Violence and Disasters

National Institute of Mental Health
6001 Executive Boulevard, Room 6200
Bethesda, MD 20892   301-443-4513
                                          866-615-6464
                                          Fax: 301-443-4279
                                          TTY: 301-443-8431
                                          e-mail: nimhinfo@nih.gov
                                          www.nimh.nih.gov

Booklet that discusses children and adolescents' reactions to violence and disasters, emphasizing the wide range of responses and the role that parents, teachers and therapists can play in the healing process.

Francis Collins, M.D., Director
Tom Insel, Director

5807 Post Traumatic Stress Disorder: A Guide
Madison Institute of Medicine
www.miminc.org/shop/store/

Comprehensive overview, diagnosis and treatment of PTSD.

2000 69 pages

5808 Post-Traumatic Stress Disorder, A Real Ill ness
National Institute of Mental Health
6001 Executive Boulevard, Room 6200
Bethesda, MD 20892   301-443-4513
                                          866-615-6464
                                          Fax: 301-443-4279
                                          TTY: 301-443-8431
                                          e-mail: nimhinfo@nih.gov
                                          www.nimh.nih.gov

An easy-to-read pamphlet of simple information about what it is, when it starts, how long it lasts and how to get help.

9 pages

Francis Collins, M.D., Director
Tom Insel, Director

5809 What Is Post Traumatic Stress Disorder?
Sidran Institute
PO Box 436
Brooklandville, MD 21022   410-825-8888
                                          888-825-8249
                                          Fax: 410-560-0134
                                          e-mail: help@sidran.org
                                          www.sidran.org

Provides an introduction of PTSD as well as symptoms, possible treatment, and other helpful resources.

Esther Giller, President and Director
Sheila Giller, Secretary/Treasurer
Tracy Howard, Book Sales/ Office Manager

Description

5810 PRADER-WILLI SYNDROME

Synonym: PWS

Involves the following Biologic System(s):

Endocrinologic Disorders,

Genetic/Chromosomal/Syndrome/Metabolic Disorders

Prader-Willi syndrome is a genetic disorder characterized by severely diminished muscle tone (hypotonia) during early infancy, short stature, unusually small hands and feet, obesity, genital abnormalities, and mental retardation. The disorder is thought to affect approximately one in 15,000 individuals. In most cases of Prader-Willi syndrome, there is decreased fetal activity during the last months of pregnancy. After birth, most affected infants experience hypotonia, have feeding difficulties due to decreased swallowing and sucking reflexes, and fail to grow and gain weight at the expected rate (failure to thrive). Starting at approximately six months to six years of age, affected infants or children begin to have an excessive appetite (polyphagia), become obsessed with eating, or lack a sense of satisfaction after a meal and often engage in binge-type eating. As a result, patients develop an abnormally increased body weight (progressive obesity) due to an excessive accumulation of body fat, particularly over the thighs, buttocks, and lower abdomen.

Infants and children with Prader-Willi syndrome also may have characteristic abnormalities of the head and face (craniofacial area), such as almond-shaped eyes, upslanting eyelid folds (palpebral fissures), abnormal deviation of one eye in relation to the other (strabismus), a thin, tented upper lip, and full cheeks. In addition, affected males and females may have insufficient secretion of certain hormones that stimulate the gonads (hypogonadotropic hypogonadism). The gonads are the reproductive glands, such as the testes or ovaries, within which the reproductive cells (sperm or ova) are produced. Affected males typically have an abnormally small penis (micropenis) and undescended testes (cryptorchidism), potentially delayed or incomplete development of secondary sexual characteristics, insufficient production of the male sex hormone testosterone, decreased or absent sperm production, and infertility. Affected females often have abnormally small underdeveloped external genitalia (i.e., hypoplastic labia minor and clitoris), absence or abnormal cessation of menstrual cycles (primary or secondary amenorrhea), and infertility. Development of female secondary sexual characteristics may be normal or incomplete. Most children with Prader-Willi syndrome also have mild to moderate mental retardation; however, in some cases, severe mental retardation may be present. Many affected children experience difficulties with speech articulation and may have an abnormally high-pitched, nasal voice. Children with Prader-Willi syndrome may have behavioral problems that become apparent during later childhood, including outbursts of anger, rage-like episodes, and stubbornness.

Some individuals with Prader-Willi syndrome may develop diabetes mellitus during or soon after puberty. Diabetes mellitus is characterized by impaired fat, protein, and carbohydrate metabolism due to insufficient production of the hormone insulin or the body's inability to appropriately utilize insulin. Associated symptoms may include excessive thirst (polydipsia) and urination (polyuria). In addition, adolescents and young adults may be prone to experiencing cardiac insufficiency, potentially resulting in life-threatening complications during the second or third decade of life.

In children with Prader-Willi syndrome, treatment typically includes measures to help prevent progressive obesity or to ensure strict weight control, such as a low-calorie diet and a proper exercise program under a physician's direction. Nutritional behavioral modification methods may be implemented that require the cooperation and support of all family members, such as ensuring regular feeding habits (e.g., having meals at the same time and location on a daily basis) and the inaccessibility of food between meals. In young males with Prader-Willi syndrome, testosterone replacement therapy may result in enlargement of micropenis; in addition, testosterone therapy during adolescence or young adulthood may have beneficial effects on the development of secondary sexual characteristics. Treatment of children with Prader-Willi syndrome also may include special education and behavioral therapies to help manage behavioral problems.

Prader-Willi syndrome is caused by deletion or disruption of certain genes (contiguous gene syndrome) located on the long arm of chromos|ome 15 (15q11-13). Most affected individualshave missing genetic material or deletion of 15q11-13 that affects the chromosome received from the father (paternally derived chromosome).

Government Agencies

5811 NIH/National Institute of Child Health and Human Development

National Institutes of Health
31 Center Drive
Bethesda, MD 20892

301-496-1333
www.nichd.nih.gov

Offers reprints, articles and various information on Prader-Willi Syndrome in children and adults.

Jay H Hoofnagle, Director
Lisa Kaeser, Program & Public Liaison

National Associations & Support Groups

5812 American Academy of Pediatrics

141 Northwest Point Boulevard
Elk Grove Village, IL 60007

847-434-4000
800-433-9016
Fax: 847-434-8000
www.aap.org

The American Academy of Pediatrics and its member pediatricians are committed to the attainment of optimal physical, mental and social health and well-being for all infants, children, adolescents, and young adults.

Sandra Hassink, MD, FAAP, President

5813 Foundation for Prader-Willi Research

6407 Bardstown Road, Suite 252
Louisville, KY 40291

502-384-8405
Fax: 502-749-9388
www.fpwr.org

Dedicated to the advancement of research on PWS. The Foundation chooses projects that are highly relevant for individuals with PWS and their families and that are scientifically sound.

Rachel Tugon, Executive Director
Alice Viroslav, President
Kathryn McGhee, Membership

5814 Genetic Alliance
4301 Connecticut Avenue NW
Washington, DC 20008
202-966-5557
800-336-4363
Fax: 202-966-8553
e-mail: info@geneticalliance.org
www.geneticalliance.org

A coalition of voluntary genetic support groups, consumers and professionals addressing the needs of individuals and families affected by genetic disorders from a national perspective.

Sharon Terry, President
Natasha Bonhomme, Vice President of Strategic Develop
Vaughn ÿEdelson, Assistant Director of Health Commun

5815 March of Dimes Birth Defects Foundation
1275 Mamaroneck Avenue
White Plains, NY 10605
914-997-4488
888-663-4637
Fax: 914-428-8203
e-mail: answers@marchofdimes.com
www.marchofdimes.com

Partnership of volunteers and professionals dedicates to improving the health of babies by preventing birth defects and infant mortality. Over 100 chapters are located across the country and can be located through the National Office.

Jennifer L Howse, President

5816 Prader-Willi Syndrome Association
8588 Potter Park Drive, Suite 500ÿ
Sarasota, FL 34238
941-312-0400
800-926-4797
Fax: 941-312-0142
e-mail: info@pwsausa.org
www.pwsausa.org

Provides educational materials, support, and advocacy for parents, caregivers, medical professionals, educators and all others involved with persons in PWS community.

Evan Farrar, Acting Executive Director
Sharon Middleton, Business Manager
Jodi O'Sullivan, Director Community Development

State Agencies & Support Groups

Alaska

5817 Prader-Willi Northwest Association
3706 29th Avenue W
Seattle, WA 98199
206-285-7679
e-mail: jlunderwood@juno.com
Joane Underwood, Co-President

Arizona

5818 Prader-Willi Syndrome Arizona Association
13839 N Bentwater Drive
Tucson, AZ 85737
520-297-7025
e-mail: p.penta@comcast.net
Tammie Penta, President

California

5819 Prader-Willi California Foundation
514 N. Prospect Avenue, Ste 110, Lower Level
Redondo Beach, CA 90277
310-372-5053
800-400-9994
Fax: 310-316-3730
e-mail: PWCF1@aol.com
www.pwcf.org

Willi Prader, Owner

Colorado

5820 Prader-Willi Colorado Association
PWSA
8290 South Yukon Way
Littleton, CO 80128
303-973-4780
e-mail: hosler@dynamicssolutions.com

Lynette Hosler, President

Connecticut

5821 Prader-Willi Connecticut Association
PWSA
35 Ansonia Drive
North Haven, CT 06473
860-204-9386
e-mail: pwsactchapter@yahoo.com
www.angelfire.com/ct/pwsctchapter/

Eileen Fletcher
Vicki Knopf

Delaware

5822 Prader-Willi Delaware Association
PWSA
300 Bethel Circle Millwood
Middletown, DE 19709
302-378-7385
e-mail: swede455@aol.com

Karen Swanson, President

Florida

5823 PWSA Florida Chapter
PWSA
694 SE Ashley Oak Way
Stuart, FL 34997
772-287-2587
e-mail: pwfa2000@aol.com
http://members.aol.com/delchert/pwsa2.htm

Dan Krauer, President

Georgia

5824 PWSA of Georgia
562 Lakeland Plaza #327
Cumming, GA 30040
770-886-2334
877-886-2334
Fax: 770-886-2335
e-mail: pwsaga@earthlink.net
www.pwsaga.org

Debbie Lange, Executive Director

Hawaii

5825 Prader-Willi Northwest Association
3706 29th Avenue W
Seattle, WA 98199
206-285-7679
e-mail: jlunderwood@juno.com

Joane Underwood, Co-President

Idaho

5826 Prader-Willi Northwest Association-Idaho
550 Lodgepole Road
Athol, ID 83801
208-683-2993
e-mail: idaho4ts@aol.com

Gene Todhunter, Contact

Illinois

5827 PWSA of Illinois
PWSA
505 Drexel Avenue
Glencoe, IL 60022
847-242-9082
e-mail: contact@pwsaillinois.org
www.pwsausa.org/IL/

Ron Bruns, President

Indiana

5828 PWSA of Indiana
Prader-Willi Syndrome Association
7536 Moonbeam Drive
Indianapolis, IN 46259
317-527-9173
e-mail: amypfeiffer@comcast.net
www.pwsausa.org/IN/

Jaque McGuire

Iowa

5829 PWSA of Iowa
15554 226th Street
Zwingle, IA 52079
319-686-4270
e-mail: Ktcaedav@netins.net
www.pwsaiowa.org

Tammy Davis, President

Kansas

5830 Prader-Willi Syndrome Advocates
14 NE Bayview Drive
Lees Summit, MO 64064
816-350-1375
Teri Douglas
Barry Douglas

Kentucky

5831 PWSA of Kentucky
Prader-Willi Syndrome Association
9213 Reigate Ct
Louisville,ÿ, KY 40222
502-339-7872
e-mail: frankandannette@fuse.net

Frank Beck, President

Maine

5832 Prader-Willi Association of New England (Maine, Mass, RI, NH, VT)
2 Ernest Street
Webster, MA 01570
508-943-1400
e-mail: sunsetrock@comcast.net
www.pwsane.org

Eileen Rullo, President
Mary Raymond, Vice President

Maryland

5833 PWSA of Maryland, Virginia & DC
Prader-Willi Syndrome Association
547 Varndell Road
Grantsville,ÿ, MD 21536
301- 89- 416
e-mail: ÿlisa@varndellengineering.com
www.pwsausa.org/MD/

Linda Keder, President
Susaie Wood, Maryland Contact

Massachusetts

5834 Prader-Willi Association of New England (Maine, Mass, RI, NH, VT)
2 Ernest Street
Webster, MA 01570
508-943-1400
www.pwsane.org

Eileen Rullo, President
Mary Raymond, Vice President

Michigan

5835 PWSA of Michigan
Prader-Willi Syndrome Association
10756 Woodbushe
Lowell, MI 49331
734-998-3507
Fax: 941-313-0142
e-mail: info@pwsami.org
www.pwsausa.org/MI/

Jon Hendrick
Chris Hendrick

Minnesota

5836 PWSA Chapter - Minnesota
Prader-Willi Syndrome Association
7691 Iverson Avenue S
Cottage Grove, MN 55016
651-768-0045
e-mail: dwestenfield@datalink.com
www.pwsausa.org/MN/

Denise Westenfield, President
Kymm Salwasser, Treasurer

Missouri

5837 PWSA Missouri Chapter
Prader-Willi Syndrome Missouri Association
3233 Hedgetree Lane Street, PO Box 410252
Creve Coeur, MO 63141
314-935-9358
Fax: 314-935-7461
e-mail: whitmanb@slu.edu
www.pwsausa.org/MO/

Judy O'Leary, President

Montana

5838 Prader-Willi Northwest Association
3706 29th Avenue W
Seattle, WA 98199
206-285-7679
e-mail: jlunderwood@juno.com

Joane Underwood, Co-President

Nebraska

5839 PWSA of Nebraska
Prader-Willi Syndrome Association
302 S 49th Avenue
Omaha, NE 68132
402-551-9168
e-mail: jvarner@cox.net
www.pwsausa.org

Jennifer Varner, Contact

Nevada

5840 PWSA Las Vegas/Nevada Support Group
PWS NV S.H.A.R.E.
www.pwsnv.org

702-526-0630
e-mail: pwsnv.org@gmail.com
www.pwsnv.org

New Jersey

5841 PWSA - New Jersey Chapter
Prader-Willi Syndrome Association
514 Gatewood Road
Cherry Hill, NJ 08003   856-795-4229
e-mail: pwsa.nj@gmail.com
www.pwsausa.org/NJ/

Sybil Cohen, President

New Mexico

5842 PWS Project for New Mexico

505-332-6700
e-mail: claroque@arc-a.org

New York

5843 Prader-Willi Alliance of New York
PWSA NY Chapter
2224 Agnew Ter
The Villages, FL 32162   585-442-1655
800-442-1655
e-mail: alliance@prader-willi.org
www.prader-willi.org

Hon. Daniel D Angiolillo, President
Rachel ÿÿÿÿ Johnson , Vice President

North Carolina

5844 PWSA of North Carolina
PWSA
4627 Mt Sinai Road
Durham, NC 27705   919-332-0621
Mary Jones Patterson

Ohio

5845 PWSA of Ohio
State Office
1087 Dover Drive
Medina, OH 44256   440-716-0552
e-mail: pwsaohio@aol.com
www.pwsaohio.org

Jennifer Bolander, President

5846 Prader-Willi Families of Ohio
4075 West 226 Street
Fairview Park, OH ÿ4412   440-716-0552
e-mail: pwfohio@aol.com
www.pwsaohio.org/

Johanna Costello, President

Oklahoma

5847 PWSA of Oklahoma
Prader-Willi Syndrome Association
3820 SE 89th Street
Oklahoma City, OK 73135   405-677-8089
Fax: 405-522-6256
e-mail: Rdmosley@swbell.net
www.pwsausa.org

Daphne Mosley, President
Curt Shacklett, Chairman

Oregon

5848 PWSA of Oregon
Prader-Willi Syndrome Association
456 Horn Lane
Eugene, OR 97404   360-609-5197
e-mail: wade175@juno.com
www.pwsausa.org

Lennae Elkington, President

Pennsylvania

5849 PWSA of Pennsylvania
Prader-Willi Syndrome Association
2415 Maryland Drive
Pittsburgh, PA 15241   412-854-8885
e-mail: pwsa_pa@verizon.net
www.pwsausa.org

Donn & John Forster, Co-Presidents

South Carolina

5850 PWSA - South Carolina
Prader-Willi Syndrome Association
912 Lake Spur Lane
Chapin, SC 29036   803-345-1379
e-mail: rleazer8@cs.com
www.pwsausa.org

Rhett Eleazer, Contact

Tennessee

5851 PWSA - Tennessee
Prader-Willi Syndrome Association
105 Foxwood Lane
Franklin, TN 37069   615-790-6659
e-mail: Tcbo333@aol.com
www.pwsausa.org

Terry Bolander

Texas

5852 Texas Prader-Willi Syndrome Association
PO Box 1542
Whitehouse, TX 75791   903-363-8680
e-mail: info@texaspwsa.com
www.pwsausa.org; www.texaspwsa.com

Derek Snitker

Utah

5853 Prader-Willi Utah Association
Prader-Willi Syndrome Association
2652 E Nottingham Way
Salt Lake City, UT 84108   801-556-8012
Fax: 801-768-3924
e-mail: sidlisathornton@aol.com
www.pwsausa.org/UT/

Lisa Thornton, President

Virginia

5854 PWSA of Maryland, Virginia & DC
Prader-Willi Syndrome Association
2601 Chriswell Place
Herndon, VA 20171   703-716-4189
e-mail: pwsamd@pwsausa.org
www.pwsausa.org/MD/

Linda Keder, President
Sherri Planton, Virginia Contact

5855 PWSA of Wisconsin
Prader-Willi Syndrome Association
2701 N Alexander Street
Appleton, WI 54911   920-882-6371
                                          866-797-2947
                              e-mail: wisonsin@pwsausa.org
                                        www.pwsausa.org/wi/

Mary Lynn Larson, Manager

Research Centers

5856 Foundation for Prader-Willi Research
5455 Wilshire Blvd, Suite 2020,
Los Angeles, CA 90036   760-536-3027
                                          888-322-5487
                                      Fax: 502-749-9388
                                          www.fpwr.org

Dedicated to the advancement of research on PWS. The Foundation chooses projects that are highly relevant for individuals with PWS and their families and that are scientifically sound.

Rachel Tugon, Executive Director
Alice Viroslav, President
Kathryn McGhee, Membership

Audio Video

5857 A Deadly Hunger
Prader-Willi Syndrome Association
8588 Potter Park Drive, Suite 500
Sarasota, FL 34238   941-312-0400
                                          800-926-4797
                                      Fax: 941-312-0142
                                  e-mail: info@pwsausa.org
                                        www.pwsausa.org

A five part series of news segments that spotlight PWS. Overview of syndrome and stresses problems associated with appetite, obesity, and behavior.

DVD

Michelle Torbert, Chair
James Koerber, Vice Chair
Ken Smith, Executive Director

5858 A Tribute to PWS Children from Around the World
Prader-Willi Syndrome Association
8588 Potter Park Road, Suite 500
Sarasota, FL 34238   941-312-0400
                                          800-926-4797
                                      Fax: 941-312-0142
                                  e-mail: info@pwsausa.org
                                        www.pwsausa.org

A video of children with PWS of all ages. The presentation is set to music.

10 Minutes

Michelle Torbert, Chair
James Koerber, Vice Chair
Ken Smith, Executive Director

5859 Food, Behavior and Beyond
Prader-Willi Syndrome Association
8588 Potter Park Drive, Suite 500
Sarasota, FL 34238   941-312-0400
                                          800-926-4797
                                      Fax: 941-312-0142
                                  e-mail: info@pwsausa.org
                                        www.pwsausa.org

Suggestions on nutrition, food and behavior, cognitive and behavioral traits and medications.

DVD

Michelle Torbert, Chair
James Koerber, Vice Chair
Ken Smith, Executive Director

5860 Maribel
Prader-Willi Syndrome Association
8588 Potter Park Drive, Suite 500
Sarasota, FL 34238   941-312-0400
                                          800-926-4797
                                      Fax: 941-312-0142
                                  e-mail: info@pwsausa.org
                                        www.pwsausa.org

Chronicles a family's struggle with their adult daughter with PWS. Helpful for families with replacement needs who need to show dramatic impact.

2004 DVD/VHS

Michelle Torbert, Chair
James Koerber, Vice Chair
Ken Smith, Executive Director

5861 PWS - The Early Years
Prader-Willi Syndrome Association
8588 Potter Park Drive, Suite 500
Sarasota, FL 34238   941-312-0400
                                          800-926-4797
                                      Fax: 941-312-0142
                                  e-mail: info@pwsausa.org
                                        www.pwsausa.org

Practical suggestions for families with a young child newly diagnosed with PWS. Includes family interviews.

2002 Video 42 Mins

Michelle Torbert, Chair
James Koerber, Vice Chair
Ken Smith, Executive Director

5862 Prader-Willi Syndrome - An Overview for He alth Professionals
Prader-Willi Syndrome Association
8588 Potter Park Drive, Suite 500
Sarasota, FL 34238   941-312-0400
                                          800-926-4797
                                      Fax: 941-312-0142
                                  e-mail: info@pwsausa.org
                                        www.pwsausa.org

A medical overview of PWS for health care professionals. It handles all the major genetics and health care issues of the child with PWS.

2004 35 Minutes

Michelle Torbert, Chair
James Koerber, Vice Chair
Ken Smith, Executive Director

Web Sites

5863 International Prader-Willi Syndrome Organi zation (IPWSO)
www.ipwso.org

                                      e-mail: info@ipwso.org
                                            www.ipwso.org

5864 Online Mendelian Inheritance in Man
National Library of Medicine, Building 38A
Bethesda, MD 20894   888-346-3656
                              e-mail: info@ncbi.nlm.nih.gov
                                    www.ncbi.nlm.nih.gov

This database is a catalog of human genes and genetic disorders.

5865 Prader-Willi Alliance of New York
244 5th Avenue, Suite D-110
New York, NY 10001   718-846-6606
                                          800-442-1655
                                      www.prader-willi.org

A chapter of the PWSA, it represents the interests of individuals in New York State with Prader-Willi Syndrome, their families, and the professionals who provide services to the Prader-Willi population.

Rachel Johnson, President
Nancy Finegold, Vice President
Tammy Reals, Vice President

5866 Prader-Willi Syndrome Association
8588 Potter Park Drive, Suite 500
Sarasota, FL 34238   941-312-0400
                                                800-926-4797
                                                Fax: 941-312-0142
                                                e-mail: info@pwsausa.org
                                                www.pwsausa.org

Dedicated to serving individuals affected by Prader-Willi Syndrome, their families, and interested professionals. To provide information, education, and support services to its members. PWSA offers a toll free telephone number for informationand referrals, a bimonthly newsletter, publications and audiovisual presentations about PWS, an annual national conference for families and professionals and a nationwide network of local chapters, parents, and professionals.

Michelle Torbert, Chair
James Koerber, Vice Chair
Ken Smith, Executive Director

Book Publishers

5867 Cookbook for the PWS Diet
Prader-Willi Syndrome Association
8588 Potter Park Drive, Suite 500
Sarasota, FL 34238   941-312-0400
                                                800-926-4797
                                                Fax: 941-312-0142
                                                e-mail: info@pwsausa.org
                                                www.pwsausa.org

Filled with low-fat, low-sugar recipes designed to be used by the whole family. Great substitution list, fun snack recipes, mealtime tips, full nutritional values calculated for each recipe. Can be used by anyone wanting to lose weight while eating nutritious, interesting food.

2003

John Heybach, Co-Chair
Ken Smith, Co-Chair
Dale Cooper, Interim Executive Directo

5868 Growth Hormone and Prader-Willi Syndrome
Linda Keder, author

Prader-Willi Syndrome Association
8588 Potter Park Drive, Suite 500
Sarasota, FL 34238   941-312-0400
                                                800-926-4797
                                                Fax: 941-312-0142
                                                e-mail: info@pwsausa.org
                                                www.pwsausa.org

Reference for families and care givers.

2001 52 pages Softcover

John Heybach, Co-Chair
Ken Smith, Co-Chair
Dale Cooper, Interim Executive Directo

5869 Management of Prader-Willi Syndrome
Prader-Willi Syndrome Association
8588 Potter Park Drive, Suite 500
Sarasota, FL 34238   941-312-0400
                                                800-926-4797
                                                Fax: 941-312-0142
                                                e-mail: info@pwsausa.org
                                                www.pwsausa.org

Latest edition of the only comprehensive textbook on PWS in print. Excellent reference tool for professionals and service providers.

550 pages 3rd Edition

John Heybach, Co-Chair
Ken Smith, Co-Chair
Dale Cooper, Interim Executive Directo

5870 Nutitional Care for Children with PWS, Inf ants and Toddlers
Prader-Willi Syndrome Association
8588 Potter Park Drive, Suite 500
Sarasota, FL 34238   941-312-0400
                                                800-926-4797
                                                Fax: 941-312-0142
                                                e-mail: info@pwsausa.org
                                                www.pwsausa.org

Provides answers to frequently asked questions about nutrition and feeding of infants and toddlers with PWS.

Revised 2004 62 pages Softcover

John Heybach, Co-Chair
Ken Smith, Co-Chair
Dale Cooper, Interim Executive Directo

5871 Overview of the Prader-Willi Syndrome
Prader-Willi Syndrome Association
8588 Potter Park Drive, Suite 500
Sarasota, FL 34232   941-312-0400
                                                800-926-4797
                                                Fax: 941-312-0142
                                                e-mail: info@pwsausa.org
                                                www.pwsausa.org

A short introduction to the syndrome for professionals and parents.

13 pages Softcover

John Heybach, Co-Chair
Ken Smith, Co-Chair
Dale Cooper, Interim Executive Directo

5872 Prader-Willi Syndrome is What I Have Not W ho I Am!
Prader-Willi Syndrome Association
8588 Potter Park Drive, Suite 500
Sarasota, FL 34238   941-312-0400
                                                800-926-4797
                                                Fax: 941-312-0142
                                                e-mail: info@pwsausa.org
                                                www.pwsausa.org

A book of feelings written by children and young adults with PWS. This book gives an important insight into lives and thoughts of our people dealing with PWS on a daily basis. A portion of the book opens the door to journal writing and an opportunity for the reader with PWS to share their feelings.

2005 70 pages softcover

John Heybach, Co-Chair
Ken Smith, Co-Chair
Dale Cooper, Interim Executive Directo

5873 Sometimes I'm Mad, Sometimes I'm Glad - A Sibling Booklet
Prader-Willi Syndrome Association
8588 Potter Park Drive, Suite 500
Sarasota, FL 34238   941-312-0400
                                                800-926-4797
                                                Fax: 941-312-0142
                                                e-mail: info@pwsausa.org
                                                www.pwsausa.org

It is in the voice of a sibling of someone with PWS. Recognizes the range of feelings that arise in having a brother or sister with the syndrome.

Revised 2005

John Heybach, Co-Chair
Ken Smith, Co-Chair
Dale Cooper, Interim Executive Directo

5874 Teacher's Handbook for the Student with PW S (Educator's Resource)
Prader-Willi Syndrome Association
8588 Potter Park Drive, Suite 500
Sarasota, FL 34238   941-312-0400
                                                800-926-4797
                                                Fax: 941-312-0142
                                                e-mail: info@pwsausa.org
                                                www.pwsausa.org

A resource book for educators. Important for all who work with these students to gain knowledge about this disorder as well as the many factors that influence their learning. This manual will provide teachers with valuable information to assist in working with students of all abilities.

2003

John Heybach, Co-Chair
Ken Smith, Co-Chair
Dale Cooper, Interim Executive Directo

5875 Tool Box of Hope - For When Your Body Does n't Feel Good
Prader-Willi Syndrome Association
8588 Potter Park Drive, Suite 500
Sarasota, FL 34238
941-312-0400
800-926-4797
Fax: 941-312-0142
e-mail: info@pwsausa.org
www.pwsausa.org

Fun and practical ways for parents and caregivers to help their child express their feelings, take medicine, get along with others, and make friends with their disability.

2003 2003 pages Ages 3-adult

John Heybach, Co-Chair
Ken Smith, Co-Chair
Dale Cooper, Interim Executive Directo

Newsletters

5876 Gathered View
Prader-Willi Syndrome Association
8588 Potter Park Drive, Suite 500
Sarasota, FL 34238
941-312-0400
800-926-4797
Fax: 941-312-0142
e-mail: info@pwsausa.org
www.pwsausa.org

The official newsletter of PWSA USA. It offers current research findings, behavior and weight management techniques, educational news and more.

Bimonthly

Michelle Torbert, Chair
James Koerber, Vice Chair
Ken Smith, Executive Director

Pamphlets

5877 Behavior Management - A Collection of Arti cles
Prader-Willi Syndrome Association
8588 Potter Park Drive, Suite 500
Sarasota, FL 34238
941-312-0400; 800-926-4797
Fax: 941-312-0142
e-mail: info@pwsausa.org
www.pwsausa.org

Includes general articles on behavior concerns, use of psychotropic medications, skin picking, and social skills teaching.

2003 49 pages softcover

Michelle Torbert, Chair
James Koerber, Vice Chair
Ken Smith, Executive Director

5878 Child With Prader-Willi Syndrome: Birth to Three
Prader-Willi Syndrome Association
8588 Potter Park Drive, Suite 500
Sarasota, FL 34238
941-312-0400
800-926-4797
Fax: 941-312-0142
e-mail: info@pwsausa.org
www.pwsausa.org

Discusses the common concerns of the first three years and offers specific recommendations for early intervention strategies. A helpful and positive resource families, physicians, early intervention worker, and other care providers.

Revised 2004 34 pages Softcover

Michelle Torbert, Chair
James Koerber, Vice Chair
Ken Smith, Executive Director

5879 Growing Up with Prader-Willi Syndrome - Pe rsonal Reflections of a Mother
Prader-Willi Syndrome Association
8588 Potter Park Drive, Suite 500
Sarasota, FL 34238
941-312-0400
800-926-4797
Fax: 941-312-0142
e-mail: info@pwsausa.org
www.pwsausa.org

A collection of seventeen articles including tips for managing family life.

Revised 2003 37 pages Booklet

Michelle Torbert, Chair
James Koerber, Vice Chair
Ken Smith, Executive Director

5880 Physical Therapy Intervention for Individu als With Prader-Willi Syndrome
Prader-Willi Syndrome Association
8588 Potter Park Drive, Suite 500
Sarasota, FL 34238
941-312-0400; 800-926-4797
Fax: 941-312-0142
e-mail: info@pwsausa.org; www.pwsausa.org

Provides general information about physical therapy intervention. Includes copies of articles by Janice Agarwal, PT and mom of a son with PWS.

11 pages softcover

Michelle Torbert, Chair
James Koerber, Vice Chair
Ken Smith, Executive Director

5881 Prader-Willi Syndrome: A Guide for Familie s & Professionals
Prader-Willi Syndrome Association
8588 Potter Park Drive, Suite 500
Sarasota, FL 34238
941-312-0400; 800-926-4797
Fax: 941-312-0142
e-mail: info@pwsausa.org
www.pwsausa.org

Contains comprehensice information about PWS including description, evaluation, genetics, diagnostic testing, management.

Revised 2005 12 pages

Michelle Torbert, Chair
James Koerber, Vice Chair
Ken Smith, Executive Director

5882 Prader-Willi Syndrome: Medical Alerts
Prader-Willi Syndrome Association
8588 Potter Park Drive, Suite 500
Sarasota, FL 34238
941-312-0400; 800-926-4797
Fax: 941-312-0142
e-mail: info@pwsausa.org; www.pwsausa.org

Important resource for parents to give their child's doctor, Er staff, cargiver, etc.

2005

Michelle Torbert, Chair
James Koerber, Vice Chair
Ken Smith, Executive Director

5883 Student with Prader-Willi Syndrome - Infor mation for Educators
Prader-Willi Syndrome Association
8588 Potter Park Drive, Suite 500
Sarasota, FL 34242
941-312-0400; 800-926-4797
Fax: 941-312-0142
e-mail: info@pwsausa.org; www.pwsausa.org

An information packet for educators of children with PWS. It includes a handbook, worksheets and brochures. Applicable for Pre-k through high school.

Michelle Torbert, Chair
James Koerber, Vice Chair
Ken Smith, Executive Director

Description

5884 PRECOCIOUS PUBERTY

Synonym: Pubertas praecox

Covers these related disorders: Gonadotropin-dependent precocious puberty, Gonadotropin-independent precocious puberty

Involves the following Biologic System(s):

Endocrinologic Disorders

Precocious puberty refers to a condition in which the onset of sexual maturation occurs before the age of eight years in girls and nine years in boys. True precocious puberty refers to the premature sexual development of the sex glands (i.e., ovaries and testes) as well as the outward appearance of the child (secondary sexual characteristics). Precocious pseudopuberty refers to the early development of only the secondary sex characteristics with no involvement of the sex glands.

True precocious puberty results from the premature production and secretion by the pituitary gland of gonadotropin, a hormone that stimulates the ovaries and the testes. Because the release of hormones from the pituitary gland is controlled by another gland, the hypothalamus, functional abnormalities of or growth of a tumor in the pituitary or the hypothalamus may also result in premature sexual development. These abnormalities may include hormone-secreting tumors of the pituitary gland, brain lesions such as a hypothalamic hamartoma, and other lesions of the central nervous system that may activate the hypothalamus. True precocious puberty may also result from an underactive thyroid gland (hypothyroidism). However, for most children with precocious puberty, the exact cause is not known. More girls are affected by precocious puberty than boys. Although most cases appear sporadically, some patients have a family history of this condition. Sexual characteristics associated with true precocious puberty are always consistent with the sex of the affected child (isosexual characteristics). Such characteristics may include the early appearance of underarm and pubic hair, facial hair in boys, and breasts and menstrual cycles in girls. The penis, testes, and ovaries enlarge and acne may develop. Although height and weight may increase rapidly, advanced bone growth may result in premature closure of the growing ends of the bone (epiphyses) and, thus, slower linear growth leading to short stature.

Precocious pseudopuberty may be caused by a tumor of the ovary, testis, or adrenal gland. Such tumors may cause excessive production of sex hormones. This form of the disorder may also be inherited as an autosomal dominant trait. In addition, precocious pseudopuberty may be associated with other disorders such as McCune-Albright syndrome, which is a condition resulting from the overproduction of hormones of multiple glands. This syndrome is characterized by premature sexual development in girls, irregularities of skin color (pigmentation) and the skeletal system, and abnormalities of various glands. Physical characteristics associated with precocious pseudopuberty are similar to those of true precocious puberty, although the testes and ovaries are not usually involved. However, children affected with this form of the disorder may develop secondary sexual characteristics associated with those of the opposite sex (heterosexual characteristics). In addition, prcocious pseudopuberty may prompt early maturation of the hormonal cycle that results in true precocious puberty.

Treatment for true precocious puberty may include the administration of gonadotropin-releasing hormones. These hormones work by diminishing the stimulatory response of the pituitary gland to the gonadotropin-releasing hormones produced naturally within the body until normal puberty begins. Treatment for precocious pseudopuberty may include the use of certain medications that reduce the levels of male and female sex hormones (i.e., testosterone and estrogen). In addition, surgery may be indicated in those patients who have precocious puberty as a result of certain types of tumors. Other treatment is symptomatic and supportive.

Government Agencies

5885 NIH/National Institute of Child Health and Human Development
31 Center Drive, Building 31
Bethesda, MD 20892   301-496-1333
                                   Fax: 301-496-1104
                                   www.nichd.nih.gov

Established in 1962 by congress, today the institute conducts and supports research on topics related to the health of children, adults, families and populations. Some of these topics include: developmental disabilities, growth and development, infant death, reproductive health and birth defects.

Jay H Hoofnagle, Director
Lisa Kaeser, Program & Public Liaison

National Associations & Support Groups

5886 American Academy of Pediatrics
141 Northwest Point Boulevard
Elk Grove Village, IL 60007   847-434-4000
                                   800-433-9016
                                   Fax: 847-434-8000
                                   www.aap.org

The American Academy of Pediatrics and its member pediatricians are committed to the attainment of optimal physical, mental and social health and well-being for all infants, children, adolescents, and young adults.

Sandra Hassink, MD, FAAP, President

5887 Genetic Alliance
4301 Connecticut Avenue NW
Washington, DC 20008   202-966-5557
                                   800-336-4363
                                   Fax: 202-966-8553
                         e-mail: info@geneticalliance.org
                                   www.geneticalliance.org

A coalition of voluntary genetic support groups, consumers and professionals addressing the needs of individuals and families affected by genetic disorders from a national perspective.

Sharon Terry, President
Natasha Bonhomme, Vice President of Strategic Develop
Vaughn ÿEdelson, Assistant Director of Health Commun

5888 MAGIC Foundation: Major Aspects of Growth in Children
6645 W North Avenue
Oak Park, IL 60302   708-383-0808
                                   800-362-4423
                                   Fax: 708-383-0899
                      e-mail: mary@magicfoundation.org
                                   www.magicfoundation.org

A national nonprofit organization providing support and education regarding growth disorders in children and related adult disorders. Provides educational information, networking, a national conference, a kids' program and an extensive medical library.

Mary Andrews, CEO
Dianne Tamburrino, Executive Director

695

Precocious Puberty / Web Sites

5889 March of Dimes Birth Defects Foundation
1275 Mamaroneck Avenue
White Plains, NY 10605   914-997-4488
888-663-4637
Fax: 914-428-8203
e-mail: answers@marchofdimes.com
www.marchofdimes.com

Partnership of volunteers and professionals dedicates to improving the health of babies by preventing birth defects and infant mortality. Over 100 chapters are located across the country and can be located through the National Office.

Jennifer L Howse, President

Web Sites

5890 KidsHealth: Precocious Puberty
www.kidshealth.org/parents/

General overview of precocious puberty including signs, causes, diagnosis and treatment.

Neil Izenberg, MD, Editor-in-Chief & Founder

5891 Online Mendelian Inheritance in Man
National Library of Medicine, Building 38A
Bethesda, MD 20894   888-346-3656
e-mail: info@ncbi.nlm.nih.gov
www.ncbi.nlm.nih.gov/entrez/dispomim.cgi?id=176400

This database contains textual information and references. It also contains copious links to MEDLINE and sequence records in the Entrez system, and links to additional related resources at NCBI and elsewhere.

5892 Society for Endocrinology
22 Apex Court, Woodlands
Bradley Stoke, BI BS32   145-464-2200
Fax: 145-464-2222
www.endocrinology.org

Aims to advance education and research in endocrinology for the benefit of the public. Lists resources such as journals, books, events, and training courses available.

5893 University of Michigan Health System
1500 E. Medical Center Drive
Ann Arbor, MI 48109   734-936-4000
e-mail: kylaboys@umich.edu
www.med.umich.edu/yourchild/topics/puberty

Information on early puberty or precocious puberty.

Pamphlets

5894 Precocious Puberty
Human Growth Foundation
997 Glen Cove Avenue, Suite 5
Glen Head, NY 11545   800-451-6434
Fax: 516-671-4055
e-mail: hgf1@hgfound.org
www.hgfound.org

Booklet

Pisit Pitukcheewanont, MD, President
Emily Germain-Lee, Vice President
Patricia D. Costa, Executive Director

696

Description

5895 PREMATURITY

Involves the following Biologic System(s):

Neonatal and Infant Disorders

Premature birth (also known as preterm birth) refers to the birth of an infant before the 37-week gestational period. Most pregnancies last for 40 weeks. About 12 percent of babies in the United States — or 1 in 8 — are born prematurely each year. Although at least 40 percent of premature births occur for unknown reasons, prematurity may result from many different factors including a condition in which the mother develops high blood pressure, large quantities of protein in the urine, and an abnormal accumulation of fluid in the body (preeclampsia); maternal heart disease, kidney disease, or diabetes; acute infection; trauma; uterine irregularities (e.g., bicornate uterus); and placental abnormalities (e.g., placenta previa). Other contributing factors may include multiple pregnancy, maternal drug use, and fetal distress. Poor nutrition and lack of appropriate prenatal care may also put the unborn child at risk for premature birth.

Premature infants usually have a characteristic appearance in addition to their small size. For example, their heads often appear too large for their bodies and their skin may be very pink, smooth, translucent, and covered with downy hair (lanugo). They may have sparse hair and very little subcutaneous fat. In girls, the genitals may be incompletely developed such that the labia majora do not cover the labia minora. In affected boys, the testes may not fully descend into the scrotum. Other findings may include the absence of the creases on the palms and soles, incomplete development of the ear, and other irregularities. In addition, the survival or health of a premature infant may be compromised as a result of the incomplete development of certain body systems. The earlier the delivery, the more immature the organs. Common irregularities associated with prematurity include inadequate development of the lungs and subsequent deficiency in the production of a substance that allows the air sacs in the lungs to remain open (surfactant). This condition may lead to respiratory distress syndrome (also called hyaline membrane disease) and associated life-threatening oxygen deficiency in the blood. Immature organ development may affect the brain, resulting in deficiencies in spontaneous breathing, inadequate sucking, and difficulty in swallowing. There is also an increased risk of bleeding in the brain (intraventricular hemorrhage). Premature infants are also particularly susceptible to serious infection resulting from incomplete placental transfer of maternal antibodies. Immature liver function may result in a temporary increase in blood levels of bilirubin causing yellowing of the eyes, skin, and mucous membranes (jaundice). Other complications of prematurity may include poor body temperature regulation, small stomach capacity, inadequacy of the intestinal tract that may result in injury or decreased blood flow to the intestines (necrotizing enterocolitis), immature kidney function, fluctuations in bloodsugar levels, reduced levels of calcium in the blood, and other irregularities related to underdevelopment of body systems. It has also been shown that premature babies are prone to developing depression as teenagers.

One of the most important steps to preventing prematurity is to receive prenatal care as early as possible in the pregnancy, and to continue such care until the baby is born. Statistics clearly show that early and good prenatal care reduces the chance of premature birth and related deaths. Two tactics are used to deal with a potential premature birth: delay the arrival of birth as much as possible, or prepare the premature fetus for arrival. Both of these tactics may be used simultaneously. Treatment for premature infants depends upon the maturity of the various organ systems at the time of birth. In many cases, these infants are cared for around the clock in a neonatal care unit where body temperature may be regulated in an incubator and respiration may be maintained through artificial ventilation, if necessary. Feeding may be accomplished through the use of intravenous feeding or through a feeding tube directly into the stomach. Nutritional supplementation may include the administration of iron and vitamins. In addition, liquids may be given to maintain fluid levels in the body. Antibiotics may be administered to help treat infection. Discharge from the hospital takes place once the infant has reached appropriate weight and certain functional criteria have been established. In addition, before discharge, parents or caregivers of these infants are given complete instructions in their proper care. Other treatment is symptomatic and supportive.

Government Agencies

5896 NIH/National Institute of Child Health and Human Development
31 Center Drive, Building 31
Bethesda, MD 20892   301-496-1333
                           Fax: 301-496-1104
                           www.nichd.nih.gov

Established in 1962 by congress, today the institute conducts and supports research on topics related to the health of children, adults, families and populations. Some of these topics include: developmental disabilities, growth and development, infant death, reproductive health and birth defects.

Jay H Hoofnagle, Director
Lisa Kaeser, Program & Public Liaison

National Associations & Support Groups

5897 Alexis Foundation - Premature Infants and Children
PO Box 1126
Birmingham, MI 48012   248-543-4169
                              877-253-9470
e-mail: thealexisfoundation@prodigy.net
www.home.vicnet.net.au/~garyh/mediarel.html

Their mission is to raise public and political awareness of the problems facing prematurely-born infants; education on the problems faced and how they can be foreseen and handled; make essential premature accessories readily available; and promote strong communication between doctors, nurses, and parents.

Elaine Sayers, Founder

5898 American Academy of Pediatrics
141 Northwest Point Boulevard
Elk Grove Village, IL 60007   847-434-4000
                                     800-433-9016
                                Fax: 847-434-8000
                                     www.aap.org

The American Academy of Pediatrics and its member pediatricians are committed to the attainment of optimal physical, mental and social health and well-being for all infants, children, adolescents, and young adults.

Sandra Hassink, MD, FAAP, President

5899 March of Dimes Birth Defects Foundation
1275 Mamaroneck Avenue
White Plains, NY 10605   914-997-4488
                                                         888-663-4637
                                                    Fax: 914-428-8203
                                        e-mail: answers@marchofdimes.com
                                                   www.marchofdimes.com

Partnership of volunteers and professionals dedicates to improving the health of babies by preventing birth defects and infant mortality. Over 100 chapters are located across the country and can be located through the National Office.

Jennifer L Howse, President

5900 National Perinatal Association
457 State Street
Binghamton, NY 13901   607-772-0468
                                                         888-971-3295
                                                    Fax: 717-920-1390
                                          e-mail: ÿnpa@nationalperinatal.org
                                                  www.nationalperinatal.org

The National Perinatal Association promotes the health and well being of mothers and infants enriching families, communities and the world.

Christine Lipoich, Manager
Mary Jo Crosby, VP Development

5901 Ropard: Association for Retinopathy of Pre maturity & Related Diseases
PO Box 250425
Franklin, MI 48025   800-788-2020
                                            e-mail: ropard@yahoo.com
                                                       www.ropard.org

Funds clinically relevant basic science and clinical research to eliminate retinopathy of prematurity and associated retinal diseases; innovative work leading directly to the development of new low vision devices and teaching techniques and services for children who are visually impaired and their families.

5902 Sidelines-National High Risk Pregnancy Sup port Network
PO Box 1808
Laguna Beach, CA 92652   888-447-4754
                                                    Fax: 949-497-5598
                                         e-mail: sidelines@sidelines.org
                                                    www.sidelines.org

Non profit organization that provides international support for women and their families experiencing premature births and complicated pregnancies.

Candace Hurley, Founder & Executive Director
Tracy Hoogenboom, Administrative Director
Nancy Veeneman, Volunteer Training Coordinator

State Agencies & Support Groups

Georgia

5903 Georgia Perinatal Association
c/o Terri Negron
5607 Walden Farm Drive
Powder Springs, GA 30127   www.georgiaperinatal.org

Works to promote perinatal health through education, collaboration and influence of state public policy. It collaborates with others to improve pregnancy and infant outcomes.

Bonnie Simmons, President
Diane Youmans, President
Margaret B. Hotz, Secretary

Texas

5904 Texas Perinatal Association
19 Cloister Parkway
Amarillo, TX 79121   e-mail: lisaplat@aol.com
                                                       www.txpa.org

Committed to achieving continuous improvement in the quality of health care to mothers and infants in the state of Texas.

Laura Street

Wisconsin

5905 Wisconsin Association for Perinatal Care
McConnell Hall
211 S. Paterson St.,ÿSuite 250
Madison, WI 53703   608-285-5858
                                                    Fax: 608-285-5004
                                         e-mail: wapc@perinatalweb.org
                                                   www.perinatalweb.org

Provides leadership and education for improved perinatal health outcomes of women, infants and their families through: increased public awareness; engaging the diverse community of perinatal health care advocates; and coordinating systems of perinatal care in Wisconsin.

Ann Conway, Executive Director
Kristine E Casto, Learning Coordinator

Libraries & Resource Centers

5906 National Center for Education in Maternal and Child Health
Georgetown University
2115 Wisconsin Ave NW, Suite 601
Washington, DC 20007   202-784-9770
                                                    Fax: 202-784-9777
                                         e-mail: mchlibrary@ncemch.org
                                                      www.ncemch.org

Information and advocacy resources for families and professionals. Includes listings of organizations providing general information and organizations focusing on more specific areas of concern to families and young adults who have disabilities.

Rochelle Mayer, Director

Research Centers

5907 NIH/National Institute of Child Health and Human Development
NICHD Clearinghouse
PO Box 3006
Rockville, MD 20847   800-370-2943
                                                    Fax: 301-984-1473
                                 e-mail: NICHDclearinghouse@mail.nih.gov
                                                     www.nichd.nih.gov

The National Institute for Child Health and Human Development conducts and supports laboratory, clinical and epidemiological research on the reproductive, neurobiologic, developmental, and behavioral processes that determine and maintain the health of children, adults, families, and populations.

5908 NIH/National Institute of Mental Health Eating Disorders Program
6001 Executive Boulevard, Room 8184
Bethesda, MD 20892   301-443-4513
                                                    Fax: 301-443-4279

Web Sites

5909 Children's Medical Ventures
3000 Minuteman Road
Andover, MA 01810   www.healthcare.philips.com/

The company offers high quality products which meet the unique needs of these special babies, including appropriately sized items, safety equipment and specialty feeding and skin care products.

5910 Newborns in Need
3323 Transou Road
Pfafftown, NC 27040   www.newbornsinneed.org

Charity organization for the care of sick and needy babies and their families.

Sam Safrit, Chairman
Connie Edwards, President
Gayle McKeethan, Vice President

5911 PREBIC-International Preterm Birth Collabo rative
www.prebic.org

Supports and enhances international networking among researchers in preterm birth.

Craig Pennell, President
Hanns Helmer, Vice President
Melanie White, Treasurer

5912 Preemie Ring
hub.familynhome.org/hub/preemie

A collection of home pages about premature infants and premature infant care, etc.

5913 Preemie Twins
PO Box 12
Pierce, NE 68767   402-606-1820
                                              Fax: 402-606-1820
                                           www.preemietwins.com

Online resource for both parents of multiples and/or premature infants.

5914 Preemie World
preemie.info

A meeting place for family and friends of preemies.

5915 Premature Baby-Premature Child
www.prematurity.org

Preemie parent support for preemie special needs.

5916 Prematurely Yours
www.prematurelyyours.com

Special products for special babies.

Kim Bryant, RN, President
Becky Meloan, RN, VP
Curtis Bryant, Treasurer/Secretary

Book Publishers

5917 Prematurely Yours
6712 Townpoint Road
Suffolk, VA 23435   757-483-9879
                                              Fax: 757-484-8267
                                   e-mail: prematurely@PreMieProducts.com
                                           www.prematurelyyours.com

Designed exclusively to record milestones for the premature infant, from birth to six years of age. Such milestones as maintaining their body temperature, nippling their feedings, and breathing without the aid of extra oxygen are, of course, taken for granted with a full term infant.

40 pages Hardcover

Kim Bryant, RN, President
Becky Meloan, RN, VP
Curtis Bryant, Treasurer/Secretary

Magazines

5918 Left Side Lines
Sidelines
PO Box 1808
Laguna Beach, CA 92652   888-447-4754
                                      e-mail: sidelines@sidelines.org
                                           www.sidelines.org

Offers articles, insights and tips related to the challange of coping with a high-risk pregnancy. Specific information is provided on prematurity, NICU, multiples, and nutrition.

80 pages

Candace Hurley, Executive Director and Founder
Tracy Hoogenboom, Managing Director
Nancy Veeneman, Operations Director

5919 Preemie Magazine
6412 Brandon Avenue, Suite 274
Springfield, VA 22150   703-468-1005
                                           www.preemiemagazine.com

Started by five preemie parents, it provides free information and an online community for preemeie parents and professionals.

Deborah A Discenza, Founder & Publisher
Nicole Hutzul, Sales & Marketing
Alicia Michaels, Director Operations/Development

Pamphlets

5920 March of Dimes-Preterm Birth Fact Sheets
March of Dimes Pregnancy & Newborn Health Edu Ctr
1275 Mamaroneck Avenue
White Plains, NY 10605   914-997-4488
                                              Fax: 914-997-4763
                                   e-mail: answers@marchofdimes.com
                                           www.marchofdimes.org

Fact sheets discuss the possible causes of preterm birth, complications associated with, and current research.

Description

5921 PREVENTABLE CHILDHOOD INFECTIONS
Involves the following Biologic System(s):
Infectious Disorders

There are several infectious diseases that typically manifest in childhood, that are preventable with proper immunizations. This chapter will cover the following: Diphtheria; Tetanus; Pertussis; Rubella (German Measles); Measles; Mumps; Polio; Chickenpox; Influenza (flu); Meningococcal; Pneumococcal; Congenital Rubella; Genital Human Papillomavirus (HPV).

Diphtheria is an acute, contagious disease characterized at its onset by sore throat and painful swallowing. One to 4 days after exposure, infected individuals may also develop a low-grade fever, headache, nausea and vomiting, chills, and a rapid heart rate. Other symptoms may include signs associated with upper respiratory tract infection. Within a few days, a grayish-brown pseudomembrane may form over the tonsils, and the throat may swell. The lymph nodes in the neck may become swollen and enlarged. Damage to the heart or nervous system may occur. Diphtheria vaccine is usually combined with those for whooping cough (pertussis) and tetanus. This DPT combination is routinely given in a series in the first few months of life. Booster doses are required. In most cases, diphtheria is transmitted through coughed or exhaled droplets. Treatment is with antibiotics and an antitoxin.

Pertussis (whooping cough) is a highly contagious infectious disease in which inflammation of the respiratory tract results from a bacterial infection, transmitted through coughing or sneezing. Pertussis usually affects infants and children, but may occur at any age. Pertussis infection lasts about 6 weeks, occurring in 3 stages: moderate cold-like symptoms (catarrhal stage); severe coughing (paroxysmal stage); cessation of symptoms (convalescent stage). Treatment typically includes bed rest, proper nutrition and fluid intake. Erythromycin or other antibiotics may be given. Pertussis vaccine is usually combined with diptheria and tetanus.

Tetanus is an infectious disease of the central nervous system caused by a toxic bacteria that acts on nerves that control muscle activity. The bacterium typically enters puncture wounds caused by dirty objects such as nails, splinters or glass fragments, or via drug injection, surgical wounds, burns, animal bites or the umbilical cord stump. Symptoms usually appear from 2 to 14 days after infection, but could take months to appear. Tetanus may be classified into general or localized. Initial symptoms of generalized tetanus often include: prolonged spasms of the muscles of the jaw (trismus or lockjaw); difficulties in opening the mouth, chewing and swallowing (dysphagia); irritability, headaches and restlessness. Prolonged spasms of facial muscles, profuse sweating, a mild fever and rapid pulse may also occur. Progressed disease includes severe muscle contractions. Treatment includes human antibodies (tetanus immune globulin) and antibiotics, surgical cleaning of the wound site, and muscle relaxants. Children should receive the DPT (diptheria, pertussis, tetanus) vaccine and booster shots, which should also be given to anyone with wounds and unknown tetanus booster status.

German measles, or rubella, is a contagious viral disease characterized by swollen lymph nodes and a fine, reddish-pink rash that persists for 1 to 3 days. It is transmitted through inhalation of droplets coughed or exhaled by infected individuals. Early symptoms may include swollen lymph nodes, especially in the neck and back of the head; joint pain (arthralgia); low-grade fever; cold symptoms; and redness and discomfort of the throat. Within 1 or 2 days, a mildly itchy rash appears on the face, spreading to the trunk, arms and legs, accompanied by a spreading red flush. The rash usually subsides after 3 days. In some cases, enlargement of the spleen may occur. Measles symptoms range from slight to severe, the latter occuring primarily in older children and adults. Pregnant women with the disease are at risk of transmitting it to their newborn (congenital rubella, see below). Protection against infection is provided through rubella immunization, usually in combination with measles and mumps vaccine. Vaccines are recommended for women of child-bearing age who have not had German measles. Treatment for rubella is symptomatic.

Measles is a highly contagious infection caused by the measles virus. Infection is characterized by a spreading rash and other sypltoms. It typically infects the young, but may develop at any age. It is spread through airborne droplets from an infected individual. Infection usually results in life-long immunity. Early symptoms develop 1 to 2 weeks after exposure and include low-grade fever; inflammation of the nasal mucous membranes; runny nose; hacking cough; conjunctivitis; and increased sensitivity to light. These symptoms are followed 2 to 3 days later by tiny, grayish-white specks surrounded by an irregular red ring (Koplik's spots), that appear on the inside of the cheeks, usually near the back teeth. A rash, accompanied by a high fever, may develop within 3 to 5 days after the onset of symptoms, characterized by faint, reddish flat spots that first appear behind the ears, at the hairline and on the neck, and then spread over the entire body. Certain lymph nodes and the spleen may become enlarged. Immunization, usually in combination with mumps and rubella vaccines provides protection; a second vaccine is usually given upon entering school. Treatment includes fever-recuding medication, antibiotics, increased fluid intake, and bed rest in a warm humidified room. Other treatment is symptomatic and supportive.

Congenital rubella is a condition caused by the German measles virus that is passed from an infected mother to the fetus. Likelihood for transmission and the potential for miscarriage, stillbirth or severe developmental abnormalities (growth retardation, heart defects, eye problems, microcephaly, skin lesions) is highest during the first trimester. Many infants with congenital rubella have inner ear and/or hearing problems. Mental retardation and motor delays may also occur, along with a risk of hepatitis, anemia, lowered blood platelets, pneumonia and bone irregularities. Prevention is directed toward immunization of women of child-bearing age via the measles vaccine.

Mumps is an acute, infectious viral disease caused by a paramyxovirus. It is characterized by enlargement of the salivary glands, particularly those that lie below and in front of the ears (parotid glands). Mumps usually affects children from 5 through 15 years. It is spread through airborne droplets or direct contact with saliva, or possibly, urine, from an infected individual. Outbreaks most often occur in late winter or early spring. Infection usually results in lifelong immunity. Symptoms appear in 14 to 24 days after exposure and include fever, neck pain, weakness, discomfort and headache. One or both parotid glands may become enlarged or tender to the touch. Chewing and swallowing may become difficult, and fever and swelling of other salivary glands and the throat may occur. Swelling of the parotid glands usually lasts 7 to 10 days. Possible complications include meningitis, and joint swelling. A vaccine to prevent the disease is given to children 12 to 15 months, and again before entering school. Treatment is symptomatic and supportive.

Polio, or polimyelitis, is an acute infectious disease caused by one of three polio viruses transmitted through fecal contamination or, occasionally, through the air. It may produce no symptoms, but will grant immunity to those infected. In young children, it is usually accompanied by only mild symptoms that appear 3 to 5 days after infection — fever, headache, sore throat, vomiting, weakness and abdominal discomfort. Recovery often occurs in 1 to 3 days. In some cases, a brief recovery is followed by additional symptoms, including brain and spinal cord involvement with neck and back stiffness and skin sensitivity. This reappearance indicates major illness, and is more common in older children and adults, and may by paralytic or nonparalytic. Immunization to prevent polio is routinely administered. Treatment for the mild form includes bedrest and pain relievers. Paralysis requires physical therapy. Other treatment is symptomatic and supportive.

Chickenpox is a common, hightly contagious viral disease caused by the varicella zoster virus. Most cases occur before the age of 10. Those who do not contract the virus during childhood remain susceptible during adulthood, when symptoms are typically more severe. Chickenpox is spread by inhalation of airborne droplets or by direct contact with fluid from skin blisters. Older children particularly may experience fever,headache, mild abdominal pain, lack of appetite and malaise. A characteristic rash develops on the chest, abdomen, face or scalp, consisting of masses of small, red, extremely itchy spots that become fluid-filled blisters. As the first lesions dry, new ones form.Complication of chickenpox may include bacterial infection of the lesions, encephalitis, and impaired control of voluntary movements. Newborns may also experience a particularly severe, progressive form of chickenpox (neonatal chickenpox). Treatment of children with mild cases of chickenpox is symptomatic and supportive. In more severe cases, the antiviral drug acyclovir may be administered. A vaccine is available to help prevent chickenpox.

Influenza (flu) is a highly contagious viral infection of the nose, throat, and lungs. Spread easily through respiratory droplets of an infected person, influenza symptoms include sudden high fever, chills, dry cough, headache, runny nose, sore throat, muscle and joint pain, and extreme fatigue, which can last up to several weeks. Influenza can be prevented by the flu vaccine of thich there are two types: the flu shot is approved for children older than six months, inlcuding healthy children and those with chronic conditions. The nasal spray flu vaccine (LAIV) is approved for use in healthy individuals two to 49 years. Minor side effects of the flu shot include soreness, redness or swelling at the shot site, low-grade fever, and aches. These may occur soon after the shot and last one to two days. On rare occasions, flu vaccinations can cause severe allergic reactions. Side effects of the nasal spray can include runny nose, wheezing, headache, vomiting, muscle aches, and fever. A flu vaccine is needed every year to keep

up with the changing flu virus. Also, studies show that the body's immunity to influenza viruses (either through infection or vaccination) declines over time.

Meningococcal disease is a leading cause of bacterial meningitis (infection of the covering of the brain and spinal cord) in children two to 18 years old, and can also cause blood infections. The bacteria that cause Meningococcal disease are spread through the exchange of nose and throat droplets through coughing, sneezing or kissing. Symptoms include nausea, vomiting, sensitivity to light, confusion and sleepiness. One of every 10 cases result in death. Meningococcal disease may leave patients limbless, with hearing and nervous system problems, developmental disabilities, and seizures or strokes. It is most common in infants less than one year, and in those 16 to 21 years. Children with certain medical conditions (i.e. no spleen), are at increased risk, as are college students living in dormitories. Meningococcal disease can be prevented by the MCV4 vaccine, which is recommended for those at risk, or who travel to countries where the disease is prevalant. The vaccine is given at age 11 to 12 years, and a booster dose at 16 years.

Genital human papillomavirus (HPV) is the most common sexually transmitted infection (STI) in the U.S. There are more than 40 types of HPV; some cause genital warts; some cause various cancers; some infect the mouth and throat. Aproximately 20 million Americans, including those 11-18 years, are currently infected with HPV, and about 6 million more are infected each year. The HPV virus can live for years in infected individuals, sometimes without symptoms. In rare cases, an infected pregnant woman can pass the HPV virus onto her newborn. HPV can be passed between straight and gay partners, even when the infected person has no symptoms. HPV can cause cervical cancer in women, and it is associated with other, less common cancers. HPV can be prevented by HPV vaccine which is given in three doses over six months. Children 11 to 12 years have the best protection from the vaccines. Two vaccines (Cervariz and Gardasil) are considered effective in protecting women against cancer and genital warts. Gardasil is considered effective in protecting men against genital warts and anal cancer; men at risk should receive the vaccine through 26 years. There is no cure for HPV.

Pneumococcal is an infection of the lungs that is caused by pneumococcus bacteria, which can also cause ear infections, sinus infections, meningitis, bacteremia and blood stream infection. In some cases pneumococcal disease can be fatal or result in brain damage, or hearing or limb loss. The bacteria is spread through infected respiratory droplets from the nose or mouth. It is common for children to carry the bacteria in their throats without becomming symptomatic. Children under two years, in group child care, or who have certain illnesses are at higher risk for pneumococcal disease, as are those with cochlear implants or cerebrospinal fluid (CSF) leaks. Pneumococcal disease is more common among certain ethnic groups, including Alaska Natives, American Indians, and African Americans. Meningitis is the most severe type of pneumococcal disease. Of children under five years with the disease, 5% will die from it, and others may have long-term effects, such as vision or hearing loss. Pneumococcal conjugate vaccine (PCV) prevents the infection. Treatment includes antibiotics which may slow or reverse emerging drug resistance found among pneumococcal infections. It is recommended that the vaccine be given to infants at two, four, and six months, followed by a booster dose at 12 to 15 months.

Hepatitis A and Hepatitis B also fall into the category of preventable childhood infections and are covered in depth in a separate chapter on Hepatitis.

Government Agencies

5922 Centers for Disease Control and Prevention
1600 Clifton Rd
Atlanta, GA 30333   800-232-4636
                                              TTY: 888-232-6348
                                              www.cdc.gov/vaccines

The CDC provides health and safety information. Many CDC publications are available to download, view online, or order at no cost.

5923 Department of Health
899 North Capitol St, NE
Washington, DC 20002   202-442-5955
                                              Fax: 202-442-4795
                                              e-mail: doh@dc.gov
                    www.doh.dc.gov/page/vaccine-preventable-diseases

The DOH conducts investigations, tracking and reporting of vaccine preventable diseases.

Saul M. Levin, MD, MPA, Interim Director, DC Dept of Health

5924 NIH/National Institute of Allergy and Infectious Diseases
6610 Rockledge Drive, MSC 6612
Bethesda, MD 20892   301-496-5717
                                                  866-284-4107
                                              Fax: 301-402-3573
                                              TDD: 800-877-8339
                                    e-mail: ocposoffice@niaid.nih.gov
                                              www.niaid.nih.gov

Conducts and supports basic and applied research to better understand, treat, and ultimately prevent infectious, immunologic, and allergic diseases.

Anthony S Fauci MD, Director

National Associations & Support Groups

5925 American Academy of Pediatrics
141 Northwest Point Boulevard
Elk Grove Village, IL 60007   847-434-4000
                                                  800-433-9016
                                              Fax: 847-434-8000
                                              www.aap.org

The American Academy of Pediatrics and its member pediatricians are committed to the attainment of optimal physical, mental and social health and well-being for all infants, children, adolescents, and young adults.

Sandra Hassink, MD, FAAP, President

5926 American Association for Respiratory Care
9425 N. MacArthur Blvd. Suite 100
Irving, TX 75063   972-243-2272
                                              e-mail: info@aarc.org
                                              www.aarc.org

The AARC encourages and promotes professional excellence, advances the science and practice of respiratory care, and serves as an advocate for patients and their families, the public, the profession and the respiratory therapist.

5927 American Association for Thoracic Surgery
500 Cummings Center, Suite 4550
Beverly, MA 1915   978-927-8330
                                              Fax: 978-524-8890
                                              aats.org

The American Association for Thoracic Surgery is an international organization of over 1,300 of the world's foremost cardiothoracic surgeons representing 41 countries.

Pedro J. del Nido, President
Thoralf M. Sundt, III, Vice President
Marc R. Moon, Secretary

5928 American Medical Association
AMA Plaza, 330 North Wabash Ave., Suite 39300
Chicago, IL 60611   800-262-3211
                                              www.ama-assn.org/ama

AMA is dedicated to ensuring sustainable physician practices that result in better health outcomes for patients.

James L. Madara, MD, CEO/ EVP
Bernard L. Hengesbaugh, Chief Operating Officer
Kenneth J. Sharigian, SVP/ Chief Strategy Officer

5929 American Nurses Association
8515 Georgia Avenue, Suite 400
Silver Spring, MD 20910   800-274-4262
                                              Fax: 301-628-5001
                                              e-mail: anf@ana.org
                                              www.nursingworld.org

The American Nurses Association (ANA) is the only full-service professional organization representing the interests of the nation's 3.1 million registered nurses through its constituent and state nurses associations and its organizational affiliates.

Pamela F. Cipriano, PhD, President
Marla J. Weston, PhD, RN, FAAN, Chief Executive Officer
Cindy R. Balkstra, Vice President

5930 American Pregnancy Association
1425 Greenway Drive, Suite 440
Irving, TX 75038   e-mail: info@americanpregnancy.org
                                              americanpregnancy.org

The American Pregnancy Association is a 501(c)(3) nonprofit organization committed to promoting pregnancy wellness through education, advocacy and community awareness.

5931 American Public Health Association
800 I Street, NW
Washington, DC 20001   202-777-2742
                                              Fax: 202-777-2534
                                              TTY: 202-777-2500
                                              www.apha.org

APHA champions the health of all people and all communities. They aim to strengthen the public health profession and speak out for public health issues and policies backed by science.

Georges C. Benjamin, MD, Executive Director
Kemi Oluwafemi, MBA, CPA, Chief Financial Officer
Susan Polan, PhD, Associate Executive Director

5932 American Society For Microbiology
1752 N Street, N.W.
Washington, DC 20036   202-737-3600
                                              Fax: 202-942-9333
                                              e-mail: service@asmusa.org
                                              www.asm.org

he American Society for Microbiology is a life science membership organization. Membership has grown from 59 scientists in 1899 to more than 39,000 members today, with more than one third located outside the United States. The members represent 26 disciplines of microbiological specialization plus a division for microbiology educators.

Nancy Sansalone, Interim Executive Director
Timothy Donohue, President
Joseph M. Campos, Secretary

5933 American Thoracic Society
25 Broadway
New York, NY 10004   212-315-8600
                                              Fax: 212-315-6498
                                              e-mail: ATSInfo@Thoracic.org
                                              www.thoracic.org

The American Thoracic Society improves global health by advancing research, patient care, and public health in pulmonary disease, critical illness, and sleep disorders. Founded in 1905 to combat TB, the ATS has grown to tackle asthma, COPD, lung cancer, sepsis, acute respiratory distress, and sleep apnea, among other diseases.

Thomas W. Ferkol, MD, President
Atul Malhotra, MD, President-elect
Stephen C. Crane, PhD, MPH, Executive Director

5934 Association of Immunization Managers
620 Hungerford Dr. Suite 29
Rockville, MD 20850
301-424-6080
Fax: 301-424-6081
www.immunizationmanagers.org

The Association of Immunization Managers (AIM) was created in 1999 to enable immunization managers to work together to effectively prevent and control vaccine-preventable diseases and improve immunization coverage in the United States and its territories.

Pejman Talebian, Chair
Claire Hannan, Executive Director
Katelyn Wells, Research and Development Director

5935 Every Child By Two
1233 20th Street NW, Suite 403
Washington, DC 20036
202-783-7034
Fax: 202-783-7042
e-mail: info@ecbt.org
www.ecbt.org

Rosalynn Carter, President & Co-Founder
Betty Bumpers, Vice President & Co-Founder

5936 Immunization Action Coalition
2550 University Avenue West, Suite 415 North
Saint Paul, MN 55114
651-647-9009
Fax: 651-647-9131
e-mail: admin@immunize.org
www.immunize.org

The Immunization Action Coalition (IAC) works to increase immunization rates and prevent disease by creating and distributing educational materials for health professionals and the public that enhance the delivery of safe and effective immunization services. The Coalition also facilitates communication about the safety, efficacy, and use of vaccines within the broad immunization community of patients, parents, health care organizations, and government health agencies.

Deborah L. Wexler, MD, Executive Director
Litjen Tan, MS, PhD, Chief Strategy Officer
Robin VanOss, Operations Manager

5937 Infectious Diseases Society of America
1300 Wilson Blvd, Suite 300
Arlington, VA 22209
703-299-0200
Fax: 703-299-0204
www.idsociety.org

The Infectious Diseases Society of America (IDSA) represents physicians, scientists and other health care professionals who specialize in infectious diseases. IDSA's purpose is to improve the health of individuals, communities, and society by promoting excellence in patient care, education, research, public health, and prevention relating to infectious diseases.

Stephen B. Calderwood, MD, FIDSA, President
Johan S. Bakken, MD, PhD, FIDSA, President-Elect
William G. Powderly, MD, FIDSA, Vice President

5938 National Association of Pediatric Nurse Practitioners
5 Hanover Square, Suite 1401
New York, NY 10004
917-746-8300
877-662-7627
Fax: 212-785-1713
www.napnap.org

National Association of Pediatric Nurse Practitioners (NAPNAP) is the professional association for pediatric nurse practitioners (PNPs) and other advanced practice nurses who care for children.

Mary Chesney, PhD, President
Cate Brennan, Executive Director
Michele Stickel, Dir of Mrktng & Strategic Projects

5939 National Association of School Nurses
1100 Wayne Avenue Suite 925
Silver Spring, MD 20910
240-821-1130
866-627-6767
Fax: 301-585-1791
www.nasn.org

The mission is to advance school nurse practice to keep students healthy, safe and ready to learn.

Donna J. Mazyck, Executive Director
Nichole K. Bobo, Nursing Education Director
Margaret Cellucci, Director of Communications

5940 National Foundation for Infectious Diseases
7201 Wisconsin Avenue, Suite 750
Bethesda, MD 20814
301-656-0003
Fax: 301-907-0878
www.nfid.org

The National Foundation for Infectious Diseases (NFID) is a non-profit, tax-exempt 501(c)(3) organization founded in 1973 dedicated to educating the public and healthcare professionals about the causes, treatment, and prevention of infectious diseases across the lifespan.

5941 National Healthy Mothers, Healthy Babies Coalition
Post Office Box 3360
Alexandria, VA 22302
703-837-4792
Fax: 703-664-0485
e-mail: info@hmhb.org
www.hmhb.org

The National Healthy Mothers, Healthy Babies Coalition (HMHB) is a recognized leader and resource in maternal and child health, reaching an estimated 10 million health care professionals, parents, and policymakers through its membership of over 100 local, state and national organizations.

Janice Frey-Angel, CEO
Andrea Goodman, MCH Director
Jennifer Sharp, Deputy Director

5942 National Meningitis Association
P.O. Box 60143
Ft. Myers, FL 33906
866-366-3662
www.nmaus.org

The National Meningitis Association (NMA) is a nonprofit organization founded by parents whose children have died or live with permanent disabilities from meningococcal disease.

5943 National Tuberculosis Controllers Association
2452 Spring Rd, SE
Smyrna, GA 30080
678-503-0503
877-503-0806
Fax: 678-503-0805
e-mail: dhwegener@tbcontrollers.org
www.tbcontrollers.org

The NTCA was created in 1995 to bring together the leaders of tuberculosis control programs in all states and territories, as well as many counties and city health departments that organize their own TB control activities.

Donna Hope Wegener, Executive Director
Jennifer Kanouse, Director of Comm. & Member Services
Eva Forest, Executive Assistant

5944 Pediatric Infectious Diseases Society
1300 Wilson Boulevard, Suite 300
Arlington, VA 22209
703-299-6764
Fax: 703-299-0473
e-mail: cphillips@idsociety.org
www.pids.org

PIDS is the world's largest organization of professionals dedicated to the treatment, control and eradication of infectious diseases affecting children. Membership is comprised of physicians, doctoral-level scientists and others who have trained or are in training in infectious diseases or its related disciplines, and who are identified with the discipline of pediatric infectious diseases or related disciplines through clinical practice, research, teaching and/or administration activities.

David W. Kimberlin, MD, President
Terri Christene Phillips, Executive Director
Faith Ham, Membership and Comm. Assistant

5945 Polio Society
4200 Wisconsin Avenue NW, #106273
Washington, DC 20016
301-897-8180
Fax: 202-994-3153
e-mail: jsh1@mhg.edu

A chartered nonprofit organization primarily for polio survivors and family members. It provides educational resources and support group services.

5946 Polio Survivors Association
12720 La Reina Avenue
Downey, CA 90242
562-862-4508
Fax: 562-862-5018
e-mail: info@polioassociation.org
www.polioassociation.org

Nonprofit organization dedicated to education, advocacy, and support to promote the well being and improve the quality of life for severely disabled polio survivors.

Richard Dagget, President

5947 Post-Polio Health International
4207 Lindell Boulevard, Suite 110
Saint Louis, MO 63108
314-534-0475
Fax: 314-534-5070
e-mail: info@post-polio.org
www.post-polio.org

Provides information to Polio survivors, their families and the health care community and promotes networking among the post-polio community.

Joan L Headley, Editor & Executive Director

5948 Shot At Life
www.shotatlife.org

202-862-6303
e-mail: info@shotatlife.org
www.shotatlife.org

This organization aims to decrease vaccine-preventable childhood deaths and give every child a chance at a healthy life, by encouraging individuals to learn about, advocate for, and donate to vaccines to protect children worldwide.

5949 Shots For Tots
4747 Earhart Blvd - Ste 107
New Orleans, LA 70125
504-483-1900
800-251-2229
Fax: 504-483-1909
e-mail: info@shotsfortots.com
www.shotsfortots.com

This organization provides up-to-date information for both parents and providers in order to ensure the highest level of immunizations for children.

Gina Deris, Coodinator

5950 World Health Organization
Avenue Appia 20
CH-1211 Geneva 27,
Switzerland
www.who.int

WHO is the directing and coordinating authority for health within the United Nations system.

Dr Margaret Chan, Director General

State Agencies & Support Groups

Arizona

5951 Maricopa Co Childhood Immunization Program
PO Box 44283
Phoenix, AZ 85064
602-262-2447
e-mail: info@mcchip.org
www.mcchip.org

5952 The Arizona Partnership for Immunization
320 E. McDowell Rd
Phoenix, AZ 85004
602-253-0090
Fax: 602-262-2654
e-mail: tapi@aachc.org
www.whyimmunize.org

Arkansas

5953 Arkansas Department of Health Div. of Comm Diseases/Immunizations
4815 West Markham St - Slot 48
Little Rock, AR 72205
501-661-2723
www.health.state.ar.us

California

5954 All Kids By Two Health Services Agency
1060 Emeline Ave - Bldg F
Santa Cruz, CA 95061
831-454-5477
Fax: 831-454-5049
e-mail: katie.lebaron@health.co.santa-cruz.ca.us
www.santacruzhealth.org

5955 California Department of Health Services Immunization Branch
2151 Berkeley Way - Rm 712
Berkeley, CA 94704
510-540-2065
www.dhs.ca.gov

5956 Community Health Improvement Partners - Immunize San Diego (CHIP-ISD)
707 Broadway - Ste 905
San Diego, CA 92101
619-515-2858
Fax: 619-544-0888
e-mail: tdanos@hasdic.org
www.sdchip.org

5957 Immunization Partnership of Alameda County
2000 Mowry Avenue
Fremont, CA 94538
510-494-7053
Fax: 510-791-3496
e-mail: ruth_young@whhs.com
www.whhs.com

Colorado

5958 Colorado Dept. of Public Heand & Environme nt: Immunization Program, DCEED-IMM-A3
4300 Cherry Creek Drive South
Denver, CO 80222
303-692-2669
www.cdphe.state.co.us/health-h.asp

District of Columbia

5959 Commission of Public Health Immunization Program
1131 Spring Road, NW
Washington, DC 20010
202-576-7130

5960 Department of Health Division of Immunization
6323 Georgia Ave, NW - Ste 305
Washington, DC 20011
202-576-7130

Florida

5961 Florida Department of Health Immunization Program
2020 Capital Circle SE
Tallahassee, FL 32399
904-487-2755
www.doh.state.fl.us

Hawaii

5962 Hawaii Department of Health Immunization Program
1250 Punchbowl Street
Honolulu, HI 96813
808-586-4400
Fax: 808-586-4444
www.hawaii.gov/health

Idaho

5963 Idaho Dept. of Health & Welfare Immunizati on Program
PO Box 83720
Boise, ID 83720
208-334-5500
800-554-2922
Fax: 208-334-5942
e-mail: idahovfc@idhw.state.id.us
www.healthandwelfare.idaho.gov

Indiana

5964 Indiana State Dept. of Health Immunization
2 North Meridian St
Indianapolis, IN 46204
317-233-1325
www.in.gov/isdh

Iowa

5965 Iowa Department of Public Health Bureau of Immunization
321 East 12th St - Lucas State Office Bldg
Des Moines, IA 50319
515-281-5787
www.idph.state.ia.us

Kansas

5966 Kansas Department of Health & Environment Immunization Program
109 SW 9th St - Ste 606
Topeka, KS 66612
785-296-5591
Fax: 785-296-6510
e-mail: info@kdhe.state.ks.us
www.kdhe.state.ks.us/index.html

Maine

5967 Maine Dept. of Human Services: Bureau of Health Immunization Program
2 Bangor Street
Augusta, ME 04330 www.maine.gov/dhhs/boh/mip/index_home.htm

Maryland

5968 Dept. of Health & Mental Hygiene-Immunizat ion
201 West Preston St
Baltimore, MD 21201
410-767-6860
TDD: 800-735-2258
ww.dhmh.state.md.us

Mississippi

5969 Mississippi Dept. of Health Bureau of Preventative Health Immunization
2423 N State St - PO Box 1700
Jackson, MS 39215
601-576-7751
Fax: 601-576-7686
www.msdh.state.ms.us/msdhhome.htm

Nebraska

5970 Nebraska Dept. of Health Immunization Prog ram
PO Box 95044
Lincoln, NE 68509
402-471-3727
e-mail: grey.borden@hhss.state.ne.us
www.hhs.state.ne.us

Nevada

5971 Nevada State Health Division Bureau of Com munity Health - Immunization Program
4150 Technology Way
Carson City, NV 89706
775-684-5900
http://health.nv.gov/immunization.htm

New Hampshire

5972 NH Dept. of Health & Human Services Immunization Program
28 Hazen Drive
Concord, NH 03301
603-271-4482
800-852-3345
www.dhhs.state.nh.us/dhhs/immunization/default.htm

New Jersey

5973 New Jersey Department of Health Immunizations Program
PO Box 369
Trenton, NJ 08625
609-588-7512
Fax: 609-588-7431
www.state.nj.us/health

New Mexico

5974 New Mexico Department of Health Immunization Program
1190 St. Francis Dr - S1260
Santa Fe, NM 87505
505-827-2463
ww.health.state.nm.us/immunize

New York

5975 New York State Department of Health Immunization Program
Corning Tower Building - Rm 649
Albany, NY 12237
518-473-4437
www.health.state.ny.us

Ohio

5976 Ohio Department of Health Immunization Program
246 N High St, PO Box 118
Columbus, OH 43216
614-466-0302
www.odh.state.oh.us

Oklahoma

5977 Oklahoma State Department of Health Immunization Division
1000 North East 10th St
Oklahoma City, OK 73117
405-271-5600
www.health.state.ok.us

Rhode Island

5978 Rhode Island Department of Health Immunization Program
3 Capitol Hill
Providence, RI 02908
401-222-2231
Fax: 401-222-6548
TTY: 800-745-5555
www.health.state.ri.us

South Carolina

5979 SC Dept. of Health & Environmental Control Immunization Division
1751 Calhoun St
Columbia, SC 29201
803-898-3432
www.scdhec.gov/health/disease/immunization

South Dakota

5980 South Dakota Department of Health Office of Disease Prevention
Health Building, 600 E. Capitol
Pierre, SD 57501   605-773-3737
e-mail: doh.info@state.sd.us
www.state.sd.us/state/executive/doh/doh.html

Tennessee

5981 Tennessee Department of Health Immunization
Cordell Hull Building, 425 5th Ave, North - 3rd Fl
Nashville, TN 37247   615-741-3111
Fax: 615-741-3491
www.state.tn.us/health

Texas

5982 Texas Department oF Health Immunization Division
1100 West 49th Street
Austin, TX 78756   512-458-7284
ww.tdh.state.tx.us

Utah

5983 Utah Department of Health
PO Box 1010
Salt Lake City, UT 84114   801-538-6101
http://hlunix.ex.state.ut.us

Vermont

5984 Vermont Department oF Health State Immunication Program
108 Cherry Street
Burlington, VT 05402   800-464-4343
TDD: 802-863-7200
www.healthyvermonters.info

Virginia

5985 Virginia Department of Health Bureau of Immunization
1500 East Main Street
Richmond, VA 23219   804-786-6246
www.vdh.state.va.us

Washington

5986 Washington State Department of Health Immunization Program
1112 SE Quince St, PO Box 47890
Olympia, WA 98504   360-236-4010
www.doh.wa.gov

Web Sites

5987 Canadian Task Force on Preventive Health C are
3280 Hospital Drive Northwest
Calgary, AL T2N 4   e-mail: info@canadiantaskforce.ca
canadiantaskforce.ca

This website is designed to serve as a practical guide to health care providers, planners and consumers for determining the inclusion or exclusion, content and frequency of a wide variety of preventive health interventions, using the evidence based recommendations of the Canadian Task Force on Preventice Health Care.

Marcello Tonelli, Chair
Richard Birtwhistle, Vice Chair
C. Maria Bacchus, Board Member

5988 Centers for Disease Control-Infection Cont rol
1600 Clifton Rd
Atlanta, GA 30333   800-232-4636
www.cdc.gov/hai/

Promotes health and quality of life by preventing and controlling disease, injury, and disability.

5989 Health Research Project (HaRP)
www.harpnet.org

A program by USAID, the project strives to improve the health status of infants, children, mothers and families through the development and research of new tools, technologies, policies and approaches.

5990 KidsHealth - Measles
kidshealth.org/parent/infections/lung/measles.html

KidsHealth provides doctor-approved health information about children from before birth through adolescence. KidsHealth provides families with accurate, up to date and jargon free health information they can use.

Neil Izenberg, MD, Editor-in-Chief & Founder

5991 KidsHealth - Rubella (German Measles)
kidshealth.org/parent/

KidsHealth provides doctor-approved health information about children from before birth through adolescence. KidsHealth provides families with accurate, up to date and jargon free health information they can use.

Neil Izenberg, MD, Editor-in-Chief & Founder

5992 KidsHealth - Tetanus
kidshealth.org/parent/

KidsHealth provides doctor-approved health information about children from before birth through adolescence. KidsHealth provides families with accurate, up to date and jargon free health information they can use.

Neil Izenberg, MD, Editor-in-Chief & Founder

5993 Pan American Health Organization (PAHO)
525 Twenty-third Street, N.W.
Washington, DC 20037   202-974-3000
Fax: 202-974-3663
www.paho.org

The mission is to strengthen national and local health systems and improve the health of the peoples of the Americas, in collaboraton with Ministries of Health, other government and international agencies, nongovernmental organizations, universities, social security agencies, community groups, and many others. Health topics include measles, mumps, rubella and diptheria.

5994 Polio Connection of America
www.geocities.com/w1066w/

For survivors of the Polio Survivors to chat and the site offers links to other polio sites.

5995 Polio Experience Network
825 Sherbrook Street
Winnipeg, MB R3A 1   204-975-3037
Fax: 204-975-3027
e-mail: postpolionetwork@gmail.com
www.postpolionetwork.ca/pps

Offers information, inspiration, ideas and resources to help patients understand polio and post-poli syndrome, and to confidently manage life with it. Also helps loved ones cope with the effects of polio. Resources are also offered for students doing research on the disease as well as general resources available.

Cheryl Currie, President
Kathryn Harper, Vice President
Estelle Boissonneault, Secretary

5996 Post Polio Awareness & Support Society of British Columbia
#102-9775-4th Street
Sidney, BC V8L 2
250-665-8849
Fax: 250-665-8859
e-mail: ppass@ppassbc.com
www.ppassbc.com

A non profit society formed as a network for polio survivors, those affected by polio, and any interested in polio.

Joan Toone, President

5997 Slack Incorporated
6900 Grove Road
Thorofare, NJ 8086
856-848-1000
Fax: 856-848-6091
e-mail: email@slackinc.com
www.slackinc.com

A leading provider of healthcare information, educational programs, and meeting and exhibit management services worldwide.

5998 Virtual Pediatric Hospital
www.virtualpediatrichospital.org

A digital library of pediatric information including resources for patients and health care professionals.

Book Publishers

5999 Everything You Need to Know About Measles and Rubella

Trisha Hawkins, author

Rosen Publishing/PowerKids Press
29 E 21st Street
New York, NY 10010
212-777-3017
800-237-9932
Fax: 888-436-4643
e-mail: rosenpub@tribeca.ios.com
www.rosenpublishing.com

Examines the continuing threat of these highly infectious respiratory diseases. Grades 7-12.

2001 64 pages
ISBN: 0-823933-22-9

Roger Rosen, President

6000 IVUN Resource Directory
4207 Lindell Boulevard, Suite 110
Saint Louis, MO 63108
314-534-0475
Fax: 314-534-5070
e-mail: info@post-polio.org
www.post-polio.org

A networking tool for health professionals and both long-term and new ventilator users. Sections include health professionals, ventilator users, equipment and aids, manufacturers, service and repair, organizations, etc. Published annually in October.

34 pages Annually

Joan L Headley, Executive Director & Editor

6001 Let's Talk About Having Chicken Pox

Elizabeth Weitzman, author

Rosen Publishing/PowerKids Press
29 E 21st Street
New York, NY 10010
212-777-3017
800-237-9932
Fax: 888-436-4643
e-mail: rosenpub@tribeca.ios.com
www.rosenpublishing.com

Highly contagious chicken pox is one of the childhood illnesses that few kids escape. This book tells kids how to handle the illness, where it comes from and how long it will take to recover. Grades K-5.

24 pages
ISBN: 0-823950-31-X

Roger Roger, President

6002 Measles

Maxine Rosaler, author

Rosen Publishing/PowerKids Press
29 E 21st Street
New York, NY 10010
212-777-3017
800-237-9932
Fax: 888-436-4643
e-mail: rosenpub@tribeca.ios.com
www.rosenpublishing.com

An examination of the history of this once thought to be harmless disease, from its ancient origins to near eradication.

2005 64 pages
ISBN: 1-404202-56-0

Roger Roger, President

6003 Post-Polio Directory
4207 Lindell Boulevard, Suite 110
Saint Louis, MO 63108
314-534-0475
Fax: 314-534-5070
e-mail: info@post-polio.org
www.post-polio.org

Over 32 pages of post polio clinics, health professionals, support groups, and other useful contacts. The directory includes international listings. Published annually in March.

Joan L Headley, Executive Director & Editor

Newsletters

6004 Infectious Diseases in Children
Slack Incorporated
6900 Grove Road
Thorofare, NJ 08086
856-848-1000
800-257-8290
e-mail: editor@healio.com
www.healio.com/footer/healio-dot-com

Pediatric news source.
Monthly
Philip A Brunell MD, Chief Medical Editor

6005 Post-Polio Health
4207 Lindell Boulevard, Suite 110
Saint Louis, MO 63108
314-534-0475
Fax: 314-534-5070
e-mail: info@post-polio.org
www.post-polio.org

Provides information to polio survivors, their families, and the health care community and promotes networking among the post-polio community.

12 pages Quarterly
ISSN: 1066-5331

William G. Stothers, President/Chairperson
Saul J. Morse, Vice President
Joan L Headley, Editor & Executive Director

Pamphlets

6006 Tetanus and Diptheria Vaccine
Centers for Disease Control & Prevention
1600 Clifton Road
Atlanta, GA 30333
404-639-3311
800-232-4636
www.cdc.gov/vaccines/pubs/vis/downloads/vis-td.pdf

Factsheet about the diseases and the vaccines.

Description

6007 PROTEIN C DEFICIENCY

Synonyms: PC deficiency, PROC deficiency

Covers these related disorders: Protein C deficiency Type I, Protein C deficiency Type II

Involves the following Biologic System(s):

Hematologic and Oncologic Disorders

Protein C deficiency is a blood clotting (thrombotic) disorder characterized by the recurrent formation of blood clots within the veins of the body (venous thrombosis). Protein C, which is formed in the liver, is a specialized protein that helps to prevent the formation of blood clots. When activated, protein C helps to dissolve fibrin, the semisolid portion of blood clots, thus inhibiting the formation of a clot. A deficiency of this protein, therefore, results in abnormal clot formation. Some signs of this disorder may become apparent during adolescence. Associated symptoms depend upon the organ or tissue affected by clot formation that leads to reduced or absent blood flow. Affected individuals may develop blood clots and inflammation in the veins of the legs (thrombophlebitis). This can occur when the blood moves slowly in the veins, such as from prolonged bed rest during an illness, surgery, or hospital stay. In some patients, these clots may dislodge from the vein and travel through the blood stream (embolus) to different parts of the body including the heart, lungs, or brain, potentially leading to life-threatening complications. However, not all patients with protein C deficiency experience all the signs associated with this disorder.

In the event of a blood clotting episode, the antithrombin factor heparin may be administered through injection into a vein (intravenous) or under the skin (subcutaneous). Other treatment may include continuing oral administration of the anti-coagulant drug warfarin to prevent a recurrence of thrombotic activity

Two types of protein C deficiency have been described in the general population. The more common form is Type I in which both protein C levels and activity are deficient. In the less common Type II, the amount of protein is normal but its activity or performance is impaired. The inherited form of protein C deficiency may be transmitted as an autosomal dominant trait. The gene for this disorder is located on the long arm of chromosome 2 (2q13-14). Protein C deficiency may also be acquired in connection with infection.

Government Agencies

6008 NIH/National Heart, Lung and Blood Institu te

National Institute of Health
31 Center Dr MSC 2486, Bldg 31, Room 5A48
Bethesda, MD 20892

301-592-8573
Fax: 240-629-3246
TTY: 240-629-3255
e-mail: NHLBIinfo@nhlbi.nih.gov
www.nhlbi.nih.gov

Primary responsibility of this organization is the scientific investigation of heart, blood vessel, lung and blood disorders. Oversees research, demonstration, prevention, education, control and training activities in these fields and emphasizes the prevention and control of heart diseases.

Elizabeth G Nabel, MD, Director
Susan Shurin, MD, Deputy Director
Sheila Pohl, Chief of Staff

National Associations & Support Groups

6009 American Academy of Pediatrics

141 Northwest Point Boulevard
Elk Grove Village, IL 60007

847-434-4000
800-433-9016
Fax: 847-434-8000
www.aap.org

The American Academy of Pediatrics and its member pediatricians are committed to the attainment of optimal physical, mental and social health and well-being for all infants, children, adolescents, and young adults.

Sandra Hassink, MD, FAAP, President

6010 Genetic Alliance

4301 Connecticut Avenue NW
Washington, DC 20008

202-966-5557
800-336-4363
Fax: 202-966-8553
e-mail: info@geneticalliance.org
www.geneticalliance.org

A coalition of voluntary genetic support groups, consumers and professionals addressing the needs of individuals and families affected by genetic disorders from a national perspective.

Sharon Terry, President
Natasha Bonhomme, Vice President of Strategic Develop
Vaughn ÿEdelson, Assistant Director of Health Commun

6011 March of Dimes Birth Defects Foundation

1275 Mamaroneck Avenue
White Plains, NY 10605

914-997-4488
888-663-4637
Fax: 914-428-8203
e-mail: answers@marchofdimes.com
www.marchofdimes.com

Partnership of volunteers and professionals dedicates to improving the health of babies by preventing birth defects and infant mortality. Over 100 chapters are located across the country and can be located through the National Office.

Jennifer L Howse, President

6012 Med Help International

6300 North Wickham Road, Suite 130
Melbourne, FL 32940

321-259-7505
Fax: 321-751-0858
e-mail: office@medhelp.org
www.medhelp.org

A not-for-profit organization dedicated to helping patients find the highest quality medical information in the world today. Patients are offered the tools necessary to make informed treatment decisions within the short time lines dictated by their illness or disease.

Cynthia ThompsonD, President & Co-Founder
Philip A Garfinkel, VP & Co-Founder

State Agencies & Support Groups

6013 Vitamin C Foundation

PO Box 130130
Spring, TX 77393

281-255-2679
800-849-9025
Fax: 630-416-1309
e-mail: ascorbade@aol.com
www.vitamincfoundation.org

A Texas nonprofit organization devoted to preserving and distributing knowledge about ascorbic acid and its vital role in the life process.

Owen R Fonorow, Co-Founder
M S Till Sr, Co-Founder

Web Sites

6014 Factor V Leiden: Thrombophilia Support Pag e
www.fvleiden.org

Factor V Leiden is the most common hereditary blood coagulation disorder in the US. It is present in 3-7% of the population in Europe and America. It is associated with Venous thrombosis, DVT, unexplained miscarriage, blood clots in the lungs, gall bladder dysfunction, preeclampsia and/or eclapsia, stroke and/or heart attack.

6015 HealthCentral.com
750 Third Avenue, 6th Floor
New York, NY 10017
212-695-2223
Fax: 212-695-2936
www.healthcentral.com

Offering information on health issues for children, women, men and seniors. Information on Protein C Deficiency includes a description, causes, symptoms, diagnosis, treatment and questions that can be asked of the doctor.

Micheael Cunnion, Chief Executive Officer
Jim Curtis, Chief Revenue Officer
Rebecca Farwell, Chief Content Officer

6016 MedicineNet
www.medicinenet.com

An online, healthcare media publishing company. It provides easy to read, in-depth, authoritative medical information for consumers via an interactive web site.

6017 Merck
2000 Galloping Hill Road
Kenilworth, NJ 7033
908-740-4000
www.merck.com

A site that offers research driven pharmaceutical products and services to improve human and animal health, directly and through its joint ventures.

Kenneth C. Frazier, Chairman & CEO
Robert M. Davis, EVP & CFO
Willie A. Deese, EVP & President

6018 Online Mendelian Inheritance in Man
National Library of Medicine, Building 38A
Bethesda, MD 20894
888-346-3656
e-mail: info@ncbi.nlm.nih.gov
www.ncbi.nlm.nih.gov

This database is a catalog of human genes and genetic disorders.

Book Publishers

6019 Merck Manual of Diagnosis and Therapy
Merck Publishing Group
PO Box 2000 RY84-15
Rahway, NJ 07065
732-594-4600
Fax: 732-388-3610
www.merckbooks.com

Since it was first published in 1899, The Merck Manual has set the standard for excellence in the medical community for current, complete, and comprehensive information for all healthcare professionals. Written by more than 300 medical experts in all fields of medicine from around the world.

2006 18th Ed 2832 pages Hardcover
ISBN: 0-911910-18-2

Mark H Beers MD, Editor-in-Chief
Robert S Porter MD, Editor

6020 Protein Deficiency and Pesticide Toxicity
Eldon M Boyd, author

Charles C Thomas
2600 South First Street
Springfield, IL 62704
217-789-8980
800-258-8980
Fax: 217-789-9130
e-mail: books@ccthomas.com
www.ccthomas.com

Discusses the approaches for analyzing Protein Deficiency and Pesticide Toxicity.
468 pages Hardcover
ISBN: 0-398024-76-6

Description

6021 PSORIASIS

Involves the following Biologic System(s):

Dermatologic Disorders

Psoriasis is a common, chronic skin disease characterized by red patches of skin that are covered by dry, thick, silvery scales. This disorder may occur at any age, but most commonly appears from the ages of 10 to 40 years. Although males and females are affected equally, females are more prone to development of this disorder when it appears during childhood. In addition, approximately half of those individuals who develop psoriasis in childhood have a family history of the disorder, but the pattern of transmission has not been determined. Individuals with psoriasis appear to produce new skin cells at a greatly accelerated rate while shedding their old cells at a normal rate. The subsequent buildup of new cells produces thickened areas of new skin that are covered by old skin, thus forming the characteristic dry, thickened, silvery patches associated with psoriasis.

Psoriatic lesions may appear anywhere on the body, but most commonly form on the scalp, elbows, knees, back, buttocks, navel area, and genitalia. In addition, relatively smaller lesions may appear on the face and pitting may develop on the nails. Peeling away a scale produces specks of bleeding from the capillaries (Auspitz's sign). Itching of the skin (pruritus) is common and scratching leads to more lesions (Koebner's phenomenon). On rare occasions, severe psoriasis may develop in newborns, accompanied by lesion formation in the diaper area.

There are different types of psoriasis. The most common form is called discoid psoriasis and is characterized by patches that form mainly on the elbows, knees, scalp, and other areas of the arms, legs, and trunk. Other findings may include nail irregul|arities such as pitting, thickening, and separation from the nail beds. In addition, psorasis is sometimes accompanied by painful swelling of the joints (arthritis). Guttate psoriasis occurs primarily in children and young adults and is characterized by the sudden appearance of small, oval, drop-like lesions on the trunk and upper portions of the arms and legs. Guttate psoriasis often develops following a streptococcal infection, viral infection, or sunburn. In addition, this form of the disorder sometimes follows the conclusion or withdrawal of corticosteroid treatment. Pustular psoriasis may be localized or generalized. In its localized form, eruptions of pustules develop over individual reddish patches that are present, usually, on the palms of the hands and the soles of the feet. Psoriasis is usually apparent on other parts of the body. Affected individuals may also experience localized discomfort. Generalized pustular psoriasis is an acute, severe, sometimes life-threatening form of the disorder that is characterized by the widespread eruption of small pustules in individuals with mild, moderate, or other types of psoriasis. Generalized pustular psoriasis is sometimes accompanied by high fever, pain in the joints, elevated levels of white blood cells (leukocytosis), low levels of blood calcium (hypocalcemia), and other irregularties.

Treatment of psoriasis is dependent upon age, area of involvement, and the type and severity of the disease. Many treatment protocols that are effective for adults may be too toxic for children; therefore, most treatment for children with psoriasis is conservative and mainly directed toward comfort and alleviation of pain. Such treatment may include the use of tar preparations in the form of gels, ointments, or bath emulsions. Additional topical treatments may include the cautious use of corticosteroid preparations, vitamin D analogs, and other ointments. Treatment for scalp lesions may include the use of a phenol and saline solution followed by tar shampoo and, when lesions are reduced, the application of a corticosteroid preparation. Severe psoriasis in children may indicate the use of various drugs such as methotrexate and certain oral retinoids; however, this therapy may be accompanied by severe side effects. Other treatment is symptomatic and supportive.

National Associations & Support Groups

6022 American Academy of Pediatrics
141 Northwest Point Boulevard
Elk Grove Village, IL 60007

847-434-4000
800-433-9016
Fax: 847-434-8000
www.aap.org

The American Academy of Pediatrics and its member pediatricians are committed to the attainment of optimal physical, mental and social health and well-being for all infants, children, adolescents, and young adults.

Sandra Hassink, MD, FAAP, President

6023 National Psoriasis Foundation
6600 SW 92nd Avenue, Suite 300
Portland, OR 97223

503-244-7404
800-723-9166
Fax: 503-245-0626
e-mail: getinfo@psoriasis.org
www.psoriasis.org

Promotes awareness and understanding of psoriasis and psoriatic arthritis through education and advocacy. The foundation also ensures access to treatment and supports research that leads to effective management of the condition.

Pam Field, CEO
Pam Field, VP Operations
Paula Fasano, Director Marketing/Communications

Research Centers

6024 University of California, San Francisco Dermatology Drug Research
515 Spruce Street
San Francisco, CA 94115

415-476-4701
Fax: 415-502-4126
e-mail: ÿcommunications@cc.ucsf.edu
cc.ucsf.edu/people

Conducts clinical testing of new or existing pharmalogic agents used in the treatment of skin disorders.

John Koo, MD, Director

Audio Video

6025 National Library of Dermatologic Teaching Slides
American Academy Of Dermatology
PO Box 94020
Palatine, IL 60094

847-330-0230
Fax: 847-330-0050
www.aad.org/store/product/

A collection of dermatologic teaching slides offering the most comprehensive series ever assembled. Each set offers a realistic presentation of classic clinical skin conditions encountered by the dermatologist.

Brett M. Coldiron, President
Elise A. Olsen, MD, Vice President
Suzanne M. Olbricht, Secretary-Treasurer

Web Sites

6026 American Academy of Dermatology (AAD)
www.aad.org/aadpamphrework/Psoriasis.html

The American Academy of Dermatoloy is dedicated to achieving the highest quality of dermatologic care for everyone. Acheivement of this vision requires a dynamic organization whose mission embodies: Excellence in patient care, education and research, adherence to eithical conduct, respinsiveness to its members and to the public unification and representation of the specialty.

Brett M. Coldiron, President
Elise A. Olsen, MD, Vice President
Suzanne M. Olbricht, Secretary-Treasurer

6027 National Psoriasis Foundation
6600 SW 92nd Ave., Ste. 300
Portland, OR 97223
800-723-9166
e-mail: getinfo@psoriasis.org
www.psoriasis.org

Promotes awareness and understanding of psoriasis and psoriatic arthritis through education and advocacy. The foundation also ensures access to treatment and supports research that leads to effective management of the condition.

Krista Kellogg, Chair
Pete Redding, Vice Chair
Randy Beranek, President/ CEO

6028 Psoriasis Association
Dick Coles House, 2 Queensbridge
Northampton, NN4 7
845-676-0076
Fax: 160-425-1621
e-mail: mail@psoriasis-association.org.uk
www.psoriasis-association.org.uk

Formed with these aims in view: to raise awareness of psoriasis; support those who have psoriasis; and fund research into the causes of and treatments for psoriasis.

4000 members

Ray Jobling, MBE, Chairman
Jonathan Swift, Vice Chairman
John Ford, MBE, Treasurer

6029 Psoriasis Connections
Thousand Oaks, CA 91320
www.psoriasisconnect.com

Connects people with medical experts on psoriasis, those affected by the condition, family and friends, and other relevant resources.

6030 Skin Page
pinch.com/skin/
e-mail: skinpage-0907-admin@pinch.com
pinch.com/skin/

Noncommercial site that provides shortcuts to search past messages in the skin diseases newsgroups and other databases. Includes a psoriasis information page and other resources.

6031 UnderstandingPsoriasis.org by Healthology
www.understandingpsoriasis.org

Current information on psoriasis gathered and presented by leaders in the field of dermatology.

Book Publishers

6032 Handbook of Psoriasis
Charles Camisa, author

Blackwell Publishing
Commerce Place, 350 Main Street
Malden, MA 02148
781-388-8200
800-216-2522
Fax: 781-388-8210
www.wiley.com

Reference for health care professionals, easy to read, yet detailed information.
2005 2nd Ed Paperback
ISBN: 1-405109-27-7

Peter B. Wiley, Chairman
Stephen M. Smith, President & CEO
Ellis E. Cousens, Executive Vice President, Chief Fin

6033 Psychological Approaches to Dermatology
Linda Papadopoulos, author

Blackwell Publishing
Commerce Place, 350 Main Street
Malden, MA 02148
781-388-8200
800-216-2522
Fax: 781-388-8210
www.wiley.com

References all the main skin conditions - psoriasis, eczema, vitiligo, dermatitis, alopecia, and others. The book blends theory and practical experience, making it a highly recommended read.
1999 176 pages Paperback
ISBN: 1-854332-92-9

Peter B. Wiley, Chairman
Stephen M. Smith, President & CEO
Ellis E. Cousens, Executive Vice President, Chief Fin

6034 Textbook of Psoriasis
Peter Van de Kerkhof, author

Blackwell Publishing
Commerce Place, 350 Main Street
Malden, MA 02148
781-388-8200
800-216-2522
Fax: 781-388-8210
www.wiley.com

Written for dermatologists, it is a concise and clinical account of psoriasis, divided into three sections: morphology of the skin, etiology and pathogenesis, and current treatments.
2003 2nd Ed Hardback
ISBN: 1-405107-17-4

Peter B. Wiley, Chairman
Stephen M. Smith, President & CEO
Ellis E. Cousens, Executive Vice President, Chief Fin

Magazines

6035 International Journal of Dermatology
International Society of Dermatology
2323 North State Street #30
Bunnell, FL 32110
386-437-4405
Fax: 386-437-4427
e-mail: info@intsocderm.org
www.intsocderm.org

Focuses on information for dermatologists and the whole specialty of dermatology research and education.
10 times a year

Evangeline Handog, MD, President
Luca Borradori, Vice President
Paulo Rowilson Cunha, Vice President

6036 Journal of Dermatologic Surgery and Oncology
International Society for Dermatologic Surgery
930 N Meachan Road
Schaumburg, IL 60173   847-330-9830
                                   Fax: 847-330-1135

Focuses on medical updates and information on dermatology.
Monthly

6037 Psoriasis Advance
National Psoriasis Foundation
6600 SW 92nd Avenue, Suite 300
Portland, OR 97223   503-244-7404
                                        800-723-9166
                                   Fax: 503-245-0626
                            e-mail: getinfo@psoriasis.org
                                     www.psoriasis.org

Member magazine that evolved from two formerly published
newsletters (Bulletin & Psoriasis Resource) connecting the psoriasis community.
36 pages Bi-monthly
Krista Kellogg, Chair
Pete Redding, Vice Chair
Randy Beranek, President/ CEO

Journals

6038 Psoriasis Forum
National Psoriasis Foundation
6600 SW 92nd Avenue, Suite 300
Portland, OR 97223   503-244-7404
                                        800-723-9166
                                   Fax: 503-245-0626
                            e-mail: getinfo@psoriasis.org
                                     www.psoriasis.org

Journal for professional members of the foundation. It is dedi-
cated to providing up-to-date, practical information to health care
providers on the front line of psoriasis treatment.
Krista Kellogg, Chair
Pete Redding, Vice Chair
Randy Beranek, President/ CEO

Newsletters

6039 Awareness
NAPVI
PO Box 317
Watertown, MA 2471   617-972-7441
                                        800-562-6265
                                   Fax: 617-972-7444
                            www.spedex.com/napvi

Newsletter offering regional news, sports and activities, conferences, camps, legislative updates, book reviews, audio reviews,
professional question and answer column and more for the visually impaired and their families.
Quarterly

6040 Bulletin
National Psoriasis Foundation
6600 SW 92nd Avenue, Suite 300
Portland, OR 97223   503-244-7404
                                        800-723-9166
                                   Fax: 503-245-0626
                            e-mail: getinfo@psoriasis.org
                                     www.psoriasis.org

Published for 35 years by the National Psoriasis Foundation, past
issues are available online in pdf form. It covered both traditional
and alternative treatments, self-help techniques, research and a
wide variety of human-interest topics. Please refer to the foundation's magazine Psoriasis Advance for updated information and
resources.
Krista Kellogg, Chair
Pete Redding, Vice Chair
Randy Beranek, President/ CEO

6041 DVH Quarterly
University of Arkansas at Little Rock
2801 S University Avenue
Little Rock, AR 72204   Fax: 501-663-3536

Offers information on upcoming events, conferences and workshops on and for visual disabilities. Book reviews, information
on the newest resources and technology, educational programs,
want ads and more.
Quarterly
Bob Brasher, Editor

6042 Dermatology Focus
Dermatology Foundation
1560 Sherman Avenue, Suite 870
Evanston, IL 60201   847-328-2256
                                   Fax: 847-328-0509
                    e-mail: dfgen@dermatologyfoundation.org
                             dermatologyfoundation.org

Includes membership activities, research articles and lists recipi-
ents of foundation awards.
Quarterly
Bruce U. Wintroub, Chairman
Michael D. Tharp, M.D., President
Staurt R. Lessin, M.D., Vice President

6043 Dermatology World
American Academy of Dermatology
PO Box 94020
Palatine, IL 60094   847-330-0230
                                   Fax: 847-330-0050
                                        www.aad.org

Offers Academy members information outside the clinical realm.
It carries news of government actions, reports of socioeconomic
issues, societal trends and other events which impinge on the
practice of dermatology.
Monthly
Brett M. Coldiron, President
Elise A. Olsen, MD, Vice President
Suzanne M. Olbricht, Secretary-Treasurer

6044 Progress in Dermatology
Dermatology Foundation
1560 Sherman Avenue, Suite 870
Evanston, IL 60201   847-328-2256
                                   Fax: 847-328-0509
                    e-mail: dfgen@dermatologyfoundation.org
                             dermatologyfoundation.org

Bulletin offering information on research reports and clinical
trials.
Quarterly
Bruce U. Wintroub, Chairman
Michael D. Tharp, M.D., President
Staurt R. Lessin, M.D., Vice President

6045 Psoriasis Resource
National Psoriasis Foundation
6600 SW 92nd Avenue, Suite 300
Portland, OR 97223   503-244-7404
                                        800-723-9166
                                   Fax: 503-245-0626
                            e-mail: getinfo@psoriasis.org
                                     www.psoriasis.org

Published from 1999 to 2002, three times a year, by the National
Psoriasis Foundation, past issues are available online in pdf form.
It helped people make educated decisions about medication, ther-
apy and product choices available for skin and joints. Please refer
to the foundation's magazine Psoriasis Advance for updated
information and resources.
Krista Kellogg, Chair
Pete Redding, Vice Chair
Randy Beranek, President/ CEO

Pamphlets

6046 Alternative Approaches
National Psoriasis Foundation
6600 SW 92nd Avenue, Suite 300
Portland, OR 97223

503-244-7404
800-723-9166
Fax: 503-245-0626
e-mail: getinfo@psoriasis.org
www.psoriasis.org

Non-traditional therapies and treatments for both psoriasis and
psoriatic arthritis including stress management, topical preparations and Chinese medicine.

2005 13 pages

Krista Kellogg, Chair
Pete Redding, Vice Chair
Randy Beranek, President/ CEO

6047 Conception, Pregnancy and Psoriasis
National Psoriasis Foundation
6600 SW 92nd Avenue, Suite 300
Portland, OR 97223

503-244-7404
800-723-9166
Fax: 503-245-0626
e-mail: getinfo@psoriasis.org
www.psoriasis.org

Overview of the effect of pregnancy on psoriasis and treatment,
risks and other considerations during conception.

2006 9 pages

Krista Kellogg, Chair
Pete Redding, Vice Chair
Randy Beranek, President/ CEO

6048 Phototherapy: Light Treatment for Psoriasi s
National Psoriasis Foundation
6600 SW 92nd Avenue, Suite 300
Portland, OR 97223

503-244-7404
800-723-9166
Fax: 503-245-0626
e-mail: getinfo@psoriasis.org
www.psoriasis.org

Light treatment options: PUVA, lasers, broad-band UVB, and
narrow-band UVB.

2006 13 pages

Krista Kellogg, Chair
Pete Redding, Vice Chair
Randy Beranek, President/ CEO

6049 Psoriasis 101: Learning to Live in the Ski n You're In
National Psoriasis Foundation
6600 SW 92nd Avenue, Suite 300
Portland, OR 97223

503-244-7404
800-723-9166
Fax: 503-245-0626
e-mail: getinfo@psoriasis.org
www.psoriasis.org

Designed to educate young people, teens and college-age young
adults about psoriasis. It is written from a young person's stand-
point with bytes of information.

2006 12 pages

Krista Kellogg, Chair
Pete Redding, Vice Chair
Randy Beranek, President/ CEO

6050 Psoriasis Research: Progress & Promise
National Psoriasis Foundation
6600 SW 92nd Avenue, Suite 300
Portland, OR 97223

503-244-7404
800-723-9166
Fax: 503-245-0626
e-mail: getinfo@psoriasis.org
www.psoriasis.org

Overview of present research and the foundation's role in supporting it. Includes new treatments and progress being made in
genetics.

2004 11 pages

Krista Kellogg, Chair
Pete Redding, Vice Chair
Randy Beranek, President/ CEO

6051 Psoriasis on Specific Skin Sites
National Psoriasis Foundation
6600 SW 92nd Avenue, Suite 300
Portland, OR 97223

503-244-7404
800-723-9166
Fax: 503-245-0626
e-mail: getinfo@psoriasis.org
www.psoriasis.org

Information on the disease affecting nails, ears, eyelids, face,
mouth and lips, hands, feet and skin folds.

2005 9 pages

Krista Kellogg, Chair
Pete Redding, Vice Chair
Randy Beranek, President/ CEO

6052 Psoriasis: How it Makes You Feel
National Psoriasis Foundation
6600 SW 92nd Avenue, Suite 300
Portland, OR 97223

503-244-7404
800-723-9166
Fax: 503-245-0626
e-mail: getinfo@psoriasis.org
www.psoriasis.org

Living with psoriasis and the emotional impact.

Krista Kellogg, Chair
Pete Redding, Vice Chair
Randy Beranek, President/ CEO

6053 Psoriatic Arthritis
National Psoriasis Foundation
6600 SW 92nd Avenue, Suite 300
Portland, OR 97223

503-244-7404
800-723-9166
Fax: 503-245-0626
e-mail: getinfo@psoriasis.org
www.psoriasis.org

Overview of the joint disease that affects about 10-30% of psoriasis sufferers. Includes diagnosis and treatment details.

2005 11 pages

Krista Kellogg, Chair
Pete Redding, Vice Chair
Randy Beranek, President/ CEO

6054 Questions and Answers About Psoriasis
NAMSIC, National Institutes of Health
1 AMS Circle
Bethesda, MD 20892

301-495-4484
877-226-4267
Fax: 301-718-6366
TTY: 301-565-2966
e-mail: NIAMSinfo@mail.nih.gov
www.niams.nih.gov

Offers various information for the psoriasis patient and their family regarding treatments, risks, nutrition and more.

2003 22 pages

Stephen I. Katz, M.D., Ph.D., Director

6055 Scalp Psoriasis
National Psoriasis Foundation
6600 SW 92nd Avenue, Suite 300
Portland, OR 97223

503-244-7404
800-723-9166
Fax: 503-245-0626
e-mail: getinfo@psoriasis.org
www.psoriasis.org

Possible treatment, tips and regimens for psoriasis of the scalp.

2005 9 pages

Krista Kellogg, Chair
Pete Redding, Vice Chair
Randy Beranek, President/ CEO

6056 Specific Forms of Psoriasis
National Psoriasis Foundation
6600 SW 92nd Avenue, Suite 300
Portland, OR 97223

503-244-7404
800-723-9166
Fax: 503-245-0626
e-mail: getinfo@psoriasis.org
www.psoriasis.org

Plaque, Pustular, guttate, inverse, and erythrodermic: overview
and treatment considerations for each type of the disease.

2006 7 pages

Krista Kellogg, Chair
Pete Redding, Vice Chair
Randy Beranek, President/ CEO

6057 Sun and Water Therapy
National Psoriasis Foundation
6600 SW 92nd Avenue, Suite 300
Portland, OR 97223

503-244-7404
800-723-9166
Fax: 503-245-0626
e-mail: getinfo@psoriasis.org
www.psoriasis.org

Provides information on climatotherapy sites as well as an overview of natural sunlight and water treatment options.

2005 11 pages

Krista Kellogg, Chair
Pete Redding, Vice Chair
Randy Beranek, President/ CEO

6058 Things to Consider
National Psoriasis Foundation
6600 SW 92nd Avenue, Suite 300
Portland, OR 97223

503-244-7404
800-723-9166
Fax: 503-245-0626
e-mail: getinfo@psoriasis.org
www.psoriasis.org

Discusses making treatment decisions, talking with your physician and knowing your rights.

Krista Kellogg, Chair
Pete Redding, Vice Chair
Randy Beranek, President/ CEO

6059 Your Diet & Psoriasis
National Psoriasis Foundation
6600 SW 92nd Avenue, Suite 300
Portland, OR 97223

503-244-7404
800-723-9166
Fax: 503-245-0626
e-mail: getinfo@psoriasis.org
www.psoriasis.org

An overview of diet-related research and therapies.

2005 9 pages

Krista Kellogg, Chair
Pete Redding, Vice Chair
Randy Beranek, President/ CEO

Camps

6060 Camp Discovery
American Academy of Dermatology
930 E Woodfield Road
Schaumburg, IL 60173

847-240-1737
Fax: 847-330-8907
e-mail: jmueller@aad.org
www.aad.org/dermatology-a-to-z/for-kids/camp-discove

A camp for young people with chronic skin conditions. There is
no fee and transportation is provided. Three locations: Camp Horizon in Millville, PA, Camp Knutson in Crosslake, MN, and
Camp Dermadillo in Burton, TX.

Brett M. Coldiron, President
Elise A. Olsen, MD, Vice President
Suzanne M. Olbricht, Secretary-Treasurer

Description

6061 PTOSIS

Synonym: Blepharoptosis

Covers these related disorders: Acquired ptosis, Congenital ptosis

Involves the following Biologic System(s):

Neurologic Disorders, Ophthalmologic Disorders

Ptosis, or blepharoptosis, refers to a condition in which one or both of the upper eyelids droop or sag as a result of an irregularity that is present at birth or an acquired weakness in the muscles of the upper eyelid that are responsible for movement. This condition may also be the result of irregularities of the nerve response for regulating muscle movements of the upper eyelids (third cranial nerve or oculomotor nerve). Congenital ptosis varies in severity; therefore, treatment depends upon the extent of the defect. If the eyelid droop is sufficient to cover the pupil, the ability to see is impaired. In some infants and children, the development of the affected eye may be slowed, resulting in reduced or lost vision (amblyopia) in that eye. In such cases, early intervention through surgery may aid in preventing the development of impaired vision. However, surgery to correct ptosis strictly for cosmetic reasons is often postponed until the affected child reaches the age of three or four years.

In some cases, ptosis is accompanied by an abnormality of certain eye muscles, resulting in irregular movements of the eyes. Other ocular irregularities often associated with congenital ptosis include misalignment of the eyes in relation to each other (strabismus) or an imbalance in the way each eye deflects light (anisometropia). Medical specialists recommended early treatment of any accompanying abnormalities to avert complications. Ptosis may also occur as a characteristic feature of several syndromes including congenital fibrosis syndrome, Horner syndrome, or Sturge-Weber syndrome. Congenital ptosis is transmitted as an autosomal dominant trait.

Acquired ptosis may develop secondary to several disorders or conditions including myasthenia gravis, a muscular disorder; botulism, a severe type of food poisoning; progressive lesions within the skull that impact on the third cranial nerve; inflammation or growths that impact the eye orbit or lid. Treatment for acquired ptosis depends upon and may be directed toward the underlying cause.

Government Agencies

6062 NIH/National Eye Institute
31 Center Drive MSC 2510
Bethesda, MD 20892
301-496-5248
e-mail: 2020@nei.nih.gov
www.nei.nih.gov

Conducts and supports research that helps prevent and treat eye diseases and other disorders of vision. This research leads to sight-saving treatments, reduces visual impairment and blindness, and improves the quality of life for people of all ages. NEI-supported research has advanced our knowledge of how the eye functions in health and disease.

Paul A Sieving M.D., Ph.D., Director

National Associations & Support Groups

6063 American Academy of Pediatrics
141 Northwest Point Boulevard
Elk Grove Village, IL 60007
847-434-4000
800-433-9016
Fax: 847-434-8000
www.aap.org

The American Academy of Pediatrics and its member pediatricians are committed to the attainment of optimal physical, mental and social health and well-being for all infants, children, adolescents, and young adults.

Sandra Hassink, MD, FAAP, President

6064 Genetic Alliance
4301 Connecticut Avenue NW
Washington, DC 20008
202-966-5557
800-336-4363
Fax: 202-966-8553
e-mail: info@geneticalliance.org
www.geneticalliance.org

A coalition of voluntary genetic support groups, consumers and professionals addressing the needs of individuals and families affected by genetic disorders from a national perspective.

Sharon Terry, President
Natasha Bonhomme, Vice President of Strategic Develop
Vaughn ÿEdelson, Assistant Director of Health Commun

6065 March of Dimes Birth Defects Foundation
1275 Mamaroneck Avenue
White Plains, NY 10605
914-997-4488; 888-663-4637
Fax: 914-428-8203
e-mail: answers@marchofdimes.com; www.marchofdimes.com

Partnership of volunteers and professionals dedicates to improving the health of babies by preventing birth defects and infant mortality. Over 100 chapters are located across the country and can be located through the National Office.

Jennifer L Howse, President

6066 National Association for Visually Handicapped
111 E 59th St,ÿ
New York, NY 10022
212-889-3141; 800-829-0500
Fax: 212-727-2931
e-mail: navh@navh.org; www.navh.org

Serves as a clearinghouse for information about all services available to the partially-sighted from public and private sources. Conducts self-help groups. Provides information on large print books, textbooks and educational tools.

Lorianie Marchi, CEO

Web Sites

6067 National Association for Visually Handicapped
111 E 59th St
New York, NY 10022
800-284-4422
lighthouse.org/navh

Helps to cope with the difficulties of vision impairment.

6068 Online Mendelian Inheritance in Man
National Library of Medicine, Building 38A
Bethesda, MD 20894
888-346-3656
e-mail: info@ncbi.nlm.nih.gov; www.ncbi.nlm.nih.gov

This database is a catalog of human genes and genetic disorders.

6069 Royal National Institute of the Blind
105 Judd Street
London, WC1H
303-123-9999
e-mail: helpline@rnib.org.uk; www.rnib.org.uk

A leading UK charity offering information, support and advice to over two million people with sight problems.

Lesley-Anne Alexander , Chief Executive
Wanda Hamilton, Group Director
Fazilet Hadi, Managing Director

Description

6070 PULMONARY HYPERTENSION

Covers these related disorders: Persistent fetal circulation (PFC)

Involves the following Biologic System(s):

Cardiovascular Disorders, Respiratory Disorders

Primary pulmonary hypertension is a condition in which the blood pressure within the pulmonary artery is abnormally high (hypertension). The pulmonary artery arises from the base of the lower right chamber of the heart (ventricle) and carries oxygen-poor blood to the lungs, where the exchange of oxygen and carbon dioxide occurs. When this occurs in newborn infants, it is known as persistent fetal circulation or more appropriately, persistent pulmonary hypertension in the newborn (PPHN).

PPHN is a condition in newborns in which blood continues to circulate through certain fetal openings or channels which usually close shortly after birth. These include the fetal opening between the left and right upper chambers of the heart (foramen ovale) and the fetal channel that joins the major artery of the body (aorta) and the pulmonary artery (ductus arteriosus). PPHN may occur in newborns for unknown reasons (idiopathic) or may result from a lack of oxygen during the birth process (birth asphyxia); certain abnormalities during pregnancy (e.g., amniotic fluid leak); certain birth defects (e.g., underdevelopment of the lungs seen in a diaphragmatic hernia); or other conditions, such as meconium aspiration, polycythemia (excess number of red blood cells, etc. PPHN affects approximately one in 500 t0 700 newborns.

Newborns with PPHN often experience symptoms immediately after birth or within the first 12 hours of life. Some may have bluish discoloration of the skin and mucous membranes (cyanosis) and increasing difficulties breathing (respiratory distress). Symptoms associated with respiratory distress may include rapid breathing (tachypnea), grunting upon exhalation, drawing in of the chest wall during inhalation, and a rapid heart rate (tachycardia).

In newborns with PPHN, immediate measures may be necessary to prevent or treat potentially life-threatening complications. Additional therapy is directed toward treating the underlying cause of the condition and providing ongoing supportive measures to increase the supply of oxygen to bodily tissues. Oxygen therapies may include the use of measures to mechanically assist breathing (mechanical ventilation), administration of certain medications (e.g., surfactant therapy; inhalation of nitric oxide to help widen pulmonary blood vessels), or use of a device known as an extracorporeal membrane oxygenator (ECMO). This device delivers oxygen to an infant's blood as it is circulated outside of the body and then returns the oxygenated blood to the body.

In contrast to PPHN, primary pulmonary hypertension is a progressive condition that often becomes apparent between the ages of 10 to 20 years. Females appear to be slightly more affected than males. Researchers suspect that th|e condition may be the result of the interactions of different genes, possibly in association with the involvement of certain environmental factors (multifactorial inheritance).

In patients with primary pulmonary hypertension, abnormal thickening and loss of elasticity of pulmonary arterial walls may cause abnormal obstruction and increased resistance of the blood flow from the right ventricle to the lungs. Consequently, the heart muscle must pump harder and at a higher pressure to adequately propel blood through the pulmonary artery, leading to enlargement of the right ventricle. Affected individuals may experience exercise intolerance (inability to do physical exercise at the level that would be expected of someone in his or her general physical condition), easy fatigability, and, in some cases, dizziness, fainting episodes (syncope), headaches, and chest pain. In addition, as the right ventricle begins to weaken in its ability to pump blood efficiently (right ventricular failure), patients may experience cyanosis, coldness of the affected limbs, enlargement of the liver (hepatomegaly), and an abnormal accumulation of fluid in body tissues (edema). Patients with severe pulmonary hypertension may experience sudden abnormalities in the rhythm or rate of the heartbeat (arrhythmias), resulting in life-threatening complications. Supportive therapies for the treatment of primary pulmonary hypertension may include intravenous administration of the medication prostacyclin to help widen pulmonary arteries (vasodilation) and increase blood flow. In addition, in some patients, the administration of calcium channel blocking agents by mouth may be beneficial. In many patients with severe primary pulmonary hypertension, heart-lung or lung transplantation may be required.

Government Agencies

6071 NIH/National Heart, Lung and Blood Institu te
National Institute of Health
PO Box 30105
Bethesda, MD 20824
301-592-8573
Fax: 240-629-3246
TTY: 240-629-3255
e-mail: nhlbiinfo@nhlbi.nih.gov
www.nhlbi.nih.gov

Primary responsibility of this organization is the scientific investigation of heart, blood vessel, lung and blood disorders. Oversees research, demonstration, prevention, education, control and training activities in these fields and emphasizes the prevention and control of heart diseases.

Elizabeth G Nabel, MD, Director
Susan Shurin, MD, Deputy Director
Sheila Pohl, Chief of Staff

6072 NIH/National Institute of Child Health and Human Development
31 Center Drive, Building 31
Bethesda, MD 20892
301-496-1333
Fax: 301-496-1104
www.nichd.nih.gov

Established in 1962 by congress, today the institute conducts and supports research on topics related to the health of children, adults, families and populations. Some of these topics include: developmental disabilities, growth and development, infant death, reproductive health and birth defects.

Jay H Hoofnagle, Director
Lisa Kaeser, Program & Public Liaison

National Associations & Support Groups

6073 American Academy of Pediatrics
141 Northwest Point Boulevard
Elk Grove Village, IL 60007
847-434-4000
800-433-9016
Fax: 847-434-8000
www.aap.org

The American Academy of Pediatrics and its member pediatricians are committed to the attainment of optimal physical, mental and social health and well-being for all infants, children, adolescents, and young adults.

Sandra Hassink, MD, FAAP, President

6074   American Heart Association
7272 Greenville Avenue
Dallas, TX 75231   214-373-6300
                                                    800-242-8721
                                               Fax: 214-706-1341
                                        e-mail: inquire@amhrt.org
                                             www.americanheart.org

Supports research, education and community service programs with the objective of reducing premature death and disability from cardiovascular diseases and stroke; coordinates the efforts of health professionals, and others engaged in the fight against heart and circulatory disease.

M Cass Wheeler, CEO

6075   American Lung Association
1301 Pennsylvania Ave. NW, Suite 800,ÿ
Washington, DC 20004   202-785-3355
                                                    800-586-4872
                                               Fax: 202-452-1805
                                                   www.lungusa.org

The American Lung Association fights lung disease in all its forms, with special emphasis on asthma, tobacco control and environmental health. The American Lung Association is funded with contributions from the public, along with gifts and grants from corporations, foundations and government agencies. The association achieves its many successes through the work of thousands of committed volunteers and staff.

Terri E Weaver, PhD RN CS FAAN, Chairman

6076   Genetic Alliance
4301 Connecticut Avenue NW
Washington, DC 20008   202-966-5557
                                                    800-336-4363
                                               Fax: 202-966-8553
                                     e-mail: info@geneticalliance.org
                                            www.geneticalliance.org

A coalition of voluntary genetic support groups, consumers and professionals addressing the needs of individuals and families affected by genetic disorders from a national perspective.

Sharon Terry, President
Natasha Bonhomme, Vice President of Strategic Develop
Vaughn ÿEdelson, Assistant Director of Health Commun

6077   March of Dimes Birth Defects Foundation
1275 Mamaroneck Avenue
White Plains, NY 10605   914-997-4488
                                                    888-663-4637
                                               Fax: 914-428-8203
                                   e-mail: answers@marchofdimes.com
                                            www.marchofdimes.com

Partnership of volunteers and professionals dedicates to improving the health of babies by preventing birth defects and infant mortality. Over 100 chapters are located across the country and can be located through the National Office.

Jennifer L Howse, President

6078   Pulmonary Hypertension Association
801 Roeder Road, Ste 1000
Silver Spring, MD 20910   301-565-3004
                                                    800-748-7274
                                               Fax: 301-565-3994
                                      e-mail: pha@phassociation.org
                                             www.phassociation.org

PHA's mission is to seek a cure; provide hope, support and education; promote awareness, and advocate for the pulmonary hypertension community.

Rino Aldrighetti, Owner
Adrienne Dern, VP
Debbie Castro, Director Volunteer Services

Web Sites

6079   MayoClinic.com - Pulmonary Hypertension
13400 E. Shea Blvd.
Scottsdale, AZ 85259   480-301-8000
                                                    800-446-2279
            mayoclinic.com/health/pulmonary-hypertension/DS00430

Introduction to the disorder, signs, symptoms, treatment, etc.

Samuel A. Di Piazza, Jr., Chairman
John H. Noseworthy, M.D., CEO and President
Jeffrey W. Bolton, CAO and Vice President

Description

6080 PULMONARY VALVE STENOSIS

Covers these related disorders: Critical pulmonic stenosis
Involves the following Biologic System(s):
Cardiovascular Disorders

Pulmonary valve stenosis is a congenital heart defect characterized by abnormal narrowing (stenosis) of the valve between the lower right-sided, pumping chamber of the heart (right ventricle) and the pulmonary artery. Situated where the pulmonary artery arises from the base of the right ventricle, the pulmonary valve enables blood to flow from the right ventricle to the lungs while preventing the backward flow of blood. The pulmonary artery carries oxygen-depleted (deoxygenated) blood to the lungs, where the exchange of oxygen and carbon dioxide occurs. In infants and children with pulmonary valve stenosis, narrowing of the pulmonary valve opening increases resistance of the blood flow from the right ventricle to the pulmonary artery. As a result, the heart muscle must pump harder and at a higher pressure to propel blood to the pulmonary artery, potentially leading to thickening of the heart muscle (hypertrophy) of the right ventricle. Pulmonary valve stenosis affects approximately one in 1,250 individuals in the general population, comprising approximately 10 percent of all heart defects that are present at birth (congenital heart defects). Less commonly, pulmonary stenosis may be due to structural abnormalities other than a restricted valvular opening, such as narrowing within the upper region of the right ventricle or a portion of the pulmonary artery (e.g., isolated infundibular stenosis, branch pulmonary artery stenosis).

In infants and children with pulmonary valve stenosis, the severity of associated symptoms may vary, depending on the size of the restricted valvular opening and, in some patients, the presence of additional heart defects. For example, some affected children may also have relatively small septal defects, such as an abnormal opening in the fibrous partition (septum) that divides the ventricles or the two upper chambers (atria) of the heart (ventricular or atrial septal defects). Infants and children with mild pulmonary valve stenosis usually have no associated symptoms (asymptomatic), do not experience hypertrophy of heart muscle, and have normal growth and development. In such patients, the condition is usually initially suspected due to detection of characteristic, abnormal heart sounds (heart murmurs) during a physician's examination with a stethoscope. In patients with moderate pulmonary valve stenosis, the right ventricle may be of normal size or mildly thickened. Although such patients are usually asymptomatic, others may experience some symptoms, such as easy fatigability and exercise intolerance.

In newborns or young infants with severe pulmonary valve stenosis, the right ventricle may be unable to pump blood adequately (right ventricular failure) and become moderately or severely enlarged. Findings associated with right ventricular failure may include poor feeding, enlargement of the liver (hepatomegaly), an abnormal accumulation of fluid in body tissues (edema) or other abnormalities. In addition, blood may begin to circulate through a previously closed fetal opening in the heart (foramen ovale) between the left and right atria that closes shortly after birth. Abnormal opening of the foramen ovale in those with pulmonary valve stenosis may cause oxygen-depleted blood to pass from the right to the left side of the atria (right-to-left shunting), into the left ventricle and into the aorta for transport to the body's tissues. Because this oxygen-depleted blood bypasses the lungs and instead recirculates throughout the body, bodily tissues receive less oxygenated blood (hypoxia). In such cases, affected newborns or infants are said to have critical pulmonic stenosis. In addition, in some infants, certain associated heart (cardiac) defects, such as atrial or ventricular septal defects, may also allow some mixing of oxygen-poor and oxygen-rich blood. Due to recirculation of oxygen-poor blood to the body's tissues, affected newborns or infants may experience mild to moderate bluish discoloration of the skin and mucous membranes (cyanosis), shortness of breath (dyspnea), and other serious symptoms and findings.

In these newborns or infants, emergency procedures are performed to widen the restricted valvular opening. Such procedures may include inflation of a balloon-tipped cathet|er (valvuloplasty) or surgical correction or resection of the valve (valvotomy). Although corrective measures may not be required in those with mild stenosis, such patients should receive regular follow-up evaluations. Such monitoring is necessary to ensure appropriate intervention for patients who may potentially experience increasing obstruction across the pulmonary valve or increasing hypertrophy of the right ventricle requiring surgical intervention. Other treatment is symptomatic and supportive.

Pulmonary valve stenosis may occur as a spontaneous, isolated finding; with other congenital heart defects; or in association with certain underlying disorders (e.g., Noonan syndrome). In some patients, the condition is thought to be determined by the interactions of several different genes, possibly in association with the involvement of certain environmental factors (multifactorial inheritance).

Government Agencies

6081 NIH/National Heart, Lung and Blood Institu te
National Institute of Health
31 Center Dr MSC 2486, Bldg 31, Room 5A48
Bethesda, MD 20892
301-592-8573
Fax: 240-629-3246
TTY: 240-629-3255
e-mail: NHLBIinfo@nhlbi.nih.gov
www.nhlbi.nih.gov

Primary responsibility of this organization is the scientific investigation of heart, blood vessel, lung and blood disorders. Oversees research, demonstration, prevention, education, control and training activities in these fields and emphasizes the prevention and control of heart diseases.

Elizabeth G Nabel, MD, Director
Susan Shurin, MD, Deputy Director
Sheila Pohl, Chief of Staff

6082 NIH/National Institute of Child Health and Human Development
31 Center Drive, Building 31
Bethesda, MD 20892
301-496-1333
Fax: 301-496-1104
www.nichd.nih.gov

Established in 1962 by congress, today the institute conducts and supports research on topics related to the health of children, adults, families and populations. Some of these topics include: developmental disabilities, growth and development, infant death, reproductive health and birth defects.

Jay H Hoofnagle, Director
Lisa Kaeser, Program & Public Liaison

National Associations & Support Groups

6083 American Academy of Pediatrics
141 Northwest Point Boulevard
Elk Grove Village, IL 60007   847-434-4000
                                      800-433-9016
                                 Fax: 847-434-8000
                                      www.aap.org

The American Academy of Pediatrics and its member pediatricians are committed to the attainment of optimal physical, mental and social health and well-being for all infants, children, adolescents, and young adults.

Sandra Hassink, MD, FAAP, President

6084 American Heart Association
7272 Greenville Avenue
Dallas, TX 75231   214-373-6300
                                      800-242-8721
                                 Fax: 214-706-1341
                          e-mail: inquire@amhrt.org
                                 www.americanheart.org

Supports research, education and community service programs with the objective of reducing premature death and disability from cardiovascular diseases and stroke; coordinates the efforts of health professionals, and others engaged in the fight against heart and circulatory disease.

M Cass Wheeler, CEO

6085 Division of Pediatric Pulmonology
New York Medical College
Pediatric Specialty Ctr, 19 Bradhurst Avenue
Hawthorne, NY 10532   914-372-3010
                                 Fax: 914-594-4336
                          e-mail: pedpulm@nymc.edu
                                 www.nymc.edu

The division is dedicated to teaching and patient care.

6086 Genetic Alliance
4301 Connecticut Avenue NW
Washington, DC 20008   202-966-5557
                                      800-336-4363
                                 Fax: 202-966-8553
                      e-mail: info@geneticalliance.org
                                 www.geneticalliance.org

A coalition of voluntary genetic support groups, consumers and professionals addressing the needs of individuals and families affected by genetic disorders from a national perspective.

Sharon Terry, President
Natasha Bonhomme, Vice President of Strategic Develop
Vaughn ÿEdelson, Assistant Director of Health Commun

6087 March of Dimes Birth Defects Foundation
1275 Mamaroneck Avenue
White Plains, NY 10605   914-997-4488
                                      888-663-4637
                                 Fax: 914-428-8203
                     e-mail: answers@marchofdimes.com
                                 www.marchofdimes.com

Partnership of volunteers and professionals dedicates to improving the health of babies by preventing birth defects and infant mortality. Over 100 chapters are located across the country and can be located through the National Office.

Jennifer L Howse, President

Web Sites

6088 Congenital Heart Information Network
www.tchin.org

An international organization that provides reliable information, support services and resources to families of children with congenital heart defects and acquired heart disease, adults with congenital heart defects, and the professionals who work with them.

6089 Southern Illinois University School of Medicine
PO Box 19658
Springfield, IL 62794   217-545-8000
                                      800-342-5748
                          www.siumed.edu/peds/index.htm

The mission of SUI School of Medicine is to assist the people of central and southern Illinois in meeting their present and future health care needs through education, clinical service and research.

Book Publishers

6090 Congenital Disorders Sourcebook
Omnigraphics
PO Box 625
Holmes, PA 19043   800-234-1340
                                 Fax: 800-875-1340
                       e-mail: info@omnigraphics.com
                                 www.omnigraphics.com

Basic consumer health information on disorders aquired during gestation, including spina bifida, hydrocephalus, cerebral palsy, heart defects, craniofacial abnormalities and fetal alcohol syndrome.

650 pages
ISBN: 0-780809-45-9

Peter Ruffner, Publisher

Description

6091 PYLORIC STENOSIS

Synonym: Infantile pyloric stenosis

Involves the following Biologic System(s):

Gastrointestinal Disorders

Pyloric stenosis refers to a condition in which the passageway (pyloric canal) that leads from the stomach to the first part of the small intestine known as the duodenum is narrowed or obstructed due to the thickening of the muscle that surrounds this opening (pyloric sphincter). Although the specific cause for this thickening is not known, many factors may be responsible, including breast-feeding, irregularities in nerve distribution to the muscle, and certain disorders such as Turner syndrome, Cornelia de Lange syndrome, trisomy 18 syndrome, and eosinophilic gastroenteritis. Pyloric stenosis is also commonly associated with certain birth defects of the gastrointestinal tract such as tracheoesophageal fistula.

Symptoms and findings associated with this disorder may develop as early as the first week of life; however, in some infants, this abnormality does not cause noticeable symptoms until the fourth or fifth month. At about the third week of life, episodes of forceful and explosive vomiting (projectile vomiting) may occur. After eating, rhythmic, wave-like movements (peristalsis) may be visible in the infant's abdominal area. Prolonged vomiting may result in excessive fluid loss (dehydration) and loss of essential elements known as electrolytes in the fluid portion of the blood (e.g., sodium, potassium, and calcium).

Treatment for infantile pyloric stenosis includes the administration of fluids to counteract the effects of dehydration. Once body fluids andelectrolytes stabilize, a surgical procedure known as a pyloromyotomy may be performed. During this procedure, a lengthwise incision is made along the thickened pyloric muscle to correct the defect.

Pyloric stenosis affects approximately three in every 1,000 infants in the United States. Boys are more often affected than girls by a ratio of four to one. Children of parents who had pyloric stenosis are approximately 10 to 20 percent more likely to be affected. Infants with types B or O blood develop this defect more often than those with other blood types.

National Associations & Support Groups

6092 American Academy of Pediatrics
141 Northwest Point Boulevard
Elk Grove Village, IL 60007
847-434-4000
800-433-9016
Fax: 847-434-8000
www.aap.org

The American Academy of Pediatrics and its member pediatricians are committed to the attainment of optimal physical, mental and social health and well-being for all infants, children, adolescents, and young adults.

Sandra Hassink, MD, FAAP, President

6093 American College of Gastroenterology
PO Box 342260
Bethesda, MD 20827
301-263-9000
www.acg.gi.org

Founded to advance the scientific study and medical practice of diseases of the gastrointestinal (GI) tract.

Jack A DiPalma, President
Amy E Foxx-Orenstein, VP

6094 Cyclic Vomiting Syndrome Association
10520 W Bluemound Road, Suite #106
Milwaukee, WI 53226
414-342-7880
Fax: ÿ41- 34- 898
e-mail: ÿcvsa@cvsaonline.org
www.cvsaonline.org

A volunteer organization serving the needs of CVS patients, their families around the world and the growing medical community studying CVS. The network has grown to over 37 medical advisors and over 90 volunteers in over 32 countries.

$75/year

Kathleen Adams, President/Research Liaison

6095 Digestive Disease National Coalition
507 Capitol Court NE, Suite 200
Washington, DC 20002
202-544-7497
Fax: 202-546-7105
www.ddnc.org

Advocacy organization comprised of 22 voluntary and professional societies concerned with the many diseases of the digestive tract and liver.

Dale Dirks, Administrator
James DeGerome, President
Dr. Henry Parkman, VP

6096 International Foundation for Functional Gastrointestinal Disorders
700 W. Virginia St., #201
Milwaukee, WI 53204
414-964-1799
888-964-2001
Fax: 414-964-7176
e-mail: iffgd@iffgd.org
www.iffgd.org

Nonprofit education and research organization founded in 1991. IFFGD addresses the issues surrounding life with gastrointestinal (GI) functional and mobility disorders and increases the awareness about these disorders among the general public, researchers and the clinical care community.

Nancy J Norton, Founder
William Norton, VP

6097 March of Dimes Birth Defects Foundation
1275 Mamaroneck Avenue
White Plains, NY 10605
914-997-4488
888-663-4637
Fax: 914-428-8203
e-mail: answers@marchofdimes.com
www.marchofdimes.com

Partnership of volunteers and professionals dedicates to improving the health of babies by preventing birth defects and infant mortality. Over 100 chapters are located across the country and can be located through the National Office.

Jennifer L Howse, President

6098 North American Society for Pediatric Gastroenterology/Hepatology/Nutrition
PO Box 6
Flourtown, PA 19031
215-233-3918
Fax: 215-233-3918
e-mail: naspghan@naspghan.org
www.naspghan.org

Strives to improve the care of infants, children and adolescents with digestive disorders by promoting advances in clinical care of children with chronic abdominal pain, diarrhea, constipation, vomiting, bleeding from the GI tract, inflammatory bowel disease, liver diseases, diseases of the pancreas, poor weight gain and nutritional problems.

Philip Sherman, President
Margaret K Stallings, Executive Director

6099 Pediatric/Adolescent Gastroesophageal Reflux Association (PAGER)
PO Box 7728
Silver Spring, MD 20907 301-601-9541
e-mail: GERGROUP@aol.com
www.reflux.org

Non profit organization providing information and support to parents and children dealing with gastroesophageal reflux.

Beth Anderson, Director
Jan Gambino-Burns, Associate Director

Libraries & Resource Centers

6100 National Digestive Diseases Information Clearinghouse
2 Information Way
Bethesda, MD 20892 301-654-3810
800-891-5389
Fax: 703-738-4929
e-mail: nddic@info.niddk.nih.gov
www2.niddk.nih.gov

The National Institute of Diabetes and Digestive and Kidney Diseases conducts and supports research on many of the most serious diseases affecting public health. The Institute supports much of the clinical research on the diseases of internal medicine and related subspecialty fields as well as many basic science disciplines.

Griffin P. Rodgers, M.D, Chairman, Executive Board
Brent B. Stanfield, Executive Secretary
Camille M. Hoover, M.S.W, Executive Officer

Web Sites

6101 American Pediatric Surgical Association
111 Deer Lake Road, Suite 100
Deerfield, IL 60015 847-480-9576
Fax: 847-480-9282
e-mail: eapsa@eapsa.org
www.eapsa.org/parents/pyloric.htm

For parents: an overview of Pyloric Stenosis including synptoms, treatment and complications.

Michael D. Klein, President
Mary L. Brandt, Secretary
Daniel von Almen, Treasurer

6102 Dr. Koop
750 Third Avenue, 6th Floor
New York, NY 10017 212-695-2223
Fax: 212-695-2936
www.healthcentral.com

Information on the condition, causes, symptoms, tests and treatment.

Micheael Cunnion, Chief Executive Officer
Jim Curtis, Chief Revenue Officer
Rebecca Farwell, Chief Content Officer

6103 KidsHealth-Pyloric Stenosis
www.kidshealth.org/parent/

Definition, causes, symptoms, treatment and complications.

Neil Izenberg, MD, Editor-in-Chief & Founder

6104 MEDLINEplus Medical Encyclopedia: Pyloric Stenosis
8600 Rockville Pike
Bethesda, MD 20894 .nlm.nih.gov/medlineplus/ency/article/000970.htm

Definitions, causes, symptoms, treatment, prognosis and complications.

Donald A.B. Lindberg, Director

6105 National Digestive Diseases Information Clearinghouse
Bethesda, MD 20892 301-496-3583
www.digestive.niddk.nih.gov

The National Institute of Diabetes and Digestive and Kidney Diseases conducts and supports research on many of the most serious diseases affecting public health. The Institute supports much of the clinical research on the diseases of internal medicine and related subspecialty fields as well as many basic science disciplines.

Griffin P. Rodgers, M.D., M.A.C.P., Director

6106 Online Mendelian Inheritance in Man
National Library of Medicine, Building 38A
Bethesda, MD 20894 888-346-3656
e-mail: info@ncbi.nlm.nih.gov
www.ncbi.nlm.nih.gov

This database is a catalog of human genes and genetic disorders.

6107 Southern Illinois University School of Medicine
PO Box 19658
Springfield, IL 62794 217-545-8000
800-342-5748
www.siumed.edu/peds/index.htm

The mission of SUI School of Medicine is to assist the people of central and southern Illinois in meeting their present and future health care needs through education, clinical service and research.

Journals

6108 Journal of Pediatric Gastroenterology and Nutrition

NASPGHAN, author

Lippincott Williams & Wilkins
530 Walnut Street
Philadelphia, PA 19106 215-521-8300
Fax: 215-521-8902
www.lww.com

Publication of the North American Society for Pediatric Gastroenterolgy, Hepatology and Nutrition, which strives to improve the care of infants, children and adolescents with digestive disorders by promoting advances in clinical care of children with chronic abdominal pain, diarrhea, constipation, vomiting, bleeding from the GI tract, inflammatory bowel disease, liver diseases, diseases of the pancreas, poor weight gain and nutritional problems.

Newsletters

6109 NASPGHAN News
PO Box 6
Flourtown, PA 19031 215-233-0808
Fax: 215-233-3918
e-mail: naspghan@naspghan.org
www.naspgn.org

Publication of the North American Society for Pediatric Gastroenterolgy, Hepatology and Nutrition, which strives to improve the care of infants, children and adolescents with digestive disorders by promoting advances in clinical care of children with chronic abdominal pain, diarrhea, constipation, vomiting, bleeding from the GI tract, inflammatory bowel disease, liver diseases, diseases of the pancreas, poor weight gain and nutritional problems.

Margaret K. Stallings, Executive Director
Kim Rose, Associate Director
Ben Zaitz, Director of Meetings

Description

6110 REFRACTION DISTURBANCES

Synonym: Ametropia

Disorder Type: Vision

Covers these related disorders: Anisometropia, Astigmatism, Hyperopia (Farsightedness), Myopia (Nearsightedness)

Involves the following Biologic System(s):

Ophthalmologic Disorders

Refraction abnormalities are defects in the cornea and the lens of the eye to focus visual images appropriately on the nerve-rich membrane at the back of the eye (retina). The cornea is the convex, transparent area in front of the eye. The lens, which is located behind the pupil, is held in place by a circular muscle that changes the shape of the lens to make appropriate adjustments in focus (ciliary muscle). As light passes through the cornea and the lens, it is bent (refracted) so that it is properly focused on the retina, which contains millions of tiny nerve cells that respond to light (photoreceptors). However, in individuals with refraction defects, light rays are not properly focused on the retina (ametropia) due to abnormalities of the cornea, the lens, or the size of the eye. These refraction defects lead to visual abnormalities.

There are three primary types of refraction abnormalities: namely, farsightedness (hyperopia), nearsightedness (myopia), and astigmatism. In farsightedness, parallel light rays come to focus behind rather that on the retina. This may be due to shortness of the eyeball from front to back, abnormally reduced refractive power of the cornea or lens, or backward displacement of the lens. If farsightedness is mild or moderate, affected children may be able to clearly visualize near and far objects due to accommodation, a process by which the shape of the lens changes and brings the area of focus forward. The range and extent of accommodation is highest durign childhood and gradually decreases with age. With greater degrees of farsightedness, affected children may experience blurring of vision, eyestrain, fatigue, and recurrent headaches. They may also engage in repeated eye rubbing and squinting and appear uninterested in reading or schoolwork. Children with farsightedness may achieve clear vision with glasses or contact lenses with convex lenses.

In children with nearsightedness (myopia), parallel light rays come to focus in front of the retina due to increased length of the eyeball from front to back, abnormally increased refractive power of the cornea or lens, or forward displacement of the lens. Affected children experience blurring of vision when focusing on distant objects, tend to hold reading material and other objects close to their face, and often squint in an effort to improve clearness and clarity of vision. Nearsightedness usually becomes apparent during school age, particularly in the years prior to and up to adolescence. The degree of nearsightedness typically becomes more severe until early adulthood, when it tends to stabilize. Many affected children have a hereditary predisposition for nearsightedness; in addition, the condition may occur in association with the other eye abnormalities (e.g., glaucoma, keratoconus) or other underlying disorders. Clear vision may be attained with glasses or contact lenses with concave lenses. Until the degree of nearsightedness stabilizes, prescriptions may need to be periodically increased in strength (e.g., varying from every few months to once every one or two years).

In children with astigmatism, parallel light rays are not clearly focused in a point on the retina due to unequal curvature of refractive surfaces of the eye. Astigmatism may result from irregularities in curvature of the cornea or, in some cases, abnormalities of the lens. Many individuals have minor degrees of astigmatism and have no associated symptoms. With more severe degrees of astigmatism, affected children may experience blurring and distortion of vision, fatigue, eyestrain, and recurrent headaches. In many cases, they may also engage in frequent eye rubbing, squint in an attempt to improve clearness and clarity of vision, hold reading materials and other objects close, and appear uninterested in schoolwork. In children with astigmatism, visual correction may be achieved with the part-time or ongoing use of glasses with cylindric or spherocylindric lenses. In some cases, contact lenses may be used to help correct vision.

Some children may also have a visual condition known as anisometropia in which the refractive or focusing ability of one eye significantly differs from the other. For example, one eye may have normal focusing ability, whereas the other may be affected by nearsightedness, farsightedness, and astigmatism. For proper vision to develop during infancy and early childhood, corresponding visual images mustform on both retinas to ensure the transmission of compatible nerve impulses (via the optic nerves) to the brain. If the images from one eye differ dramatically from the other, one may be suppressed, causing impaired visual development in one eye (amblyopia). Therefore, in infants and children with anisometropia, prompt detection and appropriate visual correction is essential to ensure proper visual development in both eyes.

Government Agencies

6111 NIH/National Eye Institute
31 Center Drive MSC 2510
Bethesda, MD 20892

301-496-5248
e-mail: 2020@nei.nih.gov
www.nei.nih.gov

Conducts and supports research that helps prevent and treat eye diseases and other disorders of vision. This research leads to sight-saving treatments, reduces visual impairment and blindness, and improves the quality of life for people of all ages. NEI-supported research has advanced our knowledge of how the eye functions in health and disease.

Paul A Sieving MD, PhD, Director

National Associations & Support Groups

6112 American Academy of Pediatrics
141 Northwest Point Boulevard
Elk Grove Village, IL 60007

847-434-4000
800-433-9016
Fax: 847-434-8000
www.aap.org

The American Academy of Pediatrics and its member pediatricians are committed to the attainment of optimal physical, mental and social health and well-being for all infants, children, adolescents, and young adults.

Sandra Hassink, MD, FAAP, President

6113 Division on Visual Impairments
Council for Exceptional Children
1110 North Glebe Road, Suite 300
Arlington, VA 22201 · · · · · · · · · · · · 800-224-6830
Fax: 703-264-9494
TTY: 866-915-5000
www.ed.arizona.edu/dvi/welcome.htm; www.cec.sped.org

A division within the CEC, it handles concerns for Federal, state and local issues and policies related to education of youths, children and infants with visual impairments.

Ellyn Ross, President
Shirley J Wilson, Secretary
Phyllis T Simmons, President Elect

6114 Lighthouse International
111 E 59th Street
New York, NY 10022 · · · · · · · · · · · · 212-821-9200
800-829-0500
Fax: 212-821-9707
TTY: 212-821-9713
e-mail: info@lighthouse.org
www.lighthouse.org

Provides services, information, resource contacts, education and research related to the needs of children who are visually impaired and their families.

Tara Cortes, CEO
Cynthia Stuen, Senior VP Services/Education
Bruce Rosenthal OD, Chief Low Vision Programs

6115 National Alliance of Blind Students
c/o Terry Pacheco
1155 15th Street NW, Suite 1004
Washington, DC 20005 · · · · · · · · · · · · 202-467-5081
800-424-8666
Fax: 202-467-5085
e-mail: rj.hodson@verizon.net
www.blindstudents.org

An advocacy and consumer organization for high school and college students who are blind or visually impaired. It works to facilitate progress toward full accessibility of college programs and facilities, provides opportunities for discussion of issues important to students and assists with National Student Seminars.

Rebecca Hodson, President

6116 National Association for Parents of Childr en with Visual Impairments
PO Box 317
Watertown, MA 02471 · · · · · · · · · · · · 617-972-7441
800-562-6265
Fax: 617-972-7444
e-mail: napvi@perkins.org
www.spedex.com/napvi/

Offers emotional support for parents of blind or visually impaired children. Provides information, training and assistance, and help in understanding and using available resources.

6117 National Association for Visually Handicapped
22 W 21st Street, 6th Floor
New York, NY 10010 · · · · · · · · · · · · 212-889-3141
888-205-5951
Fax: 212-727-2931
e-mail: navh@navh.org
www.navh.org

Serves as a clearinghouse for information about all services available to the partially-sighted from public and private sources. Conducts self-help groups. Provides information on large print books, textbooks and educational tools.

Lorianie Marchi, CEO

State Agencies & Support Groups

Alabama

6118 Alabama Institute for the Deaf & Blind
PO Box 698
Talladega, AL 35161 · · · · · · · · · · · · 256-761-3331
Fax: 256-761-3344
www.aidb.org

Services include central directory, representatives of agencies, service providers, families, and coordinators of infant, toddler, and preschool special education programs.

Terry Graham, President

Arizona

6119 National Association for Parents of the Visually Impaired
PO Box 317
Watertown, MA 02471 · · · · · · · · · · · · 617-972-7441
800-562-6265
Fax: 617-972-7444
www.spedex.com/napvi

Mary Ellen Simmons

California

6120 Blind Childrens Center
4120 Marathon Street
Los Angeles, CA 90029 · · · · · · · · · · · · 323-664-2153
Fax: 323-665-3828
www.blindchildrenscenter.org

Family-centered agency that serves children with visual impairments from birth to school age. The center-based programs and services help the children acquire skills and build their independence.

Midge Horton, Executive Director

Connecticut

6121 Region 1 of the National Association for Parents of the Visually Impaired
252 Rye Street
Broad Brook, CT 06016 · · · · · · · · · · · · 860-623-4129
Susan Ellsworth

Georgia

6122 Southeastern Region-Helen Keller National Center
1003 Virginia Avenue, Suite 104
Atlanta, GA 30354 · · · · · · · · · · · · 404-766-9625
Fax: 404-766-3447
TTY: 404-766-2820

Susan Lascek, Supervisor of Reg Representatives

Illinois

6123 National Association for Parents of the Visually Impaired
PO Box 317
Watertown, MA 02471 · · · · · · · · · · · · 617-972-7441
800-562-6265
Fax: 617-972-7444
www.spedex.com/napvi

Mary Ellen Simmons

6124 Region 3 of the National Association for Parents of the Visually Impaired
16 Thornfield Lane
Hawthorn Woods, IL 60047 · · · · · · · · · · · · 847-438-0705
Kevin O'Connor

Kansas

6125 Great Plains Region-Helen Keller National Center
4330 Shawnee Mission Parkway, suite 108
Shawnee, KS 66205
913-677-4562
Fax: 913-677-1544
e-mail: beth.jordan@hknc.org
www.helenkeller.org

Services are free and offer client advocacy, consultation and technical assistance to schools and agencies; assistance in developing local services information and referral; public education and awareness; maintenance of the National Registry.

Beth Jordan, Regional Representative

Maryland

6126 National Organization of Parents of Blind Children
350 Ignacio Blvd., Suite 200
Novato,, CA 94949
415-382-2530
Fax: 410-685-5653
e-mail: nfb@iamdiyrx.net
www.nfh.org

Informational and emotional support to parents who have a child, adolescent, or adult family member with blindness or visual impairment.

Massachusetts

6127 New England Region-Helen Keller National Center
313 Washington Street
Newton, MA 02458
617-630-1580
Fax: 617-630-1579
e-mail: hkncmeb@aol.com

New Mexico

6128 Region 5 of the National Association for Parents of the Visually Impaired
PO Box 1337
Alamogordo, NM 88311
505-682-2693

Ohio

6129 Region 2 of the National Association for Parents of the Visually Impaired
3910 Pocahontas Avenue
Cincinnati, OH 45227
513-561-8542
Victoria Gorman Miller

Pennsylvania

6130 East Central Region-Helen Keller National Center
4351 Garden City Drive
New Carrollton, MD 20785
301-459-5474
Fax: 301-459-5070
e-mail: hkncreg3cl@aol.com
www.helenkeller.org

South Carolina

6131 Region 4 of the National Association for Parents of the Visually Impaired
1032 Trail Road
Belton, SC 29627
864-338-9593

Washington

6132 Northwestern Region-Helen Keller National Center
2366 Eastlake Avenue E
Seattle, WA 98102
206-324-9120
e-mail: nwhknc@juno.com

Libraries & Resource Centers

Alabama

6133 Mobile Association for the Blind
2440 Gordon Smith Drive
Mobile, AL 36617
251-473-3585
Fax: 251-470-8622
www.mobileblind.org

Offers work adjustment training, activities of daily living, mobility, communication skills and sheltered employment for adults and children who are visually impaired.

Jim Bullock, Executive Director

Arizona

6134 Educational Services for the Visually Impaired
2402 Wildwood Avenue Suite 112
Sherwood, AR 72120
501-371-5448

Offers textbooks, Braille books and more to the visually impaired grades K-12 in the Arkansas area.

David Beavers, Director

Arkansas

6135 Arkansas Regional Library for the Blind and Physically Handicapped
1 Capitol Mall
Little Rock, AR 72201
501-682-1527
Fax: 501-682-1533
TDD: 501-682-1002
e-mail: mindy@library.arkansas.gov
www.asl.lib.ar.us/ASL_LBPH.htm

Public library books in recorded or Braille format. Popular fiction and nonfiction books for all ages, books and players are on free loan, sent to patrons by mail and may be returned postage free. Anyone who cannot see well enough to read regular print with glasses on or who has a disability that makes it difficult to hold a book or turn the pages is eligible.

John D Hall, Director

California

6136 American Action Fund for Blind Children and Adults
18440 Oxnard Street
Tarzana, CA 91356
818-343-2022
Fax: 818-343-3219
e-mail: lucyabba@aol.com
www.actinfund.org

A lending library for the visually impaired. We send out a weekly Braille newspaper for the deaf-blind (worldwide), we also send out pocket-sized Braille calendars. Our lending library is for pre-school thru high school. All of our services are free.

Lucille Abbazia, Manager

6137 Blind Children's Center
4120 Marathon Street
Los Angeles, CA 90029
323-664-2153
Fax: 323-665-3828
www.blindchildrenscenter.org

Offers support and informational groups.

Scott E. Schaldenbrand, President, Executive Committee
Danette M. Jones, Vice President
Lisa D. Hansen, Secretary

6138 Braille Institute Desert Center
70-251 Ramon Road
Rancho Mirage, CA 92270
760-321-1111
Fax: 760-321-9715
e-mail: dc@brailleinstitute.org
www.brailleinstitute.org

Dedicated to providing blind and visually impaired men, women
and children with the training, programs and services they need to
enjoy productive lives. Services offered include child development, youth programs, library services and adult education.

Lester M Sussman, Chairman
James B. Boyle Jr., Director
Thomas K. Callister, Director

6139 Braille Institute Sight Center
741 N Vermont Avenue
Los Angeles, CA 90029
323-663-1111
Fax: 323-663-0867
e-mail: la@brailleinstitute.org
www.brailleinstitute.org

Offers help, programs, services and information to the blind and
visually impaired children and adults.

Lester M Sussman, Chairman
James B. Boyle Jr., Director
Thomas K. Callister, Director

6140 Braille Institute Youth Center
741 N Vermont Avenue
Los Angeles, CA 90029
323-663-1111
Fax: 323-663-0867
e-mail: la@brailleinstitute.org
www.brailleinstitute.org

Offers various youth programs and services for the blind and visually impaired youngster.

Lester M Sussman, Chairman
James B. Boyle Jr., Director
Thomas K. Callister, Director

6141 New Beginnings - Blind Children's Center
4120 Marathon, Street
Los Angeles, CA 90029
323-664-2153
800-222-3566
Fax: 323-665-3828

Helps children and their families become independent by creating
a climate of safety and trust. Services include an infant stimulation program, educational preschool, interdisciplinary assessment
services, family services, correspondence program, toll-free national hotline and a publication and research service.

6142 San Francisco Public Library for the Blind and Print Disabled
100 Larkin Street
San Francisco, CA 94102
415-557-4400
Fax: 415-557-4252
e-mail: lbphmgr@sfpl.lib.ca.us
www.library.ca.us

Foreign-language books on cassette, children's books on cassettes
and more.

Luis Herrera, Manager

6143 Variety Audio
PO Box 5731
San Jose, CA 95150
408-277-4839

Summer reading programs, Braille writer, magnifiers, closed-circuit TV, large-print photocopier, cassette books and magazines,
children's books on cassette, home visits and other reference materials on blindness and other handicaps.

Louisa Griehshammer

6144 Council of Families with Visual Impairment
1155 15th Street NW
Washington, DC 20005
202-467-5081

Members are sighted parents of blind or visually impaired children. Offers a forum for support and outreach, sharing of experiences in parent-child relationships, and educational and cultural
information about child development. Monitors developments in
technical and legislative arenas.

Nola Webb, President

6145 Florida Bureau of Braille and Talking Book Library Services
1185 Dunn Avenue
Daytona Beach, FL 32114
386-254-3800
Fax: 386-239-6069
TDD: 800-226-6079
e-mail: mike_gunde@dbs.doe.state.fl.us
www.state.fl.us/dbs/lswel.html

Discs, cassettes, closed-circuit TV, large-print photocopier, films,
children's books on cassettes and more.

Michael Gunde, Librarian

6146 Talking Book Library, Jacksonville Public Library
2233 Park Avenue, Suite 402
Orange Park, FL 32073
904-278-5620
Fax: 904-278-5625
TDD: 904-768-7822
e-mail: office@neflin.org
www.neflin.org

Discs, cassettes and reference materials on blindness and other
disabilities.

Elizabeth Curry, President
Julie Sieg, Vice-President
Janet Loveless, Secretary

6147 Talking Book Service - Manatee County Central Library
6081 26th Street W
Bradenton, FL 34207
941-742-5914
Fax: 941-751-7089
TDD: 941-742-5951
e-mail: patricia.schubert@co.manatee.fl.us
www.co.manatee.fl.us

Offers children's books on disc and cassette and more reference
materials for the blind and physically handicapped.

Patricia Schubert, Librarian

6148 Albany Library for the Blind and Physical Handicapped
300 Pine Avenue
Albany, GA 31701
229-420-3220
Fax: 229-420-3215
e-mail: sinquefk@mail.dougherty.public.lib.ga.us
www.docolib.org/LBPH/index.html

Offers discs, cassettes, reference materials on blindness and other
handicaps, large-print photocopiers, summer reading programs,
cassette books and more.

Katy Sinquefield, Manager

6149 Bainbridge Subregional Library for the Blind and Physically Handicapped
301 S Monroe Street
Bainbridge, GA 39819
229-248-2665
800-795-2680
Fax: 229-248-2670
TDD: 912-248-2665
e-mail: lbph@mail.deccatur.public.lib.ga.us
www.swgrl.org

Discs, cassettes, summer reading programs, closed-circuit TV,
magnifiers and more.

Shelley Sudderth, Branch Manager
Susan Whittle, Director
Debbie Worthington, Administrative Secretary

6150 CEL Subregional Library for the Blind and Physically Handicapped
2708 Mechanics
Savannah, GA 31404
912-354-5864
Fax: 912-354-5534
TDD: 912-652-3635
e-mail: stokesl@cel.co.chatman.ga.us

Summer reading programs, Braille writer, magnifiers, closed-circuit TV, large-print photocopier, cassette books and magazines, children's books on cassette, home visits and other reference materials on blindness and other handicaps.

Linda Stokes, Librarian

Idaho

6151 Idaho State Talking Book Library
325 W State Street
Boise, ID 83702
208-334-2150
Fax: 208-334-4016
TDD: 800-377-1363
e-mail: tblbooks@isl.state.id.us
www.lili.org/isl/tblinfo.htm

Summer reading programs, Braille writer, magnifiers, closed-circuit TV, large-print photocopier, cassette books and magazines, children's books on cassette, home visits and other reference materials on blindness and other handicaps.

Sue Walker, Manager

Illinois

6152 Chicago Library Service for the Blind
400 S State Street
Chicago, IL 60605
312-747-4300

Summer reading programs, Braille writer, magnifiers, closed-circuit TV, large-print photocopier, cassette books and magazines, children's books on cassette, home visits and other reference materials on blindness and other handicaps.

Carol Pellish, Librarian

6153 Illinois State Library, Talkng Book and Braille Service
213 State Capitol
Springfield, IL 62756
217-785-3000
Fax: 217-558-4723
TDD: 800-665-5576
e-mail: isltbbs@ilsos.net
www.cyberdriveillinois.com

Summer reading programs, Braille writer, magnifiers, closed-circuit TV, large-print photocopier, cassette books and magazines, descriptive videos, children's books on cassette, home visits and other reference materials on blindness and other handicaps.

Anne Craig, Executive Director

6154 Mid Illinois Talking Book System
515 York Street
Quincy, IL 62301
217-224-6619
Fax: 217-224-9818

Summer reading programs, Braille writer, magnifiers, closed-circuit TV, large-print photocopier, cassette books and magazines, children's books on cassette, home visits and other reference materials on blindness and other handicaps.

6155 Mid-Illinois Talking Book Center
600 High Point Lane #2
East Peoria, IL 61611
309-694-9200
800-426-0709
Fax: 309-799-7916
e-mail: hitbc@darkstar.rsa.lib.il.us
www.mitbc.org

Summer reading programs, Braille writer, magnifiers, closed-circuit TV, large-print photocopier, cassette books and magazines, children's books on cassette, home visits and other reference materials on blindness and other handicaps.

Rose Chenoweth, Director
Valerie Brandon, Administrator

6156 Talking Book Center of Northwest Illinois
601 High Point Lane #2
East Peoria, IL 61612
309-694-9201
800-426-0710
Fax: 309-799-7917
e-mail: hitbc@darkstar.rsa.lib.il.us
www.mitbc.org

Summer reading programs, Braille writer, magnifiers, closed-circuit TV, large-print photocopier, cassette books and magazines, children's books on cassette, home visits and other reference materials on blindness and other handicaps.

Rose Chenoweth, Director
Valerie Brandon, Administrator

Indiana

6157 Northwest Indiana Subregional Library for Blind and Physically Handicapped
1919 W 81st Street
Merrillville, IN 46410
219-769-3541
Fax: 219-756-9358

Summer reading programs, Braille writer, magnifiers, closed-circuit TV, large-print photocopier, cassette books and magazines, children's books on cassette, home visits and other reference materials on blindness and other handicaps.

Renee Lewis

Iowa

6158 Iowa Library for the Blind and Physically Handicapped
Iowa Department for the Blind
524 4th Street
Des Moines, IA 50309
515-281-1333
800-362-2587
Fax: 515-281-1263
TTY: 515-281-1355
e-mail: contact@idbonline.org
www.blind.state.ia.us

Summer reading programs, magnifiers, closed-circuit TV, large-print photocopier, children's books on cassette, children's books in Braille and Print Braille, cassette magazines, home visits and reference materials on blindness and other handicaps.

Richard Sorey, Director
Bruce Snethen, Deputy Director

Kansas

6159 CKLS Headquarters
PO Box 515
Northampton, MA 01061
316-792-2393
888-622-8527
Fax: 316-792-5495
e-mail: cenks@ink.org
www.macular.org

Summer reading programs, Braille writer, magnifiers, closed-circuit TV, large-print photocopier, cassette books and magazines, children's books on cassette, home visits and other reference materials on blindness and other handicaps.

Chip Goehring, President
Mark E. Torrey, Vice President
Paul F. Gariepy, Secretary

6160 Services for the Visually Disabled
629 Poyntz Avenue
Manhattan, KS 66502
785-776-4741
Fax: 785-776-1545
e-mail: marionr@manhattan.lib.ks.us

Summer reading programs, Braille writer, magnifiers, closed-circuit TV, large-print photocopier, cassette books and magazines, children's books on cassette, home visits and other reference materials on blindness and other handicaps.

Marion Rice, Librarian

Kentucky

6161 Kentucky Library for the Blind and Physically Handicapped
PO Box 818
Frankfort, KY 40602

502-564-8300
800-372-2968
Fax: 502-564-5773
e-mail: richard.feindel@kdla.net
www.kdla.net/libserv/ktbl.htm

Large-print photocopier, cassette books and magazines, children's books on cassette, and other reference materials on blindness and other handicaps.

5,200 members

Richard Feindel, Librarian

Maryland

6162 Maryland State Library for the Blind and Physically Handicapped
415 Park Avenue
Baltimore, MD 21201

410-230-2424
Fax: 410-333-2095
TTY: 800-934-2541
TDD: 410-333-8679
e-mail: recept@lbta.lib.md.us
www.lbph.lib.md.us

Summer reading programs, Braille writer, magnifiers, large-print photocopier, cassette books and magazines, children's books on cassette, and other reference materials on blindness and other handicaps.

Jill Lewis, Manager

6163 Prince George's County Memorial Library Talking Book Center
6532 Adelphi Road
Hyattsville, MD 20782

301-699-3500

Summer reading programs, Braille writer, magnifiers, closed-circuit TV, large-print photocopier, cassette books and magazines, children's books on cassette, home visits and other reference materials on blindness and other handicaps.

Shirley Tuthill, Librarian

Massachusetts

6164 Braille and Talking Book Library Perkins School for the Blind
175 N Beacon Street
Watertown, MA 02472

617-924-3434
Fax: 617-972-7315
e-mail: info@perkins.org
www.perkins.org

C. Richard Carlson, Chairman
Leslie Nordin, Vice Chairman
Michael Schnitman, Secretary

6165 Carroll Center for the Blind
770 Centre Street
Newton, MA 02458

617-969-6200
800-852-3131
Fax: 617-969-6204
www.carroll.org

Assists blind and visually impaired adults and adolescents to adjust to loss of vision. The goal of this dynamic program is to help the person become more independent, to restore self-confidence, prepare for employment and improve the quality of life. Programs of individual counseling are offered as part of the program.

Rachel Rosenbaum, President

Michigan

6166 Downtown Detroit Subregional Library for the Blind and Handicapped
5201 Woodward Avenue
Detroit, MI 48202

313-481-1300
Fax: 313-965-1977
TDD: 313-224-0584
e-mail: deveans@cms.xx.wayne.edu
www.detroit.lib.mi.us

Summer reading programs, Braille writer, magnifiers, closed-circuit TV, large-print photocopier, cassette books and magazines, children's books on cassette, home visits and other reference materials on blindness and other handicaps.

Russell Bellant, President
Gregory Hicks, vice President
Jonathan C. Kinloch, Secretary

6167 Kent County Library for the Blind
775 Ball Avenue NE
Grand Rapids, MI 49503

616-336-3250
Fax: 616-336-3201
e-mail: kdlem@lakeland.lib.mi.us

Summer reading programs, Braille writer, magnifiers, closed-circuit TV, large-print photocopier, cassette books and magazines, children's books on cassette, home visits and other reference materials on blindness and other handicaps.

Claudya Muller, Librarian

6168 Library of Michigan Service for the Blind
PO Box 30007
Lansing, MI 48909

517-373-5614
Fax: 517-373-5865
e-mail: BTBL@michigan.gov

Summer reading programs, Braille writer, magnifiers, closed-circuit TV, large-print photocopier, cassette books and magazines, children's books on cassette, home visits and other reference materials on blindness and other handicaps.

Nancy Robertson, Manager

6169 Macomb Library for the Blind and Physically Handicapped
16480 Hall Road
Clinton Township, MI 48038

586-286-1580
Fax: 586-286-0634
TDD: 810-869-40
e-mail: macbld@libcoop.net
www.macomb.lib.mi.us/macspe/

Summer reading programs, Braille writer, closed-circuit TV, cassette books and magazines, children's books on cassette, reference materials on blindness and other handicaps.

Beverlee Babcock, Executive Director

6170 Mideastern Michigan Library Co-op
503 S Saginaw Street Suite 711
Flint, MI 48502

810-232-7119
Fax: 810-232-6639
e-mail: cnash@genesse.freeret.org
www.fakon.edu/gdl/talking.htm

Summer reading programs, Braille writer, magnifiers, closed-circuit TV, large-print photocopier, cassette books and magazines, children's books on cassette, home visits and other reference materials on blindness and other handicaps.

Carolyn Nash, Librarian

6171 Muskegon County Library for the Blind
4845 Airline Road
Muskegon, MI 49444

231-737-6310
Fax: 231-724-6675
TDD: 231-722-4103
www.muskcolib.org

Summer reading programs, Braille typewriter, magnifiers, closed-circuit TV, large-print photocopier, cassette books and magazines, children's books on cassette, home visits and other reference materials on blindness and other handicaps, The Reading Edge, Perkins Braille and large print books.

Linda Clapp, Librarian

6172   Upper Peninsula Library for the Blind Physically Handicapped
1615 Presque Isle Avenue
Marquette, MI 49855   906-228-7697
                                               Fax: 906-228-5627
                                   e-mail: rruff@uproc.lib.mi.us
                                     www.upesc.lib.mi.us/uplbph

Summer reading programs, Braille writer, magnifiers, closed-circuit TV, large-print photocopier, cassette books and magazines, children's books on cassette, home visits and other reference materials on blindness and other handicaps.

Suzanne Dees, Executive Director

6173   Washtenaw County Library
PO Box 8645
Ann Arbor, MI 48107   734-222-6850
                                               Fax: 734-222-6715
                                  e-mail: mcdaniev@ewashtenaw.org
                                              www.ewashtenaw.org

Summer reading programs, Braille writer, magnifiers, closed-circuit TV, large-print photocopier, cassette books and magazines, children's books on cassette, home visits and other reference materials on blindness and other handicaps.

Verna J. Mcdaniel, Administrator

6174   Washtenaw County Library for the Blind and Physically Disabled
PO Box 8645
Ann Arbor, MI 48107   734-222-6850
                                               Fax: 734-222-6715
                                  e-mail: mcdaniev@ewashtenaw.org
                                              www.ewashtenaw.org

Book lovers club. adaptive technology, cassette equipment, cassette books and magazines, described videos, low vision aids reference and referral services.

Verna J. Mcdaniel, Administrator

6175   Wayne County Regional Library for the Blind
30555 Michigan Avenue
Westland, MI 48186   734-727-7300
                                                    888-968-2737
                                               Fax: 734-727-7333
                                               TTY: 734-727-7330
                                   e-mail: werlbph@tln.lib.mi.us
                                     www.wayneregional.lib.mi.us

Summer reading programs, Braille writer, magnifiers, closed-circuit TV, large-print photocopier, cassette books and magazines, children's books on cassette, home visits and other reference materials on blindness and other handicaps.

Reginald Williams, Wayne County Librarian

Minnesota

6176   Minnesota Library for the Blind & Physically Handicapped
Highway 298, PO Box 68
Fairbault, MN 55021   507-333-4828
                                                    800-722-0550
                                               Fax: 507-333-4832
                                     e-mail: libblnd@state.mn.us

Summer reading programs, Braille writer, magnifiers, closed-circuit TV, large-print photocopier, cassette, large print, Braille books and magazines, children's books on cassette, and other reference materials on blindness and other handicaps.

Catherine A Durivage, Program Director

Missouri

6177   Adriene Resource Center for Blind Children
1445 Boonville Avenue
Springfield, MO 65802   417-831-8000
                                                    800-641-4310
                                               Fax: 800-328-0294
                                         e-mail: blind@ag.org
                                      www.gospelpublishing.com

Offers Braille and cassette lending library, Braille and cassette Sunday school materials for all ages, Braille and cassette periodicals and resource assistance, and resources for blind children and children of blind parents.

Paul Weingariner, Director

6178   Assemblies of God National Center for the Blind
1445 Boonville Avenue
Springfield, MO 65802   417-831-8001
                                                    800-641-4311
                                               Fax: 800-328-0295
                                         e-mail: blind@ag.org
                                      www.gospelpublishing.com

Offers Braille and cassette lending library, Braille and cassette Sunday school materials for all ages, Braille and cassette periodicals and resource assistance, and resources for blind children and children of blind parents.

Thomas Trask, Manager

6179   Wolfner Memorial Library for the Blind
PO Box 387
Jefferson City, MO 65102   573-751-8720
                                               Fax: 573-526-2985
                                               TDD: 800-347-1379
                                   e-mail: wolfner@sos.mo.gov

Summer reading programs, Braille writer, magnifiers, closed-circuit TV, large-print photocopier, cassette books and magazines, children's books on cassette, home visits and other reference materials on blindness and other handicaps.

Richard J Smith, Executive Director

Nebraska

6180   Nebraska Library Commission Talking Book & Braille Services
1200 N Street
Lincoln, NE 68508   402-471-2045
                                                    800-307-2665
                                               Fax: 402-471-2083
                                               TDD: 402-471-4038
                                   e-mail: doertli@nlc.state.ne.us
                                       www.nlc.state.ne.us

Free loan of books and magazines on cassette and in Braille, including children's materials, along with specially designed playback equipment. Summer reading program for children, Braille embossing, closed circuit TV, large-print copier. Reference materials on blindness and other disabilities.

David Oerti, Librarian

New Jersey

6181   New Jersey State Library Talking Book and Braille Center
185 West State Street
Trenton, NJ 08625   609-278-2640
                                                    800-792-8322
                                               Fax: 609-278-2647
                                               TDD: 877-882-5593
                                   e-mail: njlbh@njstatelib.org
                                              www.njstatelib.org

Free home delivery of large-print, audio, and Braille books and magazines, children's books on cassettes in Braille and other reference materials on blindness and other handicaps. Services are for New Jersey residents with print disabilities.

Adanrah Szczepaniak, Director
Anne McArthur, Head of Outreach and Audiovision

New Mexico

6182   New Mexico State Library for the Blind and Physically Handicapped
1209 Camino Carlos Ray
Santa Fe, NM 87507   505-476-9700
                                               Fax: 505-476-9761
                                   e-mail: jbrewstr@stlib.state.nm.us
                                       www.stlib.state.nm.us

Summer reading programs, Braille writer, magnifiers, closed-circuit TV, large-print photocopier, cassette books and magazines, children's books on cassette, home visits and other reference materials on blindness and other handicaps.

Susan Overland, Manager

New York

6183 New York State Talking Book & Braille Library
Empire State Plaza, CEC
Albany, NY 12230
518-474-5935
Fax: 518-486-1957
TDD: 518-474-7121
e-mail: tbbl@mail.nysed.gov
www.suffolk.lib.ny.us

Books on audio cassette, cassette players, Braille books, summer reading programs, Braille writer, magnifiers, closed-circuit TV, large-print photocopier, cassette books and magazines, children's books on cassette, reference materials on blindness and other handicaps.

Jane Somers, Director

North Carolina

6184 North Carolina Library for the Blind
1841 Capital Boulevard
Raleigh, NC 27635
919-733-4376
Fax: 919-733-6910
TDD: 919-733-1462
e-mail: nclbph@ncder.gov

Summer reading programs, Braille writer, magnifiers, closed-circuit TV, large-print photocopier, cassette books and magazines, children's books on cassette, home visits and other reference materials on blindness and other handicaps.

Francine Martin, Manager

Ohio

6185 American Council of Blind Parents
34400 Cedar Road, Apartment 108
University Heights, OH 44121
800-424-8666

Members are sighted parents of blind or visually impaired children. Offers a forum for support and outreach, sharing of experiences in parent-child relationships, and educational and cultural information about child development. Monitors developments in technical and legislative arenas.

Nola Webb, President

Oregon

6186 Oregon State Library, Talking Book and Braille Services
250 Winter Street NW
Salem, OR 97310
503-378-3849
Fax: 503-585-8059
TDD: 503-378-4276
e-mail: tbabs@sparkie.osl.state.or.us
www.tbabs.org

Cassette books and magazines, children's books on cassette, home visits and other reference materials on blindness and other handicaps.

Susan Westin, Manager

Virginia

6187 Alexandria Library Talking Book Service
5005 Duke Street
Alexandria, VA 22304
703-746-1760
Fax: 703-519-5916
TDD: 703-838-4568
e-mail: emccaffr@lea.eda
www.alexandria.lib.va.us

Summer reading programs, Braille writer, magnifiers, closed-circuit TV, large-print photocopier, cassette books and magazines, children's books on cassette, home visits and other reference materials on blindness and other handicaps.

Karen Russell, Manager

6188 Division for the Visually Handicapped
1920 Association Drive
Reston, VA 20191
703-620-3660

Members are teachers, college faculty members, administrators, supervisors and others concerned with the education and welfare of visually handicapped and blind children and youth. This is a division of the Council For Exceptional Children.

Dr. Kay Ferrell, President

6189 Division on Visual Impairments
Council for Exceptional Children
1110 North Glebe Road, Suite 300
Arlington, VA 22201
800-224-6830
Fax: 703-264-9494
TTY: 866-915-5000
www.ed.arizona.edu/dvi/welcome.htm; www.cec.sped.org

A division within the CEC, it handles concerns for Federal, state and local issues and policies related to education of youths, children and infants with visual impairments.

Ellyn Ross, President
Shirley J Wilson, Secretary
Phyllis T Simmons, President Elect

6190 Virginia State Library for the Visually and Physically Handicapped
1901 Roane Street
Richmond, VA 23222
804-367-0014

Summer reading programs, Braille writer, magnifiers, closed-circuit TV, large-print photocopier, cassette books and magazines, children's books on cassette, home visits and other reference materials on blindness and other handicaps.

Mary Ruth Halapatz, Librarian

Washington

6191 Washington Library for the Blind and Physically Handicapped
1000 Fourth Ave.
Seattle, WA 98104
206-386-4636
Fax: 206-386-4685
e-mail: wtbbl@spl.lib.wa.us
www.spl.lib.wa.us

Summer reading programs, Braille writer, magnifiers, closed-circuit TV, large-print photocopier, cassette books and magazines, children's books on cassette, home visits and other reference materials on blindness and other handicaps.

Marcellus Turner, Librarian

West Virginia

6192 West Virginia School for the Blind
301 E Main Street
Romney, WV 26757
304-822-4801
Fax: 304-822-3370
e-mail: cjohn@access.mountain.net

Summer reading programs, Braille writer, magnifiers, closed-circuit TV, large-print photocopier, cassette books and magazines, children's books on cassette, home visits and other reference materials on blindness and other handicaps.

Patsy Shank, Administrator

Research Centers

6193 Arlene R Gordon Research Institute
Lighthouse International
111 E 59th Street
New York, NY 10022   212-821-9525
                                            800-829-0500
                                        Fax: 212-821-9707
                                        TTY: 212-821-9713
                              e-mail: research@lighthouse.org
                                          www.lighthouse.org

The institute is the only research institute within a vision rehabilitation agency. Trainees can come and acquire research skills in both laboratory and field settings. It is comprised on these major divisions: Evaluation research; Vision research; and Psychosocial research.

Amy Horowitz, Director
Joann P Reinhardt PhD, Director Psychosocial Research

6194 Center for the Partially Sighted
6101 W Centinela Ave, Suite 150
Los Angeles, CA 90230   310-988-1970
                                        Fax: 310-988-1980
                             e-mail: info@low-vision.org
                                          www.low-vision.org

Provides professional, comprehensive vision rehabilitation services to visually impaired people of all ages. For those whose sight is severely limited due to macular degeneration, diabetic retinopathy, glaucoma, retinal detachment, stroke or other conditions not correctable medically or surgically.

La Donna Ringering, Executive Director
Herbert Ruderman, Psychiatrist
Marc Gerberick, IT Manager

6195 Mobile Association for the Blind
2440 Gordon Smith Drive
Mobile, AL 36617   251-473-3585
                                            877-292-5463
                                        Fax: 251-470-8622
                              e-mail: sales@mobile.blind.com

Offers work adjustment training, activities of daily living, mobility, communication skills and sheltered employment for adults and children who are visually impaired.

Jim Bullock, Executive Director

6196 New Beginnings - The Blind Children's Center
4120 Marathon Street
Los Angeles, CA 90029   323-664-2153

The purpose of the Center is to turn initial fears into hope. Helps children and their families become independent by creating a climate of safety and trust. Children learn to develop self confidence and to master a wide range of skills. Services include an infant stimulation program, educational preschool, interdisciplinary assessment services, family services, correspondence program, toll free national hotline and a publication and research service.

6197 Research to Prevent Blindness
645 Madison Avenue
New York, NY 10022   212-752-4333
                                            800-621-0026
                                        Fax: 212-688-6231
                                          www.rpbusa.org

Provides research grants to scientists interested in eye disease and vision disorders.

Diane Swift, President

Audio Video

6198 Heart to Heart
Blind Children's Center
4120 Marathon Street
Los Angeles, CA 90029   323-644-2153
                                        Fax: 323-665-3828
                                          www.blindcntr.org

Parents of blind and partially sighted children talk about their feelings.

Videotape

6199 Let's Eat
Blind Children's Center
4120 Marathon Street
Los Angeles, CA 90029   213-664-2153
                                        Fax: 213-665-3828

Teaches competent feeding skills to children with visual impairments.

Videotape

6200 See What I Feel
Britannica Film Co.
345 4th Street
San Francisco, CA 94107   415-597-5555

A blind child tells her friends about her trip to the zoo. Each experience was explained as a blind child would experience it. A teacher's guide comes with this video.

Films

Web Sites

6201 Lighthouse International
111 E 59th St
New York, NY 10022   800-284-4422
                                          www.lighthouse.org

The mission is to overcome vision impairment for people of all ages through worldwide leadership in rehabilitation services, education, research, prevention and advocacy.

6202 National Alliance of Blind Students
nabslink.org

The leading national advocacy and consumer organization for students in high school or college who are blind or visually impaired.

Sean Whalen, President
Karen Anderson, Vice President
Gabe Cazares, Vice President

6203 National Association for Visually Handicapped
111 E 59th St
New York, NY 10022   800-284-4422
                                          lighthouse.org/navh

Helps to cope with the difficulties of vision impairment.

Book Publishers

6204 Children with Visual Impairments: A Parents' Guide
Peytral Publications
PO Box 1162
Minnetonka, MN 55345   952-949-8707
                                            877-739-8725
                                        Fax: 952-906-9777
                              e-mail: help@peytral.com
                                          www.peytral.com

Covers visual impairments ranging from low vision to total blindness. Offers authoritative information and empathy, parental insight on diagnosis and treatment, orientation and mobility, literacy, legal issues and more. Valuable to parents, educators and support staff.

395 pages

M Cay Holbrook PhD, Editor

6205 Mainstreaming the Visually Impaired Child: Blind & Partially Sighted Students
Michael D Oralnsky PhD, author

Nat'l Assn for Parents of Children with Visual
PO Box 317
Watertown, MA 02471

617-972-7441
800-562-6265
Fax: 617-972-7444
www.spedex.com/napvi

121 pages

6206 Ophthalmic Disorders Sourcebook
Omnigraphics
615 Griswold
Detroit, MI 48226

313-961-1340
800-234-1340
Fax: 800-875-1340
e-mail: info@omnigraphics.com
www.omnigraphics.com

Basic consumer information about glaucoma, cataracts, macular degeneration, strabismus, refractive disorders and more.

1996 631 pages
ISBN: 0-780800-81-8

Magazines

6207 Journal of Visual Impairment and Blindness
American Foundation for the Blind
2 Penn Plaza, Suite 1102
New York, NY 10121

212-502-7600
Fax: 212-502-7777
e-mail: afbinfo@afb.net
www.afb.org

Published in braille, regular print and on cassette this journal contains a wide variety of subjects including rehabilitation, psychology, education, legislation, medicine, technology, employment, sensory aids and childhood development as they relate to visual impairments.

10x Year

Carl R. Augusto, President & CEO
Kelly Bleach, Chief Administrative Officer
Rick Bozeman, Chief Financial Officer

6208 NAVH UPDATE
National Association for Visually Handicapped
111 E 59th St
New York, NY 10022

800-284-4422
Fax: 212-727-2931
e-mail: navh@navh.org
lighthouse.org/navh

Free, large-print newsletter providing information about vision as well as general information to the partially sighted.

quarterly

6209 Reaching, Crawling, Walking - Let's Get Moving
Blind Children's Center
4120 Marathon Street
Los Angeles, CA 90029

323-664-2153
Fax: 323-665-3828
e-mail: info@blindchildrenscenter.org
www.blindchildrenscenter.org

Orientation and mobility for visually impaired preschool children.

24 pages

6210 Tactic
Clovernook Home and School for the Blind
7000 Hamilton Avenue
Cincinnati, OH 45231

513-522-3860
Fax: 513-728-3950
e-mail: clovernook@aol.com

Quarterly

Newsletters

6211 Awareness
Nat'l Assn for Parents of Children with Visual
PO Box 317
Watertown, MA 2471

617-972-7441
800-562-6265
Fax: 617-972-7444
www.spedex.com/napvi/awareness.html

Contains NAPVI regional news, commentary, letters to the editor, legislative updates, and information on conferences and events.

32 pages Quarterly

6212 National Library Service for the Blind & Physically Handicapped
Library of Congress Reference Section
1291 Taylor Street NW
Washington, DC 20542

202-707-5100
800-424-8567
Fax: 202-707-0712
TTY: 202-707-0744
TDD: 202-707-0744
e-mail: nls@loc.gov
www.loc.gov/nls

Provides information and advocacy resources for families and professionals, including listings of organizations focusing on more specific areas of concern to families and young adults who have disabilities. Administers a natural library service that provides recorded and braille reading materials to eligible children and adults who cannot read standard print.

12 pages Quarterly
ISSN: 1046-1663

Vicki Fitzpatrick, Editor

6213 Talking Book Topics
National Library Services for the Blind
1291 Taylor Street NW
Washington, DC 20542

202-707-5100
Fax: 202-707-0712
e-mail: nls@loc.gov
www.loc.gov/nls

Offers hundreds of listings of books, fiction and nonfiction, for adults and children on cassette. Also offers listings on foreign language books on cassette, talking magazines and reviews.

Bimonthly

Pamphlets

6214 Dancing Cheek to Cheek
Blind Children's Center
4120 Marathon Street
Los Angeles, CA 90029

213-664-2153
Fax: 213-665-3828
www.blindchildrenscenter.org

Discusses beginning social, play and language interactions.

33 pages

6215 Family Guide - Growth and Development of the Partially Seeing Child
National Association for Visually Handicapped
111 E 59th St
New York, NY 10022

800-284-4422
Fax: 888-305-9511
e-mail: info@navh.org
lighthouse.org/navh

Offers information for parents and guidelines in raising a partially seeing child.

6216 Family Guide to Vision Care
American Optometric Association
243 N Lindbergh Boulevard
Saint Louis, MO 63141
314-991-4100
Fax: 314-991-4101
www.aoanet.org

Offers information on the early developmental years of your vision, finding a family optometrist and how to take care of your eyesight through the learning years, the working years and the mature years.

6217 Heart to Heart
Blind Children's Center
4120 Marathon Street
Los Angeles, CA 90029
213-664-2153
Fax: 213-665-3828
www.blindchildrenscenter.org

Parents of blind and partially sighted children talk about their feelings.

12 pages

6218 Learning to Play
Blind Children's Center
4120 Marathon Street
Los Angeles, CA 90029
213-664-2153
Fax: 213-665-3828
www.blindchildrenscenter.org

Discusses how to present play activities to the visually impaired preschool child.

12 pages

6219 Let's Eat
Blind Children's Center
4120 Marathon Street
Los Angeles, CA 90029
213-664-2153
Fax: 213-665-3828
www.blindchildrenscenter.org

Teaches competent feeding skills to children with visual impairments.

28 pages

6220 Move with Me
Blind Children's Center
4120 Marathon Street
Los Angeles, CA 90029
213-664-2153
Fax: 213-665-3828
www.blindchildrenscenter.org

A parent's guide to movement development for visually impaired babies.

12 pages

6221 Selecting a Program
Blind Children's Center
4120 Marathon Street
Los Angeles, CA 90029
213-664-2153
Fax: 213-665-3828
www.blindchildrenscenter.org

A guide for parents of infants and preschoolers with visual impairments.

28 pages

6222 Standing on My Own Two Feet
Blind Children's Center
4120 Marathon Street
Los Angeles, CA 90029
323-664-2153
Fax: 323-665-3828
e-mail: info@blindchildrenscenter.org
www.blindchildrenscenter.org

A step-by-step guide to designing and constructing simple, individually tailored adaptive mobility devices for preschool-age children who are visually impaired.

36 pages

6223 Talk to Me
Blind Children's Center
4120 Marathon Street
Los Angeles, CA 90029
213-664-2153
Fax: 213-665-3828
www.blindchildrenscenter.org

A language guide for parents of deaf children.

11 pages

6224 Talk to Me II
Blind Children's Center
4120 Marathon Street
Los Angeles, CA 90029
213-664-2153
Fax: 213-665-3828
www.blindchildrenscenter.org

A sequel to Talk To Me, available in English and Spanish.

15 pages

Camps

6225 Bloomfield
5300 Angeles Vista Boulevard
Los Angeles, CA 90043
323-295-4555
800-352-2290
Fax: 323-296-0424
e-mail: info@juniorblind.org
www.junoirblind.org

This camp is dedicated to serving blind and developmentally disabled children and adults.

6226 Florida School-Deaf and Blind Summer Camp
207 San Marco Avenue
Saint Augustine, FL 32084
904-827-2200
800-800-344
e-mail: info@fsdb.k12.fl.us
www.fsdb.k12.fl.us

The Florida School for the Deaf and the Blind hosts summer campers from all over teh state of Florida for a week of fun and adventure. FSDB's 80 acre campus is where campers participate in a variety of activities including rock climbing, archery, swimming, kayaking, team games, arts and crafts, dance music, and much more.

L Daniel Hutto, President
Cindy Day, Executive Director of Parent Svcs
Terri Wiseman, Administrator of Business Services

6227 National Camps for Blind Children
Christian Record
4444 S 52nd Street
Lincoln, NE 68516
402-488-0981
Fax: 402-488-7582
e-mail: info@christianrecord.org
www.christianrecord.org

Camps throughout the US and Canada are offered at no cost to the legally blind, ages 9-65. Activities include archery, beeper basketball, water sports, hiking and rock climbing and horseback riding.

Dan Jackson, Chair
Tom Lemon, Vice Chair
Larry Pitcher, Secretary

6228 VISIONS/Vacation Camp for the Blind
500 Greenwich Street, 3rd Floor
New York, NY 10013
212-625-1616; 888-245-8333
Fax: 212-219-4078
e-mail: info@visionsvcb.org
www.visionvcb.org

Family programs at Vacation Camp for the Blind in Rockland County, NY for children who are blind, severely visually impaired or multi-handicapped. Parent or guardian must attend winter weekends and summer session.

Nancy T. Jones, President
Richard P. Simon, Vice President
Burton M. Strauss, Treasurer

Description

6229 RESPIRATORY DISTRESS SYNDROME OF THE NEWBORN

Synonyms: Hyaline membrane disese (HMD), RDS

Covers these related disorders: Meconium aspiration syndrome

Involves the following Biologic System(s):

Neonatal and Infant Disorders, Respiratory Disorders

Respiratory distress syndrome of the newborn (RDS) is a breathing disorder characterized by insufficient production of surfactant, which consists of substances produced by certain cells in the lungs. Surfactant contributes to the elasticity of lung (pulmonary) tissue and enables the air sacs (alveoli) of the lungs to remain open between breaths. The exchange of oxygen and carbon dioxide takes place across the thin walls of the air sacs. Due to insufficient surfactant in newborns with RDS, greater pressure is required to expand the lungs' airways and air sacs. As a result, the air sacs may collapse and the lungs may become unable to properly provide oxygenated blood to the body.

Surfactant is produced as the lungs mature during fetal development. Sufficient levels of surfactant are often present after approximately 35 weeks of pregnancy (gestation). RDS primarily occurs in newborns who are born prior to 37 weeks of gestation (premature newborns), affecting up to 80 percent of those who are born before 28 weeks' gestation and up to 30 percent of infants born between 32 and 36 weeks' gestation. The condition also occurs with increased frequency in infants who are born to mothers with diabetes or those who are delivered by Cesarean section. In other newborns, RDS may occur in the absence of known predisposing factors or may be due to certain birth defects or other conditions, such as meconium aspiration syndrome.rome, or persistent fetal circulation. Respiratory distress syndrome of the newborn is sometimes referred to as hyaline membrane disease, because insufficient surfactant production may cause the formation of a fibrous membrane known as hyaline membrane lining the lungs' small airways (bronchioles), ducts (alveolar ducts), and air sacs (alveoli).

Symptoms associated with RDS usually occur within minutes of birth, although they may not be recognized for several hours. These symptoms may vary in severity, depending upon the degree of prematurity or other underlying causes responsible for the condition. Newborns may experience increasing difficulty breathing (dyspnea), characterized by rapid, labored, shallow breaths (tachypnea); grunting upon exhalation; drawing in of the chest wall during inhalation; and bluish discoloration of the skin and mucous membranes (cyanosis) due to lack of sufficient oxygen supply to bodily tissues (hypoxia). Air may leak into the chest cavity surrounding the lungs (pneumothorax), causing collapse of the lungs and further breathing difficulties. Without appropriate treatment, cyanosis and breathing difficulties may progressively worsen and body temperature and blood pressure may fall. As infants with severe RDS tire, grunting upon exhalation may subside, breathing becomes irregular, and life-threatening complications may result. Depending upon the severity of the condition, infants with RDS may begin to gradually improve in about three days or may experience life-threatening symptoms within approximately two to seven days after birth.

Meconium aspiration syndrome is characterized by blockage and irritation of the airways of the lungs due to passage of meconium before birth and inhalation of meconium before or during delivery. Meconium is the thick, sticky material that forms a newborn's first stools, and is typically passed during the first 24 to 48 hours after birth. In some cases, a fetus may pass meconium into the amniotic fluid before birth and then inhale this into the lungs before or right after birth. The skin of newborns with meconium aspiration is usually stained with meconium. In severe cases, symptoms include diminished muscle tone, an abnormally slow heartbeat, or absence of spontaneous respiration at birth.

In newborns with meconium aspiration syndrome, treatment may include immediate suctioning of an affected infant's mouth, throuat, and nose and placement of a tube into the windpipe to remove meconium from the airways. In most affected newborns, imporvement usually occurs in approximately three days.

If physicians suspect that a newborn may be born prematurely, steps may be taken to delay delivery in order to help decrease the risk of RDS. If delivery cannot be delayed, some women may be given certain corticosteroid medications (e.g., dexamethasone or betamethasone) approximately 48 to 72 hours before the delivery of premature newborns to help stimulate the production of surfactant before birth. In addition, an artificial surfactant may be administered into the windpipe of affected newborns immediately after birth or within 24 hours, to help reduce the severity of RDS and associated symptoms or complications. Additional treatment may include symptomatic and supportive measures, such as use of an oxygen hood or support with a ventilator.

Government Agencies

6230 NIH/National Heart, Lung and Blood Institu te
National Institute of Health
31 Center Dr, Bldg 31 Rm 5A48
Bethesda, MD 20892

301-496-3245
Fax: 301-629-3246
TTY: 240-629-3255
e-mail: NHLBIinfo@nhlbi.nih.gov
www.nhlbi.nih.gov

Primary responsibility of this organization is the scientific investigation of heart, blood vessel, lung and blood disorders. Oversees research, demonstration, prevention, education, control and training activities in these fields and emphasizes the prevention and control of heart diseases.

Elizabeth G Nabel, MD, Director
Susan Shurin, MD, Deputy Director
Sheila Pohl, Chief of Staff

6231 NIH/National Institute of Child Health and Human Development
31 Center Drive, Building 31
Bethesda, MD 20892

301-496-1333
Fax: 301-496-1104
www.nichd.nih.gov

Established in 1962 by congress, today the institute conducts and supports research on topics related to the health of children, adults, families and populations. Some of these topics include: developmental disabilities, growth and development, infant death, reproductive health and birth defects.

Jay H Hoofnagle, Director
Lisa Kaeser, Program & Public Liaison

National Associations & Support Groups

6232 American Academy of Pediatrics
141 Northwest Point Boulevard
Elk Grove Village, IL 60007

847-434-4000
800-433-9016
Fax: 847-434-8000
www.aap.org

The American Academy of Pediatrics and its member pediatricians are committed to the attainment of optimal physical, mental and social health and well-being for all infants, children, adolescents, and young adults.

Sandra Hassink, MD, FAAP, President

6233 American Lung Association
61 Broadway, 6th Floor
New York, NY 10006

646-756-8100
800-586-4872
www.lungusa.org

The American Lung Association fights lung disease in all its forms, with special emphasis on asthma, tobacco control and environmental health. The American Lung Association is funded with contributions from the public, along with gifts and grants from corporations, foundations and government agencies. The association achieves its many successes through the work of thousands of committed volunteers and staff.

Hallema Sharif Clyburn, Director Media Relations

6234 Genetic Alliance
4301 Connecticut Avenue NW
Washington, DC 20008

202-966-5557
800-336-4363
Fax: 202-966-8553
e-mail: info@geneticalliance.org
www.geneticalliance.org

A coalition of voluntary genetic support groups, consumers and professionals addressing the needs of individuals and families affected by genetic disorders from a national perspective.

Sharon Terry, President

6235 March of Dimes Birth Defects Foundation
1275 Mamaroneck Avenue
White Plains, NY 10605

914-997-4488
888-663-4637
Fax: 914-428-8203
e-mail: answers@marchofdimes.com
www.marchofdimes.com

Partnership of volunteers and professionals dedicates to improving the health of babies by preventing birth defects and infant mortality. Over 100 chapters are located across the country and can be located through the National Office.

Jennifer L Howse, President

Web Sites

6236 American Lung Association
55 W. Wacker Drive, Suite 1150
Chicago, IL 60601

Fax: 202-452-1805
www.lung.org

The American Lung Association fights lung disease in all its forms, with special emphasis on asthma, tobacco control and environmental health.

Kathryn A. Forbes, Chair
John F. Emanuel, Vice Chair
Harold Wimmer, President/ CEO

6237 KidsHealth
www.kidshealth.org

KidsHealth provides doctor-approved health information about children from before birth through adolescence.

Neil Izenberg, MD, Editor-in-Chief & Founder

6238 RSV Info Center
www.rsvinfo.com

A comprehensive overview about the most common cause of lower respiratory tract infections in children.

Description

6239 RESPIRATORY SYNCYTIAL VIRUS INFECTION

Synonym: RSV infection

Involves the following Biologic System(s):

Infectious Disorders, Respiratory Disorders

The respiratory syncytial virus (RSV) is the most common cause of lower respiratory tract infections in infants and young children. RSV is primarily spread by the inhalation of virus-containing airborne droplets. The virus is present worldwide and causes annual epidemics of RSV infection in late autumn, winter, or as late as May or June. Such outbreaks typically peak from January through March. Nearly every child is affected by RSV infection by age two, and many experience recurrent reinfection throughout childhood.

In older children and adults, RSV infection may cause no apparent symptoms (asymptomatic) or may result in mild to moderate lung infection and associated cold-like symptoms. However, RSV infection may be severe in others, particularly infants, young children, children with heart or lung disease, or individuals with compromised immune systems. In such patients, RSV infection may lead to inflammation of the lungs' small airways (bronchiolitis), inflammation of the airways and lung tissue (bronchopneumonia), or, in extremely severe cases, potentially life-threatening complications. RSV infection is known to be the leading cause of bronchiolitis or bronchopneumonia in children younger than one year of age.

In infants and young children with RSV infection, symptoms typically begin approximately four days after infection. Initial symptoms include a runny nose (rhinorrhea) and sore throat (pharyngitis). Patients may then develop a low fever, begin to cough and sneeze, and soon experience wheezing, which is the production of a whistling sound during breathing due to inflammation and associated narrowing of the airways. If RSV infection progresses, patients may develop additional symptoms, including increasing wheezing and coughing, an abnormally rapid rate of breathing (tachypnea), drawing in of the chest wall during inhalation, and bluish discoloration of the skin and mucous membranes (cyanosis). Patients with extremely severe disease progression may develop increasingly rapid breathing, temporary cessation of breathing (apnea), listlessness, and potentially life-threatening complications. In other infants or young children with RSV infection, initial running of the nose and coughing may be followed by poor feeding, listlessness, and difficulties breathing (dyspnea) with little or no wheezing.

As mentioned above, many children experience reinfection with RSV. Reinfection usually causes less severe symptoms than those associated with initial disease. However, depending upon the age of patients and other factors, secondary infections may also sometimes be associated with severe lower respiratory tract infections. Older children who experience reinfection with RSV generally have more mild symptoms.

In children with mild or moderate RSV infection without associated bronchiolitis or bronchopneumonia, treatment typically includes symptomatic and supportive measures. Affected infants, young children, children with heart or lung disease, or those with compromised immune systems may require hospitalization. Treatment may include providing respiratory therapy with humidified air to help supply adequate oxygen to bodily tissues; ensuring an adequate intake of fluids; or administering certain medications to relax the smooth muscles of the small airways (bronchodilators). Certain infants and children are at high risk for severe RSV disease, such as those with lung disease, congenital heart disease, or immunodeficiency. In these children, certain preventive or prophylactic therapies such as RSV-specific antibodies may be recommended to help reduce (or even prevent) the severity of RSV infection in these at-risk infants and young children.

Government Agencies

6240 NIH/National Institute of Allergy and Infectious Diseases
6610 Rockledge Drive, MSC 6612
Bethesda, MD 20892

301-496-5717
866-284-4107
Fax: 301-402-3573
TDD: 800-877-8339
e-mail: ocposfoffice@niaid.nih.gov
www.niaid.nih.gov

Conducts and supports basic and applied research to better understand, treat, and ultimately prevent infectious, immunologic, and allergic diseases.

Anthony S Fauci MD, Director

6241 NIH/National Institute of Child Health and Human Development
31 Center Drive, Building 31
Bethesda, MD 20892

301-496-1333
Fax: 301-496-1104
www.nichd.nih.gov

Established in 1962 by congress, today the institute conducts and supports research on topics related to the health of children, adults, families and populations. Some of these topics include: developmental disabilities, growth and development, infant death, reproductive health and birth defects.

Jay H Hoofnagle, Director
Lisa Kaeser, Program & Public Liaison

National Associations & Support Groups

6242 American Academy of Pediatrics
141 Northwest Point Boulevard
Elk Grove Village, IL 60007

847-434-4000
800-433-9016
Fax: 847-434-8000
www.aap.org

The American Academy of Pediatrics and its member pediatricians are committed to the attainment of optimal physical, mental and social health and well-being for all infants, children, adolescents, and young adults.

Sandra Hassink, MD, FAAP, President

6243 American Lung Association
21 W 38th Street
New York, NY 10018

212-889-3370
www.lungusa.org

Founded in 1904 to fight tuberculosis, the American Lung Association today fights lung disease in all its forms, with special emphasis on asthma, tobacco control and environmental health.

Hallema Sharif Clyburn, Director Media Relations

6244 World Health Organization
Avenue Appia 20
CH-1211 Geneva 27,
Switzerland

www.who.int

WHO is the directing and coordinating authority for health within the United Nations system.

Dr Margaret Chan, Director General

Web Sites

6245 American Lung Association
55 W. Wacker Drive, Suite 1150
Chicago, IL 60601
Fax: 202-452-1805
www.lung.org

Information regarding lung disease in all its forms, with special emphasis on asthma, tobacco control and environmental health.

Kathryn A. Forbes, Chair
John F. Emanuel, Vice Chair
Harold Wimmer, President/ CEO

6246 KidsHealth
www.kidshealth.org/parent/infections/lung/rsv.html

Provides an explanation of the disorder as well as treatment and prevention.

Neil Izenberg, MD, Editor-in-Chief & Founder

6247 RSV Info Center
www.rsvinfo.com

An information center where anyone can find a comprehensive overview about the most common cause of lower respiratory tract infections in children.

Description

6248 RETINITIS PIGMENTOSA

Synonym: RP

Involves the following Biologic System(s):

Ophthalmologic Disorders

Retinitis pigmentosa (RP) refers to a group of inherited disorders in which changes occur in the light-sensitive, nerve-rich tissue membrane (retina) at the rear of the eye. This process is a slow, progressive degeneration leading to blindness. Changes in the retina include clumping (aggregation) or scattering (dispersion) of the retinal pigment, thinning or weakening of the vessels that supply the retina with oxygen-rich blood, and shrinking of the retina and the area where the optic nerve enters the retina (optic disk). Characteristic findings and symptoms of RP include difficulty in seeing at night or in dim light (night blindness; nyctalopia), a progressive reduction in the visual field with gradual loss of central vision, tunnel vision associated with loss of the peripheral visual field, and accompanying reduction of retinal function. Retinitis pigmentosa usually becomes apparent in childhood, progressing to blindness during middle age. However, the onset, severity, and rate of this progressive degeneration are widely variable.

Leber congenital retinal amaurosis (amaurosis congenita; congenital amaurosis) is a form of retinitis pigmentosa that occurs at birth or shortly thereafter and is characterized by shrinking of the optic disk (optic atrophy), thinning or weakening of the blood vessels of the retina, and widespread irregularities of retinal pigmentation. Leber congenital retinal amaurosis is transmitted as an autosomal recessive trait. In addition, retinitis pigmentosa-like degenerative changes may be associated with several metabolic, neurodegenerative, and multifold disorders.

Treatment for retinitis pigmentosa is supportive and may include the use of visual devices to enhance remaining vision. This disorder may appear as a sporadic occurrence or may be inherited, usually as an autosomal dominant disorder. There is also evidence of autosomal recessive and X-linked genetic transmission.

Government Agencies

6249 NIH/National Eye Institute
31 Center Drive MSC 2510
Bethesda, MD 20892
301-496-5248
e-mail: 2020@nei.nih.gov
www.nei.nih.gov

Conducts and supports research that helps prevent and treat eye diseases and other disorders of vision. This research leads to sight-saving treatments, reduces visual impairment and blindness, and improves the quality of life for people of all ages. NEI-supported research has advanced our knowledge of how the eye functions in health and disease.

Paul A Sieving M.D., Ph.D., Director

National Associations & Support Groups

6250 American Academy of Pediatrics
141 Northwest Point Boulevard
Elk Grove Village, IL 60007
847-434-4000
800-433-9016
Fax: 847-434-8000
www.aap.org

The American Academy of Pediatrics and its member pediatricians are committed to the attainment of optimal physical, mental and social health and well-being for all infants, children, adolescents, and young adults.

Sandra Hassink, MD, FAAP, President

6251 National Association for Visually Handicapped
22 W 21st Street, 6th Floor
New York, NY 10010
212-889-3141
888-205-5951
Fax: 212-727-2931
e-mail: navh@navh.org
www.navh.org

Serves as a clearinghouse for information about all services available to the partially-sighted from public and private sources. Conducts self-help groups. Provides information on large print books, textbooks and educational tools.

Lorianie Marchi, Ceo

6252 National Eye Health Education Program
National Eye Institute
31 Center Drive, MSC 2510
Bethesda, MD 20892
301-496-5248
Fax: 301-496-1065
www.nei.nih.gov/nehep

A program conducted by the National Eye Institute for large-scale professional and public education programs in partnership with national organizations.

Rosemary Janiszewski, Director
Karen Silver, Health Education Coordinator

6253 RP International
PO Box 900
Woodland Hills, CA 91365
818-992-0500
800-344-4877
Fax: 818-992-3265
e-mail: info@rpinternational.org
www.rpinternational.org

Dedicated to promoting and supporting research to find effective treatments and cures for retinitis pigmentosa, macular degeneration, and other degenerative diseases. Provides referrals to genetic counselors and support groups and offers a variety of educational materials including a regular newsletter and brochures.

Helen Harris, President

Research Centers

6254 UIC Eye Center
Department of Ophthalmology & Visual Sciences
1855 W Taylor Street
Chicago, IL 60612
312-996-4356
Fax: 312-996-7770
e-mail: eyeweb@uic.edu
www.uic.edu/com/eye/department

Offers help, support, information and research for persons with vision problems, including retinitis pigmentosa.

Gerald A Fishman

Web Sites

6255 British Retinitis Pigmentosa Society
PO Box 350
Buckingham, MK18
128-082-1334
Fax: 128-081-5900
e-mail: info@rpfightingblindness.org.uk
www.rpfightingblindness.org.uk

Website aims to provide a better understanding of the inherited retinal disorders. The content of this website has been written by people who have many years experience of living with RP and by very knowledgeable professionals in the field of opththalmology.

David Head, Chief Executive Officer

6256 Foundation Fighting Blindness
7168 Columbia Gateway Drive, Suite 100
Columbia, MD 21046
410-423-0600
800-683-5555
TDD: 800-683-5551
e-mail: info@FightBlindness.org
www.blindness.org

Searches for treatments and cures for macular degeneration, retinitis pigmentosa (RP), usher syndrome and the entire spectrum of retinal degenerative diseases.

William T. Schmidt, Chief Executive Officer
Stephen M. Rose, Ph.D., Chief Research Officer
Annette Hinkle, CPA, Chief Financial Officer

6257 National Association for Visually Handicapped
111 E 59th St
New York, NY 10022
800-284-4422
lighthouse.org/navh

Helps to cope with the difficulties of vision impairment.

6258 Retina South Africa - Fighting Blindness
www.rpsa.org.za/retinitis.htm

Represents retinitis pigmentosa, macular degeneration, usher syndrome and over 200 other rare conditions. Offers supports, education and counseling to affected people and their families. Self employment skills are also provided by unemployed sufferers to encourage financial independence and self esteem.

6259 Royal National Institute of the Blind
105 Judd Street
London, WC1H
303-123-9999
www.rnib.org.uk

A leading UK charity offering information, support and advice to over two million people with sight problems.

Lesley-Anne Alexander , Chief Executive
Wanda Hamilton, Group Director
Fazilet Hadi, Managing Director

6260 Texas Association of Retinitis Pigmentosa
www.geocities.com/HotSprings/7815/front.htm

Nonprofit organization based in Texas serving as a national information-sharing center to provide human services to persons with progressive vision loss from retinitis pigmentosa and other retinal degenerative disorders.

Book Publishers

6261 Children with Visual Impairments: A Parents' Guide
Peytral Publications
PO Box 1162
Minnetonka, MN 55345
952-949-8707
877-739-8725
Fax: 952-906-9777
e-mail: help@peytral.com
www.peytral.com

Covers visual impairments ranging from low vision to total blindness. Offers authoritative information and empathy, parental insight on diagnosis and treatment, orientation and mobility, literacy, legal issues and more. Valuable to parents, educators and support staff.

395 pages

M Cay Holbrook PhD, Editor

Newsletters

6262 RP Messenger
Texas Association of Retinitis Pigmentosa
PO Box 8388
Corpus Christi, TX 78468
512-852-8515
Fax: 361-852-8515
www.jwen.com/rp

A biannual newsletter offering information on retinitis pigmentosa.

Biannual

Description

6263 RETINOBLASTOMA

Involves the following Biologic System(s):

Hematologic and Oncologic Disorders, Ophthalmologic Disorders

Retinoblastoma is a malignant tumor of the nerve-rich membrane at the back of the eye known as the retina. This membrane converts light waves into nerve impulses and transmits them to the brain via the optic nerve (the second cranial nerve), resulting in vision. Retinoblastoma occurs in approximately one in 18,000 live births. In most cases, one eye is affected (unilateral). However, both eyes may be involved (bilateral) in about 30 percent of affected children. In some severe cases, the tumor may spread to other parts of the body (metastasize), particularly when there is tumor invasion of the middle layer of the eye (choroid) or the optic nerve. If tumor growth occurs along the optic nerve, the brain may be affected. However, in most children with retinoblastoma, metastasis rarely occurs before the tumor is detected.

Unilateral retinoblastoma is usually detected at approximately 21 months to two years of age, whereas bilateral retinoblastoma is typically diagnosed at about 11 to 12 months. Rarely, the tumor may be detected at birth, during later childhood or adolescence, or adulthood. In most cases, the first sign associated with retinoblastoma is the appearance of a yellowish-white mass in the pupil area (leukokoria) due to the presence of the tumor behind the lens of the eye and reflection of light off the tumor. Additional symptoms and findings often include abnormal deviation of the affected eye in relation to the other (strabismus) and impaired or absent vision. In some cases, affected children experience secondary complications, such as detachment of the retina or abnormally increased pressure of the fluid of the eye (glaucoma). Children who have more advanced retinoblastoma may also experience bleeding (hemorrhaging) within the chamber of the eye in front of the iris (hyphema), irregularities of the pupil, pain, or other symptoms. In cases of severely advanced disease or metastasis, associated findings may include protusion of the eye ball (proptosis) and abnormally increased pressure within the skull (intracranial pressure).

A gene responsible for retinoblastoma (RB gene) has been located on the long arm chromosome 13 (13q14). Many cases of unilateral retinoblastoma are thought to be due to deletions or abnormal changes (mutations) of the gene that occur randomly, for unknown reasons (sporadic). In familial cases, the exact mechanisms of inheritance are not understood. However, bilateral retinoblastoma and some cases of unilateral disease are thought to result from deletion of the gene from one chromosome and inheritance of one mutated disease gene (hemizygous state) or inheritance of two mutated RB genes (homozygous state of RB gene). Individuals with familial retinoblastoma may also have an increased risk for other malignancies. About one percent of children treated for familial retinoblastoma eventually develop a malignant bone tumor (osteosarcoma) by 10 years of age. In addition, estimates in medical literature indicate that about 30 percent of those with familial retinoblastoma are affected by a second malignancy within 30 years after their initial diagnosis.

In some rare cases, affected children may have retinoblastoma in association with an underlying chromosomal deletion syndrome (chromosome 13, monosomy 13q syndrome) that is characterized by deletion (monosomy) of a portion of chromosome 13q including the RB gene at band 13q14. Although associated symptoms and findings may vary, affected children may have characteristic abnormalities of the head and facial (craniofacial) area including a high forehead, prominent eyebrows, a rounded (bulbous) tip of the nose and broad nasal bridge, prominent earlobes, a large mouth, and a thin upper lip.

The treatment of children with retinoblastoma is directed toward preserving vision. In children with unilateral retinoblastoma, treatment typically includes surgical removal of the affected eye and a portion of the optic nerve. However, if the tumor is very small, other measures may be indicated, such as the use of radiation or extremely cold temperatures (cryotherapy) to destroy the tumor. In children with bilateral retinoblastoma, treatment is directed toward preserving useful vision in at least one eye. Therefore, initial therapy may include cryotherapy or radiotherapy of one or both eyes. Bilateral therapy may be recommended since there have been cases in which the more severely affected eye has responded more dramatically to such measures. When one eye has no remaining vision or is affected by painful complications, removal of the eye may be advised. If tumor growth has begun to extend beyond the eye, radiation therapy may also be conducted. Therapy with anticancer drugs, such as cyclophosphamide and doxorubicin, may be considered with radiation therapy. Children and adults who have been affected by familial retinoblastoma should be carefully monitored for secondary malignancies. In addition, family members of affected children should be examined by an eye specialist to detect or help rule out the presence of retinoblastoma.

Government Agencies

6264 NIH/National Cancer Institute
9609 Medical Center Drive
Bethesda, MD 20892   800-422-6237
                                      www.cancer.gov

The National Cancer Institute coordinates the National Cancer Program, which conducts and supports research, training, health information dissemination, and other programs with respect to the cause, diagnosis, prevention, and treatment of cancer, rehabilitation from cancer, and the continuing care of cancer patients and the families of cancer patients.

John E Niederhuber MD, Director

National Associations & Support Groups

6265 American Academy of Pediatrics
141 Northwest Point Boulevard
Elk Grove Village, IL 60007   847-434-4000
                                      800-433-9016
                                      Fax: 847-434-8000
                                      www.aap.org

The American Academy of Pediatrics and its member pediatricians are committed to the attainment of optimal physical, mental and social health and well-being for all infants, children, adolescents, and young adults.

Sandra Hassink, MD, FAAP, President

6266 Candlelighters Childhood Cancer Foundation
PO Box 498
Kensington, MD 20895
301-962-3520
800-366-2223
Fax: 310-962-3521
e-mail: staff@candlelighters.org
www.candlelighters.org

The Candlelighters Childhood Cancer Foundation National Office was founded in 1970 by concerned parents of children with cancer. Today our membership of over 50,000 members of the national office and more than 100,000 members across the across the country, including Candlelighters affiliate groups, includes, parents of children who are being treated or have been treated for cancer.

Ruth Hoffman, Executive Director

6267 Division on Visual Impairments
Council for Exceptional Children
1110 N Glebe Road, Suite 300
Arlington, VA 22201
800-224-6830
Fax: 703-264-9494
TTY: 866-915-5000
www.ed.arizona.edu/dvi/welcome.htm; www.cec.sped.org

A division within the CEC, it handles concerns for Federal, state and local issues and policies related to education of youths, children and infants with visual impairments.

Ellyn Ross, President
Shirley J Wilson, Secretary
Phyllis T Simmons, President Elect

6268 Genetic Alliance
4301 Connecticut Avenue NW
Washington, DC 20008
202-966-7955
800-336-4363
Fax: 202-966-8553
e-mail: info@geneticalliance.org
www.geneticalliance.org

A coalition of voluntary genetic support groups, consumers and professionals addressing the needs of individuals and families affected by genetic disorders from a national perspective.

Sharon Terry, President
Natasha Bonhomme, Vice President of Strategic Develop
Vaughn ÿEdelson, Assistant Director of Health Commun

6269 Institute for Families
4650 Sunset Blvd, MS#111
Los Angeles, CA 90027
323-669-4649
Fax: 323-665-7869
e-mail: info@instituteforfamilies.org
www.instituteforfamilies.org

A non-profit organization providing free of charge support and services to professionals and families of visually impaired children.

6270 Lighthouse International
111 E 59th Street
New York, NY 10022
212-821-9200
800-829-0500
Fax: 212-821-9707
TTY: 212-821-9713
e-mail: info@lighthouse.org
www.lighthouse.org

Provides services, information, education, resource contacts and research related to the needs of children who are visually impaired and their families.

Tara Cortes, CEO
Cynthia Stuen, Senior VP Services/Education

6271 National Alliance of Blind Students
c/o Terry Pacheco
1155 15th Street NW, Suite 1004
Washington, DC 20005
202-467-5081
800-424-8666
Fax: 202-467-5085
e-mail: rj.hodson@verizon.net
www.blindstudents.org

An advocacy and consumer organization for high school and college students who are blind or visually impaired. It works to facilitate progress toward full accessibility of college programs and facilities, provides opportunities for discussion of issues important to students and assists with National Student Seminars.

Rebecca Hodson, President

6272 National Association for Parents of Childr en with Visual Impairments
PO Box 317
Watertown, MA 02471
617-972-7441
800-562-6265
Fax: 617-972-7444
e-mail: napvi@perkins.org
www.spedex.com/napvi/

Offers emotional support for parents of blind or visually impaired children. Provides information, training and assistance, and help in understanding and using available resources.

6273 National Childhood Cancer Foundation
4600 East West Highway, Suite 600
Bethesda, MD 20814
301-718-0042
800-458-6223
Fax: 301-718-0047
e-mail: info@curesearch.org
www.curesearch.org

CureSearch unites the world's largest childhood cancer research organization, the Children's Oncology Group, and the National Childhood Cancer Foundation through our mission to cure childhood cancer. Research is the key to the cure.

Stacy Haller, Executive Director

6274 National Support & Information Network
NAPVI
PO Box 317
Watertown, MA 02471
617-972-7441
800-562-6265
www.spedex.com/napvi/network.html

Nationwide support group that provides direct support, information and referral services for parents of children with vision impairments and or multiple related disabilities.

6275 Retinoblastoma International
18030 Brookhurst Street, Box 408ÿ
Fountain Valley, CA 92708
323-669-2299
Fax: 323-660-8541
e-mail: info@retinoblastoma.net
www.retinoblastoma.net

Retinoblastoma information for parents, family and friends of retinoblastoma patients, as well as online medical education and training for health care professionals.

Christina S Ashford, President
Robin Einstein, Treasurer

State Agencies & Support Groups

Connecticut

6276 Parents Association of Connecticut Childre n with Visual Impairments (PACVI)
PO Box 455
Newtown, CT 06470
203-364-1450
www.spedex.com/napvi/chapters.html

Sabeena Ali, Co-President
Jean Loberg,, President

Florida

6277 Florida Families of Children with Visual I mpairments
Ormond Beach, FL 32174
386-677-7760
e-mail: ffcvi@yahoo.com

Sue Townsend, President

6278 Massachusetts Association for Parents of t he Visually Impaired (MAPVI)
Maynard, MA 01754   978-897-3005
e-mail: mapvi-info@viguide.com
www.mapvi.org

Anita Sullivan, President
Susan Rawlay, Regional Represenative
Chris Pine, Treasurer

6279 New England Retinoblastoma Support Group (NERSG)
Salem, NH 03079   603-893-3908
Tom Gelinas, Treasurer

Web Sites

6280 A Parent's Guide to Understanding Retinobl astoma
1275 York Avenue
New York, NY 10065   212-639-2000
800-525-2225
www.mskcc.org

Craig B. Thompson, President
John Gunn, Chief Operating Officer
Kerry Bessey, Senior Vice President

6281 Children's Cancer Web
www.cancerindex.org/ccw

An independent nonprofit site, established to provide a directory of childhood cancer resources.

6282 Life With Retinoblastoma
www.mrmegabyte.net/rb/retino.html

A support site written by the parent of a child with retinoblastoma.

6283 Online Mendelian Inheritance in Man
National Library of Medicine, Building 38A
Bethesda, MD 20894   888-346-3656
e-mail: info@ncbi.nlm.nih.gov
www.ncbi.nlm.nih.gov

This database is a catalog of human genes and genetic disorders.

6284 Retinoblastoma Solutions
1100 Bennett Road - Unit 4
Bowmanville, ON L1C 3   647-478-4902
877-624-9769
Fax: 905-697-9786
e-mail: info@impactgenetics.com
impactgenetics.com

Dedicated to advancing retinoblastoma research and making available molecular diagnostic tests to families that cannot afford it.

Franny Jewett, CEO
David McDonald, CTO
Diane Rushlow, Scientific Director

Book Publishers

6285 Children with Visual Impairments: A Parents' Guide
Peytral Publications
PO Box 1162
Minnetonka, MN 55345   952-949-8707
877-739-8725
Fax: 952-906-9777
e-mail: help@peytral.com
www.peytral.com

Covers visual impairments ranging from low vision to total blindness. Offers authoritative information and empathy, parental insight on diagnosis and treatment, orientation and mobility, literacy, legal issues and more. Valuable to parents, educators and support staff.

395 pages

M Cay Holbrook PhD, Editor

6286 Let's Talk About Going to the Hospital
Rosen Publishing Group's PowerKids Press
29 E 21st Street
New York, NY 10010   212-777-3017
800-237-9932
Fax: 888-436-4643
e-mail: rosenpub@tribeca.ios.com
www.rosenpublishing.com

If a child has to check into the hospital, chances are he or she is already upset about being ill. Knowing how a hospital functions and what the procedures are, such as when family members can visit, will help in what is already a stressful situation. Grades K-5.

24 pages
ISBN: 0-823950-36-0

Roger Rosen, President

6287 Let's Talk About When Kids Have Cancer

Melanie Apel Gordon, author

Rosen Publishing Group's PowerKids Press
29 E 21st Street
New York, NY 10010   212-777-3017
800-237-9932
Fax: 888-436-4643
e-mail: customerservice@rosenpub.com
www.rosenpublishing.com

In a straightforward yet comforting way, this book explains what cancer is, what kinds of treatments surround the disease and how to cope if a child or the friend of a child has cancer.

24 pages Paperback
ISBN: 0-823951-95-2

Roger Rosen, President

6288 My Fake Eye, The Story of My Prosthesis
Institute for Families
4650 Sunset Blvd, MS#111
Los Angeles, CA 90027   323-361-4649
Fax: 323-665-7869
e-mail: info@instituteforfamilies.org
www.instituteforfamilies.org

A full color book and comforting tool for children, siblings and parents dealing with eye enucleation. Available in Spanish.

Peggy Yoshino, Chairman
Eric Dahl, CFO
Joni Dahl, Secretary

6289 My New Eye Patch
Institute for Families
4650 Sunset Blvd, MS#111
Los Angeles, CA 90027   323-361-4650
Fax: 323-665-7870
e-mail: info@instituteforfamilies.org
www.instituteforfamilies.org

A book for describing the feelings and experiences surrounding wearing an eye patch, for children and parents. Available in Spanish.

Peggy Yoshino, Chairman
Eric Dahl, CFO
Joni Dahl, Secretary

6290 Surviving Childhood Cancer: A Guide for Families
New Harbinger Publications
5674 Shattuck Avenue
Oakland, CA 94609   510-652-0215
800-748-6273
Fax: 800-652-1613
e-mail: customerservice@newharbinger.com
www.newharbinger.com

Cancer in a child is an overwhelming experience for a family. This book explains common medical procedures and offers readers practical advice about how to cope with emotions and stress during this time.

232 pages Paperback
ISBN: 1-572241-02-0

Newsletters

6291 Awareness
NAPVI
PO Box 317
Watertown, MA 2272

617-972-7441
800-562-6265
www.spedex.com/napvi/awareness.html

Contains regional NAPVI news and announcements, legislative updates, upcoming events and conferences and articles and letters to the editor.

32 pages Quarterly

6292 DVI Quarterly
Division on Visual Impairments (CEC)
2900 Crystal Drive, Suite 1000
Arlington, VA 22202

888-232-7733
TTY: 866-915-5000
www.cec.sped.org/mb/

News on the Division of Visual Impairments, articles and announcements having to do with the education of students with visual impairmnets.

1000+ Quarterly

James P. Heiden, President
Sharon Raimondi, Treasurer
Joni L. Baldwin, Associate Professor

6293 Retinoblastoma Support News
Institute for Families
4650 Sunset Blvd, MS#111
Los Angeles, CA 90027

323-669-4649
Fax: 323-665-7869
e-mail: info@instituteforfamilies.org
www.instituteforfamilies.org

Newsletter for educational professionals and the families of children with retinoblastoma.

Quarterly

Peggy Yoshino, Chairman
Eric Dahl, Chief Financial Officer
Joni Dahl, Secretary

Pamphlets

6294 A Parent's Guide to Understanding Retinobl astoma
IRIS Medical Instruments/IRIDEX Corp
1275 York Avenue
New York, NY 10065

212-639-2000
800-525-2225
www.mskcc.org

Craig B. Thompson, President
John Gunn, Chief Operating Officer
Kerry Bessey, Senior Vice President

6295 Early Detection
Retinoblastoma International
18030 Brookhurst Street, Box 408
Fountain Valley, CA 92708

323-669-2299
Fax: 323-660-8541
e-mail: info@retinoblastoma.net
www.retinoblastoma.net

A brochure promoting the early detection and treatment of retinoblastoma.

2 pages

Description

6296 RETINOPATHY OF PREMATURITY

Synonym: ROP

Involves the following Biologic System(s):

Neonatal and Infant Disorders, Ophthalmologic Disorders

Retinopathy of prematurity (ROP) is a condition characterized by improper development of blood vessels within the retinas of both eyes. The retinas are the nerve-rich membranes at the back of the eyes that contain specialized, light-sensitive nerve cells (rods and cones). The rods and cones convert visual images into nerve impulses that are transmitted to the brain via the optic nerve (second cranial nerve). ROP primarily occurs in newborns of low birth weight who are born at less than 37 weeks after conception (premature newborns). Premature infants who weigh less than approximately three pounds, are delivered before 33 weeks of pregnancy, and develop abnormally high levels of oxygen in the blood (hyperoxia) as a result of oxygen therapy for breathing difficulties are considered to be particularly at risk for retinopathy of prematurity. Less commonly, other factors may play some role in contributing to the condition, such as heart disease, infection, abnormally low levels of circulating red blood cells (anemia), or other conditions. Generally, the lower an infant's birthweight and the greater the degree of prematurity, the higher the risk for the development of ROP.

During fetal development, the blood vessels that will supply the retinas grow from the center of the retinas, gradually extending to their outer edges shortly after birth. However, in premature newborns, the retinal blood vessels are incompletely developed, potentially causing abnormalities in subsequent retinal growth and function. In infants with ROP, associated findings may range from mild or temporary changes of the outer edges of the retina to severe abnormalities affecting the entire retina. During the active or acute stage of ROP, which typically occurs within the first month or so of life, associated findings may include abnormal narrowing of certain retinal blood vessels and subsequent widening or abnormal twisting of other retinal vessels. In addition, there is an apparent lack of blood vessel growth in certain areas of the retina, particularly of the outer rim. There may also be a gradual development of new blood vessels outside the normal area of retinal blood vessel growth, such as over the surface of the retina or into the jelly-like fluid behind the lens of the eye (vitreous humor). These vessels may tend to bleed (hemorrhage) into the retina, and some patients may develop retinal scarring as well as the formation of retinal folds or breaks or detachment of the outer portion of the retina. In severe cases, patients may undergo chronic disease progression, leading to complete retinal detachment and progressive retinal degeneration. The retina may eventually appear as an abnormal whitish membrane behind the lens of the eye (leukokoria). As the condition continues to progress, infants may develop increased fluid pressure within the eye (glaucoma), gradual degeneration and shrinkage of the eye (phthisis bulbi), and associated visual impairment leading to blindness.

In many infants with ROP, the condition spontaneously subsides and regresses. Such children may have an increased risk of progressive nearsightedness (myopia) or other eye abnormalities. However, in fewer than 10 percent, there may be ongoing disease progression, potentially causing total retinal

detachment and severe visual impairment or blindness. In fact, it is retinal detachment that is the main cause of visual impairment and blindness in ROP.

The prevention of ROP depends upon proper prenatal care and other measures to help prevent premature births. In addition, infants who are born prematurely are monitored closely to ensure prompt detection of ROP and appropriate treatment as required. In severe cases of ROP, a technique that freezes affected areas of the retina (cryotherapy) may help to reduce potentially severe complications. Laser therapy can "burn away" the periphery of the retina, which has no normal blood vessels. Both laser treatment and cryotherapy, only used in infants with advanced ROP, destroy the peripheral areas of the retina, slowing or reversing the abnormal growth of blood vessels. Unfortunately, the treatments also destroy some side vision but saves central vision. In some patients with total retinal detachment, surgical techniques may be used to help reattach the retina.

Government Agencies

6297 NIH/National Eye Institute
31 Center Drive MSC 2510
Bethesda, MD 20892
301-496-5248
e-mail: 2020@nei.nih.gov
www.nei.nih.gov

Conducts and supports research that helps prevent and treat eye diseases and other disorders of vision. This research leads to sight-saving treatments, reduces visual impairment and blindness, and improves the quality of life for people of all ages. NEI-supported research has advanced our knowledge of how the eye functions in health and disease.

Paul A Sieving M.D., Ph.D., Director

6298 NIH/National Institute of Child Health and Human Development
31 Center Drive, Building 31
Bethesda, MD 20892
301-496-1333
Fax: 301-496-1104
www.nichd.nih.gov

Established in 1962 by congress, today the institute conducts and supports research on topics related to the health of children, adults, families and populations. Some of these topics include: developmental disabilities, growth and development, infant death, reproductive health and birth defects.

Jay H Hoofnagle, Director
Lisa Kaeser, Program & Public Liaison

National Associations & Support Groups

6299 American Academy of Pediatrics
141 Northwest Point Boulevard
Elk Grove Village, IL 60007
847-434-4000
800-433-9016
Fax: 847-434-8000
www.aap.org

The American Academy of Pediatrics and its member pediatricians are committed to the attainment of optimal physical, mental and social health and well-being for all infants, children, adolescents, and young adults.

Sandra Hassink, MD, FAAP, President

6300 Association for Retinopathy of Prematurity and Related Diseases
PO Box 250425
Franklin, MI 48025
800-788-2020
e-mail: ropard@yahoo.com
www.ropard.org

Funds clinically relevant basic science and clinical research to eliminate retinopathy of prematurity and associated retinal diseases.

Susan Campbell, Administrative Director
Paula Korelitz, Outreach Director

6301 Division on Visual Impairments
Council for Exceptional Children
1110 North Glebe Road, Suite 300
Arlington, VA 22201　　　　　800-224-6830
　　　　　　　　　　　　Fax: 703-264-9494
　　　　　　　　　　　　TTY: 866-915-5000
www.ed.arizona.edu/dvi/welcome.htm; www.cec.sped.org

A division within the CEC, it handles concerns for Federal, state and local issues and policies related to education of youths, children and infants with visual impairments.

Ellyn Ross, President
Shirley J Wilson, Secretary
Phyllis T Simmons, President Elect

6302 Lighthouse International
111 E 59th Street
New York, NY 10022　　　　　212-821-9200
　　　　　　　　　　　　800-829-0500
　　　　　　　　　　　　Fax: 212-821-9707
　　　　　　　　　　　　TTY: 212-821-9713
　　　　　　　　e-mail: info@lighthouse.org
　　　　　　　　　　　　www.lighthouse.org

Provides information, services, education, resource contacts and research related to the needs of children who are visually impaired and their families.

Tara Cortes, Ceo
Cynthia Stuen, Senior VP Services/Education

6303 National Alliance of Blind Students
c/o Terry Pacheco
1155 15th Street NW, Suite 1004
Washington, DC 20005　　　　202-467-5081
　　　　　　　　　　　　800-424-8666
　　　　　　　　　　　　Fax: 202-467-5085
　　　　　　e-mail: rj.hodson@verizon.net
　　　　　　　　　www.blindstudents.org

An advocacy and consumer organization for high school and college students who are blind or visually impaired. It works to facilitate progress toward full accessibility of college programs and facilities, provides opportunities for discussion of issues important to students and assists with National Student Seminars.

Rebecca Hodson, President

6304 National Association for Parents of Childr en with Visual Impairments
PO Box 317
Watertown, MA 00247　　　　617-972-7441
　　　　　　　　　　　　800-562-6265
　　　　　　　　　　　　Fax: 617-972-7444
　　　　　　　e-mail: napvi@perkins.org
　　　　　　　　www.spedex.com/napvi/

Offers emotional support for parents of blind or visually impaired children. Provides information, training and assistance, and help in understanding and using available resources.

6305 National Association for Visually Handicapped
111 E 59th St,
New York, NY 10022　　　　　212-889-3141
　　　　　　　　　　　　800-829-0500
　　　　　　　　　　　　Fax: 212-727-2931
　　　　　　　　e-mail: navh@navh.org
　　　　　　　　　　　www.navh.org

Serves as a clearinghouse for information about all services available to the partially-sighted from public and private sources. Conducts self-help groups. Provides information on large print books, textbooks and educational tools.

Lorianie Marchi, Ceo

Audio Video

6306 Management of Retinopathy of Prematurity V ideo
ROPARD
PO Box 250425
Franklin, MI 48025　　　　　800-788-2020
　　　　　　　　e-mail: ropard@yahoo.com
　　　　　　　　　　　www.ropard.org

Information on ROP related diseases including long term treatment considerations.

Web Sites

6307 National Association for Visually Handicapped
111 E 59th St
New York, NY 10022　　　　　800-284-4422
　　　　　　　　　　　lighthouse.org/navh

Helps to cope with the difficulties of vision impairment.

Book Publishers

6308 Children with Visual Impairments: A Parents' Guide
Peytral Publications
PO Box 1162
Minnetonka, MN 55345　　　　952-949-8707
　　　　　　　　　　　　877-739-8725
　　　　　　　　　　　　Fax: 952-906-9777
　　　　　　　　e-mail: help@peytral.com
　　　　　　　　　　　www.peytral.com

Covers visual impairments ranging from low vision to total blindness. Offers authoritative information and empathy, parental insight on diagnosis and treatment, orientation and mobility, literacy, legal issues and more. Valuable to parents, educators and support staff.
395 pages
M Cay Holbrook PhD, Editor

Newsletters

6309 Sight Lines
ROPARD
PO Box 250425
Franklin, MI 48025　　　　　800-788-2020
　　　　　　　　e-mail: ropard@yahoo.com
　　　　　　　　　　　www.ropard.org

Susan Campbell, Editor

Pamphlets

6310 Looking Ahead:A Parents Guide to the Devel opment Child w/ Retinopathy Prematurity
ROPARD
PO Box 250425
Franklin, MI 48025　　　　　800-788-2020
　　　　　　　　e-mail: ropard@yahoo.com
　　　　　　　　　　　www.ropard.org

Visual stimulation activity suggestions for the development of children up to five years of age with retinopathy of prematurity.

Description

6311 RHINITIS

Synonyms: Hay Fever, Allergic Rhinitis, Non-Allergic Rhinitis

Involves the following Biologic System(s):

Immunologic and Rheumatologic Disorders, Respiratory Disorders

Rhinitis is a condition in which plant pollens, chemicals, and certain other substances irritate the membranes that line the nose, throat, sinuses, and eyelids, causing them to become swollen and inflamed, with resulting nasal stuffiness and runniness (rhinorrhea), sneezing, burning and tearing of the eyes, and soreness of the throat. It falls into two categories — allergic and non-allergic rhinitis.

Allergic rhinitis is either seasonal (tending to recur in a particular season of every year), or perennial (likely to occur or persist regardless of season). It occurs when pollens, dust, animal dander, house dust mites, and other protein substances, known collectively as allergens, prompt the body cells named plasma cells to secrete an antibody named immunoglobulin E (IgE). The IgE secreted by these cells reacts with specialized structures known as IgE receptors, which exist both on the surfaces of the cells known as mast cells, in the mucous membranes of the nose, throat, and some other parts of the body, and also on the cells known as basophils, which circulate through the body in the blood and lymphatic fluid. The reaction between IgE and its receptors on mast cells and basophils causes these cells to release histamine, a substance that triggers inflammation and swelling in surrounding tissues. The reaction of IgE with its receptors also prompts mast cells and basophils to secrete other substances, known as inflammatory mediators, that promote inflammation in various ways. Allergic rhinitis often accompanies other disorders that affect the respiratory system, eyes, or ears, such as sinusitis, asthma, and inflammation of the ear (otitis), and its effects can interfere with sleep, alertness, and schoolwork. It typically begins from childhood through early adulthood, and in most cases develops by the age of 20 years.

Non-allergic rhinitis is typically caused by smoke, fumes, cold or heat, viral and other respiratory infections, and other sources of inflammation of the nose, throat, and eyes. Moreover, although the symptoms of non-allergic rhinitis often resemble those of allergic rhinitis, it is not triggered by IgE, as is allergic rhinitis, but rather by direct irritation of mucous membranes and other tissues, by effects of cold, heat, or other factors on the nervous system, and by other mechanisms. In the condition known as non-allergic rhinitis with eosinophilia syndrome (NARES), rhinitis and other symptoms of allergy recur without being traceable to any specific allergen, and nasal secretions contain the cells known as eosinophils, which are important members of the body's immune defense system.

Although it can be difficult to distinguish allergic from non-allergic rhinitis, the distinction can be important in terms of preventing and treating these conditions. The diagnosis of allergic rhinitis is based on symptoms that recur upon exposure to seasonal pollens and other specific substances, and by tests in which exposure of a small area of skin to various allergens results in reddening or swelling. A laboratory test known as the radioallergosorbent test (RAST), in which a small sample of blood is withdrawn and IgE in the blood serum is exposed to various allergens, can also show which specific allergens are responsible for a patient's rhinitis.

Because of its more generalized nature and lack of seasonality, non-allergic rhinitis can be difficult to diagnose. Its diagnosis is usually based on its particular symptoms and on linking its occurrence to a particular chemical or other causative agent.

A first step in controlling both allergic and non-allergic rhinitis is to prevent or avoid the allergens or other substances that cause these disorders. The medicines known as antihistamines, which block the inflammatory effects of histamine in the nose, eyes, and other parts of the body, are useful in preventing or easing the symptoms of allergic rhinitis, but are much less effective for non-allergic rhinitis. Although conventional antihistamines can cause drowsiness and other undesirable effects, such effects are often less severe with newer or second-generation antihistamines, which are in some cases also useful for non-allergic rhinitis. Nasal sprays containing corticosteroid drugs are sometimes prescribed for easing nasal swelling, stuffiness, rhinorrhea, and itching in rhinitis. Nasal decongestants, which reduces swelling in the mucous membranes of the nose, may also be effective.

National Associations & Support Groups

6312 American Academy of Allergy, Asthma & Immu nology
555 E. Wells Street, Suite 1100
Milwaukee, WI 53202

414-272-6071
Fax: 414-272-6070
e-mail: mbrown@aaaai.org
www.aaaai.org

The American Academy of Allergy, Asthma & Immunology is the largest professional medical organization in the United States devoted to the allergy/immunology specialty.

Megan Brown, Communications Manager

6313 American Academy of Pediatrics
141 Northwest Point Boulevard
Elk Grove Village, IL 60007

847-434-4000
800-433-9016
Fax: 847-434-8000
www.aap.org

The American Academy of Pediatrics and its member pediatricians are committed to the attainment of optimal physical, mental and social health and well-being for all infants, children, adolescents, and young adults.

Sandra Hassink, MD, FAAP, President

6314 American College of Allergy, Asthma & Immu nology
85 West Algonquin Road, Suite 550
Arlington Heights, IL 60005

847-427-1200
Fax: 847-427-1294
e-mail: mail@acaai.org
www.acaai.org

The American College of Allergy, Asthma & Immunology is a professional association of 5,500 allergists/immunologists and allied health professionals. Established in 1942, the College is dedicated to improving the quality of patient care in allergy and immunology through research, advocacy and professional and public education.

6315 Asthma and Allergy Foundation of America
8201 Corporate Drive, Ste 1000
Landover, MD 20785

800-727-8462
www.aafa.org

AAFA provides practical information, community based services and support to people through a network of regional chapters, educational support groups and other local partners througout the United States.

6316 World Allergy Organization
555 East Wells Street, Ste 1100
Milwaukee, WI 53202
414-276-1791
Fax: 414-276-3349
e-mail: info@worldallergy.org
www.worldallergy.org

A world-wide alliance of national and regional allergy and clinical immunology societies and organizations dedicated to raising awareness and advanceing excellence in clinical education, research and training in the field of allergy and pediatric allergy.

State Agencies & Support Groups

Colorado

6317 Parents of Asthmatic/Allergic Children, In c.
1024 S. Lemay Avenue
Fort Collins, CO 80524
970-495-8153
Fax: 970-495-7608
e-mail: cmc@pvhs.org
www.coloradoallergy.com

Support group for parents and children ages 6 and older, focusing on asthma, and issues such as allergic and non-allergic rhinitis.

Cindy Coopersmith, Coordinator

Illinois

6318 Mothers of Children with Allergies (MOCHA)
Highland Park Hospital
777 Park Avenue West
Highland Park, IL 60035
847-735-8244
e-mail: supportgroups@aafa.org
www.mochallergies.org

Support group serving Chicago & the Northern suburbs for parents and children having allergies associated with the environment, food, and Asthma.

Anne Thompson, Coordinator
Denise Bunning, Coordinator

New Jersey

6319 Allergy and Asthma Support Group of Centra l New Jersey
www.allergyfriendsnj.org
e-mail: ainserro@allergyfriendsnj.org
www.allergyfriendsnj.org

The support group is for adults and parents of children with food allergies, environmental allergies, asthma, or a combination. The Allergy & Asthma Support Group of Central New Jersey supports families and friends afflicted by life threatening food allergies and other conditions such as environmental and non-environmental allergies.

Allison Inserro, Co-Facilitator

Libraries & Resource Centers

6320 The University of Iowa Libraries
100 Main Library (LIB)
Iowa City, IA 52242
319-335-5299
www.guides.lib.uiowa.edu/allergyimmunology

The libraries at the University of Iowa contain a collection of clinical resources on allergy and immunology.

6321 University of South Florida
12901 Bruce B. Downs Boulevard
Tampa, FL 33612
727-553-3533
Fax: 727-553-1295
e-mail: sborst@health.usf.edu
www.health.usf.edu

Available libraries include ACH Medical Library, Bayfront Medical Center Library, and several libraries at USF such as: Hinks and Elaine Shimberg Health Sciences Library, Tampa Campus Library and many others. All libraries have access to MEDLINE.

Stacy Borst, Training Program Coordinator

Research Centers

6322 Allergy and Asthma Medical Group and Resea rch Center
9610 Granite Ridge Drive, Suite B
San Diego, CA 92123
858-268-2368
Fax: 858-268-5147
www.allergyandasthma.com

The Allergy and Asthma Medical Group and Research Center provide quality care given by a highly-trained team of physicians, nurse practitioners, nurses, medical assistants and office personnel with an understanding of the impact of these disorders on patients and their families.

6323 Children's National Medical Center
111 Michigan Avenue NW
Washington, DC 20010
202-476-5000
TTY: 800-855-1155
www.childrensnational.org

Children's National Medical Center's recognized staff of pediatric healthcare professionals deliver sophisticated care to thousands of families throughout the region and around the world.

George Zalzal, MD, Division Chief, Otolaryngology

6324 Duke University School of Medicine Pediatr ic and Allergy Immunology
T901/Children's Health Center
Durham, NC 27710
919-681-4080
Fax: 919-681-2714
http://pediatrics.duke.edu

Thd Division of Pediatric Allergy and Immunology and its faculty and staff ar committed to excellence in patient care, research, education and advocacy. Areas of expertise include all allergic diseases, anaphylaxis, primary immunodeficiency, asthma, rhinitis and others.

George Zalzal, MD, Division Chief, Otolaryngology

6325 Johns Hopkins Division of Allergy and Clin ical Immunology
5501 Hopkins Bayview Circle
Baltimore, MD 21224
410-550-2300
e-mail: jhuallergy@jhmi.edu
www.hopkinsmedicine.org/allergy

The faculty and staff at the Johns Hopkins Division of Allergy and Clinical Immunology are working to meet the demand for advances in the treatment of allergies, asthma, and related disorders.

6326 The University of Chicago Comer Children's Hospital
5271 S. Maryland Avenue
Chicago, IL 60637
773-702-1000
888-824-0200
www.uchicagokidshospital.org/allergy

Doctors at Chicago Comer Children's Hospital are experts on a wide variety of childhood allergies, and specialize in diagnosing and treating the full range of allergic and immune disorders of infancy and childhood.

Web Sites

6327 American Academy of Pediatrics
141 Northwest Point Boulevard
Elk Grove Village, IL 60007
847-434-4000
800-433-9016
Fax: 847-434-8000
www.aap.org

The American Academy of Pediatrics and its member pediatricians are committed to the attainment of optimal physical, mental and social health and well-being for all infants, children, adolescents, and young adults.

Sandra Hassink, MD, FAAP, President

6328 http://children.webmd.com
WebMD
www.webmd.com/children

Includes comprehensive health information on pediatric allergic rhinitis, plus a variety of other pediatric health conditions. This site includes news, videos, FAQs, the opportunity to chat with other patients and parents, a glossary, and parenting topics. Users can search by condition, age, symptoms, and more.

Kristy Hammam, Senior Vice President
Denise Dym, Senior Director
Annic Jobin, Senior Director

6329 www.Nasal-Allergies.com
www.nasal-allergies.com/nasx

This web site offers education about pediatric and adult nasal allergies, inlcuding treatment and resources.

6330 www.aap.org
American Academy of Pediatrics
141 Northwest Point Boulevard
Elk Grove Village, IL 60007   847-434-4000
                                     800-433-9016
                                  Fax: 847-434-8000
                           e-mail: webeditor@aap.org
                                         www.aap.org

This site includes a variety of resources to help deal with allergic rhinitis, including a parenting corner, publications, advocacy, and recommendations on treatment.

Sandra Hassink, MD, FAAP, President
Benard P. Dreyer, MD, FAAP, President-Elect
Errol R. Alden, MD, FAAP, Executive Director/ CEO

6331 www.acaai.org
85 West Algonquin Road, Suite 550
Arlington Heights, IL 60005   847-427-1200
                                  Fax: 847-427-1294
                            e-mail: mail@acaai.org
                                         acaai.org

The American College of Allergy, Asthma & Immunology is a professional association of 5,500 allergists/immunologists and allied health professionals. Established in 1942, the College is dedicated to improving the quality of patient care in allergy and immunology through research, advocacy and professional and public education.

James L. Sublett, MD, President
Stephen A. Tilles, MD, Vice President
Bradley E. Chipps, MD, Treasurer

6332 www.pediatriccareonline.org
American Academy of Pediatrics
pediatriccare.solutions.aap.org/Pediatric-Care

This online publication includes definitions, clinical features, complications, laboratiory findings, differential diagnosis, treatment, prognosis, tools, and references for a number of pediatric conditions, including allergic rhinitis. Users can also search for other relevant American Academy of Pediatrics publications.

6333 www.wrongdiagnosis.com
www.localhealth.com

WrongDiagnosis.com provides a free health information service to help people understand their health better. The site offers factual health information that is otherwise difficult to find. Topics include allergic rhinitis and the signs and symptoms associated with the allergy.

Richard G Grower, MD, President

6334 yourtotalhealth.ivillage.com

Contains information on numerous medical topics including pediatric allergies and asthma.

Richard G Grower, MD, President

Book Publishers

6335 Fast Facts: Rhinitis
Glenis K Scadding & Wytske J Fokkens, author

Health Press
30 Amberwood Parkway
Ashland, OH 44805   800-247-6553
                                  Fax: 419-281-6883
                         e-mail: info@atlasbooks.com
                                     www.fastfacts.com

This short and very practical book has been written for the individuals who are not seen by specialists for treatment of rhinitis, so treatment can be optimized and referral decisions are made easier.

6336 Immunology and Allergy Clinics of North Am erica
1600 John F Kennedy Boulevard, Suite 1800
Philadelphia, PA 19103   314-447-8871
                                     800-654-2452
                  e-mail: ElsevierClinics@elsevier.com
                         www.immunology.theclinics.com

Comprehensive, state-of-the-art reviews by experts in the field of allergy and pediatric allergy provide current, practical information on the diagnosis and treatment of conditions affecting the respiratory system. Each issue focuses on a single topic.

Journals

6337 AAP News
American Academy of Pediatrics
141 Northwest Point Boulevard
Elk Grove Village, IL 60007   847-434-4000
                                     800-433-9016
                                  Fax: 847-434-8000
                           e-mail: webeditor@aap.org
                                         www.aap.org

A resource of product recall alerts, pediatric medication warnings, and key advancements in pediatric medicine, including allergies and related conditions.

Sandra Hassink, MD, FAAP, President
Benard P. Dreyer, MD, FAAP, President-Elect
Errol R. Alden, MD, FAAP, Executive Director/ CEO

6338 Ear, Nose and Throat Journal
www.entjournal.com

Monthly journal with articles on pediatric and adult conditions that affect the ear, nose and throat, including allergic rhinitis.

Robert T. Sataloff, MD, DMA, FACS, Editor-in-Chief
Linda Zinn, Managing Director
Mark C. Horn, Sales Manager

6339 Journal of Allergy and Clinical Immunology
www.elsevier.com

Includes articles written by experts in the fields of allergy, pediatric allergy and immunology that discuss current research, causes, diagnosis, treatments, and clinical studies relating to pediatric rhinitis and a varity of other allergic conditions. Also includes listings of new health products and medical equipment.

Youngsuk Chi, Chairman
Ron Mobed, Chief Executive Officer
Stuart Whayman, Chief Financial Officer

6340 Pediatrics
American Academy of Pediatrics
141 Northwest Point Boulevard
Elk Grove Village, IL 60007   847-434-4000
                                     800-433-9016
                                  Fax: 847-434-8000
                           e-mail: webeditor@aap.org
                                         www.aap.org

The flagship journal of the AAP, whose authoritative content has been recognized by medical experts for 60 years. Includes information on a variety of pediaric conditions, including allergic rhinitis.

Sandra Hassink, MD, FAAP, President
Benard P. Dreyer, MD, FAAP, President-Elect
Errol R. Alden, MD, FAAP, Executive Director/ CEO

6341 Pediatrics in Review
American Academy of Pediatrics
141 Northwest Point Boulevard
Elk Grove Village, IL 60007   847-434-4000
                                               800-433-9016
                                               Fax: 847-434-8000
                                        e-mail: webeditor@aap.org
                                               www.aap.org

Features real-life cases, best practices, and review articles mapped to ABP content specifications for maintenance of certification-pediatrics. Conditions covered include pediatric allergy rhinitis and related conditions.

Sandra Hassink, MD, FAAP, President
Benard P. Dreyer, MD, FAAP, President-Elect
Errol R. Alden, MD, FAAP, Executive Director/ CEO

6342 World Allergy Organization Journal
236 Gray's Inn Road
London, WC1X   203-192-2009
                                               Fax: 203-192-2010
                                       e-mail: waoj@worldallergy.org
                                               www.waojournal.org

The official journal of the World Allergy Organization whose goals include to: be a premier journal of original scientific and clinically relevant information for practicing allergists/immunologists; to publish state-of-the-art review articles and editorials on translational and clincal medicine in the field of allergy, pediatric allergy and immunology; and to present a forum for scientific interaction between allergists, pediatric allergists and immunologists worldwide.

Alessandro Fiocchi, Editor-in-Chief
Johannes Ring, Executive Editor
Erika Jensen-Jarolim, Deputy Director

Newsletters

6343 AAP Grand Rounds
American Academy of Pediatrics
141 Northwest Point Boulevard
Elk Grove Village, IL 60007   847-434-4000
                                               800-433-9016
                                               Fax: 847-434-8000
                                        e-mail: webeditor@aap.org
                                               www.aap.org

Features evidence-based summaries of clinical content from 100 journals. A key feature, 'Weighing the Evidence,' provides medical literature interpretation assistance.

Sandra Hassink, MD, FAAP, President
Benard P. Dreyer, MD, FAAP, President-Elect
Errol R. Alden, MD, FAAP, Executive Director/ CEO

6344 ACAAI eNews
85 West Algonquin Road, Suite 550
Arlington Heights, IL 60005   847-427-1200; Fax: 847-427-1294
                                            e-mail: enews@acaai.org
                                                    acaai.org

The ACAAI eNews is a monthly aggregated news service provided by the American College of Allergy, Asthma & Immunology.

Richard G Grower, MD, President

6345 Allergy & Asthma Issues
American Academy of Allergy Asthma & Immunology
555 E. Wells Street, Suite 1100
Milwaukee, WI 53202   414-272-6071; Fax: 414-272-6070
                                               www.aaaai.org

A quarterly member publication produced by the AAAAI.

Megan Brown, Communications Manager

Description

6346 SARCOIDOSIS

Synonyms: Sarcoid of Boeck, Schaumann's disease

Involves the following Biologic System(s):

Connective Tissue Disorders

Sarcoidosis is a multisystem disorder that is characterized by the abnormal development of inflammatory growths or nodules (i.e., epithelioid granulomas) in various organs in the body. The cause of this inflammatory disorder is unknown; however, it is believed that granuloma formation associated with sarcoidosis may result from infection or an exaggerated immune response to specific agents (antigens). In addition, researchers believe that some people may be genetically predisposed to sarcoidosis and develop the disease only if triggered by environmental or other factors. Although this disorder most commonly occurs during young adulthood, it may occur in children and in the elderly. Symptoms and physical findings associated with sarcoidosis are dependent upon the organ(s) involved and, in children, the age of onset. Most affected children, however, share the common symptoms of fatigue, weight loss, cough, pain in the bones and joints, and abnormally low levels of circulating red blood cells (anemia).

The nodules or granulomas associated with sarcoidosis may develop in almost any organ of the body, but most commonly affect the lungs, upper respiratory tract, lymph nodes, skin, eyes, liver, bones, joints, bone marrow, skeletal muscles, heart, liver, spleen, or the central and peripheral nervous systems. In older children and adults, the lungs are most often affected (90 percent of patients), while younger children experience less lung involvement. Characteristic findings in older children may include swelling of the lymph nodes near the blood vessels that enter and exit the lungs (hilar lymphadenopathy) as well as the lymph nodes near the windpipe (paratracheal lymphadenopathy) and those under the skin (peripheral lymphadenopathy). In addition, nodule formation may cause inflammations in the eye (e.g., uveitis and iritis) and other eye lesions, skin lesions, and liver changes. Younger children may develop a reddish, combination-type rash consisting of waxy pimples and flat, discolored lesions (maculopapular erythematous rash) as well as inflammation of the joints (arthritis).

Diagnosis of sarcoidosis is usually a challenge as it is often difficult to distinguish from other disorders with similar symptoms and findings. Therefore, differential diagnosis often involves a physical examination, medical and environmental history, and the comprehensive evaluation of laboratory tests and chest x-rays, biopsy of tissue samples, and specialized testing. Laboratory findings may show excessive levels of calcium in the blood (hypercalcemia) and in the urine (hypercalciuria), abnormally high levels of protein in the blood (hyperproteinemia), excessive levels of certain granular white cells in the blood (eosinophilia), and other blood irregularities. For example, the cells of the nodules secrete a substance called angiotensin-converting enzyme, which, in some patients, is elevated to detectable levels in the blood. Testing for this enzyme may also be employed to measure disease activity. In addition, pulmonary function tests may be used to measure progress of the disease in those children with lung involvement, and repeat chest x-rays may also be indicated to monitor progress.

In some children, sarcoidosis may resolve spontaneously within a period of months or years; however, some children may have a more chronic form of the disease that may result in progressive lung involvement, eye disease that may cause blindness, and other prolonged symptoms and findings. Treatment for sarcoidosis may include the use of corticosteroid drops or ointments to alleviate eye inflammations and oral corticosteroids to alleviate acute symptoms such as resistant inflammatory lesions of the eyes, joint pain, fever, shortness of breath, and other symptoms. Approximately 90 percent of cases are responsive to corticosteroids and can be controlled with modest maintenance doses. If no symptoms are present, corticosteroid treatment is usually not advised. Other treatment is symptomatic and supportive.

National Associations & Support Groups

6347 American Academy of Pediatrics
141 Northwest Point Boulevard
Elk Grove Village, IL 60007
847-434-4000
800-433-9016
Fax: 847-434-8000
www.aap.org

The American Academy of Pediatrics and its member pediatricians are committed to the attainment of optimal physical, mental and social health and well-being for all infants, children, adolescents, and young adults.

Sandra Hassink, MD, FAAP, President

6348 American Autoimmune Related Diseases Association
22100 Gratiot Avenue
East Detroit, MI 48021
586-776-3900
800-598-4668
Fax: 586-776-3903
e-mail: aarda@aarda.org
www.aarda.org

Dedicated to the eradiction of autoimmune diseases and the alleviation of suffering and the socio-economic impact of autoimmunity through fostering and facilitating collaboration in the areas of education, public awareness, research and patient services in an effective, ethical and efficient manner.

Virginia Ladd, Executive Director

6349 National Sarcoidosis Resource Center and Networking Program
PO Box 1593
Piscataway, NJ 08855
732-463-0497
Fax: 732-463-0497
www.nsrc-global.net

Formed to heighten public awareness and to educate people about this often chronic and disabling disease; offers information and support. The center serves the United States, Canada, Europe.

Sandra Conroy, President

6350 Sarcoid Networking Association
12619 S. Wilderness Way
Molalla, OR 97308
541-905-2092
e-mail: ÿsarcoidinformation@sarcoidosisnetwork.o
www.sarcoidosisnetwork.org

A nonprofit organization dedicated to improving the lives of those affected by sarcoidosis through providing support, eduation and other resources.

Kristi Anderson, Executive Director

6351 Sarcoid Registry
5239 SW Lance St
Roseburg, OR 97471
541-905-2092
e-mail: admin@snaregistry.org
www.snaregistry.org

Operates under the laedership of SNA-Sarcoid Networking Association to bring the Sarcoidosis community together.

Kristi Anderson, Director

6352 Sarcoidosis Network Foundation
11428 E Artesia Blvd, Suite 10
Artesia, CA 90701   562-809-8500
                                            Fax: 562-809-8182
                                        www.sarcoid-network.org

A nonprofit organization that promotes awareness and education; supports research to find a cure; and supports those affected by sarcoidosis and their families.

Ruth Jacobs, President
Charles Walker, VP
Jean Johnson-Bell, Treasurer

6353 Sarcoidosis Research Institute
3475 Central Avenue
Memphis, TN 38111   901-219-6883
                                            Fax: 901-774-7294
                                    e-mail: sarcoidosis@bellsouth.net
                                        www.sarcoidosisresearch.org

Provides patient and professional education that will result in enhanced methods of diagnosis and treatment of the disease; information that will assist patients and their support network in the management of the disease; and engages in research initiatives that will result in a cure for the debilitating disease.

State Agencies & Support Groups

California

6354 REACH - Sarcoidosis Support
10843 Kenney St
Norwalk, CA 90650   714-739-4023
Ruth Jacobs

Colorado

6355 Denver Sarcoidosis Awareness Support Group
4351 Ireland St
Denver, CO 80249   303-375-9376
                    e-mail: contacts@denversarcoidosisawareness.org
                            www.denversarcoidosisawareness.org

Provides support through sharing of experiences, discussing feeling and emotions, and sharing coping strategies.

Shirley R Holley, President

Georgia

6356 Sarcoidosis Support Group
St Joseph's/Chandler Health System
5353 Reynolds St
Savannah, GA 31405   912-819-8032
                                        e-mail: balkstra@sjchs.org
Cindy Balkstra RN

Indiana

6357 Central Indiana Sarcoidosis Support Group
Kindred Hospital
1700 W 10th St
Indianapolis, IN 46222   317-809-7011
                                        e-mail: cissg@usa.com
                                        www.indysarcoid.org

The Central Indiana Sarcoidosis Support Group was started in 1998 to offer hope and support to those diagnosed with Sarcoidosis.

Gloria Hooks, President
Kelisa Walker, Vice President
Mary Wineglass, Secretary

Maryland

6358 Sarcoidosis Awareness Network
10313 Farrar Avenue
Cheltenham, MD 20623   301-372-2885
                            e-mail: info@sarcoidosisawareness.org
                                www.sarcoidosisnetwork.net

The Sarcoidosis Awareness Network is a nonprofit organization established to increase and expand the public awareness of sarcoidosis; enhance the quality of life of sarcoidosis survivors; develop and implement a sarcoidosis registry; and to disseminate current literature on the disease so the general public is better informed about sarcoidosis and its impact on the lives of those afflicted with the disease.

Linda D. Lanier, Founder

Michigan

6359 Sarcoidosis Awareness Foundation
14540 Whitcomb St
Detroit, MI 48227   e-mail: SarcoidAwareness@aol.com
Janie L Chuney

6360 Sarcoidosis Resource Support Group
PO Box 3231
Highland Park, MI 48203   315-575-4852
                        e-mail: pmullins@detroitsworkplace.org
                            www.sarcoidosisnetwork.org/groups.htm
Pam Mullins
Dot Lawrence

6361 Sarcoidosis Support - Beaumont
William Beaumont Hospital
300 W 13 Mile Rd
Royal Oak, MI 48073   248-545-0320
                                e-mail: lagalbrith@yahoo.com
                            www.sarcoidosisnetwork.org/groups.htm
Victoria Rice
Laura Galbraith, Contact
Sylvia Johnson, Contact

New Jersey

6362 Sarcoidosis Support Resource Central New Jersey
National Sarcoidosis Resource Center
PO Box 1593
Piscataway, NJ 08855   732-699-0733
                                            Fax: 732-699-0882
                            www.sarcoidosisnetwork.org/groups.htm
Sandra Conroy

New York

6363 Long Island Sarcoidosis Support
1989 N Jerusalem Rd
E Meadow, NY 11554   516-483-2666
                            www.sarcoidosisnetwork.org/groups.htm
Robert Schoenfeld, Facilitator

North Carolina

6364 Sarcoidosis Support Group
1021 Fitzgerald Dr
Wilmington, NC 28405   910-395-0154
                            www.sarcoidosisnetwork.org/groups.htm
Uldridge Galloway

6365 University of North Carolina Sarcoidosis Support Group
Div. of Pulmonary Medicine
130 Mason Farm Rd, CB# 7020
Chapel Hill, NC 27599   919-966-5296
                                        e-mail: juliem@med.unc.edu
                                            www.unceye.org

Ricky Bass, Manager

Pennsylvania

6366 Sarcoidosis Self-Help
2112 Highland Avenue
New Castle, PA 16105
412-652-6089
www.sarcoidosisnetwork.org/groups.htm
Della Emmanuel

South Carolina

6367 Sarcoidosis Support
MUSC Medical Center
171 Ashley Ave
Charleston, SC 29425
803-792-0280
Kathy Lanza

Tennessee

6368 Middle Tennessee Sarcoidosis Support Group
PO Box 1342
Cookesville, TN 38503
931-528-7826
www.sarcoidosisnetwork.org/groups.htm
Becky Robertson

6369 Sarcoidosis Patient Forum
Sarcoidosis Research Institute-SRI
3475 Central Avenue
Memphis, TN 38111
901-219-6883
Fax: 901-774-7294
Paula Polite, President

Virginia

6370 Sarcoidosis Support Group
704 Woodnote Land
Newport News, VA 23608
804-988-3065
www.sarcoidosisnetwork.org/groups.htm
Beverly Moses

Libraries & Resource Centers

6371 National Sarcoidosis Resource Center
PO Box 1593
Piscataway, NJ 08855
732-463-0497
Fax: 732-463-0467
www.nsrc-global.net

Provides general information about special services for
sarcoidosis patients; strives to increase public awareness about
this unknown disease, and to generate interest in sarcordosis and
support research, leading to easy diagnosis, better treatments and,
ultimately, a cure.
Sandra Conroy

6372 Sarcoidosis Center
Baptist Hospital East
6005 Park Avenue, Suite 501
Memphis, TN 38119
901-761-5877
Fax: 901-761-2280
e-mail: sarcoid@sarcoidcenter.com
www.sarcoidcenter.com

A nonprofit organization providing an exchange of information
regarding sarcoidosis for patients and professionals.
Norman T Soskel MD

Research Centers

6373 National Jewish Medical & Research Center
1400 Jackson St
Denver, CO 80206
303-388-4461
800-222-5864
www.nationaljewish.org/disease-info

Information on ongoing sarcoidosis research and available treatment programs at the center.
Russell P Bowler, Vice Chair/Associate Professor

6374 Sarcoidosis Research Institute
3475 Central Avenue
Memphis, TN 38111
901-219-6883
Fax: 901-774-7294
e-mail: sarcoidosis@bellsouth.net
www.sarcoidosisresearch.org

Provides patient and professional education that will result in enhanced methods of diagnosis and treatment of the disease; information that will assist patients and their support network in the
management of the disease; and engages in research initiatives
that will result in a cure for the debilitating disease.

Audio Video

6375 Dialogue with Doris
PC Publications
PO Box 1593
Piscataway, NJ 8855
732-699-0733
Fax: 732-699-0882
www.webmd.com

Kristy Hammam, Senior Vice President
Denise Dym, Senior Director
Annic Jobin, Senior Director

6376 Help with a Hidden Disease Update
PC Publications
PO Box 1593
Piscataway, NJ 8855
732-699-0733
800-223-6429
Fax: 732-699-0882
www.webmd.com

Kristy Hammam, Senior Vice President
Denise Dym, Senior Director
Annic Jobin, Senior Director

**6377 International World Conference on Sarcoidosis-Patient
Symposium**
PC Publications
PO Box 1593
Piscataway, NJ 8855
732-699-0733
Fax: 732-699-0882
www.webmd.com

Cassette.
Kristy Hammam, Senior Vice President
Denise Dym, Senior Director
Annic Jobin, Senior Director

6378 Of Their Own-Person To Person Show
PC Publications
PO Box 1593
Piscataway, NJ 8855
732-699-0733
Fax: 732-699-0882
www.webmd.com

Kristy Hammam, Senior Vice President
Denise Dym, Senior Director
Annic Jobin, Senior Director

6379 Sarcoidosis Conference 2
PC Publications
PO Box 1593
Piscataway, NJ 8855
732-699-0733
Fax: 732-699-0882
www.webmd.com

Kristy Hammam, Senior Vice President
Denise Dym, Senior Director
Annic Jobin, Senior Director

6380 Sarcoidosis Conference 3
PC Publications
PO Box 1593
Piscataway, NJ 8855
732-699-0733
Fax: 732-699-0882
www.webmd.com

Kristy Hammam, Senior Vice President
Denise Dym, Senior Director
Annic Jobin, Senior Director

6381 Sarcoidosis and Lyme Disease
PC Publications
PO Box 1593
Piscataway, NJ 8855
732-699-0733
Fax: 732-699-0882
www.webmd.com

Kristy Hammam, Senior Vice President
Denise Dym, Senior Director
Annic Jobin, Senior Director

6382 Sarcoidosis-What's That?
PC Publications
PO Box 1593
Piscataway, NJ 8855
732-699-0733
Fax: 732-699-0882
www.webmd.com

Kristy Hammam, Senior Vice President
Denise Dym, Senior Director
Annic Jobin, Senior Director

Web Sites

6383 American Autoimmune Related Diseases Association
www.aarda.org

Dedicated to the eradication of autoimmune diseases and the alleviation of suffering and the socio-economic impact of autoimmunity through fostering and facilitating collaboration in the areas of education, public awareness, research and patient services in an effective, ethical and efficient manner.

Betty Diamond, M.D., Chairman
Stanley M. Finger, Vice Chairman
Virginia T. Ladd, President/ CEO

6384 Foundation for Sarcoidosis Research
1820 W. Webster Ave., Ste 304
Chicago, IL 60614
866-358-5477
www.stopsarcoidosis.org

Takes the lead as a nonprofit organization in funding research in finding a cure for sarcoidosis and improving patient care.

Andrea Wilson, Chairwoman
Anjan Chatterji, President
Reading Wilson, Treasurer

6385 Health Answers
410 Horsham Road
Horsham, PA 19044
215-442-9010
e-mail: Michael.tague@healthanswers.com
www.healthanswers.com

HealthAnswers offers a breadth of services in medical education, sales force training, patient support solutions, professional promotion and consumer solutions.

Michael Tague, Managing Director

6386 NIH/National Heart, Lung and Blood Institu te
P.O. Box 30105
Bethesda, MD 20824
301-592-8573
e-mail: nhlbiinfo@nhlbi.nih.gov
www.nhlbi.nih.gov/health/dci/Index/s.html

A part of the National Institutes of Health, this NHLBI site offers general information and answers to questions about Sarcoidosis.

Gary H. Gibbons, Director

6387 National Sarcoidosis Resource Center
www.nsrc-global.net

The center provides information to people throughout the U.S., Canada, and Europe. They have an ongoing research study of the symptoms and demographics of Sarcoidosis patients.

6388 Online Mendelian Inheritance in Man
National Library of Medicine, Building 38A
Bethesda, MD 20894
888-346-3656
e-mail: info@ncbi.nlm.nih.gov
www.ncbi.nlm.nih.gov

This database is a catalog of human genes and genetic disorders.

Christine E. Seidman, M.D., Chair
David J. Lipman, M.D., Executive Secretary

6389 Sarcoid Life
www.sarcoidlife.org

6390 Sarcoidosis
www.epler.com/wsarc.html

General information and answers to questions about Sarcoidosis.

6391 Sarcoidosis Center
www.sarcoidcenter.com

A nonprofit corporation designed to provide information for patients and physicians regarding sarcoidosis. The site includes a list of sarcoidosis experts by country.

6392 Sarcoidosis Research Institute
www.sarcoidosisresearch.org

Provides patient and professional education that will result in enhanced methods of diagnosis and treatment of the disease.

Book Publishers

6393 Sarcoidosis Resource Guide and Directory
PC Publications
PO Box 1593
Piscataway, NJ 08855
732-699-0733
Fax: 732-699-0882

1993 304 pages Paperback
ISBN: 0-963122-25-8

Newsletters

6394 Online Sarcoidosis Newsletter
National Sarcoidosis Resource Center
PO Box 1593
Piscataway, NJ 8855
732-699-0733
Fax: 732-699-0882

Offers information on the center's activities and events, medical and legislative updates for the patients and their families.

Quarterly

6395 Sarcoidosis Networking
Sarcoid Networking Association
6424 151st Avenue E
Sumner, WA 98390
253-891-6886
e-mail: sarcoidosis_network@prodigy.net
www.sarcoidnetwork.org

Helps those affected by sarcoidosis network with one another and the medical community.

Quarterly

Dolores O'Leary, Executive Director

Pamphlets

6396 A Sarcoidosis Questionnaire: Demographics and Symptomatology-Patients Respond
PC Publications
PO Box 1593
Piscataway, NJ 8855
732-699-0733
800-223-6429
Fax: 732-699-0882

6397 Anemia of Sarcoidosis
PC Publications
PO Box 1593
Piscataway, NJ 8855
732-699-0733
Fax: 732-699-0882

6398 Bronchoalveolar Lymphocytes in Sarcoidosis
PC Publications
PO Box 1593
Piscataway, NJ 8855
732-699-0733
Fax: 732-699-0882

6399 Case Report-MR Imaging of Myocardial Sarcoidosis
PC Publications
PO Box 1593
Piscataway, NJ 8855
732-699-0733
Fax: 732-699-0882

6400 Case Report-Osseous Sarcoidosis and Chronic Polyarthritis
PC Publications
PO Box 1593
Piscataway, NJ 8855
732-699-0733
Fax: 732-699-0882

6401 Coping with Sarcoidosis
National Sarcoidosis Resource Center
PO Box 1593
Piscataway, NJ 8855
732-699-0733
Fax: 732-699-0882

A pamphlet offering information on how to manage and live with sarcoidosis.

6402 Drugs That Have Been Used for the Treatment of Sarcoidosis
PC Publications
PO Box 1593
Piscataway, NJ 8855
732-699-0733
Fax: 732-699-0882

6403 Effects of Sarcoid and Steroids on Angiotensin-Converting Enzyme
PC Publications
PO Box 1593
Piscataway, NJ 8855
732-699-0733
Fax: 732-699-0882

6404 Masqueraders of Sarcoidosis
PC Publications
PO Box 1593
Piscataway, NJ 8855
732-699-0733
Fax: 732-699-0882

6405 Multidisciplinary Clinico-Pathologic Conference
PC Publications
PO Box 1593
Piscataway, NJ 8855
732-699-0733
Fax: 732-699-0882

6406 National Sarcoidosis Resource Center
PC Publications
PO Box 1593
Piscataway, NJ 8855
732-699-0733
Fax: 732-699-0882
www.nsrc-global.net

A booklet offering a brief introduction to the illness and information on the role of the Center in finding a cure and educating the public on Sarcoidosis.

6407 Neurosarcoidosis
PC Publications
PO Box 1593
Piscataway, NJ 8855
732-699-0733
Fax: 732-699-0882

6408 Neurosarcoidosis or Multiple Sclerosis?
National Sarcoidosis Resource Center
PO Box 1593
Piscataway, NJ 8855
732-699-0733
Fax: 732-699-0882

6409 Paranoid Psychosis Due to Neurosarcoidosis
PC Publications
PO Box 1593
Piscataway, NJ 8855
732-699-0733
800-223-6429
Fax: 732-699-0882

6410 Patient Information Package
National Sarcoidosis Resource Center
PO Box 1593
Piscataway, NJ 8855
732-699-0733
Fax: 732-699-0882

Contains various brochures and pamphlets offering information about sarcoidosis.

6411 Presidential Proclamation-National Sarcoidosis Awareness Day
PC Publications
PO Box 1593
Piscataway, NJ 8855
732-699-0733
Fax: 732-699-0882

6412 Psychological Factors in Sarcoidosis
PC Publications
PO Box 1593
Piscataway, NJ 8855
732-699-0733
Fax: 732-699-0882

6413 Pulmonary Sarcoidosis: Evaluation with High Resolution
PC Publications
PO Box 1593
Piscataway, NJ 8855
732-699-0733
Fax: 732-699-0882

6414 Pulmonary Sarcoidosis: What We Are Learning
PC Publications
PO Box 1593
Piscataway, NJ 8855
732-699-0733
Fax: 732-699-0882

6415 Right & Left Ventricular Function At Rest In Patients with Sarcoidosis
PC Publications
PO Box 1593
Piscataway, NJ 8855
732-699-0733
Fax: 732-699-0882

6416 Sarcoidosis
PC Publications
PO Box 1593
Piscataway, NJ 8855
732-699-0733
Fax: 732-699-0882

Offers information on the illness, causes, symptoms and treatments.

6417 Sarcoidosis Questionnaire: Demographics and Symptomatology-The Patients Respond
PC Publications
PO Box 1593
Piscataway, NJ 8855
732-699-0733
Fax: 732-699-0882

6418 Sarcoidosis and Other Granulatomous
PC Publications
PO Box 1593
Piscataway, NJ 8855   732-699-0733
                                                800-223-6429
                                         Fax: 732-699-0882

6419 Sarcoidosis and You-A Listing of Possible Symptoms
PC Publications
PO Box 1593
Piscataway, NJ 8855   732-699-0733
                                         Fax: 732-699-0882

6420 Sarcoidosis-International Review
PC Publications
PO Box 1593
Piscataway, NJ 8855   732-699-0733
                                         Fax: 732-699-0882

6421 Sarcoidosis-Pleural Involvement Mimicking a Coin Lesson
PC Publications
PO Box 1593
Piscataway, NJ 8855   732-699-0733
                                         Fax: 732-699-0882

6422 Sarcoidosis: A Multisystem Disease
PC Publications
PO Box 1593
Piscataway, NJ 8855   732-699-0733
                                         Fax: 732-699-0882

Explains the effects of the illness on the lungs and joints.

6423 Sarcoidosis: Usual and Unusual Manifestations
PC Publications
PO Box 1593
Piscataway, NJ 8855   732-699-0733
                                         Fax: 732-699-0882

6424 Seasonal Clustering of Sarcoidosis
National Sarcoidosis Resource Center
PO Box 1593
Piscataway, NJ 8855   732-699-0733
                                         Fax: 732-699-0882

6425 Successful Treatment of Myocardial Sarcoidosis with Steriods
PC Publications
PO Box 1593
Piscataway, NJ 8855   732-699-0733
                                         Fax: 732-699-0882

6426 Support Group Listing
PC Publications
PO Box 1593
Piscataway, NJ 8855   732-699-0733
                                         Fax: 732-699-0882

6427 World Association Sarcoidosis Other Granulatomous
PC Publications
PO Box 1593
Piscataway, NJ 8855   732-699-0733
                                         Fax: 732-699-0882

Description

6428 SCLERODERMA

Covers these related disorders: Linear scleroderma, Morphea, Systemic sclerosis

Involves the following Biologic System(s):
Connective Tissue Disorders

Scleroderma is a connective tissue disease characterized by the build up of collagen (connective tissue) resulting in thickening and hardening of the skin and underlying tissues or, in some forms of scleroderma, other organs of the body. In patients with morphea, a form of the disease that primarily affects the skin and its underlying (subcutaneous) tissues, lesions appear as limited or localized patches. In linear scleroderma, lesions appear in a band-like pattern. In other patients, particularly in adults, scleroderma may occur as a generalized, systemic disease affecting the skin and subcutaneous tissues, blood vessels, and internal organs, such as the heart, lungs, kidneys, and certain parts of the digestive tract. Although the underlying cause of scleroderma is not known, some researchers speculate that it may be an autoimmune disease in which there is an abnormal immune response against the body's own tissues. During childhood, scleroderma is more common in girls than boys.

Children with scleroderma are primarily affected by morphea or linear scleroderma. Associated symptoms and findings usually become apparent at age two or older. Patients initially develop patchy skin lesions that are dry, red or violet, and shiny in appearance. These lesions may cause associated pain or unusual sensations, such as prickling feelings in affected areas. In some children, the lesions may have a linear distribution and develop primarily on one side of the body. The lesions gradually become hard (indurated) and develop waxy, pale centers and elevated borders. As the disease continues to progress, the lesions become larger and merge, potentially involving a large area, such as an entire arm or leg. Affected areas may eventually develop deep scar tissue and firmly bind to underlying tissues, potentially resulting in pain and permanent bending of affected joints in fixed postures (joint contractures). In children with morphea or linear scleroderma, active disease may spontaneously subside over months or years or may slowly progress over many years.

Rarely, children may develop generalized, systemic scleroderma (systemic sclerosis). In such cases, associated symptoms and findings usually become apparent at age four or older. Children with systemic sclerosis often initially experience Raynaud's phenomenon, a condition characterized by sudden contraction of blood vessels supplying the fingers or toes, causing an interruption of blood flow and a subsequent excess of blood in affected areas following the restoration of blood flow (reactive hyperemia). Such episodes are usually triggered by exposure to cold temperatures and are characterized by numbness, tingling, and bluish or whitish discoloration of the fingers or toes (cyanosis) due to lack of blood flow and subsequent reddening and pain.

Children with systemic sclerosis also often develop skin lesions on the hands and feet and, in some cases, the torso and facial area. These lesions may include groups of permanently widened (dilated) blood vessels (telangiectasias). As the disease progresses, skin lesions typically become hard, develop unusually light or dark pigmentation, and gradually bind to underlying tissues and structures. Children may also experience joint swelling, discomfort, and inflammation (arthritis) as well as degenerative changes of various organs, including those of the digestive tract, particularly the esophagus; the heart; the lungs and the kidneys. Associated symptoms may be extremely variable, depending upon the rate of disease progression and the specific bodily tissues and organs affected. In some patients, such abnormalities may include difficulty swallowing (dysphagia); chronic inflammation of the lungs due to unintended inhalation of foreign matter into the airways (aspiration pneumonia); high blood pressure (hypertension); or respiratory, heart, or kidney failure. Active disease may be gradually progressive or include periods during which symptoms temporarily subside (remit).

The treatment of children with scleroderma is symptomatic and supportive. Such measures may include the use of steroids, such as cortisone or prednisone, to decrease inflammation in muscles, joints or rarely in the skin itself. Non-steroidal anti-inflammatory drugs (NSAIDs) such as ibuprofen and naproxen are sometimes used for children who have arthritis to decrease joint inflammation early physical therapy to help prevent or minimize the development of joint contractures; systemic therapy with methotrexate or other medications (e.g., cytotoxic drugs), if appropriate; careful control of high blood pressure in those with systemic disease; and other measures as required. In addition, patients with Raynaud's phenomenon should avoid cold temperatures whenever possible and dress warmly before such exposure. Scleroderma is a chronic and slowly progressive disease, lasting for months or years. The outlook depends on the type of scleroderma, where and how much skin is involved and whether or not internal organs are affected.

Government Agencies

6429 NIH/National Institute of Arthritis and Mu sculoskeletal and Skin Diseases
1AMS Circle
Bethesda, MD 20892

301-402-4484
877-226-4267
Fax: 301-718-6366
TDD: 301-565-2966
e-mail: niamsinfo@mail.nih.gov
www.niams.nih.gov

The mission of the NIAMS, a part of the NIH, is to support research into the causes, treatment, and prevention of arthritis and musculoskeletal and skin diseases, the training of basic and clinical scientists to carry out this research, and the dissemination of information on research progress in these diseases.

Stephen I Katz MD PhD, Director
Robert H Carter MD, Deputy Director
Gahan Breithaupt, Assoc Dir for Management & Operatio

National Associations & Support Groups

6430 American Academy of Pediatrics
141 Northwest Point Boulevard
Elk Grove Village, IL 60007

847-434-4000
800-433-9016
Fax: 847-434-8000
www.aap.org

The American Academy of Pediatrics and its member pediatricians are committed to the attainment of optimal physical, mental and social health and well-being for all infants, children, adolescents, and young adults.

Sandra Hassink, MD, FAAP, President

6431 American Autoimmune Related Diseases Association
22100 Gratiot Avenue
East Detroit, MI 48021
586-776-3900
800-598-4668
Fax: 586-776-3903
e-mail: aarda@aarda.org
www.aarda.org

Dedicated to the eradiction of autoimmune diseases and the alleviation of suffering and the socio-economic impact of autoimmunity through fostering and facilitating collaboration in the areas of education, public awareness, research and patient services in an effective, ethical and efficient manner.

Virginia T. Ladd, R.T., President/Executive Director
Stanley M. Finger, Ph.D., Chairman
John Kaiser, CPA, Treasurer

6432 International Scleroderma Network
7455 France Ave S, #266
Edina, MN 55435
952-831-3091
800-564-7099
e-mail: isn@sclero.org
www.scerlo.org

Nonprofit organization for the research, education, support, and awareness for scleroderma and related illnesses. Website available in 20 languages.

Kevin Lenue Billups, Founder/President

6433 Juvenile Scleroderma Network
1204 W 13th Street
San Pedro, CA 90731
310-519-9511
866-338-5892
Fax: 800-369-8309
e-mail: outreachJSDN@aol.com
www.jsdn.org

A nonprofit organization that provides support and friendship to children who have Juvenile Scleroderma.

Thomas J.A. Lehman, M.D., Chief, Pediatric Rheumatologist
Ronald Laxer, M.D., Chief, Pediatric Rheumatologist
Bernice Krafchik, M.D., Pediatric Dermatology

6434 Scleroderma Foundation
300 Rosewood Dr, Suite 105
Danvers, MA 01923
978-750-4950
800-722-4673
Fax: 978-463-5809
e-mail: sfinfo@scleroderma.org
www.scleroderma.org

Nonprofit national organization for people with scleroderma and their family and friends. Provides support and promotes education and research.

Robert J. Riggs, Ceo
Kerri Connolly, Director of Programs and Services
Tracey O. Sperry, Director of Development and Researc

State Agencies & Support Groups

Florida

6435 Scleroderma Foundation Southeast Florida Chapter
3930 Oaks Clubhouse Drive, Suite 206
Pompano Beach, FL 33069
954-798-1854
e-mail: sclerodermasefl@gmail.com
www.scleroderma.org/site/PageServer?pagename=sefl_ho
Ferne Robin, Executive Director
Jerry Lance, President
Ruth Greenspan, Vice President

Illinois

6436 Scleroderma Foundation Chicago Chapter
134 N. LaSalle St. Suite 1360
Chicago, IL 60602
312-660-1131
Fax: 312-660-1133
e-mail: GCchapter@scleroderma.org
www.scleroderma.org/site/PageServer?pagename=gc_home

We provide assistance to patients with scleroderma adhering to our three-fold mission of support, education and research.

Ann Peterson, Executive Director
Mike Robbins, President
Julie L. Drewniak, Secretary

Nevada

6437 Scleroderma Foundation Nevada Chapter
Vegas TV Building, 6760 Surrey Street
Las Vegas, NV 89118
702-368-1572
Fax: 702-368-1582
e-mail: NVchapter@scleroderma.org
http://www.scleroderma.org/site/PageServer?pagename=
Sheila Gray, President
Sheila Gray, VP, Support Group

New Jersey

6438 Scleroderma Foundation New Jersey Chapter
PO Box 285
Haddon Heights, NJ 08035
856-547-5010
866-675-5545
Fax: 856-547-5010
e-mail: sfdv1@verizon.net
Liz Van Dzura, Executive Director

New York

6439 Scleroderma Foundation Tri-State, Inc (NY, NJ, CT)
59 Front St
Binghamton, NY 13905
607-723-2239
800-867-0885
Fax: 607-723-2039
e-mail: sdtristate@aol.com
www.scleroderma.org/chapter/tristate

The mission of the Scleroderma Foundation/Tri State, Inc. Chapter is three fold: To provide educational and emotional support to people with scleroderma and their families; to stimulate and support research designed to identify the cause and cure of scleroderma as well as improve methods of treatment; and to enhance the public's awareness of this disease.

Jay Peak, Executive Director
Tom Knapp, Office Manager

Rhode Island

6440 Rhode Island Scleroderma Support Group
Roger Williams Medical Ctr
825 Chalkstone Ave
Providence, RI 02908
401-781-5013
e-mail: scleroderma@hotmail.com
www.ri.sclerodermasupportgroup.net
Carole Cowell, Contact
Frank L. Fitzpatrick, Webmaster

Texas

6441 Scleroderma Foundation Texas Bluebonnet Ch apter
101 W. McDermott Dr. Suite 115
Allen, TX 75013
972-396-9400
866-532-7673
Fax: 972-649-7910
e-mail: TXchapter@scleroderma.org
www.scleroderma.org/site/PageServer?pagename=tx_home
Emily Woods, President
Amber Paris, Vice President
Virginia Browne, Secretary

6442 Scleroderma Foundation Greater Washington DC Chapter
2010 Corporate Ridge, 7th Fl, PMB 126
McLean, VA 22102   202-999-4562
888-233-4779
e-mail: GWDCchapter@scleroderma.org
www.scleroderma.org/site/PageServer?pagename=dc_invo
Carol Sodetz, Contact

Washington

6443 Scleroderma Foundation Evergreen Chapter
PO Box 84506
Seattle, WA 98124   206-285-9822
e-mail: WAchapter@scleroderma.org
www.scleroderma.org/site/PageServer?pagename=wa_home
Bunny Garthe, President
Nic Evans, Vice President
Gloria Blanco-Duque, Secretary

Research Centers

Alabama

6444 University of Alabama - Birmingham Arthrit is Clinical Intervention Program
1717 6th Avenue South SRC 076
Birmingham, AL 35249   205-934-7727
866-876-2247
Fax: 205-975-5554
e-mail: rand1951@uab.edu
www.uab.edu/medicine/acip/

Since 1990, the Arthritis Clinical Intervention Program (ACIP) has conducted over 300 rheumatology trials (Phase I-IV). All our doctors are Board Certified Rheumatologists with many years of research experience. Dr. Jeffrey Curtis is our Medical Director.

Randall Parks, MBA, RN, Program Director
David J. Mackey, MPH, Regulatory Manager
Martha R. Sanderson, MSN, NP, Nurse Practitioner

Arizona

6445 Mayo Clinic Scleroderma Service
13400 E Shea Blvd
Scottsdale, AZ 85259   480-301-8000
Fax: 480-301-8673
www.mayoclinic.org/rheumatology-sct/
Heidi Garcia, Research Info

California

6446 Scleroderma Research Foundation
220 Montgomery St, Suite 1411
San Francisco, CA 94104   415-834-9444
800-441-2873
Fax: 415-834-9177
e-mail: info@sclerodermaresearch.org
www.srfcure.org

The Scleroderma Research Foundation's mission is to find a cure for scleroderma, a life-threatening and degenerative illness, by funding and facilitating the most promising, highest quality research and placing the disease and its need for a cure in the public eye.

Luke Evnin, PhD, Chairman
Charles Spaulding, Vice President, Communications
Jill Wayne, Director, Cure Advocate Program

District of Columbia

6447 Georgetown University
Dept of Rheumatology
PHC Bldg, 3800 Reservoir Rd, 6th Fl
Washington, DC 20007   202-784-6671
Fax: 202-784-4332
e-mail: memory@georgetown.edu
www.memory.georgetown.edu/

For adult and pediatric patients with localized and systemic scleroderma.

Raoul L Wientzen, President
R. Scott Turner, MD, PhD, Program Director
Carolyn Ward, MSPH, Program Coordinator

Pennsylvania

6448 National Registry for Childhood Onset Scleroderma (NRCOS)
University of Pittsburgh School of Medicine
M240 Scaife Hall, 3550 Terrace Street
Pittsburge, PA 15261   412-383-8674
800-603-8960
e-mail: jablonj@msx.dept-med.pitt.edu
www.sctc-online.org/studies/nrcos.htm

This registry provides a unique opportunity for researchers to study a variety of aspects of scleroderma. The registry will include systemic sclerosis and various forms of localized scleroderma such as morphea, linear scleroderma, and eosinophilic fasciitis.

Jennifer Jablon, Research Coordinator
Thomas A Medsger Jr, MD, Principal Investigator

Web Sites

6449 American Autoimmune Related Diseases Association
22100 Gratiot Ave.
Eastpointe, MI 48021   586-776-3900
800-598-4668
Fax: 586-776-3903
www.aarda.org

Dedicated to the eradication of autoimmune diseases and the alleviation of suffering and the socio-economic impact of autoimmunity through fostering and facilitating collaboration in the areas of education, public awareness, research and patient services in an effective, ethical and efficient manner.

Betty Diamond, M.D., Chairperson
Virginia T. Ladd, President/ Executive Director
Patricia Barber, Asst. Director

6450 Health Answers
410 Horsham Road
Horsham, PA 19044   215-442-9010
e-mail: Michael.tague@healthanswers.com
www.healthanswers.com

HealthAnswers offers a breadth of services in medical education, sales force training, patient support solutions, professional promotion and consumer solutions.

Michael Tague, Managing Director

6451 Online Mendelian Inheritance in Man
www.omim.org

This database is a catalog of human genes and genetic disorders.

6452 Scleroderma A to Z
7455 France Ave So #266
Edina, MN 55435   952-831-3091
800-564-7099
e-mail: isn@sclero.org
www.sclero.org

Presented by the International Scleroderma Network, it has over 1000 pages of scleroderma and scleroderma related information, resources, and links in over 20 languages.

Shelley Ensz, Founder and President
Sid Strong, Vice President
Gene Ensz, Treasurer

6453 Scleroderma Foundation
300 Rosewood Drive, Suite 105
Danvers, MA 1923

978-463-5843
800-722-4673
Fax: 978-463-5809
e-mail: sfinfo@scleroderma.org
www.scleroderma.org

The national organziation for people with scleroderma and their families and friends.

Joseph Camerino, Ph.D., Chair
Carol Feghali-Bostwick, Ph.D., Vice Chair
Robert J. Riggs, Chief Executive Officer

6454 Scleroderma Message Board
disc.server.com/Indices/7571.html

An online message board about scleroderma and related conditions.

6455 Scleroderma Support
health.groups.yahoo.com/group/sclerodermasupport2/

A place where people who live with scleroderma can talk online.

Book Publishers

6456 Cooking Up A Storm for Scleroderma: Recipe s from the Scleroderma Foundation
Scleroderma Foundation
300 Rosewood Dr, Suite 105
Danvers, MA 01923

978-463-5843
800-722-4673
Fax: 978-463-5809
e-mail: info@scleroderma.org
www.scleroderma.org

Over 480 recipes contributed by the foundations members, including patients, friends and family.

6457 It's Not Just Growing Pains

Thomas J.A. Lehman, PhD, author

Oxford University Press
198 Madison Ave
New York, NY 10016

212-726-6000
800-445-9714
Fax: 919-677-1303
e-mail: custserv.us@oup.com
www.oup.com/usa

2004 Hardback
ISBN: 0-195157-28-1

6458 Let's Talk About Going to the Hospital
Rosen Publishing Group's PowerKids Press
29 E 21st Street
New York, NY 10010

212-777-3017
800-237-9932
Fax: 888-436-4643
e-mail: rosenpub@tribeca.ios.com
www.rosenpublishing.com

If a child has to check into the hospital, chances are he or she is already upset about being ill. Knowing how a hospital functions and what the procedures are, such as when family members can visit, will help in what is already a stressful situation. Grades K-5.

24 pages
ISBN: 0-823950-36-0

Roger Rosen, President

6459 Medifocus Guidebook on Scleroderma
Medifocus.com, Inc
11529 Daffodil Lane, Suite 200
Silver Spring, MD 20902

301-649-9300
800-965-3002
Fax: 301-649-7809
e-mail: info@medifocus.com
www.medifocus.com

This guidebook has four sections: an overview for patients; a guide to medical literature; research centers; and a resource and organization guide. Updates are available online for a year with purchase of the book. Also available in electronic format.

105 pages

Ovadia Abulafia, Board Member
William I. Bensinger, M.D., Board Member
Glenn D. Braunstein, M.D., Board Member

6460 Scleroderma Book (The)

Maureen Mayes, MD, author

Oxford University Press
198 Madison Ave
New York, NY 10016

212-726-6000
800-445-9714
Fax: 919-677-1303
e-mail: custserv.us@oup.com
www.oup.com/usa

2005 Hardback
ISBN: 0-195169-40-9

Magazines

6461 Scleroderma Voice
Scleroderma Foundation
300 Rosewood Dr, Suite 105
Danvers, MA 1923

978-463-5843
800-722-4673
Fax: 978-463-5809
e-mail: sfinfo@scleroderma.org
www.scleroderma.org

Includes articles and stories, answers to medical questions, updates on research and treatments, and advice on dealing with scleroderma.

Quarterly

Joseph Camerino, Ph.D., Chair
Carol Feghali-Bostwick, Ph.D., Vice Chair
Robert J. Riggs, Chief Executive Officer

Journals

6462 Scleroderma Care and Research
Scleroderma Clinical Trials Consortium
715 Albany St, E-5
Boston, MA 2118

617-638-4486
e-mail: trials@blackmule.com
www.sclero.org/medical/journals/scar/a-to-z.html

Published by a group of international scleroderma researchers, it covers topics of interest to rheumatologists and others involved in scleroderma care, worldwide.

Pamphlets

6463 Handout on Health: Scleroderma
NIAMS, National Institutes of Health
31 Center Dr, Bldg 31, Rm 4C02
Bethesda, MD 20892

301-496-8190
Fax: 301-480-2814
www.niams.nih.gov/hi

Information including current research efforts for scleroderma.

Revised 7/2006
Stephen I. Katz, M.D., Ph.D., Director
Robert H Carter, Deputy Director
Gahan Breithaupt, Ass Dir for Management & Operations

Camps

6464 Camp Discovery
American Academy of Dermatology
930 E Woodfield Road
Schaumburg, IL 60173

847-240-1737
Fax: 847-330-8907
e-mail: jmueller@aad.org
www.campdiscovery.org

A camp for young people with chronic skin conditions. There is no fee and transportation is provided. Three locations: Camp Horizon in Millville, PA, Camp Knutson in Crosslake, MN, and Camp Dermadillo in Burton, TX.

Brett M. Coldiron, MD, President
Janine Mueller, Program Coordinator
Elise A. Olsen, MD, Vice President

6465 Camp Wonder
Children's Skin Disease Foundation
712 Bancroft Rd, #511
Walnut Creek, CA 94598

925-947-3825
Fax: 866-236-6474
www.csdf.org

Established by the CSDF for young people who suffer from skin diseases. Medically staffed camps are free to children, ages 7-17 with skin diseases that are serious or life threatening.

Christine Tenconi, Vice-President
Christine Clakley, Executive Director

Description

6466 SCOLIOSIS

Synonym: Rachioscoliosis

Covers these related disorders: Compensatory scoliosis, Congenital scoliosis, Idiopathic kyphosis (Scheuermann's disease), Idiopathic scoliosis, Kyphosis, Neuromuscular scoliosis, Syndrome-associated scoliosis

Involves the following Biologic System(s):
Orthopedic and Muscle Disorders

The term scoliosis refers to a condition characterized by a sideward (lateral) curvature of the spine. Idiopathic scoliosis is the most common form of this disorder and occurs for no known reason in otherwise healthy individuals who range in age from infancy to adolescence. Adolescent scoliosis is the most common form and accounts for 80 percent of idiopathic scoliosis. Approximately 20 percent of people with scoliosis report at least one other affected family member. Therefore, in these cases, scoliosis is thought to have a genetic component. Idiopathic scoliosis that develops during infancy often corrects itself, but it may become progressive in older children. Treatment is dependent upon age and the degree of curvature progression. Mild curvatures may require little or no treatment, while more severe involvement may require surgery or the use of braces, etc. (orthotics). Although men and women are affected in about equal numbers, women are more at risk for more significant curvature progression. Girls between onset of puberty growth spurt and cessation of spinal growth are at the greatest risk for idiopathic scoliosis. Physical examination reveals asymmetry in the height of the shoulder and hip, with forward bending.

Congenital scoliosis, apparent at birth or soon thereafter, results from the improper or incomplete development of the vertebrae during the first trimester of pregnancy. This condition may appear singularly or in association with abnormalities of other systems of the body including the heart (i.e., congenital heart disease) and genitourinary tract (e.g., absence of one kidney, duplication of the tubes that carry urine, horseshoe kidney, and other malformations). Congenital scoliosis is often accompanied by other spinal cord defects (spinal dysraphism) that may range from mild to severe. In addition, children born with certain genetic disorders such as Klippel-Feil syndrome may experience associated scoliosis. The progression of the curvature is dependent upon the specific underlying vertebral malformation, its particular growth potential, and its location. About one quarter of affected children experience no progression of the curvature and, therefore, require no treatment. Approximately half of those remaining may require early treatment, such as spinal fusion of the affected area, to stop progression of the curvature.

Neuromuscular scoliosis is associated with certain childhood diseases (e.g., cerebral palsy, Duchenne muscular dystrophy, polio, and other disorders). This type of scoliosis tends to be progressive, with the degree of deformity dependent upon many factors. Those affected children who are unable to walk (nonambulatory) often develop additional skeletal irregularities involving the pelvis and spine. In severe cases, respiratory difficulties may develop. Early evaluation and intervention through surgery and other means help to alter the progression of the spinal deformity and its associated complications.

Kyphosis is characterized by an exaggerated backward curvature of the spine. Children with poor posture resulting in mild kyphosis who have no associated spinal irregularities may be treated by maintaining good posture. Congenital kyophosis, however, results from various malformations in the spinal column and may range from mild to severe deformity. Scoliosis also is present in one-third of patients with kyphosis. When several vertebrae are involved, there is a round back appearance; when only one vertebra is involved, there is an angular curve. As affected children grow, progression of the spinal abnormality may continue until growth is complete, possibly resulting in partial paralysis. Idiopathic kyphosis or Scheuermann's disease is common to both adolescent boys and girls; cause remains unknown. Examination and x-ray screening may determine whether kyphosis is postural or a result of a spinal malformation. Symptoms of Scheuermann's disease may include mild but chronic back pain and a round-shouldered appearance.

Children with mild kyphosis may be advised to refrain from strenuous activities, while those with more severe symptoms may benefit from sleeping on a very firm mattress, or using a brace or cast. Surgery is rarely indicated.

Certain syndromes (e.g., Marfan syndrome, neurofibromatosis) place affected children at risk for spinal irregularities such as scoliosis and kyphosis. Treatment for these children includes regular orthopedic examination and intervention to prevent progression of the irregularity.

Scoliosis sometimes results from unequal leg length resulting from an irregular tilt (obliquity) of the pelvis. Treatment for this compensatory scoliosis may include the use of special orthopedic shoes.

Government Agencies

6467 **NIH/National Institute of Arthritis and Mu sculoskeletal and Skin Diseases**
1AMS Circle
Bethesda, MD 20892

301-402-4484
877-226-4267
Fax: 301-718-6366
TDD: 301-565-2966
e-mail: niamsinfo@mail.nih.gov
www.niams.nih.gov

The mission of the NIAMS, a part of the NIH, is to support research into the causes, treatment, and prevention of arthritis and musculoskeletal and skin diseases, the training of basic and clinical scientists to carry out this research, and the dissemination of information on research progress in these diseases.

Stephen I Katz MD PhD, Director
Robert H Carter MD, Deputy Director
Gahan Breithaupt, Assoc Dir for Management & Operatio

National Associations & Support Groups

6468 **American Academy of Pediatrics**
141 Northwest Point Boulevard
Elk Grove Village, IL 60007

847-434-4000
800-433-9016
Fax: 847-434-8000
www.aap.org

The American Academy of Pediatrics and its member pediatricians are committed to the attainment of optimal physical, mental and social health and well-being for all infants, children, adolescents, and young adults.

Sandra Hassink, MD, FAAP, President

6469 National Dissemination Center for Children with Disabilities
1825 Connecticut Ave NW
Washington, DC 20009
202-884-8200
800-695-0285
Fax: 202-884-8441
e-mail: nichcy@fhi360.org
www.nichcy.org

A national information and referral center for families, educators and other professionals on: disabilities in children and youth; programs and services; IDEA, the nation's special education law; and research-based information on effective practices.

Suzanne Ripley, Executive Director

6470 National Scoliosis Foundation
5 Cabot Place
Stoughton, MA 02072
781-341-6333
800-673-6922
Fax: 781-341-8333
e-mail: nsf@scoliosis.org
www.scoliosis.org

Promotes school screening, offers public awareness materials to promote public education, maintains a resource center for professional information, conducts scoliosis conferences, and offers support groups to people affected by the disease.

Joseph O'Brien, President/CEO
Dennis J. Fusco, CPA, Treasurer
Laura B. Gowen, LHD, Founder & President Emeritus

6471 Scoliosis Association
PO Box 811705
Boca Raton, FL 33481
561-994-4435
800-800-0669
Fax: 561-994-2455
e-mail: scolioassn2@aol.com
www.scoliosis-assoc.org

Sponsors and encourages spinal screening programs. Disseminates information throughout the country, and raises funds for scoliosis research. Membership fee of $20.00 includes subscription to newsletter. Videos and printed information available.

Stanley Sacks, Ceo

Libraries & Resource Centers

6472 Johns Hopkins Department of Orthopaedics Surgery
601 N Caroline Street
Baltimore, MD 21287
410-955-5000
Fax: 410-955-1719
www.hopkinsinteractive.com

Scoliosis is a three-dimensional curvature of the spine, best appreciated on an anteroposterior radiograph and physical examination. Many different causes have been identified. The most common type is idiopathic scoliosis.

Claudia L Thomas

Research Centers

6473 Scoliosis Research Society
555 E Wells Street, Suite 1100
Milwaukee, WI 53202
414-289-9107
Fax: 414-276-3349
e-mail: info@srs.org
www.srs.org

An international society that is committed to research and education for health care professionals in the field of spinal deformities. It is recognized as one of the world's premier spine societies. Current membership includes over 1000 of the world's leading spine surgeons as well as researchers, physician assistants and orthotists.

Tressa Goulding, Executive Director
Kamal N. Ibrahim, MD, FRCS(C), MA, President
John P. Dormans, MD, Vice President

6474 Shriners Hospital for Children
Headquarters
2900 Rocky Point Drive
Tampa, FL 33607
813-281-0300
800-237-5055
Fax: 813-281-8113
e-mail: patientreferrals@shrinenet.org
www.shrinershospitalsforchildren.org/

Shrine's official philanthropy is Shriners Hospital for Children, a network of 22 hospitals that provide expert, no-cost orthopaedic and burn care to children under 18.

Alan W. Madsen, Chairman of the Board
John McCabe, Executive Vice President
Kenneth Guidera, M.D., Chief Medical Officer

Audio Video

6475 Cutting Edge Medical Report
National Scoliosis Foundation
5 Cabot Place
Stoughton, MA 2072
781-341-6333
800-673-6922
Fax: 781-341-8333
e-mail: nsf@scoliosis.org
www.scoliosis.org

As seen on the Discovery Channel, this video is an in-depth examination of the latest developments in the diagnosis and treatment of scoliosis.

18 Minutes

6476 Dealing with Scoliosis: A Patient Guide to Diagnosis and Treatment
National Scoliosis Foundation
5 Cabot Place
Stoughton, MA 2072
781-341-6333
800-673-6922
Fax: 781-341-8333
e-mail: nsf@scoliosis.org
www.scoliosis.org

An upbeat video featuring Miss North Carolina Michelle Mauney and that explains diagnosis and treatment of scoliosis through the experience of several teenagers and young adults.

20 Minutes

6477 Ellie's Back
National Scoliosis Foundation
5 Cabot Place
Stoughton, MA 2072
781-341-6333
800-673-6922
Fax: 781-341-8333
e-mail: nsf@scoliosis.org
www.scoliosis.org

An eight-year-old, and her mother team up together to produce a film that portrays life with scoliosis through the eyes of a young child.

15 Minutes

6478 Growing Straighter and Stronger
National Scoliosis Foundation
5 Cabot Place
Stoughton, MA 2072
781-341-6333
800-673-6922
Fax: 781-341-8333
e-mail: nsf@scoliosis.org
www.scoliosis.org

Produced for the pre-screening education of students in grades 5-9. It emphasizes the importance of follow-up screening, encourages peer support and prescribed follow-up treatment. Video is also available on loan for a refundable deposit plus shipping and handling.

15 Minutes

6479 Preparing Yourself for Spinal Surgery (For Teenagers with Severe Scoliosis)
National Scoliosis Foundation
5 Cabot Place
Stoughton, MA 2072
781-341-6333
800-673-6922
Fax: 781-341-8333
e-mail: nsf@scoliosis.org
www.scoliosis.org

Patient educational video helping to reduce the anxiety for teenagers facing surgery by giving a sense of what to expect before, during, and after surgery.

18 Minutes

6480 School Screening with Dr. Robert Keller
National Scoliosis Foundation
5 Cabot Place
Stoughton, MA 2072
781-341-6333
800-673-6922
Fax: 781-341-8333
e-mail: nsf@scoliosis.org
www.scoliosis.org

A training video that teaches the proper technique for doing spinal screening. Defines scoliosis and kyphosis. Four teenagers, three with curves and one without, are examined and the findings explained.

60 Minutes

6481 Sharing Scoliosis: You're Not Alone
National Scoliosis Foundation
5 Cabot Place
Stoughton, MA 2072
781-341-6333
800-673-6922
Fax: 781-341-8333
e-mail: nsf@scoliosis.org
www.scoliosis.org

The Missouri chapter of the NSF, shares their experience with scoliosis including diagnosis, wearing a brace, surgery, and recovery. It is a good source of support for patients of all ages and their families.

26 Minutes

6482 Taking the Mystery Out of Spinal Deformities
Children's Hospital of LA, Div. of Orthopaedics
4650 Sunset Boulevard
Los Angeles, CA 90027
323-660-2450
888-631-2452
www.childrenshospitalla.org

Answers questions most often asked by screeners, patients and parents.

Videotape

Richard D. Cordova, FACHE, President/ CEO
Rodney B. Hanners, SVP/ COO
Barry L. Mangels, MS, CPHRM, Chief Compliance & Privacy Officer

6483 Understanding Scoliosis
National Scoliosis Foundation
5 Cabot Place
Stoughton, MA 2072
781-341-6333
800-673-6922
Fax: 781-341-8333
e-mail: nsf@scoliosis.org
www.scoliosis.org

A Kaiser Permanente educational video that clearly and positively addresses the patient community. In this video four teenagers at various stages of treatment talk about their life with scoliosis.

8 Minutes

6484 What's This Thing Called Scoliosis
Dr Charles Ray, author

National Scoliosis Foundation
5 Cabot Place
Stoughton, MA 2072
781-341-6333
800-673-6922
Fax: 781-341-8333
e-mail: nsf@scoliosis.org
www.scoliosis.org

A comprehensive overview of scoliosis using the latest computer technology. The anatomical spine and animated model work together to truly show the 3D aspects of scoliosis and the corresponding impact on the patient.

17 Minutes

Web Sites

6485 American Academy of Orthopaedic Surgeons
9400 West Higgins Road
Rosemont, IL 60018
847-823-7186
Fax: 847-823-8125
e-mail: custserv@aaos.org
www.aaos.org

Provides an informational fact sheet on scoliosis in children and adolescents.

Frederick M Azar, MD, President
Karen L. Hackett, FACHE, CAE, Chief Executive Officer
William Bruce, Chief Technology Officer

6486 Health Answers
410 Horsham Road
Horsham, PA 19044
215-442-9010
e-mail: Michael.tague@healthanswers.com
www.healthanswers.com

HealthAnswers offers a breadth of services in medical education, sales force training, patient support solutions, professional promotion and consumer solutions.

Michael Tague, Managing Director

6487 John Hopkins Department of Orthopaedics Surgery
601 N. Caroline Street, JHOC #5215
Baltimore, MD 21287
443-997-2663
e-mail: hopkinsortho@jhmi.edu
www.hopkinsmedicine.org/orthopedicsurgery/

The orthopaedics faculty works together as a team to provide optimum patient care, seeking out a role in patient care as both educators and treating physicians working together with you and your community health care providers to offer you the best possible medical and surgical care available.

6488 Natalie's Brace
www.nataliesbrace.com/scoliosis/

Personal website offering personal details and photos on scoliosis braces, general information and support.

6489 North Ameerican Spine Society
7075 Veterans Blvd.
Burr Ridge, IL 60527
630-230-3600
www.spine.org

Provides information on adolescent idiopathic scoliosis, including a description of, common problems associated with the curvature, and possible treatments.

Heidi Prather, DO, President
Christopher Bono, MD, First Vice President
Eric Muehlbauer, Executive Director

6490 Online Mendelian Inheritance in Man
www.omim.org

This database is a catalog of human genes and genetic disorders.

6491 Scoliosis Help
www.scoliosishelp.org

6492 Scoliosis Message Forum
www.scoliosis.org/forum/index.php

e-mail: jpobrien@scoliosis.org
www.scoliosis.org/forum/index.php

An independent list maintained by people who have scoliosis. You can find people with whom you can share your experiences and ask questions.

6493 Scoliosis Research Society
555 East Wells Street, Suite 1100
Milwaukee, WI 53202

414-289-9107
Fax: 414-276-3349
e-mail: info@srs.org
www.srs.org

An international society that is committed to research and education for health care professionals in the field of spinal deformities. It is recognized as one of the world's premier spine societies. Current membership includes over 1000 of the world's leading spine surgeons as well as researchers, physician assistants and orthotists.

John P. Dormans, MD, President
Tressa Goulding, CAE, CMP, Executive Director
Ashtin Neuschaefer, Administrative Manager

6494 Wheeless' Textbook of Orthopaedics
www.wheelessonline.com

Derives from a variety of sources, including journals, articles, national meetings lectures and other textbooks.

Clifford R. Wheeless III, MD, Editor-in-Chief
James A. Nunley, II, MD, Managing Editor
James R. Urbaniak, MD, Managing Editor

Book Publishers

6495 Deenie
Simon & Schuster/Atheneum Books
100 Front Street
Riverside, NJ 08075

856-461-6500
800-488-4308
Fax: 800-943-9831
www.simonandschuster.com

Deenie, a beautiful thirteen-year-old girl, had a mother who was pushing her to become a model. The agency representatives told Deenie she had the looks but walked differently. Deenie's main wish was to become a cheerleader. Her close friend, Janet, made the cheerleading squad but Deenie didn't make the finalist list. After this her gym teacher noticed her posture and called her family. After seeing therapists, the diagnosis of adolescent idiopathic scoliosis was made.

159 pages Hardcover
ISBN: 0-689866-10-0

Carolyn Reidy, President/CEO
Liz Perl, Senior Vice President, Marketing
Dennis Eulau, Executive Vice President, Operation

6496 Getting Ready, Getting Well
Mary Knapp, author

National Scoliosis Foundation
5 Cabot Place
Stoughton, MA 02072

781-341-6333
800-673-6922
Fax: 781-341-8333
e-mail: nsf@scoliosis.org
www.scoliosis.org

A guide for those anticipating surgery; divided into three sections: Making Up Your Mind, Taking Charge, and Home Again.

73 pages

Laura B. Gowen, Founder & President
W.Hugh M. Morton, Chairman
Joseph P. O'Brien, President & CEO

6497 Growing Up with Scoliosis: A Young Girl's Story
Michelle Spray, author

National Scoliosis Foundation
5 Cabot Place
Stoughton, MA 02072

781-341-6333
800-673-6922
Fax: 781-341-8333
e-mail: nsf@scoliosis.org
www.scoliosis.org

A personal account of growing up with scoliosis and the different stages of treatment, progression and surgery.

Laura B. Gowen, Founder & President
W.Hugh M. Morton, Chairman
Joseph P. O'Brien, President & CEO

6498 Handbook of Scoliosis
Scoliosis Research Society
555 East Wells Street, Suite 1100
Milwaukee, WI 53202

414-289-9107
Fax: 414-276-3349
e-mail: info@srs.org
www.srs.org

Kamal N. Ibrahim, MD, President
John P. Dormans, MD, Vice President
Hubert Labelle, MD, Secretary

6499 Nothing Hurts But My Heart
Linda Barr, author

National Scoliosis Foundation
5 Cabot Place
Stoughton, MA 02072

781-341-6333
800-673-6922
Fax: 781-341-8333
e-mail: nsf@scoliosis.org
www.scoliosis.org

For every boy, girl, and their parents who learn that bracing may be needed to treat their scoliosis. The story is of a young gymnast dealing with the issues of wearing a brace.

Laura B. Gowen, Founder & President
W.Hugh M. Morton, Chairman
Joseph P. O'Brien, President & CEO

6500 Scoliosis Surgery, The Definitive Patient' s Reference: Second Edition
Dave Wolpert, author

National Scoliosis Foundation
5 Cabot Place
Stoughton, MA 02072

781-341-6333
800-673-6922
Fax: 781-341-8333
e-mail: nsf@scoliosis.org
www.scoliosis.org

For all those contemplating surgery or that know someone who is; it explains in detail everything you need to know, written in layman's terms by someone who has gone through it.

Laura B. Gowen, Founder & President
W.Hugh M. Morton, Chairman
Joseph P. O'Brien, President & CEO

6501 Scoliosis: What Young People and Parents N eed to Know
American Physical Therapy Association
1111 N Fairfax Street
Alexandria, VA 22314

703-684-2782
800-999-2782
Fax: 703-706-8556
TDD: 703-683-6748
www.apta.org

A physical therapist's perspective about what scoliosis is and what parents and young people should look for to detect scoliosis. Also available in Spanish.

12 pages Packet of 25

Paul Rocker, President
Sharon l. Dunn, Vice President
Laurita M. Hack, Secretary

6502 Stopping Scoliosis

Nancy Schommer, author

National Scoliosis Foundation
5 Cabot Place
Stoughton, MA 02072

781-341-6333
800-673-6922
Fax: 781-341-8333
e-mail: nsf@scoliosis.org
www.scoliosis.org

Filled with accurate, currently researched information for adults concerned with their condition or that of a young person.

Laura B. Gowen, Founder & President
W.Hugh M. Morton, Chairman
Joseph P. O'Brien, President & CEO

6503 There's an S on My Back: S is for Scoliosi s

Mary Mahony, author

National Scoliosis Foundation
5 Cabot Place
Stoughton, MA 02072

781-341-6333
800-673-6922
Fax: 781-341-8333
e-mail: nsf@scoliosis.org
www.scoliosis.org

The medical journey of a fifth grader diagnosed with idiopathic scoliosis at a school screening. A realistic fiction, the story gives us a day-by-day account of what a preadolescent experiences.

Laura B. Gowen, Founder & President
W.Hugh M. Morton, Chairman
Joseph P. O'Brien, President & CEO

6504 Twenty Years At Hull House

Jane Addams, author

New American Library/Penguin Group
375 Hudson Street
New York, NY 10014

212-366-2372
Fax: 212-366-2933
e-mail: online@us.penguingroup.com
us.penguingroup.com

336 pages
ISBN: 0-451527-39-4
John Makinson, CHAIRMAN
Coram Williams, CFO
David Shanks, CEO

6505 What Can I Give You?

Mary Mahony, author

National Scoliosis Foundation
5 Cabot Place
Stoughton, MA 02072

781-341-6333
800-673-6922
Fax: 781-341-8333
e-mail: nsf@scoliosis.org
www.scoliosis.org

A wounderful story of a loving mother's care for her daughter. The medical saga of Erin and Mary offers insight and inspiration to families living with congenital scoliosis and valuable guidance to the physicians who treat them.

Laura B. Gowen, Founder & President
W.Hugh M. Morton, Chairman
Joseph P. O'Brien, President & CEO

Newsletters

6506 Backtalk

Scoliosis Association
PO Box 811705
Boca Raton, FL 33481

561-994-4435
Fax: 561-994-2455
e-mail: normlipin@aol.com
www.scoliosis-assoc.org

Information for families, patients and health care professionals. Includes a section for pen pals, an Ask the Doctor column, and a highlighted personal story.
3-4/yr

6507 Spinal Connection

National Scoliosis Foundation
5 Cabot Place
Stoughton, MA 2072

781-341-6333
800-673-6922
Fax: 781-341-8333
e-mail: nsf@scoliosis.org
www.scoliosis.org

Offers updated information, the latest medical advances, and new research studies in the area of abnormal spinal curvatures.
8 pages Bi-annual

Pamphlets

6508 1 in Every 10 Persons Has Scoliosis

National Scoliosis Foundation
5 Cabot Place
Stoughton, MA 2072

781-341-6333
800-673-6922
Fax: 781-341-8333
e-mail: nsf@scoliosis.org
www.scoliosis.org

Explains what scoliosis is and illustrates how to screen for it. It also contains facts about the Foundation.

6509 Adolescent Idiopathic Scoliosis-Prevalence ,Natural History, Treatments

National Scoliosis Foundation
5 Cabot Place
Stoughton, MA 2072

781-341-6333
800-673-6922
Fax: 781-341-8333
e-mail: nsf@scoliosis.org
www.scoliosis.org

6510 Boston Bracing System for Idiopathic Scoli osis

National Scoliosis Foundation
5 Cabot Place
Stoughton, MA 2072

781-341-6333
800-673-6922
Fax: 781-341-8333
e-mail: nsf@scoliosis.org
www.scoliosis.org

6511 Brace & Her Brace is No Handicap

National Scoliosis Foundation
5 Cabot Place
Stoughton, MA 2072

781-341-6333
800-673-6922
Fax: 781-341-8333
e-mail: nsf@scoliosis.org
www.scoliosis.org

Contains two illustrated short stories, each about a teenage girl coping successfully with scoliosis.

6512 Getting a Second Opinion

National Scoliosis Foundation
5 Cabot Place
Stoughton, MA 2072

781-341-6333
800-673-6922
Fax: 781-341-8333
e-mail: nsf@scoliosis.org
www.scoliosis.org

Reprinted from Health Tips.

6513 Medical Update Column
National Scoliosis Foundation
5 Cabot Place
Stoughton, MA 2072

781-341-6333
800-673-6922
Fax: 781-341-8333
e-mail: nsf@scoliosis.org
www.scoliosis.org

Reprints from past issues of the Spinal Connections Medical Update Column available on various topics.

6514 NSF Packets
National Scoliosis Foundation
5 Cabot Place
Stoughton, MA 2072

781-341-6333
800-673-6922
Fax: 781-341-8333
e-mail: nsf@scoliosis.org
www.scoliosis.org

Packet contains information for parents and young people, adults, and health care professionals.

6515 Postural Screening Program
National Scoliosis Foundation
5 Cabot Place
Stoughton, MA 2072

781-341-6333
800-673-6922
Fax: 781-341-8333
e-mail: nsf@scoliosis.org
www.scoliosis.org

Guidelines for physicians and school nurses.

6516 Questions Most Often Asked the NSF
National Scoliosis Foundation
5 Cabot Place
Stoughton, MA 2072

781-341-6333
800-673-6922
Fax: 781-341-8333
e-mail: nsf@scoliosis.org
www.scoliosis.org

Answers the most frequently asked questions about scoliosis and the foundation in general.

6517 Questions and Answers About Scoliosis
Federal Citizen Information Center
Pueblo, CO 81009

719-295-2675
888-878-3256
e-mail: pueblo@gpo.gov
publications.usa.gov/USAPubs.php

6518 Scoliosis and Kyphosis
Scoliosis Research Society
555 East Wells Street, Suite 1100
Milwaukee, WI 53202

414-289-9107
Fax: 414-276-3349
e-mail: info@srs.org
www.srs.org

Information and advice from parents.

John P. Dormans, MD, President
Tressa Goulding, CAE, CMP, Executive Director
Ashtin Neuschaefer, Administrative Manager

6519 Scoliosis: A Handbook for Patients
National Scoliosis Foundation
5 Cabot Place
Stoughton, MA 2072

781-341-6333
800-673-6922
Fax: 781-341-8333
e-mail: nsf@scoliosis.org
www.scoliosis.org

Information on detection and treatment of adolescent scoliosis, kyphosis and lordosis and adult scoliosis.

6520 When the Spine Curves
National Scoliosis Foundation
5 Cabot Place
Stoughton, MA 2072

781-341-6333
800-673-6922
Fax: 781-341-8333
e-mail: nsf@scoliosis.org
www.scoliosis.org

Camps

6521 Hemlocks Easter Seals Recreation
85 Jones Street
Hebron, CT 6248

860-228-9496
800-832-4409
Fax: 860-228-2091
e-mail: info@eastersealscamphemlocks.org
www.eastersealscamphemlocks.org

Accepts campers, ages 6 and under, whose major disability is orthopedic. First preference is given to Connecticut residents. A computer camp is also available.

Carl Larson

Description

6522 SEIZURES

Synonyms: Convulsions, Epilepsy

Covers these related disorders: Absence (petit mal) seizures, Complex partial seizures, Generalized (grand mal) tonic-clonic seizures, Simple partial seizures, Epilepsy

Involves the following Biologic System(s):

Neurologic Disorders

Seizures are a neurologic condition characterized by sudden episodes of uncontrolled electrical activity in the brain. These electrical disturbances may cause abnormal motor activities, lost or impaired consciousness, impaired control of certain involuntary functions (autonomic dysfunction), or sensory or behavioral abnormalities. Seizures are a common neurologic condition of childhood, affecting approximately six in 1,000 children. Approximately 70 percent of children who experience one seizure never experience another, whereas about 30 percent develop recurring seizures, which is referred to as epilepsy. Seizures may result from many different causes, including fever, head injury, infection or inflammation of the brain, insufficient oxygen supply to the brain, or certain metabolic imbalances. Seizures may also be caused by brain tumors, particular degenerative metabolic or neurological diseases, abnormal reactions to certain medications, or drug intoxication. There are also a number of syndromes and genetic disorders in which seizures are a primary feature. In many children, the exact underlying cause of recurrent seizures cannot be determined and the disorder is termed idiopathic epilepsy.

The specific form that a seizure takes and its associated symptoms may depend upon a number of factors, including the region of the brain in which the electrical disturbance arises and how widely it spreads from its point of origin. Epileptic seizures may be broadly classified into two groups: partial and generalized seizures. Partial seizures often result due to damage or impairment of a limited area of the brain, whereas generalized seizures may affect a wide area of the brain. In addition, some partial seizures may begin in a particular brain region but spread to affect most of the brain, ultimately becoming a generalized seizure. Because different seizure types may cause similar symptoms, specialized techniques that record brain wave activity (electroencephalography or EEG) and other neurologic imaging tests (such as MRI or CT scans) may play an important role in classifying certain seizure disorders.

Partial seizures, which may account for up to 40 percent of childhood seizures, may be subdivided into simple partial seizures, during which consciousness is retained, and complex partial seizures, during which consciousness is impaired. Simple partial seizures are characterized by abnormal, rhythmic muscle contractions and relaxations (clonic activity) and increased muscle tone and rigidity (tonic activity), particularly affecting muscles of the neck, face, arms, and legs. Simple partial seizures, which usually last about 10 to 20 seconds, are frequently associated with abnormal eye movements and head turning. In many children, simple partial seizures may be preceded by an aura consisting of headache, chest discomfort, and a feeling of anxiety, fear, or dread.

Complex partial seizures are characterized by a sudden pause in activity and a blank stare and may be preceded by an aura that consists of a vague feeling of fear or unpleasantness, headache, and chest discomfort. Most patients also perform certain involuntary actions following loss of consciousness. In infants, such actions may include lip smacking, swallowing, or chewing, whereas older children may conduct incoordinated, semipurposeful actions, such as rubbing objects or pulling at clothing. Such seizures may last approximately one to two minutes.

Generalized seizures may be subdivided into nonconvulsive (petit mal, absence) seizures and convulsive (grand mal or tonic-clonic) seizures. Absence seizures, which rarely occur before the age of five, usually last from a few seconds up to half a minute. During an episode, children experience a momentary loss of consciousness during which they cease speaking or performing other motor activities. They typically have a blank facial expression, their eyelids may flicker, and the head may fall forward. Patients typically have no awareness of the episode and resume the activity they were performing before the seizure.

Generalized tonic-clonic seizures may be preceded by an aura and occasionally begin with a shrill cry as patients lose consciousness. During an episode, the eyes roll back, muscles of the entire body stiffen, and all muscle groups begin to rhythmically contract and relax. If temporary cessation of breathing (apnea) occurs, patients may quickly develop an abnormal, bluish discoloration of the skin and mucous membranes (cyanosis). Bladder and bowel control may be temporarily lost. After an episode, patients are typically semiconscious and disoriented and may remain in a deep sleep for up to two hours (postictal state). During such a seizure episode, patients should be placed on one side, tight clothing around the neck should be loosened, and the jaw should be gently extended to enhance breathing. However, the mouth should not be forcibly opened nor should an object be placed between the teeth.

Generalized seizures also include a form of epilepsy known as infantile spasms, which typically begin between the ages of four and eight months and continue to approximately 18 months. Infantile spasms are characterized by sudden, brief, symmetric contractions of the arms and legs, neck, and torso. Spasms may occur for several minutes with brief intervals between each spasm. Episodes tend to occur when children are drowsy or immediately upon awakening. Depending upon the underlying cause, the condition may evolve into different forms of epilepsy later in life and may be associated with an increased risk of mental retardation.

Seizures that occur in association with a rapidly rising fever, known as febrile seizures, are the most common seizure disorder of childhood. Febrile seizures most commonly occur between nine months to five years of age and may affect up to four percent of all children. This type of seizure rarely develops into epilepsy. In many cases, there is a history of such seizures among siblings and parents, indicating that genetic factors may play some causative role. Febrile seizures often occur in association with certain upper respiratory infections and acute inflammation of the middle ear (otitis media). However, because convulsions may result from serious infections of the brain (e.g., meningitis), a thorough medical evaluation must be conducted to determine the cause of the fever. Febrile seizures are typically characterized by muscle rigidity followed by abnormal, rhythmic contractions and relaxations of muscle groups (generalized tonic-clonic seizures). The seizure may last from seconds up to about 10 minutes and is often followed by a brief period of drowsiness.

Generalized or partial seizures that continue for more than 30 minutes without a return to consciousness are known as status epilepticus. Such seizures may occur due to underlying metabolic abnormalities, neurologic disorders, congenital brain malformations, or inflammation of the brain. They may also represent prolonged febrile seizures, develop due to sudden withdrawal of antiseizure (anticonvulsant) medication, or result from unknown causes. Status epilepticus may result in life-threatening complications and is considered a medical emergency, requiring hospitalization. Treatment may include supplemental oxygen, intravenous fluids, physical and neurologic evaluations, intravenous medications including appropriate antiseizure drugs, and other measures as required. Children affected by the condition before one year of age are more likely to have mental retardation and other long-term effects, secondary to an underlying CNS disorder.

The treatment of seizures depends on the underlying cause, the type of seizure present, and other factors. If a treatable condition or disorder is identified, such as a fever, abnormal blood sugar levels, or certain tumors, measures are taken as required to treat the underlying cause. For example, in the case of febrile seizures, thorough evaluations are conducted to determine the fever's cause and measures are then taken as necessary to control the fever. If an underlying cause cannot be identified or adequately treated or controlled, treatment typically includes the administration of antiseizure (anticonvulsant) medications to help prevent, reduce, or control seizures. The specific anticonvulsant medication prescribed may depend on several factors, including the classification of the seizure, patient history, and possible side effects. Anticonvulsant drugs used to treat certain types of seizures may include carbamazepine, phenobarbital, primidone, phenytoin, gabapentin, or valproate. In addition, adrenocorticotropic hormone (ACTH) is often used to treat children with infantile spasms. If seizure control is not obtained with a particular medication, other anticonvulsants may be substituted. In some patients, combination drug therapy may be necessary to adequately control seizures. If seizure control is not obtained with anticonvulsant medications, surgery may be considered. Additional treatment is symptomatic and supportive.

National Associations & Support Groups

6523 American Academy of Pediatrics
141 Northwest Point Boulevard
Elk Grove Village, IL 60007

847-434-4000
800-433-9016
Fax: 847-434-8000
www.aap.org

The American Academy of Pediatrics and its member pediatricians are committed to the attainment of optimal physical, mental and social health and well-being for all infants, children, adolescents, and young adults.

Sandra Hassink, MD, FAAP, President

6524 American Epilepsy Society
342 N Main Street
W Hartford, CT 06117

860-586-7505
Fax: 860-568-7550
www.aesnet.org

A society of clinicians, researchers, and health care professionals which promotes education and research of epilepsy.

M. Suzanne C. Berry, MBA, CAE, Executive Director
Jacqueline A. French, M.D., President
Elson So, M.D., Vice President

6525 Cleveland Clinic Children's Hospital & Epilepsy Center
9500 Euclid Avenue
Cleveland, OH 44195

216-445-8585
800-223-2273
Fax: 216-445-7792
TTY: 216-444-0261
cms.clevelandclinic.org/childrenshospital/

Provides innovative care for infants, children, and adolescents with complex medical problems. Includes medical, surgical, rehabilitation, psychiatric and intensive care, latest technology, including a computerized epilepsy monitoring unit, a consolidated pediatric intensive care unit and operating suites. Physicians are known for their expertise in treating major medical problems, such as cardiovascular disease, cancer, digestive disorders, musculoskeletal problems and neurosensory disorders.

Gene Altus, Executive Director
Prakash Kotagal MD, Pediatric Epilepsy Head

6526 Epilepsy Foundation
8301 Professional Place
Landover, MD 20785

301-459-3700
800-332-1000
Fax: 301-459-1569
e-mail: ContactUs@efa.org
www.epilepsyfoundation.org

A national, charitable, nonprofit, volunteer agency dedicated to the welfare of people with epilepsy and their families. Its goals are the prevention and cure of seizure disorders, the alleviation of their effects, and the promotion of independence and optimal quality of life for people who have these disorders. The organization offers education, advocacy, service and research support groups, and has a network of local affiliates serving nearly 100 communities.

Phil Gattone, President/CEO
Ty Broadway, Director Web Design and Development
Dawn Leeks, Program Coordinator

6527 Epilepsy Institute
65 Broadway, Ste. 505
New York, NY 10006

212-677-8550
Fax: 212-677-5825
e-mail: info@efmny.org
www.epilepsyinstitute.org

Program services are available to residents of NYC and Westchester County. The institute is a nonprofit social service organization with information available in Spanish, French, Chinese and Russian.

Pamela Conford, Executive Director

6528 FACES: Finding a Cure for Epilepsy & Seizures
223 East 34th Street
New York, NY 10016

646-558-0900
Fax: 646-385-7163
e-mail: FACESinfo@nyumc.org
www.nyufaces.org

Nonprofit organization affiliated with NYU Medical Center and its Comprehensive Epilepsy Center. It strives to accomplish its mission through research, clinical programs, awareness, and community education and events.

Orrin Devinsky, MD, Founder
Orrin Devinsky, MD, Chair
Pamela B. Mohr, Executive Director

6529 Genetic Alliance
4301 Connecticut Avenue NW, Suite 404
Washington, DC 20008

202-966-5557
800-336-4363
Fax: 202-966-8553
e-mail: info@geneticalliance.org
www.geneticalliance.org

A coalition of voluntary genetic support groups, consumers and professionals addressing the needs of individuals and families affected by genetic disorders from a national perspective.

Sharon Terry, MA, President/CEO
Natasha Bonhomme, Vice President of Strategic Develop
Vaughn Edelson, Assistant Director of Health Commun

6530 National Association of Epilepsy Centers
5775 Wayzata Blvd, Suite 200
Washington, DC 20024
202-484-1100
888-525-6232
Fax: 202-484-1244
e-mail: info@naec-epilepsy.org
www.naecepilepsy.org

A nonprofit organization that encourages and supports professional and technical education in the treatment of epilepsy. Over 120 centers nationwide are members of the trade association, which will make referrals to its member centers.

Robert J Gumnit, MD, President
Gregory L Barkley MD, VP

6531 Parents Against Childhood Epilepsy (PACE)
7 E 85th St, Suite A3
New York, NY 10028
212-327-3070
Fax: 212-327-3075
e-mail: pacenyemail@aol.com
www.paceusa.org

Research and education fund for severe seizure disorders and epilepsy.

Susan Fahey, Manager
Lauren Beck, President
Elizabeth Aquino, VP

State Agencies & Support Groups

Arkansas

6532 Epilepsy Education Association of Arkansas
2902 E Kiehl, Suite 1B
Sherwood, AR 72120
501-833-8680
e-mail: sharon@epilepsyarkansas.com
www.epilepsyarkansas.com

A resource and provider of support and education in Arkansas for those with epilepsy.

Sharon Wingo McGinn, Director
Judy Hess RN, Co-Director

California

6533 Epilepsy Foundation of Northern California
155 Montgomery Street, Suite 309
San Francisco, CA 94104
415-677-4011
800-632-3532
Fax: 415-677-4190
e-mail: tiffany@epilepsynorcal.org
www.epilepsynorcal.org

Nonprofit center serving families affected by epilepsy since 1953.

Katherine Keeney, President
Mary Cascino, Program Manager
Tiffany Manning, Events and Communications Manager

Florida

6534 Epilepsy Association of the Big Bend
1215 Lee Ave, Suite M-4
Tallahassee, FL 32303
850-222-1777
866-778-4583
Fax: 850-222-7440
e-mail: epilepsyassoc@embarqmail.com
www.epilepsyassoc.org

Services include: case management, prevention education, counseling and advocacy, information and referral.

Scott Mehle, Executive Director

6535 Epilepsy Foundation of Florida
1200 NW 78 Ave, Suite 400
Miami, FL 33126
305-670-4949
877-553-7453
Fax: 305-670-0904
www.epilepsyfla.org

The Epilepsy Foundation of Florida (EFOF) leads the fight to stop seizures, find a cure, and overcome challenges created by epilepsy.

Karen Basha Egozi, CEO
Ivonne Anton, VP Director of Operations
Jesus Barraque, Director of Finance

6536 Florida Epilepsy Services Providers Associ ation
11200 NW 8th Avenue
Gainesville, FL 32601
352-392-6449
800-330-9746
Fax: 352-392-5792
e-mail: fespa@floridaepilepsy.org
www.floridaepilepsy.org

A nonprofit membership organization of epilepsy services providers in the state of Florida, that serve the needs of those with epilepsy and their families. Local offices for services can be found for different regions and counties of Florida.

Jim Lyons, Program Director

New Jersey

6537 Epilepsy Foundation New Jersey
1 AAA Drive, Suite 203
Trenton, NJ 08691
609-392-4900
800-336-5843
Fax: 609-392-5621
TDD: 800-852-7899
e-mail: aracioppi@efnj.com
www.efnj.com

A nonprofit organization providing support services for those with seizure disorders and their families.

Eric M Joice, Executive Director
Liza Grundell, Deputy Director
Jessica Goldsmith Barzilay, Assistant Director

New York

6538 Chrissy & Friends
930 Willowbrook Rd
Staten Island, NY 10302
718-698-1800
e-mail: info@chrissyandfriends.org
www.chrissyandfriends.org

Offers children with epilepsy an opportunity to develop friendships through a variety of activities and tutoring programs.

RoseAnne DeRenzo, President
RoseAnne Zielechowski, VP
Joan DeRenzo, Secretary

6539 Epilepsy Foundation of Long Island
506 Stewart Avenue
Garden City, NY 11530
516-739-7733
888-672-7154
Fax: 516-739-1860
e-mail: info@efli.org
www.efli.org

The Epilepsy Foundation of Long Island was founded in 1953 by a small group of parents who were determined to see their children lead productive and satisfying lives.

Jeffrey L. Nagel, President
Henry E. Klosowski, Vice President
Robert C. Creighton, Secretary

Pennsylvania

6540 Epilepsy Foundation Eastern Pennsylvania
919 Walnut Street, Suite 700
Philadelphia, PA 19107   215-629-5003
                                      800-887-7165
                                  Fax: 215-629-4997
                             e-mail: efepa@efepa.org
                                       www.efepa.org

The mission of the EPEA is to lead the fight to stop seizures, find a cure and overcome challenges created by epilepsy. They choose to fulfill the mission by meeting the non-medical needs for people affected by epilepsy/seizure disorder to enhance their lives and build supportive communities.

Frank Kotulka, Board President
Allison McCartin, Executive Director
Sue Livingston, Education Coordinator

6541 Epilepsy Foundation Western/Central Pennsy lvania
1501 Reedsdale Street, Suite 3002
Pitsburgh, PA 15219   412-261-5880
                                       800-316-5585
                                  Fax: 412-322-7885
                              e-mail: staff@efwp.org
                                        www.efwp.org

The EFWCP is a private, non-profit service organization providing public education and supportive services to individuals and families affected by epilepsy/seizure disorders. The mission is to lead the fight to stop seizures, find a cure and overcome challenges created by epilepsy.

Judith K. Painter, Executive Director
Peggy Beem, Associate Director
Colleen K Fulkerson, Special Events Coordinator

Washington

6542 Epilepsy Foundation Northwest
2311 N. 45th St., #134
Seattle, WA 98103   206-547-4551
                                       800-752-3509
                                  Fax: 206-547-4557
                          e-mail: mail@epilepsynw.org
                                    www.epilepsynw.org

Serves all of Oregon & Washington.

Michael Reeves, Chair
Brent Herrmann, President/CEO
Rose Cain, Administrative Assistant

Libraries & Resource Centers

6543 EFWCP Resource Library
Epilepsy Foundation Western/Central Pennsylvania
1501 Reedsdale Street, Suite 3002
Pitsburgh, PA 15233   412-322-5880
                                       800-361-5585
                                  Fax: 412-322-7885
                              e-mail: staff@efwp.org
                                        www.efwp.org

For people with epilepsy and their families, comprehensive information on the disorder is often a valuable, yet hard-to-find asset. Living with epilepsy often requires special services to help better understand what epilepsy is and to learn how to deal with it. EFWCP can provide information beyond what is available in physician offices and in most cases the public library. The EFWCP maintains an Epilepsy Resource Library of brochures, books, reference manuals, videos and professional articles.

Judith Painter, Executive Director
Peggy Beem, Associate Director
Colleen K Fulkerson, Special Events Coordinator

Research Centers

California

6544 EpiCenter
University of California, Irvine
Irvine, CA 92697   949-824-5011
             www.ucihs.uci.edu/epilepsyresearch/index.htm

Researchers, scientists and physicians studying the mechanisms and consequences of epilepsies through a variety of scientific approaches and research.

Tallie Z Baram, Chair

Illinois

6545 Citizens United for Research in Epilepsy (CURE)
223 W. Erie, Suite 2SW
Chicago, IL 60654   312-255-1801
                                       800-765-7118
                                  Fax: 312-255-1809
                        e-mail: info@CUREepilepsy.org
                                   www.cureepilepsy.org

Citizens United for Research in Epilepsy is a nonprofit organization dedicated to finding a cure for epilepsy by raising funds for research and by increasing awareness of the prevalence and devastation of this disease.

Susan Axelrod, Chair
Bogdan Ewendt, Executive Director
Samantha Kreindel, Director of Communications

Maryland

6546 Epilepsy Research Laboratory, Department o f Neurology
Johns Hopkins University
Meyer 2-147, 600 N Wolfe St
Baltimore, MD 21287   410-276-8560
                                  Fax: 410-563-0559
                           e-mail: pfranasz@jhimi.edu
                               www.erl.neuro.jhmi.edu/

The Epilepsy Center evaluates and cares for seizure disorder patients from pediatric through adult.

Gregory K. Bergey, M.D., Professor/Director Epilepsy Center/
Christophe Jouny, Ph.D., Assistant Professor/Co-Director Epi
Joanne Barnett, Senior Medical Office Coordinator

Missouri

6547 Pediatric Epilepsy Center
St Louis Children's Hospital
One Children's Place, Suite 12E47
St Louis, MO 63110   314-454-6120
                                  Fax: 314-454-4225
                                   www.neuro.wustl.edu/

A comprehensive and one of the largest centers for epilespy and seizure disorder care and research in the nation. It includes dedicated staff and an inpatient Epilepsy Monitoring Unit.

W. Edwin Dodson, M.D., Professor of Neurology & Pediatrics
Mary Bertrand, M.D., Associate Professor of Neurology
Christina Gurnett, M.D., Ph.D., Assistant Professor of Neurology an

New York

6548 Center for Neural Recovery & Rehabilitatio n Research
Helen Hayes Hospital
Route 9W
West Haverstraw, NY 10993   845-786-4225
                                       888-707-3422
                                  Fax: 845-947-3097
                     www.helenhayeshospital.org/research/

Helen E Scharfman PhD, Director

North Carolina

6549 Duke University Comprehensive Epilepsy Cen ter
200 Trent Drive, Room 4517, Busse Building
Durham, NC 27710
919-416-3853
Fax: 919-681-7973
e-mail: koeni002@mc.duke.edu
neuro.surgery.duke.edu

Evaluation of potential surgical candidates by epilepsy specialists.

Roger L Cothran, Director
Allan H. Friedman, MD, Division Chief
Karen Koenig, Division Administrator

Tennessee

6550 Neuroscience Institute, University of Tenn essee Health Science Center
875 Monroe Ave, Suite 426
Memphis, TN 38163
901-448-5960
Fax: 901-448-4685
www.uthsc.edu/neuroscience

Epilepsy research and studies.

William E. Armstrong, Ph.D., Director
Anton J. Reiner, Ph.D., Co-Director
Shannon Guyot, Administrative Services Assistant

Texas

6551 Baylor Comprehensive Epilepsy Center
Baylor College of Medicine
Smith Tower, 18th Floor, 6550 Fannin, Suite 1801
Houston, TX 77030
713-798-8259
Fax: 713-798-7533
www.bcm.edu/neurology/epilepsy/

Individualized care for those with seizure disorders.

Richard A. Hrachovy, M.D., Director
David K. Chen, M.D., Epileptology and Neurophysiology
Alica M. Goldman, M.D., Ph.D., Epileptology and Neurophysiology

Wisconsin

6552 Regional Epilepsy Center
Aurora St. Luke's Medical Center
2801 W Kinnickic River Pkwy, Ste 570
Milwaukee, WI 53215
414-385-8780
www.aurorahealthcare.org/services/epilepsy/
Christopher Inglese, Director

Audio Video

6553 Because You Are My Friend
Epilepsy Foundation
8301 Professional Place East, Suite 200
Landover, MD 20785
866-330-2718
800-332-1000
Fax: 301-459-1569
e-mail: ContactUs@efa.org
www.epilepsyfoundation.org

Video tape for children that provides a clear explanation of epilepsy, first aid and the importance of friendship. Cartoon slide presentation with child narration.

Warren Lammert, Chair
Phil Gattone, President/ CEO
Roger Heldman, Treasurer

6554 Epilepsy: The Untold Story
Fanflight Productions
32 Court Street, 21st Floor
Brooklyn, NY 11201
718-488-8900
800-876-1710
Fax: 718-488-8642
e-mail: info@fanlight.com
www.fanlight.com

This video tells the story of six people with Temporal Lobe Epilepsy.

1993 Video - 27 mins
ISBN: 1-572951-37-0

Nicole Johnson, Publicity Coordinator

6555 How to Recognize and Classify Seizures
Epilepsy Foundation
8301 Professional Place East, Suite 200
Landover, MD 20785
866-330-2718
800-332-1000
Fax: 301-459-1569
e-mail: ContactUs@efa.org
www.epilepsyfoundation.org

Discusses the classification of seizures and epileptic syndromes.

25 minutes

Warren Lammert, Chair
Phil Gattone, President/ CEO
Roger Heldman, Treasurer

6556 Just Like You and Me
WellMe/State of the Art
2201 Wisconsin Ave NW, Ste 350
Washington, DC 20008
202-537-0818
Fax: 202-537-0828
e-mail: contact@wellme.com
wellme.stateart.com/productions/health/epilepsy/

A video/patient info guide package on successfully living with epilepsy.

6557 Rest of the Family
Epilepsy Foundation
8301 Professional Place East, Suite 200
Landover, MD 20785
866-330-2718
800-332-1000
Fax: 301-459-1569
e-mail: ContactUs@efa.org
www.epilepsyfoundation.org

Presents the feelings and concerns of other family members, including siblings, of children with epilepsy.

Videocassette

Warren Lammert, Chair
Phil Gattone, President/ CEO
Roger Heldman, Treasurer

6558 Seizure First Aid
Epilepsy Foundation
8301 Professional Place East, Suite 200
Landover, MD 20785
866-330-2718
800-332-1000
Fax: 301-459-1569
e-mail: ContactUs@efa.org
www.epilepsyfoundation.org

This video combines footage of real seizures with reenactments to demonstrate proper first aid procedures. In addition, people with epilepsy talk about how they feel when they have a seizure, and discuss how they would like friends, family and the general public to react when a seizure occurs. 10 minutes.

Video & DVD

Warren Lammert, Chair
Phil Gattone, President/ CEO
Roger Heldman, Treasurer

6559 Understanding Seizures & Epilepsy
Epilepsy Foundation
8301 Professional Place East, Suite 200
Landover, MD 20785

866-330-2718
800-332-1000
Fax: 301-459-1569
e-mail: ContactUs@efa.org
www.epilepsyfoundation.org

Provides an explanation of seizure disorders in everyday language and dispels many misconceptions about epilepsy with medically accurate information.

Videocassette

Warren Lammert, Chair
Phil Gattone, President/ CEO
Roger Heldman, Treasurer

Web Sites

6560 American Epilepsy Society
www.aesnet.org

860-586-7505
e-mail: emurray@aesnet.org
www.aesnet.org

The society promotes research and education of professionals in the field of epilepsy and related disorders. The site includes a comprehensive listing of postgraduate training opportunities in the fields related to epilepsy.

Amy Brooks-Kayal, M.D., President
Eileen M. Murray, MM, CAE, Executive Director
Jeffrey Melin, M.Ed., CMP, Director of Education

6561 Curing Epilepsy: Focus on the Future/Bench marks for Epilepsy Research
P.O. Box 5801
Bethesda, MD 20824

301-496-5751
800-352-9424
www.ninds.nih.gov/funding/research/epilepsyweb/

Summary of March 2000, White House-initiated conference.

Walter J. Koroshetz, M.D., Acting Director
Alan L. Willard, Ph.D., Acting Deputy Director
Caroline Lewis, Executive Officer

6562 Epilepsy Foundation of America
8301 Professional Place East, Suite 200
Landover, MD 20785

866-330-2718
800-332-1000
Fax: 301-459-1569
e-mail: ContactUs@efa.org
www.epilepsyfoundation.org

Through its efforts the organization ensures that people with seizures are able to participate in all life experiences. Its goals are to eventually prevent, control and cure epilepsy through research, education, advocacy, and services.

Warren Lammert, Chair
Phil Gattone, President/ CEO
Roger Heldman, Treasurer

6563 Epilepsy.com
8301 Professional Place East, Suite 200
Landover, MD 20785

866-330-2718
800-332-1000
Fax: 301-459-1569
e-mail: ContactUs@efa.org
www.epilepsy.com

Epilepsy resources made available through an initiative by the Epilepsy Therapy Development Project.

Warren Lammert, Chair
Phil Gattone, President/ CEO
Roger Heldman, Treasurer

6564 HealingWell.com
www.healingwell.com/epilepsy/

e-mail: admin@healingwell.com
www.healingwell.com/epilepsy/

Offers information and resources including books, newsletters, and videos on a variety of diseases and chronic illnesses including epilepsy.

Peter Waite, Founder/ CEO

6565 NIH/National Institute of Neurological Dis orders and Stroke (NINDS)
PO Box 5801
Bethesda, MD 20824

301-496-5751
800-352-9424
www.ninds.nih.gov

The mission of NINDS is to reduce the burden of neurological disease - a burden borne by every age group, by every segment of society, by people all over the world.

Walter J. Koroshetz, M.D., Acting Director
Alan L. Willard, Ph.D., Acting Deputy Director
Caroline Lewis, Executive Officer

6566 North Pacific Epilepsy Research
The Northrup Center, 2311 NW Northrup Street, Suit
Portland, OR 97210

503-291-5300
Fax: 503-291-5303
www.seizures.net/

Provides information to the public and health care professionals.

Dr. Mark Yerby, Founder

Book Publishers

6567 Brainstorms Companion: Epilepsy in Our Vie w
Steven C Schachter MD, author

Epilepsy Foundation
8301 Professional Place
Landover, MD 20785

301-459-3700
800-332-1000
Fax: 301-577-2684
www.epilepsyfoundation.org

Family members, friends and coworkers of those with seizure disorders describe their feelings and observations.

1994 160 pages Paperback
ISBN: 0-781702-30-5

Phil Gattone, President & CEO
Michele Dawson, Manager of Executive operations
Sandy Finucane, Senior Advisor

6568 Brainstorms: Epilepsy in Our Words
Steven C Schachter MD, author

Epilepsy Foundation
8301 Professional Place
Landover, MD 20785

301-459-3700
800-662-6922
Fax: 301-577-2684
www.epilepsyfoundation.org

Patients describe their experiences with seizures. Sixty-eight in-depth personal accounts of actual seizures are followed by a short section on how epilepsy affects the lives of the patients.

1993 197 pages Paperback
ISBN: 0-802774-65-2

Phil Gattone, President & CEO
Michele Dawson, Manager of Executive operations
Sandy Finucane, Senior Advisor

6569 Children with Seizures: A Guide For Parent s, Teachers and Other Professionals
Epilepsy Foundation
8301 Professional Place
Landover, MD 20785

301-459-3700
800-332-1000
Fax: 301-577-2684
www.epilepsyfoundation.org

Phil Gattone, President & CEO
Michele Dawson, Manager of Executive operations
Sandy Finucane, Senior Advisor

6570 Dotty the Dalmatian Has Epilepsy
Tim Peters & Company, Inc
87 Main St, PO Box 370
Peapack, NJ 07977   908-234-2050
                                               800-543-2230
                                        Fax: 908-234-1961
                    e-mail: info@timpetersandcompany.com
                           www.timpetersandcompany.com

Part of the Dr. Wellbook® series, this is the story of Dotty the
Dalmatian who discovers she has epilepsy.

16 pages Softcover
ISBN: 1-879874-35-0

6571 Embrace the Dawn

Andrea Davidson, author

Epilepsy Foundation
8301 Professional Place
Landover, MD 20785   301-459-3700
                                               800-332-1000
                                        Fax: 301-577-2684
                           www.epilepsyfoundation.org

A moving biographical account of one person's lifelong experience with epilepsy.

127 pages Softcover

Phil Gattone, President & CEO
Michele Dawson, Manager of Executive operations
Sandy Finucane, Senior Advisor

6572 Epilepsy A to Z
Demos Medical Publishing
11 West 42nd Street, 15th Floor
New York, NY 10036   212-683-0072
                                               800-532-8663
                                        Fax: 212-683-0118
                    e-mail: orderdept@demosmedpub.com
                           www.demosmedpub.com

Easy reference in finding brief answers to questions regarding epilepsy terminology.

1995 322 pages Softcover
ISBN: 0-939957-75-0

Kathy Gonzalez, Order Dept/Fulfillment Coordinator
Paul Choi, Vice-President of Finance and Opera
Richard Winters, Executive Editor

6573 Epilepsy, A Guide to Balancing Your Life

Ilo E Leppik MD, author

Demos Medical Publishing
11 West 42nd Street, 15th Floor
New York, NY 10036   212-683-0072
                                               800-532-8663
                                        Fax: 212-683-0118
                    e-mail: orderdept@demosmedpub.com
                           www.demosmedpub.com

Part of the Quality of Life Guide Series from the American Academy of Neurology Press. Provides reliable and practical information for those diagnosed with epilepsy and seizure disorders.

2006 192 pages Softcover
ISBN: 1-932603-20-0

Kathy Gonzalez, Order Dept/Fulfillment Coordinator
Paul Choi, Vice-President of Finance and Opera
Richard Winters, Executive Editor

6574 Epilepsy: 199 Answers

Andrew N Wilner MD, author

Demos Medical Publishing
11 West 42nd Street, 15th Floor
New York, NY 10036   212-683-0072
                                               800-532-8663
                                        Fax: 212-683-0118
                    e-mail: orderdept@demosmedpub.com
                           www.demosmedpub.com

Helps to better understand conversations with the doctor and empowers the patient/caregiver to ask the right questions, resulting
in optimal care.

2003 180 pages Softcover
ISBN: 1-888799-70-5

Kathy Gonzalez, Order Dept/Fulfillment Coordinator
Paul Choi, Vice-President of Finance and Opera
Richard Winters, Executive Editor

6575 Epilepsy: Frequency, Causes and Consequenc es
Epilepsy Foundation
8301 Professional Place
Landover, MD 20785   301-459-3700
                                               800-332-1000
                                        Fax: 301-577-2684
                           www.epilepsyfoundation.org

Statistical study that addresses the causes, natural history, prevalence and risk factors of epilepsy in certain populations and the
impact on the community.

1990

Phil Gattone, President & CEO
Michele Dawson, Manager of Executive operations
Sandy Finucane, Senior Advisor

6576 Epilepsy: I Can Live with That

Sue Goss, author

Epilepsy Foundation
8301 Professional Place
Landover, MD 20785   301-459-3700
                                               800-332-1000
                                        Fax: 301-577-2684
                           www.epilepsyfoundation.org

The experience of epilepsy as recorded by a group of ordinary
men and women living in Australia. Each story focuses on personal growth, triumph over disability and emphasizes individual
courage and hope.

1995 Softcover

Phil Gattone, President & CEO
Michele Dawson, Manager of Executive operations
Sandy Finucane, Senior Advisor

6577 Growing Up With Epilepsy

Lynn Bennett Blackburn MD, author

Demos Medical Publishing
11 West 42nd Street, 15th Floor
New York, NY 10036   212-683-0072
                                               800-532-8663
                                        Fax: 212-683-0118
                    e-mail: orderdept@demosmedpub.com
                           www.demosmedpub.com

Guidance in raising a child with epilepsy, including navigating
the educational system, discipline, and social development.

2003 168 pages Softcover
ISBN: 1-888799-74-3

Kathy Gonzalez, Order Dept/Fulfillment Coordinator
Paul Choi, Vice-President of Finance and Opera
Richard Winters, Executive Editor

**6578 Keto Kid, Helping Your Child to Succeed on the Ketogenic
Diet**

Deborah Ann Snyder DO, author

Demos Medical Publishing
11 West 42nd Street, 15th Floor
New York, NY 10036   212-683-0072
                                               800-532-8663
                                        Fax: 212-683-0118
                    e-mail: orderdept@demosmedpub.com
                           www.demosmedpub.com

2006 176 pages Softcover
ISBN: 1-932603-29-3

Kathy Gonzalez, Order Dept/Fulfillment Coordinator
Paul Choi, Vice-President of Finance and Opera
Richard Winters, Executive Editor

6579 Lee the Rabbit with Epilepsy
Deborah M. Moss, author

Epilepsy Foundation
8301 Professional Place
Landover, MD 20785   301-459-3700
                                      800-332-1000
                                 Fax: 301-459-1569
                            www.epilepsyfoundation.org

Written for children ages three to six, this illustrated picture book follows the adventures of a small rabbit who has seizures. It follows her journey from the first seizure, the initial doctors visit through to treatment.

1989 21 pages Hardcover

Phil Gattone, President & CEO
Michele Dawson, Manager of Executive operations
Sandy Finucane, Senior Advisor

6580 Living Well with Epilepsy
Robert Gumnit MD, author

Demos Medical Publishing
11 West 42nd Street, 15th Floor
New York, NY 10036   212-683-0072
                                      800-532-8663
                                 Fax: 212-683-0118
                     e-mail: orederdept@demosmedpub.com
                              www.demosmedpub.com

Designed to help both health-care professionals and patients to understand all aspects of diagnosis and management; to enable patients to participate more knowledgeably in interactions with their health care team and to help steer them toward a more normal, fulfilling life.

1997 249 pages Soft / 2nd Ed
ISBN: 1-888799-11-0

Kathy Gonzalez, Order Dept/Fulfillment Coordinator
Paul Choi, Vice-President of Finance and Opera
Richard Winters, Executive Editor

6581 Missing Michael - A Mother's Story of Love
Epilepsy Foundation
8301 Professional Place
Landover, MD 20785   301-459-3700
                                      800-332-1000
                                 Fax: 301-459-1569
                            www.epilepsyfoundation.org

A mother's story of her struggle with raising her son with epilepsy. Deatils in dealing with the health care system, the school system, and the complications of medication.

Paperback

Phil Gattone, President & CEO
Michele Dawson, Manager of Executive operations
Sandy Finucane, Senior Advisor

6582 Mom I Have a Staring Problem
Epilepsy Foundation
8301 Professional Place
Landover, MD 20785   301-459-3700
                                      800-332-1000
                                 Fax: 301-459-1570
                            www.epilepsyfoundation.org

Tiffany, a seven-year old, describes her experiences with petit mal seizures; her feelings, wishes and fears. Written to help adults recognize a hidden problem that could be occuring with a child who has learning problems.

1994 24 pages Softcover
ISBN: 0-802774-65-2

Phil Gattone, President & CEO
Michele Dawson, Manager of Executive operations
Sandy Finucane, Senior Advisor

6583 My Friend Matty: A Story About Living with Epilepsy
Epilepsy Foundation
8301 Professional Place
Landover, MD 20785   301-459-3700
                                      800-332-1000
                                 Fax: 301-459-1571
                            www.epilepsyfoundation.org

A comic-book style publication for educating children written by parents whose 5-year old boy passed away.

Paperback

Phil Gattone, President & CEO
Michele Dawson, Manager of Executive operations
Sandy Finucane, Senior Advisor

6584 Pediatric Epilepsy
Demos Medical Publishing
11 West 42nd Street, 15th Floor
New York, NY 10036   212-683-0072
                                      800-532-8663
                                 Fax: 212-683-0118
                     e-mail: orderdept@demosmedpub.com
                              www.demosmedpub.com

Covers the diagnosis, treatment, classification and management of childhood epilepsies.

2001 666 pages Hardcover
ISBN: 1-888799-30-9

Kathy Gonzalez, Order Dept/Fulfillment Coordinator
Paul Choi, Vice-President of Finance and Opera
Richard Winters, Executive Editor

6585 Pediatric Epilepsy Resource Handbook
FACES/NYU Medical Center
223 East 34th Street
New York, NY 10016   646-558-0900
                                 Fax: 646-385-7163
                       e-mail: FACESinfo@nyumc.org
                            www.faces.med.nyu.edu

3rd Edition

Pamela Mohr, Executive Director
Nako Ishii, Project Co-ordinator
Luis L. Valero, Associate Director of Special Event

6586 School Planning
Epilepsy Foundation
8301 Professional Place
Landover, MD 20785   301-459-3700
                                      800-332-1000
                                 Fax: 301-577-2684
                                 TDD: 800-332-2070
                            www.epilepsyfoundation.org

This guide describes some epilepsy-related problems that children and youth may face in the areas of academics, school achievement and social development. Suggests ways parents can take a proactive approach to ensure appropriate testing, placement and achievement of educational goals for their children.

125 pages Hardcover
ISBN: 0-802774-65-2

Phil Gattone, President & CEO
Michele Dawson, Manager of Executive operations
Sandy Finucane, Senior Advisor

6587 Seizures and Epilepsy In Childhood: A Guid e
Johns Hopkins University Press
2715 N Charles Street
Baltimore, MD 21218   410-516-6900
                                      800-537-5487
                                 Fax: 410-516-6968
                              www.press.jhu.edu

A standard resource for parents in need of comprehensive medical information about their child with epilepsy.

2002 432 pages 3rd Ed / Hard
ISBN: 0-801870-50-x

Kathleen Keane, Director
Timothy D. Fuller, Chief Information Officer
Erik A. Smist, Director, Finance and Administratio

6588 Your Child and Epilepsy
Roger J Gumnit MD, author

Demos Medical Publishing
11 West 42nd Street, 15th Floor
New York, NY 10036   212-683-0072
                                      800-532-8663
                                  Fax: 212-683-0118
                        e-mail: orderdept@demospub.com
                                  www.demosmedpub.com

Provides information to help parents understand their child's epilepsy, suggestions on how to evaluate health care, to find better care if necessary and advice on how to help children with epilepsy to develop self-confidence and self-motivation.

1995 256 pages Softcover
ISBN: 0-939957-76-0

Kathy Gonzalez, Order Dept/Fulfillment Coordinator
Paul Choi, Vice-President of Finance and Opera
Richard Winters, Executive Editor

Magazines

6589 Epilepsy Foundation
Epilepsy Foundation
8301 Professional Place East, Suite 200
Landover, MD 20785   866-330-2718
                                      800-332-1000
                                  Fax: 301-459-1569
                         e-mail: ContactUs@efa.org
                              www.epilepsyfoundation.org

Catalog of epilepsy information materials, including pamphlets, books, manuals, videotapes and other items is available upon request.

Warren Lammert, Chair
Phil Gattone, President/ CEO
Roger Heldman, Treasurer

6590 EpilepsyUSA
Epilepsy Foundation
8301 Professional Place East, Suite 200
Landover, MD 20785   866-330-2718
                                      800-332-1000
                                  Fax: 301-459-1569
                                  TDD: 800-332-2070
                         e-mail: ContactUs@efa.org
                              www.epilepsyfoundation.org

Information on concerns about seizure disorders and epilepsy and new developments in treatment.

24 pages 6 issues/yr

Warren Lammert, Chair
Phil Gattone, President/ CEO
Roger Heldman, Treasurer

Journals

6591 Epilepsy & Behavior
Elsevier
Marquis One, 245 Peachtree Center Avenue, Suite 19
Atlanta, GA 30303   404-669-9400
                                      800-999-6274
                                  Fax: 404-669-9339
                         e-mail: usjcs@elsevier.com
                    www.journals.elsevier.com/epilepsy-and-behavior/

An international journal that offers current information on the behavioral aspects of seizures and epilepsy.

Bi-monthly
ISSN: 1525-5050

Ron Mobed, Chief Executive Officer
Stuart Whayman, Chief Financial Officer
Gavin Howe, EVP, Human Resources

Newsletters

6592 AES News
American Epilepsy Society
342 N Main Street
W Hartford, CT 6117   860-586-7505
                                  Fax: 860-568-7550
                                      www.aesnet.org

16 pages 3x/year

Deepak K Lachhwani, Editor
Amy Brooks-Kayal, M.D., President
Eileen M. Murray, MM, CAE, Executive Director

6593 Epilepsia: Journal of the International League Against Epilepsy
Blackwell Publishing
350 Main Street, Commerce Place
Malden, MA 2148   781-388-8200
                                      888-661-5800
                                  Fax: 781-388-8210
                         www.blackwellpublishing.com

A leading international journal on the epilepsies for more than 30 years, Epilepsia provides comprehensive coverage of current clinical and research results.

12 per year
ISSN: 0013-9580

Philip A Schwartzkroin, Co-Editor
Simon Shorvon, Co-Editor

6594 FACES: Finding a Cure for Epilepsy & Seizu res
223 East 34th Street (between 2nd and 3rd Avenues)
New York, NY 10016   646-558-0900
                                  Fax: 646-385-7163
                         e-mail: FACESinfo@nyumc.org
                                  faces.med.nyu.edu

Covers new studies, research, events and special interest stories.
Quarterly
Orrin Devinsky, MD, Founder
Pamela B. Mohr, Executive Director
Luis L. Valero, Associate Director

Pamphlets

6595 Child with Epilepsy at Camp
Epilepsy Foundation
8301 Professional Place East, Suite 200
Landover, MD 20785   866-330-2718
                                      800-332-1000
                                  Fax: 301-459-1569
                         e-mail: ContactUs@efa.org
                              www.epilepsyfoundation.org

Written for camp counselors, it helps parents explain to them the specific needs of children with epilepsy at camp to ensure a safe camping experience.

14 pages Pamphlet

Warren Lammert, Chair
Phil Gattone, President/ CEO
Roger Heldman, Treasurer

6596 Child's Guide To Seizure Disorders
Epilepsy Foundation
8301 Professional Place East, Suite 200
Landover, MD 20785   866-330-2718
                                      800-332-1000
                                  Fax: 301-459-1569
                         e-mail: ContactUs@efa.org
                              www.epilepsyfoundation.org

A pamphlet for children, brightly-colored and explains seizures, why medication should be taken, etc.

Warren Lammert, Chair
Phil Gattone, President/ CEO
Roger Heldman, Treasurer

6597 Epilepsy in Children: The Teacher's Role
Epilepsy Foundation
8301 Professional Place East, Suite 200
Landover, MD 20785
866-330-2718
800-332-1000
Fax: 301-459-1569
e-mail: ContactUs@efa.org
www.epilepsyfoundation.org

Provides an explanation for teachers on handling seizures in the classroom, the need for good communication between students and first aid procedures.

Warren Lammert, Chair
Phil Gattone, President/ CEO
Roger Heldman, Treasurer

6598 Epilepsy: You and Your Child
Epilepsy Foundation
8301 Professional Place East, Suite 200
Landover, MD 20785
866-330-2718
800-332-1000
Fax: 301-459-1569
e-mail: ContactUs@efa.org
www.epilepsyfoundation.org

This instructional booklet offers information on emotional aspects of epilepsy, how to handle seizures, medication, diet and nutrition, and offers referral organizations for parents.

Warren Lammert, Chair
Phil Gattone, President/ CEO
Roger Heldman, Treasurer

6599 Febrile Seizures Fact Sheet
NINDS/NIH Neurological Institute
Office of Communications and Public Liaison, NINDS
Bethesda, MD 20892
301-496-5751
800-352-9424
TTY: 301-468-5981
www.ninds.nih.gov/disorders/febrile_seizures/

Also available in Spanish.

Walter J. Koroshetz, M.D., Acting Director
Alan L. Willard, Ph.D., Acting Deputy Director
Caroline Lewis, Executive Officer

6600 Finding Out About Seizures: A Guide to Medical Tests
Epilepsy Foundation
8301 Professional Place East, Suite 200
Landover, MD 20785
866-330-2718
800-332-1000
Fax: 301-459-1569
e-mail: ContactUs@efa.org
www.epilepsyfoundation.org

Introduces adults and children with epilepsy to the types of tests they may have to undergo.

Warren Lammert, Chair
Phil Gattone, President/ CEO
Roger Heldman, Treasurer

6601 H.O.P.E. Series: Seizures in Childhood
Epilepsy Foundation
8301 Professional Place East, Suite 200
Landover, MD 20785
866-330-2718
800-332-1000
Fax: 301-459-1569
e-mail: ContactUs@efa.org
www.epilepsyfoundation.org

Provides an overview of the challenges associated with living with epilepsy and other seizure disorders, including potential hazards, first aid procedures, and overall help in daily living.

Warren Lammert, Chair
Phil Gattone, President/ CEO
Roger Heldman, Treasurer

6602 H.O.P.E. Series: Seizures in the Teen Year s
Epilepsy Foundation
8301 Professional Place East, Suite 200
Landover, MD 20785
866-330-2718
800-332-1000
Fax: 301-459-1569
e-mail: ContactUs@efa.org
www.epilepsyfoundation.org

Provides general information specifically for teens with epilepsy and seizure disorders.

Warren Lammert, Chair
Phil Gattone, President/ CEO
Roger Heldman, Treasurer

6603 Infantile Spasms
NINDS/NIH Neurological Institute
Office of Communications and Public Liaison, NINDS
Bethesda, MD 20892
301-496-5751
800-352-9424
TTY: 301-468-5981
www.ninds.nih.gov/disorders/infantilespasms/

Information sheet on infantile spasms (West Syndrome).

Walter J. Koroshetz, M.D., Acting Director
Alan L. Willard, Ph.D., Acting Deputy Director
Caroline Lewis, Executive Officer

6604 Kids and Seizures: Know the Hidden Signs
Epilepsy Foundation
8301 Professional Place East, Suite 200
Landover, MD 20785
866-330-2718
800-332-1000
Fax: 301-459-1569
e-mail: ContactUs@efa.org
www.epilepsyfoundation.org

Written for camp counselors, it helps parents explain to them the specific needs of children with epilepsy at camp to ensure a safe camping experience.

Warren Lammert, Chair
Phil Gattone, President/ CEO
Roger Heldman, Treasurer

6605 Managing Seizures, Information for Caregiv ers
Epilepsy Foundation
8301 Professional Place East, Suite 200
Landover, MD 20785
866-330-2718
800-332-1000
Fax: 301-459-1569
e-mail: ContactUs@efa.org
www.epilepsyfoundation.org

Explains seizures, routine and special care, emergency aid and first aid for caregivers. Includes a poster size chart for medicines and general guidance in handling a seizure.

Warren Lammert, Chair
Phil Gattone, President/ CEO
Roger Heldman, Treasurer

6606 Me and My World Storybook
Epilepsy Foundation
8301 Professional Place East, Suite 200
Landover, MD 20785
866-330-2718
800-332-1000
Fax: 301-459-1569
TDD: 800-332-2070
e-mail: ContactUs@efa.org
www.epilepsyfoundation.org

An excellent pamphlet for explaining epilepsy to children and their friends. It also discusses various types of epilepsy and its effects on family members. Ages 4-8.

Warren Lammert, Chair
Phil Gattone, President/ CEO
Roger Heldman, Treasurer

6607 Medicines for Epilepsy
Epilepsy Foundation
8301 Professional Place East, Suite 200
Landover, MD 20785

866-330-2718
800-332-1000
Fax: 301-459-1569
e-mail: ContactUs@efa.org
www.epilepsyfoundation.org

Offers information on medication and treatments, generic drugs, side effects, drug abuse and more. Contains a color chart with pictures of the most common medications for epilepsy.

Warren Lammert, Chair
Phil Gattone, President/ CEO
Roger Heldman, Treasurer

6608 Safety and Seizures
Epilepsy Foundation
8301 Professional Place East, Suite 200
Landover, MD 20785

866-330-2718
800-332-1000
Fax: 301-459-1569
e-mail: ContactUs@efa.org
www.epilepsyfoundation.org

Warren Lammert, Chair
Phil Gattone, President/ CEO
Roger Heldman, Treasurer

6609 Seizures and Epilepsy: Hope Through Research
NINDS/NIH Neurological Institute
Office of Communications and Public Liaison, NINDS
Bethesda, MD 20892

301-496-5751
800-352-9424
TTY: 301-468-5981
www.ninds.nih.gov/disorders/epilepsy/

Also available in Spanish.

Walter J. Koroshetz, M.D., Acting Director
Alan L. Willard, Ph.D., Acting Deputy Director
Caroline Lewis, Executive Officer

6610 Seizures, Epilepsy and Your Child
Epilepsy Foundation
8301 Professional Place East, Suite 200
Landover, MD 20785

866-330-2718
800-332-1000
Fax: 301-459-1569
e-mail: ContactUs@efa.org
www.epilepsyfoundation.org

A pamphlet for parents, providing guidance on daily life, first aid and treatment for children with epilepsy.

Warren Lammert, Chair
Phil Gattone, President/ CEO
Roger Heldman, Treasurer

6611 Surgery for Epilepsy
Epilepsy Foundation
8301 Professional Place East, Suite 200
Landover, MD 20785

866-330-2718
800-332-1000
Fax: 301-459-1569
e-mail: ContactUs@efa.org
www.epilepsyfoundation.org

Describes current surgical treatment and the testing that precedes it.

12 pages

Warren Lammert, Chair
Phil Gattone, President/ CEO
Roger Heldman, Treasurer

6612 Talking to Your Doctor About Seizure Disorders
Epilepsy Foundation
8301 Professional Place East, Suite 200
Landover, MD 20785

866-330-2718
800-332-1000
Fax: 301-459-1569
e-mail: ContactUs@efa.org
www.epilepsyfoundation.org

Designed to help the patient talk with medical personnel about treatment of epilepsy.

Warren Lammert, Chair
Phil Gattone, President/ CEO
Roger Heldman, Treasurer

6613 The ADA: Questions and Answers
Epilepsy Foundation
8301 Professional Place East, Suite 200
Landover, MD 20785

866-330-2718
800-332-1000
Fax: 301-459-1569
e-mail: ContactUs@efa.org
www.epilepsyfoundation.org

Offers a brief overview of the Americans with Disabilities Act and how it covers those with epilepsy.

Warren Lammert, Chair
Phil Gattone, President/ CEO
Roger Heldman, Treasurer

6614 What Everyone Should Know About Epilepsy
Epilepsy Foundation
8301 Professional Place East, Suite 200
Landover, MD 20785

866-330-2718
800-332-1000
Fax: 301-459-1569
e-mail: ContactUs@efa.org
www.epilepsyfoundation.org

Warren Lammert, Chair
Phil Gattone, President/ CEO
Roger Heldman, Treasurer

6615 When Seizures Don't Look Like Seizures
Epilepsy Foundation
8301 Professional Place East, Suite 200
Landover, MD 20785

866-330-2718
800-332-1000
Fax: 301-459-1569
e-mail: ContactUs@efa.org
www.epilepsyfoundation.org

Describes and helps with the subtle signs of a seizure for parents, child care providers and school personnel.

ISBN: 0-802774-65-2

Warren Lammert, Chair
Phil Gattone, President/ CEO
Roger Heldman, Treasurer

Camps

6616 Camp Achieve
Epilepsy Foundation Eastern Pennsylvania
919 Walnut Street, Suite 700
Philadelphia, PA 19107

215-629-5003
800-887-7165
Fax: 215-629-4997
e-mail: camp@efepa.org
www.efepa.org/programs-and-resources/camp-achieve

Camp Achieve is a week long, overnight, summer camp for youth with a primary diagnosis of epilepsy/seizure disorder that is held every year in August. Camp Achieve is a unique opportunity for the children ages 8-17 to connect with other individuals coping with the same day to day challenges. Many individuals with epilepsy/seizure disorder face isolation, bullying, and discrimination from their classmates, their neighbors, and the general public.

Frank Kotulka, Board President
Allison McCartin, Executive Director
Sue Livingston, Education Coordinator

6617 Camp Frog
Epilepsy Foundation Western/Central Pennsylvania
1501 Reedsdale Street, Suite 3002
Pittsburgh, PA 15233

412-261-5880
800-316-5585
Fax: 412-322-7885
e-mail: astein@efwp.org
www.efwp.org/programs/ProgramsCampFrog.xml

The EFWCP sponsors two-week long, overnight summer camping programs called Camp Frog. This nationally recognized activity allows kids with epilepsy/seizure disorders to be integrated into a typical camping experience with hundreds of other children. The overnight program is available to boys and girls with epilepsy/seizure disorders from grades 4 to 11. Campers enjoy a host of activities such as arts and crafts, campfire sing-alongs, swimming, team games, sailing, archery and horseback riding.

Peggy Beem, President/ CEO
Francine Reyher, Adult Services Coordinator
Colleen K Fulkerson, Special Events Coordinator

6618 Camp Ramah in New England Tikvah Program
39 Bennett Street
Palmer, MA 01609   413-283-9771
                                     Fax: 413-283-6661
                               e-mail: info@campramahne.org
                                       www.campramahne.org

The Tikvah program is one of the first summer programs for Jewish children with special needs. It continues to grow and evolve as it strives to serve campers with a wide range of special needs including, but not limited to, congitive impairments, autism, cerebral palsy and seizure disorder.

Howard Blas, Tikvah Program Director
Talya Kalender, Director, Camper Care
Benjamin Greene, Director of Education

6619 Camp Roehr
140 Iowa Ave # A
Belleville, IL 62220   618-236-2181
                                           866-848-0472
                                      Fax: 618-236-3654
            www.epilepsyfoundation.org/local/swillinois/camp.cfm

Seven day residential camp for children designed to meet the special needs of children diagnosed with epilepsy, providing a safe and fun camp experience.

Ellen Becker, Executive Director
Trudy Baxter, Director of Programs and Services
Jan Conder, Development Coordinator

6620 Crotched Mountain School & Rehabilitation Center
1 Verney Drive
Greenfield, NH 3047   603-547-3311
                                           800-800-966
                                      Fax: 603-547-3232
                            e-mail: info@crotchedmountain.org
                                       www.cmf.org

Currently serves children ages 6-22 with multiple-handicaps including: Cerebral Palsy, Spina Bifida, visual and hearing impairments and neurological disabilities, developmental disorders, mental retardation, autism, behavioral and emotional disorders, seizure disorders, spinal cord and head injuries. Member of the National Association of Independent Schools and accredited with the NE Association of Schools and Colleges, Independent Schools of Northern NE.

Donald L. Shumway, President/ CEO
Kathleen C. Brittan, VP, Development
Frederick R. Bruch, Jr., Medical Director

Description

6621 SICKLE CELL DISEASE

Synonyms: Homozygous Hb S, Sickle cell anemia

Involves the following Biologic System(s):

Hematologic and Oncologic Disorders

Sickle cell disease is an inherited blood disorder that primarily affects African Americans and is characterized by the presence of crescent or sickle-shaped red cells in the blood and the chronic premature destruction of red blood cells (hemolytic anemia). In this disorder, the red blood cells contain an abnormal form of the oxygen-carrying protein (hemoglobin) called hemoglobin S (Hgb S). This abnormality reduces the level of available oxygen (ischemia) in the blood cells and results in their characteristic sickle shape. These irregular cells tend to block the tiny blood vessels of various tissues and organs; they may cause restricted or obstructed blood flow resulting in tissue or organ damage (infarction). In addition, their unusual shape renders them fragile, leading to their premature destruction and thus anemia.

The symptoms of sickle cell disease tend to appear at or around six months of age and may include headaches; shortness of breath (dyspnea); paleness; fatigue; and a yellowish hue of the eyes, skin, and mucous membranes (jaundice). Any activity that would normally reduce the blood oxygen levels (e.g., exercise, exertion, illness, or high-altitude flying) may induce a sickle cell crisis or sudden worsening of the anemic condition accompanied by abdominal and bone pain, dyspnea, and vomiting. Infarction or a blocked blood vessel (vaso-occlusion) may also result in sickle cell crisis with the affected child experiencing chest pain and increased dyspnea. By adolescence most of those affected develop an|enlarged spleen (splenomegaly) that is no longer capable of assisting in fighting certain infections, leaving the body more vulnerable to certain types of infections (encapsulated organisms, notably pneumococcal pneumonia). Other symptoms may include skin changes resulting from poor circulation, stroke resulting from insufficient oxygen reaching the brain, or blood in the urine (hematuria) resulting from kidney damage. As the affected child grows to adulthood, the liver and heart may enlarge (hepatosplenomegaly) and a heart murmur may develop. The lungs, intestines, and gall bladder may also be affected. In addition, affected children may develop such distinct characteristics as a short torso with long extremities, fingers, and toes.

Because there is no known cure for sickle cell disease, treatment is geared toward prevention, control, and pain management. Such treatment may include the avoidance of activities that reduce blood oxygen levels, a full immunization regimen, and prompt medical intervention for any illness or viral infection. Other treatment may include folic acid supplementation, antibiotic medication for treatment and prevention of infection, oxygen therapy to improve the level of oxygen in the blood, and acetaminophen or other medication to relieve pain. To manage a sickle cell crisis, as well as the pain associated with it, affected children may be given intravenous fluids, pain-relieving drugs,and possibly blood transfusions. Other treatments being studied include certain drugs, gene therapy, and bone marrow transplantation.

Sickle cell dis|ease is inherited as an autosomal recessive trait. In this case, the defective gene for hemoglobin S is transmitted by both parents. If a child inherits this gene from only one parent (and one normal gene from the other parent, that child will usually be symptom-free, but will be a carrier of the sickle cell trait. The incidence of this disorder in the United States is approximately 150 African American children in 100,000; however, approximately one in 12 black children carries the sickle cell trait.

Government Agencies

6622 NIH/National Heart, Lung and Blood Institu te

National Institute of Health
31 Center Dr MSC 2486, Bldg 31, Room 5A48
Bethesda, MD 20892

301-592-8573
Fax: 301-592-8563
TTY: 240-629-3255
e-mail: NHLBIinfo@nhlbi.nih.gov
www.nhlbi.nih.gov

Primary responsibility of this organization is the scientific investigation of heart, blood vessel, lung and blood disorders. Oversees research, demonstration, prevention, education, control and training activities in these fields and emphasizes the prevention and control of heart diseases.

Gary H. Gibbons, M.D., Director
Susan Shurin, MD, Deputy Director
Sheila Pohl, Chief of Staff

6623 NIH/National Institute of Child Health and Human Development

31 Center Drive, Building 31
Bethesda, MD 20892

301-496-1333
Fax: 301-496-1104
www.nichd.nih.gov

Established in 1962 by congress, today the institute conducts and supports research on topics related to the health of children, adults, families and populations. Some of these topics include: developmental disabilities, growth and development, infant death, reproductive health and birth defects.

Jay H Hoofnagle, Director
Lisa Kaeser, Program & Public Liaison

National Associations & Support Groups

6624 American Academy of Pediatrics

141 Northwest Point Boulevard
Elk Grove Village, IL 60007

847-434-4000
800-433-9016
Fax: 847-434-8000
www.aap.org

The American Academy of Pediatrics and its member pediatricians are committed to the attainment of optimal physical, mental and social health and well-being for all infants, children, adolescents, and young adults.

Sandra Hassink, MD, FAAP, President

6625 American Sickle Cell Anemia Association

10900 Carnegie Avenue
Cleveland, OH 44106

216-229-8600
Fax: 216-229-4500
e-mail: irabragg@ascaa.org
www.ascaa.org

Provides education, testing, counseling, supportive services to the population at risk for sickle cell anemia and its hemoglobin variants. Bilingual educator on staff, educational materials and distribution of literature is provided by ASCAA. Referrals for children and families with special needs.

Ira Bragg-Grant, Executive Director

6626 Genetic Alliance
4301 Connecticut Avenue NW
Washington, DC 20008
202-966-5557
800-336-4363
Fax: 202-966-8553
e-mail: info@geneticalliance.org
www.geneticalliance.org

A coalition of voluntary genetic support groups, consumers and professionals addressing the needs of individuals and families affected by genetic disorders from a national perspective.

Sharon Terry, MA, President/CEO
Natasha Bonhomme, Vice President of Strategic Develop
Vaughn Edelson, Assistant Director of Health Commun

6627 Sickle Cell Disease Association of America
231 E Baltimore St, Suite 800
Baltimore, MD 21202
410-528-1555
800-421-8453
Fax: 410-528-1495
e-mail: scdaa@sicklecelldisease.org
www.sicklecelldisease.org

Promotes the finding of a universal cure for sickle cell disease while improving the quality of life for individuals and families where sickle cell related conditions exists. It also assists in the organization and development of local chapters.

Willarda Edwards, President
Sonya I Ross, VP Programs/Services
Asha Hamilton, Membership Services Coordinator

6628 Sickle Cell Information Center
Grady Memorial Hospital
80 Jesse Hill Jr Drive, PO Box 109
Atlanta, GA 30301
404-616-3572
Fax: 404-616-5998
e-mail: aplatt@emory.edu
www.scinfo.org

Sickle cell resources, education, news and research updates for caregivers, patients and professionals.

State Agencies & Support Groups

Alabama

6629 Sickle Cell Foundation of Greater Montgomery
3180 US Highway 80 W
Montgomery, AL 36108
334-286-9122
800-742-5534
Fax: 334-286-4804
e-mail: sickle2@aol.com
www.scfgm.org

Willie Owens, Executive Director

California

6630 Sickle Cell Disease Foundation of California
5777 W. Century Blvd. Suite 1230
Los Angeles, CA 90045
310-693-0247
877-288-2873
Fax: 310-216-0307
e-mail: info@scdfc.org
www.scdfc.org

Educates, screens and offers counsel to those at risk for having children with sickle cell disease and other hemoglobin disorders.

Mary E Brown, President
Roger Brown, Director Development/Public Affairs

Connecticut

6631 Sickle Cell Disease Association of America - Connecticut Chapter
Hartford Regional Office
231 E Baltimore St, Suite 800
Baltimore, MD 21202
410-528-1555
800-421-8453
Fax: 410-528-1495
e-mail: scdaa@sicklecelldisease.org
www.sicklecelldisease.org

Regional office loactions in Hartford, New Haven and New London.

Georgia

6632 Sickle Cell Foundation of Georgia
2391 Benjamin E Mays Drive
Atlanta, GA 30311
404-755-1641
800-326-5287
Fax: 404-755-7955
e-mail: info@sicklecellga.org
www.sicklecellga.org/

Provides education, screening, and counseling programs for sickle cell and other abnormal hemoglobins. The Foundation has a deep-rooted commitment to making strides in monitoring the occurrence of sickle cell, improving the quality of life for those with the disease and cooperating with individuals conducting research.

Jean Brannan, Executive Director
Harold Dobbs, Outreach Coordinator
Nesby Gibson, Project Director

Louisiana

6633 NE Louisiana Sickle Cell Anemia Foundation
PO Box 1165
Monroe, LA 71210
318-322-0896
Fax: 318-387-4740
e-mail: sickle@bayou.com
www.sicklecelldisease.org/index.cfm?page=chapter&id=

The Northeast Louisiana Sickle Cell Anemia Foundation is a community based tax exempt organization that assists victims with the inherited blood disease sickle cell anemia.

Christopher Hollins, Chair
Sonja L. Banks, President/Chief Operating Officer
Francis Aofolaju, Chief Financial Officer

Massachusetts

6634 Community Sickle Cell Support Group
1542 Tremont St
Roxbury, MA 02120
617-427-4100
e-mail: cscsginc@aol.com
www.cscsginc.org

Jackie Rodriguez, Executive Director

New Mexico

6635 Sickle Cell Council of New Mexico, Inc.
1300 San Pedro NE
Albuquerque, NM 87108
505-254-9550
Fax: 505-254-9642
e-mail: victoria@sicklecellnm.org
www.sicklecellnm.org

Blood screening, education, and genetic counseling.

Victoria A Jones, Executive Director

6636 Eastern North Carolina Chapter (SCDAA)
PO Box 5253
Jacksonville, NC 28540 910-346-2510
800-826-1314
Fax: 910-346-2614
e-mail: sickle@bizec.rr.com
www.sicklecelleasternnc.org/index.php?pr=Home_Page

The North Carolina Sickle Cell Program was established in 1973. It provides services to persons with sickle cell disease, a lifelong red blood cell disorder that is passed from parents to children through genes. The program focuses on early detection and treatment, which can prevent many serious health prblems. It also offers education and genetic counseling for the general public.

Marcia M Wright, Executive Director

6637 Sickle Cell Disease Association of the Piedmont
231 E Baltimore St, Suite 800
Baltimore, MD 21202 410-528-1555
800-421-8453
Fax: 410-528-1495
e-mail: scdaa@sicklecelldisease.org
www.sicklecelldisease.org/index.cfm?page=chapter&id=

Dedicated to educating the public and providing support to people affected by sickle cell disease. Serving the following counties: Alamance, Forsyth, Caswell, Guilford, Randolph, and Rockingham.

Gladys A Robinson, Executive Director

6638 Sickle Cell Regional Network
Ste 404
Charlotte, NC 28202 704-332-4184
800-435-6004
Fax: 704-332-2246
e-mail: plambright@sc-cnc.org

Patricia Lambright, Executive Director

6639 Lehigh Valley Sickle Cell Support Group
PO Box 1711
Allentown, PA 18105 610-706-0636
e-mail: SororW@aol.com
www.members.aol.com/SororW/index.html

For anyone affected/effected by Sickle Cell and all interested persons. Learn more about sickle cell disease and how you can help.

**6640 Sickle Cell Disease Association of America ,
Philadelphia/Delaware Valley Chapter**
5070 Parkside Avenue- Suite 1404
Philadelphia, PA 19139 215-471-8686
Fax: 215-471-7441
e-mail: scdaa.pdvc@verizon.net
www.sicklecelldisorder.com

A support group for parents of a child or children with sickle cell disease.

Stanley A Simpkins, Executive Director

6641 James R Clark Memorial Sickle Cell Foundation
1420 Gregg Street
Columbia, SC 29201 803-765-9916
800-506-1273
Fax: 803-799-6471
e-mail: office@jamesrclarksicklecell.org
www.jamesrclarksicklecell.org/?

The mission of the foundation is to optimize the social and psychological well being of residents with sickle cell disease within the fifteen county area of South Carolina. This mission is accomplished through the provision of comprehensive services to individuals, families, and communities and is further enhanced by collaboration with appropriate federal, state, and local resources and through the involvement of volunteers and contributors.

Melodie Helms-Desilet, Executive Director

6642 Sickle Cell Association of Austin - Marc Thomas Chapter
1 Highland Ctr, 314 E Highland Mall Blvd, Ste 108
Austin, TX 78752 512-458-9767
Fax: 512-458-9714
e-mail: sicklecellaustin@sbcglobal.net
www.sicklecellaustin.org/

To raise awareness, resources and support for clients with sickle cell disease.

Linda Thomas, Manager
Nora Bouie-Burleson, Office Manager

6643 Sickle Cell Association of the Texas Gulf Coast
501 S. Main St.
Galena Park, TX 77547 713-921-1400
888-908-2355
Fax: 713-921-4525
e-mail: mbruce@steelassociates.net
www.steelassociates.net

Michael Bruce
Zachary Kitchens
Jaime Lozano

Libraries & Resource Centers

6644 Children's Center for Cancer and Blood Disorders
University of South Carolina School of Medicine
5 Richland Memorial Park
Columbia, SC 29203 803-434-3533

Joint clinical and basic research of juvenile cancer and blood disorders.

Fauni Lowe, Manager

Research Centers

6645 Northern California Comprehensive Sickle C ell Center
Children's Hospital at Oakland
747 52nd St
Oakland, CA 94609 510-450-5647
e-mail: evichinsky@mail.cho.org

Sickle cell disease research.

Elliott Vichinsky MD, Director

6646 University of Southern California Comprehensive Sickle Cell Center
2025 Zonal Avenue, Room 304
Los Angeles, CA 90033 323-442-1259
Fax: 323-442-1255
e-mail: cagejohn@hsc.usc.edu

Cage S Johnson MD, Director

6647 Howard University Center for Sickle Cell Disease
1840 7th Street NW
Washington, DC 20000 202-865-8292
Fax: 202-806-4517
e-mail: sicklecell@howard.edu.
www.sicklecell.howard.edu

Okay H Odocha, Director

Chen Shi, Director

Georgia

6648 Comprehensive Sickle Cell Center
Medical College of Georgia
1521 Pope Ave
Augusta, GA 30904   706-721-0174
                                Fax: 706-721-2643
                        www.mcg.edu/center/sicklecell/

New York

6649 Bronx Comprehensive Sickle Cell Center
Albert Einstein College of Medicine
Ullman Bldg, 1300 Morris Park Ave
Bronx, NY 10461   718-430-2088
                                Fax: 718-824-3153
                        e-mail: nagel@aecom.yu.edu

Ronald L Nagel MD, Director

North Carolina

6650 Duke University Comprehensive Sickle Cell Center
Medical Center
Box 2615
Durham, NC 27710   919-684-5378
                                Fax: 919-681-7688
                        e-mail: telen002@mc.duke.edu
                        www.sicklecell.mc.duke.edu

Research into sickle cell disease including molecular and organ studies.

Marilyn Telen MD, Director

Ohio

6651 Comprehensive Sickle Cell Center
Cincinnati Children's Hospital Medical Ctr
3333 Burnet Avenue
Cincinnati, OH 45229   513-636-4200
                               800-344-2462
                                Fax: 513-636-5562
                               TTY: 513-636-4900
                        e-mail: blood@cchmc.org
                        www.cincinnatichildrens.org

Offers research and statistical information in the area of sickle cell disease.

Clinton Joiner MD, Pediatric Director

Texas

6652 Center for Cancer and Blood Disorders
Children Medical Center Dallas
1935 Medical District Dr.
Dallas, TX 75235   214-456-7000
                                Fax: 214-456-6133
                        e-mail: ccbdinfo@childrens.com
                        www.childrens.com/ccbd/

A comprehensive program for diagnosis, patient/family education and management of sickle cell diseases in childhood and adolescence. Offers access to state-of-the art research projects and clinical management.

George R Buchanan, Medical Director
Zora R Rogers, MD, Associate Medical Director
Shirley Miller, Community Relations

6653 Southwestern Comprehensive Sickle Cell Cen ter
UT Southwestern Medical Ctr/Pediatrics Dept
5323 Harry Hines Blvd
Dallas, TX 75390   214-648-3111
                                Fax: 214-648-3122
                        e-mail: George.Buchanan@UTsouthwestern.edu

State-of-the-art patient care, clinical and basic lab research, education and advocacy programs.

Web Sites

6654 American Sickle Cell Anemia Association
DD Bldg. at the Cleveland Clinic, Suite DD1-201, 1
Cleveland, OH 44106   216-229-8600
                                Fax: 216-229-4500
                        e-mail: irabragg@ascaa.org
                        www.ascaa.org

The mission of the American Sickle Cell Anemia Association is to ensure the availability and accessibility of quality, comprehensive sickle cell services, and promote the public professional awareness about sickle cell anemis an it's hemoglobin diseases ad trait variants.

Ira Bragg-Grant, Executive Director
Leslie Carter, Newborn Screening Coordinator
Charlotte Martin, Receptionist

6655 Information Center for Sickle Cell and Tha lassemic Disorders
sickle.bwh.harvard.edu

Free online information to the biomedical community, health care personnel and patients. The information can be of particular help to patients in enabling them to have a fuller and more knowledgeable role in their care.

6656 International Association of Sickle Cell Nurses and Physician Assistants
www.iascnapa.org

The association is made up of over 300 sickle cell nurses and physician assistants worldwide. It recognizes its responsibility to maintain high standards in the provision of quality and accessible health care services for individuals with sickle cell disease.

Coretta Jenerette, RN, PhD, President
Pat Corley, RN, Vice-President
Bonita Conley, MSN, RN, PNP-BC, Secretary

6657 Online Mendelian Inheritance in Man
www.omim.org

This database is a catalog of human genes and genetic disorders.

6658 Sickle Cell Disease Association of America
3700 Koppers Street, Suite 570
Baltimore, MD 21227   410-528-1555
                               800-421-8453
                                Fax: 410-528-1495
                        e-mail: scdaa@sicklecelldisease.org
                        www.sicklecelldisease.org

Promotes the finding of a universal cure for sickle cell disease while improving the quality of life for individuals and families where sickle cell related conditions exists.

Sonja L. Banks, President/Chief Operating Officer
Francis Aofolaju, Vice President, Business & Finance
Natasha Thomas, Director, Planning & Development

6659 Sickle Cell Disease Forum
www.sicklecelldisease.org/forum/

Online forum for sickle cell disease discussion/chat sponsored by the Sickle Cell Disease Association of America.

6660 Sickle Cell Kids
www.sicklecellkids.org

Teaches children how to stay healthy and answers questions about sickle cell disease. A joint venture of the Georgia Comprehensive Sickle Cell Center at Grady Health System and Cynthia Gentry, artist.

Book Publishers

6661 Blood & Circulatory Disorders Sourcebook
Omnigraphics
PO Box 8002
Aston, PA 19014   610-461-3548
                                   800-234-1340
                              Fax: 800-875-1340
                   e-mail: info@omnigraphics.com
                            www.omnigraphics.com

Basic consumer health information on blood and its components, anemias, leukemias, bleeding disorders, and circulatory disorders, including sickle cell disease, aplastic anemia, thalassemia, and hemophilia.

2005 659 pages 2nd Edition
ISBN: 0-780807-46-4

Peter Ruffner, Publisher

6662 Let's Talk About Going to the Hospital
Rosen Publishing Group's PowerKids Press
29 E 21st Street
New York, NY 10010   212-777-3017
                                   800-237-9932
                              Fax: 888-436-4643
                e-mail: rosenpub@tribeca.ios.com
                           www.rosenpublishing.com

If a child has to check into the hospital, chances are he or she is already upset about being ill. Knowing how a hospital functions and what the procedures are, such as when family members can visit, will help in what is already a stressful situation. Grades K-5.

24 pages
ISBN: 0-823950-36-0

Roger Rosen, President

6663 Let's Talk About Sickle Cell Anemia
Melanie Apel Gordon, author

Rosen Publishing Group's PowerKids Press
29 E 21st Street
New York, NY 10010   212-777-3017
                                   800-237-9932
                              Fax: 888-436-4643
                e-mail: rosenpub@tribeca.ios.com
                           www.rosenpublishing.com

Explains why sickle cell anemia is a disease that strikes more African Americans than any other people in the country. Describes symptoms and explains how a kid can help take care of himself during a pain crisis. Grades K-5.

24 pages
ISBN: 0-823954-17-X

Roger Rosen, President

6664 Understanding Sickle Cell Disease
Miriam Bloom PhD, author

University Press of Mississippi
3825 Ridgewood Road
Jackson, MS 39211   601-432-6205
                                   800-737-7788
                              Fax: 601-432-6217
                e-mail: press@ihl.state.ms.us
                           www.upress.state.ms.us

Part of the Understanding Health and Sickness Series. For general readers, a guide to understanding a debilitating genetic disease that affects tens of thousands who are of African heritage.

128 pages Paperback
ISBN: 0-878057-45-5

Leila W. Salisbury, Director
Cynthia Foster, Administrative Assistant
Tracey Curtis, Assistant For Development

Pamphlets

6665 Sickle Cell Disease
March of Dimes Resource Center
1275 Mamaroneck Avenue
White Plains, NY 10605   914-997-4488
                             Fax: 914-997-4763
                             TTY: 914-977-4764
             e-mail: resourcecenter@modimes.org
         www.marchofdimes.org/professionals/681_1221.asp

Fact Sheets: one to two page review written for the general public. Also available electronically from website www.modimes.org. Brochures: 3 panel color brochures written for the general public.

Camps

6666 Camp Crescent Moon
Sickle Cell Disease Foundation of California
6133 Bristol Parkway, Suite 240
Culver City, CA 90230   310-693-0247
                                  877-288-2873
                             Fax: 310-693-0266
                       e-mail: info@scdfc.org
                        www.campcrescentmoon.org

A specialized camp for children with sickle cell disease between the ages of 8 and 14 in southern & central California.

Mary E Brown, Camp Director
Deborah Green, Assistant Camp Director
Cage Johnson MD, Medical Director

6667 Camp Good Days & Special Times
1332 Pittsford-Mendon Rd, P.O. Box 665
Mendon, NY 14506   585-624-5555
                                  800-785-2135
                             Fax: 585-624-5799
                         www.campgooddays.org

Camp for children ages 8 to 17 with sickle cell anemia. The camp is dedicated to improving the quality of life for children, adults and families whose lives have been touched by cancer and other life challenges.

Gary Mervis, Chairman/ Founder
Wendy Bleier-Mervis, Executive Director
Lisa Booz, Western New York Regional Director

6668 Camp Vacamas
256 Macopin Road
West Milford, NJ   973-838-1394
                             Fax: 973-838-7534
                        e-mail: info@vacamas.org
                             www.vacamas.org

Disadvantaged children with asthma or sickle cell anemia, ages 8-16, are offered special programs in canoeing, backpacking, camping, music and leadership training. Sliding scale tuition. Year round programs for groups.

Michael Friedman, Executive Director
Philip Smith, Camp Director

Description

6669 SLEEP APNEA

Involves the following Biologic System(s):

Respiratory Disorders

Obstructive sleep apnea (OSA) is a breathing disorder that is commonly seen in the pediatric population. Specifically, it is when normal ventilation during sleep is disrupted because of upper airway obstruction. This process occurs intermittently throughout sleep and causes significant disruptions in normal sleep patterns. Although in adults this can result in excessive daytime sleepiness, children typically manifest changes in behavior or deficits in attention, thus affecting school performance.

Studies indicate that roughly 2% of children between the ages of 2-18 years are affected by this disorder. Girls and boys are equally likely to have OSA and African American children are more commonly affected than children of other ethnicities. OSA is also more common in children with obesity, craniofacial abnormalities and/or neurologic disorders. Children with Down syndrome are at especially increased risk.

The cause of obstructive sleep apnea is not well understood. Adenotonsillar (adenoids and tonsils) hypertrophy (increase in size) seems to be part of the process but even after tonsillectomy and adenoidectomy (removal of these tissues) many patients relapse, implying other processes involved.

The clinical features commonly seem with OSA include noisy breathing during sleep, prominent snoring often in a crescendo pattern that ends with a pause in respirations for performance, nocturnal enuresis (bed wetting) and frequent daytime napping. Complications of OSA can be failure to thrive or gain weight appropriately, pulmonary hypertension which cause stress on the right side of the heart and neurological sequelae.

Diagnosis should not be based solely on a history of snoring. Many children snore who do not suffer from OSA, however, a careful history focusing on some of the clinical features mentioned above should raise the suspicion of OSA and further evaluation can be considered. The physical exam of tonsillar hypertrophy may help support the diagnosis but often a polysomnography test, commonly called sleep study, is the most accurate way to diagnose OSA. The sleep study is a comprehensive diagnostic tool involving monitoring a patient during sleep using multiple parameters including the visual surveillance, monitoring of the heart rate and rhythm, monitoring of the respiratory rate, measurement of expired lung gases, oxygen saturation in the blood, chest wall rise with breathing and others. While the necessity of this study in children may be debated, it is considered a definitive way to establishthe diagnosis of OSA.

In general, nonsurgical therapy is very limited for the typical patient with OSA. Treatment of childhood OSA is primarily surgical. Removal of the tonsils and adenoids are often the first line of treatment as well as targeting weight reduction when relevant. Most children respond well to tonsillectomy and adenoidectomy, but for those who do not improve, nasal continued positive airway pressure (NCPAP) is another effective option which enhances the infant's respiratory function.

OSA is an important cause of health, emotional and behavioral problems in school aged children and effective and timely treatment can significantly improve school performance, and productivity and well-being of these children.

National Associations & Support Groups

6670 American Academy of Pediatrics
141 Northwest Point Boulevard
Elk Grove Village, IL 60007

847-434-4000
800-433-9016
Fax: 847-434-8000
www.aap.org

The American Academy of Pediatrics and its member pediatricians are committed to the attainment of optimal physical, mental and social health and well-being for all infants, children, adolescents, and young adults.

Sandra Hassink, MD, FAAP, President

6671 American Academy of Sleep Medicine
2510 North Frontage Road
Darien, IL 60561

630-737-9700
Fax: 630-737-9790
www.aasmnet.org

National not-for-profit professional membership organization dedicated to the advancement of sleep medicine. The Academy's mission is to assure quality care for patients with sleep disorders, promote the advancement of sleep research and provide public and professional education. The AASM delivers programs, information and services to and through its members and advocates sleep medicine supportive policies in the medical community and the public sector.

Jerry Barrett, Executive Director
Jennifer Markkanen, Assistant Executive Director

6672 American Sleep Apnea Association
6856 Eastern Ave, NW #203
Washington, DC 20012

888-293-3650
Fax: 888-293-3650
e-mail: asaa@sleepapnea.org
www.sleepapnea.org

Offers help and information to persons with sleep apnea and their families.

Edward Grandi, Executive Director
Dave Hargett, Chair

6673 Center for Disabilities and Development
University of Iowa Hospitals and Clinics
100 Hawkins Drive
Iowa City, IA 52242

319-353-6900
877-686-0031
Fax: 319-356-8284
e-mail: cdd-scheduling@uiowa.edu
www.uichildrens.org/cdd

A trusted resource for healthcare, training, research and information for people with disabilities that include: behavior disorders, brain injury, cerebral palsy, diabetes, down syndrome, learning disabilities, mental retardation, sleep disorders and spina bifida.

Judy Stephenson, Administrator
Amy Mikelson, Supervisor Info Resource Service

6674 National Sleep Foundation
1522 K Street NW, Suite 500
Washington, DC 20005

202-464-1308
Fax: 202-347-3472
e-mail: nsf@sleepfoundation.org
www.narap.org

An independent, nonprofit organization dedicated to improving public health and safety by achieving public understanding of sleep and sleep disorders, and by supporting public education, sleep-related research, and advocacy. Actively collaborates with sleep centers and support groups for patients with sleep disorders and safety organizations.

Richard Gelula, CEO

Libraries & Resource Centers

6675 American Academy of Somnology
PO Box 27077
Las Vegas, NV 89126   702-371-0947
e-mail: somnology@aol.com
www.hopperinstitute.com/aas_intro.html

Covers about 75 physicians, dentists, nurses, psychologists, technicians, and students and sponsoring organizations, including associations, institutions, and corporations, with a special interest in sleep. Newsletter, published yearly.

David Hopper, Director

Research Centers

6676 Sleep Disorders Center
Beth Israel Deaconess Medical Ctr
330 Brookline Avenue
Boston, MA 02215   617-667-7000
Fax: 617-975-5506
www.bidmc.harvard.edu

Provides testing and treatment for those with sleep disorders and offers educational workshops, plus support for their families.

Jean K Matheson, MD, Division Chief

Web Sites

6677 About.com on Sleep Disorders
www.sleepdisorders.about.com

Well-organized information including new developments and a chat room.

6678 American Academy of Sleep Medicine
2510 North Frontage Road
Darien, IL 60561   630-737-9700
Fax: 630-737-9790
e-mail: inquiries@aasmnet.org
www.aasmnet.org

The mission is to assure quality care for patients with sleep disorders, promote the advancement of sleep research and provide public and professional education.

Timothy I. Morgenthaler, MD, President
Ronald D. Chervin, MD, MS, Secretary/Treasurer
Jerome A. Barrett, Executive Director

6679 American Sleep Apnea Association
1717 Pennsylvania Avenue, NW Ste. 1025
Washington, DC 20006   888-293-3650
Fax: 888-293-3650
e-mail: asaa@sleepapnea.org
www.sleepapnea.org

Is dedicated to reducing injury, disbility, and death from sleep apnea and to enhancing the well being of those affected by this common disorder. The ASAA promotes education and awareness, the ASAA A.W.A.K.E. Network of voluntary mutual suport groups, research, and continuous improvement of care.

Tracy R. Nasca, Executive Director
Justine Amdur, AWAKE Program Coordinator
Adam Amdur, Chief Operating Officer

6680 MEDLINEplus on Sleep Apnea
8600 Rockville Pike
Bethesda, MD 20894   e-mail: custserv@nlm.nih.gov
www.nlm.nih.gov/medlineplus/sleepapnea.html

Offers information about Sleep Apnea.

Dr. Donald A.B. Lindberg, Director

6681 NIH/National Center on Sleep Disorders Research
www.nhlbi.nih.gov/about/org/ncsdr/

Coordinates sleep research, training and education supported by the government.

6682 National Sleep Foundation
1010 N. Glebe Road Suite 310
Arlington, VA 22201   703-243-1697
e-mail: nsf@sleepfoundation.org
www.sleepfoundation.org

Is an independent nonprofit organization dedicated to improving public health and safety by achieving understanding of sleep and slepp disorders, and by supporting education, sleep-related research, and advocacy.

Charles A. Czeisler, PhD, MD, Chairman
Max Hirshkowitz, PhD, Vice Chairman
Joseph Ojile, MD, Secretary

6683 Sleepdisorders.com
www.sleepdisorders.com

Provides a full range of internet communications and technology solutions from strategic consulting to concept design, content development, software engineering, and ongoing enhancements and maintenance. Our projects have encompassed direct-to-consumer marketing, direct-to-patient education, healthcare professional training, corporate intranets and database management systems, dynamic database-driven websites and hospital training.

John Douglas Hudson, M.D., Medical Director

6684 Sleepnet.com
www.sleepnet.com/sleepapnea2000.html

Categorizes sleep disorders for research, forums are up-dated frequently and posts are thoughtful and insightful.

Book Publishers

6685 Concise Guide to Evaluation and Management of Sleep Disorders
American Psychiatric Publishing
1000 Wilson Boulevard, Suite 1825
Arlington, VA 22209   703-907-7322
800-368-5777
Fax: 703-907-1091
e-mail: appi@psych.org
www.appi.org

Overview of sleep disorders medicine, sleep physiology and pathology, insomnia complaints, excessive sleepiness disorders, parasomnias, medical and psychiatric disorders and sleep, medications with sedative - hypnotic properties, special problems and populations.

2002 296 pages Paper 3rd Ed
ISBN: 1-585620-45-6

Robert E. Hales, M.D., Editor-in-Chief
Rebecca D. Rinehart, Publisher
John McDuffie, Editorial Director

6686 Let's Talk About Going to the Hospital
Rosen Publishing Group's PowerKids Press
29 E 21st Street
New York, NY 10010   212-777-3017
800-237-9932
Fax: 888-436-4643
e-mail: rosenpub@tribeca.ios.com
www.rosenpublishing.com

If a child has to check into the hospital, chances are he or she is already upset about being ill. Knowing how a hospital functions and what the procedures are, such as when family members can visit, will help in what is already a stressful situation. Grades K-5.

24 pages
ISBN: 0-823950-36-0

Roger Rosen, President

6687 Principles and Practice of Sleep Medicine
Elsevier Health Sciences Division
1600 John F Kennedy Blvd, Suite 1800
Philadelphia, PA 19103   215-239-3900
800-523-1649
Fax: 215-239-3990
www.us.elsevierhealth.com

Covers the recent advances in basic sciences as well as sleep pathology in adults. Encompasses developments in this rapidly advancing field and also includes topics related to psychiatry, circadian rhythms, cardiovascualr diseases and sleep apnea diagnosis and treatment. Hardcover.

2005 1552 pages 4th Edition
ISBN: 0-721607-97-7

6688 Restless Nights
Yale University Press
PO Box 209040
New Haven, CT 06520

203-432-0960
800-405-1619
Fax: 203-432-0948
e-mail: marketing@yale.edu.
yalepress.yale.edu/yupbooks

This book provides an explanation of sleep apnea symptoms, risk-factors, advice on diagnosis and consultation, and current available treatments.

2003 288 pages
ISBN: 0-300085-44-0

John Donatich, Director

6689 Sleep Disorders Sourcebook
Omnigraphics
PO Box 8002
Aston, PA 19014

800-234-1340
Fax: 800-875-1340
e-mail: info@omnigraphics.com
omnigraphics.com

Basic consumer health information about sleep and its disorders, including sleep apnea, insomnia, sleepwalking, restless leg syndrome and narcolepsy.

567 pages 2nd Edition
ISBN: 0-780807-43-0

Peter Ruffner, Publisher

6690 Sleeping Like a Baby

Avi Sadeh, author

Yale University Press
PO Box 209040
New Haven, CT 06520

203-432-0960
800-405-1619
Fax: 203-432-0948
e-mail: marketing@yale.edu.
yalepress.yale.edu/yupbooks

A practical and sensitive guide to solving your child's sleep problems.

2001 224 pages
ISBN: 0-300088-24-3

John Donatich, Director

6691 Snoring From A to Zzzz
Spencer Press
2525 NW Lovejoy Street, Suite 402
Portland, OR 97210

503-223-4959
Fax: 503-223-1608
e-mail: dereklipman@aol.com

Covers organizations, associations, support groups, and manufactorers of sleep-related medical products relevant to sleep disorders. Discussess every aspect of snoring and sleep apnea from causes to cures.

256 pages Paperback
ISBN: 0-965070-81-6

Derek S Lipman, MD, Author/Editor

6692 Snoring and Sleep Apnea
Demos Medical Publishing
386 Park Avenue S
New York, NY 10016

212-683-0072
800-532-8663
Fax: 212-683-0118
e-mail: orderdept@demosmedpub.com
www.demosmedpub.com

A straightforward, jargon-free approach to dealing with snoring and sleep problems.

286 pages 3rd Ed/Soft
ISBN: 1-888799-29-3

Kathy Gonzalez, Order Dept/Fulfillment Coordinator
Paul Choi, Vice-President of Finance and Opera
Richard Winters, Executive Editor

Pamphlets

6693 Get the Facts About Sleep Apnea
American Sleep Apnea Association
1717 Pennsylvania Avenue, NW Ste. 1025
Washington, DC 20006

202-293-3650
888-293-3650
Fax: 888-293-3650
e-mail: asaa@sleepapnea.org
www.sleepapnea.org

Brochures are also available in bulk.

Will Headapohl, Chair
Tracy R. Nasca, Executive Director
Justine Amdur, AWAKE Program Coordinator

6694 Sleep Apnea
National Sleep Foundation
1010 N. Glebe Road Suite 310
Arlington, VA 22201

703-243-1697
Fax: 202-347-3472
e-mail: nsf@sleepfoundation.org
www.sleepfoundation.org

A brochure about sleep apnea, a breathing disorder characterized by brief interruptions of breathing during sleep. Brochure explains what it is, who gets it, and how it is diagnosed and treated.

Charles A. Czeisler, PhD, MD, Chairman
Max Hirshkowitz, PhD, Vice Chairman
Joseph Ojile, MD, Secretary

Description

6695 SLEEPWALKING

Synonym: Somnambulism

Involves the following Biologic System(s):

Developmental/Behavioral/Psychiatric Disorders

Sleepwalking, also known as somnambulism, is a condition where the child engages in activities that are normally associated with wakefulness while asleep or in a sleeplike state. It occurs most commonly in children, particularly those from approximately four to six years of age. About 10 to 15 percent of children experience at least one episode of sleepwalking during childhood. In addition, approximately one in five children who sleepwalk has a family history of the condition. In many patients, sleepwalking occurs in association with bed-wetting (nocturnal enuresis) or night terrors (sleep disturbances that typically occur shortly after the onset of sleep). In some cases, a stressful event may lead to an episode of sleepwalking.

In children, sleepwalking occurs during stage four of NREM (nonrapid eye movement) sleep. NREM sleep consists of four progressively deeper stages of sleep that are typically characterized by slow, deep brain waves, muscle relaxation and slowed breathing rate, slowed heart rate, and lowered blood pressure. In contrast, REM (rapid eye movement) sleep, which is associated with dreaming, is characterized by increased levels of brain activity, rapid eye movements, and involuntary muscle jerks.

During an episode of sleepwalking, affected children may simply sit up in bed or move to the edge of the bed, without engaging in actual sleepwalking. In other cases, however, children may get out of bed and walk through their home. They may also perform certain routine acts, such as turning on a hallway light. Unless children are simultaneously experiencing night terrors, they usually do not have associated anxiety. During an episode, most children have their eyes open and are guided by their vision. Therefore, they typically move around familiar obstacles; however, some children may make no effort to avoid certain objects in their path, potentially resulting in injury. In addition, some children may mumble simple words or phrases or repeatedly perform certain acts, such as turning a doorknob back and forth. If children are urged to return to bed during such an episode, they may sometimes follow such instruction; however, they usually must be gently steered back to their beds. Sleepwalking episodes typically last only a few minutes, and children usually have little or no memory of the experience. In children, sleepwalking is rarely associated with psychologic abnormalities, and the number of episodes usually decreases by early adolescence. However, the persistence of sleepwalking episodes into adulthood is thought to be associated with a significant risk of psychiatric disease. Parents or caregivers of children who sleepwalk should take precautions to help protect them against injury. Possible obstacles or breakable objects should be removed from their paths. It may be advisable to block staircases and to have children sleep on the ground floor of the house, if possible.

Government Agencies

6696 NIH/National Institute of Mental Health
6001 Executive Boulevard, Room 8184, MSC 9663
Bethesda, MD 20892
301-443-4513
866-615-6464
Fax: 301-443-4279
TTY: 301-443-8431
e-mail: nimhinfo@nih.gov
www.nimh.nih.gov

Conducts strategic planning for specific research areas as well as for the Institute as a whole.

Dr Thomas R Insel, Director

National Associations & Support Groups

6697 American Academy of Pediatrics
141 Northwest Point Boulevard
Elk Grove Village, IL 60007
847-434-4000
800-433-9016
Fax: 847-434-8000
www.aap.org

The American Academy of Pediatrics and its member pediatricians are committed to the attainment of optimal physical, mental and social health and well-being for all infants, children, adolescents, and young adults.

Sandra Hassink, MD, FAAP, President

6698 American Academy of Sleep Medicine
2510 North Frontage Road
Darien, IL 60561
630-737-9700
Fax: 630-737-9790
www.aasmnet.org

National not-for-profit professional membership organization dedicated to the advancement of sleep medicine. The Academy's mission is to assure quality care for patients with sleep disorders, promote the advancement of sleep research and provide public and professional education. The AASM delivers programs, information and services to and through its members and advocates sleep medicine supportive policies in the medical community and the public sector.

Jerry Barrett, Executive Director
Jennifer Markkanen, Assistant Executive Director

6699 Center for Disabilities and Development
University of Iowa Hospitals and Clinics
100 Hawkins Drive
Iowa City, IA 52242
319-353-6900
877-686-0031
Fax: 319-356-8284
e-mail: cdd-scheduling@uiowa.edu
www.uichildrens.org/cdd

A trusted resource for healthcare, training, research and information for people with disabilities that include: behavior disorders, brain injury, cerebral palsy, diabetes, down syndrome, learning disabilities, mental retardation, sleep disorders and spina bifida.

Judy Stephenson, Administrator
Amy Mikelson, Supervisor Info Resource Service

6700 Federation of Families for Children's Mental Health
9605 Medical Center Drive, Suite 280
Rockville, MD 20850
240-403-1901
Fax: 240-403-1909
e-mail: ffcmh@ffcmh.org
www.ffcmh.org

The National family run organization is dedicated exclusively to helping children with mental health needs and their families achieve a better quality of life.

Sandra Spencer, Executive Director

6701 National Mental Health Consumers' Self-Help Clearinghouse
1211 Chestnut Street, Suite 1207
Philadelphia, PA 19107
215-751-1810
800-553-4539
Fax: 215-636-6312
e-mail: info@mhselfhelp.org
www.mhselfhelp.org

Offers information, support and appropriate referrals; and promotes public and professional education. Provides networking for those with special interests related to albinism. Promotes and supports research and funding that will improve diagnosis and management of albinism and hypopigmentation.

Joseph Rogers, Executive Director & Founder

6702 National Sleep Foundation
1522 K Street NW, Suite 500
Washington, DC 20005
202-464-1308; Fax: 202-347-3472
e-mail: nsf@sleepfoundation.org
www.narap.org

An independent, nonprofit organization dedicated to improving public health and safety by achieving public understanding of sleep and sleep disorders, and by supporting public education, sleep-related research, and advocacy. Actively collaborates with sleep centers, support groups for patients with sleep disorders and safety organizations.

Richard Gelula, CEO

Libraries & Resource Centers

6703 American Academy of Somnology
PO Box 27077
Las Vegas, NV 89126
702-371-0947
e-mail: somnology@aol.com
www.hopperinstitute.com/aas_intro.html

Covers about 75 physicians, dentists, nurses, psychologists, technicians, and students and sponsoring organizations, including associations, institutions, and corporations, with a special interest in sleep.

David Hopper, Director

Web Sites

6704 About.com on Sleep Disorders
www.sleepdisorders.about.com

Well-organized information including new developments and a chat room.

6705 National Sleep Foundation
1010 N. Glebe Road Suite 310
Arlington, VA 22201
703-243-1697
e-mail: nsf@sleepfoundation.org; www.sleepfoundation.org

Is an independent nonprofit organization dedicated to improving public health and safety by achieving understnading of sleep and sleep disorders, and by supporting education, sleep-related research, and advocacy.

Charles A. Czeisler, PhD, MD, Chairman
Max Hirshkowitz, PhD, Vice Chairman
Joseph Ojile, MD, Secretary

6706 Online Mendelian Inheritance in Man
www.omim.org

This database is a catalog of human genes and genetic disorders.

6707 Sleep Walking in Children
familydoctor.org/160.xml

Brief overview of possible parental concerns of sleep walking in children.

6708 SleepEducation.com
2510 North Frontage Road
Darien, IL 60561
630-737-9700; Fax: 630-737-9790
www.sleepeducation.com

Online resources on sleep related topics and sleep disorders including sleepwalking.

6709 Sleepdisorders.com
www.sleepdisorders.com

Provides a full range of internet communications and technology solutions from strategic consulting to concept design, content development, software engineering, and ongoing enhancements and maintenance. Our projects have encompassed direct-to-customer marketing, direct-to-patient education, healthcare professional training, corporate intranets and database management systems, dynamic database-driven web sites and hospital training.

John Douglas Hudson, M.D., Medical Director

Book Publishers

6710 Concise Guide to Evaluation and Management of Sleep Disorders
American Psychiatric Publishing
1000 Wilson Boulevard, Suite 1825
Arlington, VA 22209
703-907-7322; 800-368-5777
Fax: 703-907-1091
e-mail: appi@psych.org; www.appi.org

Over view of sleep disorders medicine, sleep physiology and pathology, insomnia complaints, excessive sleepiness disorders, parasomnias, medical and psychiatric disorders and sleep, medications with sedative-hypnotic properties, special problems and populations.

2002 296 pages Paper 3rd Ed
ISBN: 1-585620-45-6

Robert E. Hales, M.D., Editor-in-Chief
Rebecca D. Rinehart, Publisher
John McDuffie, Editorial Director

6711 Sleep Disorders Sourcebook
Omnigraphics
PO Box 8002
Aston, PA 19014
800-234-1340; Fax: 800-875-1340
e-mail: info@omnigraphics.com; omnigraphics.com

Basic consumer health information about sleep and its disorders, including insomnia, sleepwalking, sleep apnea, restless leg syndrome and narcolepsy.

567 pages 2nd Edition
ISBN: 0-780807-43-0

Peter Ruffner, Publisher

6712 Sleep: The Brazelton Way

T Berry Brazelton; Joshua D Sparrow, author

Perseus Books Group-Da Capo Press
250 West 57th Street, 15th Floor
New York, NY 10107   617-252-5200; www.perseusbooksgroup.com

Pediatrician provide highly effective and affordable guides to lead parents through struggles of getting babies and toddlers to sleep.

2003 Paperback
ISBN: 0-738207-82-9

David Steinberger, President & CEO

6713 Snoring From A to Zzzz
Spencer Press
2525 NW Lovejoy Street, Suite 402
Portland, OR 97210
503-223-4959; Fax: 503-223-1608
e-mail: dereklipman@aol.com

Covers organizations, associations, support groups, and manufactorers of sleep-related medical products relevant to sleep disorders. Discussess every aspect of snoring and sleep apnea from causes to cures.

256 pages Paperback
ISBN: 0-965070-81-6

Derek S Lipman, MD, Author/Editor

Description

6714 SOCIAL ANXIETY DISORDER

Synonym: Social phobia

Involves the following Biologic System(s):

Neurologic Disorders

Social Anxiety Disorder (also called social phobia) is diagnosed in individuals who are overwhelmingly anxious and excessively self-conscious in everyday social situations. Children with social anxiety disorder are usually diagnosed once they reach school age, but symptoms have been seen in children as young as two years. Symptoms include an intense, chronic fear of being watched and judged by others, and fear of doing things that will embarrass them. This fear causes anxiety for days or weeks before a dreaded situation, and may become so severe that it interferes with school and other ordinary activities, often making it difficult to make and keep friends.

Social anxiety disorder is a fear reaction to a danger that isn't actually dangerous—although the body and mind react as if the danger is real. The physical responses to fear—fast hearbeat, quick breathing actually occur as adrenaline and other chemicals prepare the body to either fight or flee the danger (fight-flight). This biological mechanism kicks in when we feel afraid, alerting us to danger so we can protect ourselves. Those with the disorder experience this response too frequently, too strongly, and in situations where it's not appropriate (dangerous). Because the physcial sensations are real, however, the danger seems real, too.

Indivduals with social anxiety disorder are often unable to do common things in front of other people, like signing a check in front of a cashier, eating or drinking in a resta urant, or using a public restroom. Most people with the disorder know they shouldn't be afraid, but can't control their fear. They usually interact easily only with their family and a few close friends. Physical symptoms often accompany the anxiety, including blushing, profuse sweating, trembling, nausea, and difficulty speaking. These symptoms increase the feeling of being watched, which intensifies the anxiety.

Like many other anxiety-based disorders, social anxiety disorder usually results from the combination of three factors: genetics; learned behaviors; and life experiences. Those who constantly receive criticism may grow to expect that reaction from everyone they meet. Children who are teased or bullied are more likely to retreat into themselves. They will be paranoid of making a mistake or disappointing someone, and be overly sensitive to criticism.

Social anxiety disorder can increase feelings of loneliness or disappointment over missed opportunities for friendship, getting the most out of school, sharing talents, and learning new skills. Some children and teens are so shy and fearful about talking to others that they exhibit selective mutism—not speaking at all to certain people (i.e. teachers or students they don't know) or in certain places (i.e. at someone else's house). These individuals have normal conversations with people and places they are comfortable with, and their selective silence is sometimes mistaken for a stuck-up attitude or rudeness. Instead, selective mutism stems from feeling uncomfortable and afraid.

Psychotherapy is a successful treatment for social anxiety disorder, and is used sometimes in combination with certain medications. A physical examination will rule out physical reasons for the symptoms being exhibited. Cognitive behavior therapy is especially useful for treating social anxiety. It teaches different ways of thinking, behaving, and reacting to situations that help reduce the feelings of anxiousness and fear. It can also help people learn and practice social skills. Sometimes anti-anxiety or anti-depressant medications are prescribed. Although safe and effective for many people, they may be risky for some, especially children, teens, and young adults. Those taking anti-depressants should be monitored closely, especially at the start of their treatment.

Family and other supportive adults are especially important to children with social anxiety disorder. It is often a supportive environment that gives those with the disorder the courage to go outside their comfort zone.

Government Agencies

6715 Center for Mental Health Services Knowledge Exchange Program

US Department of Health and Human Services
PO Box 42557
Washington, DC 20015

800-789-2647
Fax: 240-747-5470
TDD: 866-889-2647
http://mentalhealth.samhsa.gov

Supplies the public with expert responses to commonly asked questions about various mental health disorders, and directs the caller to appropriate resources.

6716 NIH/National Institute of Mental Health

6001 Executive Boulevard, Room 8184, MSC 9663
Bethesda, MD 20892

301-443-4513
866-615-6464
Fax: 301-443-4279
TTY: 301-443-8431
e-mail: nimhinfo@nih.gov
www.nimh.nih.gov

Conducts strategic planning for specific research areas as well as for the Institute as a whole.

Dr Thomas R Insel, Director

National Associations & Support Groups

6717 American Academy of Pediatrics

141 Northwest Point Boulevard
Elk Grove Village, IL 60007

847-434-4000
800-433-9016
Fax: 847-434-8000
www.aap.org

The American Academy of Pediatrics and its member pediatricians are committed to the attainment of optimal physical, mental and social health and well-being for all infants, children, adolescents, and young adults.

Sandra Hassink, MD, FAAP, President

6718 American Counseling Association

6101 Stevenson Ave
Alexandria, VA 22304

703-823-9800
800-347-6647
Fax: 703-823-0252
e-mail: webmaster@counseling.org
www.counseling.org

Represents professional counselors in various practice settings, and stands ready to serve more than 55,000 members with the resources they need to make a difference. From webinars, publications, and journals to Conference education sessions and legislative action alerts, ACA is where counseling professionals turn for powerful, credible content and support.

Robert L. Smith, President

6719 American Mental Health Foundation (AMHF)
PO Box 3
Riverdale, NY 10028   212-737-9027
e-mail: elomke@americanmentalhealthfoundation.or
americanmentalhealthfoudnation.org

Dedicated to the extensive and intensive research in the theories and techniques of treatment of emotional illness and to the implementation of reforms in the mental health system. Efforts have resulted in development of better and less expensive treatment methods. Findings are disseminated in English and other major languages.

Monroe W Spero, MD
Evander Lomke, Executive Director

6720 American Psychiatric Association
1000 Wilson Boulevard, Suite 1825
Arlington, VA 22209   703-907-7300
888-35 -7924
e-mail: apa@psych.org
www.psychiatry.org

It is a medical specialty society representing growing membership of more than 36,000 psychiatrists.

6721 American Psychological Association
750 First St. NE
Washington, DC 20002   202-336-5500
800-374-2721
TTY: 202-336-6123
www.apa.org

The mission is to advance the creation, communication and application of psychological knowledge to benefit society and improve people's lives.

Norman B. Anderson, PhD, CEO/ EVP
L. Michael Honaker, PhD, Deputy Chief Executive Officer
Ellen G. Garrison, PhD, Senior Policy Advisor

6722 American School Counselor Association
1101 King Street, Suite 310
Alexandria, VA 22314   703-683-2722
800-306-4722
Fax: 703-997-7572
e-mail: asca@schoolcounselor.org
www.schoolcounselor.org

The mission of ASCA is to represent professional school counselors and to promote professionalism and ethical practices.

Richard Wong, Executive Director
Jeff Broderson, Information Technology Admin.
Kathleen M Rakestraw, Director of Communications

6723 Anxiety Disorders Association of America
8730 Georgia Avenue, Suite 600
Silver Spring, MD 20910   240-485-1001
Fax: 240-485-1035
e-mail: information@adaa.org
www.adaa.org

Offers resources and information for persons with anxiety and stress-related disorders.

Alies Muskin, Executive Director

6724 Anxiety Disorders Institute
1 Dunwoody Park Suite 112
Atlanta, GA 30338   770-395-6845

Provides support, training, and services for those suffering from anxiety disorders, and their families.

6725 Anxiety and Phobia Treatment Center
Whire Plains Hospital Center
Davis Avenue & East Post Road
White Plains, NY 10601   914-681-1038
Fax: 914-681-2284
e-mail: jchessa@wphospital.org
phobia-anxiety.com

Treatment groups for individuals suffering from phobias. Deals with fears through contextual therapy, a treatment and study of the phobia in the actual setting in which the phobic reactions occur. Conducts Intensive Courses, Phobia Self-Help Groups, 8-week Phobia Clinics and individual treatment. Publications: PM Newsletter, bimonthly. Articles and papers. Annual conference.

Fredrick J Neumen, MD, Director

6726 Federation of Families for Children's Mental Health
9605 Medical Center Drive, Suite 280
Rockville, MD 20850   240-403-1901
Fax: 240-403-1909
e-mail: ffcmh@ffcmh.org
www.ffcmh.org

The National family run organization is dedicated exclusively to helping children with mental health needs and their families achieve a better quality of life.

Sandra Spencer, Executive Director

6727 National Anxiety Foundation
3135 Custer Drive
Lexington, KY 40517   859-281-0003
www.lexington-on-line.com/naf.html

Nonprofit organization that provides education to the public and professionals about anxiety through printed and electronic media.

Stephen Cox MD, President & Medical Director

6728 Phobia Society of America
133 Rollins Avenue, Suite 4B
Rockville, MD 20852   301-231-9350
Fax: 301-231-7392
www.adaa.org

Offers support for those suffering from phobia and panic attacks.

6729 Phobics Anonymous
PO Box 1180
Palm Springs, CA 92263   706-327-2148

Twelve-step program for panic disorders and anxiety. Publications available.

Marily Gellis PhD, Contact

6730 Selective Mutism Foundation
PO Box 25972
Tamarac, FL 33320   305-748-7714
Fax: 305-748-7714
www.selectivemutismfoundation.org

Promotes awareness and understanding for individuals and families affected by selective mutism, an inherited anxiety disorder in which children with normal or deficient language skills are unable to speak in school or social situations. SM is often mistaken for normal shyness and may go undetected for as long as two years. Encourages research and treatment. Maintains speakers' bureau. Publications: Let's Talk, annual newsletter. Selective Mutism, A Silent Cry for Help, brochure.

Sue Newman, Co-Founder & Director

6731 Social Anxiety Association
socialphobia.org

The Social Anxiety Association is a non-profit organization founded in 1997 to meet the growing needs of people with social anxiety.

Thomas A. Richards, Ph.D., President

6732 Special Interest Group on Phobias and Related Anxiety Disorders (SIGPRAD)
245 E 87th Street
New York, NY 10128

212-860-5560
Fax: 212-744-5751
e-mail: lindy@interport.net
www.cyberpsych.org

For psychologists, psychiatrists, social workers and other individuals interested in treatment of anxiety disorders. Objectives are to increase knowledge, facilitate communication, and support research and treatment of phobias and related anxiety disorders. Conducts programs at professional meetings. Affiliated with the Association for Advancement of Behavior Therapy. Periodic symposiums and workshops.

Carol Lindemann, PhD, CEO

Audio Video

6733 Acquiring Courage: Audio Cassette Program for the Rapid Treatment of Phobias
New Harbinger Publications
5674 Shattuck Avenue
Oakland, CA 94609

510-652-2002
800-748-6273
Fax: 800-652-1613
e-mail: customerservice@newharbinger.com
newharbinger.com

ISBN: 1-879237-03-2

6734 Anxiety Disorders
American Counseling Association
6101 Stevenson Ave, Suite 600
Alexandria, VA 22304

703-823-9800
800-347-6647
Fax: 800-473-2329
e-mail: webmaster@counseling.org
counseling.org

Increase your awareness of anxiety disorders, their symptoms, and effective treatments. Learn the effect these disorders can have on life and how treatment can change the quality of life for people presently suffering from these disorders. Includes 6 audiotapes and a study guide.

Robert L. Smith, President

Book Publishers

6735 Anxiety & Phobia Workbook
Edmund J Bourne, author

New Harbinger Publications
5674 Shattuck Avenue
Oakland, CA 94609

510-652-2002
800-748-6273
Fax: 510-652-5472
TTY: 800-652-1613
e-mail: customerservice@newharbinger.com
www.newharbinger.com

This comprehensive guide is recommended to those struggling with anxiety disorders. Includes step-by-step instructions for the crucial cognitive-behavioral techniques that have given real help to hundreds of thousands of readers struggling with anxiety disorders.

448 pages 4th Edition
ISBN: 1-572244-13-5

6736 Anxiety Cure: An Eight-Step Program for Ge tting Well
John Wiley & Sons
10475 Crosspoint Boulevard
Indianapolis, IN 46256

877-762-2974
Fax: 800-597-3299
www.wiley.com

A practical guide, written by a father and his two daughters, featuring a step-by-step program for curing the six main kinds of anxiety.

272 pages 2nd Edition
ISBN: 0-471464-87-2

Peter B. Wiley, Chairman
Stephen M. Smith, President & CEO
Ellis E. Cousens, Executive Vice President, Chief Fin

6737 Anxiety Disorders
Cambridge University Press
40 W 20th Street
New York, NY 10011

212-924-3900
800-872-7423
Fax: 914-937-4712
e-mail: marketing@cup.org
cup.org

This comprehensive text covers all the anxiety disorders found in the latest DSM and ICD classifications. Provides detailed information about seven principal disorders, including anxiety in the medically ill. For each disorder, the book covers diagnosis criteria, epidemiology, etiology and pathogenesis, clinical features, natural history and different diagnoses. Describes treatment approaches, both psychological and pharmacological.

354 pages

6738 Anxiety Disorders: Practioner's Guide
John Wiley & Sons
111 River Street
Hoboken, NJ 7030-

212-850-6000
Fax: 212-850-6008
e-mail: info@wiley.com
wiley.com

210 pages
ISBN: 0-471931-12-8

Stephen M. Smith, President/ CEO
John Kritzmacher, EVP/ CFO
MJ O'Leary, EVO, Human Resources

6739 Encyclopedia of Phobias, Fears, and Anxieties
Facts on File
11 Penn Plaza, Room M274
New York, NY 10001

212-290-8090
800-322-8755

500 pages

6740 Helping Your Anxious Child
New Harbinger Publications
5674 Shattuck Avenue
Oakland, CA 94609

510-652-2002
800-748-6273
Fax: 510-652-5472
TTY: 800-652-1613
e-mail: customerservice@newharbinger.com
www.newharbinger.com

Step-by-step guide for parents of anxious children to help them overcome their fears and anxieties. Detailed strategies and techniques.

168 pages Paperback
ISBN: 1-572241-91-8

6741 Psychological Trauma
American Psychiatric Press
1400 K Street, NW
Washington, DC 20005

202-682-6262
800-368-5777
Fax: 202-789-2648
e-mail: order@appi.org
www.appi.org

Epidemiology of trauma and post-tramatic stress disorder. Evaluation, neuroimaging, neuroendocrinology and pharmacology.

1998 206 pages

Robert E. Hales M.D, Editor-in-Chief
Rebecca D. Rinehart, Publisher
John McDuffie, Editorial Director

6742 **Shy Children, Phobic Adults: Nature and Treatment of Social Phobia**
American Psychological Press
1400 K Street, NW
Washington, DC 20005

202-682-6262
800-368-5777
Fax: 202-789-2648
e-mail: orders@appi.org
www.appi.org

Describes the simuliarities and differences in the syndrome across all ages. Draws from the clinical, social and developmental literatures, as well as from extensive clinical experience. Illustrates the impact of developmental stage on phenomenology, diagnosis and assessment and treatment of social phobia.

1998 321 pages

Robert E. Hales M.D, Editor-in-Chief
Rebecca D. Rinehart, Publisher
John McDuffie, Editorial Director

Pamphlets

6743 **Anxiety Disorders**
National Institute of Mental Health
6001 Executive Boulevard, Room 6200, MSC 9663
Bethesda, MD 20892

301-443-4536
866-615-6464
Fax: 301-443-4279
TTY: 301-443-8431
e-mail: NIMHpress@mail.nih.gov
www.nimh.nih.gov

This brochure helps to identify the symptoms of anxiety disorders, explains the role of research in understanding the causes of these conditions, describes effective treatments, helps you learn how to obtain treatment and work with a doctor or therapist, and suggests ways to make treatment more effective.

6744 **Anxiety Disorders Fact Sheet**
Center for Mental Health Services
PO Box 42490
Washington, DC 20015

800-789-2647
Fax: 301-984-8796
e-mail: ken@mentalhealth.org
mentalhealth.org

This fact sheet presents basic information on the symptoms, formal diagnosis, and treatment for generalized anxiety disorder, panic disorders, phobias, and post traumatic stress disorder.

3 pages

6745 **Anxiety Disorders in Children and Adolescents**
Center for Mental Health Services
PO Box 42490
Washington, DC 20015

800-789-2647
Fax: 301-984-8796
e-mail: ken@mentalhealth.org
mentalhealth.org

This fact sheet defines anxiety disorders, identifies warning signs, discusses risk factors, describes types of help available, and suggests what parents or other caregivers can do.

3 pages

6746 **Families Can Help Children Cope with Fear, Anxiety**
Center for Mental Health Services
PO Box 42490
Washington, DC 20015

800-789-2647
Fax: 301-984-8796
e-mail: ken@mentalhealth.org
mentalhealth.org

This fact sheet defines conduct disorder, identifies risk factors, discusses types of help available, and suggests what parents or other caregivers responses should be to common signs of fear and anxiety.

Description

6747 SPEECH IMPAIRMENT

Synonym: Speech dysfunction

Involves the following Biologic System(s):

Neurologic Disorders

Speech impairment refers to the decreased ability or inability to effectively communicate through vocalizations or uttered sounds. Difficulty speaking or more profound dysfunctions of speech may result from many different factors that include neurologic influences; muscular defects, injuries, or paralysis; structural irregularities of the vocal cords; psychologic influences; mental retardation; and other factors.

In some children, speech impairment may be classified as a dysfunction of articulation characterized by the inability to articulate or produce words properly (dysarthria) as a result of damage to the part of the brain responsible for regulation of the muscles that control the speech apparatus (e.g., mouth, lips, and voice box or larynx). Such damage may result from head or brain injuries, tumors, strokes, and certain diseases. Characteristic speech patterns of children with dysarthria are varied and may be described as unintelligible, slow, slurred, halting, tremulous, hoarse, or possessing a nasal quality. Additional causes of articulation dysfunction or delay include structural defects such as cleft lip or palate, hearing impairment or deafness, and other nervous system irregularities. In addition, speech impairment may result from irregularities directly related to the vocal cords that may affect the quality of the voice.

Impaired ability to communicate (aphasia or dysphasia) may also result from injury to the part of the brain responsible for language comprehension, resulting in the reduced ability or inability to express, write, or understand language. Such injury may be caused by head trauma, brain lesions, infection, or other factors. This type of impairment may be present in many different variations such as garbled sentences, extremely slow and difficult speech, absence of speech (mutism), and other irregularities. In addition, children with behavioral, emotional, or psychologic irregularities as well as those with hearing impairment may also experience delays in language comprehension and development.

It is important to identify the underlying cause of any dysfunction of speech or delay in speech development in order to allow for the most favorable educational and social outcome. Specialists in the diagnosis and treatment of these types of disorders (e.g., otolaryngologists and speech therapists) may base their treatment plans on the evaluation of family and medical histories, physical examination of essential speech structures, and specialized testing that may include speech, language, and hearing assessments. Treatment is directed toward the specific cause of impairment and may include exercises tailored to the specific patient's needs, as well as the cooperation of parents or caregivers, pediatricians, educators, and others to provide a supportive environment.

Government Agencies

6748 NIH/National Institute on Deafness and Oth er Communication Disorders (NIDCD)
31 Center Drive, MSC 2320
Bethesda, MD 20892   e-mail: nidcdinfo@nidcd.nih.gov
                                                 www.nidcd.nih.gov

A National Institute of Health, the NIDCD supports research and provides education and information on these following health topics: voice, speech, language, hearing, ear infections, deafness, balance, smell and taste.

Dr James F Battey JrD, Director
Judith A Cooper PhD, Deputy Director
W David Kerr, Executive Officer

National Associations & Support Groups

6749 Advocure NF2
P.O. Box 4118
Clearwater, FL 33758   e-mail: contact@advocurenf2.org
                                                 www.advocurenf2.org

Advocure NF2 Inc. is a working advocacy group, liaison, and 501(c)(3) public charity for the NF2 international community and NF2 Crew.

Barbara Franklin, Vice President, Interim President
Sheila Heal, Secretary
Cynthia Henrion, Treasurer

6750 American Academy of Pediatrics
141 Northwest Point Boulevard
Elk Grove Village, IL 60007   847-434-4000
                                                        800-433-9016
                                                  Fax: 847-434-8000
                                                        www.aap.org

The American Academy of Pediatrics and its member pediatricians are committed to the attainment of optimal physical, mental and social health and well-being for all infants, children, adolescents, and young adults.

Sandra Hassink, MD, FAAP, President

6751 American Board of Fluency and Fluency Disorders
563 Carter Court, Suite B
Kimberly, WI 54136   920-750-7720
                                                   Fax: 920-882-3655
                               e-mail: info@stutteringspecialists.org
                                          www.stutteringspecialists.org

The mission is to promote among speech-language pathologists the highest standards for training and service delivery to impact positively the communication skills and thereby the lives of those who demonstrate fluency disorders.

Kristin Chmela, Co-Chair
Lynne Shields, Co-Chair
June Campbell, Treasurer

6752 American Laryngological Association
www.alahns.org

Founded in 1878, the ALA is a scholarly organization of physicians and scientists who have made significant contributions to the care of patients with disorders of the larynx and upper aerodigestive tract. The ALA recognizes the accomplishments of these individuals through membership, seeks to encourage research in laryngology and elevate the standards of the fundamental teaching of laryngology in medical schools and postgraduate medical education.

6753 American School Counselor Association
1101 King Street, Suite 310
Alexandria, VA 22314   703-683-2722
                                                      800-306-4722
                                                Fax: 703-997-7572
                           e-mail: asca@schoolcounselor.org
                                        www.schoolcounselor.org

The mission of ASCA is to represent professional school counselors and to promote professionalism and ethical practices.

Richard Wong, Executive Director
Jeff Broderson, Information Technology Admin.
Kathleen M Rakestraw, Director of Communications

6754 American Speech Language Hearing Associati on (ASHA)
2200 Research Boulevard
Rockville, MD 20850   301-897-5700
                                       800-638-8255
                                  Fax: 301-571-0457
                               e-mail: pr@asha.org
                                       www.asha.org

A professional and credentialing association made up of more than 123,000 international pathologists, audiologists and scientists. The association promotes the interests of and provides services for those in the hearing, speech, and language field, and advocates for people with communication disorders.

Patricia A. Prelock, PhD, President
Elizabeth S. McCrea, PhD, CCC-SLP, President-Elect
Shelly S. Chabon, PhD, CCC-SLP, Immediate Past President

6755 Aphasia Hope Foundation
P.O. Box 79701
Houston, TX 77279   855-764-4673
                        e-mail: sandycaudell@aphasiahope.org
                                       www.aphasiahope.org

Aphasia Hope Foundation is a public 501(c) 3 non-profit foundation that has a two-fold mission: (1) to promote research into the prevention and cure of aphasia and (2) to ensure all survivors of aphasia and their caregivers are aware of and have access to the best possible treatments available.

6756 Association for Research in Otolaryngology
19 Mantua Rd.
Mt Royal, NJ 8061   856-423-0041
                                  Fax: 856-423-3420
                          e-mail: headquarters@aro.org
                                       www.aro.org

ARO Midwinter Meetings bring together over 1500 investigators from around the world to present current results in hearing, vestibular function, and related fields, as well as representatives of funding agencies, publishers, and scientific vendors.

6757 Association of Academic Physiatrists
10461 Mill Run Circle, Suite 730
Owings Mills, MD 21117   410-654-1000
                                  Fax: 410-654-1001
                         e-mail: tknowlton@physiatry.org
                                       www.physiatry.org

The Association of Academic Physiatrists (AAP) is the only academic association dedicated to the specialty of physical medicine and rehabilitation (PM&R) in the world. AAP is a community of leading physicians, researchers, in-training physiatrists, and others involved or interested in leadership, mentorship, and discovery in PM&R.

Tiffany Knowlton, JD, MBA, Executive Director
Bernadette M. Rensing, Comm. & Marketing Manager
Amy Schnappinger, Member Services Manager

6758 Association of University Centers on Disabilities
1100 Wayne Ave., Suite 1000
Silver Spring, MD 20910   301-588-8252
                                  Fax: 301-588-2842
                             e-mail: aucdinfo@aucd.org
                                       www.aucd.org

The Association of University Centers on Disabilities (AUCD) is a membership organization that supports and promotes a national network of university-based interdisciplinary programs.

Andrew J. Imparato, JD, Executive Director
Abigail (Abbey) Alberico, MPH, Project Manager
Leon Barnett, MSEd, Program Specialist

6759 Auditory-Verbal Learning Institute
7205 North Habana Ave
Tampa, FL 33614   813-227-8766
                                  Fax: 813-932-9583
                               e-mail: info@avli.org
                                       www.avli.org

Promotes and teaches Auditory-Verbal Therapy.

Pamela Sullins, Director/CEO
Alisa Jenkins, Marketing/Product Consultant
Judith Marlowe PhD, Program Development Consultant

6760 CHERAB Foundation
P.O. Box 8524
Port St. Lucie, FL 34952   772-335-5135
                               e-mail: help@cherab.org
                                       www.cherab.org

Provides communication help, eductaion, research.

6761 Center for Parent Information and Resources
35 Halsey St., Fourth Floor
Newark, NJ 7102   e-mail: malizo@spannj.org
                                       www.parentcenterhub.org

The Center for Parent Information and Resources (CPIR) serves as a central resource of information and products to the community of Parent Training Information (PTI) Centers and the Community Parent Resource Centers (CPRCs), so that they can focus their efforts on serving families of children with disabilities.

Myriam Alizo, Project Assistant
Debra Jennings, Project Director
Lisa K□pper, Product Development Coordinator

6762 Center for Speech and Language Disorders
310-D S. Main St.
Lombard, IL 60148   630-652-0200
                               e-mail: lynns@csld.org
                                       www.csld.org

Works with the mission to help children with communication disorders reach their full potential through family centered services.

Lynn Scheuer Kozak, Executive Director
Mary Catherine Brady, Operations Manager
Phyllis Kupperman, M.A., CCC-SLP, Founder

6763 Childhood Apraxia of Speech Association
416 Lincoln Avenue 2nd Fl.
Pittsburgh, PA 15209   www.apraxia-kids.org

The Childhood Apraxia of Speech Association is a 501(c)(3) non-profit publicly funded charity whose mission is to strengthen the support systems in the lives of children with apraxia so that each child is afforded their best opportunity to develop speech and communication.

Sue Freiburger, Board Secretary
Sharon Gretz, M.Ed, Executive Director
Kathy Hennessy, Education Director

6764 Council of Academic Programs in Communication
3000 South Jamaica Ct., Ste 390
Aurora, CO 80014   303-835-9089
                                  Fax: 800-805-5932
                          e-mail: mchavez@capcsd.org
                                       www.capcsd.org

CAPCSD is dedicated to promoting academic excellence, visionary leadership and collaboration among communication sciences and disorders academic programs.

Judith Vander Woude, Ph.D., President
Rich Folsom, VP for Student Development
Mary Chavez Rudolph, Ph.D., Executive Director

6765 Educational Audiology Association
700 McKnight Park Drive, Suite 708
Pittsburgh, PA 15237   800-460-7322
                                  Fax: 888-729-3489
                            e-mail: admin@edaud.org
                                       edaud.org

The Educational Audiology Association is an international organization of audiologists and related professionals who deliver a full spectrum of hearing services to all children, particularly those in educational settings.

Mike Sharp, AuD, CCC-A, President
Gary Pillow, President-Elect
Erin Schafer, PhD, Secretary

6766 National Aphasia Association
www.aphasia.org

The National Aphasia Association (NAA) is a non-profit organization founded in 1987 by Martha Taylor Sarno, MA, MD,(hon) as the 1st National organization dedicated to advocating for persons with aphasia and their families. Several of our board members, including the President, are people with Aphasia or family members.

Darlene S. Williamson, President
Daniel Martin, VP Strategic Planning
Barbara Kessler, VP, Community Outreach & Education

6767 National Black Association for Speech-Language and Hearing
700 McKnight Park Drive, Suite 708
Pittsburgh, PA 15237   855-727-2836
                                             Fax: 888-729-3489
                                       e-mail: nbaslh@nbaslh.org
                                                www.nbaslh.org

The Association was incorporated in Washington D.C., June 30, 1978. The committee wanted to establish a viable mechanism through which the professional needs of the Black professionals, students, and the communicatively handicapped community could be met.

Rachel M. Williams, PhD, CCC-SLP, Chair
Kellie E. Green, MA, CCC-SLP, Secretary, PR Co-Chair
Linda McCabe Smith, Treasurer, Membership Co-Chair

6768 National Spasmodic Dysphonia Association
300 Park Boulevard, Suite 335
Itasca, IL 60143   800-795-6732
                                             Fax: 630-250-4505
                                       e-mail: NSDA@dysphonia.org
                                                www.dysphonia.org

The National Spasmodic Dysphonia Association (NSDA) is a not-for-profit 501c(3) organization dedicated to advancing medical research into the causes of and treatments for SD, promoting physician and public awareness of the disorder, and providing support to those affected by SD through symposiums, support groups, and on-line resources.

Charlie Reavis, President
Marcia Sterling, Treasurer
Mary Bifaro, Support Services Director

6769 Voice Foundation (The)
219 N. Broad St. 10th Floor
Philadelphia, PA 19107   215-735-7999
                                             Fax: 215-762-5572
                                                voicefoundation.org

The Voice Foundation was founded in 1969 by the internationally celebrated voice specialist Wilbur James Gould, M.D.. At that time interdisciplinary care of the human voice was non-existent. Dr. Gould's groundbreaking foresight brought together physicians, scientists, speech-language pathologists, performers, and teachers to share their knowledge and expertise in the care of the professional voice user.

Robert Thayer Sataloff, Chairman
Stuart Orsher, MD, President
Michael S. Benninger, MD, Vice President

6770 Voice Health Institute
1 Bowdoin Square
Boston, MA 2114   617-720-5000
                                             Fax: 617-720-5001
                                   e-mail: info@voicehealthinstitute.org
                                             www.voicehealthinstitute.org

Since its inception and qualification as a federally-approved non-profit public charity (501-C-3), the VHI has funded educational and award-wining pioneering research programs.

Julie Andrews, Chairman
John L. Ward, Ph.D., President

State Agencies & Support Groups

New York

6771 Brooklyn College Speech and Hearing Center
2900 Bedford Ave, 4400 Boylan Hall
Brooklyn, NY 11210   718-951-5186
                                             Fax: 718-951-4363
                                   e-mail: mbergen@brooklyn.cuny.edu
                                www.brooklyn.cuny.edu/bc/spotlite/news/110804.htm

Provides diagnostic and rehabilitative services to children and adults with speech, language, hearing and voice impairments.

Christopher Kimmich, President
Susan Bohne, Assistant Director

North Carolina

6772 North Carolina Speech, Hearing and Languag e Association
PO Box 28359
Raleigh, NC 27611   919-833-3984
                                             Fax: 919-832-0445
                                       e-mail: info@ncshla.org
                                                www.ncshla.org

Promotes the professional practice of speech, language and hearing sciences and works to enhance the lives of those who are communicatively impaired, through a variety of programs and opportunities.

Louise Raleigh, President
Tracie Rice, President-Elect
Kathleen Cox, Ph.D., CCC-SLP, Past President

Ohio

6773 Cleveland Hearing and Speech Center
11635 Euclid Avenue
Cleveland, OH 44106   216-231-0787
                                             Fax: 216-795-2135
                                                www.chsc.org

A nonprofit organization in Northeast Ohio dedicated to serving the needs of those with special communication needs.

Hilary Beatrez, Director of Finance and Administrat
Susan M. Bungard, CCDHH Program Director
Michelle L. Burnett, Director of Clinical Services

6774 Speech and Hearing Clinic
Kent State University
A104 Music & Speech Bldg, PO Box 5190
Kent, OH 44242   330-672-2672
                                             Fax: 330-672-2643
                                                www.kent.edu/spa

Services provided include: full-service clinic diagnoses, therapy, treatment and hearing aid repair.

Lynn Rowan, Executive Director

Oklahoma

6775 Oklahoma Speech Language Hearing Associati on
1741 S Cleveland Ave, Suite 301
Sioux Falls, SD 57103   405-802-1630
                                             Fax: 405-271-3360
                                       e-mail: office@oslha.org
                                                www.oslha.org

Deborah Earley, President
Sarah Baker, President Elect
Tracy Grammer, Past President

6776 Reading and Speech Clinic
Unit 9
Bend, OR 97701   541-389-3302
                                        800-283-0818
e-mail: ellen@readingandspeechclinic.com
www.readingandspeechclinic.com

Provides alternate therapies for improving speech, language, spelling and reading difficulties.

Ellen Jacobs PhD, Director

Tennessee

6777 Memphis State University, Center for the Communicatively Impaired
807 Jefferson Avenue
Memphis, TN 38105   901-678-2009
                                        Fax: 901-525-1282
www.memphis.edu/csd/crisci.htm

Offers research into hearing loss, deafness, and speech impairments.

Maurice I Mendel, Director

Texas

6778 Callier Center for Communication Disorders
University of Texas at Dallas
1966 Inwood Road
Dallas, TX 75235   214-905-3000
                                        Fax: 214-905-3022
                                        TDD: 214-905-3012
e-mail: barbara.ember@utdallas.edu
www.callier.utdallas.edu

Multidisciplinary center serving infants through adults with all types of communcation disorders: diagnostic and treatment; hearing aid services; cochlear implant evelation and follow-up; N Texas Cochlear Implant Summer Listening Camp; aural rehabilitation services; assistive listening device program; tinnitus and hyperacusis clinic; speech-language pathology and psychological diagnostic and therapy services; research.

Thomas Campbell, Executive Director
Christine A Dollaghan, Child Language Development
Robert Stillman PhD, Communication Disorders

Washington

6779 Scottish Rite Centers for Childhood Langua ge Disorders
2800 16th Street, NW
Washington, DC 20009   202-232-8155
                                        Fax: 202-483-8169
www.dcsr.org/clinic.php

Association offering speech-language evaluations and treatment, hearing screening and consultation and referrals to children ages birth to 18 years with hearing or speech disorders. Seven locations/clinincs are offered throughout the state of Washington.

Tommie L. Robinson, Jr., Ph.D, Director

6780 University of Washington Department of Spe ech & Hearing Sciences
1417 NE 42nd Street
Seattle, WA 98105   206-685-7400
                                        Fax: 206-543-1093
e-mail: sphscadv@u.washington.edu
www.depts.washington.edu/sphsc/

Committed to understanding the basic processes and mechanisms involved in human speech, hearing, language, their disorders and to improving the quality of life for individuals affected by communication disorders across the life span.

Stacy Betz, Child Language Disorders

Research Centers

Arizona

6781 National Center for Neurogenic Communicati on Disorders
University of Arizona
Speech & Hearing Sciences Bldg, Rm 500
Tucson, AZ 85721   520-621-1472
cnet.shs.arizona.edu

The center is supported by a grant from the NIDCD, a National Institute of Health, and is staffed by scientists, educators and students who are concerned with speech and language disorders caused by diseases of the nervous system.

Thomas J Hixon PhD, Director
Kathryn A Bayles PhD, Associate Director

Colorado

6782 Speech, Language, and Hearing Center
University of Colorado, Boulder
2501 Kittregde Loop Rd
Boulder, CO 80309   303-492-5375
slhs.colorado.edu/clinical-services?

Focuses on communication disorders including speech and hearing impairments.

Susan M Moore, Director

Michigan

6783 University Center for the Development of L anguage & Literacy
University of Michigan
1111 E Catherine Street
Ann Arbor, MI 48109   734-764-8440
                                        Fax: 734-647-2489
www.languageexperts.org/research/

Focuses on communicative disorders including hearing impairments and speech disorders. Provides intensive language intervention for adults with aphasia as well as children with language disorders. Clinic offers residential program for adults and school liasion for children.

Carol C. Persad, PhD., ABPP, Director of the University Center f
Mimi Block, MS, CCC-SLP, Clinical Services Manager

Nebraska

6784 Boys Town National Research Hospital
555 N 30th Street
Omaha, NE 68131   402-498-6511
                                        Fax: 402-498-6638
                                        TTY: 402-498-6543
www.boystownhospital.org

An internationally recognized center for state-of-the-art research, diagnosis, treatment of patients with ear diseases, hearing and balance disorders, cleft lip and palate, and speech/language problems.

Patrick E Brookhouser, President

Nevada

6785 University of Nevada - Department of Speec h-Language Pathology
School of Medicine
Redfield Bldg, MS 152
Reno, NV 89557   775-784-4887
                                        Fax: 775-784-4095
e-mail: lgoldberg@medicine.nevada.edu
www.medicine.nevada.edu/spa/

The department includes an active clinic and nine faculty for research in language, speech and hearing.

Thomas Watterson, Chair
Leslie Goldberg, Clinical Director

New York

6786 Henry Youngerman Center for Communication Disorders
SUNY Fredonia/Dept of Comm Disorders/Sciences
Thompson Hall W123
Fredonia, NY 14063   716-673-3202
                                      Fax: 716-673-3235

Studies communications disorders including hearing and speech.
It features a newly constructed research labs and an in-house
clinic that serves as a training ground for graduate clinicians. The
clinic provides speech/language and hearing services to members
of the college, student, and local community.

Melissa A Sidor MS, CCC/SLP Clinic Director
Dr Kim Tillery PhD, CCC/Aud-Chair, Professor

North Carolina

6787 Communications Disorders Clinic
Reich College of Education
400 University Hall Drive, PO Box 32041
Boone, NC 28608   828-262-2185
                                      Fax: 828-262-6766
                                      www.cdclinic.appstate.edu

The clinic provides prevention, assessment, and treatment of
speech, language and hearing disorders for all ages. It also provides several outreach programs.

Mary Ruth Sizer, Director

Washington

6788 University of Washington Speech and Hearin g Clinic
1417 N.E. 42nd St
Seattle, WA 98105   206-685-7400
                                      Fax: 206-616-1185
                                      e-mail: shclinic@u.washington.edu
                                      depts.washington.edu/sphsc/

A center for education and research serving speech, language, and
hearing needs within the university and the community. Serves as
a teaching facility in the fields of speech-language pathology and
audiology, with state of the art technology, innovative diagnostic
and treament methods, and internationally and nationally
recognized areas of research.

Nancy Alarcon MS, CCC-SLP, Director
Joan Hanson, Manager

Wisconsin

6789 Waisman Center - Auditory Physiology Resea rch Laboratory
University of Wisconsin, Madison
1500 Highland Ave
Madison, WI 53705   608-263-1656
                                      www.physiology.wisc.edu/brugge/bruggelab.html?

The research laboratory is part of the Waisman Center which is
dedicated to advancing the knowledge about human development,
developmental disabilities, and neurodegenerative disorders.

James S Malter, Director

Web Sites

6790 Parent Pals
parentpals.com/gossamer/pages/Speech_and_Language

                                      e-mail: specialed@parentpals.co m
                       parentpals.com/gossamer/pages/Speech_and_Language

Their goal is to provide special education and gifted information,
continuing education, support, weekly tips, games, book resources, and news and views for parents and professionals.

Book Publishers

6791 Listen Little Star
Auditory-Verbal Learning Institute
7205 North Habana Ave
Tampa, FL 33614   813-227-8766
                                      Fax: 813-932-9583
                                      e-mail: info@avli.org
                                      www.avli.org

A family activity kit for parents designed to help their babies develop listening and speaking skills. It includes 12 activities, a
workbook, checklist, plush toy, and note-taking section.

**6792 Management of Motor Speech Disorders in Children and
Adults**
Pro-Ed
8700 Shoal Creek Boulevard
Austin, TX 78757   512-451-3246
                                      800-897-3202
                                      Fax: 800-397-7633
                                      e-mail: general@proedinc.com
                                      www.proedinc.com

Second edition of this popular text incorporates information
about both dysarthria and apraxia of speech in children and adults
and reviews techniques for physical and motor speech examination and treatment techniques.

618 pages Hardcover
ISBN: 0-890797-84-6

6793 Preschool Motor Speech Evaluation & Interv ention
Pro-Ed
8700 Shoal Creek Boulevard
Austin, TX 78757   512-451-3246
                                      800-897-3202
                                      Fax: 800-397-7633
                                      e-mail: general@proedinc.com
                                      www.proedinc.com

Comprehensive resource manual for evaluating and treating oral
motor and motor speech disorders in children 18 months to six
years of age.

Journals

6794 American Journal of Speech-Language Pathol ogy
American Speech Language Hearing Association
2200 Research Blvd
Rockville, MD 20850   301-296-5700
                                      800-478-2071
                                      Fax: 301-296-8580
                                      TTY: 301-296-5650
                                      TDD: 301-296-5650
                                      www.asha.org

Pertains to all aspects of clinical practice in speech-language pathology.

Quarterly

Dr Laura Justice, Editor

6795 Communication Disorders Quarterly
Hammill Institute on Disabilities/Sage Publication
2455 Teller Road
Thousand Oaks, CA 91320   800-818-7243
                                      Fax: 800-583-2665
                                      e-mail: journals@sagepub.com
                                      www.sagepub.com

Presents cutting-edge information on typical and atypical communication disorders across the continuum-from oral language development to literacy. CDQ is the official journal of the Division
for Communicaative Disabilities and Deafness of the CEC. ISSN:
Print: 1525-722; Electronic: 1538-4837; Subscriptions available:
Institutional - Print Only $141, Insitutional - Print & E-access
$144, Personal $57.

Quarterly
ISSN: 1528-7401

Judy K Montgomery, PhD, Editor

6796 Journal of Speech, Language, and Hearing R esearch
American Speech Language Hearing Association
2200 Research Blvd
Rockville, MD 20850   301-296-5700
                                          800-478-2071
                                     Fax: 301-296-8580
                                     TTY: 301-296-5650
                                     TDD: 301-296-5650
                                          www.asha.org

Pertains broadly to studies of the processes and disorders of hearing, language, and speech and to the diagnosis and treatment of such disorders.

Bi-monthly

Dr Anne Smith, Editor, Speech
Dr Karla McGregor, Editor, Language
Dr Robert Schlauch, Editor, Hearing

6797 Language, Speech, and Hearing in Schools
American Speech Language Hearing Association
2200 Research Blvd
Rockville, MD 20850   301-296-5700
                                          800-478-2071
                                     Fax: 301-296-8580
                                     TTY: 301-296-5650
                                     TDD: 301-296-5650
                                          www.asha.org

An archival journal for research and practice in educational settings. Publishes studies and articles that pertain to speech, language, and hearing disorders and differences in children and adolescents, as well as to professional issues affecting service delivery in educational settings.

Quarterly

Dr Kenn Apel, Editor

Newsletters

6798 Callier Communications
Callier Center - University of Texas at Dallas
1966 Inwood Road
Dallas, TX 75235   214-905-3000
                                     Fax: 214-905-3022
                                     TDD: 214-905-3012
                                          www.callier.utdallas.edu

W. Bennett Cullum, President
Jodelle Oakley, MS, Director, Education Division
Jan Lougeay, MA, CCC/SLP, Director of Clinical Education

6799 Communique
NCSHLA Publications
PO Box 28359
Raleigh, NC 27611   919-833-3984
                                     Fax: 919-832-0445
                                     e-mail: info@ncshla.org
                                          www.ncshla.org

The official newsletter of NCSHLA.

Quarterly

G Peyton Maynard, Executive VP
AJ Jacques, Executive Secretary
Cindy Davis Ling, President

Camps

6800 Central Michigan University Summer Clinics
444 Moore
Mount Pleasant, MI   517-774-3803

Designed for children, ages 6 and up, with speech, language and hearing disorders who can benefit from intensive clinical work. A wide range of recreational and social activities form part of the clinical program and promote the social use of skills learned in class.

6801 Meadowood Springs Speech and Hearing Camp
PO Box 1025
Pendleton, OR 97801   541-276-2752
                                     Fax: 541-276-7227
                                     e-mail: info@meadowoodsprings.org
                                          www.meadowoodsprings.org

On 143 acres in the Blue Mountains of Eastern Oregon, this camp is designed to help young people who have diagnosed clinical disorders of speech, hearing or language. A full range of activities in recreational and clinical areas is available. For cabin reservations 541-566-2191.

Rosemarie Atfield, Executive Director
Marie Story, Camp Manager
Cliff Story, Camp Manager

6802 University of Iowa - Wendell Johnson Speech and Hearing Clinic
Wendell Johnson Speech And Hearing Center
Iowa City, IA 52242   319-335-8718
                                     Fax: 319-335-8851
                                     e-mail: speech-path-aud@uiowa.edu
                                          clas.uiowa.edu/comsci/

The clinic offers assessment and remediation for disordered communication in adults and children. The clinic also offers an Intensive Summer Residential Clinic for school age children needing intervention services because of speech, language, hearing and/or reading problems.

Ruth Bentler, Professor / Department Chair
Dorothy Albright, Secretary
Vicki Jennings, Secretary

Description

6803 SPINA BIFIDA

Covers these related disorders: Encephalocele, Meningocele, Myelocele (Myelomeningocele, Meningomyelocele), Spina bifida occulta

Involves the following Biologic System(s):

Neurologic Disorders, Orthopedic and Muscle Disorders

Spina bifida, literally meaning "cleft spine," is a congenital abnormality, known as a neural tube defect, which is characterized by the failure during embryonic development of one or more of the developing vertebrae to develop completely or fuse. This frequently results in the exposure of part of the spinal cord. It is the most common neural tube defect in the United States—affecting 1,500 to 2,000 of the more than 4 million babies born in the country each year. Spina bifida occulta, the most common and least severe form of this defect, is characterized by a dimpling, dark tufts of hair, spider-like fine lines (telangiectasia), or a benign fatty tumor (lipoma) on the lower back or lumbosacral area. There is no protrusion or exposure of the spinal cord and it rarely involves problems with the nervous system. Some affected children, however, may experience weakness in the legs and feet and difficulty in bladder and bowel control resulting from an adhesion of the spinal cord to the area of the abnormality.

Meningocele occurs when the three membranes surrounding the spinal cord (meninges) protrude through the vertebral defect. Most meningoceles are covered by skin and contain cerebrospinal fluid. Although most affected children have no apparent neurologic involvement, some children may experience nerve dysfunction and associated irregularities (e.g., tethered spinal cord, diastematomyelia, and syringomyelia). If cerebrospinal fluid is leaking from the meningocele, immediate surgery is usually required to avoid infection or inflammation of the meninges (meningitis). Surgery to correct the meningocele may be performed at a later date in those children who are not at risk for such infection.

Myelocele is a severe form of spina bifida that affects one in 1,000 newborns. This form of the disorder is characterized by a protrusion of the spinal cord and meninges through the vertebral canal, covered by a raw swelling. Most myeloceles are located in the lumbosacral region. This abnormality may result in impaired function of the skeletal system, the skin, the genitourinary tract, and the peripheral and central nervous systems. Physical findings associated with myelocele are widely variable and depend upon the portion of the spinal cord affected and may include the inability to control the bladder and bowel functions, lack of muscle tone in the legs, and other irregularities of the lower extremities. Some children with myelocele develop an unusual accumulation of cerebrospinal fluid in the skull, resulting in enlargement of the head (hydrocephalus) and associated symptoms that may include choking and difficulty in feeding and breathing. The insertion of a tube or shunt is often indicated to relieve fluid buildup. Treatment of myelocele often involves a team of medical specialists working closely to manage care for the affected child. This care usually involves surgery to repair the myelocele. Other approaches to treatment are geared toward correction, alleviation, or management of symptoms. For example, training children or their parents how to empty the bladder through catheterization may help to avoid urinary tract infections and kidney disease. Also, laxatives or enemas may be used to relieve the constipation often associated with this abnormality. Other treatment may include the use of braces and canes or crutches and physical therapy to maintain joint mobility and to strengthen muscular function. Further treatment is supportive. The exact cause of myelocele is unknown; however, it is thought that environmental and nutritional influences may be contributing factors.

Encephalocele, a very severe and rare type of spina bifida, is characterized by the protrusion of the brain through a defect in the cranium. Affected children often experience visual difficulties, mental retardation, and seizures.

A common screening method used to look for spina bifida during pregnancy is a second trimester maternal serum alpha fetoprotein (MSAFP) screening. The MSAFP screen measures the level of a protein called alpha-fetoprotein (AFP), which is made naturally by the fetus and placenta. During pregnancy, a small amount of AFP normally crosses the placenta and enters the mother's bloodstream. But if abnormally high levels of this protein appear in the mother's bloodstream it may indicate that the fetus has a neural tube defect. Amniocentesis, an exam in which a sample of fluid is obtained from the amniotic sac that surrounds the fetus, may also be used to diagnose spina bifida. Research has shown that supplementation with folic acid, starting before pregnancy, reduces the risk of neural tube defects. It is recommended that all women of childbearing age consume 400 micrograms of folic acid daily.

Government Agencies

6804 NIH/National Institute of Arthritis and Musculoskeletal and Skin Diseases
1AMS Circle
Bethesda, MD 20892

301-402-4484
877-226-4267
Fax: 301-718-6366
TDD: 301-565-2966
e-mail: niamsinfo@mail.nih.gov
www.niams.nih.gov

The mission of the NIAMS, a part of the NIH, is to support research into the causes, treatment, and prevention of arthritis and musculoskeletal and skin diseases, the training of basic and clinical scientists to carry out this research, and the dissemination of information on research progress in these diseases.

Stephen I Katz MD PhD, Director
Robert H Carter MD, Deputy Director
Gahan Breithaupt, Assoc Dir for Management & Operatio

National Associations & Support Groups

6805 American Academy of Pediatrics
141 Northwest Point Boulevard
Elk Grove Village, IL 60007

847-434-4000
800-433-9016
Fax: 847-434-8000
www.aap.org

The American Academy of Pediatrics and its member pediatricians are committed to the attainment of optimal physical, mental and social health and well-being for all infants, children, adolescents, and young adults.

Sandra Hassink, MD, FAAP, President

6806 Center for Disabilities and Development
University of Iowa Hospitals and Clinics
100 Hawkins Drive
Iowa City, IA 52242
319-353-6900
877-686-0031
Fax: 319-356-8284
e-mail: cdd-scheduling@uiowa.edu
www.uichildrens.org/cdd

A trusted resource for healthcare, training, research and information for people with disabilities that include: behavior disorders, brain injury, cerebral palsy, diabetes, down syndrome, learning disabilities, mental retardation, sleep disorders and spina bifida.

Judy Stephenson, Administrator
Amy Mikelson, Supervisor Info Resource Service

6807 Easter Seals Disability Services Chicago, IL 60606

312-726-6200
800-221-6827
Fax: 312-726-1494
TDD: 312-726-4258
e-mail: extranetinfo@easterseals.com
www.extranet.easterseals.com

Helps individuals with special needs and disabilities and their families to lead better lives through a variety of services including job training, development centers, rehabilitation, and education.

Lou Lowenkron, Chairman
James E Williams Jr, President/CEO

6808 Genetic Alliance
4301 Connecticut Avenue NW
Washington, DC 20008
202-966-5557
800-336-4363
Fax: 202-966-8553
e-mail: info@geneticalliance.org
www.geneticalliance.org

A coalition of voluntary genetic support groups, consumers and professionals addressing the needs of individuals and families affected by genetic disorders from a national perspective.

Sharon Terry, MA, President/CEO
Natasha Bonhomme, Vice President of Strategic Develop
Vaughn Edelson, Assistant Director of Health Commun

6809 March of Dimes Birth Defects Foundation
1275 Mamaroneck Avenue
White Plains, NY 10605
914-997-4488
888-663-4637
Fax: 914-997-4763
e-mail: answers@marchofdimes.com
www.marchofdimes.com

Partnership of volunteers and professionals dedicated to improving the health of babies by preventing birth defects and infant mortality. Over 100 chapters are located across the country and can be located through the national office.

Jennifer L Howse, President

6810 National Center for Education in Maternal and Child Health
Georgetown University
2115 Wisconsin Ave NW, Suite 601
Washington, DC 20007
202-784-9770
Fax: 202-784-9777
e-mail: mchlibrary@ncemch.org
www.ncemch.org

Provides leadership in disseminating information, program development, and education to individuals with an interest in maternal and child health (MCH), public health policy, and systems of care.

Rochelle Mayer, Director
Olivia Pickett, Director Library Services

6811 National Dissemination Center for Children with Disabilities
1825 Connecticut Ave NW
Washington, DC 20009
202-884-8200
800-695-0285
Fax: 202-884-8441
e-mail: nichcy@fhi360.org
www.nichcy.org

A national information and referral center for families, educators and other professionals on: disabilities in children and youth; programs and services; IDEA, the nation's special education law; and research-based information on effective practices.

Suzanne Ripley, Executive Director

6812 National Rehabilitation Information Center
4200 Forbes Blvd, Suite 202
Lanham, MD 20706
301-459-5900
800-346-2742
Fax: 301-459-4263
TTY: 301-459-5984
e-mail: naricinfo@heitechservices.com
www.naric.com

An online gateway to over 70,000 disability and rehabilitation related documents and journal articles, and other resources.

Mark Odum, Director

6813 Spina Bifida Association
4590 MacArthur Boulevard NW, Suite 250
Washington, DC 20007
202-944-3285
800-621-3141
Fax: 202-944-3295
e-mail: sbaa@sbaa.org
www.spinabifidaassociation.org

Serves as the national office representing approximately 60 chapters of parents and other members of families having children born with spina bifida, individuals with spina bifida, and health professionals who work with them. Operates a national information and referral service, periodic public awareness campaigns, scholarships and an annual meeting.

Cindy Brownstein, Ceo
Caroline Alston, Director, Programs/Field Initiative
Mary E Johnson, Director Communications

State Agencies & Support Groups

Alabama

6814 Spina Bifida Association of Alabama
PO Box 13254
Birmingham, AL 35202
256-325-8600
e-mail: info@sbaofal.org
www.sbaofal.org

Providing medical, social, and financial support to those afflicted with spina bifida.

Betsy Hopson, President
Angie Pate, Executive Director
Jamie Martin, Field Service Coordinator

Arizona

6815 Arizona Spina Bifida Association
1001 E Fairmount Avenue
Phoenix, AZ 85014
602-274-3323
Fax: 602-274-7632
e-mail: office@sbaaz.org
www.sbaaz.org/?

Arlene Plouff, Manager

Arkansas

6816 Spina Bifida Association of Arkansas
4590 MacArthur Blvd., NW, Suite 250
Washington, DC 20007
202-944-3285
Fax: 202-944-3295
e-mail: sbaa@sbaa.org
www.spinabifidaassociation.org

Providing medical, social, and financial support to those afflicted with spina bifida.

Vicki Rucker, Executive Director

California

6817 Spina Bifida Association of Greater Bay Ar ea
4590 MacArthur Blvd., NW, Suite 250
Washington, DC 20007
202-944-3285
Fax: 202-944-3295
e-mail: sbaa@sbaa.org
www.spinabifidaassociation.org

Providing medical, social, and financial support to those afflicted with spina bifida.

Traci Whittemore, President

6818 Spina Bifida Association of Greater San Di ego
4590 MacArthur Blvd., NW, Suite 250
Washington, DC 20007
202-944-3285
Fax: 202-944-3295
e-mail: sbaa@sbaa.org
www.spinabifidaassociation.org

Providing medical, social, and financial support to those afflicted with spina bifida.

Mary Robbins Wade, President

Colorado

6819 Spina Bifida Association of Colorado
PO Box 22994
Denver, CO 80222
303-797-7870
e-mail: sbacolorado@gmail.com
www.coloradospinabifida.org

Providing medical, social, and financial support to those afflicted with spina bifida.

Chris Mestas, Board Chair / SBACO Website
Rev. John Anderson, Immediate Past Chair
LaVon Birney, Executive Director

Connecticut

6820 Spina Bifida Association of Connecticut
370 Osgood Avenue Suite 106
New Britain, CT 06053
860-839-0115
800-574-6274
Fax: 860-832-6260
e-mail: sbac@sbac.org
www.sbac.org

Providing medical, social, and financial support to those afflicted with spina bifida.

Carol Toomey, Chair
Rebecca Hajosy, Treasurer/Secretary
Kiley J Carlson, Executive Director

Florida

6821 Spina Bifida Association of Central Florid a
100 W. Lucerne Circle, Suite 100-M
Orlando, FL 32801
407-248-9210
Fax: 407-248-9227
e-mail: info@sbacfl.org
sbacentralflorida.org

Providing medical, social, and financial support to those afflicted with spina bifida.

Beccy Hosoda, President

6822 Spina Bifida Association of Jacksonville N emours Childrens Clinic
807 Children's Way
Jacksonville, FL 32207
904-390-3686
800-722-6355
Fax: 904-390-3466
e-mail: Sbaj@sbaj.org
www.sbaj.org

Providing medical, social, and financial support to those afflicted with spina bifida.

Stephanie King, Executive Director
Margaret Quintana, Treasurer

6823 Spina Bifida Association of Southeast Florida
4590 MacArthur Blvd., NW, Suite 250
Washington, DC 20007
202-944-3285
Fax: 202-944-3295
e-mail: sbaa@sbaa.org
www.spinabifidaassociation.org

Providing medical, social, and financial support to those afflicted with spina bifida.

Irene Ballart, President

6824 Spina Bifida Association of Tampa Bay
PO Box 16603
Tampa, FL 33687
813-933-4827
e-mail: sbatampabay@aol.com
www.sbatampabay.org

Providing medical, social, and financial support to those afflicted with spina bifida.

Dianne Gore, President

Georgia

6825 Spina Bifida Association of Georgia
5072 Bristol Industrial Way, Suite F
Buford, GA 30518
770-939-1044
Fax: 770-939-1049
e-mail: sbag@spinabifidaga.org
spinabifidaga.org

Jim Okula, Executive Director

Illinois

6826 Spina Bifida Association of Illinois
8765 W Higgins Rd, Suite 403
Chicago, IL 60631
773-444-0305
800-969-4722
Fax: 773-444-0327
e-mail: sbail@sbail.org
www.sbail.org

The Illinois Spina Bifida Association is dedicated to improving the quality of life of people with spina bifida through direct services, information and referral and public awareness. Direct services include family outreach, education advocacy and more.

Amy Maggio, Executive Director

Indiana

6827 Spina Bifida Association of Central Indian a
PO Box 19814
Indianapolis, IN 46219
317-592-1630
e-mail: membership@sbaci.org
www.sbaci.org

Providing medical, social, and financial support to those afflicted with spina bifida.

Lisa Jones, President

6828 Spina Bifida Association of Northern Indiana
4590 MacArthur Blvd., NW, Suite 250
Washington, DC 20007
202-944-3285
Fax: 202-944-3295
e-mail: sbaa@sbaa.org
www.spinabifidaassociation.org

Providing medical, social, and financial support to those afflicted with spina bifida.

Tim Yoder, President

Iowa

6829 Spina Bifida Association of Iowa
8525 Douglas Avenue Suite 39
Urbandale, IA 50322   515-964-8810
e-mail: contact@sbaia.org
www.sbaia.org

Providing support, a reimbursement program, quarterly newsletter and public awareness campaigns.

Maryanne Lorenz, Manager

Kentucky

6830 Spina Bifida Association of Kentucky
982 Eastern Parkway, Box 18
Louisville, KY 40217   502-637-7363
866-340-7225
Fax: 502-637-1010
e-mail: sbak@sbak.org
www.spinabifidakentucky.org

Providing support to those afflicted with spina bifida.

Joe O'Bryan, Board Chair/President
Eddie Brown Jr., Incoming Chair
Cris Miller, Secretary

Louisiana

6831 Spina Bifida Association of Greater New Orleans
PO Box 1346
Kenner, LA 70063   504-737-5181
e-mail: sbagno@sbagno.org
www.sbagno.org

Providing support to those afflicted with spina bifida.

Julie Johnston, Coordinator

Maryland

6832 Spina Bifida Association of Chesapeake-Pot omac
PO Box 1750
Annapolis, MD 21404   888-733-0988
Fax: 410-295-9744
e-mail: cpbs@kennedykrieger.org
www.chesapeakespinabifida.org

Providing support to those afflicted with spina bifida.

Toni Shumate, Executive Director

Massachusetts

6833 Spina Bifida Association of Massachusetts
25 Birch Street, Building B
Milford, MA 01757   888-479-1900
Fax: 504-482-5301
e-mail: edugan@sbamass.org
www.sbamass.org

SBA Mass is a community of support for a large group of Massachusetts residents who sometimes need an empathetic ear or a voice of advocacy. They are staffed entirely be volunteers dedicated to supporting their mission.

Ellen Heffernan-Dugan, LIOSOW, Operations Associate
Cara Packard, President
Matt Neal, Vice Chair and Treasurer

Michigan

6834 Spina Bifida Association of Upper Peninsula Michigan
1220 N 3rd Street
Ishpeming, MI 49849   906-485-5127
e-mail: cbengson@chartermi.net
sba-up.8m.com

Providing support to those affected by spina bifida.

Lois Bengson, President

6835 Spina Bifida Association of West Michigan
235 Wealthy SE
Grand Rapids, MI 49503   616-949-3428
e-mail: wmisbo@gmail.com
www.wmspinabifida.org/

Providing support to those afflicted with spina bifida.

Carol Carpenter, Interim President

Minnesota

6836 Spina Bifida Association of Minnesota
PO Box 29323
Brooklyn Center, MN 55429   651-222-6395
Fax: 651-228-0914
e-mail: sbamn@hotmail.com
www.sbamn.org

Providing support to those afflicted with spina bifida.

James Thayer, Executive Director

Mississippi

6837 Spina Bifida Association of Mississippi
PO Box 180594
Richland, MS 39218   601-420-0030
Fax: 601-420-0300
e-mail: sbafms@yahoo.com
www.spinabifidams.com

Providing support to those afflicted with spina bifida.

Amy Wilkinson, Executive Director

Missouri

6838 Spina Bifida Association of Greater Saint Louis
9201 Watson Road, Suite 125
Crestwood, MO 63126   314-843-2244
800-784-0983
Fax: 314-765-6246
e-mail: sbastl@charter.net
www.sbstl.com

Providing support to those afflicted with spina bifida.

Mark Abbott, Chairman

Nebraska

6839 Spina Bifida Association of Nebraska
7612 Maple St
Omaha, NE 68134   402-572-3570
Fax: 402-572-3002
e-mail: sbamom@cox.net
www.spinabifidanebraska.org

Providing support to those afflicted with spina bifida.

Megan Sorensen, President

New Jersey

6840 Spina Bifida Association of the Tri-State Region
84 Park Avenue
Flemington, NJ 08822   908-782-7475
Fax: 908-782-6102
e-mail: info@sbatsr.org
www.sbatsr.org

Serves New Jersey, New York metro area and Southern Connecticut. Providing medical, social, and financial support to those afflicted with spina bifida.

Jane Horowitz, Executive Director
Haley Hopper, Director Development

New York

6841 Spina Bifida Association of Albany/Capital District
109 Spring Road
Scotia, NY 12302
518-399-9151
e-mail: Sbaalbany102@aol.com
www.sbaalbany.org

Providing support to those afflicted with spina bifida.

Karen Wentworth, Director

6842 Spina Bifida Association of Greater Roches ter
PO Box 3
Fairport, NY 14450
585-388-7450
e-mail: pritch50@yahoo.com
www.sbaa.com

Providing support to those afflicted with spina bifida.

Mary Pritchard, Manager

6843 Spina Bifida Association of Nassau County
12 Hampton Rd
South Beach, NY 11789
631-821-9028
e-mail: kid3418@optonline.net
www.sbancny.org

Providing support to those afflicted with spina bifida.

Leslieann Sussman, President

6844 Spina Bifida Association of Western New York
137 Warner Ave
N Tonawanda, NY 14120
716-446-5595
Fax: 716-735-7561
e-mail: pmorris@sbawny.org
www.sbawny.org

Providing support to those living with spina bifida.

Cynthia Carlson, President

North Carolina

6845 Spina Bifida Association of North Carolina
3915 Grace Court
Indian Trail, NC 28079
800-847-2262
Fax: 800-847-2262
e-mail: sbanc@mindspring.com
sbanc.home.mindspring.com

Providing support to those afflicted with spina bifida. There are five regional support groups in the state.

Kim Gates, Charlotte/Piedmont Contact
Jolyne Wagner, Raleigh Area Contact

Ohio

6846 Spina Bifida Association of Canton
PO Box 9024
Canton, OH 44711
330-863-2531
e-mail: cmgriffin@neo.rr.com
www.sbacanton.org

Providing support to those afflicted with spina bifida.

Connie Griffin, President

6847 Spina Bifida Association of Central Ohio
7574 Danbridge Way
Westerville, OH 43082
614-818-3840
e-mail: lauriedvm@sbcglobal.net
www.sbaco.blogspot.com

Providing support to those afflicted with spina bifida.

Laurie Schulze, President

6848 Spina Bifida Association of Cincinnati
644 Linn Street, Suite 635
Cincinnati, OH 45203
513-923-1378
e-mail: sbacincy@excel.com
www.sbacincy.org

Providing support to those afflicted with spina bifida.

Diane Burns, President

6849 Spina Bifida Association of Greater Dayton
4801 Springfield St
Dayton, OH 45431
937-236-1122
Fax: 937-434-4899
e-mail: sbadayton@yahoo.com
www.sbadayton.org

Providing support to those afflicted with spina bifida.

David Skinner, President

6850 Spina Bifida Association of North West Ohio
302 Conant St., Suite C
Maumee, OH 43537
419-794-0561
e-mail: jobrien@sbanwo.org
www.sbaofnorthwestohio.org

Providing support to those afflicted with spina bifida.

Mindy Gallant, Chair
Christina Fulton, Vice Chair
Jennifer O'Brien, Executive Director

6851 Spina Bifida Association of Tri-County Ohio
PO Box 8701
Warren, OH 44484
330-793-8544
e-mail: jchappel@sbcglobal.net
www.spaa.org

Providing support to those living with spina bifida, from youth into adulthood. Also places an emphasis on parent support groups.

Julie Solomon, President

Pennsylvania

6852 Spina Bifida Association Pittsburgh
4590 MacArthur Blvd., NW, Suite 250
Washington, DC 20007
202-944-3285
Fax: 202-944-3295
e-mail: sbaa@sbaa.org
www.spinabifidaassociation.org

Providing medical, social, and financial support to those afflicted with spina bifida.

Shannon Williams, President

6853 Spina Bifida Association of Delaware Valley
PO Box 1235
Havertown, PA 19803
610-584-5530
800-223-0222
e-mail: info@sbadv.org
www.sbadv.org

Providing medical, social, and financial support to those living with spina bifida.

Keri Mascaro, President

6854 Spina Bifida Association of Greater Pennsy lvania
215 E State St, Suite D
Quarryville, PA 17566
717-786-9280
Fax: 717-786-8821
e-mail: SBAofPA@aol.com
spinabifidaresource.weebly.com

Providing medical, social, and financial support to those afflicted with spina bifida.

Patricia Fulvio, Executive Director

Tennessee

6855 Spina Bifida Association of Tennessee
4590 MacArthur Blvd., NW, Suite 250
Washington, DC 20007
202-944-3285
Fax: 202-944-3295
e-mail: sbaa@sbaa.org
www.spinabifidaassociation.org

Providing medical, social, and financial support to those living with spina bifida.

Lynn Hess, President

Texas

6856 Spina Bifida Association of Houston-Gulf Coast
440 Benmar Suite 3052
Houston, TX 77060
281-447-2707
Fax: 281-997-2378
e-mail: president@sbahgc.org
www.sbahgc.org

Providing medical, social, and financial support to those afflicted with spina bifida.

Jennifer Franklin, Vice President
Joan Peck, Treasurer
Michelle Lockstedt, Secretary, Fundraising

6857 Spina Bifida Association of North Texas
705 Ave B, Suite 204
Garland, TX 75040
972-238-8755
Fax: 214-703-1981
e-mail: sbnorthtexas@aol.com
www.spinabifidant.org/?

Providing medical, social, and financial support to those living with spina bifida.

Carol Barrett, Contact

6858 Spina Bifida Association of Texas
1550 NE Loop 410, Suite 224
San Antonio, TX 78209
210-826-7289
866-597-2289
e-mail: sbinfo@sbatx.org
www.sbatx.org

Providing medical, social, and financial support to those afflicted with spina bifida.

Nora Oyler, Executive Director

Utah

6859 Spina Bifida Association of Utah
900 S 1500 East, Apt C124
Clearfield, UT 84015
801-214-8070
e-mail: support@utahspinabifida.org
www.utahspinabifida.org/

Providing medical, social, and financial support to those living with spina bifida.

Ilene Hall, President

Virginia

6860 Spina Bifida Association of the Roanoke Valley
PO Box 7652
Roanoke, VA 24019
540-342-1231
Fax: 540-890-1244
e-mail: sbaroanokevalley@yahoo.com
www.sbarv.org

Providing medical, social, and financial support to those living with spina bifida.

Millie Wilson, President

Washington

6861 Evergreen Spina Bifida Association
611 2nd street, Suite A
Snohomish, WA 98290
253-589-3700
e-mail: sbaws@yahoo.com
www.sbaws.org/?

Providing medical, social, and financial support to those afflicted with spina bifida.

Ed Kennedy, President

Wisconsin

6862 Spina Bifida Association of Greater Fox Valley
4590 MacArthur Blvd., NW, Suite 250
Washington, DC 20007
202-944-3285
Fax: 202-944-3295
e-mail: sbaa@sbaa.org
www.spinabifidaassociation.org

Providing support to those living with spina bifida.

Kelly Richard

6863 Spina Bifida Association of Northern Wisconsin
PO Box 421
Schofield, WI 54476
715-359-9674
e-mail: dtackley@cheqnet.net

Providing medical, social, and financial support to those afflicted with spina bifida.

David Bouchard, President

6864 Spina Bifida Association of Wisconsin
830 N 109th Street, Suite 6
Wauwatosa, WI 53226
414-607-9061
Fax: 414-607-9602
e-mail: sbawi@sbawi.org
www.sbawi.org

SBAWI is made up of those with spina bifida, as well as family, friends and health care providers. The association is dedicated to helping its membership emotionally, educationally, and financially.

Karen Drzewiecki, President
James B. Hanley, Secretary
Alexandria Sluis, Treasurer

Conferences

6865 SBA National Conference
Spina Bifida Association
4590 MacArthur Boulevard NW, Suite 250
Washington, DC 20007
202-944-3285
800-621-3141
Fax: 202-944-3295
e-mail: sbaa@sbaa.org
www.spinabifidaassociation.org

Children and adults with Spina Bifida, their families, physicians, nurses, and other clinicians have the unique opportunity to gain information on the latest medical care and network on various issues which affect their lives and professions.

June

Cindy Brownstein, CEO

Audio Video

6866 Challenge
Spina Bifida Association
1600 Wilson Blvd., Suite 800
Arlington, VA 22209
202-944-3285
800-621-3141
Fax: 202-944-3295
e-mail: sbaa@sbaa.org
www.spinabifidaassociation.org

A human look of how people come to grips with and overcome the challenges related to living with Spina Bifida.

1992 14 minutes

Sara Struwe, President/ CEO
Elizabeth Merck, Director of Development
Lisa Raman, Director

Web Sites

6867 Association for Spina Bifida and Hydroceph alus
www.asbah.org

A UK charity that provides information and advice to those with spina bifida and their families.

6868 Children with Spina Bifida: A Resource Page for Parents
www.waisman.wisc.edu/~rowley/sb-kids/

e-mail: rowley@waisman.wisc.edu
www.waisman.wisc.edu/~rowley/sb-kids/

A resource page for parents with children with Spina Bifida.

6869 International Federation for Spina Bifida and Hydrocephalus
Cellebroersstraat 16/Rue des Alexiens 16
Brussels, B-100   32 -0 2-502
e-mail: info@ifglobal.org
www.ifglobal.org

The world-wide umbrella organization for spina bifida and hydracephalus organizations. It's primary goal is prevention through the dissemination of information and education.

Margo Whiteford, President
Jackie Bland, Treasurer
Lieven Bauwens, Secretary General

6870 LFSN: Lipomyelomeningecele Family Support Network
www.lfsn.org

A network of families providing support and information sharing to those affected by Occult Spinal Dysraphisms.

6871 March of Dimes Birth Defects Foundation
1275 Mamaroneck Avenue
White Plains, NY 10605   914-997-4488
www.marchofdimes.org

March of Dimes researchers, colunteers, educators, outreach workers and advocates work together to give all babies a fighting chance against the threats to their health: prematurity, birth defects, low birthweight.

6872 Online Mendelian Inheritance in Man
www.omim.org

This database is a catalog of human genes and genetic disorders.

6873 Spina Bifida Association of America
1600 Wilson Blvd., Suite 800
Arlington, VA 22209   202-944-3285
Fax: 202-944-3295
e-mail: sbaa@sbaa.org
www.spinabifidaassociation.org

The mission is to promote the prevention os spina bifida and to enhance the lives of all affected. The association was founded to address the specific needs of the spina bifida community and serves as the national representative of almost 60 chapters. SBAA's efforts benefit thousands of infants, children, adults, parents and professionals each year.

Sara Struwe, President/ CEO
Elizabeth Merck, Director of Development
Lisa Raman, Director

6874 Wheeless' Textbook of Orthopaedics
www.wheelessonline.com

Derives from a variety of sources, imcluding journals, articles, national meetings lectures and other textbooks.

Clifford R. Wheeless, III, M.D., Author

Book Publishers

6875 All Kinds of Friends, Even Green!
Ellen B Sensi, author

Spina Bifida Association
4590 MacArthur Boulevard NW, Suite 250
Washington, DC 20007   202-944-3285
800-621-3141
Fax: 202-944-3295
e-mail: sbaa@sbaa.org
www.spinabifidaassociation.org

Moses has spina bifida and a lot of friends. Which one will he choose to write about for his school project?

Cindy Brownstein, President & CEO
Sara Struwe, Chief Operating Officer & Director
Christopher Vance, Director of Development

6876 Answering Your Questions About Spina Bifida
Spina Bifida Association
4590 MacArthur Boulevard NW, Suite 250
Washington, DC 20007   202-944-3285
800-621-3141
Fax: 202-944-3295
e-mail: sbaa@sbaa.org
www.spinabifidaassociation.org

Provides information to help people understand the basic medical, educational and social issues which commonly affect people with Spina Bifida.

Cindy Brownstein, President & CEO
Sara Struwe, Chief Operating Officer & Director
Christopher Vance, Director of Development

6877 Bowel Continence and Spina Bifida
Spina Bifida Association
4590 MacArthur Boulevard NW, Suite 250
Washington, DC 20007   202-944-3285
800-621-3141
Fax: 202-944-3295
e-mail: sbaa@sbaa.org
www.spinabifidaassociation.org

An excellent book aimed at anyone (infant or adult) trying to attain bowel continence. Focuses on continence programs, bowel management development and includes a chart and glossary of terms.

Cindy Brownstein, President & CEO
Sara Struwe, Chief Operating Officer & Director
Christopher Vance, Director of Development

6878 Children with Spina Bifida: A Parent's Gui de
Spina Bifida Association
4590 MacArthur Boulevard NW, Suite 250
Washington, DC 20007   202-944-3285
800-621-3141
Fax: 202-944-3295
e-mail: sbaa@sbaa.org
www.spinabifidaassociation.org

Comprehensive publication provides easy-to-understand coverage of neurosurgery, physical therapy, emotional health, education, urological concerns, orthopedic concerns, childhood development and more. Valuable for parents, educators and libraries.

Cindy Brownstein, President & CEO
Sara Struwe, Chief Operating Officer & Director
Christopher Vance, Director of Development

6879 Complete IEP Guide: How to Advocate for Your Special Ed Child
Spina Bifida Association
4590 MacArthur Boulevard NW, Suite 250
Washington, DC 20007   202-944-3285
800-621-3141
Fax: 202-944-3295
e-mail: sbaa@sbaa.org
www.spinabifidaassociation.org

This all-in-one guide will help you understand special education law, identify your child's needs, prepare for meetings, develop the IEP and resolve disputes.

Cindy Brownstein, President & CEO
Sara Struwe, Chief Operating Officer & Director
Christopher Vance, Director of Development

6880 Confronting the Challenges of Spina Bifida
Spina Bifida Association
4590 MacArthur Boulevard NW, Suite 250
Washington, DC 20007 202-944-3285
800-621-3141
Fax: 202-944-3295
e-mail: sbaa@sbaa.org
www.spinabifidaassociation.org

A group curriculum addressing self-care, self-esteem, and social skills in eight to 13 year olds.

Cindy Brownstein, President & CEO
Sara Struwe, Chief Operating Officer & Director
Christopher Vance, Director of Development

6881 Congenital Disorders Sourcebook
Omnigraphics
PO Box 8002
Aston, PA 19014 800-234-1340
Fax: 800-875-1340
e-mail: info@omnigraphics.com
www.omnigraphics.com

Basic consumer health information on disorders aquired during gestation, including spina bifida, hydrocephalus, cerebral palsy, heart defects, craniofacial abnormalities and fetal alcohol syndrome.

650 pages
ISBN: 0-780809-45-9

Peter Ruffner, Publisher

6882 Featherless/Desplumado
Juan Felipe Herrera, author

Spina Bifida Association
4590 MacArthur Boulevard NW, Suite 250
Washington, DC 20007 202-944-3285
800-621-3141
Fax: 202-944-3295
e-mail: sbaa@sbaa.org
www.spinabifidaassociation.org

Tomasito, although confined to a wheelchair, feels free when on the soccer field.

Cindy Brownstein, President & CEO
Sara Struwe, Chief Operating Officer & Director
Christopher Vance, Director of Development

6883 Friends No Matter What
Rose Blivins, author

Spina Bifida Association
4590 MacArthur Boulevard NW, Suite 250
Washington, DC 20007 202-944-3285
800-621-3141
Fax: 202-944-3295
e-mail: sbaa@sbaa.org
www.spinabifidaassociation.org

The story of two boys, one in a wheelchair and one who loves to play basketball. How will it work out?

Cindy Brownstein, President & CEO
Sara Struwe, Chief Operating Officer & Director
Christopher Vance, Director of Development

**6884 Guidelines for Spina Bifida and Health Car e Services
Throughout Life**
Spina Bifida Association
4590 MacArthur Boulevard NW, Suite 250
Washington, DC 20007 202-944-3285
800-621-3141
Fax: 202-944-3295
e-mail: sbaa@sbaa.org
www.spinabifidaassociation.org

Guidelines designed to help spina bifida sufferers throughout their entire lives.

Cindy Brownstein, President & CEO
Sara Struwe, Chief Operating Officer & Director
Christopher Vance, Director of Development

6885 Introduction to Spina Bifida
Spina Bifida Association
4590 MacArthur Boulevard NW, Suite 250
Washington, DC 20007 202-944-3285
800-621-3141
Fax: 202-944-3295
e-mail: sbaa@sbaa.org
www.spinabifidaassociation.org

An aid and guide for those who care for someone with spina bifida, written in non-medical terms and language.

Cindy Brownstein, President & CEO
Sara Struwe, Chief Operating Officer & Director
Christopher Vance, Director of Development

6886 Looking for Goodwill
Patt & Scott Price, author

Spina Bifida Association
4590 MacArthur Boulevard NW, Suite 250
Washington, DC 20007 202-944-3285
800-621-3141
Fax: 202-944-3295
e-mail: sbaa@sbaa.org
www.spinabifidaassociation.org

An inspirational read, the result of a trek across the US and random interviews showing the heart and attitude of America.

Cindy Brownstein, President & CEO
Sara Struwe, Chief Operating Officer & Director
Christopher Vance, Director of Development

**6887 Negotiating the Special Education Maze: A Guide for Parents
and Teachers**
Spina Bifida Association
4590 MacArthur Boulevard NW, Suite 250
Washington, DC 20007 202-944-3285
800-621-3141
Fax: 202-944-3295
e-mail: sbaa@sbaa.org
www.spinabifidaassociation.org

An excellent aid for the development of an effective special education program.

Cindy Brownstein, President & CEO
Sara Struwe, Chief Operating Officer & Director
Christopher Vance, Director of Development

**6888 New Language of Toys: Teaching Communicati on Skills to
Children with Special Needs**
Spina Bifida Association
4590 MacArthur Boulevard NW, Suite 250
Washington, DC 20007 202-944-3285
800-621-3141
Fax: 202-944-3295
e-mail: sbaa@sbaa.org
www.spinabifidaassociation.org

A guide for parents and teachers, this reader-friendly resource guide provides a wealth of information on how play activities affect a child's language development (with a focus on special needs) and where to get the toys and materials to use in these activities.

Cindy Brownstein, President & CEO
Sara Struwe, Chief Operating Officer & Director
Christopher Vance, Director of Development

6889 Nick Joins In

Joe Lasker, author

Spina Bifida Association
4590 MacArthur Boulevard NW, Suite 250
Washington, DC 20007
202-944-3285
800-621-3141
Fax: 202-944-3295
e-mail: sbaa@sbaa.org
www.spinabifidaassociation.org

When Nick, who is in a wheelchair, enters a regular classroom, for the first time he realizes that he has much to contribute.

Cindy Brownstein, President & CEO
Sara Struwe, Chief Operating Officer & Director
Christopher Vance, Director of Development

6890 Rolling Along with Goldilocks and the Three Bears

Cindy Meyers, author

Spina Bifida Association
4590 MacArthur Boulevard NW, Suite 250
Washington, DC 20007
202-944-3285
800-621-3141
Fax: 202-944-3295
e-mail: sbaa@sbaa.org
www.spinabifidaassociation.org

The familiar folktale with a special-needs twist.

Cindy Brownstein, President & CEO
Sara Struwe, Chief Operating Officer & Director
Christopher Vance, Director of Development

6891 SPINAbilities: A Young Person's Guide to Spina Bifida

Spina Bifida Association
4590 MacArthur Boulevard NW, Suite 250
Washington, DC 20007
202-944-3285
800-621-3141
Fax: 202-944-3295
e-mail: sbaa@sbaa.org
www.spinabifidaassociation.org

Practical suggestions and tips for young people on becoming independent and managing their healthcare.

Cindy Brownstein, President & CEO
Sara Struwe, Chief Operating Officer & Director
Christopher Vance, Director of Development

6892 Sexuality and the Person with Spinabifida

Stephen Sloan PhD, author

Spina Bifida Association
4590 MacArthur Boulevard NW, Suite 250
Washington, DC 20007
202-944-3285
800-621-3141
Fax: 202-944-3295
e-mail: sbaa@sbaa.org
www.spinabifidaassociation.org

Focuses on sexuality, sexual development, sexual activity, and other important issues.

Cindy Brownstein, President & CEO
Sara Struwe, Chief Operating Officer & Director
Christopher Vance, Director of Development

6893 Steps to Independence: Teaching Everyday Skills to Children with Special Needs

Spina Bifida Association
4590 MacArthur Boulevard NW, Suite 250
Washington, DC 20007
202-944-3285
800-621-3141
Fax: 202-944-3295
e-mail: sbaa@sbaa.org
www.spinabifidaassociation.org

A guide to help parents teach life skills to their disabled child.

Cindy Brownstein, President & CEO
Sara Struwe, Chief Operating Officer & Director
Christopher Vance, Director of Development

6894 Teaching Students with Spina Bifida

BOSC Books-Books on Special Children
PO Box 3378
Amherst, MA 01004
413-256-8164
Fax: 413-256-8896
www.boscbooks.com

Explores the vital issues of concern to students with spina bifida including aspects of their social, personal and cognitive development. The book is sensitively written and abounds with useful tips covering such things as crutch storage, work space organization, etc.

460 pages Softcover

6895 Unlocking Potential: College and Other Choices for People with LD and AD/HD

Spina Bifida Association
4590 MacArthur Boulevard NW, Suite 250
Washington, DC 20007
202-944-3285
800-621-3141
Fax: 202-944-3295
e-mail: sbaa@sbaa.org
www.spinabifidaassociation.org

An indispensible tool for high school students with learning disabilities and AD/HD. Includes a comprehensive listing of resources.

Cindy Brownstein, President & CEO
Sara Struwe, Chief Operating Officer & Director
Christopher Vance, Director of Development

6896 Views from Our Shoes: Growing Up with a Brother or Sister with Special Needs

Spina Bifida Association
4590 MacArthur Boulevard NW, Suite 250
Washington, DC 20007
202-944-3285
800-621-3141
Fax: 202-944-3295
e-mail: sbaa@sbaa.org
www.spinabifidaassociation.org

A balanced view of the positives and negatives of living with a disabled sibling. Written for siblings ages nine and up.

Cindy Brownstein, President & CEO
Sara Struwe, Chief Operating Officer & Director
Christopher Vance, Director of Development

Newsletters

6897 Insights into Spina Bifida

Spina Bifida Association
1600 Wilson Blvd., Suite 800
Arlington, VA 22209
202-944-3285
800-621-3141
Fax: 202-944-3295
e-mail: sbaa@sbaa.org
www.spinabifidaassociation.org

Includes articles on the latest research, legislation, features, emotional aspects, educational information, and information on the Association's national conference.

Bimonthly

Sara Struwe, President/ CEO
Elizabeth Merck, Director of Development
Lisa Raman, Director

Pamphlets

6898 Educational Issues Among Children With Spina Bifida

Spina Bifida Association
1600 Wilson Blvd., Suite 800
Arlington, VA 22209
202-944-3285
800-621-3141
Fax: 202-944-3295
e-mail: sbaa@sbaa.org
www.spinabifidaassociation.org

Sara Struwe, President/ CEO
Elizabeth Merck, Director of Development
Lisa Raman, Director

6899 Learning Among Children with Spina Bifida
Spina Bifida Association
1600 Wilson Blvd., Suite 800
Arlington, VA 22209   202-944-3285
                                              800-621-3141
                                         Fax: 202-944-3295
                                     e-mail: sbaa@sbaa.org
                              www.spinabifidaassociation.org

Sara Struwe, President/ CEO
Elizabeth Merck, Director of Development
Lisa Raman, Director

**6900 Monetary Allowance, Health Care and Vocational Training &
Rehabilitation**
National Veterans Services Fund
PO Box 2465
Darien, CT 06820   203-656-0003
                                              800-521-0198
                                         Fax: 203-656-1957
                                     e-mail: nvsf@NVSF.org
                                               www.nvsf.org

Monetary allowance, health care, vocational training and rehabilitation for Vietnam Veterans' children with spine bifida.

Pamphlet

6901 SBAA General Information Brochure
Spina Bifida Association
1600 Wilson Blvd., Suite 800
Arlington, VA 22209   202-944-3285
                                              800-621-3141
                                         Fax: 202-944-3295
                                     e-mail: sbaa@sbaa.org
                              www.spinabifidaassociation.org

Sara Struwe, President/ CEO
Elizabeth Merck, Director of Development
Lisa Raman, Director

6902 SBAA General Information Packet
Spina Bifida Association
1600 Wilson Blvd., Suite 800
Arlington, VA 22209   202-944-3285
                                              800-621-3141
                                         Fax: 202-944-3295
                                     e-mail: sbaa@sbaa.org
                              www.spinabifidaassociation.org

Sara Struwe, President/ CEO
Elizabeth Merck, Director of Development
Lisa Raman, Director

6903 Social Development and the Person With Spina Bifida
Spina Bifida Association
1600 Wilson Blvd., Suite 800
Arlington, VA 22209   202-944-3285
                                              800-621-3141
                                         Fax: 202-944-3295
                                     e-mail: sbaa@sbaa.org
                              www.spinabifidaassociation.org

20 pages

Sara Struwe, President/ CEO
Elizabeth Merck, Director of Development
Lisa Raman, Director

6904 Urologic Care of the Child with Spina Bifida
David Joseph MD, author

Spina Bifida Association
1600 Wilson Blvd., Suite 800
Arlington, VA 22209   202-944-3285
                                              800-621-3141
                                         Fax: 202-944-3295
                                     e-mail: sbaa@sbaa.org
                              www.spinabifidaassociation.org

2001

Sara Struwe, President/ CEO
Elizabeth Merck, Director of Development
Lisa Raman, Director

Camps

6905 Camp Boggy Creek
30500 Brantley Branch Road
Eustis, FL 32736   352-483-4200
                                              866-462-6449
                                         Fax: 352-483-0589
                              e-mail: info@campboggycreek.org
                                        www.boggycreek.org

A year round camp serving seriously ill children throughout
Florida. We offer week-long summer sessions for the children
and family retreat weekends for the whole family.

June Clark, President/CEO
David Mann, Camp Director
Kimmy Lamborn, Assistant Camp Director

6906 Camp Oakhurst
111 Monmouth Road
Oakhurst, NJ 7755   732-531-0215
                                         Fax: 732-531-0292
                                     e-mail: info@nysh.org
                                     www.campoakhurst.com

A summer camp and year round respite program for children and
adults with physical disabilities.

Robert Pacenza, Executive Director
Charles Sutherland, Camp Director

6907 Mountaineer Spina Bifida Camp
350 Capital Street
Charleston, WV 800-6   304-558-7098
                                              800-800-642
                                         Fax: 304-558-2866
                                       www.kidscamps.com

The mission is to help children and teens to develop self-esteem,
social skills, and self reliance while they participate in recreational and social activities.

Description

6908 SPINAL MUSCULAR ATROPHIES
Synonym: SMA
Covers these related disorders: Fazio-Londe disease (Progressive bulbar palsy of childhood), SMA type I (Werdnig-Hoffmann disease; Acute SMA), SMA type II (Intermediate SMA), SMA type III (Kugelberg-Welander disease)
Involves the following Biologic System(s):
Neurologic Disorders, Orthopedic and Muscle Disorders

The spinal muscular atrophies (SMAs) refer to a group of progressive, inherited neuromuscular disorders characterized by the progressive degeneration of motor neurons. Motor neurons are nerves that originate in the spinal cord and stimulate and control muscle movement (motor neurons). Spinal muscular atrophy type I, also called Werdnig-Hoffmann disease, usually becomes apparent between the second and fourth month of life; however, some infants may have symptoms at birth, including difficult breathing and the inability to feed. Other characteristic symptoms and findings include lack of muscle tone (hypotonia), muscle weakness, the inability to control head movements, absence of tendon stretch reflexes, and uncontrollable twitching or small movements (fasciculations) of the tongue and possibly other muscles. Within two to three years of age, continued breathing and feeding difficulties, along with other progressive problems, may lead to life-threatening complications. Treatment is symptomatic and supportive.

Children with SMA type II usually show signs of progressive muscle weakness of the legs and, to a lesser degree, the arms during the first or second year of life. As the disease progresses, many affected children develop side-to-side curvature of the spine (scoliosis), difficulty swallowing, and a nasal quality to their speech. Children with SMA type II may be severely physically handicapped and are usually of average or above average intelligence. Affected chidren are prone to repeated respiratory infections and breathing difficulties. Life-threatening complications may occur during adolescence or early adulthood.

SMA type III or chronic spinal muscular atrophy may become apparent between the ages of two to 17 years. This is the mildest form of SMA. Progressive weakness associated with chronic SMA is most apparent in the trunk area of the body, especially in the muscles of the shoulder girdle area. There is muscle weakness and loss of muscle mass (atrophy). In addition, deep tendon reflexes may be decreased or absent and muscle twitching (fasciculations) may be present. Some affected children may also have a tremor when the hands are outstretched. Repeated respiratory infections are common.

Fazio-Londe disease, also called progressive bulbar palsy of childhood, is a rare type of spinal muscular atrophy that results from degeneration of motor neurons located, for the most part, in the brain stem. This rare disorder is characterized by progressive palsy or paralysis of the nerves that emerge from the skull (cranial nerves). Symptoms and physical findings associated with Fazio-Londe disease include progressive loss of muscle mass (atrophy) and paralysis of the muscles of the tongue, mouth, lips, throat (pharynx), and voice box (larynx).

A team approach involving specialists such as neurologists, orthopedists, and physical therapists, in cooperation with parents or caregivers, may be helpful in providing care for children with spinal muscular atrophies. Other treatment is symptomatic and supportive.

SMA is usually inherited as an autosomal recessive trait, although some cases of autosomal dominant transmission have been reported. This disorder occurs in approximately one out of every 25,000 births. The genes for SMA types I, II, and III seem to be related and are located on the long arm of chromosome 5 (5q11-13).

National Associations & Support Groups

6909 American Academy of Pediatrics
141 Northwest Point Boulevard
Elk Grove Village, IL 60007
847-434-4000
800-433-9016
Fax: 847-434-8000
www.aap.org

The American Academy of Pediatrics and its member pediatricians are committed to the attainment of optimal physical, mental and social health and well-being for all infants, children, adolescents, and young adults.

Sandra Hassink, MD, FAAP, President

6910 Families of Spinal Muscular Atrophy
925 Busse Road
Elk Grove Village, IL 60007
847-367-7620
800-886-1762
Fax: 847-357-7623
e-mail: info@fsma.org
www.fsma.org

Families of SMA was founded for the purpose of encouraging support and raising funds to promote research into the causes and cure of spinal muscular atrophy. Funds are specifically directed to scientific, educational, or literary purposes in keeping with a charitable organization. It has more than 24 chapters worldwide and over 5000 member families.

Kenneth Hobby, President
Jill Jarecki, Research Director
Karen O'Brien, General Information

6911 Fight SMA / Andrew's Buddies
1807 Libbie Ave, Suite 104
Richmond, VA 23226
804-515-0080
Fax: 804-515-0081
e-mail: heatherlennon@fightsma.com
www.fightsma.org/?

Corporation with 15 US chapters that works to raise awareness of SMA and accelerate treatment and a cure.

Martha Slay, President
Sarah Williams, Treasurer

6912 Genetic Alliance
4301 Connecticut Avenue NW
Washington, DC 20008
202-966-5557
800-336-4363
Fax: 202-966-8553
e-mail: info@geneticalliance.org
www.geneticalliance.org

A coalition of voluntary genetic support groups, consumers and professionals addressing the needs of individuals and families affected by genetic disorders from a national perspective.

Sharon Terry, MA, President/CEO
Natasha Bonhomme, Vice President of Strategic Develop
Vaughn Edelson, Assistant Director of Health Commun

6913 March of Dimes Birth Defects Foundation
1275 Mamaroneck Avenue
White Plains, NY 10605   914-428-7100
                                          888-663-4637
                                     Fax: 914-428-8203
          e-mail: resourcecenter@modimes.org
                    www.marchofdimes.com

Partnership of volunteers and professionals dedicated to improving the health of babies by preventing birth defects and infant
mortality. Over 100 chapters are located across the country and
can be located through the national office.

Jennifer L Howse, President

6914 Muscular Dystrophy Association
3300 E Sunrise Drive
Tucson, AZ 85718   520-529-2000
                                          800-572-1717
                                     Fax: 520-529-5300
                    e-mail: mda@mdausa.org
                              www.mda.org

The MDA is a voluntary health agency, and a partnership between
scientists and concerned citizens, aimed at conquering
neuromuscular diseases affecting more than 1 million Americans.
MDA works worldwide with research, medical, and community
programs, and supports more research on neuromuscular diseases
than any other private-sector organization in the world.

Robert Ross, CEO

6915 Spinal Muscular Atrophy Coalition (SMA Coa lition)
119 W 72nd Street, PO Box 187
New York, NY 10023   646-253-7100
                                     Fax: 212-247-3079
              e-mail: info@smafoundation.org
                       www.smafoundation.org

A group of nonprofit organizations that stand together to raise
awareness and advocate for progress towards the treatment and
cure of SMA.

6916 Spinal Muscular Atrophy Foundation
119 W 72nd St, #187
New York, NY 10023   646-253-7100
                                     Fax: 212-247-3079
              e-mail: info@smafoundation.org
                       www.smafoundation.org

Loren Eng, President
Cynthia Joyce, Executive Director
Yevgeniy Izrayelit, Operations Manager

State Agencies & Support Groups

Arizona

6917 Families of SMA - Arizona Chapter
P.O. Box 43861 Phoenix
Phoenix, AZ 85080   602-314-4902
                    e-mail: arizona@fsma.org
                              www.fsma.org

Angel Wolff, President

California

6918 Families of SMA - Northern California Chap ter
PO Box 9014
Santa Rosa, CA 95405   707-571-8990
                    e-mail: ncalif@fsma.org
                              www.fsma.org

David Sereni, President

Connecticut

6919 Families of SMA - Connecticut Chapter
PO Box 124
Rowayton, CT 06853   203-288-1488
                                          800-866-1762
                    e-mail: conn@fsma.org
                              www.fsma.org

Jonathan Goldsberry, President

Indiana

6920 SMA Support Inc
PO Box 6301
Kokomo, IN 46904   765-688-0247
                                     Fax: 801-460-2813
                              www.smasupport.com

Laura Stants, Contact

New York

6921 Families of SMA - Long Island NY Chapter
PO Box 322
Rockville Center, NY 11571   516-214-0348
                    e-mail: greaterny@fsma.org
                              www.fsma.org

Debbie Cuevas, President

Tennessee

6922 Families of SMA - Tennessee Chapter
PO Box 7025
Knoxville, TN 37921   865-945-7636
                    e-mail: tennessee@fsma.org
                              www.fsma.org

Sarah Boggess, President

Research Centers

6923 SMA Research Group
Stanford University School of Medicine
300 Pasteur Dr, Rm A343
Stanford, CA 94305   650-723-6469
                                     Fax: 650-320-9443
              e-mail: mitzine@stanford.edu
                       neurology.stanford.edu

SMA clinical trials.

Mitzine Wright, Resident & Fellowship Coordinator
Chris Hopkins, Clerkship & Grand Rounds Coordinato
Diane Madsen, Administrative Associate to the Cha

6924 Spinal Muscular Atrophy Clinic
Columbia Pediatric Neuromuscular Disease Ctr
180 Ft Washington Ave, Harkness Pavilion, Ste 525
New York, NY 10032   212-342-0263
                                     Fax: 212-342-2893
              e-mail: kidsmda@columbia.edu
                       www.columbiasma.org

Dr Darryl De Vivo, Director
Dr Petra Kaufmann, Associate Director
Leslie Disla, Clinic Coordinator

6925 Spinal Muscular Atrophy Project
NINDS
PO Box 5801
Bethesda, MD 20824   301-496-5751
                                          800-352-9424
              e-mail: smaproject-fd@saic.com
                       www.smaproject.org

Research program established by NINDS (National Institute of Neurological Disorders and Stroke) as a model of developing a safe and effective treatment for SMA. The program adopts the methods used by the pharmaceutical industry to carry out drug discovery according to accepted standards.

Audio Video

6926   Living with SMA
Families of SMA
925 Busse Rd
Elk Grove Village, IL 60007   847-367-7620
                                           800-886-1762
                                      Fax: 847-357-7623
                                e-mail: info@curesma.org
                                           www.curesma.org

Tapes 3 and 4 are available and are part of the Living with SMA video series. Overview of Type II and Type III/Kennedy's.

18 pages

Kenneth Hobby, President
Jill Jarecki, PhD, Research Director
Colleen McCarthy O'Toole, Family Support Director

Web Sites

6927   Families of Spinal Muscular Atrophy
925 Busse Rd
Elk Grove Village, IL 60007   800-886-1762
                                e-mail: info@curesma.org
                                           www.curesma.org

Families of SMA was founded for the purpose of encouraging support and raising funds to promote research into the causes and cure of spinal muscular atrophy.

Kenneth Hobby, President
Jill Jarecki, PhD, Research Director
Colleen McCarthy O'Toole, Family Support Director

6928   Online Mendelian Inheritance in Man
www.omim.org

This database is a catalog of human genes and genetic disorders.

6929   Spinal Muscular Atrophy Information Page
Office of Communications and Public Liaison, NINDS
Bethesda, MD 20892   301-496-5751
                                           800-352-9424
                           www.ninds.nih.gov/disorders/sma/
Walter J. Koroshetz, M.D., Acting Director
Alan L. Willard, Ph.D., Acting Deputy Director
Caroline Lewis, Executive Officer

6930   Spinal Muscular Atrophy Project
www.smaproject.org

Research program established by NINDS (National Institute of Neurological Disorders and Stroke) as a model of developing a safe and effective treatment for SMA. The program adopts the methods used by the pharmaceutical industry to carry out drug discovery according to accepted standards.

Newsletters

6931   Compass
Families of SMA
925 Busse Rd
Elk Grove Village, IL 60007   847-367-7620
                                           800-886-1762
                                      Fax: 847-357-7623
                                e-mail: info@curesma.org
                                           www.curesma.org

Newsletter dedicated solely to SMA research updates and information.

42 pages Quarterly

Kenneth Hobby, President
Jill Jarecki, PhD, Research Director
Colleen McCarthy O'Toole, Family Support Director

6932   Directions
Families of SMA
925 Busse Rd
Elk Grove Village, IL 60007   847-367-7620
                                           800-886-1762
                                      Fax: 847-357-7623
                                e-mail: info@curesma.org
                                           www.curesma.org

32 pages Quarterly

Kenneth Hobby, President
Jill Jarecki, PhD, Research Director
Colleen McCarthy O'Toole, Family Support Director

6933   SMA Newsletter
Columbia Pediatric Neuromuscular Disease Ctr
Harkness Pavilion, Floor 5, 180 Fort Washington Av
New York, NY 10032   212-342-0263
                                      Fax: 212-342-2893
                           e-mail: kidsmda@columbia.edu
                                        www.columbiasma.org

Research updates, upcoming events and conferences, news, and a kids page.

Jessica Rascoll DPT, Newsletter Contact
Dr. Darryl C. De Vivo, Director

Pamphlets

6934   Facts About Spinal Muscular Atrophy
Muscular Dystrophy Association
222 S. Riverside Plaza, Suite 1500
Chicago, IL 60606   520-529-2000
                                           800-572-1717
                                      Fax: 520-529-5300
                          e-mail: publications@mdausa.org
            mda.org/publications/facts-about-spinal-muscular-atr

Covers the four forms of the disease and outlines the characteristics and genetic patterns of the SMAs. Research efforts aimed at finding the causes, treatments, and cures are also described. On-line and in Spanish.

2003

Steven M. Derks, President/ CEO
Valerie A. Cwik, M.D., EVP/ CSO/ CMO
Julie Faber, EVP/ CFO

6935   Understanding SMA
Families of SMA
925 Busse Rd
Elk Grove Village, IL 60007   847-367-7620
                                           800-886-1762
                                      Fax: 847-357-7623
                                e-mail: info@curesma.org
                                           www.curesma.org

This booklet is for the educaton and support of those with SMA.

18 pages

Kenneth Hobby, President
Jill Jarecki, PhD, Research Director
Colleen McCarthy O'Toole, Family Support Director

Description

6936 STRABISMUS

Synonyms: Heterotropia, Manifest deviation, Squint

Covers these related disorders: Accommodation strabismus, Nonparalytic strabismus, Paralytic strabismus

Involves the following Biologic System(s):

Neurologic Disorders, Ophthalmologic Disorders, Orthopedic and Muscle Disorders

Strabismus refers to a condition in which the eyes are not aligned properly in relation to each other and are focused on different objects simultaneously. Approximately four percent of all children under six years of age are affected by some form of strabismus. The eye deviations associated with this condition are classified according to the direction of the deviation. An eye that is turned inward is considered esotropic or convergent; an eye turned outward is exotropic or divergent; an eye turned upward is hypertropic; and an eye turned downward is hypotropic. In normal vision, both eyes focus as a unit to produce a single, three-dimensional image. In children with strabismus, the divergent images sent to the brain from the eyes may produce double vision (diplopia). In many cases, the brain will compensate for this error by blocking the image from the deviated eye, often resulting in poor vision or loss of vision in that eye (suppression amblyopia).

The most common type of strabismus is nonparalytic, in which this often-inherited ocular deviation is constant and results from a defect in the actual positioning of the eyes. Approximately 50 percent of individuals with nonparalytic strabismus have one eye turned inward. These inward-turned or esotropic deviations that appear before six months of age are classified as congenital or infantile esotropia. Outward-turned or exotropic deviations, the second most common type of strabismus, usually occur in children between six months and four years of age. Some outward deviations may result from neurologic disorders and craniofacial abnormalities.

Paralytic strabismus results from dysfunction of an eye muscle as the result of ocular muscle paralysis or a deficit of the nerves that supply the muscles. This resultant muscular imbalance causes the degree of deviation in the affected eye to vary as the eyes move.

Farsighted children are at particular risk for developing accommodative strabismus (accommodative esotropia), in which the lens of the eye tries to compensate for blurred images received by the brain by focusing the eyes inward (converging). If the compensation or accommodation demands are too great, some children may develop this additional eye abnormality.

Strabismus may result from many different factors; therefore, medical specialists make every effort to determine and treat the underlying cause as soon as possible after diagnosis. Such factors may include hereditary influences; trauma; neurologic abnormalities resulting from intracranial tumors or weaknesses in the walls of blood vessels in the brain (aneurysms); infection; systemic disorders; blood vessel malformations; structural abnormalities; and association with certain syndromes such as Duane syndrome.

Permanent loss of vision can occur if strabismus and its attendant amblyopia are not treated before age 4 to 6 years. Interventions may include wearing a patch over the normal eye in order to compel the brain to receive images from the affected eye. Patching often improves the vision in the deviating eye. Upon improvement, surgery may be performed to equalize the pull of the eye muscles. Children affected with paralytic strabismus may also benefit from wearing glasses with special lenses (prisms) that deflect light, thus altering positioning of objects seen through the lenses. In addition, children with paralytic strabismus with significant ocular deviation may benefit from eye muscle surgery to improve alignment. Farsighted children with accommodative strabismus may be treated with prescription glasses that lessen the need for ocular accommodation when focusing on objects that are far away. Certain medications in the form of eye drops may also aid in focusing on objects that are nearby. Other treatment is aimed toward the underlying cause of the ocular deviation.

Government Agencies

6937 NIH/National Eye Institute

31 Center Drive MSC 2510
Bethesda, MD 20892

301-496-5248
e-mail: 2020@nei.nih.gov
www.nei.nih.gov

Conducts and supports research that helps prevent and treat eye diseases and other disorders of vision. This research leads to sight-saving treatments, reduces visual impairment and blindness, and improves the quality of life for people of all ages. NEI-supported research has advanced our knowledge of how the eye functions in health and disease.

Paul A Sieving M.D., Ph.D, Director
Dr. Deborah Carper, Deputy Director
Dr. Richard S. Fisher, Associate Director for Science Poli

National Associations & Support Groups

6938 American Academy of Pediatrics

141 Northwest Point Boulevard
Elk Grove Village, IL 60007

847-434-4000
800-433-9016
Fax: 847-434-8000
www.aap.org

The American Academy of Pediatrics and its member pediatricians are committed to the attainment of optimal physical, mental and social health and well-being for all infants, children, adolescents, and young adults.

Sandra Hassink, MD, FAAP, President

6939 Genetic Alliance

4301 Connecticut Avenue NW
Washington, DC 20008

202-966-5557
800-336-4363
Fax: 202-966-8553
e-mail: info@geneticalliance.org
www.geneticalliance.org

A coalition of voluntary genetic support groups, consumers and professionals addressing the needs of individuals and families affected by genetic disorders from a national perspective.

Sharon Terry, MA, President/CEO
Natasha Bonhomme, Vice President of Strategic Develop
Vaughn Edelson, Assistant Director of Health Commun

6940 National Association for Visually Handicapped
111 E 59th St
New York, NY 10022
212-889-3141
800-829-0500
Fax: 212-727-2931
e-mail: navh@navh.org
www.navh.org

Serves as a clearinghouse for information about all services available to the partially-sighted from public and private sources. Conducts self-help groups. Provides information on large print books, textbooks and educational tools.

Lorianie Marchi, Ceo

Research Centers

6941 Emory Eye Center - Strabismus Research
1365B Clinton Rd NE
Atlanta, GA 30322
404-778-2020
www.eyecenter.emory.edu/clinical_specialties/strabis

Clinical strabismus research.

Anastasios Costarides
Amy K Hutchinson MD

Web Sites

6942 National Association for Visually Handicapped
111 E 59th St
New York, NY 10022
212-821-9497
800-284-4422
e-mail: kcampbell@lighthouse.org
lighthouse.org

Helps to cope with the difficulties of vision impairment.

6943 Online Mendelian Inheritance in Man
www.omim.org

This database is a catalog of human genes and genetic disorders.

6944 Royal National Institute of the Blind
105 Judd Street
London, WC1H
303-123-9999
www.rnib.org.uk

A leading UK charity offering information, support and advice to over two million people with sight problems.

Wanda Hamilton, Group Director
Fazilet Hadi, Managing Director
Sally Harvey, Managing Director

Book Publishers

6945 Ophthalmic Disorders Sourcebook
Omnigraphics
615 Griswold
Detroit, MI 48226
313-961-1340
800-234-1340
Fax: 313-961-1383
e-mail: info@omnigraphics.com
www.omnigraphics.com

Basic consumer information about glaucoma, cataracts, macular degeneration, strabismus, refractive disorders and more.

1996 631 pages
ISBN: 0-780800-81-8

Journals

6946 Journal of AAPOS
Elsevier
P.O. Box 193832
San Francisco, CA 94119
415-561-8505
Fax: 415-561-8531
e-mail: aapos@aao.org
www.jaapos.org

Covers pediatric ophthalmology and strabismus as it affects all groups. Presenting important clinical information on everything from the fundamentals to the finer points of diagnostic problem-solving, the Journal provides a comprehensive view of the field.

6 issues/yr
ISSN: 1091-8531

David G Hunter MD, PhD, Editor-in-Chief
T D Kozachek PhD, Managing Editor

Description

6947 STUTTERING

Involves the following Biologic System(s):

Developmental/Behavioral/Psychiatric Disorders, Neurologic Disorders

Stuttering refers to a type of speech dysfunction that interferes with the normal flow of speech (dysfluency). This dysfunction is characterized by difficulty in uttering certain sounds, letters, syllables, words, or phrases and is usually manifested by frequent hesitations, stumbling, or delay in enunciation, as well as prolongation of certain sounds. As young children develop language skills, they typically experience hesitations in speech as a result of still-developing muscle coordination and limited vocabulary. If excessive attention is given to these temporary speech deficiencies, some children may become self-conscious, anxious, and fearful of speaking. These types of emotional reactions may be manifested as persistent and compulsive movements of certain muscle groups that interfere with the normal flow of speech. Children who stutter may have difficulty with only particular letters, sounds, or words. In addition, the severity of the stutter is often related to the amount of stress evoked by the particular situation. Some affected children and adults may have associated tremors or tics. It is estimated that over three million Americans stutter. Stuttering affects individuals of all ages but occurs most frequently in young children between the ages of 2 and 6 who are developing language. Boys are three times more likely to stutter than girls.

Although most stuttering results from psychological causes, this speech dysfunction may sometimes occur as a result of certain disorders of the central nervous system, neuromuscular abnormalities, or injury to organs related to speech. Stuttering that results from behavioral influences is often self-limited and, in 80 percent of those affected, resolves during childhood.

There are a variety of treatments available for stuttering. Any of the methods may improve stuttering to some degree, but there is at present no cure for stuttering. Stuttering therapy, however, may help prevent developmental stuttering from becoming a life-long problem. In young children, treatment for stuttering is mainly supportive. Parents or caregivers are often counseled not to place undue emphasis on speech irregularities. Additional supportive care may include recognition of accomplishments and other gestures that will contribute to the development of self-worth. If stuttering persists beyond early childhood or into adulthood, speech therapy is usually indicated.

Government Agencies

6948 NIH/National Institute on Deafness and Oth er Communication Disorders (NIDCD)
31 Center Drive, MSC 2320
Bethesda, MD 20892
800-241-1044
TTY: 800-241-1055
e-mail: nidcdinfo@nidcd.nih.gov
www.nidcd.nih.gov

Conducts and supports biomedical research and research training on normal mechanisms, as well as diseases and disorders of hearing, balance, smell, taste, voice, speech and language.

Dr James F Battey Jr, Director
Judith A Cooper PhD, Deputy Director
W David Kerr, Executive Officer

National Associations & Support Groups

6949 American Academy of Pediatrics
141 Northwest Point Boulevard
Elk Grove Village, IL 60007
847-434-4000
800-433-9016
Fax: 847-434-8000
www.aap.org

The American Academy of Pediatrics and its member pediatricians are committed to the attainment of optimal physical, mental and social health and well-being for all infants, children, adolescents, and young adults.

Sandra Hassink, MD, FAAP, President

6950 American School Counselor Association
1101 King Street, Suite 310
Alexandria, VA 22314
703-683-2722
800-306-4722
Fax: 703-997-7572
e-mail: asca@schoolcounselor.org
www.schoolcounselor.org

The mission of ASCA is to represent professional school counselors and to promote professionalism and ethical practices.

Richard Wong, Executive Director
Jeff Broderson, Information Technology Admin.
Kathleen M Rakestraw, Director of Communications

6951 American Speech Language Hearing Associati on (ASHA)
2200 Research Boulevard
Rockville, MD 20850
301-897-5700
800-638-8255
Fax: 301-571-0457
e-mail: pr@asha.org
www.asha.org

A professional and credentialing association made up of more than 123,000 international pathologists, audiologists and scientists. The association promotes the interests of and provides services for those in the hearing, speech, and language field, and advocates for people with communication disorders.

Patricia A. Prelock, PhD, President
Elizabeth S. McCrea, PhD, CCC-SLP, President-Elect
Shelly S. Chabon, PhD, CCC-SLP, Immediate Past President

6952 Genetic Alliance
4301 Connecticut Avenue NW
Washington, DC 20008
202-966-5557
800-336-4363
Fax: 202-966-8553
e-mail: info@geneticalliance.org
www.geneticalliance.org

A coalition of voluntary genetic support groups, consumers and professionals addressing the needs of individuals and families affected by genetic disorders from a national perspective.

Sharon Terry, MA, President/CEO
Natasha Bonhomme, Vice President of Strategic Develop
Vaughn Edelson, Assistant Director of Health Commun

6953 National Center for Stuttering
388 2nd Ave, Suite 136
New York, NY 10010
800-221-2483
Fax: 212-683-1372
e-mail: executivedirector@stuttering.com
www.stuttering.com

Distributes information for parents of young children showing early signs of stuttering. For older children and adults, free information is available on treatment programs nationwide.

Martin F Schwartz, Executive Director

6954 **National Stuttering Association**
119 W 40th Street, 14th Fl
New York, NY 10018
212-944-4050
800-937-8888
Fax: 212-944-8244
e-mail: info@westutter.org
www.westutter.org

A self-help support organization for people who stutter. It maintains a toll-free hotline on stuttering and a nationwide resource list for individuals seeking a speech-language pathologist who specializes in stuttering. Several publications are also directed toward medical professionals who serve the stuttering community.

Elaine Saitta, Executive Director
Katia Skowronska, Assistant Director

6955 **Speak Easy International Foundation**
233 Concord Drive
Paramus, NJ 07652
201-262-0895
Fax: 201-262-0895

A self-help support group for stutters.

Bob Gathman, Founder/President

6956 **Stuttering Foundation of America**
1805 Moriah Woods Blvd., Suite 3
Memphis, TN 38117
901-761-0343
800-992-9392
Fax: 901-761-0484
e-mail: info@stutteringhelp.org
www.stutteringhelp.org

Provides free online resources, services and support to those who stutter and their families, as well as support for research into the causes of stuttering. Extensive educational programs on stuttering for professionals are also offered.

Jane H Fraser, President

State Agencies & Support Groups

6957 **Speech, Language, & Hearing Center University of Colorado**
2501 Kittredge Loop Rd., Campus Box 409
Boulder, CO 80309
303-492-5375
Fax: 303-492-3274
e-mail: susan.moore@colorado.edu
slhs.colorado.edu/clinical-services?

Informational and emotional support to parents who have a child, adolescent, or adult family member with special needs.

Web Sites

6958 **NIH/National Institute on Deafness and Oth er Communication Disorders (NIDCD)**
www.nidcd.nih.gov/health/voice/stutter.asp

Fact sheet and information page on stuttering and other resources.

6959 **Online Mendelian Inheritance in Man**
www.omim.org

This database is a catalog of human genes and genetic disorders.

6960 **Parent Pals**
parentpals.com/gossamer/pages/Speech_and_Language
e-mail: specialed@parentpals.com
parentpals.com/gossamer/pages/Speech_and_Language

Their goal is to provide special education and gifted information, continuing education, support, weekly tips, games, book resources, and news and views for parents and professionals.

Book Publishers

6961 **Programmed Therapy for Stuttering in Child ren and Adults**
Charles C Thomas Publisher
2600 S 1st Street
Springfield, IL 62704
217-789-8980
800-258-8980
Fax: 217-789-9130
e-mail: books@ccthomas.com
www.ccthomas.com

This book highlights the systematic scientific approach to studying and treating stuttering by way of learning theory, single-subject research design and operant conditioning.

2001 360 pages 2nd Edition
ISBN: 0-398071-07-3

6962 **Straight Talk on Stuttering: Information, Encouragement, and Counsel**
Lloyd M Hulit, author

Charles C Thomas Publisher
2600 S 1st Street
Springfield, IL 62704
217-789-8980
800-258-8980
Fax: 217-789-9130
e-mail: books@ccthomas.com
www.ccthomas.com

Written for stutterers and those who interact with stutterers, including parents, caregivers, teachers, and speech-language pathologists. The author dispels myths, corrects the misperceptions and creates a message of hope for all people who have this fascinating communication disorder.

338 pages 2nd Ed/ Hard
ISBN: 0-398075-19-4

6963 **Stutter No More**
Dr Martin F Schwartz, author

National Center for Stuttering
388 2nd Ave, Suite 136
New York, NY 10010
800-221-2483
Fax: 212-683-1372
e-mail: executivedirector@stuttering.com
www.stuttering.com

The book covers a simple learning technique to stop stuttering in 9-12 months.

Martin F. Schwartz, Executive Director

Newsletters

6964 **Stuttering Foundation of America Newslette r**
Stuttering Foundation of America
1805 Moriah Woods Blvd., Suite 3
Memphis, TN 38117
901-761-0343
800-992-9392
Fax: 901-761-0484
e-mail: info@stutteringhelp.org
www.stutteringhelp.org

Quarterly newsletter available online in pdf format.

Jane H Fraser, President

Camps

6965 **Meadowood Springs Speech and Hearing Camp**
PO Box 1025
Pendleton, OR 97801
541-276-2752
Fax: 541-276-7227
e-mail: info@meadowoodsprings.org
www.meadowoodsprings.org

On 143 acres in the Blue Mountains of Eastern Oregon, this camp is designed to help young people who have diagnosed clinical disorders of speech, hearing or language. A full range of activities in recreational and clinical areas is available. For cabin reservations 541-566-2191.

Rosemarie Atfield, Executive Director
Marie Story, Camp Manager
Cliff Story, Camp Manager

6966 University of Iowa - Wendell Johnson Speech and Hearing Clinic
Wendell Johnson Speech And Hearing Center
Iowa City, IA 52242   319-335-8718
                                         Fax: 319-335-8851
                          e-mail: speech-path-aud@uiowa.edu
                                       clas.uiowa.edu/comsci/

The clinic offers assessment and remediation for disordered communication in adults and children. The clinic also offers an Intensive Summer Residential Clinic for school age children needing intervention services because of speech, language, hearing and/or reading problems.

Ruth Bentler, Professor / Department Chair
Dorothy Albright, Secretary
Vicki Jennings, Secretary

Description

6967 SUBACUTE SCLEROSING PANENCEPHALITIS (SSPE)

Synonyms: Dawson's encephalitis, Van Bogaert's encophalitis

Involves the following Biologic System(s):

Immunologic and Rheumatologic Disorders, Neurologic Disorders

Subacute sclerosing panencephalitis (SSPE) is a rare, life-threatening, slow viral infection of the brain caused by a measles-like virus. SSPE appears months or years after a typical mild or severe measles infection and occurs most frequently in children and adolescents between the ages of five and 15 years. This disease occurs more often in children who develop measles before 18 months of age and is twice as prevalent in boys as it is in girls. Symptoms develop gradually and may commence with subtle behavorial changes such as forgetfulness or outbursts of temper, deterioration in school performance, sleeplessness, and hallucinations. These symptoms are often followed by more bizarre behavior, seizures, repetitive muscular jerks (myoclonic jerks) and other abnormal movements, eye irregularities, and mental deterioration (dementia). Late findings may include muscular rigidity or, in some patients, weak muscles, difficulty swallowing, blindness, or coma. In addition, due to generalized weakness and impaired muscle control associated with SSPE, life-threatening complications such as pneumonia may occur. Subacute sclerosing panencephalitis is incompatible with life; its usual duration is from one to three years.

The diagnosis of SSPE may be confirmed through laboratory tests that detect the presence of antibodies to the measles virus in the cerebrospinal fluid and the presence of large numbers of measles antibodies in the serum. In most cases, subacute sclerosing pnencephalitis may be prevented by immunization with attenuated measles virus vaccine.

Treatment of SSPE is geared toward chronic care. Over the last decade, however, stabilization of disease and in clinical progression has been observed with medications that alter the body's immune system response to this virus (immunomodulators), such as interferon and certain antiviral drugs including ribavirin and isoprinosine. Studies of other therapeutic programs are ongoing. Other treatment is symptomatic and supportive.

Government Agencies

6968 NIH/National Institute of Allergy and Infectious Diseases
6610 Rockledge Drive, MSC 6612
Bethesda, MD 20892
301-496-5717
866-284-4107
Fax: 301-402-3573
TDD: 800-877-8339
e-mail: ocposfoffice@niaid.nih.gov
www.niaid.nih.gov

Conducts and supports basic and applied research to better understand, treat, and ultimately prevent infectious, immunologic, and allergic diseases.

Anthony S Fauci MD, Director

6969 NIH/National Institute of Neurological Dis orders and Stroke (NINDS)
PO Box 5801
Bethesda, MD 20824
301-496-5751
800-352-9424
www.ninds.nih.gov/disorders/subacute_panencephalitis

National Associations & Support Groups

6970 American Academy of Pediatrics
141 Northwest Point Boulevard
Elk Grove Village, IL 60007
847-434-4000
800-433-9016
Fax: 847-434-8000
www.aap.org

The American Academy of Pediatrics and its member pediatricians are committed to the attainment of optimal physical, mental and social health and well-being for all infants, children, adolescents, and young adults.

Sandra Hassink, MD, FAAP, President

6971 Genetic Alliance
4301 Connecticut Avenue NW
Washington, DC 20008
202-966-5557
800-336-4363
Fax: 202-966-8553
e-mail: info@geneticalliance.org
www.geneticalliance.org

A coalition of voluntary genetic support groups, consumers and professionals addressing the needs of individuals and families affected by genetic disorders from a national perspective.

Sharon Terry, MA, President/CEO
Natasha Bonhomme, Vice President of Strategic Develop
Vaughn Edelson, Assistant Director of Health Commun

6972 World Health Organization
Avenue Appia 20
CH-1211 Geneva 27,
Switzerland
e-mail: publications@who.int
www.who.int

WHO is the directing and coordinating authority for health within the United Nations system.

Dr Margaret Chan, Director General

Web Sites

6973 Encephalitis Information Resource
www.encepahlitis.info

Site is provided by the Encephalitis Society

6974 MedlinePlus
www.nlm.nih.gov/medlineplus/aboutmedlineplus.html
e-mail: custserv@nlm.nih.gov
www.nlm.nih.gov/medlineplus/aboutmedlineplus.html

Information on the condition, causes, symptoms, tests, and treatment.

Dr. Donald A.B. Lindberg, Director

6975 NIH/National Institute of Neurological Dis orders and Stroke (NINDS)
Office of Communications and Public Liaison, NINDS
Bethesda, MD 20892
301-496-5751
800-352-9424
www.ninds.nih.gov/disorders/subacute_panencephalitis

Information fact sheet on the disorder.

Walter J. Koroshetz, M.D., Acting Director
Alan L. Willard, Ph.D., Acting Deputy Director
Caroline Lewis, Executive Officer

Book Publishers

6976 Let's Talk About Going to the Hospital
Rosen Publishing Group's PowerKids Press
29 E 21st Street
New York, NY 10010
212-777-3017
800-237-9932
Fax: 888-436-4643
e-mail: rosenpub@tribeca.ios.com
www.rosenpublishing.com

If a child has to check into the hospital, chances are he or she is already upset about being ill. Knowing how a hospital functions and what the procedures are, such as when family members can visit, will help in what is already a stressful situation. Grades K-5.

24 pages
ISBN: 0-823950-36-0

Roger Rosen, President

Description

6977 SUDDEN INFANT DEATH SYNDROME

Synonyms: Cot death, Crib death, SIDS

Involves the following Biologic System(s):

Neonatal and Infant Disorders

Sudden infant death syndrome (SIDS) refers to the sudden, unexpected, and unexplained death of an apparently healthy infant. This syndrome may occur from the ages of two weeks to one year, but most commonly occurs between the ages of two to four months. Approximately 75 to 95 percent of all deaths related to SIDS occur by the age of six months. Sudden infant death syndrome is responsible for approximately half of all infant deaths that occur between the ages of 1 month and one year and, in the United States, affects approximately 1.3 of every 1,000 infants in that age group. SIDS is somewhat more common in boys and in infants born to individuals of African-American or Native American descent. In addition, sudden infant death syndrome occurs more often during the winter months.

Very little is sure about the exact cause of SIDS, but researchers believe that certain brain stem abnormalities may be a contributing factor to its occurrence. Such irregularities may affect the regulation of body temperature, cardiorespiratory function, and associated sleep and arousal mechanisms. Although the relationship is not fully understood, brain stem abnormalities, especially sleep and arousal deficit, may interact with certain other influencing factors (epidemiologic risk factors) to put infants at risk for SIDS. Such epidemiologic risk factors may include prematurity, low birth weight, bottle feeding, exposure to smoking, recent illness with fever and previous near death episodes requiring resuscitation. Also, mothers with abnormally low levels of circulating red blood cells (anemia) or those who smoke or use drugs during pregnancy may be at increased risk for having an infant with SIDS. Other factors may include insufficient prenatal care and low socioeconomic status. In addition, recent studies have shown that putting infants to sleep on their stomachs is a significant risk factor, as is the use of soft bedding or extra linens and toys (e.g., comforters, quilts, stuffed animals, etc.) in the crib.

To alleviate certain risk factors, appropriate prenatal care is essential in the possible prevention of SIDS. Also, after birth, parents are counseled to be alert to any respiratory changes or distress and to closely observe infants during and after any illness. In addition, new guidelines recommend that infants be placed in the crib on their backs, as statistics have shown declines in SIDS rates among those who have complied with this recommendation. Sleeping on the back has been recommended for some time to avoid SIDS, with the catchphrase "Back To Bed" and "Back to Sleep." Other guidelines include the advice that crib mattresses should be firm and should fit tightly within the crib frame; that comforters, quilts, pillows, toys, etc. should be removed from the crib; that, if possible, sleeper-type pajamas be used instead of blankets; that if a blanket must be used, it should be thin, should reach no further than the infant's chest, and shou ld be tucked around the infant's chest and mattress; and that the baby's head should be uncovered at all times during sleep. Infants who die from SIDS tend to have higher concentrations of nicotine and cotinine (a biological marker for secondhand smoke expo-

sure) in their lungs than those who die from other causes. Parents who smoke can significantly reduce their children's risk of SIDS by either quitting or smoking only outside and leaving their house completely smoke-free. In the event of the death of an infant from SIDS, counseling by trained specialists is strongly advised for parents and remaining siblings. In addition, support groups composed of families who have been affected by SIDS may be comforting and helpful.

Government Agencies

6978 National Center for Health Statistics
4770 Buford Hwy, NE
Atlanta, GA 30341
800-232-4636
800-311-3435
www.cdc.gov

National Associations & Support Groups

6979 American Academy of Pediatrics
141 Northwest Point Boulevard
Elk Grove Village, IL 60007
847-434-4000
800-433-9016
Fax: 847-434-8000
www.aap.org

The American Academy of Pediatrics and its member pediatricians are committed to the attainment of optimal physical, mental and social health and well-being for all infants, children, adolescents, and young adults.

Sandra Hassink, MD, FAAP, President

6980 American SIDS Institute
528 Raven Way
Naples, FL 34110
239-431-5425
800-232-7437
Fax: 239-431-5536
e-mail: prevent@sids.org
www.sids.org

A national nonprofit organization dedicated to the prevention of sudden infant death syndrome and the promotion of infant health.

Marc Peterzell, Chairman
Betty McEntire PhD, Executive Director

6981 Compassionate Friends
PO Box 3696
Oak Brook, IL 60522
630-990-0010
877-969-0010
Fax: 630-990-0246
e-mail: nationaloffice@compassionatefriends.org
www.compassionatefriends.org

Compassionate Friends assists families toward the positive resolution of grief following the death of a child of any age and provides information to help others be supportive. A national nonprofit, self-help support organization that offers friendship, understanding, and hope to bereaved parents, grandparents and siblings.

Patricia Loder, Executive Director
Ronald Haynes, VP
Patricia Loder, Executive Director

6982 Council of Guilds for Infant Survival
PO Box 3586
Davenport, IA 52808
319-322-4870

Conducts research and provides information on SIDS.
Chris Elliott

6983 First Candle/SIDS Alliance
2105 Laurel Bush Road,, Suite 201
Bel Air, MD 21015
443-640-1049
800-221-7437
Fax: 410-653-8709
e-mail: info@firstcandle.org
www.sidsalliance.org; www.firstcandle.org

First Candle started as the National SIDS Foundation focusing on supporting families that experienced SIDS. In 2002, it broadened its scope to include other areas of infant death, committing its resources in hopes of having an impact on all these areas. It's mission is to help babies survive and thrive.

Marian Sokol, President
Deborah M Boyd, Executive Director
Laura L Reno, Director Public Affairs/Marketing

6984 National Center for Education in Maternal and Child Health
Georgetown University
2115 Wisconsin Ave NW, Suite 601
Washington, DC 20007
202-784-9770
Fax: 202-784-9777
e-mail: mchlibrary@ncemch.org
www.ncemch.org

6985 National Center for the Prevention of SIDS
4770 Buford Hwy, NE
Atlanta, GA 30341
800-232-4636
Fax: 410-653-8709
www.cdc.gov/sids/?

Offers medical updates and information on prevention of SIDS and other disorders to parents and professionals.

6986 National SIDS/Infant Death Resource Center (Resource Center)
2115 Wisconson Avenue, NW, Suite 601
Washington, DC 20007
202-687-7437
866-866-7437
Fax: 202-784-9777
e-mail: info@sidscenter.org
www.sidscenter.org

NSIDRC (Resource Center) serves as a central source of information on sudden infant death and on promoting healthy outcomes for infants from birth through the first year of life and beyond.

Rochelle Mayer, Project Director

6987 National Sudden Infant Death Syndrome Foundation
31 Center Drive, Room 2A32
Bethesda, MD 20892
301-496-5133
Fax: 301-496-7101

6988 Parents Helping Parents - A Family Resource Center
1400 Parkmoor Avenue Suite 100
San Jose, CA 95126
408-727-5775
Fax: 408-727-0182
e-mail: general@php.com
www.php.com

A group of parents and professionals committed to alleviating some of the problems, hardships and concerns of families with children having special needs.

Candy Smith, Director

6989 Pregnancy and Infant Loss Center
402 Jackson St
St. Charles, MO 63301
366-437-7014
800-821-6819
e-mail: info@nationalshare.org
nationalshare.org

Offers support, resources, and education on miscarriage, stillbirth and newborn death. Nonprofit organization, membership and quarterly newsletter $20 per year.

6990 SHARE National Headquarters
Saint Elizabeth's Hospital
402 Jackson St
St. Charles, MO 63301
636-947-6164
800-821-6819
Fax: 636-947-7486
e-mail: info@nationalshare.org
nationalshare.org

Serve those whose lives are touched by the tragic death of a baby through early pregnancy loss, stillbirth, or in the first few months of life.

Cathie Lamert, Executive Director
Rose Carlson, Program Director
Megan Nichols, Outreach &Public Relatons Director

6991 SIDS Educational Services
PO Box 2426
Hyattsville, MD 20784
301-322-2620
Fax: 301-322-9822
e-mail: SIDSES@aol.com
www.sidssurvivalguide.org

Supports families grieving the loss of children to Sudden Infant Death Syndrome and other infant death causes. Information and support services are also provided to children grieving any type of death.

6992 SIDS Information and Referral Hotline
SIDS Alliance
1314 Bedord Avenue
Baltimore, MD 21208
410-653-8226
800-221-7437
Fax: 410-653-8709

24 hour information and referral line for parents who wish to discuss their concerns with a SIDS counselor, request additional information about SIDS and to receive referrals to the local SIDS affiliate in their area.

State Agencies & Support Groups

Alabama

6993 Bureau of Family Health Services-Alabama Child Death Review
Alabama Department of Public Health
43 Foundry Avenue
Waltham, MA 02453
617-618-2918
Fax: 334-206-2972
e-mail: jallison@edc.org
www.childrenssafetynetwork.org
Jennifer Allison, CSN Assistant Director, State Partn

Alaska

6994 SIDS Information & Counseling Program Alaska Department of Health
1231 Gambell Street, Suite 302
Anchorage, AK 99501
907-272-1534
Fax: 907-274-1384
sid-network.org/map
Linda D Vlastuin, RN, MPH, Program Consultant

Arizona

6995 Office of Women's & Children's Health
Arizona Department of Health Services
150 N 18th Ave, Suite 320
Phoenix, AZ 85007
602-542-1025
Fax: 602-542-0883
e-mail: newbers@azdhs.gov
www.azdhs.gov

The Unexplained Infant Death Council comes under the OWCH and assists the department to develop unexplained infant death training and educational programs.

Sheila Sjolander, Manager

Arkansas

6996 Arkansas Department of Health - SIDS Information & Counseling Program
4815 W Markham Street
Little Rock, AR 72205
501-661-2000
800-462-0599
Fax: 501-671-1450
www.healthy.arkansas.gov

Rosalind Abernathy, Project Coordinator

California

6997 California SIDS Program
11344 Coloma Road
Gold River, CA 95670
916-851-437
800-369-7437
Fax: 916-851-5937
e-mail: info@californiasids.com
www.californiasids.com

Gwen Edelstein, Program Director
Susan More MA, Grief Counselor and Educator

6998 CorStone-Children & Loss Group
CorStone
250 Camino Alto
Mill Valley, CA 94941
415-331-6161
Fax: 415-388-6165
e-mail: info@corstone.org
www.corstone.org

For children who have suffered the loss of a close loved one. Parent group meets separately at the same time.

Richard Cuadra MFT, Program Director
Melissa Mullin MFT, Program Coordinator

6999 Region IX Office Program Consultants for Maternal and Child Health
50 United Nations Plaza
San Francisco, CA 94102
415-437-8101
Fax: 415-437-8105
nrc.uchsc.edu

Lyn Headley, MD

Colorado

7000 Colorado SIDS Program
425 S Cherry Street, Suite 890
Denver, CO 80246
303-320-7771
888-285-7437
Fax: 303-320-7827
e-mail: shelia@coloradosids.org
www.angeleyes.org

Donna Buss, President
Daniel Trujillo, Vice President
Luanne Chavez, Assisstant Vice President

7001 Region VIII Office Program Consultants for Maternal and Child Health
1961 Stout Street
Denver, CO 80294
303-844-7854
Fax: 303-844-2019
e-mail: laurie.konsella@hhs.gov

Laurie Konsella, M.P.A

Delaware

7002 SIDS Information & Counseling - Division of Public Health
501 Ogletown Road
Newark, DE 19711
302-368-6840

Elaine Markell, LCSW, BCD, Program Coordinator

District of Columbia

7003 Division of Community Health Nursing
825 N Capitol Street, NE
Washington, DC 20002
202-698-0705
Fax: 202-645-7030

Mary Breach, RN, MSN, Nursing Coordinator

Florida

7004 Children's Medical Services Program Florida SIDS Program
Bin A-13 4025 Bald Cypress Way
Tallahassee, FL 32399
850-245-4444
Fax: 850-245-4047
e-mail: susann-arbor@doh.state.fl.us
www.doh.state.fl.us

Georgia

7005 Georgia Department of Human Resources Children's Health Services
2 Peach Tree Street NW
Atlanta, GA 30303
404-656-6750
dhs.georgia.gov

Linette Jackson Hunt, MD, MPH, Chief

7006 Georgia Department of Human Resources - Center for Family Resource Planning
2 Peach Tree Street NW
Atlanta, GA 30303
404-656-7660
www.dhs.georgia.gov

Provides grief support for parents.
Lee Hackel

7007 Region IV Office Program Consultants For Maternal and Child Health
Atlanta Federal Center
61 Forsyth Street, SW, Suite 3M60
Atlanta, GA 30303
404-562-7980
Fax: 404-562-7974
e-mail: kgonzalez@hrsa.gov
nrc.uchsc.edu

Dorothy Redfern, RN, MSPH

Hawaii

7008 Hawaii SIDS Information & Counseling Project
Kapiolani Children's Medical Center
1319 Punahou Street #1100
Honolulu, HI 96826
808-983-8368
Sharon Morton, RN, Nurse Consultant

Idaho

7009 Child Health Improvement Program Idaho Department of Health
211 Idaho CareLine, PO Box 83720
Boise, ID 83720
208-334-5945
800-926-2588
Fax: 208-334-5531
e-mail: careline@dhw.idaho.gov
www.idahocareline.org

Simonne deGlee, MS, PNP, SIDS Coordinator

Illinois

7010 Region V Office Program Consultants for Maternal and Child Health
233 N Michigan Avenue
Chicago, IL 60601
312-353-4042
Fax: 312-886-3770
e-mail: dparker@hrsa.gov

Kathryn Vedder, MD, MPH

7011 Statewide SIDS Program - Illinois Department of Public Health
535 W Jefferson Street
Springfield, IL 62761
217-785-4528
www.illinois.gov

Lori Bennett, Coordinator

Indiana

7012 Indiana State Board of Health - SIDS Project
2 N Meridian Street
Indianapolis, IN 46204
317-233-1325
Fax: 317-233-7394
e-mail: opac@isdh.state.in.us
www.in.gov/isdh/

Judith Monroe, Manager

Iowa

7013 Iowa SIDS Program
Iowa Department of Public Health
406 SW School St
Ankeny, IA 50023
515-965-7655
866-480-4741
www.iowasids.org

Beverly Richardson, MA, MCH Consultant

Kansas

7014 Kansas Department of Health & Environment Bureau of Family Health
1000 SW Jackson Street, Suite 220
Topeka, KS 66612
785-296-1500
800-332-6262
Fax: 785-296-1562
www.kdheks.gov

Azzie N Young, PhD, Director

Kentucky

7015 Kentucky Department of Human Resources Bureau of Health Services
700 Capitol Avenue, Suite 100
Frankfort, KY 40601
502-564-2611
governor.ky.gov

Ida Lyons, RN, SIDS Coordinator

Louisiana

7016 Public Health Services of Louisiana
628 N 4th Street
Baton Rouge, LA 70802
225-342-9500
Fax: 225-342-5568
e-mail: dhhwebinfo@la.gov
www.dhh.louisiana.gov/

Dorris Brown, Center Director
Myrra Lowe, Chief Financial Officer
Beth Scalso, Chief of Staff

Maine

7017 Department of Human Services
221 State Street
Augusta, ME 04333
207-287-3707
Fax: 207-287-3005
TTY: 800-606-0215
www.maine.gov/dhhs

Brenda Harvey, Manager
Mary Mayhew, Commisioner

Maryland

7018 Center for Infant & Child Loss
737 W. Lombard Street, Room 233
Baltimore, MD 21201
410-706-5062
800-808-7437
Fax: 410-328-4596
e-mail: caring@infantandchildloss.org
www.infantandchildloss.org

Donna C Becker, RN, MSN, Director

7019 Maryland SIDS Information & Counseling Program
2905 64th Avenue
Cheverly, MD 20785
301-773-9671
sids-network.org

Daniel Timmel, MSW, Project Director
Jodi Shaefer, Director

Massachusetts

7020 Massachusetts Chapter of SIDS Alliance
Boston Medical Center
1 Boston Medical Place
Boston, MA 02118
617-638-8000
800-641-7437
Fax: 617-414-5555
www.bmc.org

State chapter offering educational resources and information on SIDS, parent groups, support networks, monthly meetings and workshops to the community.

Mary McClain, Manager
Mary McClain, RN, MS

7021 Region I Office Program Consultants For Maternal and Child Health
John F Kennedy Building
Room 1826
Boston, MA 02203
617-565-1433
Fax: 617-565-3044
e-mail: btausey@hrsa.gov
www.mchb.hrsa.gob

Shirley A Smith, RN, MS

Michigan

7022 Apnea Identification Program
Children's Hospital of Michigan
3901 Beaubien Street
Detroit, MI 48201
313-745-5437
888-DMC-2500
www.chmkids.org

Karen Braniff, RN, MSW, Nurse Specialist

7023 Genesee County Health Department
630 S Saginaw Street
Flint, MI 48502
810-257-3612
Fax: 810-257-3147
e-mail: gchd-info@gchd.us
www.gchd.us

Robert Pestronk, Manager
Mark Valck, Health Director
Gary Johnson, Medical Director

7024 Kent County Health Department
300 Monroe Avenue NW
Grand Rapids, MI 49503
616-632-7590
Fax: 616-632-7083
www.accesskent.com

Cathy Raevsky, Executive Director

7025 Oakland County Health Division - SIDS Project
1200 N Telegraph Road
Pontiac, MI 48341
248-858-1280
Fax: 248-858-0178
www.oakgov.com/health

Rosemary Rowney, Manager

7026 SIDS LEAD - Children's Special Health Care Services
Michigan Department of Public Health
3423 N Martin Luther King Jr Boulevard
Lansing, MI 48906
517-373-3500
e-mail: arias@state.mi.us
www.mdmh.state.mi.us/

Cheryl Lauber, MSN

7027 SIDS Nursing Intervention Program
43525 Elizabeth Road
Mount Clemens, MI 48043
810-469-5520
Loretta Lindsay, RN, Coordinator

Minnesota

7028 Minnesota Sudden Infant Death Center
Minneapolis Children's Medical Center
2525 Chicago Avenue
Minneapolis, MN 55404
612-813-6285
TTY: 800-732-3812

Kathleen Farnbach, PHN, Project Coordinator

Mississippi

7029 Mississippi State Department of Health and Child Health Services
570 East Woodrow Wilson Drive
Jackson, MS 39216
601-576-7634
www.msdh.state.ms.us

Jenny Griffin, Manager

Missouri

7030 Region VII Office Program Consultants for Maternal and Child Health
Federal Building
601 E 12th Street
Kansas City, MO 64106
816-426-5291
Fax: 816-426-3633
e-mail: bappelbaum@hrsa.gov

Bradley Appelbaum, MD, MPH

7031 SIDS Resources
1120 South Sixth Street, Suite 100
Saint Louis, MO 63104
314-822-2323
800-421-3511
Fax: 314-588-0850
www.sidsresources.org

Helen Fuller, MSW, Executive Director
Laura Hillman, President
Karl Barnickol, Secretary

Montana

7032 Montana Department of Health & Environmental Sciences
Family & Maternal & Child Health Bureau
Cogswell Building
Helena, MT 59620
406-444-4740
Maxine Ferguson, RN, MN, Bureau Chief

Nebraska

7033 Nebraska SIDS Foundation
University of Nebraska Medical Center
600 S 42nd Street
Omaha, NE 68198
402-559-4212
www.nebraskasidsfoundation.org

Valerie Ciciulla, Coordinator

Nevada

7034 Nevada State Division of Health, Maternal & Child Health
505 E King Street, Room 205
Carson City, NV 89701
702-687-4885
www.health.nv.gov/MCH.htm

Luana Ritch, Health Educator

New Hampshire

7035 New Hampshire SIDS Program
New Hampshire Division of Public Health Services
6 Hazen Drive
Concord, NH 03301
603-271-4533
800-852-3345
Fax: 603-271-3745

Audrey Knight, MSN, CPNP, SIDS Coordinator

New Jersey

7036 New Jersey Department of Health - Child Health Program
CN 364, 363 W State Street
Trenton, NJ 08625
609-292-5616
Judith Hall, BSN, RNC, Evaluator

7037 New Jersey SIDS Resource Center
254 Easton Avenue
New Brunswick, NJ 08901
732-249-2160

New York

7038 NYS Center for SIDS Office
Stony Brook University
School of Social Welfare Health Science Center
Stony Brook, NY 11794
631-632-6000
Fax: 631-444-6475
e-mail: marie.chandick@stonybrook.edu
www.stonybrook.edu

Marie Chandrick, Director

7039 New York City Information & Counseling Program for SIDS
520 1st Avenue, Room 506
New York, NY 10016
212-757-1051
800-522-5006

Judith Gaines, CSW, PhD, SIDS Program Director

7040 Region II Office Program Consultants for Maternal and Child Health
26 Federal Plaza
New York, NY 10278
212-264-2571
Fax: 212-264-2673
e-mail: ssmith@hrsa.gov

Margaret Lee, MD

7041 Western New York SIDS Center
200 Fairport Village Lane
Fairport, NY 14450
716-223-5110
Gabrielle Weiss, BPS, Director

North Carolina

7042 North Carolina SIDS Information and Counseling Program
North Carolina Department Of Environmental Health
2709 Water Ridge Parkway
Charlotte, NC 28217
704-644-4200
800-868-8777
Fax: 704-644-4210
www.safetync.org

Dianne Tyson, BSW, Administrative Assistant

North Dakota

7043 North Dakota SIDS Management Program
600 E Boulevard Avenue
Bismarck, ND 58505
701-328-4464
800-472-2286
Fax: 701-328-1412
www.ndhealth.gov/SIDS

Bertie Hagberg, RN, Coordinator
Katie Schimdt, North Dakota SIDS Management Progra
Peggy Stanton, Administrative Assistant

Ohio

7044 Perinatal and Infant Health Unit - SIDS Information and Counseling Program
Ohio Department Of Health
246 N High Street
Columbus, OH 43266
614-466-4716
e-mail: webmaster@ghodh.state.oh.us
www.adh.state.oh.us/

Ben Chukwumah, MD, MPH, Project Director

Oklahoma

7045 Oklahoma State Department of Health - Maternal and Child Health Services
1000 NE 10th Street
Oklahoma City, OK 73117
405-271-5600
Fax: 405-271-3431
e-mail: webmaster@health.ok.gov.
www.ok.gov/health

Mike Crutcher, Manager

Oregon

7046 Oregon State Health Division - SIDS Information and Counseling Program
1400 SW 5th Avenue
Portland, OR 97201
503-229-6617
Sue Omel, RN, MPH, Child Coordinator

7047 SIDS Resource of Oregon
4035 NE Sandy Boulevard, Suite 209
Portland, OR 97212
503-287-8265
800-221-7437
Fax: 503-287-8693
e-mail: sidsor@teleport.com
www.teleport.com/~sidsor

Todd Llinchliffer

Pennsylvania

7048 Pennsylvania SIDS Center
Suite 250 Riverfront Place
Pittsburgh, PA 15212
412-322-5680
800-258-7437
Fax: 215-923-2989
www.sids-pa.org/

Rosanne English, RN, Executive Director

7049 Region III Office Program Consultants for Maternal and Child Health
Public Ledger Building
150 S Independence Mall West, Suite 1172
Philadelphia, PA 19106
215-861-4379
Fax: 215-861-4338
e-mail: valos@hrsa.gov

Jane Coury, MSN, RN

Rhode Island

7050 Rhode Island Department of Health National SIDS Foundation
3 Capitol Hl
Providence, RI 02908
401-222-5960
Fax: 401-444-3422
www.health.ri.gov/

Anne M Roach, RN, SIDS Coordinator

South Carolina

7051 South Carolina Department of Health & Environmental Control - SIDS Information
2600 Bull Street
Columbia, SC 29201
803-898-3300
www.scdhec.gov/administration/hplhc/health.htm
Brenda Creswell, ACSW, LMSW, SIDS Coordinator

South Dakota

7052 South Dakota Department of Health
Health Building
500 East Capitol Avenue
Pierre, SD 57501
605-773-3361
800-738-2301
Fax: 605-773-5683
e-mail: dolt.info@state.sd.us
www.doh.sd.gov

Doneen Hollingsworth, Manager

Tennessee

7053 Tennessee SIDS Program
Tennessee Department Of Health
425 5th Ave, N Cordell Hull Bldg, 3rd Fl
Nashville, TN 37243
615-741-7335
Fax: 615-741-1063
e-mail: tn.health@tn.gov
health.state.tn.us/MCH/SIDS/SIDS_program.htm
Judith Womack, RN, Director Child Health

Texas

7054 Harris County Health Department
2223 West Loop South
Houston, TX 77027
713-439-6000
e-mail: publicinfo@hd.co.harris.tx.us
www.hcphes.org

Kathleen Ingrando, RN, BSN, Program Coordinator

7055 North Texas SIDS Information And Counseling Program
5000 Harry Hines
Dallas, TX 75235
214-590-0135
Fax: 214-590-0173

Leslie U Malone, SIDS Coordinator

7056 Region VI Office Program Consultants For Maternal and Child Health
1301 Young Street 10th Floor
Dallas, TX 75202
214-767-3003
Fax: 214-767-3038
e-mail: twells@hrsa.gov

Marianne Davenport, CPNP, MPH

7057 Texas Department of Health - SIDS Information and Counseling Program
211 N. Florence, Suite 101
El Paso, TX 79901   915-532-1006
                                                  888-963-7111
                                            Fax: 512-458-7750
                             e-mail: bhc@borderhealth.org
                                          www.borderhealth.org

Eduardo J Sanchez, Manager

Utah

7058 Utah Department of Health
Child Health Bureau
PO Box 141010
Salt Lake City, UT 84114   801-538-6003
                                                  health.utah.gov

Judith Ahrano, SIDS Director

Vermont

7059 Vermont Department of Health - SIDS Information and Counseling Program
108 Cherry Street
Burlington, VT 05401   802-863-7200
                                            Fax: 802-865-7754
                        e-mail: sshepar@udh.state.ut.us
                                        www.healthvermont.gov

Wendy Davis, Manager

Virginia

7060 Virginia SIDS Program - Virginia Department of Health
Virginia Department of Health
P.O. Box 2448
Richmond, VA 23218   804-864-7001
                                            Fax: 804-864-7001
                            e-mail: schuettd@aol.com
                                          www.vdh.state.va.us

Arlethia V Rogers, RN, Nurse Consultant

Washington

7061 Region X Office Program Consultants for Maternal and Child Health
2201 6th Avenue
Seattle, WA 98121   206-553-0215
Kay Girl, RNC, MN, Acting

7062 SIDS Northwest Regional Center
Washington Department of Health
4800 Sand Point Way NE
Olympia, WA 98504   360-236-3560
                                                  800-441-4392
                                          www.doh.wa.gov

Lauren Valk Lawson, MN, Program Director

West Virginia

7063 West Virginia Department of Health and Human Services
One Davis Square, Suite 100, East
Charleston, WV 25301   304-558-0684
                                            Fax: 304-558-1130
                                          www.wvdhhr.org

Joan R Kenny, RN, SIDS Director

Wisconsin

7064 Counseling and Research Center for SIDS
2115 Wisconsin Avenue- NW Suite 601
Washington, DC 20007   202-687-7437
                                                  866-866-7437
                                            Fax: 202-784-9777
                             e-mail: info@sidscenter.org
                                          www.sidscenter.org

Rochelle Mayer, Director

Wyoming

7065 Wyoming Department of Health
Division of Health and Medical Services
401 Hathaway Building
Cheyenne, WY 82002   307-777-7656
                                            Fax: 307-777-7439
                             e-mail: wdh@state.wy.us
                                          www.health.wyo.gov

J Richard Hillman, MD, PhD, Administrator

Libraries & Resource Centers

7066 National Sudden Infant Death Syndrome Resource Center
Circle Solutions, Inc
8280 Greensboro Drive, Suite 300
McLean, VA 22102   703-893-6383
                                            Fax: 703-821-2098
                    e-mail: marketing@circlesolutions.com
                                          www.circlesolutions.com

Resource Center provides information on keeping children safe through their first year and beyond, about SIDS, and about handling the grief of losing a child to SIDS, and so much more.

Kristina Lewis, Chairman, Executive Committee
Louis Cartwright, jr., Vice President-Finance
Michael Collins, Vice President-IT

7067 Sudden Infant Death Syndrome (SIDS) Network
PO Box 520
Ledyard, CT 06339   Fax: 860-887-7309
                                          sids-network.org/

Research Centers

7068 American SIDS Institute
528 Raven Way
Naples, FL 34110   239-431-5425
                                                  800-232-7437
                                            Fax: 239-431-5536
                             e-mail: prevent@sids.org
                                          www.sids.org

A national nonprofit organization dedicated to the promotion of infant health and the prevention of sudden infant death syndrome.

Marc Peterzell, Chairman
Betty McEntire PhD, Executive Director

7069 CJ Foundation for SIDS
Don Imus WFAN Pediatric Center
30 Prospect Ave
Hackensack, NJ 07601   201-996-5111
                                                  800-620-7832
                                            Fax: 201-996-5326
                             e-mail: info@cjsids.org
                                          www.cjsids.org

Barry Bornstein, Executive Director

7070 Center for Research for Mothers & Children
National Institute of Child Health & Development
31 Center Drive, Building 31
Bethesda, MD 20892
301-496-5575
1 8-0 3-0 29
Fax: 866-760-5947
e-mail: NICHDInformationResourceCenter@mail.nih.
www.nichd.nih.gov

This institute conducts and supports research on all stages of human development, from the preconception to adulthood, to better understand the health of children, adults, families, and communities.

7071 Massachusetts Sudden Infant Death Syndrome
Boston City Hospital
818 Harrison Avenue
Boston, MA 02118
617-638-8131

A joint program of Boston City Hospital and Children's Hospital. Services provided include around-the-clock availability for consultation to health professionals and families, counseling of families, parent group meetings and supportive home visits.

7072 National Sudden Infant Death Syndrome Research Center
Circle Solutions, Inc
8280 Greensboro Drive, Suite 300
McLean, VA 22102
703-821-8955
Fax: 703-821-2098
e-mail: marketing@circlesolutions.com
www.circlesolutions.com

Provides information services and technical assistance concerning SIDS and related topics in order to promote understanding of SIDS and to comfort those affected by a SIDS loss. Offers its services to parents, family members, caregivers, counselors, medical and legal professionals, and the general public.

7073 Pathology Department SIDS/SUDC Research Project
Children's Hospital San Diego
3020 Children's Way, MC5007
San Diego, CA 92123
858-966-5944
Dr Henry Krous, Director
Amy Chadwick, Project Manager

7074 Pediatric Pulmonary Unit
Massachusetts General Hospital
55 Fruit Street
Boston, MA 02114
617-726-2000
www.massgeneral.org

Sudden infant death syndrome and childhood disorders research.

Douglas R Johnson, Associate Director

7075 Southwest SIDS Research Institute
Brazosport Memorial Hospital
100 Medical Drive
Lake Jackson, TX 77566
979-297-4411
Fax: 979-297-6682
e-mail: admin@brazosportmemorial.com
www.brazosportmemorial.com

Mari Uranga, Manager

7076 Sudden Infant Death Syndrome Institute of The University of Maryland
2105 Laurel Bush Road,, Suite 201
Bel Air, MD 21015
443-640-1049
Fax: 410-653-8709
e-mail: info@firstcandle.org
www.firstcandle.org

Debora Boyd, Executive Director

7077 USC - Neonatology Research Units
1240 Mission Road
Los Angeles, CA 90033
323-266-3813
Fax: 323-266-5049
www.usc.edu

Focuses on clinical problems of the newborn and premature infant.

Paul YK Wu, MD, Director

Conferences

7078 National Sudden Infant Death Syndrome Alliance Conference
www.healthyplace.com
210-225-4388
800-221-7437
www.healthyplace.com

Unites parents, caregivers, and researchers with government, business, and community service groups in a nationwide movement to advance the support of SIDS families and hasten the elimination of SIDS through medical research. Funds medical research and offers emotional support nationally and locally.

Gary Koplin, President
Harry Croft, M.D, Medical Director
Patricia Avila, Editor

Audio Video

7079 7 Steps to Reducing the Risk of SIDS
InJoy Productions
7107 La Vista Place
Longmont, CO 80503
303-447-2082
800-326-2082
Fax: 303-449-8788
e-mail: custserv@injoyvideos.com
www.injoyvideos.com

Shows how to dramatically lower infant's risk of using simple, important safety steps. Although SIDS is a frightening subject, this video's positive and compassionate tone will help ease parent's anxieties by showing them how to give their baby a healthy and happy first year.

14 minutes

Web Sites

7080 American SIDS Institute
528 Raven Way
Naples, FL 34110
239-431-5425
Fax: 239-431-5536
www.sids.org

A national nonprofit health care organization that is dedicated to the prevention of sudden infant death and the promotion of infant health through an aggresive, comprehensive nationwide program of: Research, Clinical Services, Education and Family Support.

Marc Peterzell, JD, Chairman
Betty McEntire, PhD, CEO/ Executive Director

7081 Center for Research for Mothers & Children
31 Center Drive, Building 31, Building 31, Room 2A
Bethesda, MD 20892
800-370-2943
Fax: 866-760-5947
TTY: 888-320-6942
e-mail: NICHDInformationResourceCenter@mail.nih.
www.nichd.nih.gov

Composed of several branches the principle NIH source of support for research and research training in maternal and child health, through grants, contracts, and cooperative agreements. Through this research, CRMC-supported scientists are advancing fundamental and clinical knowledge concerning maternal health and child development problems such as low birth wieght, mental retardation and developmental disabilities, specific learning disabilities, congenital and genetic defects and others.

Alan E. Guttmacher, M.D., Director
Lisa Kaeser, Program Analyst
Lisa Williams Simons, Senior Research Assistant

7082 Compassionate Friends
www.compassionatefriends.org

Assists families toward the positive resolution of grief following the death of a child of any age and provides information to help others be supportive.

7083 Health Answers
410 Horsham Road
Horsham, PA 19044   215-442-9010
e-mail: Michael.tague@healthanswers.com
www.healthanswers.com

HealthAnswers offers a breadth of services in medical education, sales force training, patient support solutions, professional promotion and consumer solutions.

Michael Tague, Managing Director

7084 National Center for Education in Maternal and Child Health
www.ncemch.org

202-784-9552
e-mail: rmayer@ncemch.org
www.ncemch.org

The National Center for Education in Maternal and Child Health provides national leadership to the maternal and child health community in three key areas - program development, policy analysis and education, and knowledge to improve the health and well-being of the nation's children and families.

Rochelle Mayer, Ed.D., Director

7085 Online Mendelian Inheritance in Man
www.omim.org

This database is a catalog of human genes and genetic disorders.

7086 SID Network
PO Box 520
Ledyard, CT 6339   e-mail: sidsnet1-at-sids-network-dot-org
sids-network.org/net.htm

Nonprofit voluntary agency that is dedicated to eliminate sudden infant death syndrome through the support of SIDS research projects, provide support for those who have been touched by the tragedy of sudden Infant Death Syndrome and to raise public awareness of sudden infant death syndrome through education.

Book Publishers

7087 Apparent Life - Threatening Event and Sudden Infant Death Syndrome
Circle Solutions, Inc
8280 Greensboro Drive, Suite 300
McLean, VA 22102   703-821-8955
866-866-7437
Fax: 703-821-2098
e-mail: marketing@circlesolutions.com
www.circlesolution.com

Provides information about ALTE and its relationship to SIDS.

1992 29 pages

Kristina Lewis, Chairman, Executive Committee
Louis Cartwright, jr., Vice President-Finance
Michael Collins, Vice President-IT

7088 Crib Death: The Sudden Infant Death Syndrome
Futura Publishing Company
135 Bedford Road
Armonk, NY 10504   914-273-1014
Fax: 914-273-1015
www.growinghealthcare.com

A thorough book, that discusses the theories of SIDS and their implications. Athough it is aimed at the medical professional, lay people will also gain a clearer understanding of SIDS.

1995 456 pages Hardcover

7089 Death Investigations and Sudden Infant Death Syndrome
Circle Solutions, Inc
8280 Greensboro Drive, Suite 300
McLean, VA 22102   703-821-8955
Fax: 703-821-2098
e-mail: marketing@circlesolutions.com
www.circlesolutions.com

Contains abstracts of articles on autopsies, death certification, and infant death scene investigation and SIDS.

1991 104 pages

Kristina Lewis, Chairman, Executive Committee
Louis Cartwright, jr., Vice President-Finance
Michael Collins, Vice President-IT

7090 Death of a Child, the Grief of the Parents A Lifetime Journey
Circle Solutions, Inc
8280 Greensboro Drive, Suite 300
McLean, VA 22102   703-821-8955
Fax: 703-821-2098
e-mail: marketing@circlesolutions.com
www.circlesolutions.com

1997 38 pages

Kristina Lewis, Chairman, Executive Committee
Louis Cartwright, jr., Vice President-Finance
Michael Collins, Vice President-IT

7091 Grief, Bereavement and Sudden Infant Death Syndrome
Circle Solutions, Inc
8280 Greensboro Drive, Suite 300
McLean, VA 22102   703-821-8955
Fax: 703-821-2098
e-mail: marketing@circlesolutions.com
www.circlesolutions.com

Contains abstracts of selected materials on the grief and bereavement process specific to the loss of a child to SIDS.

1991 28 pages

Kristina Lewis, Chairman, Executive Committee
Louis Cartwright, jr., Vice President-Finance
Michael Collins, Vice President-IT

7092 SIDS Research
Circle Solutions, Inc
8280 Greensboro Drive, Suite 300
McLean, VA 22102   703-821-8955
Fax: 703-821-2098
e-mail: marketing@circlesolutions.com
www.circlesolutions.com

Contains abstracts of relevant articles published during 1993.

1995 146 pages

Kristina Lewis, Chairman, Executive Committee
Louis Cartwright, jr., Vice President-Finance
Michael Collins, Vice President-IT

7093 SIDS Survival Guide
Independent Publishers Group
814 N Franklin Street
Chicago, IL 60610   312-337-0747
800-888-4741
Fax: 312-337-5985
e-mail: frontdesk@ipgbook.com
www.ipgbook.com

Offers information and comfort for grieving family, friends and professionals who seek to help them.

1994 290 pages Paperback
ISBN: 0-964121-87-5

Curt Matthews, CEO

7094 SIDS: A Parents Guide to Understanding & Preventing SIDS
Hachette Book Group USA
322 South Enterprise Blvd
Lebanon, IN 46052   800-759-0190
Fax: 800-286-9471
e-mail: customer.service@hbgusa.com
www.hachettebookgroup.biz

1995
ISBN: 0-316779-12-1

David Young, Chairman
Evan Schnittman, Executive Vice President
Jamie Raab, President & Publisher

7095 Smoking and Sudden Infant Death Syndrome
Circle Solutions, Inc
8280 Breensboro Drive, Suite 300
McLean, VA 22102
703-821-8955
Fax: 703-821-2098
TTY: 703-556-4831
e-mail: marketing@circlesolutions.com
www.circlesolutions.com

Contains abstracts of materials about tobacco use, its relationship to SIDS, and the dangers to the unborn and the newly born from passive and secondary smoking.

1992 34 pages

Kristina Lewis, Chairman, Executive Committee
Louis Cartwright, jr., Vice President-Finance
Michael Collins, Vice President-IT

7096 Sudden Death in Infancy, Childhood & Adolescence
Cambridge University Press
32 Avenue Of The Americas
New York, NY 10013
212-924-3900
Fax: 212-691-3239
e-mail: newyork@cambridge.org
www.cambridge.org/us

1994 400 pages
ISBN: 0-521420-31-8

7097 Sudden Infant Death Syndrome Risk Factors
Circle Solutions, Inc
8280 Greensboro Drive, Suite 300
McLean, VA 22102
703-821-8955
Fax: 703-821-2098
TTY: 703-556-4831
e-mail: marketing@circlesolutions.com
www.circlesolutions.com

Contains selected articles published between 1989 and 1993 on the risk factors for SIDS.

1994 131 pages

Kristina Lewis, Chairman, Executive Committee
Louis Cartwright, jr., Vice President-Finance
Michael Collins, Vice President-IT

Newsletters

7098 Illuminations
First Candle/SIDS Alliance
9 Newport Drive, Suite 200
Forest Hill, MD 21050
443-640-1049
800-221-7437
Fax: 410-653-8709
e-mail: info@firstcandle.org
www.firstcandle.org

Quarterly

Christopher Blake, CEO
Barb Himes, IBCLC, Director of Education and Training
Shannon Carswell, Creative Director

7099 Network
Parent Care
9041 Colgate Street
Indianapolis, IN 46268
317-872-9913
Fax: 317-872-0795

Offers information on support groups, meetings, organizations and resources for parents and professionals dealing with the chronically ill child.

7100 Newsletter: SIDS
Massachusetts Center For SIDS
1 Boston Medical Center Place
Boston, MA 2118
617-638-8000
www.bmc.org/program/sids/

Offers information on SIDS, articles pertaining to the latest information available on the mystery condition, latest research and fund-raising news and professional resources available.

Monthly

Pamphlets

7101 After Sudden Infant Death Syndrome
Circle Solution, Inc
8280 Greensboro Drive, Suite 300
McLean, VA 22102
703-821-8955
Fax: 703-821-2098
e-mail: marketing@circlesolutions.com
www.circlesolutions.com

1993 16 pages

Kristina Lewis, President/ Chair
Louis Cartwright, Jr., Vice President of Finance
Laura Scherzer, CMP, PMP, Vice President of Operations

7102 Bilingual Risk Reduction Brochure
First Candle/SIDS Alliance
9 Newport Drive, Suite 200
Forest Hill, MD 21050
443-640-1049
800-221-7437
Fax: 410-653-8709
e-mail: info@firstcandle.org
www.firstcandle.org

Provides an understanding of the risk of SIDS and the steps that can be taken to help the baby survive and thrive.

2 pages

Christopher Blake, CEO
Barb Himes, IBCLC, Director of Education and Training
Shannon Carswell, Creative Director

7103 Facts About Apnea and Other Apparent Life-Threatening Events
Circle Solution, Inc
8280 Greensboro Drive, Suite 300
McLean, VA 22102
703-821-8955
Fax: 703-821-2098
e-mail: marketing@circlesolutions.com
www.circlesolutions.com

Explains apparent life-threatening events in infants, their relationship to SIDS and current views on home monitoring.

1987 2 pages

Kristina Lewis, President/ Chair
Louis Cartwright, Jr., Vice President of Finance
Laura Scherzer, CMP, PMP, Vice President of Operations

7104 Facts About SIDS
Sudden Infant Death Syndrome Alliance
1314 Bedford Avenue
Baltimore, MD 21208
410-653-8226
Fax: 410-653-8709

Offers information on basic facts, answers to the most frequently asked questions about SIDS and information on numbers to call and referral centers for more help.

7105 Infant Positioning and Sudden Infant Death Syndrome
Circle Solutions, Inc
8280 Greensboro Drive, Suite 300
McLean, VA 22102
703-821-8955
Fax: 703-821-2098
e-mail: marketing@circlesolutions.com
www.circlesolutions.com

Contains abstracts of selected articles on the topic of sleep position and SIDS.

1994

Kristina Lewis, President/ Chair
Louis Cartwright, Jr., Vice President of Finance
Laura Scherzer, CMP, PMP, Vice President of Operations

7106 National SIDS Resource Center Brochure
Circle Solutions, Inc
8280 Greensboro Drive, Suite 300
McLean, VA 22102 703-821-8955
Fax: 703-821-2098
e-mail: marketing@circlesolutions.com
www.circlesolutions.com

1994

Kristina Lewis, President/ Chair
Louis Cartwright, Jr., Vice President of Finance
Laura Scherzer, CMP, PMP, Vice President of Operations

7107 Nationwide Survey of Sudden Infant Death Syndrome (SIDS) Service
Circle Solutions, Inc
8280 Greensboro Drive, Suite 300
McLean, VA 22102 703-821-8955
Fax: 703-821-2098
e-mail: marketing@circlesolutions.com
www.circlesolutions.com

Analysis of availability of SIDS services.

1994

Kristina Lewis, President/ Chair
Louis Cartwright, Jr., Vice President of Finance
Laura Scherzer, CMP, PMP, Vice President of Operations

7108 Pacifiers and SIDS: Reducing the Risk
First Candle/SIDS Alliance
9 Newport Drive, Suite 200
Forest Hill, MD 21050 443-640-1049
800-221-7437
Fax: 410-653-8709
e-mail: info@firstcandle.org
www.firstcandle.org

A brochure for parents and caregivers.

Christopher Blake, CEO
Barb Himes, IBCLC, Director of Education and Training
Shannon Carswell, Creative Director

7109 SIDS Prevention
Corporate Office
100 Enterprise Way, Suite G300
Scotts Valley, CA 95066 831-438-4060
800-620-8884
Fax: 831-438-4284
e-mail: support@etr.freshdesk.com
www.etr.org

Gives overview, risk factors, prevention of Sudden Infant Death Syndrome.

50 pamphlets

Dan McCormick, MHA, Chief Executive Officer
David Kitchen, MBA, Chief Financial Officer
Erin Cassidy-Eagle, PhD, Director, Research

7110 SIDS: Toward Prevention and Improved Infant Health
American SIDS Institute
528 Raven Way
Naples, FL 34110 239-431-5425
800-232-sids
Fax: 239-431-5536
e-mail: prevent@sids.org
www.sids.org

Practical guide for those planning a pregnancy, for parents-to-be and for new parents.

Marc Peterzell, JD, Chairman
Betty McEntire, PhD, CEO/ Executive Director

7111 Surviving the Death of a Baby
First Candle/SIDS Alliance
9 Newport Drive, Suite 200
Forest Hill, MD 21050 443-640-1049
800-221-7437
Fax: 410-653-8709
e-mail: info@firstcandle.org
www.firstcandle.org

13 pages
Christopher Blake, CEO
Barb Himes, IBCLC, Director of Education and Training
Shannon Carswell, Creative Director

Description

7112 SYNCOPE

Synonyms: Swoon, Faint

Involves the following Biologic System(s):

Cardiovascular Disorders

Syncope is a medical term describing a phenomenon more commonly known as fainting. Specifically, syncope is a brief loss of consciousness that resolves without intervention. In the pediatric population most episodes of syncope are uncomplicated without neurologic or cardiac after effects (sequelae).

The true incidence of syncope is difficult to ascertain since many episodes are not reported to a medical provider. Roughly 15-25% of all children experience at least one episode of syncope or near-syncope, although adolescents are are the most common segment of the pediatric population to experience syncope and the most likely to have recurrent episodes.

The most common cause of fainting in pediatrics is neurocardiogenic (related to a problem of the nervous system and the heart) syncope, also known as vasovagal or vasodepressor syncope. The other cases of syncope can be divided into neurologic, cardiac, metabolic, toxin (drug abuse), and psychogenic. While greater than 95% of syncopal episodes have a benign etiology (cause), such as the simple vasovagal syncope, there are several rare causes that are fatal, accounting for 4-5 deaths per 100,000 pediatric patients. The possibility of a fatal etiology necessitates the need for a thorough investigation into any syncopal episode.

An appropriate evaluation begins with a thorough history and physical exam. The history should focus on details around the event, change in position (from sitting to standing, for instance), exercise, trauma, and past history of similar events. Family history is critical when evaluating unexplained sudden deaths, hearing loss, cardiac disease, recurrent fainting, seizure disorders or arrhythmias. The physical exam should include a careful neurologic exam as well as a thorough cardiac exam looking for murmurs, clicks or gallops (unusual heart sounds) and careful blood pressure measurements including orthostatic measurements (when the patient is sitting and then stands up. In individuals who have fainted, the blood pressure can drop significantly upon standing, indicating at least one possible cause of the syncopal episode.

The diagnostic evaluation continues with an electrocardiogram looking at abnormal rhythms as well as signs of cardiomyopathy (heart disease). If the physical examination and ECG are normal and the history is consistent with a simple 'faint', no further workup may be necessary. If the history is inconsistent with vasovagal syncope or if there are any abnormalities on the physical or ECG, referral to a specialist, usually a pediatric cardiologist or adult cardiologist, is appropriate. Further testing may include a tilt table test, 24-hour holter monitor, echocardiography, exercise stress testing or electrophysiology testing.

Treatment for syncope varies depending on the etiology. For simple vasodepressor syncope, management is often focused on increasing fluid and salt intake in an effort to improve blood volume and pressure. Often discovering the triggers for these patients enables them to avoid them or anticipate their response more effectively (i.e. lying on the ground with feet up before syncope occurs). Medication is an option if the syncopal episodes are frequent and impacton the patient's lifestyle. The most widely used and successfully used medication class has been beta-blockers. More serious cardiac causes of syncope may need to be treated with antiarrhythmics, pacemakers or defibrillators. These interventions can be life-saving and allow patients to lead full productive lives.

National Associations & Support Groups

7113 American Academy of Pediatrics

141 Northwest Point Boulevard
Elk Grove Village, IL 60007

847-434-4000
800-433-9016
Fax: 847-434-8000
www.aap.org

The American Academy of Pediatrics and its member pediatricians are committed to the attainment of optimal physical, mental and social health and well-being for all infants, children, adolescents, and young adults.

Sandra Hassink, MD, FAAP, President

7114 NIH/National Heart, Lung and Blood Institu te

National Institute of Health
31 Center Dr MSC 2486, Bldg 31, Rm5A48
Bethesda, MD 20892

301-592-8573
Fax: 301-592-8563
TTY: 240-629-3255
e-mail: NHLBIinfo@nhlbi.nih.gov
www.nhlbi.nih.gov

Primary responsibility of this organization is the scientific investigation of heart, blood vessel, lung and blood disorders. Oversees research, demonstration, prevention, education, control and training activities in these fields and emphasizes the prevention and control of heart diseases.

Gary H. Gibbons, M.D., Director
Susan Shurin, MD, Deputy Director
Sheila Pohl, Chief of Staff

7115 NIH/National Institute of Neurological Dis orders and Stroke (NINDS)

PO Box 5801
Bethesda, MD 20824

301-496-5751
800-352-9424
Fax: 301-496-0296
TTY: 301-468-5981
www.ninds.nih.gov

Information and advocacy resources for families and professionals. Includes listings of organizations providing general information and organizations focusing on more specific areas of concern to families and young adults who have disabilities.

Story C Landis PhD, Director
Audrey C Penn MD, Deputy Director

Web Sites

7116 EMedicine Journal: Syncope

www.emedicine.com/med/topic3385.htm

Syncope information covering background, pathophysiology, frequency, mortality/morbidity, causes, lab studies and tests, diet, activity, drugs used in treatment, complications and patient education. Authored by Dr Jatin Dave and co-authored by Dr John Michael Gaziano.

7117 NINDS Syncope Information Page

Office of Communications and Public Liaison, NINDS
Bethesda, MD 20892

301-496-5751
800-352-9424
www.ninds.nih.gov/disorders/syncope/

Walter J. Koroshetz, M.D., Acting Director
Alan L. Willard, Ph.D., Acting Deputy Director
Caroline Lewis, Executive Officer

7118 Syncope Information Page
7272 Greenville Ave.
Dallas, TX 75231   800-242-8721
                              www.heart.org/HEARTORG/

American Heart Association information page about Syncope
such as what it is and what causes it.

Elliott Antman, President
Bernie Dennis, Chairman
Alvin Royse, Chairman-Elect

Description

7119 SYNDACTYLY

Synonyms: Syndactylia, Syndactylism

Involves the following Biologic System(s):

Orthopedic and Muscle Disorders

Syndactyly refers to an abnormality that is present at birth (congenital) and characterized by the joining together (fusing) of two or more fingers or toes. This relatively common abnormality seems to occur more frequently in boys than in girls. It is often inherited as an autosomal dominant trait. Syndactyly often results from incomplete or abnormal embryonic development of the fingers or toes. In some infants, it occurs spontaneously as the hands or feet of the developing fetus may be unnaturally constricted within the uterus. Classification of syndactyly is based on the severity of the clinical presentation. Defects associated with syndactyly may range from a simple or incomplete joining or webbing of the skin between two digits to fusion from the base to the tip of the digits, complete with fusion of the bones and nails.

Syndactyly of the foot may involve complete or incomplete webbing that usually affects the second and third toes. This simple condition is referred to as zygosyndactyly and often requires no treatment. Syndactyly may also involve webbing and bone fusion (synostosis) of the fourth and fifth toes with duplication of the fifth toe in a condition called syndactyly/polysyndactyly.

As in the foot, syndactyly of the hand may involve a simple webbing. However, in some cases, the fusion of certain fingers may be more complex and involve shared nerves and blood supply. Syndactyly of the fingers should be carefully evaluated to determine the best method of treatment, allowing for growth and dexterity of the fingers.

Syndactyly may also occur in association with several genetic disorders. Such disorders include acrocephalopolysyndactyly type II (Carpenter's syndrome), characterized by mental retardation and irregularities involving the head, hand, and genitalia; acrocephalosyndactyly type I (Apert's syndrome), characterized by craniofacial irregularities and syndactyly of the hands and feet; trisomy 18 syndrome, a chromosomal abnormality characterized by multiple craniofacial abnormalities, irregularities of the hands and feet, and severe mental retardation; and other inherited diseases. Treatment of syndactyly associated with these and other inherited disorders depends upon the nature of the underlying disorder. In itself, a minor incomplete syndactyly is not an indication for surgery if the only issue is its appearance. However, a syndactyly that prevents full range of motion in the involved fingers warrants surgical release to increase the fingers' ability to function. The timing of surgery is variable. However, as more fingers are involved and as the syndactyly becomes more complex, release should be performed earlier.

Government Agencies

7120 NIH/National Institute of Arthritis and Mu sculoskeletal and Skin Diseases
1AMS Circle
Bethesda, MD 20892

301-402-4484
877-226-4267
Fax: 301-718-6366
TDD: 301-565-2966
e-mail: niamsinfo@mail.nih.gov
www.niams.nih.gov

The mission of the NIAMS, a part of the NIH, is to support research into the causes, treatment, and prevention of arthritis and musculoskeletal and skin diseases, the training of basic and clinical scientists to carry out this research, and the dissemination of information on research progress in these diseases.

Stephen I Katz MD PhD, Director
Robert H Carter MD, Deputy Director
Gahan Breithaupt, Assoc Dir for Management & Operatio

National Associations & Support Groups

7121 American Academy of Pediatrics
141 Northwest Point Boulevard
Elk Grove Village, IL 60007

847-434-4000
800-433-9016
Fax: 847-434-8000
www.aap.org

The American Academy of Pediatrics and its member pediatricians are committed to the attainment of optimal physical, mental and social health and well-being for all infants, children, adolescents, and young adults.

Sandra Hassink, MD, FAAP, President

7122 CHERUB-Association of Families and Friends of Children with Limb Disorders
Children's Hospital of Buffalo
936 Delaware Avenue
Buffalo, NY 14209

716-762-9997

Answers the questions and problems that families of juveniles diagnosed with a disorder may be experiencing.

Sandra Richenberg
Kathy Gura

7123 Genetic Alliance
4301 Connecticut Avenue NW
Washington, DC 20008

202-966-5557
800-336-4363
Fax: 202-966-8553
e-mail: info@geneticalliance.org
www.geneticalliance.org

A coalition of voluntary genetic support groups, consumers and professionals addressing the needs of individuals and families affected by genetic disorders from a national perspective.

Sharon Terry, MA, President/CEO
Natasha Bonhomme, Vice President of Strategic Develop
Vaughn Edelson, Assistant Director of Health Commun

7124 March of Dimes Birth Defects Foundation
1275 Mamaroneck Avenue
White Plains, NY 10605

914-428-7100
888-663-4637
Fax: 914-428-8203
e-mail: askus@marchofdimes.com
www.marchofdimes.com/?

Partnership of volunteers and professionals dedicated to improving the health of babies by preventing birth defects and infant mortality. Over 100 chapters are located across the country.

Jennifer L Howse, President

7125 Shriners Hospitals for Children
Headquarters
2900 Rocky Point Drive
Tampa, FL 33607
813-281-0300
800-237-5055
Fax: 813-281-8113
www.shrinershospitalsforchildren.org

Network of 22 hospitals that provide expert, no-cost orthopedic and burn care to children under 18.

Peter F Armstrong, VP

Web Sites

7126 A-to-Z Health & Disease Information
www.hmc.psu.edu/healthinfo/pq/poly.htm

Information page on polydactyly and syndactyly provided by Penn State Medical Center. Information includes a listing of physicians who treat the disorder, causes, symptoms, a general overview, diagnosis and treatment.

7127 Online Mendelian Inheritance in Man
www.omim.org

This database is a catalog of human genes and genetic disorders.

7128 Pediatric Plastic Surgery
One Hospital Drive, MC504
Columbia, MO 65212
573-882-4158
Fax: 573-884-4585
e-mail: mumedicine@missouri.edu
medicine.missouri.edu/surgery/

Answers to questions about syndactyly and surgery provided by the University of Missouri Children's Hospital.

7129 Syndactyly
www.pncl.co.uk/~belcher/information/Syndactyly.pdf

Information sheet on syndactyly.

Description

7130 SYSTEMIC LUPUS ERYTHEMATOSUS

Synonyms: Lupus, SLE

Involves the following Biologic System(s):

Immunologic and Rheumatologic Disorders

Systemic lupus erythematosus (SLE) is a chronic, inflammatory, multisystem disorder of connective tissue that may affect many organ systems in the body including the skin, joints, membranes that line the walls of certain bodily cavities (serosal membranes), or kidneys. In children with the disorder, associated symptoms are often progressive and, without appropriate treatment, may result in life-threatening complications. However, in some patients, symptoms may spontaneously subside and periodically recur with varying levels of severity (relapsing-remitting). SLE usually becomes apparent during late adolescence or a patient's 20s or 30s. However, in up to 20 percent of patients, symptoms may begin during childhood, usually after the age of eight. Females are more commonly affected than males in all age groups.

The specific underlying cause of SLE is unknown. However, the disorder is thought to result from abnormalities in the regulating mechanisms of the immune system that normally prevent it from attacking the body's own cells and tissues. In addition, researchers speculate that certain microorganisms or other environmental factors may play some role in causing SLE. Familial cases have also been reported, suggesting potential genetic mechanisms. In some individuals, SLE-like symptoms may also occur after exposure to certain medications, such as particular antiseizure drugs or certain antibiotics known as sulfonamides. Drug-induced symptoms are usually relatively mild and subside when the responsible medication is removed.

The range and severity of associated symptoms and findings may vary. Although associated symptoms may begin suddenly or gradually, most children with SLE tend to have more acute, severe symptoms than adults. In some children, symptoms may tend to recur or worsen in association with certain infections. In addition, exposure to sunlight may worsen associated skin or other symptoms. Many children with SLE initially experience generalized symptoms, such as a fever, a general feeling of ill health (malaise), joint swelling and inflammation (arthritis) or pain (arthralgia), loss of appetite (anorexia), and weight loss. Most children also have associated skin abnormalities, including a scaly, reddish or bluish rash that is in a distinctive butterfly distribution across the cheeks and the bridge of the nose (butterfly rash). The affected area may be abnormally sensitive to sunlight (photosensitive), and the rash may gradually spread to other facial areas, the neck, scalp, chest, and arms. Additional skin symptoms may include flat, reddish, dot-like spots (punctate lesions) on the fingertips, palms, soles, arms, legs, and torso; abnormal changes of the tissues beneath t|he fingernails and toenails (nail beds); tender, reddish-purple swellings or nodules on the legs (erythema nodosum); and itchy, reddish, flat or raised lesions of the skin and mucous membranes (erythema multiforme). Patients may also develop painless sores of the mucous membranes of the mouth and nose. The hair may be abnormally coarse and dry, and some children may have patchy areas of baldness on the scalp (alopecia).

Many children with SLE may also experience joint stiffness; inflammation of muscles (myositis), causing muscle pain and weakness; abnormal changes and localized loss of bone in certain areas (aseptic necrosis), particularly the head of the thigh bone (femur); and Raynaud's phenomenon. This condition is characterized by sudden contraction of the relatively small blood vessels supplying the fingers and toes (digits), causing an interruption of blood flow to the digits and a subsequent excess of blood in affected areas following restoration of blood flow (reactive hyperemia). Such episodes are usually triggered by exposure to cold temperatures and are characterized by numbing, tingling, and bluish or whitish discoloration of the digits due to lack of blood flow and subsequent reddening and pain as blood flow is reestablished. Many children with SLE may also develop inflammation of the membranes that line the lungs and chest cavity (|pleurisy), surround the heart (pericarditis), and line the wall of the abdomen and cover the abdominal organs (peritonitis). Additional heart abnormalities may also be present, such as abnormal heart murmurs, inflammation of heart muscle (myocarditis), enlargement of the heart (cardiomegaly), a decreased ability of the heart to pump blood effectively to the lungs and the rest of the body (heart failure), and, in some severe cases, heart attacks (myocardial infarctions), potentially causing life-threatening complications.

Kidney involvement is common among children with SLE and may be the only disease manifestation. Associated inflammation of the filtering units of the kidneys (glomerulonephritis) may be mild, moderate, or severe. Symptoms and findings may range from small amounts of blood in the urine (hematuria) of mildly increased levels of protein in the urine (proteinuria) to kidney failure that causes potentially life-threatening complications. Some children with SLE may also experience symptoms due to involvement of the brain and spinal cord (central nervous system). Associated neurologic abnormalities may include personality changes, episodes of abnormally increased electrical activity in the brain (seizures), or other findings. In addition, in some children, disease progression may also affect other tissues and organs, causing additional symptoms and findings.

The treatment of SLE is individualized and based upon the severity of the disease and the specific organ systems affected. Episodes of active disease should be considered emergencies that require immediate evaluation and aggressive treatment to help prevent damage to affected tissues and organs. In addition, careful follow-up and ongoing monitoring is required to detect worsening disease and to ensure prompt, appropriate treatment as required. Therapy may include the use of nonsteroidal antiinflammatory drugs (NSAIDs)s or salicylates (aspirin) to help alleviate joint pain and antimalarial agents or topical corticosteroid creams to treat skin symptoms. In severe cases, immunosuppressive drugs may also be administered; however, such agents must be used with great caution in children. Treatment of kidney inflammation may also include the use of certain corticosteroids, such as prednisone, and in some patients, the addition of immunosuppressive agents, such as azathioprine. Children with severe kidney disease may require regular dialysis or kidney transplantation. Dialysis is a medical procedure that removes excess fluid from the body and waste products from the blood. Additional treatment is symptomatic and supportive.

National Associations & Support Groups

7131 American Academy of Pediatrics
141 Northwest Point Boulevard
Elk Grove Village, IL 60007

847-434-4000
800-433-9016
Fax: 847-434-8000
www.aap.org

The American Academy of Pediatrics and its member pediatricians are committed to the attainment of optimal physical, mental and social health and well-being for all infants, children, adolescents, and young adults.

Sandra Hassink, MD, FAAP, President

7132 American Autoimmune Related Diseases Association
22100 Gratiot Avenue
Eastpointe, MI 48021

586-776-3900
800-598-4668
Fax: 586-776-3903
e-mail: aarda@aarda.org
www.aarda.org

Dedicated to the eradication of autoimmune diseases and the alleviation of suffering and the socio-economic impact of autoimmunity through fostering and facilitating collaboration in the areas of education, public awareness, research and patient services in an effective, ethical and efficient manner.

Virginia Ladd, Executive Director

7133 American Juvenile Arthritis Organization
1330 W. Peachtree Street., Suite 100
Atlanta, GA 30309

404-872-7100
800-283-7800
Fax: 404-237-8153
e-mail: info.ga@arthritis.org
www.arthritis.org

Devoted to serving the special needs of children, teens, and young adults with childhood rheumatic diseases and their families. Offers both support and information through national and local programs that serve the needs of families, friends and health professionals. Serves as a clearinghouse of information, sponsors an annual national conference, monitors and promotes legislation, sponsors research, and offers training to both parents and health professionals.

Sage Rhodes, President

7134 Children's Hospital Boston
300 Longwood Avenue
Boston, MA 02115

617-355-6000
TTY: 617-730-0152
www.childrenshospital.org

Mission is to provide the highest quality care; be the leading source of research and discovery; educate the next generation of leaders in child health and enhance the health and well-being of the children and families in our local community.

Leslie M Higuchi, President & CEO
Sandra Fenwick, Chief Operating Officer

7135 Genetic Alliance
4301 Connecticut Avenue NW
Washington, DC 20008

202-966-5557
800-336-4363
Fax: 202-966-8553
e-mail: info@geneticalliance.org
www.geneticalliance.org

A coalition of voluntary genetic support groups, consumers and professionals addressing the needs of individuals and families affected by genetic disorders from a national perspective.

Sharon Terry, MA, President/CEO
Natasha Bonhomme, Vice President of Strategic Develop
Vaughn Edelson, Assistant Director of Health Commun

7136 Lupus Foundation of America
2000 L Street NW, Suite 710
Washington, DC 20036

202-349-1155
800-558-0121
Fax: 202-349-1156
e-mail: LupusInfo@aol.com
www.lupus.org/newsite/

The LFA mission is to educate and support those affected by lupus. It supports research into the cause and cure of lupus. Information resources are available on request, including free pamphlets, brochures (English/Spanish), and articles for people seeking an understanding of lupus. Books and materials on lupus are also available through the LFA. There are nearly 300 chapters, branches, and support groups in 32 states throughout the US.

Sandra Raymond, President
Cindy Coney, Board Secretary

Research Centers

7137 Lupus Research Institute
330 Seventh Ave, Suite 1701
New York, NY 10001

212-812-9881
Fax: 212-545-1843
e-mail: lupus@LupusNY.org
www.lupusresearchinstitute.org

Established exclusively for lupus research. It has invested almost $20 million in new research and has funded 73 studies in 22 states.

Robert J Ravitz, Co-Chair
John A Luke, Treasurer

7138 SLE Lupus Foundation
330 Seventh Ave, Suite 1701
New York, NY 10001

212-685-4118
800-745-8787
Fax: 212-545-1843
e-mail: lupus@LupusNY.org
www.lupusny.org

Purpose is to raise funds for research grants, provide information and services to lupus patients, and educate the public about lupus. Patient services include self-help groups, orientation meetings, referrals, publications, and counseling on personal and financial problems related to the disease.

Richard K DeScherer, President
Margaret G Dowd, Executive Director

Web Sites

7139 American Autoimmune Related Diseases Association
22100 Gratiot Ave.
Eastpointe, MI 48021

586-776-3900
800-598-4668
Fax: 586-776-3903
www.aarda.org

Dedicated to the eradiction of autoimmune diseases and the alleviation of suffering and the socio-economic impact of autoimmunity through fostering and facilitating collaboration in the areas of education, public awareness, research and patient services in an effective, ethical and efficient manner.

Betty Diamond, M.D., Chairperson
Virginia T. Ladd, President/ Executive Director
Patricia Barber, Asst. Director

7140 Children's Hospital Boston
300 Longwood Avenue
Boston, MA 2115

617-355-6000
800-355-7944
www.childrenshospital.org

Mission is to provide the highest quality care; be the leading source of reseach and discovery; educate the next generation of leaders in child health and enhance the health and well-being of the children and families in our local community.

Sandra L. Fenwick, President/ CEO
Kevin Churchwell, MD, EVP, Health Affairs & COO
Naomi Fried, PhD, Chief Innovation Officer

Book Publishers

7141 Are You Tired Again...I Understand

Marilyn Deutsch PhD, author

Lupus Foundation of America
PO Box 932615
Atlanta, GA 31193

866-484-3532
Fax: 770-442-9742
e-mail: orders@lupus.org
www.lupus.org

An activity workbook for children to help them understand and what to expect when living with someone with lupus.

1996 42 pages Paperback

Sandra C. Raymond, President & CEO
Mary Schwarz, COO
Seung-Ae Chung, CFO

7142 Coping with Lupus

Robert Phillips PhD, author

Lupus Foundation of America
PO Box 932615
Atlanta, GA 31193

866-484-3532
Fax: 770-442-9742
e-mail: LupusInfo@aol.com
www.lupus.org

A practicing psychologist offers sound, meaningful and compassionate advice to individuals who must live with lupus.

2001 373 pages Softcover

Sandra C. Raymond, President & CEO
Mary Schwarz, COO
Seung-Ae Chung, CFO

7143 Disability Handbook for Social Security Applicants

Douglas Smith, author

Lupus Foundation of America
PO Box 932615
Atlanta, GA 31193

866-484-3532
e-mail: LupusInfo@aol.com
www.lupus.org

The handbook also includes the Disability Evaluation Guide for People with Systemic Lupus Erythematosus: Writing Medical Reports to the Social Security Administration. It helps people get their disability benefits promptly, without unnecessary appeals. Tells what you have to prove and how to prove it.

1995 137 pages Softcover

Sandra C. Raymond, President & CEO
Mary Schwarz, COO
Seung-Ae Chung, CFO

7144 Get to Sleep! How To Sleep Well...Despite Lupus

Robert Phillips PhD, author

Lupus Foundation of America
PO Box 932615
Atlanta, GA 31193

770-280-4177
866-484-3532
Fax: 770-442-9742
e-mail: orders@lupus.org
www.lupus.org

Written in a simple, straightforward style, this easy to follow action guide teaches you the most effective strategies for enabling you to get the sleep you want and need.

1995 14 pages
ISBN: 0-895294-75-3

Sandra C. Raymond, President & CEO
Mary Schwarz, COO
Seung-Ae Chung, CFO

7145 Immune System Disorders Sourcebook

Omnigraphics
PO Box 8002
Aston, PA 19014

800-234-1340
Fax: 800-875-1340
e-mail: info@omnigraphics.com
www.omnigraphics.com

Basic information about lupus, multiple sclerosis, guillain-barre syndrome and other disorders of the immune system.

671 pages 2nd Edition
ISBN: 0-780807-48-0

Peter Ruffner, Publisher

7146 Let's Talk About Going to the Hospital

Rosen Publishing Group's PowerKids Press
29 E 21st Street
New York, NY 10010

212-777-3017
800-237-9932
Fax: 888-436-4643
e-mail: rosenpub@tribeca.ios.com
www.rosenpublishing.com

If a child has to check into the hospital, chances are he or she is already upset about being ill. Knowing how a hospital functions and what the procedures are, such as when family members can visit, will help in what is already a stressful situation. Grades K-5.

24 pages
ISBN: 0-823950-36-0

Roger Rosen, President

7147 Loopy Lupus Helps Tell Scott's Story

Lupus Foundation of America
PO Box 932615
Atlanta, GA 31193

770-280-4177
866-484-3532
Fax: 770-442-9742
e-mail: orders@lupus.org
www.lupus.org

Written by a boy named Scott and his 3rd grade class explaining what it is like to live with lupus.

2002 34 pages Paperback

Sandra C. Raymond, President & CEO
Mary Schwarz, COO
Seung-Ae Chung, CFO

7148 Lupus Book

Daniel J Wallace MD, author

Lupus Foundation of America
PO Box 932615
Atlanta, GA 31193

770-280-4177
866-484-3532
Fax: 770-442-9742
e-mail: orders@lupus.org
www.lupus.org

Packed with useful, easy to understand information and practical guidance for people with lupus, their family members, friends and physicians. This hardcover book explains virtually every aspect of the disease and will help people better manage their day to day fight with lupus.

2005 271 pages 3rd Edition
ISBN: 0-195181-81-4

Sandra C. Raymond, President & CEO
Mary Schwarz, COO
Seung-Ae Chung, CFO

7149 Lupus Erythematosus: A Patient's Guide

Lupus Foundation of America
PO Box 932615
Atlanta, GA 31193

770-280-4177
866-484-3532
Fax: 770-442-9742
e-mail: orders@lupus.org
www.lupus.org

A popular LFA publication, the handbook provides a brief but detailed overview of the disease and guide for living well with lupus.

2000 27 pages

Sandra C. Raymond, President & CEO
Mary Schwarz, COO
Seung-Ae Chung, CFO

7150 Lupus Q&A: Everything You Need To Know
Lupus Foundation of America
PO Box 932615
Atlanta, GA 31193

770-280-4177
866-484-3532
Fax: 770-442-9742
e-mail: orders@lupus.org
www.lupus.org

Resource written for patients that want to learn more about lupus than what their doctors may or may not tell them.

2004 240 pages Paperback

Sandra C. Raymond, President & CEO
Mary Schwarz, COO
Seung-Ae Chung, CFO

7151 Sick and Tired of Feeling Sick and Tired
Lupus Foundation of America
PO Box 932615
Atlanta, GA 31193

770-280-4177
866-484-3532
Fax: 770-442-9742
e-mail: orders@lupus.org
www.lupus.org

Written in simple terms, the author offers understanding and practical guidance to people who live with ICI's and those who care for and about them.

2000 304 pages New Ed/ Paper
ISBN: 0-393320-65-0

Sandra C. Raymond, President & CEO
Mary Schwarz, COO
Seung-Ae Chung, CFO

7152 When Mom Gets Sick

Rebecca Samuels, author

Lupus Foundation of America
PO Box 932615
Atlanta, GA 31193

770-280-4177
866-484-3532
Fax: 770-442-9742
e-mail: orders@lupus.org
www.lupus.org

Written and illustrated by a nine-year-old, this is a compelling story based on the experiences of a sensitive and insightful young girl who makes the best from what could be a devastating situation.

27 pages

Sandra C. Raymond, President & CEO
Mary Schwarz, COO
Seung-Ae Chung, CFO

Magazines

7153 Lupus Now®
Lupus Foundation of America
2000 L Street NW, Suite 410
Washington, DC 20036

202-349-1155
800-558-0121
Fax: 202-349-1156
e-mail: info@lupus.org
www.lupus.org/newsite/

National and official magazine of the LFA. It includes lifestyle and wellness features and articles, research news, upcoming events, and other timely information for people with lupus, their families and health professionals.

48 pages 3x/year

Sandra C. Raymond, President/ CEO
Joan T. Merrill, MD, Medical Director
Seung-Ae Chung, CPA, Chief Financial Officer

Description

7154 TAY-SACHS DISEASE

Synonyms: GM2 gangliosidosis, type I, Hexa deficiency, Hexosaminidase A deficiency, Tay-Sachs disease, infantile type, TSD

Covers these related disorders: Tay-Sachs disease, juvenile type (GM2 gangliosidosis, type III)

Involves the following Biologic System(s):
Genetic/Chromosomal/Syndrome/Metabolic Disorders

Tay-Sachs disease, also known as GM2 gangliosidosis type I or infantile type, is a progressive degenerative metabolic disorder that occurs when two copies of the disease gene are inherited from the parents (autosomal recessive trait). The disorder, which belongs to a group of diseases known as lysosomal storage disorders, results from insufficient activity of the enzyme beta-hexosaminidase A. Enzymes within lysosomes, which are the major digestive units of cells, break down particles of nutrients such as certain fats and carbohydrates. In individuals with Tay-Sachs disease, insufficient activity of the enzyme hbeta-exosaminidase A causes an abnormal accumulation of particular fats (i.e., gangliosides) in certain tissues of the body, particularly nerve cells of the brain. Tay-Sachs disease affects approximately one in 3,500 to 4,000 newborns. The disease occurs predominantly in people of Ashkenazi Jewish (i.e., northeastern European Jewish) descent. About one in 30 individuals of Ashkenazi Jewish ancestry carries a single copy of the disease gene (heterozygous carrier).

Infants with Tay-Sachs disease appear to develop as expected until approximately four to six months of age, except for a marked startle reaction to sudden noises (hyperacusis) that may be apparent soon after birth. From four to six months of age, affected infants may begin to have decreased focusing and eye contact and appear listless and irritable. As the disease progresses, infants have delays in the acquisition of skills requiing the coordination of mental and physical activities (psychomotor delays) and lose previously acquired skills. By about one year of age, most affected children lose the ability to roll over, sit, stand, or vocalize sounds. In addition, muscle tone is severely diminished (hypotonia). With continuing disease progression, children experience increasing muscle rigidity and associated restrictions of movement (spasticity); uncontrolled electrical disturbances in the brain (seizures) that may be accompanied by prolonged contractions and relaxations of certain muscles (tonic-clonic convulsions); development of abnormal red circular areas of the middle layer of the eyes (cherry-red spots or Tay's sign); blindness; deafness; and loss of cognitive abilities (dementia). In many affected children, there is also enlargement of the brain (metabolic megalencephaly) due to abnormal accumulation of gangliosides in brain cells. Life-threatening complications often develop by approximately two to four years of age.

There are also variants of Tay-Sachs disease in which the onset of symptoms occurs later in life. For example, in children with the variant known as Tay-Sachs disease, juvenile type (GM2 gangliosidosis, type III), symptoms typically become apparent during mid-childhood although they may sometimes develop as early as the second year of life. This disease variant, which is characterized by varying levels of hexosaminidase deficiency, is also inherited as an autosomal rece|ssive trait. Associated symptoms may include progressive impairment of voluntary movements (ataxia); involuntary movements characterized by rapid, jerking or slow, repetitive, writhing movements (choreoathetosis); loss of speech; seizures; and visual loss. Patients may experience life-threatening complications by approximately 15 years of age.

The disease gene responsible for Tay-Sachs disease is located on the long arm of chromosome 15 (15q23-24). Several distinct changes (mutations) in this disease gene have been identified in individuals with Tay-Sachs disease. In addition, different mutations are responsible for the infantile and juvenile forms of the disorder. Tests have been developed to help confirm carrier status in individuals who may carry a single copy of the disease gene (e.g., serum or leukocyte hexosaminidase A testing). It is recommended that individuals of Askenazi Jewish descent obtain testing prior to starting a family. In addition, genetic counseling is provided for those individuals who are heterozygous carriers and desire to start a family or have additional children. Specialized testing is also available that may confirm a diagnosis of Tay-Sachs disease before birth (e.g., chorionic villus sampling). The treatment of infants and children with Tay-Sachs disease includes symptomatic and supportive measures. Even with the best of care, children with Tay-Sachs disease usually die by age 4, from recurring infection.

Government Agencies

7155 NIH/National Institute of Child Health and Human Development
31 Center Drive, Building 31
Bethesda, MD 20892
301-496-1333
Fax: 301-496-1104
www.nichd.nih.gov

Established in 1962 by congress, today the institute conducts and supports research on topics related to the health of children, adults, families and populations. Some of these topics include: developmental disabilities, growth and development, infant death, reproductive health and birth defects.

Jay H Hoofnagle, Director
Lisa Kaeser, Program & Public Liaison

7156 NIH/National Institute of Neurological Dis orders and Stroke (NINDS)
PO Box 5801
Bethesda, MD 20824
301-496-5751
800-352-9424
Fax: 301-496-0296
TTY: 301-468-5981
www.ninds.nih.gov

Works to reduce the burden of neurological disease by conducting, fostering, coordinating and guiding research on the causes, prevention, diagnosis and treatment of neurological disorders and stroke, while supporting basic research in related scientific areas.

Story C Landis Ph.D., Director
Audrey S Penn M.D., Deputy Director

National Associations & Support Groups

7157 American Academy of Pediatrics
141 Northwest Point Boulevard
Elk Grove Village, IL 60007
847-434-4000
800-433-9016
Fax: 847-434-8000
www.aap.org

The American Academy of Pediatrics and its member pediatricians are committed to the attainment of optimal physical, mental and social health and well-being for all infants, children, adolescents, and young adults.

Sandra Hassink, MD, FAAP, President

7158 Canadian Society for Mucopolysaccharid e & Related Diseases Inc
PO Box 30034, RPO Parkgate, North Vancouver
Britich Columbia,
Canada   604-924-5130
                                                   800-667-1846
                                              Fax: 604-924-5131
                                               www.mpssociety.ca

Committed to supporting families affected with MPS and related diseases, educating medical professionals and the general public about MPS and related diseases, and raising funds for research.

Kirsten Harkins, Executive Director

7159 Chicago Center for Jewish Genetic Disorder
Ben Gurion Way, 30 South Wells Street
Chicago, IL 60606   312-357-4718
                               e-mail: jewishgeneticsctr@juf.org
                                    www.jewishgeneticscenter.org

Provides public and professional education and to empower community members to seek out information and prevention strategies. Represents the blending of science with religious, cultural and historical sensitivity and awareness.

Karen Litwack, Director
Rachel Sacks, Community Outreach Coordinator

7160 Conner's Way Foundation for Tay-Sachs Dise ase
7746 Rockburn Drive
Ellicott City, MD 21043   410-379-0568
                                               www.connersway.com

Provides support for parents and families with Tay-Sachs disease. Also, provides fundraising events.

Desiree Hopf, Co-Chair
Carl Hopf, Co-Chair

7161 Genetic Alliance
4301 Connecticut Avenue NW
Washington, DC 20008   202-966-5557
                                                   800-336-4363
                                              Fax: 202-966-8553
                                 e-mail: info@geneticalliance.org
                                          www.geneticalliance.org

A coalition of voluntary genetic support groups, consumers and professionals addressing the needs of individuals and families affected by genetic disorders from a national perspective.

Sharon Terry, MA, President/CEO
Natasha Bonhomme, Vice President of Strategic Develop
Vaughn Edelson, Assistant Director of Health Commun

7162 Genetic Alliance, Inc
4301 Connecticut Avenue NW, Suite 404
Washington, DC 20008   202-966-5557
                                              Fax: 202-966-8553
                                 e-mail: info@geneticalliance.org
                                          www.geneticalliance.org

Dedicated to improving the quality of life for everyone living with genetic conditions. Provide accuracy organizations results in measurable growth: increased funding for research, access to services, and support for emerging technologies.

Sharon Terry, MA, President/CEO
Natasha Bonhomme, Vice President of Strategic Develop
Vaughn Edelson, Assistant Director of Health Commun

7163 Jewish Genetic Disease Consortium
450 West End Avenue
New York, NY 10024   855-642-6900
                                                   866-370-4363
                           e-mail: info@jewishgeneticdiseases.org
                                    www.jewishgeneticdiseases.org

Created as a means by which a number of smaller, individual organizations could join together to heighten awareness of Jewish genetic diseases with a strong and unified voice.

Randy Yudenfriend-Glaser, Chair
Richard N. Gladstein, Co-Chair

7164 March of Dimes Birth Defects Foundation
1275 Mamaroneck Avenue
White Plains, NY 10605   914-428-7100
                                              Fax: 914-428-8203
                                             www.marchofdimes.com

Mission is to improve the health of babies by preventing birth defects, premature birth, and infant mortality. Provide research, community services, education and advocacy to save babies' lives, to give all babies a fighting chance against the threats to their health: prematurity, birth defects, low birth weight.

Jennifer L Howse, President

7165 NIH/National Institute of Neurological Dis orders and Stroke (NINDS)
PO Box 5801
Bethesda, MD 20824   301-496-5751
                                                   800-352-9424
                                              Fax: 301-496-0296
                                              TTY: 301-468-5981
                                               www.ninds.nih.gov

Mission is to reduce the burden of neurological disease - a burden borne by every age group, by every segment of society, by people all over the world.

Walter J. Koroshetz, M.D., Acting Director
Alan L. Willard, Ph.D., Acting Deputy Director
Caroline Lewis, Executive Officer

7166 National Tay-Sachs and Allied Diseases Association
2001 Beacon Street, Suite 204
Boston, MA 2135   617-277-4463
                                                   800-906-8723
                                              Fax: 617-277-0134
                                         e-mail: info@ntsad.org
                                               www.ntsad.org

Direct, fund and promote research to develop treatments and cures; provide comprehensive support services to affected families and individuals; guide prevention, education, awareness and screening through effective grassroots collaborations with chapters and affiliates; lead advocacy efforts as the recognized authority for this family of genetic diseases.

Shari Ungerleider, President
Merle Adelman, Development
Sue Kahn, Executive Director

Web Sites

7167 Chicago Center for Jewish Genetic Disorder
www.jewishgeneticscenter.org

                               e-mail: jewishgeneticsctr@juf.org
                                    www.jewishgeneticscenter.org

Provides public and professional education and to empower community members to seek out information and prevention strategies.Represents the blending of science with religious, cultural and historical sensitivity and awareness.

7168 Genetic Alliance, Inc
4301 Connecticut Ave NW, Suite 404
Washington, DC 20008   202-966-5557
                                              Fax: 202-966-8553
                                 e-mail: info@geneticalliance.org
                                          www.geneticalliance.org

Dedicated to improving the quality of life for everyone living with genetic conditions. Provide accuracy organizations results in measurable growth: increased funding for research, access to services, and support for emerging technologies.

Sharon Terry, MA, President/ CEO
Natasha Bonhomme, VP, Strategic Development
Ruth Evans, Director of Accounting

7169 Health Answers
410 Horsham Road
Horsham, PA 19044
215-442-9010
e-mail: Michael.tague@healthanswers.com
www.healthanswers.com

HealthAnswers offers a breadth of services in medical education, sales force training, patient support solutions, professional promotion and consumer solutions.

Michael Tague, Managing Director

7170 Healthfinder
1101 Wootton Parkway
Rockville, MD 20852
e-mail: healthfinder@hhs.gov
www.healthfinder.gov

A key resource for finding the best government and nonprofit health and human services information on the internet. Links to carefully selected information and web sites from over 1,500 health-related organizations.

7171 Jewish Genetic Disease Consortium
450 West End Avenue
New York, NY 10024
855-642-6900
e-mail: info@JewishGeneticDiseases.org
www.jewishgeneticdiseases.org

Created as a means by which a number of smaller, individual organizations could join together to heighten awareness of Jewish genetic diseases with a strong and unified voice.

Randy Yudenfriend-Glaser, Chair
Richard N. Gladstein, Co-Chair
Shari Ungerleider, Project Coordinator

7172 March of Dimes Birth Defects Foundation
1275 Mamaroneck Avenue
White Plains, NY 10605
914-997-4488
www.marchofdimes.org

Mission is to improve the health of babies by preventing birth defects, premature birth, and infant mortality. Provide research, community services, education and advocacy to save babies' lives, to give all babies a fighting chance against the threats to their health: prematurity, birth defects, low birthweight.

7173 NIH/National Institute of Neurological Dis orders and Stroke (NINDS)
PO Box 5801
Bethesda, MD 20824
301-496-5751
800-352-9424
www.ninds.nih.gov

Mission is to reduce the burden of neuroligical disease - a burden borne by every age group, by every segment of society, by people all over the world.

Walter J. Koroshetz, M.D., Acting Director
Alan L. Willard, Ph.D., Acting Deputy Director
Caroline Lewis, Executive Officer

7174 National Tay-Sachs and Allied Disease Foundation
2001 Beacon Street, Suite 204
Boston, MA 2135
617-277-4463
800-906-8723
e-mail: info@ntsad.org
www.ntsad.org

Dedicated to the treatment and prevention of Tay-Sachs and related diseases, and to provide information and support services to individuals and families affected by these diseases through education, research, genetic screening, family services and advocacy.

Shari Ungerleider, President
Merle Adelman, Development
Sue Kahn, Executive Director

7175 Online Mendelian Inheritance in Man
www.omim.org

This database is a catalog of human genes and genetic disorders.

7176 The Canadian Society for Mucopolysaccharid e & Related Diseases Inc
PO Box 30034, RPO Parkgate, North Vancouver
British Columbia, BC V7
604-924-5130
800-667-1846
Fax: 604-924-5131
e-mail: info@mpssociety.ca
www.mpssociety.ca

Committed to supporting families affected with MPS and related diseases, educating medical professionals and the general public about MPS and related diseases, and raising funds for research.

Bernie Geiss, Chair
Jamie Myrah, Executive Director
Karen Saxvik, Executive Assistant

Book Publishers

7177 Home Care Book
National Tay-Sachs and Allied Diseases Association
2001 Beacon Street, Suite 204
Boston, MA 02135
617-277-4463
800-906-8723
Fax: 617-277-0134
e-mail: info@ntsad.org
www.ntsad.org

Written by parents for parents and professionals, a guide to caring for children with progressive neuological disorders at home.

Kevin Romer, President
Stuart Altman, Vice President
Jayne Gershkowitz, Vice President-Finance

7178 International Quality for Adult Tay-Sachs Carrier Testing
National Tay-Sachs and Allied Diseases Association
2001 Beacon Street, Room 204
Boston, MA 02135
617-277-4463
800-906-8723
Fax: 617-277-0134
e-mail: info@ntsad.org
www.ntsad.org

Kevin Romer, President
Stuart Altman, Vice President
Jayne Gershkowitz, Vice President-Finance

7179 Let's Talk About Going to the Hospital
Rosen Publishing Group's PowerKids Press
29 E 21st Street
New York, NY 10010
212-777-3017
800-237-9932
Fax: 888-436-4643
e-mail: rosenpub@tribeca.ios.com
www.rosenpublishing.com

If a child has to check into the hospital, chances are he or she is already upset about being ill. Knowing how a hospital functions and what the procedures are, such as when family members can visit, will help in what is already a stressful situation. Grades K-5.

24 pages
ISBN: 0-823950-36-0

Roger Rosen, President

7180 Lifting of Canavan's Carrier Testing Facilities
National Tay-Sachs and Allied Diseases Association
2001 Beacon Street, Room 204
Boston, MA 02135
617-277-4463
800-906-8723
Fax: 617-277-0134
e-mail: info@ntsad.org
www.ntsad.org

Kevin Romer, President
Stuart Altman, Vice President
Jayne Gershkowitz, Vice President-Finance

7181 Monograph on Canavan's Disease
National Tay-Sachs and Allied Diseases Association
2001 Beacon Street, Room 204
Boston, MA 02135

617-277-4463
800-906-8723
Fax: 617-277-0134
e-mail: info@ntsad.org
www.ntsad.org

Kevin Romer, President
Stuart Altman, Vice President
Jayne Gershkowitz, Vice President-Finance

7182 Tay-Sachs Disease
Rosen Publishing
29 East 21st Street
New York, NY 10010

212-777-3017
800-237-9932
Fax: 888-436-4643
e-mail: rosenpub@tribeca.ios.com
www.rosenpublishing.com

With colorful graphics and photographs, and a clear presentation of a tragic genetic disease, this title looks at gentic inheritance, dominant and recessive genes, and the carrier screening programs working to prevent Tay-Sachs.

6-12 64 pages 2007
ISBN: 1-404206-97-3

Roger Rosen, President

7183 Tay-Sachs Disease-A Bibliography, Medical Dictionary, & Annotated Research Guide
ICON Health Publications/ICON Group International
9606 Tierra Grande St., Suite 205
San Diego, CA 92126

Fax: 858-635-9414
e-mail: orders@icongroupbooks.com
www.icongrouponline.com

A 3-in-1 reference book that provides a complete medical dictionary covering hundreds of terms and expressions relationg to Tay-Sachs disease. Also gives extensive lists of bibliographic citations. Provides information to users on how to update their knowledge using various internet resources.

132 pages

7184 The Official Parent's Sourcebook on Tay-Sa chs Disease
ICON Health Publications/ICON Group International
9606 Tierra Grande St., Suite 205
San Diego, CA 92126

Fax: 858-635-9414
e-mail: orders@icongroupbooks.com
www.icongrouponline.com

A comprehensive manual for anyone interested in self-directed research on tay-Sachs. Fully referenced with ample Internet listings and glossary.

128 pages

Newsletters

7185 Breakthrough
National Tay-Sachs and Allied Diseases Association
2001 Beacon Street, Room 204
Boston, MA 2135

617-277-4463
800-906-8723
Fax: 617-277-0134
e-mail: info@ntsad.org
www.ntsad.org

Annual newsletter for friends and supporters that focuses on the latest advances in research, profiles of families and individuals helped by NTSAD and disease profiles.

Shari Ungerleider, President
Merle Adelman, Development
Sue Kahn, Executive Director

7186 The Connection
The Canadian MPS Society
PO Box 30034, RPO Parkgate, North Vancouver
British Columbia, BC V7
Canada

604-924-5130
800-667-1846
Fax: 604-924-5131
e-mail: info@mpssociety.ca
www.mpssociety.ca

Members only quarterly newsletter, a valuable resource filled with information on MPS-related news, including updates on new treatments and care options, current research and clinical trials, MPS-related events, and family news.

Bernie Geiss, Chair
Jamie Myrah, Executive Director
Karen Saxvik, Executive Assistant

Pamphlets

7187 Late Onset Tay-Sachs Fact Sheet
National Tay-Sachs and Allied Diseases Association
2001 Beacon Street, Room 204
Boston, MA 2135

617-277-4463
800-906-8723
Fax: 617-277-0134
e-mail: info@ntsad.org
www.ntsad.org

Quick reference information sheet on the chronic or late onset of Tay-Sachs is available for no charge.

Shari Ungerleider, President
Merle Adelman, Development
Sue Kahn, Executive Director

7188 Services to Families
National Tay-Sachs And Allied Diseases Association
2001 Beacon Street, Room 204
Boston, MA 2135

617-277-4463
800-906-8723
Fax: 617-277-0134
e-mail: info@ntsad.org
www.ntsad.org

Offers information on the Association parent peer groups, referrals and advocacy services to families and patients.

Shari Ungerleider, President
Merle Adelman, Development
Sue Kahn, Executive Director

7189 Tay-Sachs & Sandhoff Disease
The Canadian MPS Society
PO Box 30034, RPO Parkgate, North Vancouver
British Columbia, BC V7
Canada

604-924-5130
800-667-1846
Fax: 604-924-5131
e-mail: info@mpssociety.ca
www.mpssociety.ca

Bernie Geiss, Chair
Jamie Myrah, Executive Director
Karen Saxvik, Executive Assistant

7190 What Every Family Should Know
National Tay-Sachs & Allied Diseases Association
2001 Beacon Street, Room 204
Boston, MA 2135

617-277-4463
800-906-8723
Fax: 617-277-0134
e-mail: info@ntsad.org
www.ntsad.org

50 page booklet detailing lysosomal storage and leukodystrophy disorders, with sections on Tay-Sachs, Sandhoff, Niemann-Pick, Gaucher, Canavan, Fabry, Pompe, therapeutic approaches and unique disease table.

Shari Ungerleider, President
Merle Adelman, Development
Sue Kahn, Executive Director

7191 What is Tay-Sachs?

National Tay-Sachs and Allied Diseases Association
2001 Beacon Street, Room 204
Boston, MA 2135

617-277-4463
800-906-8723
Fax: 617-277-0134
e-mail: info@ntsad.org
www.ntsad.org

Informative educational pamphlet describing Infantile tay-Sachs, its inheritance and prevention is available for no charge.

Shari Ungerleider, President
Merle Adelman, Development
Sue Kahn, Executive Director

Description

7192 TELANGIECTASIA

Synonym: Telangiectasis

Covers these related disorders: Ataxia-telangiectasia (AT), Phlebectasia, Cutis marmorata, Hereditary hemorrhagic telangiectasia, Rendu-Osler-Weber disease, Spider Angioma

Involves the following Biologic System(s):

Dermatologic Disorders

Telangiectasia refers to the permanent widening or dilation of small blood vessels near the surface of the skin (superficial capillaries, arterioles, and venules). This results in the appearance of relatively small, red, well-defined skin lesions that have fine or coarse red lines or a spider-like network of red lesions that radiate from a central point (spider telangiectasia). Telangiectasias may develop as the result of an underlying disorder such as lupus erythematosus, dermatomyositis, rosacea, or psoriasis. These skin lesions may also result from exposure to sunlight, x-rays, or other forms of radiation.

Ataxia-telangiectasia (AT) is a rare, inherited, progressive disorder of the nervous system involving degenerative changes in the central nervous system along with defects in the immune system. AT is transmitted as an autosomal recessive trait and is characterized by the appearance during early childhood of telangiectasias involving the ears, face, the membranes that line the white outer coat of the eyes (bulbar conjunctiva), or other areas. Affected children are at risk for recurrent respiratory infections. Degeneration of the cerebellum, which is the part of the brain responsible for the regulation and coordination of voluntary movement and other vital functions, also occurs in children with AT.

Congenital generalized phlebectasia, sometimes called cutis marmorata telangiectatica congenita, is a benign telangiectasia that is apparent at birth and is characterized by red or purple-hued net-like lesions that may have a somewhat marbled appearance. These telangiectasias may be localized to an arm or leg or the trunk of the body; however, sometimes these skin lesions are more widely spread. In addition, the lesions may become more prominent with changes in outside temperature, crying, or exertion. This condition often resolves spontaneously by adolescence. Treatment is supportive.

Generalized essential telangiectasia is a rare condition that may affect children or adults and is characterized by the appearance of solitary or convergent patches of network-like telangiectasias. These lesions may appear on large but localized areas of the body such as the arms or legs or may sometimes involve or progress to the entire body. This disorder is limited to the skin with no health-associated irregularities. Treatment is supportive.

Hereditary benign telangiectasia is a rare, genetic disorder that is inherited as an autosomal dominant trait and is characterized by the appearance of telangiectasias on the skin of the face, arms, and upper portion of the trunk. This progressive disorder is limited to the skin.

Hereditary hemorrhagic telangiectasia, also called

Rendu-Osler-Weber disease, is an inherited disorder that is transmitted as an autosomal dominant trait and is characterized by recurrent nosebleeds and the development of small telangiectasias of the skin and mucous membranes. These lesions range in color from red to purple and most often appear on the face, lips, and the membranes of the nose and mouth. In addition, the gastrointestinal tract, genitourinary tract, liver, brain, lungs, throat, voice box (larynx), and the membrane that lines the eyelids and whites of the eyes (conjunctiva) may be involved. Because the affected blood vessels may be fragile, they often break resulting in bleeding or hemorrhage from the gastrointestinal and genitourinary tracts, lungs, mouth, and nose.

Spider angioma, sometimes called spider nevus, is a telangiectasia characterized by the central, elevated, red lesion that is surrounded by a radiating, spider-like network of small blood vessels. Although these types of telangiectasias are often associated with conditions in which levels of circulating estrogen are elevated (e.g., pregnancy and liver disease), spider angiomas may also occur in preschool and school-age children. These lesions usually appear on the face, ears, forearms, and hands and often resolve on their own. Treatment is directed toward the removal of persistent angiomas and may include various methods such as freezing with liquid nitrogen (cryotherapy), the use of electric current to promote coagulation (electrocoagulation), or certain laser techniques such as intensed pulse light using a specially constructed flash lamp and focusing optics.

Telangiectasias can result in naevus flammeus (port-wine stain), which is a flat birthmark on the head or neck that spontaneously regresses. A port-wine stain, if present, will grow proportionally with the child. There is a high association with Sturge-Weber syndrome, a nevus formation in the skin and is associated with glaucoma, meningeal angiomas, and mental retardation. Unilateral nevoid telangiectasia refers to the appearance of telangiectasias on one side of the body in conjunction with an increase in the levels of circulating estrogen. These lesions sometimes develop in adolescent girls when they begin menstruation. Pregnancy may also prompt their development. When apparent in men, telangiectasias are the result of circulating estrogen secondary to liver disease. If this condition results from pregnancy, the lesions often fade or resolve during the postpartum period. Chronic treatment with corticosteroids may also lead to telangiectasias.

Government Agencies

7193 NIH/National Institute of Arthritis and Mu sculoskeletal and Skin Diseases

1AMS Circle

Bethesda, MD 20892

301-402-4484
877-226-4267
Fax: 301-718-6366
TTY: 301-565-2966
e-mail: niamsinfo@mail.nih.gov
www.niams.nih.gov

The mission of the NIAMS, a part of the NIH, is to support research into the causes, treatment, and prevention of arthritis and musculoskeletal and skin diseases, the training of basic and clinical scientists to carry out this research, and the dissemination of information on research progress in these diseases.

Stephen I Katz MD PhD, Director
Robert H Carter MD, Deputy Director
Gahan Breithaupt, Assoc Dir for Mngmnt & Operations

National Associations & Support Groups

7194 American Academy of Dermatology (AAD)
PO Box 4014
Schaumburg, IL 60168
847-240-1280
866-503-7546
Fax: 847-240-1859
e-mail: mrc@aad.org
www.aad.org

Dedicated to achieving high quality dermatologic care for everyone which encompasses: responsiveness, unification and representation of the specialty, and excellence in patient care, education and research.

Brett M. Coldiron, MD, President
Elise A. Olsen, MD, VP
Suzanne M. Olbricht, MD, Secretary/Treasurer

7195 American Academy of Pediatrics
141 Northwest Point Boulevard
Elk Grove Village, IL 60007
847-434-4000
800-433-9016
Fax: 847-434-8000
www.aap.org

The American Academy of Pediatrics and its member pediatricians are committed to the attainment of optimal physical, mental and social health and well-being for all infants, children, adolescents, and young adults.

Sandra Hassink, MD, FAAP, President

7196 American Skin Association
6 East 43rd Street, 28th Floor
New York, NY 10017
212-889-4858
800-499-7546
Fax: 212-889-4959
e-mail: info@americanskin.org
www.americanskin.org

The American Skin Association is the only volunteer led health organization dedicated through research, education and advocacy to saving lives and alleviating human suffering caused by the full spectrum of skin disorders.

Philip G. Prioleau, MD, President
Kathleen Reichert, Executive Vice President
Ashley R. Jutchenko, Assistant Director

7197 Ataxia-Telangiectasia Children's Project
5300 W. Hillsboro Blvd., Suite 105
Coconut Creek, FL 33073
954-481-6611
800-543-5728
Fax: 954-725-1153
e-mail: info@atcp.org
www.atcp.org

A non-profit organization that raises funds to support and coordinate biomedical research projects, scientific conferences and a clinical center aimed at finding a cure for ataxia-telagiectasia, a lethal genetic disease that attacks children, causing progressive loss of muscle control, cancer and immune system problems.

Brad Margus, Founder
Vicki Margus, Founder
Jennifer Thornton, Executive Director

7198 Children's Hospital Boston
300 Longwood Avenue
Boston, MA 2115
617-355-6000
800-355-7944
TTY: 617-355-0443
www.childrenshospital.org

Mission is to provide the highest quality care; be the leading source of research and discovery; educate the next generation of leaders in child health and enhance the health and well-being of the children and families in our local community.

Sandra L. Fenwick, President/ CEO
Kevin Churchwell, MD, EVP, Health Affairs & COO
Naomi Fried, PhD, Chief Innovation Officer

7199 Hereditary Hemorrhagic Telangiectasia (HHT) Foundation International
PO Box 329
Monkton, MD 21111
410-357-9932
800-448-6389
Fax: 410-357-0655
e-mail: hhtinfo@curehht.org
curehht.org

Dedicated to increasing public and professional awareness and understanding of hereditary hemorrhagic telangiectasia (HHT). Supports ongoing medical research into the cause, prevention, and treatment of HHT; and offers a variety of materials including informational brochures and a quarterly newsletter.

Marianne Clancy, Executive Director

7200 NIH/National Institute of Neurological Dis orders and Stroke (NINDS)
PO Box 5801
Bethesda, MD 20824
301-496-5751
800-352-9424
Fax: 301-496-0296
TTY: 301-468-5981
www.ninds.nih.gov

Mission is to reduce the burden of neurological disease - a burden borne by every age group, by every segment of society, by people all over the world.

Walter J. Koroshetz, M.D., Acting Director
Alan L. Willard, Ph.D., Acting Deputy Director
Caroline Lewis, Executive Officer

7201 National Ataxia Foundation
2600 Fernbrook Lane Suite 119
Minneapolis, MN 55447
763-553-0020
Fax: 763-553-0167
e-mail: naf@ataxia.org
www.ataxia.org

Objectives of this organization are to make an early diagnosis of ataxia by locating all potential victims and encouraging them to have an examination, public information and professional education materials and basic research on the disease.

Charlene Danielson, President
Camille Daglio, Vice-President
Michael Parent, Executive Director

7202 Society for Pediatric Dermatology
8365 Keystone Crossing, Suite 107
Indianapolis, IN 46240
317-202-0224
Fax: 317-205-9481
e-mail: info@pedsderm.net
www.pedsderm.net

Objective is to promote, develop and advance education, research and care of skin disease in all pediatric age groups.

Kent Lindeman, CMP, Executive Director
Stephanie Garwood, MTA, Meeting Manager
Barbara Case, Accounting Manager

Web Sites

7203 American Academy of Dermatology (AAD)
PO Box 4014
Schaumburg, IL 60168
847-240-1280
866-503-7546
Fax: 847-240-1859
e-mail: mrc@aad.org
www.aad.org

Dedicated to achieving high quality dermatologic care for everyone which encompasses: responsiveness, unification and representation of the specialty, and excellence in pateint care, education and research.

Brett M. Coldiron, MD, President
Elise A. Olsen, MD, VP
Suzanne M. Olbricht, MD, Secretary/Treasurer

7204 American Skin Association
6 East 43rd Street, 28th Floor
New York, NY 10017

212-889-4858
800-499-7546
Fax: 212-889-4959
e-mail: info@americanskin.org
www.americanskin.org

The American Skin Association is the only volunteer led health organization dedicated through research, education and advocacy to saving lives and alleviating human suffering caused by the full spectrum of skin disorders.

Philip G. Prioleau, MD, President
Kathleen Reichert, Executive Vice President
Ashley R. Jutchenko, Assistant Director

7205 Ataxia-Telangiectasia Children's Project
5300 W. Hillsboro Blvd., Suite 105
Coconut Creek, FL 33073

954-481-6611
800-543-5728
Fax: 954-725-1153
e-mail: info@atcp.org
www.atcp.org

A non-profit organization that raises funds to support and coordinate biomedical research projects, scientific conferences and a clinical center aimed at finding a cure for ataxia-telagiectasia, a lethal genetic disease that attacks childre, causing progressive loss of muscle control, cancer and immune system problems.

Brad Margus, Founder
Vicki Margus, Founder
Jennifer Thornton, Executive Director

7206 Children's Hospital Boston
300 Longwood Avenue
Boston, MA 2115

617-355-6000
800-355-7944
www.childrenshospital.org

Mission is to provide the highest quality care; be the leading source of reseach and discovery; educate the next generation of leaders in child health and enhance the health and well-being of the children and families in our local community.

Sandra L. Fenwick, President/ CEO
Kevin Churchwell, MD, EVP, Health Affairs & COO
Naomi Fried, PhD, Chief Innovation Officer

7207 Hereditary Hemorrhagic Telangiectasia (HHT) Foundation International
PO Box 329
Monkton, MD 21111

410-357-9932
Fax: 410-357-0655
e-mail: hhtinfo@curehht.org
curehht.org

Dedicated to increasing public and professional awareness and understanding of hereditary hemorrhagic telangiectasia (HHT). Supports ongoing medical research into the cause, prevention, and treatment of HHT; and offers a variety of materials including informational brochures and a quarterly newsletter.

7208 NIH/National Institute of Neurological Dis orders and Stroke (NINDS)
PO Box 5801
Bethesda, MD 20824

301-496-5751
800-352-9424
www.ninds.nih.gov

Mission is to reduce the burden of neuroligical disease - a burden borne by every age group, by every segment of society, by people all over the world.

Walter J. Koroshetz, M.D., Acting Director
Alan L. Willard, Ph.D., Acting Deputy Director
Caroline Lewis, Executive Officer

7209 National Ataxia Foundation
2600 Fernbrook Lane Suite 119
Minneapolis, MN 55447

763-553-0020
Fax: 763-553-0167
e-mail: naf@ataxia.org
www.ataxia.org

Objectives of this organization are to make an early diagnosis of ataxia by locating all potential victims and encouraging them to have an examination, public information and professional education materials and basic research on the disease.

Charlene Danielson, President
Camille Daglio, Vice-President
Michael Parent, Executive Director

7210 Online Mendelian Inheritance in Man
www.omim.org

This database is a catalog of human genes and genetic disorders.

7211 Society for Pediatric Dermatology
8365 Keystone Crossing, Suite 107
Indianapolis, IN 46240

317-202-0224
Fax: 317-205-9481
e-mail: info@pedsderm.net
www.pedsderm.net

Objective is to promote, develop and advance education, research and care of skin disease in all pediatric age groups.

Kent Lindeman, CMP, Executive Director
Stephanie Garwood, MTA, Meeting Manager
Barbara Case, Accounting Manager

Newsletters

7212 Hereditary Hemorrhagic Telangiectasia Foundation International Newsletter
PO Box 329
Monkton, MD 21111

410-357-9932
800-448-6389
Fax: 410-357-0655
e-mail: hhtinfo@curehht.org
curehht.org

The Foundation is dedicated to increasing public and professional awareness and understanding of hereditary hemorrhagic telangiectasia (HHT). Supports ongoing medical research into the cause, prevention, and treatment of HHT.

Quarterly

Pamphlets

7213 Ataxia-Telangiectasia and Cancer Risk
5300 W. Hillsboro Blvd., Suite 105
Coconut Creek, FL 33073

954-481-6611
800-543-5728
Fax: 954-725-1153
e-mail: info@atcp.org
www.atcp.org

Brad Margus, Founder
Vicki Margus, Founder
Jennifer Thornton, Executive Director

7214 Ataxia-Telangiectasia and Estrogen Replace ment in Females
5300 W. Hillsboro Blvd., Suite 105
Coconut Creek, FL 33073

954-481-6611
800-543-5728
Fax: 954-725-1153
e-mail: info@atcp.org
www.atcp.org

Brad Margus, Founder
Vicki Margus, Founder
Jennifer Thornton, Executive Director

7215 Ataxia-Telangiectasia and Immune Function
5300 W. Hillsboro Blvd., Suite 105
Coconut Creek, FL 33073

954-481-6611
800-543-5728
Fax: 954-725-1153
e-mail: info@atcp.org
www.atcp.org

Brad Margus, Founder
Vicki Margus, Founder
Jennifer Thornton, Executive Director

7216 Ataxia-Telangiectasia and Swallowing Probl ems
5300 W. Hillsboro Blvd., Suite 105
Coconut Creek, FL 33073

954-481-6611
800-543-5728
Fax: 954-725-1153
e-mail: info@atcp.org
www.atcp.org

Brad Margus, Founder
Vicki Margus, Founder
Jennifer Thornton, Executive Director

7217 Ataxia-Telangiectasia and X-Rays
5300 W. Hillsboro Blvd., Suite 105
Coconut Creek, FL 33073

954-481-6611
800-543-5728
Fax: 954-725-1153
e-mail: info@atcp.org
www.atcp.org

Brad Margus, Founder
Vicki Margus, Founder
Jennifer Thornton, Executive Director

Description

7218 TETRALOGY OF FALLOT

Synonym: Fallot's syndrome

Involves the following Biologic System(s):

Cardiovascular Disorders

Tetralogy of Fallot is a combination of four specific heart malformations that are present at birth (congenital heart defects). Normally, oxygen-poor blood that returns from the body to the heart into the right upper chamber of the heart (right atrium), is pumped into the right lower chamber (right ventricle), and is then pumped into the pulmonary artery and on to the lungs, where the exchange of oxygen and carbon dioxide occurs. Oxygen-rich blood returns from the lungs to the heart via the left atrium, is pumped into the left ventricle, and is subsequently pumped into the major artery of the body (aorta) for circulation to the body's tissues. However, newborns with tetralogy of Fallot typically have four coexisting cardiac defects: i.e., (1) obstruction of the normal outflow of blood from the right ventricle due to abnormal narrowing (stenosis) of the opening between the right ventricle and the pulmonary artery (pulmonary stenosis); (2) an abnormal opening in the partition (septum) that separates the ventricles of the heart (ventricular septal defect or VSD); (3) displacement or override of the aorta, allowing oxygen-poor blood to flow directly from the right ventricle into the aorta; and (4) abnormal thickness of the right ventricle (right ventricular hypertrophy). Tetralogy of Fallot is thought to affect approximately one in 1,000 infants and children.

In patients with tetralogy of Fallot, the onset and severity of associated symptoms depend, in part, upon the degree of right ventricular outflow obstruction. Primary symptoms and findings in mild cases may be only a an unusual heart sound (murmur) heard through the stethoscope. In other cases, there may be a bluish discoloration of the skin and mucous membranes (cyanosis) due to decreased levels of oxygen in the blood; an insufficient supply of oxygen to bodily cells (hypoxia); and difficulties feeding. In infants with tetralogy of Fallot, cyanosis is typically most apparent in the nail beds of the fingers and toes and in the mucous membranes of the mouth and lips. In severe cases, cyanosis may be apparent soon after birth. In such newborns, pulmonary blood flow may primarily depend upon the fetal vascular channel that joins the pulmonary artery and the aorta (ductus arteriosus). Because this fetal vascular channel closes shortly after birth, severe cyanosis may develop within the first hours or days after birth. In other patients, cyanosis may not become apparent until later during the first year of life.

Some affected infants experience periodic attacks or spells during which cyanosis worsens (hypoxic or blue spells). During such hypoxic spells, patients may become restless and cyanotic; develop extreme shortness of breath; and potentially lose consciousness (syncope). Although the onset of these attacks is unpredictable, they may tend to occur after severe crying episodes or upon awakening (Tet spells). The duration of the spells may range from a few minutes to a few hours, and they should be considered life-threatening and an indication for surgical repair.

Tetralogy of Fallot may be diagnosed based upon a complete clinical examination and patient history, detection of distinc-tive heart murmurs, and various specialized tests (e.g., x-ray studies, echocardiogram, electrocardiogram, cardiac catheterization). Surgery is performed in the first year of life, and often in the first six months of life, depending upon the severity of right ventricular outflow obstruction. Corrective open-heart surgery patches the ventricular septal defect, and enlarges the opening between the pulmonary artery and right ventricle. In many cases, corrective open-heart surgery may be recommended during the neonatal or infant period to avoid the risk of cyanotic spells later in infancy. Before and after corrective open-heart surgery, patients may be susceptible to bacterial infection of certain areas of the heart (e.g., bacterial endocarditis). Therefore, patients should be provided with antibiotic medication (antibiotic prophylaxis) with dental visits and certain surgical procedures. Additional treatment is symptomatic and supportive.

Tetralogy of Fallot may occur as an isolated condition, with other congenital heart defects, or in some cases, in association with certain chromosomal abnormalities (e.g., DiGeorge syndrome — a partial gene deletion that results in heart defects, low calcium levels, and immune deficiency — and Down syndrome.) Prenatal factors associated with higher than normal risk for this condition include maternal rubella (German measles) or other viral illnesses during pregnancy, poor prenatal nutrition, maternal alcoholism, mother over 40 years old, and diabetes. Researchers indicate that, in some patients, tetralogy of Fallot may be due to the interaction of one or more genes v(22q11). As with patients that have undergone any heart surgery, antibiotic prophylaxis (prevention) is indicated during dental treatment in order to prevent infective endocarditis, inflammation of the heart's inner lining or the heart valves.

Government Agencies

7219 NIH/National Heart, Lung and Blood Institu te

National Institute of Health
31 Center Dr MSC 2486, Bldg 31, Room 5A52
Bethesda, MD 20892

301-592-8573
Fax: 240-629-3246
TTY: 240-629-3255
e-mail: NHLBIinfo@nhlbi.nih.gov
www.nhlbi.nih.gov

Primary responsibility of this organization is the scientific investigation of heart, blood vessel, lung and blood disorders. Oversees research, demonstration, prevention, education, control and training activities in these fields and emphasizes the prevention and control of heart diseases.

Gary H. Gibbons, M.D., Director
Nakela Cook, MD, MPH, Chief of Staff
Kathleen B. O'Sullivan, Executive Officer

7220 NIH/National Institute of Child Health and Human Development

31 Center Drive, Building 31, Building 31, Room 2A
Bethesda, MD 20892

301-496-1333
800-370-2943
Fax: 866-760-5947
TTY: 888-320-6942
e-mail: NICHDInformationResourceCenter@mail.nih.
www.nichd.nih.gov

Established in 1962 by congress, today the institute conducts and supports research on topics related to the health of children, adults, families and populations. Some of these topics include: developmental disabilities, growth and development, infant death, reproductive health and birth defects.

Alan E. Guttmacher, M.D., Director
Lisa Kaeser, Program Analyst
Lisa Williams Simons, Senior Research Assistant

National Associations & Support Groups

7221 American Academy of Pediatrics
141 Northwest Point Boulevard
Elk Grove Village, IL 60007
847-434-4000
800-433-9016
Fax: 847-434-8000
www.aap.org

The American Academy of Pediatrics and its member pediatricians are committed to the attainment of optimal physical, mental and social health and well-being for all infants, children, adolescents, and young adults.

Sandra Hassink, MD, FAAP, President

7222 American Heart Association
7272 Greenville Avenue
Dallas, TX 75231
214-373-6300
800-242-8721
Fax: 214-706-1341
e-mail: inquire@amhrt.org
www.heart.org

Supports research, education and community service programs with the objective of reducing premature death and disability from cardiovascular diseases and stroke; coordinates the efforts of health professionals, and others engaged in the fight against heart and circulatory disease.

Elliott Antman, President
Nancy Brown, CEO
Suzie Upton, Chief Development Officer

7223 Children's Hospital Boston
300 Longwood Avenue
Boston, MA 2115
617-355-6000
800-355-7944
TTY: 617-355-0443
www.childrenshospital.org

Mission is to provide the highest quality care; be the leading source of research and discovery; educate the next generation of leaders in child health and enhance the health and well-being of the children and families in our local community.

Sandra L. Fenwick, President/ CEO
Kevin Churchwell, MD, EVP, Health Affairs & COO
Naomi Fried, PhD, Chief Innovation Officer

7224 Congenital Heart Anomalies, Support, Education & Resources (CHASER)
2112 N Wilkins Road
Swanton, OH 43558
419-825-5575
Fax: 419-825-2880
e-mail: chaser@compuserve.com
www.csun.edu/~hcmth011/chaser/

National organization for support, education and resources for families and patients who deal with children born with congenital heart malformations.

Anita Myers, Executive Director

7225 Genetic Alliance
4301 Connecticut Ave NW, Suite 404
Washington, DC 20008
202-966-5557
800-336-4363
Fax: 202-966-8553
e-mail: info@geneticalliance.org
www.geneticalliance.org

A coalition of voluntary genetic support groups, consumers and professionals addressing the needs of individuals and families affected by genetic disorders from a national perspective.

Sharon Terry, MA, President/ CEO
Natasha Bonhomme, VP, Strategic Development
Ruth Evans, Director of Accounting

7226 Little Hearts
110 Court Street, Suite 3A, PO Box 171
Cromwell, CT 6416
860-635-0006
866-435-4673
e-mail: info@littlehearts.org
www.littlehearts.org

Provides support, resources, networking, and hope to families affected by congenital heart defects. Membership consists of families nationwide who have or are expecting a child with a congenital heart defect.

Lenore Cameron, Director

Web Sites

7227 American Heart Association
7272 Greenville Ave.
Dallas, TX 75231
800-242-8721
www.heart.org

Supports research, education and community service programs with the objective of reducing premature death and disability from cardiovascular diseases and stroke; coordinates the efforts of health professionals, and others engaged in the fight against heart and circulatory disease.

Elliott Antman, President
Nancy Brown, CEO
Suzie Upton, Chief Development Officer

7228 Children's Hospital Boston
300 Longwood Avenue
Boston, MA 2115
617-355-6000
800-355-7944
www.childrenshospital.org

Mission is to provide the highest quality care; be the leading source of reseach and discovery; educate the next generation of leaders in child health and enhance the health and well-being of the children and families in our local community.

Sandra L. Fenwick, President/ CEO
Kevin Churchwell, MD, EVP, Health Affairs & COO
Naomi Fried, PhD, Chief Innovation Officer

7229 Congenital Heart Anomalies, Support, Education & Resources (CHASER)
2112 N Wilkins Road
Swanton, OH 43558
419-825-5575
Fax: 419-825-2880
e-mail: chaser@compuserve.com
www.csun.edu/~hcmth011/chaser/

National organization for support, education and resources for families and patients who deal with children born with congenital heart malformations.

7230 Congenital Heart Information Network
www.tchin.org

An international organization that provides reliable information, support services and resources to families of children with congenital heart defects and acquired heart disease, adults with congenital heart defects, and the professionals who work with them.

7231 Little Hearts
P.O. BOX 171
Cromwell, CT 6416
860-635-0006
866-435-4673
www.littlehearts.org

Provides support, resources, networking, and hope to families affected by congenital heart defects. Membership consists of families nationwide who have or are expecting a child with a congenital heart defect.

7232 Southern Illinois University School of Medicine
PO Box 19639
Springfield, IL 62794
217-545-8000
800-342-5748
e-mail: admin@siuhealthcare.org
www.siumed.edu/peds/index.htm

The mission of SUI School of Medicine is to assist the people of central and southern Illinois in meeting their present and future health care needs through education, clinical service and research.

Book Publishers

7233 Congenital Disorders Sourcebook
Omnigraphics
PO Box 8002
Aston, PA 19014

800-234-1340
Fax: 800-875-1340
e-mail: info@omnigraphics.com
www.omnigraphics.com

Basic consumer health information on disorders aquired during
gestation, including spina bifida, hydrocephalus, cerebral palsy,
heart defects, craniofacial abnormalities and fetal alcohol
syndrome.

650 pages
ISBN: 0-780809-45-9

Peter Ruffner, Publisher

Description

7234 THALASSEMIAS

Covers these related disorders: Alpha-thalassemia,
Beta-thalassemia, Beta-thalassemia minor, Beta-thalassemia major
Involves the following Biologic System(s):
Genetic/Chromosomal/Syndrome/Metabolic Disorders,
Hematologic and Oncologic Disorders

The term thalassemia refers to a group of inherited blood disorders that includes the alpha-thalassemias and the more common beta-thalassemias. The thalassemias are characterized by the faulty production of hemoglobin, the protein that carries oxygen within the red blood cells. Hemoglobin is composed of two pairs of amino acid chains (globins), the alpha chains and the beta chains. The improper synthesis of hemoglobin is caused by a defect within the globin genes and results in abnormal, fragile red blood cells. Beta-thalassemia minor, a less severe form of the disease, is inherited when the defective gene is transmitted by one parent, while beta-thalassemia major is inherited through the defective genes of both parents.

A mild anemia is usually present in individuals with beta-thalassemia minor; however, it is not unusual for affected individuals to be symptom-free. Symptoms of beta-thalassemia major include fatigue; shortness of breath (dyspnea); and yellowing of the skin, eyes, and mucous membranes (jaundice). Other symptoms, usually associated with the premature destruction of red blood cells (hemolytic anemia) and subsequent release of iron, may include bronzed or freckled skin and enlargement of the spleen (splenomegaly). In severe cases, iron that gets deposited in the heart, liver, and pancreas may eventually lead to impaired function. In addition, extreme activity of the bone marrow may result in thickened and enlarged bones in the skull and face, while normal growth may be retarded.

Alpha-thalassemia, far less common than beta-thalassemia, ranges in severity from a carrier state with no symptoms to the most severe form that is incompatible with life. The severity of symptoms is dependent upon the level of alpha-chain involvement. The most severe form of alpha-thalassemia involves the complete absence of alpha-chain production.

Thalassemia patients vary a lot in their treatment needs depending on the severity of their anemia. Treatment for symptomatic thalassemias includes blood transfusion therapy to ensure normal growth. However, repeated blood transfusions may exacerbate iron deposition into the internal organs (hemosiderosis), necessitating treatment with iron-chelating drugs that increase iron excretion. Other treatment may include bone marrow transplantation.

Thalassemia is inherited as an autosomal recessive trait and is most prevalent among people living in or originating from the Mediterranean, the Middle East, and Southeast Asia. As with other genetically acquired disorders, aggressive birth screening and genetic counseling is recommended.

Government Agencies

7235 NIH/National Heart, Lung and Blood Institute
National Institute of Health
31 Center Dr MSC 2486, Bldg 31, Rm5A48
Bethesda, MD 20892　　　　301-592-8573
Fax: 301-592-8563
TTY: 240-629-3255
e-mail: NHLBIinfo@nhlbi.nih.gov
www.nhlbi.nih.gov

Primary responsibility of this organization is the scientific investigation of heart, blood vessel, lung and blood disorders. Oversees research, demonstration, prevention, education, control and training activities in these fields and emphasizes the prevention and control of heart diseases.
Gary H. Gibbons, M.D., Director
Charles Peterson, MD, MBA, Director, Blood Diseases/Resources

7236 NIH/National Institute of Arthritis and Musculoskeletal and Skin Diseases
1AMS Circle
Bethesda, MD 20892　　　　301-402-4484
877-226-4267
Fax: 301-718-6366
TDD: 301-565-2966
e-mail: niamsinfo@mail.nih.gov
www.niams.nih.gov

The mission of the NIAMS, a part of the NIH, is to support research into the causes, treatment, and prevention of arthritis and musculoskeletal and skin diseases, the training of basic and clinical scientists to carry out this research, and the dissemination of information on research progress in these diseases.
Stephen I Katz MD PhD, Director
Robert H Carter MD, Deputy Director
Gahan Breithaupt, Assoc Dir for Management & Operatio

7237 NIH/National Institute of Child Health and Human Development
31 Center Drive, Building 31
Bethesda, MD 20892　　　　301-496-1333
Fax: 301-496-1104
www.nichd.nih.gov

Established in 1962 by congress, today the institute conducts and supports research on topics related to the health of children, adults, families and populations. Some of these topics include: developmental disabilities, growth and development, infant death, reproductive health and birth defects.
Jay H Hoofnagle, Director
Lisa Kaeser, Program & Public Liaison

National Associations & Support Groups

7238 AHEPA Cooley's Anemia Foundation
1909 Q Street NW, Suite 500
Washington, DC 20009　　　　202-232-6300
Fax: 202-232-2140
e-mail: ahepa@ahepa.org
www.ahepa.org

Dedicated to advancing the treatment and cure of cooley's anemia, an inherited blood disorder. Provides information, referrals to local medical sources, medical supplies to people in need, and listings of informational materials available from the Foundation.
Basil Mossaidis, Executive Director
Patricia Farish, Controller
Phil Attey, Internet Strategist and Webmaster

7239 American Academy of Dermatology (AAD)
PO Box 4014
Schaumburg, IL 60168　　　　847-240-1280
866-503-7546
Fax: 847-240-1859
e-mail: mrc@aad.org
www.aad.org

Dedicated to achieving high quality dermatologic care for everyone which encompasses: responsiveness, unification and representation of the specialty, and excellence in patient care, education and research.

Stephen P Stone MD, President
William P Coleman III, MD, VP
David M Pariser MD, Secretary/Treasurer

7240 American Academy of Pediatrics
141 Northwest Point Boulevard
Elk Grove Village, IL 60007
847-434-4000
800-433-9016
Fax: 847-434-8000
www.aap.org

The American Academy of Pediatrics and its member pediatricians are committed to the attainment of optimal physical, mental and social health and well-being for all infants, children, adolescents, and young adults.

Sandra Hassink, MD, FAAP, President

7241 American Heart Association
7272 Greenville Avenue
Dallas, TX 75231
214-373-6300
800-242-8721
Fax: 214-706-1341
e-mail: inquire@amhrt.org
www.heart.org

Supports research, education and community service programs with the objective of reducing premature death and disability from cardiovascular diseases and stroke; coordinates the efforts of health professionals, and others engaged in the fight against heart and circulatory disease.

M Cass Wheeler, CEO

7242 American Skin Association
6 East 43rd Street, 28th Floor
New York, NY 10017
212-889-4858
800-499-7546
Fax: 212-889-4959
e-mail: info@americanskin.org
www.americanskin.org

The American Skin Association is the only volunteer led health organization dedicated through research, education and advocacy to saving lives and alleviating human suffering caused by the full spectrum of skin disorders.

Joyce Weidler, Manager
George W Hambrick, Jr, President/Founder
David R Bickers, MD, Executive VP

7243 Ataxia-Telangiectasia Children's Project
5300 W. Hillsboro Blvd., Suite 105
Coconut Creek, FL 33073
954-481-6611
800-543-5728
Fax: 954-725-1153
e-mail: info@atcp.org
www.atcp.org

A non-profit organization that raises funds to support and coordinate biomedical research projects, scientific conferences and a clinical center aimed at finding a cure for ataxia-telagiectasia, a lethal genetic disease that attacks children, causing progressive loss of muscle control, cancer and immune system problems.

Brad Margus, Founder
Vicki Margus, Founder

7244 Children's Blood Foundation
333 East 38th Street, Suite 380
New York, NY 10016
212-297-4336
Fax: 212-297-4340
e-mail: info@childrensbloodfoundation.org
www.childrensbloodfoundation.org

Mission is to support the comprehensive clinical care of children living with blood disorders; to foster research to help understand the causes of childhood blood disorders; and to sponsor the fellowship training of pediatricians of the subspecialty of pediatric hematology and oncology.

1952

John Calicchio, Chairman

7245 Children's Hospital Boston
300 Longwood Avenue
Boston, MA 02115
617-355-6000
617-355-6000
Fax: 800-355-7944
TTY: 617-730-0152
www.childrenshospital.org

Mission is to provide the highest quality care; be the leading source of research and discovery; educate the next generation of leaders in child health and enhance the health and well-being of the children and families in our local community.

Leslie M Higuchi, President & CEO
Sandra Fenwick, Chief Operating Officer

7246 Congenital Heart Anomalies, Support, Education & Resources (CHASER)
2112 N Wilkins Road
Swanton, OH 43558
419-825-5575
Fax: 419-825-2880
e-mail: chaser@compuserve.com
www.csun.edu/~hcmth011/chaser/chaser-news.html?

National organization for support, education and resources for families and patients who deal with children born with congenital heart malformations.

Anita Myers, Executive Director

7247 Cooley's Anemia Foundation
330 Seventh Avenue, #900
New York, NY 10001
212-279-8090
800-522-7222
Fax: 212-279-5999
e-mail: info@cooleysanemia.org
www.thalassemia.org

Advancing the treatment and cure for this fatal blood disease, enhancing the quality of life of patients and educating the medical profession, trait carriers and the public about Cooley's anemia/thalassemia major.

1954

Gina Cioffi Esq, National Executive Director

7248 Genetic Alliance
4301 Connecticut Avenue NW
Washington, DC 20008
202-966-5557
800-336-4363
Fax: 202-966-8553
e-mail: info@geneticalliance.org
www.geneticalliance.org

A coalition of voluntary genetic support groups, consumers and professionals addressing the needs of individuals and families affected by genetic disorders from a national perspective.

Sharon Terry, MA, President/CEO
Natasha Bonhomme, Vice President of Strategic Develop
Vaughn Edelson, Assistant Director of Health Commun

7249 Hereditary Hemorrhagic Telangiectasia (HHT) Foundation International
PO Box 329
Monkton, MD 21111
410-357-9932
800-448-6389
Fax: 410-357-9931
e-mail: hhtinfo@hht.org
www.hht.org

Dedicated to increasing public and professional awareness and understanding of hereditary hemorrhagic telangiectasia (HHT). Supports ongoing medical research into the cause, prevention, and treatment of HHT; and offers a variety of materials including informational brochures and a quarterly newsletter.

Marianne Clancy, Executive Director

7250 Little Hearts
110 Court Street, Suite 3A, PO Box 171
Cromwell, CT 06416
860-635-0006
866-435-4673
e-mail: info@littlehearts.org
www.littlehearts.org

Provides support, resources, networking, and hope to families affected by congenital heart defects. Membership consists of families nationwide who have or are expecting a child with a congenital heart defect.

Lenore Cameron, Director

7251 March of Dimes Birth Defects Foundation
1275 Mamaroneck Avenue
White Plains, NY 10605   914-428-7100
                          Fax: 914-428-8203
                          www.marchofdimes.com

Mission is to improve the health of babies by preventing birth defects, premature birth, and infant mortality. Provide research, community services, education and advocacy to save babies' lives, to give all babies a fighting chance against the threats to their health: prematurity, birth defects, low birth weight.

Jennifer L Howse, President

7252 NIH/National Institute of Neurological Dis orders and Stroke (NINDS)
PO Box 5801
Bethesda, MD 20824   301-496-5751
                          800-352-9424
                          Fax: 301-496-0296
                          TTY: 301-468-5981
                          www.ninds.nih.gov

Mission is to reduce the burden of neurological disease - a burden borne by every age group, by every segment of society, by people all over the world.

Story C. Landis Ph.D., Director
Walter J. Koroshetz M.D., Deputy Director

7253 National Ataxia Foundation
2600 Fernbrook Lane Suite 119
Minneapolis, MN 55447   763-553-0020
                          Fax: 763-553-0167
                          e-mail: naf@ataxia.org
                          www.ataxia.org

Objectives of this organization are to make an early diagnosis of ataxia by locating all potential victims and encouraging them to have an examination, public information and professional education materials and basic research on the disease.

Mike Parent, Executive Director

7254 National Tay-Sachs and Allied Diseases Association
2001 Beacon Street, Suite 204
Boston, MA 02135   617-277-4463
                          800-906-8723
                          Fax: 617-277-0134
                          e-mail: info@ntsad.org
                          www.ntsad.org

Direct, fund and promote research to develop treatments and cures; provide comprehensive support services to affected families and individuals; guide prevention, education, awareness and screening through effective grassroots collaborations with chapters and affiliates; lead advocacy efforts as the recognized authority for this family of genetic diseases.

Diana Pangonis, Executive Director

7255 Society for Pediatric Dermatology
8365 Keystone Crossing, Suite 107
Indianapolis, IN 46240   317-202-0224
                          Fax: 317-205-9481
                          e-mail: spd@hp-assoc.com
                          www.pedsderm.net

Objective is to promote, develop and advance education, research and care of skin disease in all pediatric age groups.

Kent Lindeman, Executive Director

7256 Thalassemias Action Group (TAG)
330 Seventh Avenue, #900
New York, NY 10001   800-522-7222
                          e-mail: tag@cooleysanmeia.org
                          www.studygroup.com

Started by a group of young adults who realized that by helping and sharing with each other, coping with the daily struggles of life with thalassemia was made a little easier.

1985
Jesal Kapasi, President

State Agencies & Support Groups

California

7257 Cooley's Anemia Foundation-California
2629 Foothill Boulevard, #319
La Crescenta, CA 91214   800-601-2821
                          e-mail: ca_chapter@hotmail.com
                          www.thalassemia.org

Robert Yamashita, President
Christine Giannamore, Coordinator

Georgia

7258 Cooley's Anemia Foundation-Buffalo Chapter
781 Eagle Crossing Drive
Lawrenceville, GA 30044   678-357-4021
                          Fax: 678-969-0367
                          e-mail: supermom2kids@earthlink.net
                          www.thalassemia.org

Tahseen Mahmood, President

Maryland

7259 Cooley's Anemia Foundation-Capital Area (DC, VA, MD)
15321 Peach Orchard Road
Silver Spring, MD 20905   301-989-8947
                          e-mail: cvitaliti@aol.com
                          www.thalassemia.org/get-involved/chapters/capitol-ch
Carl C Vitaliti, President

Massachusetts

7260 Cooley's Anemia Foundation-Massachusetts Chapter
44 Joseph Road
Newton, MA 02460   617-332-5952
                          e-mail: rvscomi@comcast.net
                          www.thalassemia.org/get-involved/chapters/massachuse
Rudi Viscomi, President

New York

7261 Cooley's Anemia Foundation - Staten Island
16 Dreyer Ave
Staten Island, NY 10314   718-761-5380
                          e-mail: streganonaterri@aol.com
                          www.thalassemia.org/get-involved/chapters/staten-isl
Terri DiFilippo, President

7262 Cooley's Anemia Foundation-Buffalo
135 Wellington Road
Buffalo, NY 14216   716-832-3055
                          www.thalassemia.org

Dennis Locurto, President

7263 Cooley's Anemia Foundation-Long Island/Bro oklyn Chapter
PO Box 190
Franklin Square, NY 11010   516-697-5310
                          Fax: 516-358-9101
                          e-mail: findacure.caf@gmail.com
                          www.thalassemia.org/get-involved/chapters/l-i-chapte
Thomas Rotolo, President

7264 Cooley's Anemia Foundation-Queens
157-26 9th Avenue
Beachurst, NY 11357   718-746-7677
                          Fax: 718-746-7678
                          e-mail: JohnPoPs55@aol.com
                          www.thalassemia.org/get-involved/chapters/queens-cha

Paul Tucci, President
Abbey Chakalis, Events Manager
John Mancino, Contact

7265 Cooley's Anemia Foundation-Suffolk Chapter
740 Smithtown Bypass #201
Smithtown, NY 11787   631-863-0532
                                             Fax: 631-863-0535
                            e-mail: darlene@suffolkcaf.com
                www.thalassemia.org/get-involved/chapters/suffolk-ch
Tony Laurino, Executive Director

7266 Cooley's Anemia Foundation-Westchester/Roc kland Chapter
3 Sammuel Purdy Lane
Katonah, NY 10536   914-232-1808
                            e-mail: anemia@optonline.net
                www.thalassemia.org/get-involved/chapters/westcheste
Peter Chieco, President
Janet Manning, Executive Director

Texas

7267 Cooley's Anemia Foundation - Texas
1004 Field Trail
Mesquite, TX 75150   214-324-6147
                                             Fax: 214-324-0612
                                             www.thalassemia.org

Mateen Shah, President

Conferences

7268 TAG Conference
Thalassemia Action Group
330 Seventh Avenue, #900
New York, NY 10001   800-522-7222
                                             Fax: 212-279-5999
                            e-mail: info@cooleysanemia.org
                                             www.cooleysanemia.org

Held annually around March-April, look at website for more information.

Anthony J. Viola, President
Gina Cioffi, Executive Director
Amy Celento, Vice President

Web Sites

7269 Children's Blood Foundation
www.childrensbloodfoundation.org

Mission is to support the comprehenisve clinical care of children living with blood disorders; to foster research to help understand the causes of childhood blood disorders; and to sponsor the fellowship training of pediatricians of the subspecialty of pediatric hematology and oncology.

7270 Children's Hospital Boston
300 Longwood Avenue
Boston, MA 2115   617-355-6000
                                                 800-355-7944
                                             www.childrenshospital.org

Mission is to provide the highest quality care; be the leading source of reseach and discovery; educate the next generation of leaders in child health and enhance the health and well-being of the children and families in our local community.

Sandra L. Fenwick, President/ CEO
Kevin Churchwell, MD, EVP, Health Affairs & COO
Naomi Fried, PhD, Chief Innovation Officer

7271 Cooley's Anemia Foundation
330 Seventh Avenue, #200
New York, NY 10001   800-522-7222
                                             Fax: 212-279-5999
                                             www.cooleysanemia.org

The only US-based voluntary health organization that aids in patient services, medical research, education and public information to fight thalassemia, a blood disease also known as Cooley's anemia. Members of CAF work alongside the Thalassemia Action Group (TAG) to provide national support, encouragement and friendship to other patients and families.

Anthony J. Viola, President
Gina Cioffi, Esq., National Executive Director
Eileen Scott, Patient Services Manager

7272 March of Dimes Birth Defects Foundation
1275 Mamaroneck Avenue
White Plains, NY 10605   914-997-4488
                                             www.marchofdimes.org

Mission is to improve the health of babies by preventing birth defects, premature birth, and infant mortality. Provide research, community services, education and advocacy to save babies' lives, to give all babies a fighting chance against the threats to their health: prematurity, birth defects, low birthweight.

7273 NIH/National Heart, Lung and Blood Institu te
31 Center Dr MSC 2486, Bldg 31, Room 5A52
Bethesda, MD 20892   301-592-8573
                            e-mail: NHLBIinfo@nhlbi.nih.gov
                                             www.nhlbi.nih.gov

Primary responsibility of this organization is the scientific investigation of heart, blood vessel, lung and blood disorders. Oversees research, demonstration, prevention, education, control and training activities in these fields and emphasizes the prevention and control of heart diseases.

Gary H. Gibbons, M.D., Director
Nakela Cook, MD, MPH, Chief of Staff
Kathleen B. O'Sullivan, Executive Officer

7274 Online Mendelian Inheritance in Man
www.omim.org

This database is a catalog of human genes and genetic disorders.

7275 Thalassemias Action Group (TAG)
330 Seventh Avenue, #200
New York, NY 10001   800-522-7222
                                             Fax: 212-279-5999
                                             www.cooleysanemia.org

Promotes positive attidtude toward life; stresses the importance of compliance and chelation therapy; and provides patients with a channel of communication and information.

Anthony J. Viola, President
Gina Cioffi, Esq., National Executive Director
Eileen Scott, Patient Services Manager

Book Publishers

7276 Blood & Circulatory Disorders Sourcebook
Omnigraphics
PO Box 8002
Aston, PA 19014   800-234-1340
                                             Fax: 800-875-1340
                            e-mail: info@omnigraphics.com
                                             www.omnigraphics.com

Basic consumer health information on blood and its components, anemias, leukemias, bleeding disorders, and circulatory disorders, including aplastic anemia, thalassemia, sickle-cell disease and hemophilia.

2005 659 pages
ISBN: 0-780807-46-4

Peter Ruffner, Publisher

7277 Coloring Book on Thalassemia
Cooley's Anemia Foundation
330 Seventh Avenue, #200
New York, NY 10001   212-279-8090
                                                 800-522-7222
                                             Fax: 212-279-5999
                            e-mail: info@cooleysanemia.org
                                             www.cooleysanemia.org

Available in English, Italian, Greek and Chinese.

Anthony J. Viola, President
Gina Cioffi, Executive Director
Amy Celento, Vice President

7278 Cooley's Anemia 7th Annual Symposium
Cooley's Anemia Foundation
330 Seventh Avenue, #200
New York, NY 10001   800-522-7222
                                       Fax: 212-279-5999
                                 e-mail: info@cooleysanemia.org
                                    www.cooleysanemia.org

Published by the New York Academy of Sources.
1997
Anthony J. Viola, President
Gina Cioffi, Executive Director
Amy Celento, Vice President

7279 Genes, Blood & Courage
Cooley's Anemia Foundation
330 Seventh Avenue, #200
New York, NY 10001   800-522-7222
                                       Fax: 212-279-5999
                                 e-mail: info@cooleysanemia.org
                                    www.cooleysanemia.org

Anthony J. Viola, President
Gina Cioffi, Executive Director
Amy Celento, Vice President

7280 Let's Talk About Going to the Hospital
Rosen Publishing Group's PowerKids Press
29 E 21st Street
New York, NY 10010   212-777-3017
                                            800-237-9932
                                       Fax: 888-436-4643
                              e-mail: rosenpub@tribeca.ios.com
                                    www.rosenpublishing.com

If a child has to check into the hospital, chances are he or she is
already upset about being ill. Knowing how a hospital functions
and what the procedures are, such as when family members can
visit, will help in what is already a stressful situation. Grades
K-5.
24 pages
ISBN: 0-823950-36-0

Roger Rosen, President

Newsletters

7281 CAF Medical Update
Cooley's Anemia Foundation
330 Seventh Avenue, #200
New York, NY 10001   800-522-7222
                                       Fax: 212-279-5999
                                 e-mail: info@cooleysanemia.org
                                    www.cooleysanemia.org

Medical information.
Biannual
Anthony J. Viola, President
Gina Cioffi, Esq., National Executive Director
Eileen Scott, Patient Services Manager

7282 Lifeline
Cooley's Anemia Foundation
330 Seventh Avenue, #200
New York, NY 10001   800-522-7222
                                       Fax: 212-279-5999
                                 e-mail: info@cooleysanemia.org
                                    www.cooleysanemia.org

Cooley's Anemia Foundation
Biannual
Anthony J. Viola, President
Gina Cioffi, Esq., National Executive Director
Eileen Scott, Patient Services Manager

7283 TAG Newsletter
Cooley's Anemia Foundation
330 Seventh Avenue, #200
New York, NY 10001   800-522-7222
                                       Fax: 212-279-5999
                                 e-mail: info@cooleysanemia.org
                                    www.cooleysanemia.org

Anthony J. Viola, President
Gina Cioffi, Esq., National Executive Director
Eileen Scott, Patient Services Manager

Pamphlets

7284 Cooley's Anemia Fact Cards
Cooley's Anemia Foundation
330 Seventh Avenue, #200
New York, NY 10001   800-522-7222
                                       Fax: 212-279-5999
                                 e-mail: info@cooleysanemia.org
                                    www.cooleysanemia.org

Anthony J. Viola, President
Gina Cioffi, Esq., National Executive Director
Eileen Scott, Patient Services Manager

7285 Cooley's Anemia Foundation (CAF) Pamphlet
Cooley's Anemia Foundation
330 Seventh Avenue, #200
New York, NY 10001   800-522-7222; Fax: 212-279-5999
                                 e-mail: info@cooleysanemia.org
                                    www.cooleysanemia.org
Anthony J. Viola, President
Gina Cioffi, Esq., National Executive Director
Eileen Scott, Patient Services Manager

7286 Desferal Q & A
Cooley's Anemia Foundation
330 Seventh Avenue, #200
New York, NY 10001   800-522-7222; Fax: 212-279-5999
                                 e-mail: info@cooleysanemia.org
                                    www.cooleysanemia.org

Guidelines for home infusion.
Anthony J. Viola, President
Gina Cioffi, Esq., National Executive Director
Eileen Scott, Patient Services Manager

7287 Sibling Donor Cord Blood Program Pamphlet
Cooley's Anemia Foundation
330 Seventh Avenue, #200
New York, NY 10001   800-522-7222; Fax: 212-279-5999
                                 e-mail: info@cooleysanemia.org
                                    www.cooleysanemia.org
Anthony J. Viola, President
Gina Cioffi, Esq., National Executive Director
Eileen Scott, Patient Services Manager

**7288 Thalassemia Action Group (TAG) Patient Sup port Group
Brochure**
Cooley's Anemia Foundation
330 Seventh Avenue, #200
New York, NY 10001   800-522-7222; Fax: 212-279-5999
                                 e-mail: info@cooleysanemia.org
                                    www.cooleysanemia.org
Anthony J. Viola, President
Gina Cioffi, Esq., National Executive Director
Eileen Scott, Patient Services Manager

7289 What is Thalassemia Trait?
Cooley's Anemia Foundation
330 Seventh Avenue, #200
New York, NY 10001   800-522-7222
                                       Fax: 212-279-5999
                                 e-mail: info@cooleysanemia.org
                                    www.cooleysanemia.org

This booklet offers information on the thalassemia trait.
Anthony J. Viola, President
Gina Cioffi, Esq., National Executive Director
Eileen Scott, Patient Services Manager

Description

7290 THROMBOCYTOPENIAS

Covers these related disorders: Idiopathic thrombocytopenia purpura (ITP)

Involves the following Biologic System(s):
Hematologic and Oncologic Disorders

Thrombocytopenia is a term that describes a condition in which the level of circulating platelets in the blood is reduced, resulting in a tendency to bleed. By changing shape and adhering to each other and the walls of broken blood vessels, platelets, also known as thrombocytes, play an essential role in the clotting process. Normal blood levels usually demonstrate 150,000 to 350,000 platelets per microliter. When the platelet count is reduced to 30,000 per microliter or lower, abnormal bleeding under the skin may occur and result in purple bruising or spots (purpura). Nosebleeds (epistaxis), bleeding of the gums , and blood in the urine (hematuria) are also common. Often, low platelet levels do not lead to clinical problems; rather, they are picked up on a routine full blood count.

Thrombocytopenia may result from a slowdown in platelet production or the rapid destruction of these cells. Certain diseases such as anemia, leukemia, lymphoma, bone marrow disorders, or autoimmune diseases may cause thrombocytopenia. Other causes include enlargement of the spleen (splenomegaly), cirrhosis, certain drugs, viral infection, and x-ray or radiation exposure.

The treatment of thrombocytopenia is based upon its underlying cause. For example, if the low platelet count is caused by a specific underlying disease, treatment is geared toward that disease. Low platelet counts caused by a specific drug necessitate the withdrawal of that drug. If bleeding is severe, platelet transfusions may be administered.

Idiopathic thrombocytopenia purpura (ITP) is a term used to describe thrombocytopenia of unknown origin. This condition often follows a viral infection and, in children, usually disappears within a month or so with no treatment. The duration of ITP in adolescents and adults is often more prolonged, and close medical follow up and avoidance of contact sports and activities is essential.

Government Agencies

7291 NIH/National Heart, Lung and Blood Institu te
National Institute of Health
31 Center Dr MSC 2486, Bldg 31, Room 5A48
Bethesda, MD 20892
301-592-8573
Fax: 301-592-8563
TTY: 240-629-3255
e-mail: NHLBIinfo@nhlbi.nih.gov
www.nhlbi.nih.gov

Primary responsibility of this organization is the scientific investigation of heart, blood vessel, lung and blood disorders. Oversees research, demonstration, prevention, education, control and training activities in these fields and emphasizes the prevention and control of heart diseases.

Gary H. Gibbons, M.D., Director
Susan Shurin, MD, Deputy Director
Sheila Pohl, Chief of Staff

National Associations & Support Groups

7292 American Academy of Pediatrics
141 Northwest Point Boulevard
Elk Grove Village, IL 60007
847-434-4000
800-433-9016
Fax: 847-434-8000
www.aap.org

The American Academy of Pediatrics and its member pediatricians are committed to the attainment of optimal physical, mental and social health and well-being for all infants, children, adolescents, and young adults.

Sandra Hassink, MD, FAAP, President

7293 American Heart Association
7272 Greenville Avenue
Dallas, TX 75231
214-373-6300
800-242-8721
Fax: 214-706-1341
e-mail: inquire@amhrt.org
www.heart.org/HEARTORG/

Our mission is to reduce disability and death from cardiovascular diseases and stroke. Parents will find education and support to you better care for a child with arrhythmias.

Nancy Brown, CEO
Suzie Upton, Chief Development Officer
Sunder Joshi, Chief Administrative Officer & CFO

7294 Children's Blood Foundation
333 East 38th Street, Suite 380
New York, NY 10016
212-297-4336
Fax: 212-297-4340
e-mail: info@childrenscbf.org
www.childrenscbf.org

Promotes the welfare of and addresses the issues that affect people with immune or idiopathic thrombocytopenic purpura. Goals are to provide patient support, ongoing medical research to advance the knowledge and treatment and educate the public and medical communities about the disorder. Provides educational and support materials including fact sheets, brochures, and a booklet entitled 'What's It Called Again?'

Les J. Lieberman, Chairman
Ronald J. Iervolino, President
Jennifer Zaleski, Executive Director

7295 Children's Hospital Boston
300 Longwood Avenue
Boston, MA 02115
617-355-6000
TTY: 617-730-0152
www.childrenshospital.org

Mission is to provide the highest quality care; be the leading source of research and discovery; educate the next generation of leaders in child health and enhance the health and well-being of the children and families in our local community.

Dr. James Mandell, CEO
Sandra Fenwick, President & COO
James Mandell, MD, Chief Executive Officer

7296 Genetic Alliance
4301 Connecticut Avenue NW, Suite 404
Washington, DC 20008
202-966-5557
800-336-4363
Fax: 202-966-8553
e-mail: info@geneticalliance.org
www.geneticalliance.org

A coalition of voluntary genetic support groups, consumers and professionals addressing the needs of individuals and families affected by genetic disorders from a national perspective.

Sharon Terry, MA, President/CEO
Natasha Bonhomme, Vice President of Strategic Develop
Vaughn Edelson, Assistant Director of Health Commun

7297 Platelet Disorder Support Association
33 Rollins Avenue, #5
Rockville, MD 20852
301-770-6636
877-528-3538
Fax: 301-770-6638
e-mail: pdsa@pdsa.org
www.itppeople.com

Our organization is devoted to bringing you the most timely, accurate and comprehensive information about ITP and assisting you in meeting others who share your interests.

Peter Pruitt, Board Chairman
Caroline Kruse, Executive Director
Marjorie Ligelis, Chief Financial Officer

Web Sites

7298 American Heart Association
7272 Greenville Ave.
Dallas, TX 75231
800-242-8721
www.heart.org

Our mission is to reduce disability and death from cardiovascular diseases and stroke. Parents will find education and support to you better care for a child with arrhythmias.

Elliott Antman, President
Nancy Brown, CEO
Suzie Upton, Chief Development Officer

7299 Children's Blood Foundation
www.childrensbloodfoundation.org

Promotes the welfare of and addresses the issues that affect people with immune or idiopathic thrombocytopenic purpura. Goals are to provide patient support, ongoing medical research to advance the knowledge and treatment and educate the public and medical communities about the disorder. Provides educational and support materials including fact sheets, brochures, and a booklet entitled 'What's It Called Again?'

7300 Children's Hospital Boston
300 Longwood Avenue
Boston, MA 2115
617-355-6000
800-355-7944
www.childrenshospital.org

Mission is to provide the highest quality care; be the leading source of reseach and discovery; educate the next generation of leaders in child health and enhance the health and well-being of the children and families in our local community.

Sandra L. Fenwick, President/ CEO
Kevin Churchwell, MD, EVP, Health Affairs & COO
Naomi Fried, PhD, Chief Innovation Officer

7301 Online Mendelian Inheritance in Man
www.omim.org

This database is a catalog of human genes and genetic disorders.

7302 Platelet Disorder Support Association
8751 Brecksville Road, Suite 150
Cleveland, OH 44141
440-746-9003
877-528-3538
Fax: 844-270-1277
e-mail: pdsa@pdsa.org
www.pdsa.org

Our organization is devoted to bringing you the most timely, accurate and comprehensive information about ITP and assisting you in meeting others who share your interests.

Caroline Kruse, Executive Director
Marjorie Ligelis, Chief Financial Officer
Nancy Potthast, Director of Marketing

Book Publishers

7303 Harrison's Principles of Inernal Medicine 15th Edition
McGraw-Hill
PO Box 182605
Columbus, OH 43218
800-338-3987
Fax: 609-308-4480
e-mail: customer.service@mheducation.com
www.mcgraw-hill.com

Raises the bar for internal medicine references. Features over 90 new chapters, Harrison's continues to provide authoritative record of internal medicine as practiced by the leading experts in the field.

Lloyd G. Waterhouse, President & CEO
Patrick Milano, CFO
David Stafford, Senior Vice President

7304 Let's Talk About Going to the Hospital
Rosen Publishing Group's PowerKids Press
29 E 21st Street
New York, NY 10010
212-777-3017
800-237-9932
Fax: 888-436-4643
e-mail: rosenpub@tribeca.ios.com
www.rosenpublishing.com

If a child has to check into the hospital, chances are he or she is already upset about being ill. Knowing how a hospital functions and what the procedures are, such as when family members can visit, will help in what is already a stressful situation. Grades K-5.

24 pages
ISBN: 0-823950-36-0

Roger Rosen, President

Description

7305 THUMBSUCKING

Involves the following Biologic System(s):

Developmental/Behavioral/Psychiatric Disorders

Thumbsucking is a common habit that is prevalent among infants and young children. This behavior is usually used as a device for providing pleasure, amusement, comfort, oral gratification, and release of stress or tension. Sometimes a security object, such as a blanket, may become part of the thumbsucking habit. In most children, thumbsucking reaches a plateau between the ages of 18 months to two years and then slowly but steadily decreases until it disappears at about five to six years of age. One reason to encourage children to give up the habit before they enter school is to prevent the teasing they would otherwise receive. By adolescence, most normal children abandon thumbsucking because of peer pressure.

Although it is generally thought that thumbsucking does not cause any long-term developmental irregularities, thumbsucking that continues beyond age six may lead to acquired problems with the bones and tissues of the thumb and an abnormal bite or contact pattern between upper and lower teeth (malocclusion). The longer the habit persists, the more likely affected children are to develop these types of problems. Conversely, the earlier this habit comes to an end, the more likely that irregular positioning of the teeth will improve without intervention.

Many physicians agree that, as a general rule, the best treatment for thumbsucking is to ignore the behavior and wait patiently for the children to outgrow the habit or to discontinue the behavior on their own. Treatment is generally supportive as punishing or reprimanding often adds to stress levels, becomes a power struggle with the parent, and may actually worsen the problem. Other treatment may include the use of certain appliances that are fitted with small projections that alert children to their behavior when they attempt to suck their thumbs. Older children may require the use of orthodontic appliances to correct irregularities associated with malocclusion.

Government Agencies

7306 NIH/National Institute of Dental and Cranifacial Research (NIHDCR)

National Institutes of Health
31 Center Drive, MSC 2290, Building 31
Bethesda, MD 20892
301-496-4261
Fax: 301-402-2185
e-mail: nidcrinfo@mail.nih.gov
www.nidcr.nih.gov

The mission is to promote the general health of American people by improving their oral, dental and craniofacial health. Through the conduct and support of research and training of researchers, the NIDCR aims to promote health, prevent diseases and conditions, and develop new diagnostic and therapeutics.

Dr Lawrence A Tabak, Director
Thomas G Murphy, Acting Executive Director

7307 National Oral Health Information Clearinghouse

1 NOHIC Way
Bethesda, MD 20892
301-402-7364
866-232-4528
Fax: 301-480-4098
e-mail: nidcrinfo@mail.nih.gov
www.nidcr.nih.gov

Produces and distributes patient and professional education materials including fact sheets, brochures, information packets and provides referrals to other organizations dealing with special care in oral health. Special care is an approach to oral health management that is tailored to the specific needs of persons with a variety of medical, disabling or mental conditions.

National Associations & Support Groups

7308 American Academy of Pediatrics

141 Northwest Point Boulevard
Elk Grove Village, IL 60007
847-434-4000
800-433-9016
Fax: 847-434-8000
www.aap.org

The American Academy of Pediatrics and its member pediatricians are committed to the attainment of optimal physical, mental and social health and well-being for all infants, children, adolescents, and young adults.

Sandra Hassink, MD, FAAP, President

7309 American Dental Association

211 East Chicago Avenue
Chiacgo, IL 60611
312-266-7255
Fax: 312-266-9867
www.aae.org

Committed to the public's oral health, ethics, science and professional advancement; leading a unified profession through initiatives in advocacy, education, research and the development of standards.

James Drinan, Executive Director

7310 C.S. Mott Children's Hospital

1540 East Hospital Drive
Ann Arbor, MI 48109
734-936-4000
www.mottchildren.org

Provides information on how to handle a child's thumb sucking. Why they do it; how long it will last; how to help overcome the issue?

7311 Children's Hospital Boston

300 Longwood Avenue
Boston, MA 02115
617-355-6000
TTY: 617-730-0152
www.childrenshospital.org

Mission is to provide the highest quality care; be the leading source of research and discovery; educate the next generation of leaders in child health and enhance the health and well-being of the children and families in our local community.

Leslie M Higuchi, President & CEO
Sandra Fenwick, Chief Operating Officer

Web Sites

7312 American Dental Association

211 East Chicago Ave.
Chicago, IL 60611
312-440-2500
e-mail: affiliates@ada.org
www.ada.org

Committed to the public's oral health, ethics, science and professional advancement; leading a unified profession through initiatives in advocacy, education, research and the development of standards.

Dr. Maxine Feinberg, President
Dr. Carol Gomez Summerhays, President-Elect
Dr. Kathleen T. O'Loughlin, Executive Director

7313 C.S. Mott Children's Hospital
1540 East Hospital Drive
Ann Arbor, MI 48109   734-936-6641
e-mail: mottchildren@umich.edu
www.mottchildren.org

Provides information on how to handle a child's thumbsucking.
Why they do it; how long it will last; how to help overcome the
issue?

Paul King, Executive Director
John M. Park, M.D., Associate Professor
Chris Dickinson, Chief Medical Officer

7314 Children's Hospital Boston
300 Longwood Avenue
Boston, MA 2115   617-355-6000
800-355-7944
www.childrenshospital.org

Mission is to provide the highest quality care; be the leading
source of reseach and discovery; educate the next generation of
leaders in child health and enhance the health and well-being of
the children and families in our local community.

Sandra L. Fenwick, President/ CEO
Kevin Churchwell, MD, EVP, Health Affairs & COO
Naomi Fried, PhD, Chief Innovation Officer

**7315 NIH/National Institute of Dental and Crani ofacial Research
(NIHDCR)**
Bethesda, MD 20892   301-496-4261
866-232-4528
Fax: 301-480-4098
e-mail: nidcrinfo@mail.nih.gov
www.nidcr.nih.gov

The mission is to promote the general health of American people
by improving their oral, dental and craniofacial health. Through
the conduct and support of research and training of researchers,
the NIDCR aims to promote health, prevent diseases and conditions, and develop new diagnostic and therapeutics.

Martha J. Somerman, DDS, PhD, Director
Kathleen G. Stephan, Executive Officer
Michelle A. Culp, Director

7316 National Oral Health Information Clearinghouse
Bethesda, MD 20892   301-496-4261
866-232-4528
Fax: 301-480-4098
e-mail: nidcrinfo@mail.nih.gov
www.nidcr.nih.gov

Produces and distributes patient and professional education materials including fact sheets, brochures, information packets and
provides referrals to other organizations dealing with special care
in oral health. Special care is an approach to oral health management that is tailored to the specific needs of persons with a variety of medical, disabling or mental conditions.

Martha J. Somerman, DDS, PhD, Director
Kathleen G. Stephan, Executive Officer
Michelle A. Culp, Director

Pamphlets

7317 A Healthy Mouth for Your Baby
National Oral Health Information Clearinghouse
1 NOHIC Way
Bethesda, MD 20892   301-496-4261
866-232-4528
Fax: 301-480-4098
e-mail: nidcrinfo@mail.nih.gov
www.nidcr.nih.gov

Martha J. Somerman, DDS, PhD, Director
Kathleen G. Stephan, Executive Officer
Michelle A. Culp, Director

7318 Seal Out Tooth Decay
National Oral Health Information Clearinghouse
1 NOHIC Way
Bethesda, MD 20892   301-496-4261
866-232-4528
Fax: 301-480-4098
e-mail: nidcrinfo@mail.nih.gov
www.nidcr.nih.gov

Martha J. Somerman, DDS, PhD, Director
Kathleen G. Stephan, Executive Officer
Michelle A. Culp, Director

Description

7319 TICS

Covers these related disorders: Chronic motor tic disorder, Tourette syndrome, Transient tics of childhood
Involves the following Biologic System(s):
Neurologic Disorders

Tics are repetitive or stereotypical, compulsive, abrupt (spasmodic) movements of a muscle or muscle groups. Although any muscle may be affected, tics most commonly involve muscles of the eyes, face, neck, or shoulders. Movements may include blinking, sniffing, facial grimacing, lip smacking, tongue thrusting, or shoulder shrugging. Tics may begin as intentional movements to relieve perceived tension. However, they may rapidly become unintentional or involuntary in nature. Although tics are extremely difficult to suppress, most patients are able to do so for short periods. Tics are often worsened by stress or any perceived attention to the condition; in contrast, they typically disappear during sleep.

In most patients, tics become apparent between approximately five to 10 years of age. According to some estimates, as many as 25 percent of children may be affected. Most children may experience a spontaneous disappearance of tics within a few weeks or less than one year after onset. In such patients, the condition is referred to as transient tics of childhood. Supportive measures that may be helpful in alleviating transient tics include providing children with a tranquil environment as well as additional rest.

Some children may experience chronic motor tics that persist throughout adult life. In such patients, the condition is known as chronic motor tic disorder. Chronic motor tics may simultaneously affect muscles in up to three different muscle groups.

In contrast to transient tics of childhood and chronic motor tics, which are considered relatively benign, restricted tic disorders, a genetic, neurologic disorder known as Tourette syndrome is characterized by multiple, chronic, complex tics. Tourette syndrome usually becomes apparent in children between the ages of two to 14 years. Initial symptoms typically include motor tics of the face, eyelids, shoulders, and neck. Movements may include grimacing, excessive eye blinking, or stretching of the neck. Vocal (phonic) tics, such as involuntary coughing, grunting, barking, or throat clearing, are also common. Additional symptoms may include involuntary repetition of obscene words (coprolalia) or words spoken by other individuals (echolalia); aggressive behaviors; the performance of repetitive actions or impulses in response to recurrent, persistent thoughts (obsessive-compulsive behaviors); and secondary learning, emotional, or social difficulties. Researchers suggest that variable expression of the disease gene responsible for Tourette syndrome may cause transient tics of childhood or chronic motor tics in other individuals, indicating possible overlap between the conditions. Several studies have demonstrated that immediate (first-degree) relatives of patients with Tourette syndrome have an increased frequency of such tic conditions.

In some patients with severe chronic motor tic disorder, treatment may include therapy with certain medications (e.g., certain benzodiazepines or haloperidol). The treatment of

Tourette syndrome is symptomatic and supportive and may include therapy with certain medications, such as haloperidol, pimozide, clonidine, clonazepam, or carbamazepine. In addition, for those with learning, behavioral, and social difficulties, multidisciplinary management and the provision of special social, academic, and vocational services may be important in helping patients achieve their potential. (Please refer to the section entitled Tourette Syndrome for further information on this disorder.)

Government Agencies

7320 NIH/National Institute of Neurological Disorders and Stroke (NINDS)
PO Box 5801
Bethesda, MD 20824
301-496-5751
800-352-9424
Fax: 301-496-0296
TTY: 301-468-5981
www.ninds.nih.gov

Works to reduce the burden of neurological disease by conducting, fostering, coordinating and guiding research on the causes, prevention, diagnosis and treatment of neurological disorders and stroke, while supporting basic research in related scientific areas.
Story C Landis Ph.D., Director
Audrey S Penn M.D., Deputy Director

National Associations & Support Groups

7321 American Academy of Child & Adolescent Psychiatry
3615 Wisconsin Avenue NW
Washington, DC 20016
202-966-7300
Fax: 202-966-2891
e-mail: clinical@aacap.org
www.aacap.org

Mission is to promote mentally healthy children, adolescents and families through research, training, advocacy, prevention, comprehensive diagnosis and treatment, peer support and collaboration.
Elizabeth Hughes, Asst. Director of Education & Recer
Quentin Bernhard III, CME Coordinator
Alan Ezagui, Deputy Director of Development

7322 American Academy of Pediatrics
141 Northwest Point Boulevard
Elk Grove Village, IL 60007
847-434-4000
800-433-9016
Fax: 847-434-8000
www.aap.org

The American Academy of Pediatrics and its member pediatricians are committed to the attainment of optimal physical, mental and social health and well-being for all infants, children, adolescents, and young adults.
Sandra Hassink, MD, FAAP, President

7323 American School Counselor Association
1101 King Street, Suite 310
Alexandria, VA 22314
703-683-2722
800-306-4722
Fax: 703-997-7572
e-mail: asca@schoolcounselor.org
www.schoolcounselor.org

The mission of ASCA is to represent professional school counselors and to promote professionalism and ethical practices.
Richard Wong, Executive Director
Jeff Broderson, Information Technology Admin.
Kathleen M Rakestraw, Director of Communications

7324 Genetic Alliance
4301 Connecticut Avenue NW
Washington, DC 20008
202-966-7955
800-336-4363
Fax: 202-966-8553
e-mail: info@geneticalliance.org
www.geneticalliance.org

A coalition of voluntary genetic support groups, consumers and professionals addressing the needs of individuals and families affected by genetic disorders from a national perspective.

Sharon Terry, MA, President/CEO
Natasha Bonhomme, Vice President of Strategic Develop
Vaughn Edelson, Assistant Director of Health Commun

7325 NADD: National Association for the Dually Diagnosed
132 Fair Street
Kingston, NY 12401
845-331-4336
800-331-5362
Fax: 845-331-4569
e-mail: info@thenadd.org
www.thenadd.org

Nonprofit organization designed to promote the interests of professional and parent development with resources for individuals who have the coexistence of mental illness and mental retardation. Provides conferences, educational services and training materials to professionals, parents, concerned citizens and service organizations.

Dr Robert Fletcher, CEO

7326 WE MOVE (Worldwide Education and Advocacy for Movement Disorders)
5731 Mosholu Avenue
Bronx, NY 10024
212-875-8312
800-437-6682
Fax: 212-875-8389
e-mail: wemove@wemove.org
www.wemove.org

Provides movement disorder information and education materials to physicians, patients, the media and the public via its comprehensive web sites, training courses, and more. It's goal is to make early diagnosis, up-to-date treatment and patient support a reality for all people living with movement disorders.

Susan Bressman, President
Mo Moadeli, Vice President
Wendy Borow-Johnson, Secretary

Audio Video

7327 Dakota
Tourette Syndrome Association
42-40 Bell Boulevard
Bayside, NY 11361
718-224-2999
888-486-8738
Fax: 718-279-9596
e-mail: ts@tsa-usa.org
tsa-usa.org

A happy eleven year old baseball playing, video game whiz, Dakota is diagnosed with Tourette's Syndrome and ADHD.

7 minutes

7328 Family Life with Tourette Syndrome... Personal Stories
Tourette Syndrome Association
42-40 Bell Boulevard
Bayside, NY 11361
718-224-2999
888-486-8738
Fax: 718-279-9596
e-mail: ts@tsa-usa.org
tsa-usa.org

In extended, in-depth interviews, all the people engagingly profiled in After the Diagnosis...The Next Steps, reveal the individual ways they developed to deal with TS. Each shows us that the key to leading a successful life in spite of having TS, is having a loving, supportive network of family and friends. Available in its entirety or as separate vignettes.

58 minutes

7329 Ryan
Tourette Syndrome Association
42-40 Bell Boulevard
Bayside, NY 11361
718-224-2999
888-486-8738
Fax: 718-279-9596
e-mail: ts@tsa-usa.org
tsa-usa.org

Ryan's family first thought his behavior was a deliberate way to get attention, lateer educate themselves and others about Ryan's Tourette's Syndrome.

11 minutes

7330 The Turners
Tourette Syndrome Association
42-40 Bell Boulevard
Bayside, NY 11361
718-224-2999
888-486-8738
Fax: 718-279-9596
e-mail: ts@tsa-usa.org
tsa-usa.org

Three of the four Turner daughters have Tourette's Syndrome in varying degress.

12 minutes

Web Sites

7331 American Academy of Child & Adolescent Psychiatry
3615 Wisconsin Avenue, N.W.
Washington, DC 20016
202-966-7300
Fax: 202-966-2891
e-mail: communications@aacap.org
www.aacap.org

Mission is to promote mentally healthy children, adolescents and families through research, training, advocacy, prevention, comprehensive diagnosis and treatment, peer support and collaboration.

Paramjit T. Joshi, M.D., President
Gregory K. Fritz, M.D., President-Elect
Aradhana Sood, M.D., Secretary

7332 NADD: National Association for the Dually Diagnosed
132 Fair Street
Kingston, NY 12401
845-331-4336
800-331-5362
Fax: 845-331-4569
e-mail: info@thenadd.org
www.thenadd.org

Nonprofit organization designed to promote the interests of professional and care providers for individuals who have the coexistence of mental illness and mental retardation. NADD provides conferences, educational services and training materials to professionals, parents, concerned citizens and service organizations.

Robert J. Fletcher DSW, Chief Executive Officer
Donna McNelis, Ph.D., President
Dan Baker, Ph.d., Vice President

7333 NIH/National Institute of Neurological Dis orders and Stroke (NINDS)
PO Box 5801
Bethesda, MD 20824
301-496-5751
800-352-9424
www.ninds.nih.gov

Works to reduce the burden of neurological disease by conducting, fostering, coordinating and guiding research on the causes, prevention, diagnosis and treatment of neurological disorders and stroke, while supporting basic research in related scientific areas.

Walter J. Koroshetz, M.D., Acting Director
Alan L. Willard, Ph.D., Acting Deputy Director
Caroline Lewis, Executive Officer

7334 Online Mendelian Inheritance in Man
www.omim.org

This database is a catalog of human genes and genetic disorders.

7335 Parents Helping Parents
Sobrato Center For Nonprofits-San Jose, 1400 Parkm
San Jose, CA 95126   408-727-5775
                                        855-727-5775
                                   Fax: 408-286-1116
                                             php.com

Mission is to help children with special needs revive the resources, love, hope, respect, health care, education, and other services they need to reach their full potential by providing them
with strong families, dedicated professionals and responsive systems to serve them.

Mary Ellen Peterson, M.A., Executive Director/CEO
Nancy O'Rourke, Chief Development Officer
Jane Floethe-Ford, Director of Education Services

7336 Tourette Syndrome Online
www.tourette-syndrome.com

Devoted to children and adults with Tourette syndrome disorder
and their families, friends, teachers and medical professionals.

**7337 WE MOVE (Worldwide Education and Advocacy for
Movement Disorders)**
www.wemove.org

Provides movement disorder information and education materials
to physicians, patients, the media and the public via its comprehensive web sites, training courses, and more. It's goal is to make
early diagnosis, up-to-date treatment and patient support a reality
for all people living with movement disorders.

Book Publishers

7338 Cognitive-Behavioral Management of Tic Dis orders
John Wiley & Sons
111 River Street
Hoboken, NJ 07030   201-748-6000
                                   Fax: 201-748-6088
                                e-mail: info@wiley.com
                                        www.wiley.com

Provides a comprehensive review of what is known about the
occurance and diagnosis of Tics.

2005 Paperback
ISBN: 0-470093-80-1

Peter B. Wiley, Chairman
Stephen M. Smith, President & CEO
Ellis E. Cousens, Executive Vice President, Chief Fin

7339 Hi, I'm Adam
Hope Press
PO Box 188
Duarte, CA 91009   800-321-4039
                                   Fax: 626-358-3520
                          e-mail: dcomings@earthlink.net
                                      www.hopepress.com

Adam Buehrens is ten years old and has Tourette syndrome.
Adam wrote and illustrated this book because he wants everyone
to know he and other children with Tourette syndrome are not
crazy. They just hava a common neurological disorder. If you
know a child that has tics, temper tantrums, unreasonable fears, or
problems dealing with school, you will find this a reassuring
story.

7340 Teaching the Tiger
Hope Press
PO Box 188
Duarte, CA 91009   800-321-4039
                                   Fax: 626-358-3520
                          e-mail: dcomings@earthlink.net
                                      www.hopepress.com

A handbook for individuals involved in the education of students
with Attention Deficit Disorder, Tourette Syndrome, or Obsessive
Compulsive Disorder.

ISBN: 1-878267-34-5

David E Comings MD, Presenter

**7341 Tourette's Syndrome - Tics, Obsession, Com pulsions:
Developmental Psychopathology**
John Wiley & Sons
111 River Street
Hoboken, NJ 07030   201-748-6000
                                   Fax: 201-748-6088
                                e-mail: info@wiley.com
                                        www.wiley.com

Once thought to be rare, Tourette's Syndrome is now seen as a
relatively common childhood disorder either in its complete or
partial incarnations. Drawing on the work of contributors hailing
from the prestigeous Yale University Child Psychiatry Department, this edited volume explores the disorder from many perspectives, mapping out the diagnosis, genetics, phenomenology,
natural history, and treatment of Tourette's syndrome.

1998 600 pages Hardcover
ISBN: 0-471160-37-7

Peter B. Wiley, Chairman
Stephen M. Smith, President & CEO
Ellis E. Cousens, Executive Vice President, Chief Fin

7342 What Makes Ryan Tic?
Hope Press
PO Box 188
Duarte, CA 91009   800-321-4039
                                   Fax: 626-358-3520
                          e-mail: dcomings@earthlink.net
                                      www.hopepress.com

Covers Ryan's very difficult adolescent years-a period when his
symptoms were so severe he had to be placed in a residential
treatment facility-and the subsequent period of returning home
and pursuing a virtually normal life following his excellent response to the right combination of medication, family and school
support.

Susan Hughes, Author

Journals

7343 Movement Disorders
John Wiley & Sons
111 River Street
Hoboken, NJ 7030-   201-748-6000
                                   Fax: 201-748-6088
                                e-mail: info@wiley.com
                                        www.wiley.com

Publishes reviews, viewpoints, full length articles, historical reports, brief reports, clinical/scientific notes, videotape briefs, pa-
tient/imaging briefs, and letters. ISSN: 0885-3185

Vol 22 13 Issues

Stephen M. Smith, President/ CEO
John Kritzmacher, EVP/ CFO
MJ O'Leary, EVO, Human Resources

Pamphlets

7344 Matthew and Tics
Tourette Syndrome Association
42-40 Bell Boulevard
Bayside, NY 11361   718-224-2999
                                        888-486-8738
                                   Fax: 718-279-9596
                               e-mail: ts@tsa-usa.org
                                          tsa-usa.org

A story for young children with Tourette's Syndrome and their
peers; promotes acceptance and understanding.

7345 Tics and Tourette's Syndrome Fact Sheet
Movement Disorder Resource Center - WE MOVE
204 E 84th Street
New York, NY 10024   212-241-8567
                                        800-437-6682
                                   Fax: 212-987-7363
                                   www.life-in-motion.org

Provides overviews of both diseases.

Description

7346   TOURETTE SYNDROME

Synonyms: Gilles de la Tourette syndrome, GTS

Involves the following Biologic System(s):

Neurologic Disorders

Tourette syndrome is a neurologic disorder that typically becomes apparent in children between the ages of two to 14 years, with approximately 50 percent of cases occurring before seven years of age. The disorder, which is thought to affect about one in 2,000 individuals, is approximately three times more prevalent in males than females and is more common among Caucasians than other populations. In children with Tourette syndrome, associated symptoms and findings vary greatly in range and severity. Initial symptoms may include involuntary, repetitive (stereotypical) muscle movements (motor tics) of the face, eyelids, shoulders, and neck, such as grimacing, abrupt head turning, excessive eye blinking, or stretching of the neck. In some patients with severe symptoms, motor tics may evolve to include self-mutilating behaviors, such as nail biting, lip biting, or facial punching. Children with Tourette syndrome may also develop vocal tics, such as involuntary coughing, grunting, barking, sniffling, or throat clearing. As the disease progresses, additional symptoms may develop including involuntary repetition of obscene words (coprolalia), words spoken by other individuals (echolalia), or one's own words (palilalia) or imitation of other individuals' behaviors (echokinesis or echopraxia). The symptoms associated with Tourette syndrome may periodically decrease or increase in intensity; may subside during high levels of concentration, such as when reading or studying; and may worsen with stress. Tourette syndrome is considered a life-long disorder; however, in approximately 50 to 66 percent of patients, symptoms significantly decrease about 10 to 15 years after initial diagnosis and treatment.

Children with Tourette syndrome may also experience associated behavioral abnormalities, such as aggressive behavior or the performance of repetitive actions or impulses in response to recurrent, persistent thoughts (obsessive-compulsive behaviors). Obsessive-compulsive behaviors are typically performed to help neutralize obsessive thoughts and relieve anxieties. Many affected children may also develop learning, emotional, or social difficulties. The treatment of Tourette syndrome is symptomatic and supportive and may include therapy with certain medications, such as haloperidol, pimozide, clonidine, clonazepam, or carbamazepine. In addition, for those with learning, behavioral, and social difficulties, multidisciplinary management and the provision of special social, academic, and vocational services may be important in helping patients achieve their potential.

Although the exact cause of Tourette syndrome is unknown, studies suggest that the disorder may result due to abnormalities of neurotransmitter (dopamine) activity within a certain area of the brain (basal ganglia). In most cases, Tourette syndrome is thought to be inherited as an autosomal dominant trait that occurs as the result of changes (mutations) in a gene located on the long arm (q) of chromosome 18 (18q22.1). Some children with mutations of this disease gene may not have symptoms associated with the disorder (incomplete penetrance). In addition, in those children with the defective gene who do have symptoms associated with Tourette syndrome, such symptoms may vary in range and severity from case to case (variable expressivity). Such variability of gene expression and penetrance may be suggested by the fact that immediate (first-degree) relatives of patients have an increased frequency of Tourette syndrome, tic conditions, and obsessive-compulsive disorder. In addition, some researchers suspect that Tourette syndrome may result from inheritance of a disease gene in combination with certain environmental factors that may trigger the gene's expression (multifactorial inheritance). Research suggests that individuals who have two copies of a disease gene for Tourette syndrome (homozygotes) typically express the disorder, whereas some who inherit one disease gene (heterozygotes) may not develop the disorder unless particular environmental factors (e.g., infection, such as due to exposure to Group A beta-hemolytic streptococcus) trigger its expression. Tourette syndrome is associated with a vary of misconceptions, for instance, that people with Tourette syndrome are mentally disturbed and that they always exhibit coprolalia. Tourette's is a neurological condition that (according to the most recent research) is primarily genetic in nature. Although there may be learning disabilities associated with Tourette's, the brain is wholly undamaged in respect to intellectual functioning. Statistically, coprolalia is present in less than 5% of TS patients.

Government Agencies

7347   Centers for Disease Control and Prevention Division: Tuberculosis Elimination
1600 Clifton Road NE, MS E-10
Atlanta, GA 30323   404-639-8813
                                                             800-232-4636
                                                   TTY: 888-232-6348
                                             e-mail: cdcinfo@cdc.gov
                                       www.cdc.gov/nchstp/tb/contact.html
Raymond Strikas, Director
Tom Frieden, MD, MPH, Director, Centers for Disease Contr
Linda C. Degutis, DrPH, MSN, Director, National Center for Injur

7348   NIH/National Heart, Lung and Blood Institu te
31 Center Dr MSC 2486, Bldg 31, Room 5A52
Bethesda, MD 20892   301-592-8573
                                                   Fax: 240-629-3246
                                                   TTY: 240-629-3255
                                       e-mail: NHLBIinfo@nhlbi.nih.gov
                                                    www.nhlbi.nih.gov

Primary responsibility of this organization is the scientific investigation of heart, blood vessel, lung and blood disorders. Oversees research, demonstration, prevention, education, control and training activities in these fields and emphasizes the prevention and control of heart diseases.

Elizabeth G Nabel, MD, Director
Susan Shurin, MD, Deputy Director
Sheila Pohl, Chief of Staff

7349   NIH/National Heart, Lung, and Blood Instit te
31 Center Dr MSC 2486, Bldg 31, Room 5A52
Bethesda, MD 20892   301-592-8573
                                                   Fax: 301-629-3246
                                                   TTY: 240-629-3255
                                        e-mail: nhlbinfo@nhlbi.nih.gov
                                                    www.nhlbi.nih.gov

Provides leadership for a national program in diseases of the heart, blood vessels, lungs, and blood; blood resources; and sleep disorders.

Elizabeth G Nabel MD, Director
Susan Shurin, MD, Deputy Director
Sheila Pohl, Chief of Staff

7350 NIH/National Institute of Allergy and Infectious Diseases
6610 Rockledge Drive, MSC 6612
Bethesda, MD 20892
301-496-5717
866-284-4107
Fax: 301-402-3573
TDD: 800-877-8339
e-mail: ocposfoffice@niaid.nih.gov
www.niaid.nih.gov

Conducts and supports basic and applied research to better understand, treat, and ultimately prevent infectious, immunologic, and allergic diseases.

Anthony S Fauci MD, Director
Hugh Auchincloss, M.D., Principal Deputy Director
John J. McGowan, Ph.D., Deputy Director for Science Managem

7351 NIH/National Institute of Allergy and Infectious Diseases
6610 Rockledge Drive, MSC 6612
Bethesda, MD 20892
301-496-5717
866-284-4107
Fax: 301-402-3573
TDD: 800-877-8339
e-mail: ocposfoffice@niaid.nih.gov
www.niaid.nih.gov

Conducts and supports basic and applied research to better understand, treat, and ultimately prevent infectious, immunologic, and allergic diseases.

Anthony S Fauci MD, Director
Hugh Auchincloss, M.D., Principal Deputy Director
John J. McGowan, Ph.D., Deputy Director for Science Managem

7352 NIH/National Institute of Child Health and Human Development
31 Center Drive, Building 31, Room 2A32
Bethesda, MD 20892
301-496-1333
800-370-2943
Fax: 866-760-5947
TTY: 888-320-6942
e-mail: NICHDInformationResourceCenter@mail.nih.
www.nichd.nih.gov

Established in 1962 by congress, today the institute conducts and supports research on topics related to the health of children, adults, families and populations. Some of these topics include: developmental disabilities, growth and development, infant death, reproductive health and birth defects.

Jay H Hoofnagle, Director
Lisa Kaeser, Program & Public Liaison

7353 New York City Department of Health Bureau of Tuberculosis Control
125 Worth Street
New York, NY 10013
212-346-7572
www.nyc.gov/html

Michael R Bloomberg, Mayor
Desiree Kim, Executive Director

National Associations & Support Groups

7354 American Academy of Child & Adolescent Psychiatry
3615 Wisconsin Avenue NW
Washington, DC 20016
202-966-7300
Fax: 202-966-2891
e-mail: clinical@aacap.org
www.aacap.org

Mission is to promote mentally healthy children, adolescents and families through research, training, advocacy, prevention, comprehensive diagnosis and treatment, peer support and collaboration.

Elizabeth Hughes, Asst. Director of Education & Recer
Quentin Bernhard III, CME Coordinator
Alan Ezagui, Deputy Director of Development

7355 American Academy of Pediatrics
141 Northwest Point Boulevard
Elk Grove Village, IL 60007
847-434-4000
800-433-9016
Fax: 847-434-8000
www.aap.org

The American Academy of Pediatrics and its member pediatricians dedicate their efforts and resources to the health, safety and well-being of infants, children, adolescents and young adults.

Sandra Hassink, MD, FAAP, President

7356 American Heart Association
7272 Greenville Avenue
Dallas, TX 75231
214-373-6300
800-242-8721
Fax: 214-706-1341
e-mail: inquire@amhrt.org
www.heart.org

Supports research, education and community service programs with the objective of reducing premature death and disability from cardiovascular diseases and stroke; coordinates the efforts of health professionals, and others engaged in the fight against heart and circulatory disease.

Nancy Brown, CEO
Suzie Upton, Chief Development Officer
Sunder Joshi, Chief Administrative Officer/CFO

7357 American Lung Association
1301 Pennsylvania Ave. NW, Suite 800
Washington, DC 20004
202-785-3355
800-548-8252
Fax: 202-452-1805
e-mail: info@lung.org
www.lung.org

The American Lung Association fights lung disease in all its forms, with special emphasis on asthma, tobacco control and environmental health. The American Lung Association is funded by contributions from the public, along with gifts and grants from corporations, foundations and government agencies. The association achieves its many successes through the work of thousands of committed volunteers and staff.

Ross P. Lanzafame, Board Chair
Harold Wimmer, President/CEO
John F. Emanuel, J.D., Secretary/Treasurer

7358 American School Counselor Association
1101 King Street, Suite 310
Alexandria, VA 22314
703-683-2722
800-306-4722
Fax: 703-997-7572
e-mail: asca@schoolcounselor.org
www.schoolcounselor.org

The mission of ASCA is to represent professional school counselors and to promote professionalism and ethical practices.

Richard Wong, Executive Director
Jeff Broderson, Information Technology Admin.
Kathleen M Rakestraw, Director of Communications

7359 American Society for Reproductive Medicine
1209 Montgomery Highway
Birmingham, AL 35216
205-978-5000
Fax: 205-978-5005
e-mail: asrm@asrm.org
www.asrm.org

The American Society for Reproductive Medicine is an organization devoted to advancing knowledge and expertise in infertility, reproductive medicine and biology. The ASRM is a voluntary nonprofit organization.

Linda C. Giudice, President
Rebecca Sokol, M.D., Vice President
Robert W. Rebar, M.D, Executive Director

7360 Arc of the United States
1660 L Street, NW, Suite 301
Washington, DC 20036
202-534-3700
800-433-5255
Fax: 202-534-3731
e-mail: info@thearc.org
www.thearc.org

The Arc of the United States works to include all children and adults with cognitive, intellectual, developmental disabilities in every community. We are a national organization of and for the people with mental retardation and related developmental disabilities and their families. It is devoted to promoting and improving supports and services for people with mental retardation and their families. The ARC was founded by a small group of parents and other concerned individuals.

Peter V. Berns, CEO
Karen Wolf-Branigin, Senior Program Officer
Amy Goodman, Co-Director, Autism NOW

7361 Children's Hospital Boston
300 Longwood Avenue
Boston, MA 02115
617-355-6000
800-355-7944
TTY: 617-730-0152
www.childrenshospital.org

Mission is to provide the highest quality care; be the leading source of research and discovery; educate the next generation of leaders in child health and enhance the health and well-being of the children and families in our local community.

Sandra Fenwick, President/Chief Operating Officer
James Mandell, MD, Chief Executive Officer
Dick Argys, Senior Vice President and Chief Adm

7362 Chromosome 18 Registry & Research Society
7155 Oakridge Drive
San Antonio, TX 78229
210-657-4968
Fax: 210-657-4968
e-mail: office@chromosome18.org
www.chromosome18.org

The purpose of the Chromosome 18 Registry & Research Society is to offer support to patients and families, to educate the public about different available treatments and to connect families and doctors to the research community.

Jannine Cody, President
Ben Flowe Jr, VP Public Relations
Claudia Traa, Executive Director

7363 Congenital Heart Anomalies, Support, Education & Resources (CHASER)
2112 N Wilkins Road
Swanton, OH 43558
419-825-5575
Fax: 419-825-2880
e-mail: chaser@compuserve.com
www.csun.edu/~hcmth011/chaser/

National organization for support, education and resources for families, patients and professionals who deal with children born with congenital heart malformations. Information on hospitals, medical assistance, and schooling. Offers Chaser News, an international newsletter and Chaser's Pediatric Heart Surgeons Facility Directory.

Anita Myers, Executive Director

7364 Congenital Heart Information Network
PO Box 3397
Margate City, NJ 08402
609-823-4507
Fax: 215-627-4036
e-mail: mb@tchin.org
www.tchin.org

CHIN is an international organization that provides reliable information, support services and resources to families of children with congenital heart defects and acquired heart disease.

Mona Barmash, President

7365 Epilepsy Foundation
8301 Professional Place
Landover, MD 20785
866-330-2718
800-332-1000
Fax: 301-459-1569
e-mail: ContactUs@efa.org
www.epilepsyfoundation.org

An organization works to ensure that people with seizures are able to participate in all life experiences; and to prevent, control and cure epilepsy through research, education, advocacy and services.

Phil Gattone, President/CEO
Sandy Finucane, Senior Advisor
Priscilla Burton, Senior Advisor

7366 Family Support Network
7514 Big Bend Blvd.
Saint Louis, MO 63119
314-644-5055
800-255-6872
Fax: 314-644-5057
e-mail: info@familysupport.org
www.familysupportnet.org/

The Support Network is an organized partnership of individuals whose lives have been affected by Tuberous Sclerosis. Across the nation, the Support Network is providing the latest medical information, education and support to those individuals who are seeking understanding about the genetic disease and offering them words of encouragement and empowerment.

Susan Didier, MSW, LCSW, Director of Family Services
Julia Pickup, MSW, LCSW, Lead Therapist
Ayriel Hadley, BA, Office Manager

7367 Genetic Alliance
4301 Connecticut Avenue NW, Suite 404
Washington, DC 20008
202-966-7955
800-336-4363
Fax: 202-966-8553
e-mail: info@geneticalliance.org
www.geneticalliance.org

A coalition of voluntary genetic support groups, consumers and professionals addressing the needs of individuals and families affected by genetic disorders from a national perspective.

Sharon Terry, President/CEO
Lisa Wise, MA, Chief Operating Officer
Natasha Bonhomme, Vice President of Strategic Develop

7368 MUMS: National Parent to Parent Network
150 Custer Street
Green Bay, WI 54301
920-336-5333
877-336-5333
Fax: 920-339-0995
e-mail: mums@netnet.net
www.netnet.net/mums

A national parent-to-parent organization for parents or care providers of a child with any disability, rare or not so rare disorder, chromosomal abnormality or health condition.

Julie J Gordon, Director

7369 National Dissemination Center for Children with Disabilities
1825 Connecticut Ave NW
Washington, DC 20009
202-884-8200
800-695-0285
Fax: 202-884-8441
TTY: 800-695-0285
e-mail: nichcy@aed.org
www.nichcy.org

A national information and referral center for families, educators and other professionals on: disabilities in children and youth; programs and services; IDEA, the nation's special education law; and research-based information on effective practices.

Suzanne Ripley, Executive Director

7370 National Tuberculosis Center at New Jersey Medical School
185 South Orange Avenue, MSB C-696
Newark, NJ 07107
973-972-4300
Fax: 973-972-3268
e-mail: njmsadmiss@umdnj.edu
www.umdnj.edu

The National Tuberculosis Center was established in 1993 in response to the resurgence of tuberculosis in the United States. The center operates under the direction of Lee B. Reichmann, MD, MPH. The center operates a toll-free information line to provide state-of-the-art information to health care professionals and the public. Senior medical staff and nurses are available to respond to calls Monday-Friday from 9am-5pm.

Kevin M. Barry, M.D., MBA, Chairperson
Mary Ann Christopher, RN, MSN, Vice-Chairperson
Bradford W. Hildebrandt, Secretary

7371 National Tuberous Sclerosis Association
801 Roeder Road, Suite 750
Landover, MD 20785   301-562-9890
800-225-6872
Fax: 301-562-9870
e-mail: info@tsalliance.org
www.tsalliance.org

Nonprofit organization.

Matt Bolger, Chair
Kari Luther Rosbeck, President/CEO
Keith Hall, Vice Chair

7372 Support Organization for Trisomy 18, 13, and Related Disorders (SOFT)
2982 S Union Street
Rochester, NY 14624   585-594-4621
800-716-7638
e-mail: barbsoft@rochester.rr.com
www.trisomy.org

SOFT is a network of families and professional dedication to providing support and understanding to families involved in the issue and decision surrounding the diagnosis and care in related chromosome disorders. Support is provided throughout pre-natal diagnosis, the child's life and after their passing. It is committed to the support of families personal decision in alliance with a parent-professional partnership. Site includes a listing of local chapters in 25 states.

Barb Vanherreweghe, President
Steve Wagner, Board Member
Raquel Wagner, Board Member

7373 Trisomy 18 Foundation
4491 Cheshire Station Plaza, Suite 157
Dale City, VA 22193   810-867-4211
e-mail: t18info@trisomy18.org
www.trisomy18.org

The foundation's mission is to search for a cure and treatments; to educate and support medical professionals; and to create a worldwide caring community for those affected.

Victoria Miller, Executive Director
Sean Brown, Vice-President of Development
Kris Shaughnessy, M.A., Community Affairs Program Office

7374 Tuberous Sclerosis Alliance
801 Roeder Road, Suite 750
Silver Spring, MD 20910   301-562-9890
800-225-6872
Fax: 301-562-9870
e-mail: info@tsalliance.org
www.tsalliance.org

The Tuberous Sclerosis Alliance is dedicated to finding a cure for Tuberous Sclerosis complex while improving the lives of those affected. TSC is a genetic disease causing tumors to grow throughout the body and is the leading cause of epilepsy and autism.

Matt Bolger, Chair
Kari Luther Rosbeck, President/CEO
Keith Hall, Vice Chair

7375 United Network for Organ Sharing
700 N 4th Street, PO Box 2484
Richmond, VA 23219   804-782-4800
Fax: 804-782-4816
www.unos.org

Our mission is to advance organ availability and transplantation by uniting and supporting our communities for the benefit of patients through education, technology and policy development.

Walter K Graham, CEO
Vicki F Sauer, Executive VP/COO
Marcia D Manning, Director Community Affairs

7376 WE MOVE (Worldwide Education and Advocacy for Movement Disorders)
5731 Mosholu Avenue
Bronx, NY 10024   212-875-8312
800-437-6682
Fax: 212-875-8389
e-mail: wemove@wemove.org
www.wemove.org

A nonprofit organization dedicated to educating and informing patients, professionals and the public about the latest clinical advances, management and treatment options for neurologic movement disorders.

Susan Bressman, President
Mo Moadeli, Vice President
Wendy Borow-Johnson, Secretary

7377 World Health Organization
Avenue Appia 20
CH-1211 Geneva 27,   www.who.int

WHO is the directing and coordinating authority for health within the United Nations system.

Dr Margaret Chan, Director General
Dr Anarfi Asamoa-Baah, Deputy Director-General
Hans Troedsson, Executive Director of the Director-

State Agencies & Support Groups

Arizona

7378 Tourette Syndrome Association - Arizona Chapter
6501 E. Greenway Pkwy, PO Box 103-414
Scottsdale, AZ 85254   520-620-2288
800-203-7490
e-mail: info@tsa-az.org
www.tsa-az.org

The Arizona chapter of the Tourette Syndrome Association was established to serve the community touched by Touretty Syndrome.

Kelly Medlyn, President
Marci Frantz, Vice President
Teri Mendenhall, Secretary

California

7379 Tourette Syndrome Association - Northern California/Hawaii Chapter
www.tsanorcal-hawaii.org

925-548-3605
e-mail: gibsonohare@sbcglobal.net
www.tsanorcal-hawaii.org

A voluntary organization dedicated to providing assistance and support for individuals with Tourette Syndrome, their families, friends & loved ones.

Sandy Gibson-O'Hare, Chair
Sandra Brackett, Vice Chair
Samantha Phillips, Secretary

7380 Tourette Syndrome Association - Southern California Chapter
PO Box 3778
Cerritos, CA 90703   866-478-1935
e-mail: bcourdy@ca.rr.com
www.tourettesyndrome-sca.org

The TSA of Southern California is an all volunteer, non-profit organization whose missions is to support the needs of families affected by Tourette Syndrome. The goal is to advocate for individuals with TS, educate the public and professionals about TS, and promote awareness.

Colorado

7381 Tourette Syndrome Association - Rocky Mountain Region
992 S 4th Avenue, Suite 100, PMB 198
Brighton, CO 80601
720-212-7535
e-mail: support@tsa-rmr.org
www.tsa-rmr.org

The TSARMR serves Colorado, Montana, Wyoming, and Nevada.

Sally Mescher Allen, Chair
Donna Davies, Vice Chair
Lorraine Alcott, Secretary

Connecticut

7382 Tourette Syndrome Association - Connecticut Chapter
PO Box 185883
Hamden, CT 06518
203-980-4215
e-mail: joytavo@tsact.org
www.tsact.org

The mission of the Connecticut chapter of the Tourette Syndrome Association, Inc. is to educate the general public about Touretty Syndrome and further the acceptance of people with Tourette Syndrome in all settings.

Peter Tavolacci, Vice-Chairman
Paul Nazario, Treasurer
Jeanette Nazario, Board Member

Florida

7383 Tourette Syndrome Association of Florida
PO Box 411416
Melbourne, FL 32941
727-418-0240
e-mail: support@tsa-fl.org
www.tsa-fl.org

The TSA of Florida is a voluntary organization dedicated to helping individuals with Tourette Syndrome and their families by gathering and distributing information, promoting local self-help and professional services, and providing local TS support groups and meetings.

Donna Sakuta, Executive Director

Hawaii

7384 Tourette Syndrome Association - Northern California/Hawaii Chapter
www.tsanorcal-hawaii.org
925-548-3605
e-mail: gibsonohare@sbcglobal.net
www.tsanorcal-hawaii.org

A voluntary organization dedicated to providing assistance and support for individuals with Tourette Syndrome, their families, friends & loved ones.

Sandy Gibson-O'Hare, Chair
Sandra Brackett, Vice Chair
Samantha Phillips, Secretary

Illinois

7385 Tourette Syndrome Association of Illinois
800 Roosevelt Road, Suite A-10
Glen Ellyn, IL 60137
630-790-8083
877-TSA-IL55
Fax: 630-790-8084
e-mail: tsaillinois@yahoo.com
www.tsa-illinois.org

TSA of Illinois' mission is to serve and support those whose lives are affected by Tourette Syndrome. TSA-IL promotes awareness, advocates, and educates the public, health care providers, and educators about Tourette Syndrome. TSA-IL supports medical and scientific research about Tourette Syndrome.

Sande S Shamash, President
Jen Johnson, Vice President, Membership
Joan Lindauer, Vice President, Government Relation

Indiana

7386 Tourette Syndrome Association of Indiana
PO Box 3797
West Lafayette, IN 47996
765-714-9880
e-mail: tsaofindiana@gmail.com
www.tsaindiana.org

One of TSA of Indiana's many priorities is to establish access to current information and easy communication for its members. The leaders are committed to serving and supporting those whose lives are affected by Tourette Syndrome.

Michele Lehman, President
Brenda Leopold, Youth Ambassador Program Coordin.
John Leopold, Youth Ambassador Program Coordin.

Maine

7387 Tourette Syndrome Association - Maine/New Hampshire Chapter
www.tsa-maine.org
207-699-4258
e-mail: info@tsa-maine.org
www.tsa-maine.org

The Tourette Syndrome Association is a non-profit organization aimed at identifying the cause of, finding the cure for, and controlling the effects of this disorder. TSA also seeks to broaden awareness of Tourette Syndrome and provide support for families and individuals who deal with it.

Maryland

7388 Tourette Syndrome Association of Greater Washington
5851 Deale Churchton Road, Suite 4
Deale, MD 20751
410-867-1151
877-295-2148
Fax: 301-576-4527
e-mail: info@tsagw.org
www.tsagw.org

The TSA of Greater Washington is a non-profit organization comprised of an all volunteer Board of Directors, two paid Staff and numerous unaffiliated volunteers. The mission is to improve the quality of life in those affected by Tourette Syndrome through education, advocacy and awareness in Maryland, Virginia and Washington D.C.

Marla Shea Gabala, Chairman
Judy Krauthamer, Vice Chair/Treasurer
Mark Etzel, Secretary

Massachusetts

7389 Tourette Syndrome Association of Massachusetts
39 Godfrey Street
Taunton, MA 02780
617-277-7589
e-mail: info@tsa-ma.org
www.tsa-ma.org

The Tourette Syndrome Association of Massachusets is an all volunteer, non-profit organization whose mission is to support the needs of families affected by Tourette Syndrome. The goal is to advocate for individuals with TS, educate the public and professionals about TS, and promote awareness.

Chrissy Joyal, President
Liliane Larsen, Vice President/Treasurer
Judy Storeygard, Education Specialist

Minnesota

7390 Tourette Syndrome Association - Minnesota Chapter
2233 University Avenue, Suite 338
St. Paul, MN 55114
651-646-0099
Fax: 952-918-0350
e-mail: director@tsa-mn.org
www.tsa-mn.org

The mission is to assist Minnesotan's with Tourette syndrome in achieving their fullest potential through education, support and public awareness programs.

Lee Baker, Executive Director

Missouri

7391 Tourette Syndrome Association - Greater Missouri Chapter
6526 Parkwood Place
St. Louis, MO 63116
314-984-9019
e-mail: lmchd52@gmail.com
www.missouritsa.org

Serves individuals and families in the St. Louis and Kansas City metropolitan areas and beyond. In concert with the national TSA, they provide information about Tourette Syndrome (TS) and the resources available to help affected families throughout the service area.

Lynn Dunlap, Chair
Pete Abel, Co-Chair/ Government Liaison
Marty Guise, Secretary

Montana

7392 Tourette Syndrome Association - Rocky Mountain Region
992 S 4th Avenue, Suite 100, PMB 198
Brighton, CO 80601
720-212-7535
e-mail: support@tsa-rmr.org
www.tsa-rmr.org

The TSARMR serves Colorado, Montana, Wyoming, and Nevada.

Sally Mescher Allen, Chair
Donna Davies, Vice Chair
Lorraine Alcott, Secretary

Nevada

7393 Tourette Syndrome Association - Rocky Mountain Region
992 S 4th Avenue, Suite 100, PMB 198
Brighton, CO 80601
720-212-7535
e-mail: support@tsa-rmr.org
www.tsa-rmr.org

The TSARMR serves Colorado, Montana, Wyoming, and Nevada.

Sally Mescher Allen, Chair
Donna Davies, Vice Chair
Lorraine Alcott, Secretary

New Jersey

7394 Tourette Syndrome Association of New Jersey
50 Division Street, Suite 205
Somerville, NJ 08876
732-972-4459
e-mail: info@tsanj.org
www.tsanj.org

The Tourette Syndrome Association of New Jersey, Inc., a chapter of the national Tourette Syndrome Association, is a non-profit organization whos membership includes individuals with Tourette Syndrome, their families and friends, and interested professionals.

New Mexico

7395 Tourette Syndrome Association - New Mexico Chapter
42-40 Bell Boulevard
Bayside, NY 11361
718-224-2999
e-mail: info@tsanm.org
www.tsanm.org

The purpose is to provide information, support, and assistance to adults, children, and families affected by Tourette Syndrome. The hope is to provide education and to encourage an understanding and acceptance of this disorder.

Jennifer Johns, President
Helen Gutierrez, Secretary
Tanya Mueller, Treasurer

New York

7396 Tourette Syndrome Association - Greater Rochester and Finger Lakes Area
92 Windmere Road
Rochester, NY 14617
585-752-6190
e-mail: info@rochestertourette.org
www.rochestertourette.org

The TSA of Greater Rochester and the Finger Lakes, Inc. is a non-profit organization whose mission is to provide support, information and advocacy to people with TS and their families in friends. The chapter serves the community at large with support groups, in-services, and public awareness programs to the local, educational, and medical communities.

Diana Pratt, Chair
Patrick Scanlon, Vice Chair
Bob Gleason, Treasurer

7397 Tourette Syndrome Association - Greater New York State Chapter
20 Thomas Jefferson Lane
Synder, NY 14226
716-839-4430
Fax: 716-839-1956
e-mail: info@tsa-gnys.org
www.tsa-gnys.org

The Tourette Syndrome Association of Greater New York State is an affiliate chapter of the TSA, Inc. The chapter serves an area from Buffalo to the Pennsylvania border to the south. There is a Greater Rochester TSA chapter that serves greater Rochester, NY. TSA-GNYS then picks up from Rochester and continues east to serve Syracuse and all of the central NY area.

Susan Conners, President
Marge Henning, Co-Chair
John Silverwood, Co-Chair

7398 Tourette Syndrome Association - Hudson Valley Chapter
PO Box 517
Ardsley, NY 10502
914-378-5025
e-mail: info@tsa-nyhv.org
www.tsa-nyhv.org

The mission of the Hudson Valley Chapter is; to provide service, information, and support to people with TS and their families; to educate medical and educational professionals in order to increase their understanding of TS; and to promote a greater understanding of TS in the community at large.

Shelly Cooler, President
Marilyn Trichon, Vice President
Richard Yannetti, Executive Director

7399 Tourette Syndrome Association - Long Island Chapter
PO Box 615
Jericho, NY 11753
516-876-6947
e-mail: longisland.tsa@gmail.com
www.li-tsa.org

The Long Island TSA's mission is to provide help (at the community level) to families affected by Tourette Syndrome by providing services to its members in Nassau and Suffolk counties.

Lisa Filippi, Co Chair
Kate Callan, Co-Vice Chair
Jane Zwilling, 1st Vice Chair and Chair, Education

7400 Tourette Syndrome Association - New York City Chapter
www.tsa-nyc.org

646-395-0162
e-mail: chapter@tsa-nyc.org
www.tsa-nyc.org

The New York city chapter offers a variety of services to people with Tourette Syndrome, their families, educators, and professionals.

Chelsea White, Chairperson
Linda McAndrew, Secretary
Jonathan Marks, Treasurer

Ohio

7401 Tourette Syndrome Association of Ohio
PO Box 40163
Cincinnatti, OH 45240

513-320-7161
800-543-2675
e-mail: admin@tsaohio.org
www.tsaohio.org

The Tourette Syndrome Association of Ohio is a nonprofit organization whose membership includes individuals with Tourette Syndrome, their families, friends, and interested professionals.

Coreen Brown, Chair of the Board
Joleah Dean, Executive Director of the Board

Oregon

7402 Tourette Syndrome Association - Washington and Oregon Chapter
318 West Galer Street
Seattle, WA 98119

718-224-2999
e-mail: tsawashingtonchapter@yahoo.com
www.tsa-waor.org

This chapter exists to offer information, support and resources regarding Tourette Syndrome and its related conditions. They work together with the medical community, the schools and families whose lives are touched by TS.

Todd Henry, Chair
Erin Farrar, Vice Chair
Bernadette Witty, Secretary

Pennsylvania

7403 PA Tourette Syndrome Alliance
PO Box 148
McSherrystown, PA 17344

717-337-1134
800-990-3300
Fax: 717-698-1420
e-mail: info@patsainc.org
www.patsainc.org

The services provided by PA-TSA are focused on increasing understanding of the disorder and providing proven accommodations and strategies so the child or adult can succeed.

Melinda Bowling, President
Lesley Geye, Vice-President
Susan Lutz, Treasurer

Rhode Island

7404 Tourette Syndrome Association of Rhode Island
6946 Post Road, Suite 402
North Kingstown, RI 00285

401-886-0887
e-mail: info@oshean.org
www.ri.net/tsari

TSARI tries to define the needs of Rhode Islanders with TS and their families and design services for them. They offer support and education to families with TS.

Susan Cerrone Abely, Chair
John Smithers, Vice-Chair
Michael Pickett, Treasurer

Utah

7405 Tourette Syndrome Association - Utah Chapter
PO Box 701312
West Valley City, UT 84170

801-967-2125
866-274-0700
e-mail: chair@tsa-utah.org
www.tsa-utah.org

The local chapter of the national TSA organization, serving as a resource for individuals who have Tourette Syndrome and their families. Membership is open to anyone who is interested in Tourette Syndrome.

Kelsey Brown, Chairman
Adam Westwood, Treasurer
Gerri Harper, Secretary

Washington

7406 Tourette Syndrome Association - Washington and Oregon Chapter
318 West Galer Street
Seattle, WA 98119

718-224-2999
e-mail: tsawashingtonchapter@yahoo.com
www.tsa-waor.org

This chapter exists to offer information, support and resources regarding Tourette Syndrome and its related conditions. They work together with the medical community, the schools and families whose lives are touched by TS.

Todd Henry, Chair
Erin Farrar, Vice Chair
Bernadette Witty, Secretary

Wyoming

7407 Tourette Syndrome Association - Rocky Mountain Region
992 S 4th Avenue, Suite 100, PMB 198
Brighton, CO 80601

720-212-7535
e-mail: tsarmr@att.net
www.tsa-rmr.org

The TSARMR serves Colorado, Montana, Wyoming, and Nevada.

Sally Mescher Allen, Chair
Donna Davies, Vice Chair
Lorraine Alcott, Secretary

Research Centers

7408 Tourette Syndrome Clinic
Cincinnati Children's Hospital Medical Center
333 Burnet Avenue
Cincinnati, OH 45229

513-636-4200
800-344-2462
TTY: 513-636-4900
e-mail: tics@cchmc.org
www.cincinnatichildrens.org

Clinic that specializes in evaluating, diagnosing and treating kids, adolescents and adults with Tourette's Syndrome symptoms, including tics, hyperactivity, attention deficits, obsessive compulsive behaviors and other symptoms of Tourette Syndrome.

Donald L Gilbert, MD, MS, Director
Libby Cox, Care Manager, Movement Disorder Cen
Tara Lipps, Staff Nurse and Study Coordinator

7409 Trisomy 18 Foundation
4491 Cheshire Station Plaza, Suite 157
Dale City, VA 22193

810-867-4211
e-mail: t18info@trisomy18.org
www.trisomy18.org

The foundation's mission is to search for a cure and treatments; to educate and support medical professionals; and to create a worldwide caring community for those affected.

7877 American Academy of Child and Adolescent Psychiatry
3615 Wisconsin Avenue NW
Washington, DC 20016 202-966-7300
Fax: 202-966-2891
e-mail: clinical@aacap.org
www.aacap.org

The AACAP (American Academy of Child and Adolescent Psychiatry) is the leading national professional medical association dedicated to treating and improving the quality of life for children, adolescents, and families affected by these disorders. The AACAP is a 501 (c)(3) nonprofit organization established in 1953.

Martin J. Drell, M.D, President
Paramjit T. Josh, President-Elect
David R. DeMaso, M.D., Secretary

7878 American Academy of Dermatology (AAD)
PO Box 4014
Schaumburg, IL 60168 847-240-1280
866-503-7546
Fax: 847-240-1859
e-mail: MRC@aad.org
www.aad.org

Largest, most influential and most representative of all dermatologic associations. Committed to the highest quality standards in continuing medical education. Developed a platform to promote and advance the science and art of medicine and surgery related to the skin; promotes the highest possible standards in clinical practice, education and research in dermatology and related disciplines; and supports and enhances patient care and promotes the public interest relating to dermatology.

Dirk M. Elston, MD, President
Lisa A. Garner, VP
Suzanne M. Olbricht, Secretary/Treasurer

7879 American Academy of Pediatrics
141 Northwest Point Boulevard
Elk Grove Village, IL 60007 847-434-4000
800-433-9016
Fax: 847-434-8000
www.aap.org

The American Academy of Pediatrics and its member pediatricians dedicate their efforts and resources to the health, safety and well-being of infants, children, adolescents and young adults.

Sandra Hassink, MD, FAAP

7880 American Amputee Foundation
P.O. Box 94227
North Little Rock, AR 72190 501-835-9290
Fax: 501-835-9292
e-mail: info@americanamputee.org
www.americanamputee.org

AAF empowers amputees, their families, and care providers to make informed decisions be providing them information, referral, peer counseling, literature, and education.

Catherine J. Walden, Executive Director
Shelly Soderlund, Executive Assistant

7881 American Association for Leisure and Recreation
1900 Association Drive
Reston, VA 20191 703-476-3400
800-213-7193
Fax: 703-476-9527
e-mail: aair@aahperd.org
www.aahperd.org

American Association for Leisure and Recreation serves recreation professionals practitioners, educators, and students who advance the profession and enhance the quality of life of all Americans through creative and meaningful leisure and recreation experiences.

E. Paul Roetert, Chief Executive Officer
Gale Wiedow, President
Dolly D. Lambdin, President-Elect

7882 American Association of Children's Residential Centers (AACRC)
11700 W. Lake Park Drive
Milwaukee, WI 53224 877-332-2272
877-332-2272
Fax: 877-332-2272
e-mail: info@aacrc-dc.org
www.aacrc-dc.org

The American Association of Children's Residential Centers brings professionals together to advance the frontiers of knowledge pertaining to the spectrum of therapeutic living environments for children and adolescents with behavioral health disorders.

Richard Altman, MSW, ACSW, Chief Executive Officer
William Powers, Chief Executive Officer
Christopher Bellonci, President

7883 American Association of the Deaf-Blind
8630 Fenton Street, Suite 121
Silver Spring, MD 20910 301-495-4403
Fax: 301-495-4404
TTY: 301-495-4402
e-mail: aadb-info@aadb.org
www.aadb.org

The American Association of the Deaf-Blind is a national consumer organization of, by, and for deaf-blind Americans. Deaf-blind does not necessarily mean totally deaf and totally blind. It is a broad term that describes people who have varying degrees and types of both vision and hearing loss together. Our mission is to endeavor to enable deaf-blind persons to achieve their maximum potential through increased independence, productivity and integration into the community.

600 Members

Jill Gaus, President
Lynn Jansen, VP
Debby Lieberman, Secretary

7884 American Association on Intellectual and D evelopmental Disabilities
501 3rd Street, NW Suite 200
Washington, DC 20001 202-387-1968
800-424-3688
Fax: 202-387-2193
e-mail: aamr@access.digex.net
www.aamr.org

American Association on Intellectual and Developmental Disabilities' mission is to promote progressive policies, sound research, effective practices, and universal human rights for people with intellectual disabilities.

Marc J. Tass,, PhD, President
Amy S. Hewitt, PhD, Vice President
Margaret Nygren, EdD, Executive Director

7885 American Auditory Society
PO Box 779
Pennsville, NJ 08070 877-746-8315
Fax: 650-763-9185
e-mail: amaudsoc@comcast.net
www.amauditorysoc.org

The primary aims of the Society are to increase knowledge and understanding of the ear, hearing and balance; disorders of the ear, hearing and balance, and preventions of these disorders; and habilitation and rehabilitation of individuals with hearing and balance dysfunction.

Linda Hood, President
Wayne J Staab, PhD, Executive Director
Harvey Abrams, Board of Director

7886 American Autoimmune Related Diseases Association
22100 Gratiot Avenue
Eastpointe, MI 48021 586-776-3900
800-598-4668
Fax: 586-776-3903
e-mail: aarda@aarda.org
www.aarda.org

Dedicated to the eradication of autoimmune diseases and the alleviation of suffering and the socio-economic impact of autoimmunity through fostering and facilitating collaboration in the areas of education, public awareness, research and patient services in an effective, ethical and efficient manner.

Betty Diamond, M.D, Chair
Noel R. Rose, M.D., Ph.D, Chairman Emeritus
Virginia Ladd, Executive Director

7887 American Blind Bowling Association
3319 W. Parkridge Drive
Peoria, IL 61604   919-621-1707
                        e-mail: keithedg2@yahoo.com
                                www.abba1951.org

Information on adaptive bowling activities for people who are blind.

Keith Edgerton, Chair
Rozella Campbell, Secretary/Treasurer
Wilbert Turner, Public Relations Committee Chair

7888 American Blind Skiing Foundation
1831 Mission Hills Rd., Unit 203
Northbrook, IL 60062   312-409-1605
                            e-mail: ABSF@absf.org
                                    www.absf.org

ABSF is committed to serving visually impaired children and adults, giving them the opportunities and experiences that build confidence and independence.

Nate Magit, President
Ron Klein, Vice President
Jim Hynan, Treasurer

7889 American Board of Dermatology
Henry Ford Health System
1 Ford Place
Detroit, MI 48202   313-874-1088
                                     Fax: 313-872-3221
                              e-mail: abderm@hfhs.org
                                     www.abderm.org

Sole mission is to ensure competence for patients with cutaneous diseases through board representation.

Terry L. Barrett, President
Christopher J. Arpey, Vice President
Thomas D. Horn, Executive Director

7890 American Board of Pediatrics
111 Silver Cedar Court
Chapel Hill, NC 27514   919-929-0461
                                     Fax: 919-929-9255
                              e-mail: abpeds@abpeds.org
                                       www.abp.org

The American Board is Pediatrics certifies general pediatricians and pediatric subspecialists based on standards of excellence that lead to high quality health care for infants, children and adolescents.

Dr. David G. Nichols, President/CEO

7891 American Camping Association
5000 State Road, 67 N
Martinsville, IN 46151   765-342-8456
                                           800-428-2267
                                     Fax: 765-342-2065
                         e-mail: Wo.turner5@sbcglobal.net
                                    www.acacamps.org

The American Camping Association is a community of camp professionals who, for nearly 100 years, have joined together to share our knowledge and experience and to ensure the quality of camp program.

Wilbert Turner, Chair
Peg Smith, CEO
Tisha Bolger, President

7892 American Cancer Society
250 Williams Street NW
Atlanta, GA 30303   800-227-2345
                                     Fax: 404-315-9348
                       e-mail: angelina.veal@cancer.org
                                     www.cancer.org

The American Cancer Society is a nationwide, community-based voluntary health organization. Headquartered in Atlanta, Georgia, the ACS has state divisions and more than 3,400 local offices. For more than 80 years, ACS has led the way in cancer research. The goal is to prevent cancer, save lives, and diminish suffering from cancer.

Gary M. Reedy, Chair
Robert E. Youle, Vice Chair
Vincent T. DeVita, President

7893 American Canoe Association
108 Hanover St
Fredricksburg, VA 22401   540-907-4460
                                     Fax: 888-229-3792
                      e-mail: aca@americancanoe.org
                                  www.americancanoe.org

The mission of the American Canoe Association is to promote the health, social and personal benefits of canoeing, kayaking and rafting and to serve the needs off all paddlers for safe, enjoyable and quality paddling opportunities.

Wade Blackwood, Executive Director
Cireena Katto, Office Manager
Kelsey Bracewell, Safety Education, Instruction, & Ou

7894 American Dermatological Association
PO Box 551301
Davie, FL 33355   954-452-1113
                                     Fax: 305-945-7063
                      e-mail: info@amer-derm-assn.org
                                www.amer-derm-assn.org

Professional society of physicians specializing in dermatology. Promotes teaching, practice, public education and research into dermatology.

Rex Amonette, President
John Wolf, Vice President
Julie Odessky, Executive Manager

7895 American Epilepsy Society
342 N Main Street
W Hartford, CT 06117   860-586-7505
                                           800-332-1000
                                     Fax: 860-568-7550
                                       www.aesnet.org

A society of clinicians, researchers, and health care professionals which promotes education and research of epilepsy.

Suzanne C Berry, Executive Director
Cheryl-Ann Tubby, Assistant Executive Director
Elizabeth Kunsey, Senior Meeting Planner

7896 American Hearing Research Foundation
8 South Michigan Avenue, Suite #1205
Chicago, IL 60603   312-726-9670
                                     Fax: 312-726-9695
                    e-mail: ahrf@american-hearing.org
                               www.american-hearing.org

A nonprofit foundation serving two vital roles — funding significant research in hearing and balance disorders and helping educate the public.

Richard G. Muench, Chair
Alan G. Micco, M.D, President
Mark R. Muench, Vice President

7897 American Heart Association
7272 Greenville Avenue
Dallas, TX 75231   214-373-6300
                                           800-242-8721
                                     Fax: 214-706-1341
                           e-mail: inquire@amhrt.org
                                     www.heart.org

Supports research, education and community service programs with the objective of reducing premature death and disability from cardiovascular diseases and stroke; coordinates the efforts of health professionals, and others engaged in the fight against heart and circulatory disease.

Nancy Brown, CEO
Suzie Upton, Chief Development Officer
Sunder Joshi, Chief Administrative Officer/CFO

7898   American Juvenile Arthritis Organization
1330 W. Peachtree Street., Suite 100
Atlanta, GA 30309   404-872-7100
                                          800-933-7023
                                     Fax: 404-237-8153
                          e-mail: info.ga@arthritis.org
                                       www.arthritis.org

Devoted to serving the special needs of children, teens, and
young adults with childhood rheumatic diseases and their families. Offers both support and information through national and local programs that serve the needs of families, friends and health
professionals. Serves as a clearinghouse of information, sponsors
an annual national conference, monitors and promotes legislation,
sponsors research, and offers training to both parents and health
professionals.

Daniel T. McGowan, Chair
John H. Klippel, President
Michael V. Ortman, Secretary

7899   American Liver Foundation
39 Broadway, Suite 2700
New York, NY 10006   212-668-1000
                                          800-465-4837
                                     Fax: 212-483-8179
                      e-mail: info@liverfoundation.org
                                  www.liverfoundation.org

National, voluntary, nonprofit organization dedicated to the prevention, treatment and cure of liver diseases. The foundation offers support groups, advocacy, medical research support and
education.

Thomas F. Nealon III, Chair
David Ticker, Chief Financial Officer
Cynthia Gardner, Vice President, Field Development

7900   American Lung Association
1301 Pennsylvania Ave. NW, Suite 800
Washington, DC 20004   202-785-3355
                                          800-586-4872
                                     Fax: 202-452-1805
                           e-mail: info@lungusa.org
                                          www.lung.org

The American Lung Association fights lung disease in all its
forms, with special emphasis on asthma, tobacco control and environmental health. The American Lung Association is funded
with contributions from the public, along with gifts and grants
from corporations, foundations and government agencies. The association achieves its many successes through the work of thousands of committed volunteers and staff.

Bruce A Herring, Board Chair
Harold Wimmer, President/CEO
John F. Emanuel, J.D., Secretary/Treasurer

7901   American Pediatrics Society
3400 Research Forest Drive, Suite B-7
The Woodlands, TX 77381   281-419-0052
                                     Fax: 281-419-0082
                             e-mail: info@aps-spr.org
                                        www.aps-spr.org

The objects of the Society shall be to bring together men and
women for the advancement of the study of children and their diseases, for the prevention of illness and the promotion of health in
childhood, for the promotion of pediatric education and research,
and to honor those who, by their contributions to pediatrics, have
aided in its advancement.

Debbie Anagnostelis, Executive Director
Kathy Cannon, Associate Executive Director
Kate Culliton, Accounting Manager

7902   American Red Cross
2025 E Street NW
Washington, DC 20006   202-303-4498
                                          800-733-2767
                                     Fax: 202-303-0044
                       e-mail: info@usa.redcross.org
                                        www.redcross.org

The American Red Cross has been the nation's premier emergency response organization. As part of a worldwide movement
that offers neutral humanitarian care to the victims of war, the
American Red Cross distinguished itself by also aiding victims of
devastating natural disasters.

Bonnie McElveen-Hunter, Chair
Gail J. McGovern, President and CEO
Brian J. Rhoa, Chief Financial Officer

7903   American Skin Association
6 East 43rd Street, 28th Floor
New York, NY 10017   212-889-4858
                                          800-499-7546
                                     Fax: 212-889-4959
                       e-mail: info@americanskin.org
                                      www.americanskin.org

The American Skin Association is the only volunteer led health
organization dedicated through research, education and advocacy
to saving lives and alleviating human suffering caused by the full
spectrum of skin disorders.

Howard P. Milstein, Chair
George W Hambrick, Jr, President/Founder
David R Bickers, MD, Executive VP

7904   American Society for Deaf Children
800 Florida Ave NE, #2047
Washington, DC 20002   800-942-2732
                                     Fax: 410-795-0965
                       e-mail: asdc@deafchildren.org
                                       www.deafchildren.org

A nonprofit, parent-helping-parent organization promoting a positive attitude toward signing and deaf culture. Also provides support, encouragement, and current information about deafness to
families with deaf and hard of hearing children.

Jodee Crace, President
Avonne Brooker-Rutowski, Vice President
Timothy G. Frelich, Treasurer

7905   American Speech Language Hearing Associati on (ASHA)
2200 Research Boulevard
Rockville, MD 20850   301-296-5700
                                          800-498-2071
                                     Fax: 301-296-8580
                                     TTY: 301-296-5650
                       e-mail: actioncenter@asha.org
                                          www.asha.org

A professional organization made up of over 123,000 hearing,
speech and language professionals. It is a credentialing organization as well promotes the interests of provides services and information for those with communication disorders.

Arlene A. Pietranton, PhD, CAE, Chief Executive Officer
Patricia A. Prelock, President
Neil T. Shepard, PhD, CCC-A (Bio, Vice President for Academic
Affairs

7906   American Wheelchair Table Tennis Association
P.O. Box 5266
Kendall Park, NJ 08824   732-266-2634
                                     Fax: 732-355-6500
                 e-mail: johnsonjennifer@yahoo.com
                                          www.wsusa.org

AWTTA is the National Governing Body of Wheelchair Sports,
U.S.A., for table tennis. Information on adaptive table tennis activities for people of many abilities. Includes local chapters, referrals, fun and social interaction and support groups.

Barbara Chambers, Chairperson
Jessica Galli, Secretary
Mike Burns, Treasurer

7907   Association for Children's Mental Health
6017 W. St. Joseph Hwy., Suite #200
Lansing, MI 48917   517- 37- 401
                                          888-226-4543
                                     Fax: 517-372-4032
                                         www.acmh-mi.org

ACMH is a family organization with statewide staff and membership who support activities to enhance the system or services which address the needs of children with serious emotional disorders and their families. ACMH is a statewide chapter of the national Federation of families for Children's Mental Health and our membership of over 1200 individuals is comprised of family members, professionals and concerned.

Malisa Pearson, Executive Director
Mary Porter, Business Manager
Terri Henrizi, Training Coordinator and Family Sup

7908 Association for Education & Rehabilitation of the Blind & Visually Impaired
1703 N Beauregard Street, Suite 440
Alexandria, VA 22311
703-671-4500
877-492-2708
Fax: 703-671-6391
e-mail: markr@aerbvi.org
www.aerbvi.org

This association is the only international membership organization dedicated to rendering all possible support and assistance to the professionals who work in all phases of education and rehabilitation of blind and visually impaired children and adults.

Jim Adams, President
Susan Jay Spungin, Secretary
Lou Tutt, Executive Director

7909 Association for Persons with Severe Handicaps (TASH)
1001 Connecticut Avenue, NW, Suite 235
Washington, DC 20036
202-540-9020
Fax: 202-540-9019
e-mail: info@tash.org
www.tash.org

An international association of people with disabilities, their family members, other advocates, and professionals fighting for a society in which inclusion of all people in all aspects of society is the norm.

David Westling, President
Jean Trainor, Vice President
Barbara Trader, Executive Director

7910 Association for the Gifted Child
Council for Exceptional Children
2900 Crystal Drive, Suite 1000
Arlington, VA 22202
703-620-3660
888-232-7733
Fax: 703-264-9494
TTY: 866-915-5000
e-mail: service@cec.sped.org
www.cec.sped.org

Focuses on the delivery of information to both professionals and parents about gifted and talented children and their needs.

Lynda Van Kuren, Contact

7911 Association for the Handicapped
350 5th Avenue, Suite 3304
New York, NY 10118
212-868-1217
Fax: 212-868-1219

Information on adaptive sports and recreation activities for people of many abilities. Includes local chapters, referrals, fun and social interaction and support groups.

7912 Association for the Help of Retarded Children
83 Maiden Lane
New York, NY 10038
212-780-2690
800-662-1220
Fax: 212-777-5893
e-mail: ahrcnyc@dti.net
www.ahrcnyc.org

Developmentally disabled children and adults, their families, and interested individuals. Provides support services, training programs, clinics, schools and residential facilities to the developmentally disabled. Publications: The Chronicle, quarterly newsletter.

Amy West, Chief Financial Officer
Laura J. Kennedy, President
Gary Lind, Executive Director

7913 Association of Blind Athletes
1 Olympic Plaza
Colorado Springs, CO 80909
719-630-0422
Fax: 719-630-0616
e-mail: usaba@usa.net
www.usaba.org

The mission of the United States Association of Blind Athletes is to increase the number and quality of grassroots through competitive, world-class athletic opportunities for Americans who are blind or visually impaired. We value the life enhancing aspects of sports and the opportunity to demonstrate the abilities of people who are blind and visually impaired.

Dave Bushland, President
Tracie Foster, Vice President
Mark A. Lucas, MS, Executive Director

7914 Association of Children's Prosthetic/ Orthotic Clinics
6300 N River Road, Suite 727
Rosemont, IL 60018
847-698-1637
Fax: 847-823-0536
e-mail: acpoc@aaos.org
www.acpoc.org

An association of professionals who are involved in clinics which provide prosthetic-orthotic care for children with limb loss or orthopedic disabilities.

J Ivan Krajbich, MD, President
David B Rotter, CPO, Vice President
Jorge Amelio Fabregas, MD, Secretary-Treasurer

7915 Association of University Centers on Disabilities
1100 Wayne Ave., Suite 1000
Silver Spring, MD 20910
301-588-8252
800-424-3410
Fax: 301-588-2842
TTY: 301-588-3319
e-mail: aucdinfo@aucd.org
www.aucd.org

The Association of University Centers on Disabilities (formerly the American Association of University Affiliated Programs) is a nonprofit organization that promotes and supports the national network of university centers on disabilities, which includes University Centers for Excellence in Developmental Disabilities Education, Research, and Service Leadership Education in Neurodevelopment and Related Disabilities Programs and Developmental Disabilities Research Centers.

Julie Fodor, PhD, President
George S. Jesien, PhD, Executive Director
Laura Martin, MA, Director of Operations

7916 Barbara DeBoer Foundation
79 Fifth Avenue/16th Street
New York, NY 10003
212-620-4230
800-424-9836
Fax: 212-807-3677
e-mail: order@foundationcenter.org
www.foundationcenter.org

Offers a variety of programs that include advocacy services, donor awareness, referral information, medication and medical center information.

Bradford K. Smith, President
Lisa Philp, Vice President for Strategic Philan
Lawrence T. McGill, Vice President for Research

7917 Beneficial Designs
2240 Meridian Boulevard, Suite C
Minden, NV 89423
425-373-5787
Fax: 775-783-8823
e-mail: hello@beneficialdesign.com
www.beneficialdesign.com

Beneficial Designs works towards universal access through research, design, and education. We believe all individuals should have access to the physical, intellectual, and spiritual aspects of life. We seek to enhance the quality of life for people of all abilities, and work to achieve this aim by developing and marketing technology for daily living, vocational, and leisure activities.

Peter Axelson, Founder/Research Director
Denise Yamada Axelson, Research Coordinator

7918 Benetech
480 S California Avenue, Suite 201
Palo Alto, CA 94306   650-644-3400
                                  Fax: 650-475-1066
                            e-mail: info@benetech.org
                                  www.benetech.org

Benetech (formerly Arkenstone) is a nonprofit venture that combines the impact of technological solutions with the social entrepreneurship business model to help disadvantaged communities in our society and across the world.

Jim Fruchterman, President/CEO
Marc Levine, Senior Project Manager
Jane Simchuk, Administration Manager

7919 Birth Defect Research for Children
976 Lake Baldwin Lane, Suite 104
Orlando, FL 32814   407-895-0802
                                  Fax: 407-895-0824
                        e-mail: staff@birthdefects.org
                              www.birthdefects.org

A nonprofit organization that provides information about birth defects of all kinds to parents and professionals. Offers a library of medical books and files of information on less common categories of birth defects and is involved in research to discover possible links between environmental exposures and birth defects.

Betty Mekdeci, Executive Director

7920 Boundless Playgrounds
401 Chestnut St, Suite 410
Chattanooga, TN 37402   423-648-5619
                                       877-268-6353
                                  Fax: 860-243-5854
                 e-mail: info@boundlessplaygrounds.org
                          www.boundlessplaygrounds.org

Boundless Playgrounds helps communities create extraordinary playgrounds where all children, with and without disabilities, can develop essential skills for life as they learn together through play.

Frederick Leone, Chief Executive Officer
Monique Farias, Technical Services Manager
Antonio Mulkusack, Director of Technical Services

7921 Boy Scouts of America National Council
9190 Rockville Pike
Bethseda, MD 20814   301-530-9360
                                  Fax: 301-564-9513
                              www.boyscouts-ncac.org

The mission of the Boy Scouts of America is to prepare young people to make ethical and moral choices over their lifetimes by instilling in them the values of the values of the Scouts Oath and Law.

Hugh Redd, Council President
Ed Yarbrough, Council Commissioner
Les Baron, Scout Executive

7922 Braille Revival League
American Council of the Blind
1155 15th Street NW, Suite 1004
Washington, DC 20005   202-467-5081
                                       800-424-8666
                                  Fax: 202-467-5085
                                e-mail: info@acb.org
                                       www.acb.org

Encourages blind people to read and write in Braille, advocates for mandatory Braille instruction in educational facilities for the blind, strives to make available a supply of Braille materials from libraries and printing houses and more.

7923 Brass Ring Society
500 Macaw Lane, #5
Fern Park, FL 32730   407-339-6188
                                       800-666-9474
                                  Fax: 407-339-6369
                                    www.brassring.org

Society that seeks to fulfill the dreams of children with life-threatening illnesses.

Ray Esposito, Director

7924 Breckenridge Outdoor Education Center
PO Box 697
Breckenridge, CO 80424   970-453-6422
                                       800-383-2632
                                  Fax: 970-453-4676
                              e-mail: boec@boec.org
                                      www.boec.org

The Breckenridge outdoor Education Center is a non-profit organization whose mission is to expand the potential of people with disabilities and special needs through meaningful, educational, and inspiring outdoor experiences.

Tim Casey, Chairman
John Ebright, Vice-Chairman
Bruce Fitch, Executive Director

7925 CANDU Parent Group
Riverwalk Community Center
2100 Manchester Rd., Bldg. B, Suite. 925
Wheaton, IL 60187   630-752-0066
                                  Fax: 630-752-1064
                         e-mail: il@namidupage.org
                               www.namidupage.org

Support and advocacy group for parents of children with serious emotional disturbance, behavioral disorders, or mental illness.

Tony Davis, President
Cora Corley, Secretary
Bob Barger, Treasurer

7926 CHERUB-Association of Families and Friends of Children with Limb Disorders
Children's Hospital of Buffalo
936 Delaware Avenue
Buffalo, NY 14209   716-762-9997

Answers the questions and problems that families of juveniles diagnosed with a disorder may be experiencing.

Sandra Richenberg
Kathy Compliance Officer

7927 Cancer Information Service
National Cancer Institute
6116 Executive Boulevard, Suite 3036A
Bethesda, MD 20892   800-422-6237
                                  Fax: 301-330-7968
                                  TTY: 800-332-8615
                               www.cis.nic.nih.gov

The Cancer Information Service provides the latest and most accurate cancer information to patients, their families, the public, and health professionals. Through its network of regional offices, the CIS serves the United States, Puerto Rico, the U.S. Virgin Islands, and the Pacific Islands.

Andrew C Von Eschenback, Director

7928 Candlelighters Childhood Cancer Foundation
10920 Connecticut Ave., Suite A, PO Box 498
Kensington, MD 20895   301-962-3520
                                       800-366-2226
                                  Fax: 301-962-3521
                          e-mail: staff@candlelighters.org
                                      www.acco.org

The Candlelighters Childhood Cancer Foundation was founded by concerned parents of children with cancer. The foundation is a national nonprofit membership organization whose mission is to educate, support, serve, and advocate for families of children with cancer, survivors of childhood cancer, and the professionals who care for them.

Naomi Bartley, President
Janine Lynne, Vice President
Ruth I. Hoffman, Executive Director

7929 Center for Best Practices in Early Childhood
College of Education and Human Services
1 University Circle
Macomb, IL 61455   309-298-1634
                                  Fax: 309-298-2305
                          e-mail: jk-johanson@wiu.edu
                                 www.wiu.edu/thecenter

Operates the following: Early Childhood Interactive Technology Literacy Curriculum Project; Disseminating and Replicating an Effective Early Childhood Comprehensive Technology System; Expressive Arts Outreach; ECCSPLOR-IT; LiTECH Interactive Outreach; STARNET Regions I and III; and Provider Connections.

Joyce Johanson, Associate Director
Linda Robinson, Assistant Director
Patricia Hutinger, Director

7930 Center for Literacy and Disability Studies
321 South Columbia Street Suite 1100 Bondurant Hal
Chaple Hill, NC 27599   919-966-8566
Fax: 919-843-3250
e-mail: clds@unc.edu
www.med.unc.edu

The Center for Literacy and Disability Studies is a unit within the Department of Allies Health Sciences, school of Medicine, at the University of North Carolina at Chapel Hill.

Karen Erickson

7931 Center for Mental Health Services Knowledge Exchange Network
US Department of Health and Human Services
PO Box 42557
Washington, DC 20015   800-789-2647
Fax: 240-747-5470
TDD: 866-889-2647
www.mentalhealth.samhsa.gov

Supplies the public with responses to their commonly asked questions about mental health issues and services.

7932 Chai Lifeline/Camp Simcha National Office
151 W 30th Street
New York, NY 10001   212-465-1300
800-242-4543
Fax: 212-465-0949
e-mail: info@chailifeline.org
www.chailifeline.org

Chai Life is a not for profit organization dedicated to helping children suffering from serous illness as well as their family members. We offer a comprehensive range is services to address the multiple needs of patients, parents, and siblings.

Esther Schwartz, Director of Hospital Services

7933 Child Abuse Prevention Association
503 E 23rd Street
Independence, MO 64055   816-252-8388
Fax: 816-252-1337
e-mail: capa@childabuseprevention.org
www.childabuseprevention.org

Mission is to prevent and treat all forms of child abuse by creating changes in individuals, families and society which strengthen relationships and promote healing.

Shelly Hall, Chairman
Jeanetta Issa, CEO
Karen Costa, Clinical Director

7934 Child Care Plus+
Univ. of Montana Rural Institute on Disabilities
634 Eddy Avenue
Missoula, MT 59812   406-243-6355
800-235-4122
Fax: 406-243-4730
TDD: 406-243-5467
e-mail: ccplus@selway.umt.edu
www.ccplus.org

Provides inclusion information and resources for child care providers and other professionals: written materials (newsletter, curriculum, articles), training, workshops, technical assistance and various other resources.

Sandra L. Morris, Center Co-Director
Susan Harper-Whalen, Consultant
Karen Martin, Inclusion I and II Instructor

7935 Children's Defense Fund
25 E Street NW
Washington, DC 20001   202-628-8787
800-233-1200
Fax: 202-662-3510
e-mail: cdfinfo@childrensdefense.org
www.childrensdefense.org

Information and advocacy resources for families and professionals. Includes listings of organizations providing general information and organizations focusing on more specific areas of concern to families and young adults who have disabilities.

Geoffrey Canada, Chairman
Kenneth Troshinsky, Chief Financial Officer
Marian Wright Edelman, President

7936 Children's Hopes and Dreams
138 Cloudland Road
Dahlonega, GA 30533   706-482-2248
Fax: 706-482-2289
e-mail: chdfdover@juno.com
www.helpingnow.org

Three programs: Dream fulfillment program is for children age four through seventeen with life threatening illness who have not received a dream before; Pen Pal Program matches children five through seventeen with chronic or life threatening illnesses, conditions, disabilities or major trauma to other ill children by their age, sex and illness category; Kid's Kare Package program supplies new donated items to children through Pen Pal Program and/or health care professionals.

Luke Oswald, Program Director

7937 Children's Hopes and Dreams Foundation
Wish Fulfillment Foundation
138 Cloudland Road
Dahlonega, GA 30533   706-482-2248
Fax: 706-482-2289
e-mail: chdfdover@juno.com
www.helpingnow.org

Children's Hopes & Dreams Foundation has been serving children with serious childhood illnesses since 1983.

10,000 Members

Luke Oswald, Program Director

7938 Children's Hospice International
1101 King Street Suite 360
Alexandria, VA 22314   703-684-0330
800-242-4453
Fax: 703-684-0330
e-mail: info@chionline.org
www.chionline.org

This nonprofit organization works to improve hospice care for children. Free services include information and referral service for child care, counseling, support groups, pain management, professional education, and research. This is a membership group, with a membership fee for other services.

Ann Armstrong-Dailey, Founding Director/CEO
Richard Larkin, Secretary/Treasurer
Rebecca Brant, Directors

7939 Children's Hospital Boston
300 Longwood Avenue
Boston, MA 02115   617-355-6000
Fax: 617-277-4832
TTY: 617-730-0152
e-mail: webteam@tch.harvard.edu
www.childrenshospital.org

Children's Hospital Boston is a 325 bed comprehensive center for pediatric health care. As the largest pediatric medical center in the United States, Children's offers a complete range of health care services for children from 15 weeks gestation through 21 years of age (and older in some cases).

James Mandell, MD, Chief Executive Officer
Sandra Fenwick, President and Chief Operating Offic
Naomi Fried, PhD, Chief Innovation Officer

7940 Children's Organ Transplant Association
2501 Cota Drive
Bloomington, IN 47403   800-366-2682
                                    Fax: 812-336-8885
                                    e-mail: cota@cota.org
                                    www.cota.org

The association provides fundraising assistance for children needing life-saving transplants and promotes organ, marrow and tissue
donation.

Rick Lofgren, President/CEO
Lisa Fulkerson, VP/CFO
Judy Sutton, Administrative Assisstant

7941 Children's Wish Foundation International
8615 Roswell Road
Atlanta, GA 30350   770-393-9474
                                         800-323-9474
                                    Fax: 770-393-0683
                                    e-mail: wish@childrenswish.org
                                    www.childrenswish.org

A nonprofit organization that fulfills wishes for children with life
threatening illnesses. The criteria for wish fulfillment are: The
child must be under the age of eighteen, and have been diagnosed
with a life threatening illness.

Arthur Stein, President
Linda Dozoretz, Founder/Executive Director

7942 Chill: Straight Talk About Stress
Childs Work/Childs Play
303 Crossways Park Drive
Woodbury, NY 11797   516-349-5520
                                         800-962-1141
                                    Fax: 800-262-1886
                                    e-mail: info@Childswork.com
                                    www.Childswork.com

Childswork/Childsplay uses a prevention and intervention model
when creating its high-quality products. These programs focus on
the behavioral, social, and emotional issues children deal with at
home and at school. Through the use of games, print materials
and visual media, counselors and educators have a superior array
of counseling tools at their disposal.

7943 Christian Horizons
25 Sportsworld Crossing Road
Kitchener, ON N2P 0   519-650-0966
                                         866-362-6810
                                    Fax: 519-650-8984
                                    e-mail: info@christian-horizons.org
                                    www.christian-horizons.org

Devoted to assisting individuals, with developmental disabilities,
on a day-to-day basis.

Nigel Wilford, Chair
Janet Nolan, CEO
Claire Lebold, Vice Chair

7944 Compassionate Friends
PO Box 3696
Oak Brook, IL 60522   630-990-0010
                                         877-969-0010
                                    Fax: 630-990-0246
                                    e-mail: nationaloffice@compassionatefriends.org
                                    www.compassionatefriends.org

Compassionate Friends assists families toward the positive resolution of grief following the death of a child of any age and provides information to help others be supportive. A national
nonprofit, self-help support organization that offers friendship,
understanding, and hope to bereaved parents, grandparents and
siblings.

Rick Yotti, President
Ronald Haynes, VP
Patricia Loder, Executive Director

7945 Cooperative Wilderness Handicapped Outdoor Group
Idaho State University
921 South 8th Avenue
Pocatello, ID 83209   208-282-3912
                                    Fax: 208-282-2127
                                    e-mail: krindavi@isu.edu
                                    www.isu.edu

A regional self-help group to provide recreational opportunities
for people of all disabilities. The program is part of the Idaho
State University.

Dr. Michael McCurry, Professor Of Geosciences
Dr. Leslie Devaud, Associate Professor Of Ph Sciences

7946 Council for Educational Diagnostic Services (CEDS)
Council for Exceptional Children
1664 N. Virginia Street
Reno, NV 89557   775-784-1110
                                         888-232-7733
                                    Fax: 775-784-6429
                                    TTY: 703-264-9446
                                    www.unr.edu

Promotes the highest quality of diagnostic and prescriptive procedures involved in the education of individuals with disabilities
and/or who are gifted. Members include educational diagnosticians, psychologists, social workers, speech and language specialists, physicians, and other professionals and related service
professionals.

Dr. Marc Johnson, President
Patricia Richard, Assistant Vice President for Consti
Janet Sanderson, Executive Assistant to the Presiden

7947 Council for Exceptional Children
2900 Crystal Drive, Suite 1000
Arlington, VA 22202   703-620-3660
                                         888-232-7733
                                    Fax: 703-264-9494
                                    TTY: 866-915-5000
                                    e-mail: service@cec.sped.org
                                    www.cec.sped.org

Advocates appropriate policies, standards and development for
students with special needs.

Lynda Van Kuren, Contact

7948 Council of Administrators of Special Education
Council for Exceptional Children
101 Katelyn Circle, Suite E
Warner Robins, GA 31088   478-333-6892
                                         888-232-7733
                                    Fax: 478-333-2453
                                    TTY: 703-264-9446
                                    e-mail: lpurcell@casecec.org
                                    www.casecec.org

A international professional educational organization which is affiliated with the Council for Exceptional Children (CEC) whose
members are dedicated to the enhancement of the worth, dignity,
potential, and uniqueness of each individual in society. The mission is to provide leadership and support to members by shaping
policies and practices which impact the quality of education.

Laurie VanderPloeg, President
Tom Adams, Finance Committee Chairman
Dr. Luann Purcell, Executive Director

7949 Council of Families with Visual Impairments
American Council of the Blind
6686 Capricorn Lane N.E.
Bremerton, WA 98311   360-698-0827
                                         800-424-8666
                                    Fax: 202-467-5085
                                    e-mail: cindybur@comcast.net
                                    www.cfvi.info/keep.html

A network of parents with blind or visually impaired children
that offers support and outreach, shares experiences in par-
ent/child relationships, exchanges educational, cultural and medical information about child development and more.

7950 Courage Center
3915 Golden Valley Road
Minneapolis, MN 55422   763-588-0811
888-846-8253
Fax: 612-520-0577
TTY: 763-520-0245
e-mail: Information@CourageCenter.org
www.couragecenter.org

The mission of Courage Center is to empower people with physical disabilities to reach for their full potential in every aspect of life. We are guided by the vision that one day, all people will live, work, learn and play in a community based on abilities, not disabilities.

John Church, Chair
Kathy Connors, Treasurer
Jan Malcolm, Secretary

7951 CureSearch: The National Childhood Cancer Foundation
4600 East West Highway, Suite 600
Bethseda, MD 20814   800-458-6223
Fax: 301-718-0047
e-mail: info@curesearch.org
www.curesearch.org

Cure Search unites the Children's Oncology Group (COG) and the National Childhood Center Foundation (NCCF) through a shared mission to cure and prevent childhood and adolescent cancer through scientific discovery and compassionate care.

Stuart Siegel, Chair
Laura Thrall, President and CEO
Christine Bor, Chief Development Officer

7952 Deafness Research Foundation
363 Seventh Avenue, 10th Floor
New York, NY 10001   212-257-6140
866-454-3924
e-mail: info@hearinghealthfoundation.org
www.hearinghealthfoundation.org

The nation's largest voluntary health organization entirely committed to public awareness and support for basic and clinical research into deafness and hearing disabilities. Sponsors a broad program of innovative research and education into the causes, treatments and prevention of nerve deafness, increases the number of young scientists entering and engaged in otologic studies, increases the nation's awareness and creates an understanding of serious hearing dysfunctions.

Shari Eberts, Chairman
Mark Angelo, President
Andrea Boidman, Executive Director

7953 Developmental Delay Resources
5801 Beacon St.
Pittsburgh, PA 15217   800-497-0944
Fax: 412-422-1374
www.devdelay.org

A nonprofit organization dedicated to meeting the needs of those working with children who have developmental delays in sensory motor, language, social, and emotional areas. DDR provides a network for parents and professionals and current information after the diagnosis to support children with special needs.

Patricia S. Lemer, Executive Director
Teresa Badillo, Executive Board
Margaret Britt, Executive Board

7954 Developmental Disabilities Nurses Association
Po Box 536489
Orlando, FL 32853   407-835-0642
800-888-6733
Fax: 407-426-7440
e-mail: ddnahq@aol.com
www.ddna.org

A nonprofit professional nursing organization founded to meet the professional needs of nurses serving individuals with developmental disabilities.

Kathleen Brown, President
Wendy Herbers, Vice President
Richanne Cunningham, Secretary

7955 Disability Rights Education & Defense Fund
2212 6th Street
Berkeley, CA 94710   510-644-2555
Fax: 510-841-8645
e-mail: dredf@dredf.org
www.dredf.org

Nonprofit law and public policy center that specializes in laws affecting more than 45 million Americans with disabilities. DREDF was founded 16 years ago to challenge the barriers that exclude people with disabilities from participating in all aspects of society.

Jenny Kern, President/Chair
Susan Henderson, Executive Director
Arlene B. Mayerson, Directing Attorney

7956 Disabled Shooting Services
National Rifle Association of America
11250 Waples Mill Road
Fairfax, VA 22030   703-267-1495
800-672-3888
e-mail: info@nrpa.org
www.compete.nra.org

Information on adaptive shooting activities for people of many abilities. Includes local chapters, referrals, fun and social interaction and support groups.

Dave Baskin, Department Head

7957 Disabled Sports USA
451 Hungerford Drive, Suite 100
Rockville, MD 20850   301-217-0960
Fax: 301-217-0968
e-mail: info@dsusa.org
www.dsusa.org

A national nonprofit, organization established in 1967 by disabled Vietnam veterans to serve the war injured. DS/USA now offers nationwide sports rehabilitation programs to anyone with a permanent disability.

Kirk Bauer, Executive Director
Cheryl Collins, Administrative Services Manager
Orlando Gill, Field Representative

7958 Division for Early Childhood
27 Fort Missoula Road, Suite 2
Missoula, MT 59804   406-543-0872
Fax: 406-543-0887
TTY: 703-264-9446
e-mail: dec@dec-sped.org
www.dec-sped.org

This division is one of seventeen divisions of the Council for Exceptional Children, the largest international professional organization dedicated to improving educational outcomes for individuals with exceptionalities, students with disabilities, and/or the gifted.

Leah Weiner, Executive Director
Cynthia Wood, Associate Executive Director

7959 Division for Physical and Health Disablities
Council for Exceptional Children
1110 N Glebe Road, Suite 300
Arlington, VA 22201   703-620-3660
888-232-7733
Fax: 703-264-9474
TTY: 703-264-9446
www.education.gsu.edu

Advocates for quality education for individuals with physical disabilities and special health care needs in schools, hospitals, or home settings.

Pam DeLoach, President
Blanche Jackson Glimps, Vice President
Peggy Allgood, Interim Secretary

7960 Division of Birth Defects & Developmental Disabilities
National Center for Environmental Health
4770 Buford Highway NE
Atlanta, GA 30341   770-488-7150
888-232-6789
Fax: 770-488-7156
www.cdc.gov

Information and advocacy resources for families and professionals dealing with children with birth defects and developmental disabilities.

Raymond Strikas, Director
Tom Frieden, MD, MPH, Director, Centers for Disease Contr
Linda C. Degutis, DrPH, MSN, Director, National Center for Injur

7961 Division on Career Development and Transition
Council for Exceptional Children
1110 N Glebe Road, Suite 300
Arlington, VA 22201
703-620-3660
888-232-7733
Fax: 703-264-9474
TTY: 866-915-5000
www.dcdt.org

Focuses on the career development of individuals with disabilities and their transition from school to adult life.

Audrey Trainor, President
Joseph W. Madaus, Vice President
Darlene Unger, Treasurer

7962 ERIC Clearinghouse on Disabilities & Gifted Children
Council for Exceptional Children
1110 N Glebe Road Suite 300
Arlington, VA 22201
703-620-3660
888-232-7733
Fax: 703-264-9494
TTY: 866-915-5000
e-mail: ericec@cec.sped.org
www.cec.sped.org/ericec.htm

Information and advocacy resources for families and professionals. Includes listings of organizations providing general information and organizations focusing on more specific areas of concern to families and young adults who have disabilities.

7963 Easter Seals Disability Services
233 South Wacker Drive, Suite 2400
Chicago, IL 60606
205-759-1211
800-221-6827
Fax: 312-726-1494
TDD: 312-726-4258
e-mail: info@easterseals.com
www.easterseals.com

Easter Seals mission is to create solutions that change lives for children and adults with disabilities and to provide appropriate developmental and rehabilitation services. Services provided include early intervention, after-school programs, preschool, tutoring, medical rehabilitation, vocational services, adult and senior day services, respite and in home care, camping and recreation, residential housing, support services, support groups, transportation and referrals.

Stephen F. Rossman, Chairman
Richard W. Davidson, 1st Vice Chairman
James E Williams Jr, President/CEO

7964 Endocrine Society
8401 Connecticut Avenue, Suite 900
Chevy Chase, MD 20815
301-941-0200
Fax: 301-941-0259
e-mail: endostaff@endo-society.org
www.endo-society.org/

To advance excellence in endocrinology and promote its essential role as an integrative force in scientific research and medical practice.

William F. Young, Jr., M.D., M.Sc., President
Ursula Kaiser, M.D., Vice President (Basic Scientist)
Margaret E. W ierman, M.D., Vice President (Clinical Scientist)

7965 Family Caregiver Alliance
180 Montgomery Street Suite 900
San Francisco, CA 94104
415-434-3388
800-445-8016
Fax: 415-434-3508
e-mail: info@caregiver.org
www.caregiver.org

Good information with resources and hotline numbers.

Ping Hao, MBA, President
Jacquelyn Kung, Vice President
Kathleen Kelly, MPA, Executive Director

7966 Family Voices
3701 San Mateo Blvd NE, Suite 200
Albuguerque, NM 87110
505-872-4774
888-835-5669
Fax: 505-872-4780
e-mail: kidshealth@familyvoices.org
www.familyvoices.org

Family Voices, a national grassroots network of families and friends, advocates for health care services that are famliy-centered, community-based, comprehensive. coordinated and culturally competent for all children and youth with special health care needs; promotes the inclusion of all families as decision makers at all levels of health care; and supports essential partnerships between families and professionals.

Molly Cole, President
Marcia O'Malley, Vice-President
Lynn Pedraza, Executive Director

7967 Federation for Children with Special Needs Center
529 Main Street, Suite 1102
Boston, MA 02129
617-236-7210
800-331-0688
Fax: 617-241-0330
e-mail: fcsninfo@fcsn.org
www.fcsn.org

The Federation is a center for parents and parent organizations to work together on behalf of children (up to age 22) with special needs and their families. The Federation operates a Parent Center in Massachusetts that offers a variety of services to parents, parent groups and others who are concerned with children with special needs.

James F. Whalen, President
Michael Weiner, Treasurer
Kate Brewe, Information Specialist

7968 Federation of Families for Children's Mental Health
9605 Medical Center Drive, Suite 280
Rockville, MD 20850
240-403-1901
Fax: 240-403-1909
e-mail: ffcmh@ffcmh.org
www.ffcmh.org

The National family run organization is dedicated exclusively to helping children with mental health needs and their families achieve a better quality of life.

Teka Dempson, President
Sherri Luthe, Vice President
Sandra Spencer, Executive Director

7969 Foundation for Exceptional Children
16 Lake Shore Road
Grosse Poimte Farm, MI 48236
313-885-8660

To improve the well-being of children and families by providing theapeutic, social and educational services.

7970 Friends' Health Connection
PO Box 114
New Brunswick, NJ 08903
732-418-1811
800-483-7436
Fax: 732-249-9897
e-mail: info@friendshealthconnection.org
www.friendshealthconnection.org

Organization Mission Friends' Health Connection is a nonprofit organization that connects people who are currently experiencing or who have overcome the same disease, illness, handicap or injury in order to communicate for mutual support.
1989

Roxanne Black-Weisheit, FHC Founder and Executive Director

7971 Genetic Alliance
4301 Connecticut Avenue NW, Suite 404
Washington, DC 20008
202-966-7955
800-336-4363
Fax: 202-966-8553
e-mail: info@geneticalliance.org
www.geneticalliance.org

A nonprofit tax exempt organization founded in 1986 as a national coalition of consumers, professionals and genetic support groups to voice the common concerns of children and adults and families living with, and at risk of, genetic conditions. The Alliance builds partnerships among consumers and professionals and the private and public sectors to promote optimum healthcare and enhanced quality of life for individuals identified with genetic conditions.

Sharon Terry, President/CEO
Natasha Bonhomme, Vice President of Strategic Develop
Lisa Wise, MA, Chief Operating Officer

7972   Girl Scouts of the USA
Membership and Program Group
420 5th Avenue
New York, NY 10018   212-852-8000
800-478-7248
Fax: 212-852-6515
www.girlscouts.org

Girl Scout of the USA is the world's preeminent organization dedicated solely to girls-all girls-where, in an accepting and nurturing environment, girls build character and skills for success in the real world.

Anna Maria Ch vez, CEO
Nhadine Leung, Chief of Staff
Connie L. Lindsey, Chairman

7973   Handicapped Scuba Association
1104 El Prado
San Clemente, CA 92672   949-498-4540
800-673-5084
Fax: 949-498-6128
e-mail: hsa@hsascuba.com
www.hsascuba.com

Information on adaptive scuba diving activities for people of many abilities. Includes local chapters, referrals, fun and social interaction and support groups.

7974   Handle with Care
184 McKinstry Road
Gardnier, NY 12525   845-255-4031
888-590-5049
Fax: 845-256-0094
e-mail: info@handlewithcare.com
www.handlewithcare.com

Information and advocacy resources for families and professionals. Includes listings of organizations providing general information and organizations focusing on more specific areas of concern to families and young adults who have disabilities.

Bruce Chapman, Founder/President
Hilary Adler, Vice President
Jeanette Smith, Accounting Dept. & Office Manager

7975   Heriditary Disease Foundation
3960 Broadway, 6th Floor
New York, NY 10032   212-928-2121
Fax: 212-928-2172
e-mail: cures@hdfoundation.org
www.hdfoundation.org

Conducts interdisciplinary workshop program that recruits scientists to develop and apply new technologies, supports basic research on genetic illness through grant and postdoctoral fellowship programs at major universities, and provides research tissue to medical investigators.

Nancy Wexler, President
Frank O. Gehry, Vice President
Alice Wexler, Secretary

7976   Houston Challengers TIRR Sports
1475 W Gray
Houston, TX 77019   713-521-3737

Information on adaptive sports and recreation activities for people of many abilities. Includes local chapters, referrals, fun and social interaction and support groups.

7977   Human Growth Foundation
997 Glen Cove Avenue, Suite 5
Glen Head, NY 11545   516-671-4041
800-451-6434
Fax: 516-671-4055
e-mail: hgfl@hgfound.org
www.hgfound.org

Provides referrals to support groups, services, and genetic counseling on its toll-free telephone line. Encourages communication among support groups and continuing education.

Pisit Pitukcheewanon, President
Emily Germain-Lee, Vice President
Patti D Costa, Executive Director

7978   Independent Living Research Utilization Program
2323 S Shepard, Suite 1000
Houston, TX 77019   713-520-0232
Fax: 713-520-5785
TTY: 713-520-5136
e-mail: ilru@ilru.org
www.ilru.org

Information and advocacy resources for families and professionals on independent living for people with disabilities.

Lex Frieden, Director, ILRU
Linda CoVan, Grant Coordinator
Maria Del Bosque, Project Associate

7979   Indian Health Service
Mental Health/Social Service Programs Branch
801 Thompson Avenue, Suite 400
Rockville, MD 20852   301-443-1083

Includes listings of organizations providing general information and organizations focusing on more specific areas of concern to Native American families and young adults who have disabilities.

7980   Institute for Families of Blind Children
4650 Sunset Blvd, Mail Stop 111
Los Angeles, CA 90027   213-669-4649
800-669-4549
Fax: 323-665-7869
e-mail: info@instituteforfamilies.org
www.instituteforfamilies.org

Offers support and information to families of blind children. Provides direct counseling and nation-wide telephone counseling.

Peggy Yoshino, Chairman
Eric Dahl, Chief Financial Officer
Joni Dahl, Secretary

7981   International Braille and Technology Center for the Blind
National Federation of the Blind
1800 Johnson Street
Baltimore, MD 21230   410-659-9314
Fax: 410-685-5653
e-mail: nfb@nfb.org
www.nfb.org

World's largest and most complete evaluation and demonstration center of all assistive technology used by the blind from around the world. Includes all Braille, synthetic speech, print-to-speech scanning, internet and portable devices and programs. Available for tours by appointment to blind persons, employers, technology manufacturers, teachers, parents and those working in the assistive technology field.

Curtis Chong, President, Computer Science

7982   International Society of Dermatology
2323 North State Street #30
Bunnell, FL 32110   386-437-4405
Fax: 386-437-4427
e-mail: info@IntSocDermatol.org
www.intsocderm.org

Promotes interest, education and research in dermatology.

Francisco Kerdel, President
Mark D P Davis, MD, Vice President
Martin Kassir, MD, Vice President

7983 International Wheelchair Aviators
82 Corral Drive
Keller, TX 76244   817-229-4634
e-mail: wheelchairaviators@yahoo.com
www.wheelchairaviators.org

Provides information for pilots or future pilots who have a disability.

Mike Smith, President

7984 Iron Overload Diseases Assocation
525 Mayflower Rd.
West Palm Beach, FL 33405   561-586-8246
Fax: 561-842-9881
e-mail: iod@ironoverload.org
www.ironoverload.org

Committed to providing information and support to affected individuals and their families, educating the general public, promoting and supporting research, and pressing for earlier diagnosis and more effective treatment. Acts as a clearinghouse for affected individuals and family members, provides telephone consultations, offers referrals to genetic counseling and support groups. Provides a variety of educational and support materials including books, newsletters, pamphlets, and fact sheets.

7985 Jewish Children's Adoption Network
PO Box 147016
Denver, CO 80214   303-573-8113
Fax: 303-893-1447
e-mail: jcan@qwest.net
www.jcan.qwestoffice.net

Information and advocacy resources for families and professionals. Includes listings of organizations providing general information.

Stephen Krausz, PhD, President

7986 Job Opportunities for the Blind
1800 Johnson Street
Baltimore, MD 21230   410-659-9314
Fax: 410-685-5653
e-mail: nfb@nfb.org
www.nfb.org

Information and resources for those with visual impairments.

Curtis Chong, President, Computer Science

7987 Just One Break
570 Seventh Avenue, 6th Floor
New York, NY 10018   212-785-7300
Fax: 212-785-4513
TTY: 212-785-4515
e-mail: justonebreak@interactive.net
www.justonebreak.com

Information and advocacy resources for families and professionals dealing with families and young adults who have disabilities.

C. Jeffrey Knittel, Chairman
Russ Cusick, Chief People Officer
John D. Kemp, President

7988 Learning Disabilities Association of Ameri ca
4156 Library Road
Pittsburgh, PA 15234   412-341-1515
888-300-6710
Fax: 412-344-0224
e-mail: info@LDAAmerica.org
www.ldaamerica.org

Helps families of the affected individual through information and referral to professionals in their area. A membership organization with affiliates across the country.

Sheila Buckley, Executive Director

7989 MUMS: National Parent to Parent Network
150 Custer Street
Green Bay, WI 54301   920-336-5333
877-336-5333
Fax: 920-339-0995
e-mail: mums@netnet.net
www.netnet.net/mums/

Matches parents of children with rare disorders. Provides information and advocacy resources for families and professionals. Includes listings of organizations providing general information and organizations focusing on more specific areas of concern to families and young adults who have disabilities.

Julie Gordon, Director

7990 Make Today Count
101 1/2 S Union Street
Alexandria, VA 22314   703-548-9674

An organization that helps patients and their families cope with cancer and other serious diseases and improve their quality of life.

7991 March of Dimes Birth Defects Foundation
1275 Mamaroneck Avenue
White Plains, NY 10605   914-997-4488
888-663-4637
Fax: 914-428-8203
e-mail: resourcecenter@modimes.org
www.marchofdimes.com

Partnership of volunteers and professionals dedicated to the mission of the March of Dimes to improve the health of babies by preventing birth defects and infant mortality. Chapters are situated across the country and can be located through the web site, National Office, or telephone book. The Resource Center answers questions relating to preconception health, pregnancy, childbirth and birth defects.

Dr Jennifer Howse, President

7992 March of Dimes Nursing Modules
1275 Mamaroneck Avenue
White Plains, NY 10605   914-997-4488
888-663-4637
Fax: 914-428-8203
e-mail: productquestions@marchofdimes.com
www.marchofdimes.com/catalog

Nursing modules are self-directed learning monographs designed for registered nurses and nurse-midwives. Created to help nurses meet the challenges posed by a rapidly changing world of technological advances, evolving demographics and greater cultural diversity, they focus on effective care delivery during the pre-conceptional, prenatal, intrapartum, postpartum and inter-conceptional periods.

Dr Jennifer Howse, President

7993 NADD: National Association for the Dually Diagnosed
132 Fair Street
Kingston, NY 12401   845-331-4336
800-331-5362
Fax: 845-331-4569
e-mail: info@thenadd.org
www.thenadd.org

Nonprofit organization designed to promote the interests of professional and parent development with resources for individuals who have the coexistence of mental illness and mental retardation. Provides conferences, educational services and training materials to professionals, parents, concerned citizens, and service organizations.

Dr Robert Fletcher, CEO
Michelle Jordan, Office Manager
Lisa Christie, Conference Planner

7994 NAEYC: National Association for the Education of Young Children
1313 L Street, NW, Suite 500
Washington, DC 20005   202-232-8777
800-424-2460
Fax: 202-328-1846
e-mail: pubaff@aeyc.org
www.naeyc.org

Information and advocacy resources for families and professionals. Includes listings of organizations providing general information and organizations focusing on more specific areas of concern to families and young adults who have disabilities.

Gera Jacobs, President
Roberta Schomburg, Vice President
Jerlean E. Daniel, Executive Director

7995 National Ability Center
PO Box 682799, 1000 Ability Way
Park City, UT 84068
435-649-3991
Fax: 435-658-3992
TDD: 435-649-3991
e-mail: info@DiscoverNAC.org
www.discovernac.org

Information on adaptive sports and recreation activities for people of many abilities. Includes local chapters, referrals, fun and social interaction and support groups.

Gail Loveland, Executive Director
Ellen Hall Adams, Program Director
Kristi Brangle, Executive Assistant - Resource Deve

7996 National Academy for Child Development (NACD)
549 25th Street
Ogden, UT 84401
801-621-8606
Fax: 801-621-8389
e-mail: info@nacd.org
www.nacd.org

International organization of parents and professionals dedicated to helping children and adults reach their full potential.

Julian Neil, Director of Health

7997 National Adoption Center
1500 Walnut Street, Suite 701
Philadelphia, PA 19102
215-735-9988
800-862-3678
Fax: 215-735-9410
e-mail: nac@nationaladoptioncenter.org
www.adopt.org

Information and advocacy resources for families and professionals interested in or dealing with adoption. Includes listings of organizations providing general information and organizations focusing on specific areas of concern.

Ken Mullner, Executive Director
Gloria Hochman, Director of Communications
Christine Jacobs, Program Director

7998 National Alliance for the Mentally Ill
3803 N. Fairfax Dr., Ste. 100
Arlington, VA 22203
703-524-7600
800-950-6264
Fax: 703-524-9094
TDD: 703-516-7227
e-mail: info@nami.org
www.nami.org

NAMI is a nonprofit, grassroots, self-help, support and advocacy organization of consumers, families and friends of people with severe mental illness, such as schizophrenia, bipolar disorder, major depressive disorder, obsessive compulsive disorder, anxiety disorders, autism and other severe and persistent mental illnesses that affect the brain.

David Levy, Chief Financial Officer
Lynn Borton, Chief Operating Officer
Jean-Michel Texier, Chief Information Officer

7999 National Amputee Golf Association
11 Walnut Hill Road
Amherst, NH 03031
603-672-6444
800-633-6242
Fax: 603-672-2987
e-mail: webmaster@nagagolf.org
www.nagagolf.org

Information on adaptive golf activities for people of many abilities. Includes local chapters, referrals, fun and social interaction and support groups.

Kenny Greene, Executive Director
Virgil Price, Treasurer
Bob Wilson, Consultant

8000 National Archery Association
4065 Sinton Road, Suite 110
Colorado Springs, CO 80907
719-578-4576
Fax: 719-632-4733
e-mail: dparker@usarchery.org
www.usarchery.org

Information on adaptive archery activities for people of many abilities. Includes local chapters, referrals, fun and social interaction and support groups.

Denise Parker, Chief Executive Officer
Cindy Clark, Office/Finance Manager
Amber Hildebrand, Accounting Assistant

8001 National Arts and Disability Center
760 Westwood Plaza
Los Angeles, CA 90095
310-794-1141
800-UCL- MD1
Fax: 310-794-1143
TTY: 310-267-2356
e-mail: oraynor@mednet.ucla.edu
www.semel.ucla.edu

Information and advocacy resources for families and professionals. Includes listings of organizations providing general information on art and disabilities.

Olivia Raynor, Director
Beth Stoffmacher, Technical Assisstance Coordinator
Peter Whybrow, Director

8002 National Association for Parents of Childr en with Visual Impairments
PO Box 317
Watertown, MA 02471
617-972-7441
800-562-6265
Fax: 617-972-7444
e-mail: napvi@perkins.org
www.spedex.com/napvi/

Julie Urban, President
Venetia Hayden, Vice President
Susan LaVenture, Executive Director

8003 National Association of Blind Students
National Federation of the Blind
1800 Johnson Street
Baltimore, MD 21230
410-659-9314
Fax: 410-685-5653
www.nabslink.org

Provides support, information and encouragement to blind college and university students. Leads the way in offering resources for national testing, accessible textbooks and materials, overcoming negative attitudes about blindness from school personnel, developing new techniques of accomplishing laboratory or field assignments and many other college experiences. Offers strong advocacy and motivational support.

Sean Whalen, President
Shelby Ball, Treasurer
Cindy Bennett, Secretary

8004 National Association of Protection and Advocacy Systems
900 2nd Street NE, Suite 211
Washington, DC 20002
202-408-9514
Fax: 202-408-9520
TTY: 202-408-9521
e-mail: NAPAS@earthlink.net
www.napas.org

Information and advocacy resources for families and professionals. Includes listings of organizations providing general information and organizations focusing on more specific areas of concern to families and young adults who have disabilities.

Curtis L Decker, Executive Director

8005 National Association of the Dually Diagnosed
132 Fair Street
Kingston, NY 12401
845-331-4336
800-331-5362
Fax: 845-331-4569
e-mail: info@thenadd.org
www.thenadd.org

Seeks to stimulate the public and professional awareness regarding the dually diagnosed population, and to encourage the exchange of pertinent information, promoting educational and training programs, advocating for appropriate governmental policies, supporting research focusing on identification, diagnosis, and treatment.

Robert J. Fletcher DSW, Chief Executive Officer
Michelle Jordan, Office Manager
Lisa Christie, Conference Planner

8006 National Center for Learning Disabilities
381 Park Avenue S, Suite 1401
New York, NY 10016   212-545-7510
                                      888-575-7373
                                      Fax: 212-545-9665
                                      www.ncld.org

Works to ensure that the nation's 15 million children, adolescents
and adults with learning disabilities have every opportunity to
succeed in school, work and life. NCLD provides essential information to parents, professionals and individuals with learning disabilities, promotes research and programs to foster effective
learning and advocates for policies to protect and strengthen
educational rights and opportunities.

Sheldon Horowitz MD, LD Resources/Essential Information
James H Wendorf, Executive Director
Alan Bendich, Director, Finance & Operations

8007 National Center for Sight
National Society To Prevent Blindness
500 Remington Road
Schaumburg, IL 60173   847-843-2020
                                      Fax: 847-843-8458

A toll-free line offering information on a broad range of vision,
eye health and safety topics including sports eye safety, lazy eye,
diabetic retinopathy, glaucoma, cataracts, children's eye disorders, and more.

8008 National Center for Vision and Child Development
Lighthouse
111 E 59th Street
New York, NY 10022   212-821-9200
                                      800-829-0500
                                      Fax: 212-821-9707
                                      TTY: 212-821-9713
                                      e-mail: info@lighthouse.org
                                      www.lighthouse.org

The mission is to overcome vision impairment for people of all
ages through worldwide leadership in rehabilitation services, education, research, prevention and advocacy.

Joseph A. Ripp, Chairman
Mark G. Ackermann, President/Chief Executive Officer
Robert P. Hoak Jr., Chief Development Officer

8009 National Center on Accessbility
University of Indiana
501 North Morton Street, Suite 109
Bloomington, IN 47404   812-856-4422
                                      800-424-1877
                                      Fax: 812-856-4480
                                      TTY: 812-856-4421
                                      e-mail: nca@indiana.edu
                                      www.ncaonline.org

Information on adaptive activities for people of many abilities.
Includes local chapters, referrals, fun and social interaction and
support groups.

Sherril York, Director
Ray Bloomer, Director of Education & Technical A
Jennifer Skulski, Director of Marketing and Special P

8010 National Children's Cancer Society
One South Memorial Drive, Suite 800
Saint Louis, MO 63102   314-241-1600
                                      800-532-6459
                                      Fax: 314-241-6949
                                      e-mail: nccs@children-cancer.com
                                      nationalchildrenscancersociety.com

NCCS offers a multifaceted outreach program, which includes financial assistance, education, information, and emotional support.
They provide financial assistance for bone marrow transplantation, donor harvest, donor search, donor recruitment, and family
emergency expenses (such as travel, hotel, food). They also have
an active advocacy program to help families with insurance
companies and hospitals.

Mark Stolze, President
Julie Komanetsky, Director Patient/Family Services

8011 National Christian Resource Center
Bethesda Lutheran Homes
300 N. Kanawha Street, Suite 100
Beckley, WV 25801   304-252-9494
                                      800-369-4636
                                      Fax: 304-252-9004
                                      e-mail: ernie@CRCbeckley.com
                                      www.crcbeckley.com

Information and advocacy resources for families and professionals. Includes listings of organizations providing general information and organizations focusing on more specific areas of concern
to families and young adults who have disabilities.

Ernie Drumheller, CRC Director
Mike Carter, WOAY Operations Manager
Jim Hale, CRC Director of Communications

8012 National Disability Sports Alliance
4101 W. Green Oaks, Suite 305, #149
Arlington, TX 76016   401-792-7130
                                      Fax: 401-792-7132
                                      e-mail: info@ndsaonline.org
                                      www.chasa.org

Nonprofit organization. Coordinates sports, recreation and fitness
activities for individuals with physical disabilities. Main focus is
on cerebral palsy, traumatic brain injury and stroke.

Nancy Atwood, Executive Director
Jana Smoot White, Board Director
Julie Ring, Board Director

8013 National Dissemination Center for Children with Disabilities
1825 Connecticut Ave NW
Washington, DC 20009   202-884-8200
                                      800-695-0285
                                      Fax: 202-884-8441
                                      TTY: 800-695-0285
                                      e-mail: nichcy@aed.org
                                      www.nichcy.org

A national information and referral center that provides information on disabilities and disability-related issues for families, educators and other professionals.

Suzanne Ripley, Executive Director

8014 National Early Childhood Technical Assistance System
500 NationsBank Plaza, 137 East Franklin Street
Chapel Hill, NC 27514   919-962-2001
                                      Fax: 919-966-7463
                                      TDD: 919-966-4041
                                      e-mail: nectas@unc.edu
                                      www.unc.edu

Assists states and other designated governing jurisdictions as
they develop multidisciplinary, coordinated and comprehensive
services for children with special needs.

8015 National Family Caregivers Association
10400 Connecticut Avenue, Suite 500
Kensington, MD 20895   301-942-6430
                                      800-896-3650
                                      Fax: 301-942-2302
                                      e-mail: info@caregiveraction.org
                                      www.caregiveraction.org

The only not-for-profit organization dedicated to making life
better for all of America's family caregivers. Services include information support and validation, public awareness and advocacy; NFCA strives to minimize the disparity between a
caregivers quality of life and that of mainstream Americans.

Jon Shanfield, Chair
John Schall, CEO
Lisa Winstel, Chief Operating Officer

8016 National Father's Network
Kindering Center
16120 NE 8th Street
Bellevue, WA 98008   425-653-4286
                                      800-224-6827
                                      Fax: 425-747-1069
                                      e-mail: jmay@fathersnetwork.org
                                      www.fathersnetwork.org

935

Information and advocacy resources for fathers. Includes listings of organizations providing general information and organizations focusing on more specific areas of concern to fathers and young adults who have disabilities.

Greg Schell, Director

8017 National Foundation for Facial Reconstruction
333 East 30th Street, Lobby Unit
New York, NY 10016
212-263-6656
Fax: 212-263-7534
e-mail: info@nffr.org
www.nffr.org

The National Foundation for Facial Reconstruction, founded in 1951 by the late Dr. John Marquis Converse, to enable patients with facial deformities to lead productive fulfilling lives. NFFR lends its support to the multidisciplinary craniofacial team at the Institute of Reconstructive Plastic Surgery at NYU Medical Center. An assembly of world-renowned surgeons, mental health professionals, research specialists and staff, give their time and expertise, using the latest reconstructive techniques

Whitney Burnett, Executive Director
Kelly Strantz, Director of Development and Events
Deborah Malkoff, Pediatric Dietitian

8018 National Foundation for Transplants
5350 Poplar Avenue, Suite 430
Memphis, TN 38119
901-684-1697
800-489-3863
Fax: 901-684-1128
e-mail: info@transplants.org
www.transplants.org

Nonprofit organization that assists transplant candidates and recipients nationwide when public or private insurance does not cover all their transplant-related costs. Offers a fund raising program for patients who need to raise $10,000 or more, and grant program that helps patients with smaller, one-time needs.

Jackie D. Hancock, Jr., President/CEO
Kristin Clay, Database Coordinator
Annalisa Daughety, Online Marketing and Database Manag

8019 National Foundation of Wheelchair Tennis
70 West Red Oak Lane
White Plains, NY 10604
914-696-7000
Fax: 714-361-6603
e-mail: nfwt@aol.com
www.usta.com

Information on adaptive tennis for people of many abilities. Includes local chapters, referrals, fun and social interaction and support groups.

Jon Vegosen, Chairman of the Board/President
Geoffrey Russell, Manager, Talent ID and Development
Joe Ceriello, Manager, USTA Training Center

8020 National Handicapped Sports
451 Hungerford Drive, Suite 100
Rockville, MD 20850
301-217-0960
Fax: 301-217-0968
e-mail: dsusa@dsusa.org
www.disabledsportsusa.org

Information on adaptive sports and recreation activities for people of many abilities, including local chapters, referrals, fun and social interaction and support groups.

Kirk Bauer, Executive Director
Cheryl Collins, Administrative Services Manager
Orlando Gill, Field Representative

8021 National Hospice Organization
1731 King Street, Suite 100
Alexandria, VA 22314
703-837-1500
800-338-8898
Fax: 703-837-1233
e-mail: nhpco_info@nhpco.org
www.nhpco.org

The nation's only advocate for terminally ill children, patients and their families. Provides member programs, represents hospice care interests in Congress, regulatory agencies and the public.

Ronald Fried, Chair
J. Donald Schumacher, PsyD, President/CEO
Galen Miller, PhD, Executive Vice President

8022 National Industries for the Blind
1310 Braddock Place
Alexandria, VA 22314
703-310-0500
Fax: 703-998-8268
e-mail: communications@nib.org
www.nib.org

A nonprofit organization that represents over 100 associated industries serving people who are blind in thirty-six states. These agencies serve people who are blind or visually impaired and help them to reach their full potential. Services include job and family counseling, job skills training, instruction in Braille and other communication skills, children's programs and more.

Gary J. Krump, Chairperson
Kevin A. Lynch, President and Chief Executive Offic
Claudia Knott, Chief Operating Officer

8023 National Industries for the Severely Handicapped
2235 Cedar Lane
Vienna, VA 22182
703-560-6800
Fax: 703-849-8916
e-mail: info@nish.org
www.nish.org

Information and advocacy resources for families and professionals. Includes listings of organizations providing general information and organizations focusing on more specific areas of concern to families and young adults who have disabilities.

8024 National Mental Health Consumers' Self-Help Clearinghouse
1211 Chestnut Street, Suite 1207
Philadelphia, PA 19107
267-507-3810
800-553-4539
Fax: 215-636-6312
e-mail: info@mhselfhelp.org
www.mhselfhelp.org

Offers information, support, and appropriate referrals and promotes public and professional education. Provides networking for those with special interest related to albinism and management of albinism and hypopigmentation.

Joseph Rogers, Executive Director
Susan Rogers, Director
Christa Burkett, Technical Assistance Coordinator

8025 National Organization for Rare Disorders
55 Kenosia Avenue, PO Box 1968
Danbury, CT 06810
203-744-0100
800-999-6673
Fax: 203-798-2291
TDD: 203-797-9590
e-mail: orphan@rarediseases.org
www.rarediseases.org

The National Organization for Rare Disorders (NORD), a 501(c)(3) organization, is a unique federation of voluntary health organization dedicated to helping with rare 'orphan' diseases and assisting the organization that serve them. NORD is committed to the identification, treatment, and cure of rare disorders through programs of education, advocacy, research, and service.

Peter L Saltonstall, President & CEO
Pamela Gavin, Chief Operating Officer
Mary Cobb, SVP Membership & Organiz. Strategy

8026 National Organization on Disability
77 Water Street, Suite 204
New York, NY 10005
646-505-1191
Fax: 646-505-1184
TDD: 202-293-5968
e-mail: info@nod.org
www.nod.org

The mission of the National Organization on Disability (N.O.D.) is to expand the participation and contribution of America's 54 million men, women and children with disabilities in all aspects of life, by raising awareness through programs and information.

Thomas J. Ridge, Chairman
Cory Olicker Henkel, Chief Operating Officer
Miranda Pax, Chief of Staff

8027 National Parent Network on Disabilities
1130 17th Street NW, Suite 400
Washington, DC 20036   202-463-2299
                                     Fax: 202-463-9403
                                        www.npnd.org

Information and advocacy resources for families and professionals. Includes listings of organizations providing general information and organizations focusing on more specific areas of concern
to families and young adults who have disabilities.

8028 National Parent Resource Center
Federation for Children with Special Needs
95 Berkeley Street, Suite 104
Boston, MA 02116   617-482-2915
                                        800-695-2939
                                     Fax: 617-572-2094
                                   e-mail: fcsninfo@fcsn.org
                                        www.fcsn.org

A parent-run resource system designed to further the needs and
goals of family-centered, community-based coordinated care for
children with special health needs and their families. Offers written materials, training packages, workshops and presentations for
parents and professionals on special education, health care
financing and other topics.

8029 National Parent to Parent Support and Information System
457 State Street
Binghamton, NY 13901   706-632-8822
                                        888-971-3295
                                     Fax: 607-772-0468
                                 e-mail: npa@nationalperinatal.org
                                    www.nationalperinatal.org

NPPSIS is a nonprofit organization established to support,
strengthen, and empower families through one-on-one parent contacts. Links families nationally whose children have special
health care needs and rare disorders, and provides parents with
heath care information, resources and referrals to allow them to
identify appropriate services.

Bernadette Hoppe, MA, JD, MPH, President
Karen D'Apolito, PH.D., APN, N, VP of Programs
Mona Liza Hamlin, BSN, RN, IB, VP of Development

8030 National Perinatal Association (NPA)
457 State Street
Binghamton, NY 13901   813-971-1008
                                        888-971-3295
                                     Fax: 607-772-0468
                                 e-mail: npa@nationalperinatal.org
                                    www.nationalperinatal.org

Information and advocacy resources for families and professionals. Includes listings of organizations providing general information and organizations focusing on more specific areas of concern
to families and young adults who have disabilities.

Bernadette Hoppe, MA, JD, MPH, President
Karen D'Apolito, PH.D., APN, N, VP of Programs
Mona Liza Hamlin, BSN, RN, IB, VP of Development

8031 National Rehabilitation Information Center
8400 Corporate Drive, Suite 500
Landover, MD 20785   301-459-5900
                                        800-346-2742
                                     Fax: 301-459-4263
                                     TTY: 301-459-5984
                             e-mail: naricinfo@heitechservices.com
                                        www.naric.com

NARIC is a library and information center focusing in disability
and rehabilitation research. Information specialists provide quick
information and referrals free of charge. Other services include
customized searches of REHABDATA, the premier database of
disability and rehabilitation literature, and documents from
NARIC's collection of more than 70,000 documents are available
for nominal fee.

Mark X. Odum, Project Director
Jessica H. Chaiken, Media and Information Services Mana
Natalie J. Collier, Library and Acquisitions Manager

8032 National Respite Locator Service
800 Eastowne Drive, Suite 105
Chapel Hill, NC 27514   919-490-5577
                                        800-773-5433
                                     Fax: 919-490-4905
                                  e-mail: mmathers@chtop.org
                                        www.chtop.org

Information for families and professionals interested in repite
care. Includes listings of organizations that provide respite services to families.

Patricia Parker, Board Chair
Angela Poole, Treasurer
Mike Mathers, Executive Director

8033 National Self-Help Clearinghouse
365 5th Avenue, Suite 3300
New York, NY 10016   212-817-1822
                                  e-mail: info@selfhelpweb.org
                                      www.selfhelpweb.org

Information and advocacy resources for families and professionals. Includes listings of organizations providing general information and organizations focusing on more specific areas of concern
to families and young adults who have disabilities.

Frank Riessman, Executive Director

8034 National Skeet & Sporting Clay Headquarters
5931 Roft Road
San Antonio, TX 78253   210-688-3371
                                        800-877-5338
                                     Fax: 210-688-3014

Information on adaptive skeet and sporting clay activities for
people of many abilities.

8035 National Sleep Foundation
1010 N. Glebe Road, Suite 310
Arlington, VA 22201   703-243-1697
                                     Fax: 202-347-3472
                                 e-mail: nsf@sleepfoundation.org
                                     www.sleepfoundation.org

Works to improve the quality of life for millions of Americans
who suffer from sleep disorders, and to prevent the catastrophic
accidents that are related to poor or disordered sleep through research, education and the dissemination of information towards
the cause of Narcolepsy Project. Seeks patients to aid new research project targeting the cause of the disorder.

Russell Rosenberg, PhD, Chairman
David M. Cloud, MBA, CEO
Amy Wolfson, PhD, Secretary

**8036 National Technical Assistance Center for Children's Mental
Health**
Georgetown University Child Development Center
PO Box 571485
Washington, DC 20007   202-687-5000
                                     Fax: 202-687-8899
                                 e-mail: gucdc@georgetown.edu
                                    www.gucchd.georgetown.edu

Provides services to children experiencing emotional and mental
problems.

Phyllis R. Magrab, Ph.D., Principal Investigator
James R. Wotring, M.S.W., A.C.S.W, Director of the National TA
Center
Bruno Anthony, Ph.D., Senior Policy Associate

8037 National Vaccines Information Center
407 Church Street, Suite H
Vienna, VA 22180   703-938-0342
                                     Fax: 703-938-5768
                                 e-mail: contactNVIC@gmail.com
                                        www.nvic.org

Information and advocacy resources for families and professionals. Includes listings of organizations providing general information and organizations focusing on more specific areas of concern
to families and young adults who have disabilities.

Barbara Loe Fisher, Co-Founder and President
Kathi Williams, Co-Founder and Vice President
Paul Arhtur, Director of Operations

8038 National Wheelchair Racquetball Association
2380 McGinley Road
Monroeville, PA 15146   412-856-2400
                                        Fax: 412-856-2437

Information on adaptive racquetball activities for people of many abilities.

8039 National Wheelchair Shooting Federation
102 Park Avenue
Rockledge, PA 19111   215-379-2359
                                        Fax: 215-663-9662

Information on adaptive shooting activities for people of many abilities.

8040 National Wheelchair Softball Association
13414 Paul Street
Omaha, NE 68145   402-305-5020
                                        Fax: 612-437-3889
                                 e-mail: bfroendt@cox.net
                                 www.wheelchairsoftball.org

Information on adaptive softball activities for people of many abilities.

Brian Chavez, President
Bruce Froendt, Commissioner
Thomas Dodd, 1st Director at Large

8041 National Youth Crisis Hotline
5331 Mount Alifan Drive
San Diego, CA 92111   800-448-4663

Information and referral for runaways; also youth and parents with problems.

8042 New England Center for Children
33 Turnpike Road
Southborough, MA 01772   508-481-1015
                                        Fax: 508-485-3421
                                    e-mail: info@necc.org
                                    www.necc.org

Serving students between the ages of 3 and 22 diagnosed with autism, learning disabilities, language delays, mental retardation, behavior disorders and related disabilities; educational curriculum encompasses both the teaching of functional life skills and traditional academics; communication skills are taught throughout all activities in the school, residence, and community. Tuition and fees are set by the state. Consulting services also available.

Lisel Macenka, Chair
Vincent Strully, Chief Executive Officer & Founder
Katherine E. Foster, MEd., Chief Operating Officer

8043 NineLine
460 W 41st Street
New York, NY 10036   212-613-0300
                                        800-999-9999
                                    www.covenanthouse.org

Nationwide crisis/suicide hotline.

Andrew P. Bustillo, Board Chair
Kevin Ryan, President/CEO
Daniel C. McCarthy, Senior Vice President/Chief Financi

8044 North American Riding for the Handicapped
7475 Dakin Street, Suite 600
Denver, CO 80223   303-452-1212
                                        800-369-7433
                                        Fax: 303-252-4610
                                    e-mail: narha.org
                                    www.pathintl.org

Information on adaptive riding activities for people of many abilities. Includes local chapters, referrals, fun and social interaction and support groups. NARHA is a membership organization that promotes and supports equine activities for the disabled. Membership dues are $50 - $150.

Kay Green, Chief Executive Officer
Carolyn Malcheski, Director of Human Resource and Fina
Kaye Marks, Director of Marketing and Communica

8045 Oak-Leyden Developmental Services
411 Chicago Avenue
Oak Park, IL 60302   708-524-1050
                                        Fax: 708-524-2469
                                 e-mail: vplomin@oak-leyden.org
                                 www.oak-leyden.org

The mission of Oak-Leyden Developmental Services is to help people with developmental disabilities meet life's challenges and reach their highest potential.

Bob Atkinson, President & CEO
Valerie Plomin, Director of Development
Darlene Ehling, Director of Development

8046 Pan American Health Organization (PAHO)
525 23rd Street NW
Washington, DC 20037   202-974-3000
                                        Fax: 202-974-3663
                                 e-mail: postmaster@paho.org
                                 www.paho.org

Acts as the directing and co-ordinating authority on international health work; aids in the prevention and control of epidemic, endemic and other diseases; promotes the improvement of nutrition, housing, sanitation, recreation, economic or working conditions; promotes improved standards of teaching and training in the health, medical and related professions; and fosters activities in the field of mental health.

Mirta Roses Periago, Director

8047 Parents Information Network FFCMH
1926 1700th Avenue
Lincoln, IL 62656   217-735-1662
                                    ffcmh.org/local.htm

Bridget Schneider

8048 Pathways Awareness Foundation
150 N Michigan Avenue, Suite 2100
Chicago, IL 60601   800-955-2445
                                        Fax: 888-795-8154
                                        TTY: 800-326-8154
                                 e-mail: friends@pathwaysawareness.org
                                 www.pathwaysawareness.org

Established in 1988, Pathways Awareness Foundation is a national, nonprofit organization dedicated to raising awareness about the gift of early detection and early therapy for infants and children with physical movement differences. PAF provides informational materials to raise awareness of subtle indicators of physical development problems in infants and young children. We also have a parent answered toll-free phone. Our activities are based upon the expertise of our Medical Round Table.

Shirley W. Ryan, President
Sarah Kerndt, Education Director
Kathy O'Brien, Resource Director

8049 Pharmaceutical Manufacturers Association
1100 15th Street NW
Washington, DC 20005   800-762-4636
                                    www.pharmindex.com

Many drug companies have programs to provide free medicines (including chemotherapy) to needy patients. Eligibility requirements vary, but most are available to those not covered by private or public insurance programs. Ask your physician to request, on letterhead, a free copy of the Directory of Pharmaceutical Indigent Programs.

8050 Pike Institute on Law and Disability
Boston University School of Law
765 Commonwealth Avenue
Boston, MA 02115   Fax: 617-353-2906
                                        TTY: 617-353-2904
                                 e-mail: pikeinst@bu.edu
                                 www.sph.bu.edu

Information and advocacy resources for families and professionals. Includes listings of organizations providing general information and organizations focusing on more specific areas of concern to families and young adults who have disabilities.

Edi Ablavs, Communications Specialist
Meg Comeau, Project Director
Cara Frigand, Project Director

8051   Pilot Parents (PP)
1941 S 42nd Street, Suite 122
Omaha, NE 68105   402-346-5220
                                        Fax: 402-346-5253
                            e-mail: aadamson@olliewebb.org
                                        www.olliewebb.org

Parents, professionals and others concerned with providing emotional and peer support to new parents of children with special needs. Sponsors a parent-matching program which allows parents who have had sufficient experience and training in the care of their own children to share their knowledge and expertise with parents of children recently diagnosed as disabled. Publications: The Gazette, newsletter, published 6 times a year.

Laurie Ackermann, Executive Director
Jennifer Varner, Coordinator

8052   Pioneers Division of CEC
Council for Exceptional Children
2900 Crystal Drive, Suite 1000
Arlington, VA 22202   703-620-3660
                                             888-232-7733
                                        Fax: 703-264-9474
                                        TTY: 866-915-5000
                                        www.cec.sped.org

Promotes activities and programs to increase awareness of the educational needs of children with disabilities and/or who are gifted, and the services that are available to them.

Lynda Van Kuren, Contact

8053   Planetree Health Information Service
2040 Webster Street
San Francisco, CA 94115   415-923-3680

A nonprofit consumer-oriented resource for health information, including relaxation and visualization techniques. Write or call for a catalog and price list.

8054   Prevent Blindness America
211 W Wacker Drive #1700
Chicago, IL 60606   800-331-2020
                                        Fax: 312-363-6001
                        e-mail: info@preventblindness.org
                                   www.preventblindness.org

A volunteer eye health and safety organization dedicated to fighting blindness and saving sight. Focused on promoting a continuum of vision care, Prevent Blindness America touches the lives of millions of people each year through public and professional education, advocacy, certified vision screening training, community and patient service programs and research.

Hugh R Parry, President/CEO
Jeff Todd, COO
Arzu Bilazer, Creative Director

8055   Rainbows
1111 Tower Road
Schaumburg, IL 60173   708-310-1880

Peer support groups for adults and children who are grieving.

8056   Resources for Children with Special Needs
116 E 16th Street, 5th Floor
New York, NY 10003   212-677-4650
                                        Fax: 212-254-4070
                           e-mail: info@resourcesnyc.org
                                      www.resourcesnyc.org

A not for profit agency providing information, referrals, advocacy, training and support for New York City parents of children with learning, developmental, emotional and physical disabilities and special needs and the professionals who serve them. Publishers of The Comprehensive Directory: Programs and Services for Children and Youth with Disabilities and their Families in the Metro New York Area, Camps 2004, Schools and services for Children with Autism Spectrum Disorders.

Rachel Howard, Executive Director
Stephen Stern, Director of Finance and Administrat
Todd Dorman, Director of Communications and Outr

8057   Roeher Institute
York University
Kinsmen Building, 4700 Keele Street
North York, ON, M3J
Canada   416-661-9611
                                        Fax: 416-661-5701
                                        TDD: 416-661-2023
                                 e-mail: info@roeher.ca
                                   www.indie.ca/roeher

Conducts research for various pediatric disabilities.

8058   Ronald McDonald Houses
One Kroc Drive
Oak Brook, IL 60523   603-623-7048
                                        Fax: 630-623-7488
                                   e-mail: info@rmhc.org
                                        www.rmhc.org

Provides national programs, funding and other support to network of 150 local Ronald McDonald Houses, homes-away-from-homes for families of seriously ill children

Martin J Coyne Jr, President and CEO
Aggie Dentice, Friends of Ronald McDonals House Ch
Linda Dunham, Ronald McDonald House Charities Boa

8059   Rural Institute on Disabilities
University of Montana
52 Corbin Hall
Missoula, MT 59812   406-243-5467
                                             800-732-0323
                                        Fax: 406-243-4730
                                        TTY: 403-243-5467
                        e-mail: rural@ruralinstitute.umt.edu
                                   www.ruralinstitute.umt.edu

Information and advocacy resources for families and professionals. Includes listings of organizations providing general information and organizations focusing on more specific areas of concern to families and young adults who have disabilities.

8060   Sexuality Information and Education Council of the US (SIECUS)
90 John Street, Suite 402
New York, NY 10038   212-819-9770
                                        Fax: 212-819-9776
                                e-mail: siecus@siecus.org
                                        www.siecus.org/

Information and advocacy resources for families and professionals. Includes listings of organizations providing general information and organizations focusing on more specific areas of concern to families and young adults who have disabilities.

Monica Rodriguez, President/CEO
Jason I. Osher, Chief Operating Officer
Kurt Conklin, MPH, MCHES, Program Director

8061   Sibling Support Project
Children's Hospital and Regional Medical Center
4800 Sand Point Way NE
Seattle, WA 98105   206-987-2000
                                        Fax: 206-527-5705
                                        TTY: 206-987-2280
                                 e-mail: dmeyer@chmc.org
                                   www.seattlechildrens.org

Information and advocacy resources for families and professionals. Includes listings of organizations providing general information and organizations focusing on more specific areas of concern to families and young adults who have disabilities.

8062   Ski for Light
1455 West Lake Street
Minneapolis, MN 55408   612-827-3232
                                    e-mail: info@sfl.org
                                        www.sfl.org

Nonprofit organization founded in 1975 to promote the physical fitness of visually and mobility impaired adults.

8063 Society for Pediatric Dermatology
8365 Keystone Crossing, Suite 107
Indianapolis, IN 46240

317-202-0224
Fax: 317-205-9481
e-mail: spd@hp-assoc.com
www.pedsderm.net

Objective is to promote, develop and advance education, research and care of skin disease in all pediatric age groups.

Sheila Friedlander, MD, President
Anthony Mancini, MD, Secreatary/Treasurer
Kent Lindeman, Executive Director

8064 Sparrow Foundation
1110 East Michigan Avenue
Seattle, WA 48912

517-364-5680
Fax: 517-364-5698
e-mail: foundation@sparrow.org
www.sparrow-fdn.org

This nonprofit charitable and educational organization was started by the family of a child who needed a bone marrow transplant, for which their insurance carrier refused to pay. The foundation provides seed money to schools, youth organizations, service clubs, and churches which help persons with medical needs.

John Pirich, Chair
Ron Simon, Vice Chair
Charles Blockett, Secretary/Treasurer

8065 Spaulding for Children
16250 Northland Drive, Suite 100
Southfield, MI 48075

248-443-7080
Fax: 248-443-7099
e-mail: sfc@spaulding.org
www.spaulding.org

Information and advocacy resources for families and professionals. Includes listings of organizations providing general information and organizations focusing on more specific areas of concern to families and young adults who have disabilities.

8066 Special Needs Advocate for Parents (SNAP)
1801 Avenue of the Stars #401
Century City, CA 90067

310-452-3759
888-310-9889
Fax: 310-450-5769
TTY: 310-201-9889
e-mail: info@spapinfo.org
www.icdri.org

Nonprofit organization with advisors nationwide and information and advocacy resources for families and professionals. Includes listings of organizations providing general information and organizations focusing on more specific areas of concern to families and young adults who have disabilities, support groups, educational advocates and medical insurance problem solving. Quarterly newsletter with articles of interest.

Marla Kraus, Executive Director

8067 Special Olympics
1133 19th Street, NW
Washington, DC 20036

202-628-3630
800-700-8585
Fax: 202-824-0200
e-mail: info@specialolympics.org
www.specialolympics.org

Information on adaptive sports and recreation activities and related health issues for people of many abilities. Including local chapters, referrals, fun and social interaction and support groups.

Timothy P. Shriver, Ph.D., Chairman/Board of Directors/Chief E
J. Brady Lum, President & Chief Operating Officer
Peter Wheeler, Chief Strategic Properties

8068 Specialized Training of Military Parents (STOMP)
Washington PAVE
6316 S 12th Street
Tacoma, WA 98465

253-565-2266
800-572-7368
Fax: 253-566-8052
TTY: 253-565-2266
e-mail: stomp@washingtonpave.com
www.stompproject.org

Information and advocacy resources for military families who have children with special education or health needs. Includes listings of organizations providing general information and organizations focusing on more specific areas of concern and family to family connections.

Heather Hedbon, Founder & Director
Luz Adriana Martinez, Parent Education Coordinator
Valerie Patterson, Parent Education Coordinator

8069 Starbright
5757 Wilshire Boulevard, Suite M100
Los Angeles, CA 90036

310-479-1212
800-315-2580
Fax: 310-479-1235

The Foundation is dedicated to the development of projects that empower seriously ill children to combat the medical and emotional challenges they face on a daily basis. STARBRIGHT projects do more then educate and entertain, address the core issues that accompany illness, the pain, fear and loneliness and depression that can be as damaging as the sickness itself.

8070 Tech Connection
Family Resource Associates
1421 Park Ave., Ste. 100
Chico, CA 95928

732-747-5310
Fax: 732-747-1896
e-mail: techhorin@aol.com
www.techconnection.us

Tech Connection is a resource center to help children and adults who have disabilities gain access to the benefits of technology. Includes nationwide network of community-based assistive technology, resource centers, hands on consultants and product demonstrations and evaluations.

8071 Technology Assistance for Special Consumers
1856 Keats Drive
Huntsville, AL 35810

256-859-8300
Fax: 256-859-4332
TDD: 256-532-5996
e-mail: tasc@ucphuntsville.org
www.ucptasc.org

Technology group of parents, consumers and professionals; provides resources to help children and adults who have disabilities gain access to the benefits of technology. Includes nationwide network of community-based assistive technology, resource centers, hands on consultants and product demonstrations.

Laura Parks, M.Ed., Assistive Technology Specialist
Julie Yockel, M.S., CCC-SLP, AAC Specialist
Mark Pepper, STAR Reutilization Specialist

8072 US Paralympics
U.S. Olympic Committee
1 Olympic Plaza, 30 Cimino Drive
Colorado Springs, CO 80903

719-866-2030
Fax: 719-866-2029
e-mail: alison.nicholas@usoc.org
www.teamusa.org

A division of the United States Olympic Committee, we focus our efforts on enhancing programs, funding and opportunities for persons with physical disabilities to participate in Paralympic sport. The Paralympic Games are the second largest sporting event in the world, conceding top honors only to the Olympics. The multi-sport competition showcases the talents and abilities of the world's most elite athletes with physical disabilities.

Alison Nicholas, Program Coordinator
Beth Bason, Communications Coordinator
Joe Walsh, Director

8073 Vision of Children Foundation
11975 El Camino Real, Suite 104
San Diego, CA 92130

858-314-7917
Fax: 858-314-7920
e-mail: info@visionofchildren.org
www.visionofchildren.org

Provides information, promotes research and assists the families of blind and visually impaired children in locating organizations and service providers who can give support.

Samuel A Hardage, Chairman
Elizabeth Dole, Senator, Honorary Co-Chair
Andria Kinnear, Executive Director

8074 WE MOVE (Worldwide Education and Advocacy for Movement Disorders)
Mt. Siani Medical Center
5731 Mosholu Avenue
Bronx, NY 10471

212-241-8567
800-437-6682
Fax: 212-875-8389
e-mail: wemove@wemove.org
www.wemove.org

WE MOVE provides movement disorder information and educational materials to physicians, patients, the media, and the public via its comprehensive web site, training courses, patient support group and more. Its goal is to make early diagnosis, up-to-date treatment and patient support a reality for all people living with movement disorders.

Mark Stacy, MD, Chair, Education Committee
Susan Bressman, President
Mo Moadeli, Vice President

8075 World Institute on Disability
3075 Adeline Street, Suite 280
Berkeley, CA 94703

510-225-6400
Fax: 510-225-0477
TTY: 510-225-0478
e-mail: wid@wid.org
www.wid.org

Information and advocacy resources for families and professionals. Includes listings of organizations providing general information and organizations focusing on more specific areas of concern to families and young adults who have disabilities.

Stanley K Yarnell MD, Chairman
Martin B Schulter, Vice Chair

8076 World Research Foundation
41 Bell Rock Plaza
Sedona, AZ 86351

928-284-3300
Fax: 928-248-3530
e-mail: info@wrf.org
www.wrf.org

Nonprofit organization. Your global source of information on illnesses and therapies used around the world.

LaVerne Ross, Co-Founder
Steven Ross

8077 Young Adult Institute
460 West 34th St.
New York, NY 2382

212-273-6100
TDD: 212-290-2787
www.yai.org

A nonprofit professional organizations serving developmentally disabled children and adults in many programs throughout the New York metropolitan area. Provides over 50 program sites for thousands of participants.

Stephen E. Freeman, L.C.S.W., Chief Executive Officer
Thomas A. Dern, L.C.S.W., Chief Operating Officer
Sanjay Dutt, Chief Financial Officer

8078 Zero to Three
1255 23rd Street, NW, Suite 350
Washington, DC 20037

202-638-1144
800-899-4301
Fax: 202-638-0851
e-mail: webhelp@zerotothree.org
zerotothree.org

The mission is to promote the healthy development of our nation's infants and toddlers by supporting and strengthening families, communities and those who work on their behalf. We are dedicated to advancing current knowledge , promoting beneficial policies and practices and providing training, technical assistance, and leadership development. A nonprofit organization.

Janice Im, Chief Program Officer
Laura Shiflett, Chief Financial/Administrative Offi
Matthew E Melmed, Executive Director

State Agencies & Support Groups

Alabama

8079 ARC of Morgan County
401 14th Street, Suite 4-E
Decatur, AL 35601

205-355-6192
Fax: 256-350-4502
e-mail: arc@hiwaay.net
www.arcofmorgancounty.org

Informational and emotional support to parents who have a child, adolescent, or adult family member with special needs.

Lisa English, President
Sherry Stephenson, Vice President
Ireta Hogan, Secretary

8080 Early Intervention Program
2129 East South Blvd
Montgomery, AL 36111

334-281-8780
800-441-7607
Fax: 334-281-1973
e-mail: oholder@rehab.state.al.us
www.rehab.state.al.us

Services include central directory, representatives of agencies, service providers, families, and coordinators of infant, toddler, and preschool special education programs.

Stephen G. Kayes, Board of Director
Jimmie Varnado, Board of Director

8081 Friends for Life Auburn United Methodist Church
99 South Street
Auburn, NY 13021

315-253-6295
www.auburnunitedmethodist.org

Informational and emotional support to parents who have a child, adolescent, or adult family member with special needs.

Richelle Duchaner, Pastor
Geri Jackson, Administrative Assisstant
Mary Howard, Coordinator of Congregational Life

8082 Special Education Action Committee Huntsville Outreach Office
3322 S Memorial Parkway, Suite 25
Huntsville, AL 35801

256-882-3911
Fax: 256-882-3974
e-mail: seach@traveler.com
www.hsv.tis.net/~seachsv

Informational and emotional support to parents who have a child, adolescent, or adult family member with special needs.

8083 Special Education Services
Department of Education
PO Box 302101
Montgomery, AL 36130

334-242-8114
800-392-8020
Fax: 334-242-9192
e-mail: jwaid@sdenet.alsde.edu
www.alsde.edu

Services include central directory, representatives of agencies, service providers, families, and coordinators of infant, toddler, and preschool special education programs.

Robert J. Bentley, President
Thomas R. Bice, Ed.D., Secretary/Executive Officer
Stephanie Bell, Vice President

8084 Statewide Technology Access & Response System for Alabamians with Disabilities
2125 E South Boulevard, PO Box 20752
Montgomery, AL 36120
334-613-3480
800-782-7656
Fax: 334-613-3485
TDD: 334-613-3519
e-mail: tgannaway@rehab.state.al.us
www.mindspring.com/alstar/

State assisted programs and support group information for people of many abilities. Includes local chapters, referrals, fun and social interaction and support groups.

Alaska

8085 Alaska Department of Education
801 W 10th Street, Suite 200, PO Box 110500
Juneau, AK 99811
907-465-2800
Fax: 907-465-4156
TTY: 907-465-2815
e-mail: eed.webmaster@alaska.gov
www.eed.state.ak.us

Individuals with Disabilities Education Act requires early intervention and preschool special education for children with disabilities and special health care needs. Services include central directory, representatives of agencies, service providers, families, and coordinators of infant, toddler, and preschool special education programs.

Steven J. Hostetter, President

8086 Assistive Technologies of Alaska
3330 Arctic Blvd., Suite 101
Anchorage, AK 99503
907-563-2599
800-723-2852
Fax: 907-563-0699
TTY: 907-561-2592
TDD: 907-269-3569
e-mail: mystie@atlaak.org
www.atlaak.org

State assisted programs and support group information for people of many abilities. Includes local chapters, referrals, fun and social interaction and support groups.

8087 Maternal, Child & Family Health, Early Intervention/Infant Learning Program
State of Alaska Department of Health
1231 Gambell Street
Anchorage, AK 99501
907-269-3419
Fax: 907-269-3465
e-mail: jbatuk@health.state.ak.us

Early intervention and preschool special education for children with disabilities and special health care needs. Services include administration of statewide early intervention programs for infants and toddlers with developmental delays or disabilities and their families.

Jane Atuk, Part C Coordinator
Karen Martinek, Special Needs Services Unit

8088 PARENTS
4743 E Northern Lights Boulevard
Anchorage, AK 99508
907-337-7678
800-478-7678
Fax: 907-337-7671
TDD: 907-337-7678
e-mail: parentsss@alaska.com
www.parentsinc.org

Parent Training and Information (PTI) programs help parents to understand their children's specific needs, communicate more effectively with professionals, participate in the educational planning process, and obtain information about relevant programs, services and resources.

Arizona

8089 Arizona Early Intervention Program/ Department of Economic Security
3839 N. 3rd St, Suite 304 Site Code No. 801 A-6
Phoenix, AZ 85012
602-532-9960
888-439-5609
Fax: 602-200-9820
e-mail: allazeip2@azdes.gov
www.azdes.gov/azeip

Early intervention and preschool special education for children with disabilities and special health care needs. Services include central directory, representatives of agencies, service providers, families, and coordinators of infant, toddler, and preschool special education programs.

8090 Arizona Technology Access Program Institute for Human Development
2400 N. Central Avenue, Suite 300
Pheonix, AZ 85004
602-728-9534
800-477-9921
Fax: 602-728-9353
TTY: 602-728-9536
e-mail: Daniel.Davidson@nau.edu
www.nau.edu/ihd/aztap

State assisted programs and support group information for people of many abilities. Includes local chapters, referrals, fun and social interaction and support groups.

8091 Blake Foundation Children's Achievement Center
3825 E 2nd Street
Tucson, AZ 85716
520-325-0611
Fax: 520-327-5414
www.nectas.unc.edu

Services include central directory, representatives of agencies, service providers, families, and coordinators of infant, toddler, and preschool special education programs.

Annabell Rose, Interagency Coordinating Council

8092 Division of Special Education State Department of Education
1535 W Jefferson
Phoenix, AZ 85007
602-542-3852
Fax: 602-542-5404
e-mail: lbusenb@mail1.ade.state.az.us
www.nectas.unc.edu

Individuals with Disabilities Education Act requires all states and territories to provide early intervention and preschool special education for children with disabilities and special health care needs. Services include central directory, representatives of agencies, service providers, families, and coordinators of infant, toddler, and preschool special education programs.

Lynn Busenbark, Preschool Special Ed. Coordinator

8093 Pilot Parents of Southern Arizona
2600 N Wyatt Drive
Tucson, AZ 85712
520-324-3150
877-365-7220
Fax: 520-324-3152
e-mail: ppsa@pilotparents.org
www.pilotparents.org

Parent Training and Information (PTI) programs help parents to understand their children's specific needs, communicate more effectively with professionals, participate in the educational planning process, and obtain information about relevant programs, services and resources.

Lynn Kallis, Executive Director
Robert Snyder, Director of Education & Training
Cheryl McKenzie, Administrative Assistant

8094 Raising Special Kids
5025 E Washington Street, Suite 204
Phoenix, AZ 85034
602-242-4366
800-237-3007
Fax: 602-242-4306
e-mail: info@specialkids.org
www.raisingspecialkids.org

Provides support and training to families of children who have disabilities and special health needs, helps parents communicate more effectively with professionals, participate in the educational planning process and obtain information about programs and resources available to them. Offers training to professionals in health, education and social services.

Paula Banahan, President
Joyce Millard-Hoie, Executive Director
Janna Murrell, Director of Family Support and Educ

8095 Southwest Human Development
PO BOX 28487
Austin, TX 78755 512-467-7916
800-369-9082
Fax: 512-467-1453
TTY: 888-467-1455
e-mail: info@swhuman.org
www.swhuman.org

Services include central directory, representatives of agencies, service providers, families, and coordinators of infant, toddler, and preschool special education programs.

Blake Stanford, President/CEO

Arkansas

8096 Arkansas Disability Coalition
1501 N. University Avenue, Suite 268
Little Rock, AR 72207 501-614-7020
800-223-1330
Fax: 501-614-9082
TDD: 501-614-7020
e-mail: adc@alltel.net
www.adcpti.org

Parent Training and Information (PTI) programs help parents to understand their children's specific needs, communicate more effectively with professionals, participate in the educational planning process, and obtain information about relevant programs, services and resources.

Wanda Horton, Executive Director
Karen Lutrick, Parent Educator
Bryan Cozart, Project Director

8097 Arkansas Disability Coalition Parent Train ing and Information Center
1501 N. University Avenue, Suite 268
Little Rock, AR 72207 501-614-7020
800-223-1330
Fax: 501-614-9082
TDD: 501-614-7020
e-mail: adc@alltel.net
www.adcpti.org

The Arkansas Parent Training and Information Center (PTI) is a project of the Arkansas Disability Coalition. It is funded through a federal grant from the US Department of Education that serves families of children ages birth through 26 years of age who have a disability, but not yet diagnosed.

Wanda Horton, Executive Director
Karen Lutrick, Parent Educator
Bryan Cozart, Project Director

8098 DD Services, Department of Human Services
PO Box 1437, Slot 2520
Little Rock, AR 72203 501-682-8699
Fax: 501-682-8890
e-mail: dds1@aristotle.net
www.chasa.org

Individuals with Disabilities Education Act requires all states and territories to provide early intervention and preschool special education for children with disabilities and special health care needs. Services include central directory, representatives of agencies, service providers, families, and coordinators of infant, toddler, and preschool special education programs.

Sherrill Archer, Coordinator

8099 FOCUS
305 W Jefferson Avenue
Jonesboro, AR 72401 870-935-2750
Fax: 870-931-3755
e-mail: focusinc@ipa.net
www.taalliance.org

Parent Training and Information (PTI) programs help parents to understand their children's specific needs, communicate more effectively with professionals, participate in the educational planning process, and obtain information about relevant programs, services and resources.

8100 Family-2-Family Health Information Center of Arkansas
1501 N. University Avenue, Suite 268
Little Rock, AR 72207 501-614-7020
800-223-1330
Fax: 501-614-9082
TDD: 501-614-7020
e-mail: adc@alltel.net
www.adcpti.org

The Family-2-Family Health Information Center of Arkansas (F2F HIC) is a nonprofit family-run organization that assists families of children and youth with special health care needs and the professionals who serve them. They provide health-related support, information, resources and training.

Bryan Cozart, Project Director
Karen Lutrick, Parent Educator
Wanda Horton, Executive Director

8101 Increasing Capabilities Access Network
Dept of Education/Arkansas Rehabilitation Services
525 W. Capitol
Little Rock, AR 72201 501-666-8868
800-828-2799
Fax: 501-666-5319
TTY: 501-666-8868
TDD: 800-828-2799
e-mail: Barbara.Gullett@arkansas.gov
www.ar-ican.org

State assisted programs and support group information for people of many abilities. Includes local chapters, referrals, fun and social interaction and support groups.

Barry Vuletich, Program Administrator

8102 Parent to Parent Arc of Arkansas
2004 South Main Street
Little Rock, AR 72206 501-375-7770
Fax: 501-372-4621

Informational and emotional support to parents who have a child, adolescent, or adult family member with special needs.

8103 Special Education Section State Department of Education
4 Capitol Mall, Room 105-C
Little Rock, AR 72201 501-682-4225
Fax: 501-682-4313
e-mail: sreifeiss@arkedu.k12.ar.us
www.unc.edu

Individuals with Disabilities Education Act requires all states and territories to provide early intervention and preschool special education for children with disabilities and special health care needs. Services include central directory, representatives of agencies, service providers, families, and coordinators of infant, toddler, and preschool special education programs.

Sandra Reifeissk, Preschool Special Ed. Coordinator

California

8104 ARC Family Resource Project
2421 Lomitas Avenue, PO Box 219
Santa Rosa, CA 95402 877-694-4335
Fax: 707-578-8601
e-mail: arcsoco@sonic.net

943

Parent Training and Information (PTI) programs help parents to understand their children's specific needs, communicate more effectively with professionals, participate in the educational planning process, and obtain information about relevant programs, services and resources.

Traci N Turner, Program Coordinator
Elvis Bozarth, President

8105 CARE Family Resource Center
1350 Arnold Drive, Suite 203
Martinez, CA 94553
925-313-0999
800-281-3023
Fax: 925-370-8651

Informational and emotional support to parents who have a child, adolescent, or adult family member with special needs.

8106 Carolyn Kordich Family Resource Center
1135 W. 257th Street
Harbor City, CA 90710
310-325-7288
Fax: 310-325-7288
e-mail: ckfrc@worldnet.att.net

Informational and emotional support to parents who have a child, adolescent, or adult family member with special needs.

8107 Challenged Family Resource Center
827 West 20th Street
Merced, CA 95340
209-385-5314
Fax: 209-385-5317
e-mail: dkuneck@aol.com
www.challengedfrc.org

Informational and emotional support to parents who have a child, adolescent, or adult family member with special needs.

8108 Children Living with Illness
The Center for Attitudinal Healing
33 Buchanan Drive
Sausalito, CA 94965
415-331-6161
Fax: 415-331-4545

For children who are ill, have an ill sibling, or an ill parent. Parent group meets separately at the same time.

Jimmy Pete

8109 Comfort Connection Family Resource Center
12361 Lewis Street, Suite 101
Garden Grove, CA 92840
714-748-7491
Fax: 714-748-8149

Informational and emotional support to parents who have a child, adolescent, or adult family member with special needs.

8110 Department of Developmental Services of Early Start Program
1600 9th Street, PO Box 944202
Sacramento, CA 94244
916-654-1690
800-515-2229
Fax: 916-654-2054
TTY: 916-654-2054
TDD: 916-654-2054
e-mail: earlystart@dds.ca.gov
www.dds.ca.gov

Individuals with Disabilities Education Act requires all states and territories to provide early intervention and preschool special education for children with disabilities and special health care needs. Services include central directory, representatives of agencies, service providers, families, and coordinators of infant, toddler, and preschool special education programs.

Mark Hutchinson, Chief Deputy Director
Terri Delgadillo, Director
Rick Ingraham, Quality Management/Development Bran

8111 Early Start Family Resource Network
1425 S. Waterman Ave.
San Bernadino, CA 92408
909-890-4794
800-974-5553
Fax: 909-890-4709
www.esfrn.org

Informational and emotional support to parents who have a child, adolescent, or adult family member with special needs.

8112 Exceptional Family Resource Center
9245 Sky Park Court, Suite 130
San Diego, CA 92123
619-594-7416
800-281-8252
Fax: 858-268-4275
e-mail: efro@cybergate.com
www.efrconline.org

Informational and emotional support to parents who have a child, adolescent, or adult family member with special needs.

Sherry Torok, Executive Director
Susan Carlton-Bahm, Manager
Joyce Clark, Manager

8113 Exceptional Family Support, Education and Advocacy Center
6402 Skyway
Paradise, CA 95969
530-876-8321
Fax: 530-876-0346
e-mail: sea@sunset.net
www.taalliance.org

Parent Training and Information (PTI) programs help parents to understand their children's specific needs, communicate more effectively with professionals, participate in the educational planning process, and obtain information about relevant programs, services and resources.

8114 Exceptional Parents
Family Resource Center
4440 N 1st Street
Fresno, CA 93726
559-229-2000
Fax: 559-229-2956
TTY: 559-225-6059
e-mail: epu1@cybergate.com
www.exceptionalparents.org

Informational and emotional support to parents who have a child, adolescent, or adult family member with special needs.

Suzanne Ellis, Chief Financial Officer
Kyle Loreto, President
Marion Karian, Executive Director

8115 Families Caring for Families
Family Resource Center
113 W Pillsbury Street, Suite A1
Lancaster, CA 93534
661-949-1746
Fax: 661-948-7266

Informational and emotional support to parents who have a child, adolescent, or adult family member with special needs.

8116 Family First Program Alpha Resource Center
4501 Cathedral Oaks Road, Suite A1
Santa Barbara, CA 93110
805-683-2145
Fax: 805-967-3647
e-mail: arcofsb@slcom.com

Informational and emotional support to parents who have a child, adolescent, or adult family member with special needs.

8117 Family Focus Resource Center
18111 Nordhoff Street
Northridge, CA 91330
818-677-6854
Fax: 818-677-5574
e-mail: family.focus@csun.edu
www.familyfocusresourcecenter.org

Informational and emotional support to parents who have a child, adolescent, or adult family member with special needs.

Ivor Weiner, Principal Investigator
Victoria Berrey, Program Manager
Stacie Anderle, PRRS, Coordinator

8118 Family Resource Center
5828 North Clark Street
Chicago, IL 60660
773-334-2300
800-676-2229
Fax: 773-334-8228
www.f-r-c.org

Informational and emotional support to parents who have a child, adolescent, or adult family member with special needs.

Debbie Frisch, Board President
Richard Pearlman, Executive Director
Jane Turner, Associate Director

8119 H.E.A.R.T.S. Connection Family Resource Center
3101 N Sillect Avenue, Suite 115
Bakersfield, CA 93308   661-328-9055
                                         800-210-7633
                                    Fax: 661-328-9940
                          e-mail: heartsfrc@igalaxy
                                   www.heartsfrc.org

Informational and emotional support to parents who have a child,
adolescent, or adult family member with special needs.

Susan Graham, Director
Ana Gomez, Family Resource Specialist
Ana Gomez, Family Resource Specialist

**8120 Harbor Regional Center Family and Professional Resource
Center**
21231 Hawthorne Boulevard
Torrance, CA 90503   310-543-0691
                                    Fax: 310-316-8843
                  e-mail: familyresourcecntr@hddf.com
                                    www.harborrc.org

Informational and emotional support to parents who have a child,
adolescent, or adult family member with special needs.

8121 MATRIX: Parent Network and Family Resource Center
94 Galli Drive, Suite C
Novato, CA 94949   415-884-3535
                                         800-578-2592
                                    Fax: 415-884-3555
                       e-mail: info@matrixparents.org
                                 www.matrixparents.org

Informational and emotional support to parents who have a child,
adolescent, or adult family member with special needs.

Lee Cox, Chief Financial Officer
Rhanda Dunn, Board President
Nora Thompson, Executive Director

8122 Matrix Parents Network and Resource Center
94 Galli Drive, Suite C
Novato, CA 94949   415-884-3535
                                         800-578-2592
                                    Fax: 415-884-3555
                       e-mail: info@matrixparents.org
                                 www.matrixparents.org

Matrix is a nonprofit agency that serves families of children with
special needs and disabilities. Provides information and referral,
individual support, technical assistance, support groups, training
about special education and services, and direction to appropriate
early start services.

Lee Cox, Chief Financial Officer
Rhanda Dunn, Board President
Nora Thompson, Executive Director

8123 Parents Helping Parents of San Francisco
4752 Mission St Ste 100
San Francisco, CA 94112   415-841-8820
                                    Fax: 415-841-8824
                           www.parentcenternetwork.org

Parent Training and Information (PTI) programs help parents to
understand their children's specific needs, communicate more effectively with professionals, participate in the educational planning process, and obtain information about relevant programs,
services and resources.

Paula Goldberg, National ALLIANCE PTAC Co-Director
Sue Folger, National ALLIANCE PTAC Co-Director
Debbie Andrews, Communications Coordinator

8124 Parents Helping Parents of Santa Clara
3041 Olcott Street
Santa Clara, CA 95054   408-727-5775
                                    Fax: 408-727-0182
                               e-mail: info@php.com
                                        www.php.com

Informational and emotional support to parents who have a child,
adolescent, or adult family member with special needs.

Mary Ellen Peterson, M.A., Executive Director/CEO
Nancy O'Rourke, Chief Development Officer
Paul Schutz, Chief Financial Officer

8125 Peaks and Valleys Family Resource Center
20 Sherwood Place No. 4
Salinas, CA 93906   831-755-1450
                                         800-400-2937
                                    Fax: 831-755-1470
                       e-mail: peaks@montereyk12.ca.us

Informational and emotional support to parents who have a child,
adolescent, or adult family member with special needs.

8126 San Gabriel/Pomona Parents' Place
1500 S Hyacinth Avenue # B
West Covina, CA 91791   626-919-1091
                                         800-422-2022
                                    Fax: 626-337-2736
                           e-mail: empower@gte.net
                               www.parentsplacefrc.com

Family Resource Center committed to supporting, promoting and
enhancing family focused services in a parent driven atmosphere
for families who have children with special needs. Family Resource Centers are part of the California Early Start Program
which addresses the unique and individual needs of families raising a child with a disability. The Parent's Place is dedicated to
empowering families through information/education, referrals
and parent to parent support.

Sona Baghdassarian, Director
Judy Kyne, Administrative Secretary
Elena Sanchez, Parent Resource Specialist

**8127 South Central Los Angeles Regional Center for
Devlopmentally Disabled Persons**
6500 W Adams Boulevard
Los Angeles, CA 90007   213-744-7000
                                    Fax: 213-744-8494
                                    TTY: 213-763-5634

Informational and emotional support to parents who have a child,
adolescent, or adult family member with special needs.

8128 Special Connections Family Resource Center
400 Encinal Street
Santa Cruz, CA 95060   831-464-0669
                                    Fax: 831-465-9177
                             e-mail: frcedp@aol.com

Informational and emotional support to parents who have an infant or toddler (birth to 36 months) with special needs.

Leslie Burnham, Program Supervisor

8129 Special Education Division State Department of Education
PO Box 944272
Sacramento, CA 94244   916-327-3696
                                    Fax: 916-327-8878
                     e-mail: cbourne@mail515a.cde.ca.gov
                                   www.nectas.unc.edu

Individuals with Disabilities Education Act requires all states and
territories to provide early intervention and preschool special education for children with disabilities and special health care
needs. Services include central directory, representatives of agencies, service providers, families, and coordinators of infant, toddler, and preschool special education programs.

Constance J Bourne, Preschool Special Ed. Coordinator

8130 Starlight Children's Foundation
2049 Century Park East. Suite 4320
Los Angeles, CA 90067   310-479-1212
                                         800-274-7827
                                    Fax: 323-634-0090
                          e-mail: Jenny@starlight.org
                                    www.starlight.org

International nonprofit organization dedicated to improving the
quality of life for seriously ill children and their families. Working with more than 850 hospitals worldwide, the Foundation provides an impressive menu of both in-hospital and outpatient
programs and services. A leader in delivering distractive entertainment therapies, over 85,000 children benefit from Starlight's
programs each month.

Jacqueline Hart-Ibrahim, Chief Executive Officer
Clifford R. Ball, CFO/CTO
Denise Muniz, Development Director

8131 Support for Families of Children with Disabilities
1663 Mission Street, 7th Floor
San Francisco, CA 94103

415-282-7494
Fax: 415-282-1226
TTY: 415-920-5040
e-mail: info@supportforfamilies.org
www.supportforfamilies.org

Parent Training and Information (PTI) programs help parents to understand their children's specific needs, communicate more effectively with professionals, participate in the educational planning process, and obtain information about relevant programs, services and resources.

Christian Dauer, SFCD, Board President
Laura Lanzone, SFCD, Vice President
Juno Duenas, SFCD, Executive Director

8132 Team Advocates for Special Kids, Anaheim
100 W. Cerritos Ave
Anaheim, CA 92805

714-533-8275
866-828-8275
Fax: 714-533-2533
e-mail: taskca@yahoo.com
www.taskca.org

Programs help parents to understand their children's specific needs, communicate more effectively with professionals, participate in the educational planning process, and obtain information about relevant programs, services and resources.

Marta Anchondo, Executive Director/CEO

8133 Team Advocates for Special Kids, San Diego
4550 Kearney Villa Road, #102
San Diego, CA 92123

858-874-2386
Fax: 858-874-2375

Programs help parents to understand their children's specific needs, communicate more effectively with professionals, participate in the educational planning process, and obtain information about relevant programs, services and resources.

8134 Warmline Family Resource Center
6960 Destiny Dr., Suite 106
Rocklin, CA 95677

916-632-2100
800-660-7995
Fax: 916-632-2103
e-mail: warmlinefrc@warmlinefrc.com
www.warmlinefrc.org

Informational and emotional support to parents who have a child, adolescent, or adult family member with special needs.

Heather Green, Contact
Amber Johnson, Contact

Colorado

8135 Assistive Technology Partners
601 E 18th Avenue, Suite 130
Denver, CO 80203

303-315-1280
800-255-3477
Fax: 303-837-1208
TTY: 303-837-8964
e-mail: GeneralInfo@AT-Partners.org
www.ucdenver.edu

State assisted programs and support group information for people of many abilities. Focuses on assistive technology devices and services for persons with disabilities, training and technical assistance available.

8136 Colorado Consortium of Intensive Care Nurseries United Parents (UP)
1056 E 19th Avenue, B535
Denver, CO 80218

303-861-6557
Fax: 303-764-8092
e-mail: McGinley.Pandora@ex.tchden.org

Informational and emotional support to parents who have a child, adolescent, or adult family member with special needs.

8137 Delta/Montrose Parent to Parent
2091 E Locust Road
Montrose, CO 81401

970-249-2878
Fax: 970-252-0544
e-mail: children@gi.net

Informational and emotional support to parents who have a child, adolescent, or adult family member with special needs.

8138 Denver Early Childhood Connections
2727 W 92nd Avenue
Denver, CO 80204

303-458-0852
Fax: 303-744-9502

Provides resource coordination for children eligible for Part C services and referrals to other agencies for children with needs outside of the Part C realm. Parent to parent support, parent education and community playgroups are some of the services that are conducted. Forums are hosted on varied topics relevant to parents of young children as well as in-service and pre-service workshops on child development. IFSP development, parent's rights under IDEA, and other resource packets are available

Newsletter

Judith Persoff, Executive Director

8139 Disability Connection and RAFT, Larimer County's Early Childhood Connection
PO Box 270714
Fort Collins, CO 80527

970-229-0224
Fax: 970-229-0242
e-mail: bstuts@fornet.org

Informational and emotional support to parents who have a child, adolescent, or adult family member with special needs.

8140 Effective Parent Project
255 Main Street
Grand Junction, CO 81501

970-241-4068
Fax: 970-241-3725

Informational and emotional support to parents who have a child, adolescent, or adult family member with special needs.

8141 El Groupo Vida
P.O. Box 11096
Denver, CO 80211

303-904-6073
Fax: 303-296-4105
e-mail: info@elgrupovida.org
www.elgrupovida.org

Informational and emotional support to parents who have a child, adolescent, or adult family member with special needs.

Gabriela Perez, Board President
Italia Cortes-Santillan, Vice President
Gabriela Perez, Interim (Volunteer) Executive Direc

8142 Help Parent Support Group Hope & Education for Loving Parents
378 S Falcon
Pueblo West, CO 81007

719-545-2282
Fax: 719-547-1282
e-mail: fastgram@aol.com

Informational and emotional support to parents who have a child, adolescent, or adult family member with special needs.

8143 Oasis
1120 N Circle Drive, Suite 19
Colorado Springs, CO 80909

719-635-8722
Fax: 719-577-9482
e-mail: oasis@juno.com

Informational and emotional support to parents who have a child, adolescent, or adult family member with special needs.

8144 PEAK Parent Center
611 N Weber, Suite 200
Colorado Springs, CO 80903

719-531-9400
800-284-0251
Fax: 719-531-9452
TDD: 719-531-9403
e-mail: info@peakparent.org
www.peakparent.org

Parent Training and Information (PTI) programs help parents to understand their children's specific needs, communicate more effectively with professionals, participate in the educational planning process, and obtain information about relevant programs, services and resources.

Kent Willis, President
Sarah Billerbeck, Vice President
Barbara Buswell, Executive Director

8145 Parent Support Group of Littleton & Auora
7600 E Arapahoe, Suite 219
Englewood, CO 80112
303-773-0044
Fax: 303-773-8780

Informational and emotional support to parents who have a child, adolescent, or adult family member with special needs.

8146 Parents Supporting Parents of Eagle County
PO Box 2656
Vail, CO 81658
970-926-6015
Fax: 970-926-6015

Informational and emotional support to parents who have a child, adolescent, or adult family member with special needs.

8147 Parents Supporting Parents of Garfield and Pitkin County
PO Box 784
Silt, CO 81652
970-876-5768
Fax: 970-876-5204

Informational and emotional support to parents who have a child, adolescent, or adult family member with special needs.

8148 Prevention Initiatives State Department of Education
210 E Colfax, Room 301
Denver, CO 80203
303-866-6600
Fax: 303-866-0793
e-mail: smith_s@cde.state.co.us
www.cde.state.co.us

Provides early intervention and preschool special education for children with disabilities and special health care needs. Services include central directory, representatives of agencies, service providers, families, and coordinators of infant, toddler, and preschool special education programs.

Susan Smith, Infant/Toddler Program Coordinator
Marie Huchton, Senior Consultant
Dan Jorgensen, Principal Consultant

8149 Resources for Young Children and Families
1120 N Circle Drive, Suite 19
Colorado Springs, CO 80909
719-577-9190
Fax: 719-577-9482
e-mail: partc@rycf.org

Informational and emotional support to parents who have a child, adolescent, or adult family member with special needs.

8150 Wilderness on Wheels Foundation
PO Box 1007
Wheat Ridge, CO 80034
303-403-1110
www.wildernessonwheels.org

State assisted programs and support group information for people of many abilities. Includes local chapters, referrals, fun and social interaction and support groups.

Connecticut

8151 A.J. Pappanikou Center for Developmental D isabilities
263 Farmington Avenue, MC 6222
Farmington, CT 06030
860-679-1500
866-623-1315
Fax: 860-679-1571
TTY: 860-679-1502
e-mail: contact.us.ucedd@uchc.edu
www.uconnucedd.org

Individuals with Disabilities Education Act requires all states and territories to provide early intervention and preschool special education for children with disabilities and special health care needs. Services include central directory, representatives of agencies, service providers, families, and coordinators of infant, toddler, and preschool special education programs.

Mary Beth Bruder, Director
Tierney Giannotti, Associate Director
Linda Procko, Program Coordinator

8152 Assistive Technology Project
Department of Social Services, BRS
25 Sigourney Street, 11th Floor
Hartford, CT 06106
860-424-4881
800-537-2549
Fax: 860-424-4850
TDD: 860-424-4850
e-mail: cttap@aol./com
www.tachact.uconn.edu

State assisted programs and support group information for people of many abilities. Includes local chapters, referrals, fun and social interaction and support groups.

8153 CPAC
338 Main Street
Niantic, CT 06357
860-739-3089
Fax: 860-739-7460
e-mail: cpac@cpacinc.org
www.cpacinc.org

Programs help parents to understand their children's specific needs, communicate more effectively with professionals, participate in the educational planning process, and obtain information about relevant programs, services and resources.

8154 Department of Mental Retardation
460 Capital Avenue
Hartford, CT 06106
860-418-6134
Fax: 860-418-6003
e-mail: lbgood993@aol.com
www.birth23.org

Individuals with Disabilities Education Act requires all states and territories to provide early intervention and preschool special education for children with disabilities and special health care needs. Services include central directory, representatives of agencies, service providers, families, and coordinators of infant, toddler, and preschool special education programs.

Linda Goodman, Part C Director
Lynn.S Johnson, Assistant Director
Karyn Pitt, Administrative Assistant

8155 Parent to Parent Network of Connecticut the Family Center
Dept. of Connecticut Children's Medical Center
282 Washington
Hartford, CT 06106
860-545-9021
Fax: 860-545-9201
TTY: 860-545-9002
e-mail: mcole@ccmckids.org
www.ccmckids.org

Informational and emotional support to parents who have a child, adolescent, or adult family member with special needs.

8156 State Department of Education
25 Industrial Park Road
Middletown, CT 06457
860-632-1485
Fax: 860-807-2062
www.unc.edu

Individuals with Disabilities Education Act requires all states and territories to provide early intervention and preschool special education for children with disabilities and special health care needs. Services include central directory, representatives of agencies, service providers, families, and coordinators of infant, toddler, and preschool special education programs.

Leslie Averna, Acting Bureau Chief

Delaware

8157 Delaware Assisstive Technology Initiative (DATI)
University of Delaware
461 Wyoming Road
Newark, DE 19716

302-831-0354
800-870-3284
Fax: 302-831-4690
TDD: 302-651-6794
e-mail: dati@asel.udel.edu
www.dati.org

The Delaware Assistive Technology Initiative (DATI) connects Delawareans who have disabilities with the tools they need in order to learn, work, play and participate in community life safely and independently. DATI services include: Equipment demonstration center in each county; no-cost, short-term equipment loans that let you try before you buy; Equipment Exchange Program; AT workshops and other training sessions; advocacy for improved AT access policies and funding and several more.

Beth Mineo, Director
Bob Piech, Project Coordinator
Ron Sibert, Funding Specialist

8158 Department of Public Instruction
PO Box 1402
Dover, DE 19903

302-739-5471
Fax: 302-739-2388
e-mail: mbrooks@state.de.us
www.unc.edu

Individuals with Disabilities Education Act requires all states and territories to provide early intervention and preschool special education for children with disabilities and special health care needs. Services include central directory, representatives of agencies, service providers, families, and coordinators of infant, toddler, and preschool special education programs.

Martha Brooks, Director

8159 Parent Information Center of Delaware
6 Larch Avenue, Suite 404, Larch Corporate Center
Wilmington, DE 19804

302-999-7394
888-547-4412
Fax: 302-999-7637
e-mail: PEP700@aol.com
www.picofdel.org

Programs help parents to understand their children's specific needs, communicate more effectively with professionals, participate in the educational planning process, and obtain information about relevant programs, services and resources.

Verna Hensley, President
Marie-Anne Aghazadian, Executive Director
Mindy Cox, Office Manager

District of Columbia

8160 Advocates for Justice and Education
1012 Pennsylvania Ave SE
Washington, DC 20020

202-678-8060
888-327-8060
Fax: 202-678-8062
e-mail: aje.qpg.com
www.aje-dc.org

Programs help parents to understand their children's specific needs, communicate more effectively with professionals, participate in the educational planning process, and obtain information about relevant programs, services and resources.

Tracey Davis, Board Chair
Kim Y. Jones, Executive Director & Member
Antoinette C. Bush, Board Secretary

8161 DC Arc
900 Vamum Street, NE
Washington, DC 20017

202-636-2950
Fax: 202-636-2996
www.taalliance.org

Programs help parents to understand their children's specific needs, communicate more effectively with professionals, participate in the educational planning process, and obtain information about relevant programs, services and resources.

8162 DC-EIP Services
717 14th Street, NW, Suite 730
Washington, DC 20002

202-727-1839
Fax: 202-727-8166
TDD: 202-727-2114
www.chasa.org

Provides early intervention and preschool special education for children with disabilities and special health care needs. Services include central directory, representatives of agencies, service providers, families, and coordinators of infant, toddler, and preschool special education programs.

Joan Christopher, Infant/Toddler Program Coordinator

8163 Georgetown University Child Development Center
National Early Childhood Technical Assistance Ctr
3700 O St., N.W.
Washington, DC 20057

202-687-0100
Fax: 202-687-8899
www.georgetown.edu

Individuals with Disabilities Education Act requires all states and territories to provide early intervention and preschool special education for children with disabilities and special health care needs. Services include central directory, representatives of agencies, service providers, families, and coordinators of infant, toddler, and preschool special education programs.

Paul Tagliabue, Chair
Chris Augostini, Senior Vice President and Chief Ope
John J. DeGioia, Ph.D., President

8164 Giddings School Special Education Division
National Early Childhood Technical Assistance Ctr
Campus Box 8040 Unc-Ch
Chapel Hill, NC 27599

919-962-2001
Fax: 919-966-7463
TDD: 919-843-3269
www.nectas.unc.edu

Services include central directory, representatives of agencies, service providers, families, and coordinators of infant, toddler, and preschool special education programs.

Ann Palmore, Preschool Special Ed. Coordinator

8165 Partnership for Assistive Technology
220 I Street NE, Suite 202
Washington, DC 20002

202-547-0198
Fax: 202-547-2662
TDD: 202-547-2657

State assisted programs and support group information for people of many abilities. Includes local chapters, referrals, fun and social interaction and support groups.

Florida

8166 Alliance for Assistive Service and Technology (FAAST)
325 John Knox Road, Building 400, Suite 402
Tallahassee, FL 32301

850-487-3278
888-788-9216
Fax: 850-487-2805
TDD: 850-922-5951
e-mail: faast@faast.org
www.faast.org

State assisted programs and support group information for people of many abilities. Includes local chapters, referrals, fun and social interaction and support groups.

2-8 pages Newsletter

Gayle Miller, Esq., Chair
Karen M. Clay, Chair-Elect
Lisa Taylor, Treasurer

8167 Early Intervention Unit, Division of Children's Medical Services
1309 Winewood Boulevard
Tallahassee, FL 32399
850-488-6005
Fax: 850-921-5241
e-mail: Fran_L_Wilber@dcf.state.fl.us
www.nectas.unc.edu

Individuals with Disabilities Education Act requires all states and territories to provide early intervention and preschool special education for children with disabilities and special health care needs. Services include central directory, representatives of agencies, service providers, families, and coordinators of infant, toddler, and preschool special education programs.

Fran Wilber, Infant/Toddler Program Coordinator

8168 Family Network on Disabilities
2735 Whitney Road
Clearwater, FL 33760
727-523-1130
800-825-5736
Fax: 727-523-8687
TDD: 727-523-1130
e-mail: fnd@gate.net
www.fndfl.org

Parent Training and Information (PTI) programs help parents to understand their children's specific needs, communicate more effectively with professionals, participate in the educational planning process, and obtain information about relevant programs, services and resources.

Richard La Belle, Executive Director
Christine Goulbourne, Director of Programs
Joseph Hecker, Director of Finance

8169 Florida Department of Education
325 W Gaines Street
Tallahassee, FL 32399
850-245-0505
Fax: 850-245-9667
e-mail: westc@mail.doe.state.fl.us
www.fldoe.org

Individuals with Disabilities Education Act requires all states and territories to provide early intervention and preschool special education for children with disabilities and special health care needs. Services include central directory, representatives of agencies, service providers, families, and coordinators of infant, toddler, and preschool special education programs.

Carale Chu, Chief of Staff
Will Krebs, Deputy Chief of Staff
Dr. Tony Bennett, Commissioner, Florida Department of

8170 Florida's Collaboration for Young Children and their Families Head State
1310 Cross Creek Circle, Suite A
Tallahassee, FL 32301
850-487-8871
Fax: 850-487-0045
e-mail: kkamiya@com1.med.usf.edu
www.nectas.unc.edu

Provides early intervention and preschool special education for children with disabilities and special health care needs. Services include central directory, representatives of agencies, service providers, families, and coordinators of infant, toddler, and preschool special education programs.

Katherine Kamiya, Interagency Coordinator

8171 US Blind Golfers Association
3093 Shamrock Street N
Tallahassee, FL 32308
904-893-4511
Fax: 904-893-4511
e-mail: nightgolf@concentric.net
www.usblindgolf.com

State assisted programs and support group information for people of many abilities. Includes local chapters, referrals, fun and social interaction and support groups.

David Meador, President
Phil Hubbard, Vice President
Bill McMahon, Board Members

Georgia

8172 DHR/Division of Public Health - Babies Can t Wait Program
2 Peachtree Street NE, Room 7-315
Atlanta, GA 30303
404-657-2700
888-651-8224
Fax: 404-657-2763
e-mail: skmoss@dhr.state.ga.us
www.health.state.ga.us/programs/bcw

Babies Can't Wait (BCW) Program is Georgia's Part C Early Intervention Program under Part C of the federal Individuals with Disabilities Education Improvement Act (IDEA). Services include a comprehensive, coordinated, multidisciplinary, interagency system of early intervention supports for infants and toddlers with disabilities from birth to age 3 and their families.

Janie Brodnax, Chief Operating Officer DHP
Brenda Fitzgerald, M.D., Commissioner, Georgia Department of
Russell Crutchfield, Deputy Chief of Staff

8173 Department for Exceptional Students Georgia Department of Education
205 Jessie Hill Jr. Drive, SE, Suite 1870
Atlanta, GA 30334
404-657-9965
Fax: 404-651-6457
e-mail: tbowen@doe.k12.ga.us
www.nectas.unc.edu

Provides early intervention and preschool special education for children with disabilities and special health care needs. Services include central directory, representatives of agencies, service providers, families, and coordinators of infant, toddler, and preschool special education programs.

Toni Waylor Bowen, Preschool Special Ed. Coordinator

8174 Department of Counseling and Educational Leadership-Columbus State University
4225 University Avenue, Suite 754
Columbus, GA 31907
706-568-2222
Fax: 706-569-3134
www.nectas.unc.edu

Individuals with Disabilities Education Act requires all states and territories to provide early intervention and preschool special education for children with disabilities and special health care needs. Services include central directory, representatives of agencies, service providers, families, and coordinators of infant, toddler, and preschool special education programs.

Katherine McCormick, Interagency Coordinating Council

8175 Parent to Parent of Georgia
3070 Presidential Parkway, Suite 130
Atlanta, GA 30340
770-451-5484
800-229-2038
Fax: 770-458-4091
e-mail: parenttoparent@fga.org
www.p2pga.org

Statewide informational and emotional support to families and individuals affected by disability.

8176 Parents Educating Parents and Professional for All Children (PEPPAC)
8318 Durelee Lane, Suite 101
Douglasville, GA 30134
770-577-7771
Fax: 770-577-7774
e-mail: peppac@bellsouth.net
www.taalliance.org

Parent Training and Information (PTI) programs help parents to understand their children's specific needs, communicate more effectively with professionals, participate in the educational planning process, and obtain information about relevant programs, services and resources.

8177 Tools for Life Division of Rehabilitation Services
1700 Century Circle B-4
Atlanta, GA 30345

404-894-4960
800-578-8665
Fax: 404-894-9320
TDD: 404-657-3085
e-mail: 102476.1737@compuserve.com
www.gatfl.org

State assisted programs and support group information for people of many abilities. Includes local chapters, referrals, fun and social interaction and support groups.

Hawaii

8178 AWARE
200 N Vineyard Boulevard, Suite 310
Honolulu, HI 96817

808-536-9684
Fax: 808-537-6780
e-mail: LDAH@gte.net
www.taalliance.org

Parent Training and Information (PTI) programs help parents to understand their children's specific needs, communicate more effectively with professionals, participate in the educational planning process, and obtain information about relevant programs services, and resources.

8179 Assistive Technology Resource Centers of H awaii (ATRC)
414 Kuiwii Street, Suite 104
Honolulu, HI 96817

808-532-7110
800-645-3007
Fax: 808-532-7120
e-mail: atrc-info@atrc.org
www.atrc.org

State assisted programs and support group information for people of many abilities. Includes local chapters, referrals, fun and social interaction and support groups.

8180 Parents and Children Together (PACT) Honolulu, HI 96819

808-847-3285
Fax: 808-841-1485
e-mail: admin@pacthawaii.org
www.pacthawaii.org

Individuals with Disabilities Education Act requires all states and territories to provide early intervention and preschool special education for children with disabilities and special health care needs. Services include central directory, representatives of agencies, service providers, families, and coordinators of infant, toddler, and preschool special education programs.

David Shibata, Chair
Dana Ann Takushi, Vice Chair
Lowell Kalapa, Treasurer

8181 Special Needs Branch Department of Education
637 18th Avenue, Building C, Room 101
Honolulu, HI 96816

808-733-4900
Fax: 808-733-4841
e-mail: michael_fahley@notes.k12.hi.us
www.unc.edu

Individuals with Disabilities Education Act requires all states and territories to provide early intervention and preschool special education for children with disabilities and special health care needs. Services include central directory, representatives of agencies, service providers, families, and coordinators of infant, toddler, and preschool special education programs.

Michael Fahey, Preschool Special Ed. Coordinator

8182 Zero-To-3 Hawaii Project
1600 Kapiolani Boulevard, Suite 1401
Honolulu, HI 96814

808-957-0066
Fax: 808-946-5222
e-mail: jeanj@hawaii.edu
www.chasa.org

Services include central directory, representatives of agencies, service providers, families, and coordinators of infant, toddler, and preschool special education programs.

Jean Johnson, Infant/Toddler Program Coordinator

Idaho

8183 Assistive Technology Project
1 West Old State Capitol Plaza, Suite 100
Springfield, ID 62701

217-522-7985
800-852-5110
Fax: 217-522-8067
TTY: 217-522-9966
TDD: 208-855-3559
e-mail: seile861@uidaho.edu
www.iltech.org

State assisted programs and support group information for people of many abilities. Includes local chapters, referrals, fun and social interaction and support groups.

8184 Department of Education
PO Box 83720
Boise, ID 83720

208-332-6917
Fax: 208-334-4664
e-mail: jkbrenn@sde.state.id.us
www.unc.edu

Individuals with Disabilities Education Act requires all states and territories to provide early intervention and preschool special education for children with disabilities and special health care needs. Services include central directory, representatives of agencies, service providers, families, and coordinators of infant, toddler, and preschool special education programs.

Nolene Weaver, Supervisor

8185 Idaho Parents Unlimited
500 S 8th Street
Boise, ID 83702

208-342-5884
800-242-4785
Fax: 208-342-1408
TDD: 208-342-5884
e-mail: parents@ipulidaho.org
www.ipulidaho.org

Parent Training and Information (PTI) programs help parents to understand their children's specific needs, communicate more effectively with professionals, participate in the educational planning process, and obtain information about relevant programs services, and resources.

Angela Lindig, Executive Director

8186 Infant/Toddler Program
PO Box 83720
Boise, ID 83720

208-334-5523
Fax: 208-334-6664
e-mail: jonesm@dhw.state.id.us
www.idahochild.org

Services include central directory, representatives of agencies, service providers, families, and coordinators of infant, toddler, and preschool special education programs.

Mary Jones, Infant/Toddler Program Coordinator

8187 Palouse Area Parent To Parent
317 17th Avenue
Lewiston, ID 83501

208-746-8599
TTY: 208-746-8599
e-mail: irel102w@wonder.em.cdc.gov

Informational and emotional support to parents who have a child, adolescent, or adult family member with special needs.

8188 Parent Reaching Out to Parents
2195 Ironwood Court
Coeur d'Alene, ID 83814

208-769-1409
Fax: 208-769-1430
parentsreachingout.com

Informational and emotional support to parents who have a child, adolescent, or adult family member with special needs.

Lorena Freund, Coordinator
Kathy Dalberg, Secretary/Treasurer

Illinois

8189 Archway
PO Box 1180, 2751 W Main
Carbondale, IL 62903
618-549-4442
Fax: 618-549-0231

Informational and emotional support to parents who have a child, adolescent, or adult family member with special needs.

8190 Assistive Technology Project
1 W Old State Capitol Plaza, Suite 100
Springfield, IL 62701
217-522-7985
800-852-5110
Fax: 217-522-8067
TTY: 217-522-9966
TDD: 217-522-9966
e-mail: iatp@iltech.org
www.ittech.org

State assisted programs and support group information for people of many abilities. Includes local chapters, referrals, fun and social interaction and support groups.

Wilhelmina Gunther, Executive Director
Shelly Lowe, Finance/Personnel Manager
Theresa Ganci, Finance/Personnel Assistant

8191 Child and Family Connections
PO Box 741280
Boynton Beach, FL 33474
773-233-1799
800-554-1802
Fax: 773-233-2011
www.cfcpbc.org

Informational and emotional support to parents who have a child, adolescent, or adult family member with special needs.

8192 Developmental Services Center
1304 W Bradley
Champaign, IL 61821
217-356-9176
Fax: 217-356-9851
e-mail: jmcateer@dsc-illinois.org
www.dsc-illinois.org

Informational and emotional support to parents who have a child, adolescent, or adult family member with special needs.

Dale Morrissey, Chief Executive Officer
Danielle Matthews, Executive Vice President of Support
Patty Walters, Executive Vice President of Consume

8193 Family Resource Center on Disabilities
11 E. Adams St. Suite 1002
Chicago, IL 60603
312-939-3513
800-952-4199
Fax: 312-854-8980
TTY: 312-939-3519
TDD: 312-939-3519
e-mail: info@frcd.org
www.frcd.org

Parent Training and Information (PTI) programs help parents to understand their children's specific needs, communicate more effectively with professionals, participate in the educational planning process, and obtain information about relevant programs, services and resources.

Karen Aguilar, Coalition Director
Melody Musgrove, Director, Special Education Program

8194 Family T.I.E.S. Network
830 S Spring Street
Springfield, IL 62704
217-544-5809
800-865-7842
Fax: 217-544-6018
e-mail: FTIESN@aol.com
www.taalliance.org

Parent Training and Information (PTI) programs help parents to understand their children's specific needs, communicate more effectively with professionals, participate in the educational planning process, and obtain information about relevant programs, services and resources.

8195 Greater Interagency Council Parent to Parent Support Network
925 W 175th Street
Homewood, IL 60430
708-799-2718
Fax: 708-799-7974

Informational and emotional support to parents who have a child, adolescent, or adult family member with special needs.

8196 Leukemia Research Foundation
3520 Lake Avenue, Suite #202
Wilmette, IL 60091
847-424-0600
888-558-5385
Fax: 847-424-0606
e-mail: info@lrfmail.org
www.leukemia-research.org

Founded to conquer leukemia by funding research into the causes and cures of the disease and to enrich the quality of life by those touched by leukemia.

Kevin Radelet, Executive Director
Cindy Kane, Senior Director of Development
Carl Alston, Director of Communications

8197 National Center for Latinos with Disabilities
1921 S Blue Island Avenue
Chicago, IL 60608
312-666-3393
800-532-3393
Fax: 312-666-1787
TTY: 312-666-1788
e-mail: ncld@ncld.com
homepage.interaccess.com/~ncld/

Parent Training and Information (PTI) programs help parents to understand their children's specific needs, communicate more effectively with professionals, participate in the educational planning process, and obtain information about relevant programs, services and resources.

Everardo Franco, Executive Director
Nancy Perez, Coordinator Info and Referral

8198 Next Steps - Parents Reaching Parents
100 W Randolph, Suite 8-100
Chicago, IL 60601
312-814-4042
Fax: 708-799-7974
TTY: 312-814-4042
e-mail: caroldors@aol.com

Informational and emotional support to parents who have a child, adolescent, or adult family member with special needs.

8199 Office of Community Health and Prevention Bureau of Early Intervention, DHR
222 South College, 2nd Floor
Springfield, IL 62704
217-782-9260
Fax: 217-782-7849
www.dhs.state.il.us/ei

Provides early intervention and preschool special education for children with disabilities and special health care needs. Services include central directory, representatives of agencies, service providers, families, and coordinators of infant, toddler, and preschool special education programs.

Mary Miller, Infant/Toddler Program Coordinator
Brian Bond, Contact

8200 Parent to Parent Network
1530 Lincoln Avenue
Charleston, IL 61920
217-348-0127
Fax: 217-348-0740

Informational and emotional support to parents who have a child, adolescent, or adult family member with special needs.

8201 Southern IL Child and Family Connections
2751 W Main Street
Carbondale, IL 62903
888-340-6702
Fax: 618-549-8137

Informational and emotional support to parents who have a child, adolescent, or adult family member with special needs.

8202 State Board of Education Department of Special Education
National Early Childhood Technical Assistance Ctr
100 N 1st Street, Suite 233
Springfield, IL 62777 217-782-5589
Fax: 217-782-7849
e-mail: preising@smtp.isbe.state.il.us
www.unc.edu

Individuals with Disabilities Education Act requires all states and territories to provide early intervention and preschool special education for children with disabilities and special health care needs. Services include central directory, representatives of agencies, service providers, families, and coordinators of infant, toddler, and preschool special education programs.

Jack Shook, Division Administrator

Indiana

8203 ATTAIN: Assistive Technology Through Action in Indiana
32 E Washington Street, Suite 1400
Indianapolis, IN 46204 317-486-8808
800-527-8246
Fax: 317-486-8809
TDD: 800-743-3333
e-mail: attaininfo@attaininc.org
www.attanic.org

State assisted programs and support group information for people of many abilities. Includes local chapters, referrals, fun and social interaction and support groups.

8204 About Special Kids (ASK)
7172 Graham Road, Suite 100
Indianapolis, IN 46250 317-257-8683
800-964-4746
Fax: 317-251-7488
e-mail: familynetw@aboutspecialkids.org
www.aboutspecialkids.org

Helping children with special needs live better lives by education, empowering and connecting their families.

Cindy Robinson, Director of Education and Informati
Jane Scott, Director of Family Support
Joe Brubaker, Executive Director

8205 Assistive Technology Training and Information Center
3354 Pine Hill Drive, PO Box 2441
Vincennes, IN 47591 812-886-0575
800-962-8842
Fax: 812-886-1128
e-mail: inattic1@aol.com
www.theattic.org

Technology group of parents, consumers and professionals that provides resources to help children and adults who have disabilities gain access to the benefits of technology. Includes nationwide network of community-based assistive technology, resource centers, hands on consultants and product demonstrations.

8206 Division of Exceptional Learners Indiana Department of Education
State House, Room 229
Indianapolis, IN 46204 317-232-0570
Fax: 317-232-0589
e-mail: scochran@doe.state.in.us
www.doe.state.in.us/exceptional

Individuals with Disabilities Education Act requires all states and territories to provide preschool special education for children with disabilities. Special Education and related services are provided through the public schools.

Sheron Cochran, Preschool Special Ed Coordinator

8207 Down Syndrome Association of Central Indiana
10792 Downing Street
Carmel, IN 46033 317-574-9757
Fax: 317-574-9757
e-mail: MKaye62801@aol.com

Provides informational and emotional support to parents who have a child, adolescent, or adult family member with special needs. Program offers an important connection for a parent who is seeking support for a special disability issue, by matching him or her with a trained veteran parent.

8208 Family Resource Center of Southeast Indiana
4101 Timberview Road
West Harrison, IN 47060 812-637-1445

Informational and emotional support to parents who have a child, adolescent, or adult family member with special needs.

8209 First Direction
PO Box 4234
Lafayette, IN 47903 765-423-1460

Informational and emotional support to parents who have a child, adolescent, or adult family member with special needs.

8210 First Steps
402 W Washington Street, Suite W-386
Indianapolis, IN 46204 317-233-9229
Fax: 317-232-7948
e-mail: mgreer@fssa.state.in.us
www.chasa.org

Individuals with Disabilities Education Act requires all states and territories to provide early intervention and preschool special education for children with disabilities and special health care needs. Services include central directory, representatives of agencies, service providers, families, and coordinators of infant, toddler, and preschool special education programs.

Maureen Greer, Part C Director

8211 First Steps for Families
500 8th Avenue
Terre Haute, IN 47804 812-231-8419
Fax: 812-231-8208
e-mail: famnetwork@aol.com

Informational and emotional support to parents who have a child, adolescent, or adult family member with special needs.

8212 First Steps, Early Interventions, New Horizons Rehabilitation
PO Box 98
Batesville, IN 47006 812-934-4528
Fax: 812-934-2522
TTY: 812-934-4528

Informational and emotional support to parents who have a child, adolescent, or adult family member with special needs.

8213 Future Choices
309 N High Street
Muncie, IN 47305 765-741-3494
Fax: 765-741-8333
e-mail: futurechoicesinc@aol.com

Informational and emotional support to parents who have a child, adolescent, or adult family member with special needs.

8214 Knox County Advocates
1805 Indiana Avenue
Vincennes, IN 47591 812-882-0375
Fax: 812-886-1128
e-mail: INATTIC1@aol.com

Informational and emotional support to parents who have a child, adolescent, or adult family member with special needs.

8215 NEO Fight
PO Box 17715
Indianapolis, IN 46217 317-446-3013
e-mail: info@neofight.org
www.neofight.org

Informational and emotional support to parents who have a child, adolescent, or adult family member with special needs.

Michie Sebree, R.N., President
Kathleen Smith, Secretary
Amanda Blann, Board Member

8216 Project Special Care
4755 Kinsway Drive, Suite 105
Indianapolis, IN 46205   317-257-8683
                                     Fax: 317-251-7488
                                     www.ipin.org

Informational and emotional support to parents who have a child,
adolescent, or adult family member with special needs.

8217 US Rowing Assocation
2 Wall Street
Princeton, NJ 08540   609-751-0700
                                          800-314-4769
                                     Fax: 609-924-1578
                              e-mail: members@usrowing.org
                                     www.usrowing.org

State assisted programs and support group information for people
of many abilities. Includes local chapters, referrals, fun and social
interaction and support groups.

Brian Klausner, Chief Financial Officer
Glenn Merry, Chief Executive Officer
Beth Kohl, Chief Marketing Officer

Iowa

8218 ARC of East Central Iowa Pilot Parents
680 2nd Street SE, Suite 200
Cedar Rapids, IA 52404   319-365-0487
                                          800-843-0272
                                     Fax: 319-365-9938

Informational and emotional support to parents who have a child,
adolescent, or adult family member with special needs.

8219 Bureau of Children, Family, and Community Services
Grimes State Office Building, 3rd Floor
Des Moines, IA 50319   515-281-7145
                                     Fax: 515-242-6019
                         e-mail: dee.gethman@ed.state.ia.us
                                     www.chasa.org

Individuals with Disabilities Education Act requires all states and
territories to provide early intervention and preschool special education for children with disabilities and special health care
needs. Services include central directory, representatives of agencies, service providers, families, and coordinators of infant, toddler, and preschool special education programs.

Lynda Pletcher, Preschool Special Ed. Coordinator

8220 Family & Educator Connection - Cedar Falls /Waterloo Region
3706 Cedar Heights Drive
Cedar Falls, IA 50613   219-273-8265
                                          800-542-8375
                                     Fax: 319-273-8275
                                     TTY: 319-273-8291
                         e-mail: dpaton@aea267.k12.ia.us
                                     www.aea267.k12.ia.us

The Family & Educator Connection is part of the Parent & Educator Connection, a statewide network of families and educators
working together to serve children and young adults with special
needs. They work together in positive ways to improve educational programs for children and youth with disabilities.

Rod Ball, Administrator
Edie Penno, Special Education Coordinator and T
Sandy Lichty, Consultant for Challenging Behavior

**8221 Family & Educator Connection - Clear Lake/ Mason City
Region**
Mason City Airport Grounds, 9184 B 265th Street
Clear Lake, IA 50428   641-357-6125
                                          800-392-6640
                         e-mail: skraschel@aea27.k12.ia.us
                                     www.aea267.k12.ia.us

The Family & Educator Connection is part of the Parent & Educator Connection, a statewide network of families and educators
working together to serve children and young adults with special
needs. They work together in positive ways to improve educational programs for children and youth with disabilities.

Roberta Kraft-Abrahamson, Director District 1 - Vice Presiden
Sandy Kraschel, Administrator

8222 Family & Educator Connection - Marshalltow n Region
909 South 12th Street
Marshalltown, IA 50158   641-844-2469
                                          800-735-1539
                                     Fax: 641-752-0075
                         e-mail: alawler@aea267.k12.ia.us
                                     www.aea267.k12.ia.us

The Family & Educator Connection is part of the Parent & Educator Connection, a statewide network of families and educators
working together to serve children and young adults with special
needs. They work together in positive ways to improve educational programs for children and youth with disabilities.

Andy Lawler, Administrator
David Giese, Director District 5

8223 Iowa Program for Assistive Technology
University Hospital School
303A CDD, 100 Hawkins Drive
Iowa City, IA 52242   319-353-6108
                                          800-331-3027
                                     Fax: 319-356-8284
                                     TDD: 800-331-3027
                         e-mail: jane_gay@uiowa.edu
                                     www.uiowa.edu

State assisted programs and support group information for people
of many abilities. Includeslocal chapters, referrals, fun and social
interaction and support groups.

Linda Monroe, Contact

8224 Iowa's System of EI Services
Grimes State Office Building, 3rd Floor
Des Moines, IA 50319   515-281-7145
                                     Fax: 515-242-6019
                         e-mail: lynda.pletcher@ed.state.ia.us
                                     www.chasa.org

Individuals with Disabilities Education Act requires all states and
territories to provide early intervention and preschool special education for children with disabilities and special health care
needs. Services include central directory, representatives of agencies, service providers, families, and coordinators of infant, toddler, and preschool special education programs.

Lynda Pletcher, Infant/Toddler Program Coordinator

8225 Parent Educator Connection
Grimews State Office Bldg
Des Moines, IA 50318   515-242-5295
                                          800-572-5073
                                     Fax: 712-722-1643
                         e-mail: bjones@aea5.k12.ia.uss

Informational and emotional support to parents who have a child,
adolescent, or adult family member with special needs.

8226 Parent Educator Connection Program
Heartland AEA 11, 6500 Corporate Drive
Johnston, IA 50131   515-270-9030
                                          800-362-2720
                                     Fax: 515-270-5383
                         www.aea11.k12.ia.us/parents/PEC/

Provides informational and emotional support to parents who
have a child, adolescent, or adult family member with special
needs. Program offers an important connection for a parent who
is seeking support for special disability issue, by matching him or
her with a trained veteran parent.

Paula Vincent, Chief Administrator
David King, Chief Financial Officer
Kevin Fangman, Director of District Services

Kansas	**Kentucky**

8227 Assistive Technology for Kansas Project
2601 Gabriel, PO Box 738
Parsons, KS 67357
316-421-8367
800-526-3648
Fax: 620-421-8367
TDD: 316-421-0954
e-mail: ssack@parsons.lsi.ukans.edu
www.atk.ku.edu/kansas/

State assisted programs and support group information for people of many abilities. Includes local chapters, referrals, fun and social interaction and support groups.

Sara Sack, ATK Director
Sheila Simmons, ATK Coordinator
Sarah Walters, Kansas Infant Toddler Services

8228 Department of Health & Environment
1000 Sw Jackson
Topeka, KS 66612
785-296-1500
Fax: 785-368-6368
e-mail: info@kdheks.gov
www.kdheks.gov

Individuals with Disabilities Education Act requires all states and territories to provide early intervention and preschool special education for children with disabilities and special health care needs. Services include central directory, representatives of agencies, service providers, families, and coordinators of infant, toddler, and preschool special education programs.

Nathan Bainbridge, Senior Executive Policy Analyst
Tim Keck, Deputy Chief Counsel
Glen Yancey, Information Technology Director

8229 Families Together
3033 West 2nd, Suite 106
Wichita, KS 67203
316-945-7747
888-815-6364
Fax: 316-945-7795
e-mail: wichita@familiestogetherinc.org
www.familiestogetherinc.org

Parent Training and Information (PTI) programs help parents to understand their children's specific needs, communicate more effectively with professionals, participate in the educational planning process, and obtain information about relevant programs, services and resources.

Linda Peterson, President
Eric Morrison, Vice President
Jill Elkins, Secretary

8230 Families Together/Parent to Parent of KS
501 Jackson, Suite 400
Topeka, KS 66603
785-233-4777
800-264-6343
Fax: 756-233-4787
TTY: 785-233-4777
e-mail: family@inlandnet.net

Informational and emotional support to parents who have a child, adolescent, or adult family member with special needs.

8231 Special Education Administration Kansas St ate Department of Education
120 E 10th Avenue
Topeka, KS 66612
785-296-3201
Fax: 785-296-7933
e-mail: tsmith@ksde.org
www.ksde.org/Default.aspx?tabid=4745

Individuals with Disabilities Education Act requires all states and territories to provide early intervention and preschool special education for children with disabilities and special health care needs. Services include central directory, representatives of agencies, service providers, families, and coordinators of infant, toddler, and preschool special education programs.

Tiffany Smith, Consultant
Colleen Riley, Team Director
Gayle Stuber, Early Learning & Preschool Coord.

8232 Assistive Technology Services Network
8412 Westport Road
Louisville, KY 40242
502-429-4484
800-327-5287
Fax: 502-429-7114
TDD: 502-327-9855
www.katsnet.org

State assisted programs and support group information for people of many abilities. Includes local chapters, referrals, fun and social interaction and support groups.

Stephen M. Johnson, Executive Director

8233 College of Education - Western Kentucky University
Interdisciplinary Early Childhood Education
#1 Big Red Way, Western Kentucky University
Bowling Green, KY 42101
270-745-5414
Fax: 270-745-6474
e-mail: vicki.stayton@wku.edu
www.nectas.unc.edu

Individuals with Disabilities Education Act requires all states and territories to provide early intervention and preschool special education for children with disabilities and special health care needs. Services include central directory, representatives of agencies, service providers, families, and coordinators of infant, toddler, and preschool special education programs.

Vicki Stayton, Interagency Coordinating Council

8234 Division of Preschool Services
1711 Capotol Plaza Tower
Frankfort, KY 40601
502-564-7056
Fax: 502-564-6771
e-mail: bsinglet@kde.state.ky.us
www.nectas.unc.edu

Provides early intervention and preschool special education for children with disabilities and special health care needs. Services include central directory, representatives of agencies, service providers, families, and coordinators of infant, toddler, and preschool special education programs.

Barbara Singleton, Preschool Special Ed. Coordinator

8235 Infant-Toddler Program, Division of Mental Retardation
275 E Main Street
Frankfort, KY 40621
502-564-7722
Fax: 502-564-0438
e-mail: jhenson@mail.state.ky.us
www.nectas.unc.edu

Individuals with Disabilities Education Act requires all states and territories to provide early intervention and preschool special education for children with disabilities and special health care needs. Services include central directory, representatives of agencies, service providers, families, and coordinators of infant, toddler, and preschool special education programs.

Jim Henson, Infant/Toddler Program Coordinator

8236 Special Parent Involvement Network
10301-B Deering Road
Louisville, KY 40272
502-937-6894
800-525-7746
Fax: 502-937-6464
e-mail: spininc@kyspin.com
www.kyspin.com

Parent Training and Information (PTI) programs help parents to understand their children's specific needs, communicate more effectively with professionals, participate in the educational planning process, and obtain information about relevant programs, services and resources.

Crump Caroline, Director

Louisiana

8237 Division of Special Populations
PO Box 94064
Baton Rouge, LA 70804
225-342-3633
800-737-2958
Fax: 225-342-5880
e-mail: Vberidon@mail.doe.state.la.us
www.doe.state.la.us

Individuals with Disabilities Education Act requires all states and territories to provide early intervention and preschool special education for children with disabilities and special health care needs. Services include central directory, representatives of agencies, service providers, families, and coordinators of infant, toddler, and preschool special education programs.

Evelyn Johnson, Infant/Toddler Program Coordinator
Virginia C. Beridon, Director

8238 Families Helping Families of Greater New Orleans
1323 Division Street, Suite 110
Metairie, LA 70002
504-888-9111
800-766-7736
Fax: 504-888-0246
e-mail: fhfgno@ix.netcom.com
www.fhfgno.org

Informational and emotional support to parents who have a child, adolescent, or adult family member with special needs.

8239 Louisiana Assistive Technology Access Network
3042 Old Forge Drive, Suite D
Baton Rouge, LA 70898
225-925-9500
800-270-6185
Fax: 225-925-9560
TDD: 225-925-9500
e-mail: latanstate@aol.com
www.latan.org

State assisted programs and support group information for people of many abilities. Includes local chapters, referrals, fun and social interaction and support groups.

Charles Tate, Board Chair
Jim Parks, Vice Chair
Julie Nesbit, ATP, President/CEO

8240 Preschool Programs - Division of Special Populations
PO Box 94064
Baton Rouge, LA 70804
225-342-3633
800-737-2958
Fax: 225-342-5880
e-mail: Vberidon@mail.doe.state.la.us
www.doe.state.la.us

Individuals with Disabilities Education Act requires all states and territories to provide early intervention and preschool special education for children with disabilities and special health care needs. Services include central directory, representatives of agencies, service providers, families, and coordinators of infant, toddler, and preschool special education programs.

Evelyn Johnson, Infant/Toddler Program Coordinator
Virginia C. Beridon, Director

8241 Project PROMPT
4323 Division Street, Suite 110
Metairie, LA 70002
504-888-9111
800-766-7736
Fax: 504-888-0246
e-mail: thsgno@ix.netcom.com
www.taalliance.org

Parent Training and Information (PTI) programs help parents to understand their children's specific needs, communicate more effectively with professionals, participate in the educational planning process, and obtain information about relevant programs, services and resources.

Maine

8242 CDC Lincoln County
PO Box 1114
Damariscotta, ME 04543
207-563-1411
Fax: 207-563-6312
www.nectas.unc.edu

Individuals with Disabilities Education Act requires all states and territories to provide early intervention and preschool special education for children with disabilities and special health care needs. Services include central directory, representatives of agencies, service providers, families, and coordinators of infant, toddler, and preschool special education programs.

Jean Eaton, Interagency Coordinating Council

8243 Child Department Services
146 State House Station
Augusta, ME 04333
207-287-3272
Fax: 207-287-5900
e-mail: jaci.holmes@state.me.us

Provides early intervention and preschool special education for children with disabilities and special health care needs. Services include central directory, representatives of agencies, service providers, families, and coordinators of infant, toddler, and preschool special education programs.

Joanne C Holmes, Infant/Toddler Program Coordinator

8244 Child Department Services, Department of Education
23 State House Station
Augusta, ME 04333
207-287-5950
Fax: 207-287-2550
e-mail: Debbie.Violette@state.me.us
www.unc.edu

Provides early intervention and preschool special education for children with disabilities and special health care needs. Services include central directory, representatives of agencies, service providers, families, and coordinators of infant, toddler, and preschool special education programs.

Joanne C Holmes, Preschool Special Ed. Coordiantor

8245 Consumer Information and Technology Training Exchange (Maine CITE)
46 University Drive
Augusta, ME 04330
207-621-3195
Fax: 207-629-5429
TDD: 207-621-3195
e-mail: powers@maine.maine.edu
www.mainecite.org

State assisted programs and support group information for people of many abilities. Includes local chapters, referrals, fun and social interaction and support groups.

Kathleen Powers, Program Director
Kathy Adams, OTR/L, ATP, Training Coordinator
Darcy York, Administrative Assistant

8246 Special Needs Parent Info Network
PO Box 2067
Augusta, ME 04338
207-623-2144
800-870-7746
Fax: 207-623-2148
e-mail: parentconnect@mpf.org
www.startingpointsforme.org

Parent Training and Information (PTI) programs help parents to understand their children's specific needs, communicate more effectively with professionals, participate in the educational planning process, and obtain information about relevant programs, services and resources.

Lorraine Christensen, President
Steve Ocean, Vice President/Treasurer
Janice LaChance, Executive Director

8247 York County Parent Awareness
150 Main Street, Midtown Mall
Sanford, ME 04027
207-324-2337
Fax: 207-324-5621
e-mail: ycpa@mmp.org

Informational and emotional support to parents who have a child, adolescent, or adult family member with special needs.

Maryland

8248 ARC Family Connection Parent to Parent Program
11600 Nebel Street
Rockville, MD 20852   301-984-5777
                                           Fax: 301-816-2429

Informational and emotional support to parents who have a child, adolescent, or adult family member with special needs.

8249 Developmental Pediatrics School of Medicine, University of Maryland
630 W Fayette Street, Room 5686
Baltimore, MD 21201   410-706-3542
                                           Fax: 410-706-0835
                                           www.nectas.unc.edu

Individuals with Disabilities Education Act requires all states and territories to provide early intervention and preschool special education for children with disabilities and special health care needs. Services include central directory, representatives of agencies, service providers, families, and coordinators of infant, toddler, and preschool special education programs.

Renee Wachtel, Interagency Coordinating Council

8250 MD Infant/Toddler/Preschool Services Division
200 W Baltimore Street
Baltimore, MD 21201   410-767-0238
                                           800-535-0182
                                           Fax: 410-333-2661
                                           TDD: 410-333-0781
                                           e-mail: cbaglin@msde.state.md.us
                                           www.msde.state.md.us

Individuals with Disabilities Education Act requires all states and territories to provide early intervention and preschool special education for children with disabilities and special health care needs. Services include central directory, representatives of agencies, service providers, families, and coordinators of infant, toddler, and preschool special education programs.

Carol Ann Baglin, Assstant State Superintendent

8251 Maryland Infant and Toddlers Program Family Support Network
200 W Baltimore, 4th Floor
Baltimore, MD 21201   410-767-0652
                                           Fax: 410-333-8165

Informational and emotional support to parents who have a child, adolescent, or adult family member with special needs.

8252 Parents Place of Maryland
801 Cromwell Park Drive, Suite 103
Glen Burnie, MD 21061   410-768-9100
                                           Fax: 410-768-0830
                                           TDD: 410-768-9100
                                           e-mail: info@ppmd.org
                                           www.ppmd.org

Parent Training and Information (PTI) programs help parents to understand their children's specific needs, communicate more effectively with professionals, participate in the educational planning process, and obtain information about relevant programs, services and resources.

Josie Thomas, Executive Director
Suzie Shannon, Administration
Mary Baskar, Health Projects Coordinator

8253 Partners in Intensive Care
PO Box 41043
Bethesda, MD 20824   301-681-2708
                                           Fax: 301-681-2707

Informational and emotional support to parents who have a child, adolescent, or adult family member with special needs.

8254 Technology Assistance Program Maryland Rehabilitation Center
2301 Argonne Drive, Room T-17
Baltimore, MD 21218   410-554-9230
                                           800-832-4827
                                           Fax: 410-554-9237
                                           TTY: 866-881-7488
                                           e-mail: mdtap.org
                                           www.mdtap.org

State assisted programs and support group information for people of many abilities. Includes local chapters, referrals, fun and social interaction and support groups.

Tony Rice, Loan Program Director
Tanya Goodman, Loan Program Assistant Director
Lori Markland, Director of Communications, Outreac

Massachusetts

8255 Bureau of Early Childhood Programs
350 Main Street
Malden, MA 02148   781-388-3300
                                           Fax: 781-388-3394
                                           e-mail: eschaefer@doe.mass.edu
                                           www.doe.mass.edu

Individuals with Disabilities Education Act requires all states and territories to provide early intervention and preschool special education for children with disabilities and special health care needs. Services include central directory, representatives of agencies, service providers, families, and coordinators of infant, toddler, and preschool special education programs.

David P. Driscoll, Commissioner

8256 Children's Happiness Foundation
PO Box 266
Marshfield, MA 02050   781-837-9609
                                           Fax: 781-837-5229
                                           e-mail: rsvpmktg@aol.com

Serves New England children ages three to eighteen with life-threatening or chronic degenerative diseases.

8257 Early Intervention Services
250 Washington Street
Boston, MA 02108   617-624-5969
                                           Fax: 617-624-5990
                                           e-mail: Ron.Benham@state.ma.us

Individuals with Disabilities Education Act requires all states and territories to provide early intervention and preschool special education for children with disabilities and special health care needs. Services include central directory, representatives of agencies, service providers, families, and coordinators of infant, toddler, and preschool special education programs.

Ron Benham, Infant/Toddler Program Coordinator

8258 Education Development Center - EDC
43 Foundry Avenue
Waltham, MA 02453   617-969-7100
                                           800-225-4276
                                           Fax: 617-969-5979
                                           TTY: 617-964-5448
                                           e-mail: pprintz@edc.org
                                           www.edc.org

One of the largest nonprofit education and health organizations. With programs for children and families combining research and practice, promoting professional development and systematic change, forging community links, and influencing the policies and legislation that affect the lives of children. The New England RAP incorporates proven strategies to enhance the efforts of organizations servicing children with disabilities and their families.

Luther Luedtke, President and Chief Executive Offic
Cheryl Hoffman-Bray, Vice President/Chief Financial Offi
Robert Spielvogel, Vice President/Chief Technology Off

8259   Family Ties at Massachusetts Department of Public Health
5 Randolph Street
Canton, MA 02021
781-774-6736
Fax: 781-774-6618
TTY: 781-774-6619
TDD: 508-947-0977
e-mail: mcsummers@fcsn.org
www.massfamilyties.org

Informational and emotional support to parents who have a child, adolescent, or adult family member with special needs.

Mary Castro Summers, Program Director

8260   Federation for Children with Special Needs
1135 Tremont Street Suite 420
Boston, MA 02120
617-236-7210
800-331-0688
Fax: 617-572-2094
TDD: 617-482-2915
e-mail: fcsninfo@fcsn.org
www.fcsn.org/

Parent Training and Information (PTI) programs help parents to understand their children's specific needs, communicate more effectively with professionals, participate in the educational planning process, and obtain information about relevant programs, services and resources.

James F. Whalen, President
Maureen Jerz, Director of Development
Tom Hamel, Director of Finance

8261   Greater Boston Arc Parent Support
1505 Commonwealth Avenue
Boston, MA 02135
617-783-3900
Fax: 617-783-9190
e-mail: bostonarc@aol.com
gbarc.org

Informational and emotional support to parents who have a child, adolescent, or adult family member with special needs.

8262   Massachusetts Assistive Technology Partnership
1295 Boylston Street, Suite 310
Boston, MA 02215
617-355-7153
Fax: 617-355-6345
TDD: 617-355-7301
e-mail: matp@matp.net
www.matp.org

State assisted programs and support group information for people of many abilities. Includes local chapters, referrals, fun and social interaction and support groups.

8263   National Birth Defects Center
40 2nd Avenue, Suite 520
Waltham, MA 02451
781-466-9555
Fax: 781-487-2361

Treats patients with birth defects, mental retardation and genetic diseases.

Michigan

8264   CAUSE
2365 Woodlake Frive, Suite 100
Okemos, MI 48864
517-347-2283
800-221-9105
Fax: 517-886-9366
TTY: 517-347-2283
TDD: 517-886-9167
www.causeonline.org

Parent Training and Information (PTI) programs help parents to understand their children's specific needs, communicate more effectively with professionals, participate in the educational planning process, and obtain information about relevant programs, services and resources.

8265   Early on Michigan
PO Box 30008
Lansing, MI 48909
517-335-4865
Fax: 517-373-7504
e-mail: banfieldj@state.mi.us
www.1800earlyon.org

Provides early intervention and preschool special education for children with disabilities and special health care needs. Services include central directory, representatives of agencies, service providers, families, and coordinators of infant, toddler, and preschool special education programs.

Julie Banfield, Infant/Toddler Program Coordinator

8266   Family Support Network of Michigan Parent Participation Program-MDCH
200 6th Street, 3rd Fl., S Tower, Suite 315
Detroit, MI 48226
517-373-3740
Fax: 313-256-2605
TDD: 517-373-3573

Informational and emotional support to parents who have a child, adolescent, or adult family member with special needs.

8267   Livingston County CMH Services
2280 East Grand River
Howell, MI 48843
517-546-4126
Fax: 517-546-1300
www.nectas.unc.edu

Provides early intervention and preschool special education for children with disabilities and special health care needs. Services include central directory, representatives of agencies, service providers, families, and coordinators of infant, toddler, and preschool special education programs.

Mac Miller, Interagency Coordinating Council

8268   Office of Special Education
608 W. Allegan Street, PO Box 30008
Lansing, MI 48909
517-373-9433
Fax: 517-373-7504
e-mail: webmaster@oses.mde.state.mi.us
www.michigan.gov

Individuals with Disabilities Education Act requires all states and territories to provide early intervention and preschool special education for children with disabilities and special health care needs. Services include central directory, representatives of agencies, service providers, families, and coordinators of infant, toddler, and preschool special education programs.

Sally Vaughn, Deputy Superintendent, Chief Academ
Jacqueline Thompson, Director
Mike P. Flanagan, Superintendent of Public Instructio

8269   Parents are Experts
23077 Greenfield Road, Suite 205
Southfield, MI 48075
248-557-5070
800-827-4843
Fax: 248-557-4456
TDD: 248-557-5070
e-mail: ucp@ameritech.net
www.taalliance.org

Parent Training and Information (PTI) programs help parents to understand their children's specific needs, communicate more effectively with professionals, participate in the educational planning process, and obtain information about relevant programs, services and resources.

8270   TECH 2000 Project-Michigan Disability Rights Coalition
740 W Lake Lansing Road, Suite 400
East Lansing, MI 48823
517-333-2477
800-760-4600
Fax: 517-333-2677
TDD: 517-333-2477
e-mail: roanne@match.org
www.discoalition.org

State assisted programs and support group information for people of many abilities. Includes local chapters, referrals, fun and social interaction and support groups.

8271 ARC Suburban
1526 E 122nd Street
Burnsville, MN 56337
612-890-3057
Fax: 612-890-3527

Informational and emotional support to parents who have a child, adolescent, or adult family member with special needs.

8272 Department of Children, Family, & Learning
1500 Highway 36 W
Roseville, MN 55113
651-582-8200
Fax: 651-582-8872
e-mail: michael.eastman@state.mn.us

Individuals with Disabilities Education Act requires all states and territories to provide early intervention and preschool special education for children with disabilities and special health care needs. Services include central directory, representatives of agencies, service providers, families, and coordinators of infant, toddler, and preschool special education programs.

Michael Eastman, Preschool Special Ed. Coordinator

8273 Family to Family Network ARC of Hennepin County
4301 Highway 7, Suite 104
Minneapolis, MN 55416
612-920-0855
Fax: 612-920-1480

Informational and emotional support to parents who have a child, adolescent, or adult family member with special needs.

8274 Interagency Early Intervention Project
550 Cedar Street
Saint Paul, MN 55101
612-296-7032
Fax: 612-296-5076
e-mail: jan.rubenstein@state.mn.us
www.pediatricservices.com

Individuals with Disabilities Education Act requires all states and territories to provide early intervention and preschool special education for children with disabilities and special health care needs. Services include central directory, representatives of agencies, service providers, families, and coordinators of infant, toddler, and preschool special education programs.

Jan Rubenstein, Infant/Toddler Program Coordinator

8275 Parents for Parents
345 N Smith Avenue, MS 70-403
Saint Paul, MN 55102
651-220-6731
Fax: 651-220-6125
e-mail: pat.schaffner@childrenshc.org

Informational and emotional one-to-one support to parents who have a child or adolescent with special needs.

Pat Schaffner, Parent to Parent Specialist

8276 Pilot Parents in Anoka and Ramsey Counties
1201 89th Avenue NE, Suite 305
Blaine, MN 55434
612-783-4958
Fax: 612-783-4900

Informational and emotional support to parents who have a child, adolescent, or adult family member with special needs.

8277 Pilot Parents of Northeast Minnesota
201 Ordean Building
Duluth, MN 55802
218-726-4725
Fax: 218-726-4722

Informational and emotional support to parents who have a child, adolescent, or adult family member with special needs.

8278 Vinland Center
PO Box 308
Loretto, MN 55357
763-479-3555
Fax: 763-479-2605
e-mail: vinland@vinlandcenter.org
www.vinlandcenter.org

State assisted programs and support group information for people of many abilities. Includes local chapters, referrals, fun and social interaction and support groups.

Gerald Seck, President
Mary Roehl, Executive Director
Duane Reynolds, Associate Director

8279 Voyageur Outward Bound School
101 E Chapman, Suite 120
St. Ely, MN 55731
218-365-7790
800-321-4453
Fax: 218-365-7079
www.vobs.com

State assisted programs and support group information for people of many abilities. Includes local chapters, referrals, fun and social interaction and support groups.

Jack Lee, Executive Director
Suellen Sack, Program Director
Poppy Potter, Director of Operations

8280 Wilderness Inquiry
808 14th Avenue SE
Minneapolis, MN 55414
612-676-9400
800-728-0719
Fax: 612-676-9475
TTY: 800-728-0719
e-mail: info@wildernessinquiry.org
www.wildernessinquiry.org

State assisted programs and support group information for people of many abilities. Includes local chapters, referrals, fun and social interaction and support groups.

Tom Nelson, Chair
Greg Lais, Executive Director
Beth Dooley, Communications Director

8281 First Steps Program
570 East Woodrow Wilson
Jackson, MS 39215
601-576-7816
Fax: 601-576-7540
www.nectas.unc.edu

Individuals with Disabilities Education Act requires all states and territories to provide early intervention and preschool special education for children with disabilities and special health care needs. Services include central directory, representatives of agencies, service providers, families, and coordinators of infant, toddler, and preschool special education programs.

Roy Hart, Infant/Toddler Program Coordinator

8282 Office of Special Education
359 NW Street, Suite 337, PO Box 771
Jackson, MS 39205
601-359-3498
Fax: 601-359-2078
e-mail: dbowman@mdek12.state.ms.us
www.nectas.unc.edu

Individuals with Disabilities Education Act requires all states and territories to provide early intervention and preschool special education for children with disabilities and special health care needs. Services include central directory, representatives of agencies, service providers, families, and coordinators of infant, toddler, and preschool special education programs.

Dot Bowman, Preschool Special Ed. Coordinator

8283 Parent Partners
5 Old River Place, Suite 101
Jackson, MS 39202
601-354-3302
800-366-5707
Fax: 601-354-2426
e-mail: ptiofms@misnet.com
www.parentpartners.org

Parent Training and Information (PTI) programs help parents to understand their children's specific needs, communicate more effectively with professionals, participate in the educational planning process, and obtain information about relevant programs, services and resources.

8284 Project Start
PO Box 1698
Jackson, MS 39215

601-987-4872
800-852-8328
Fax: 601-364-2349
e-mail: dyoung@mdrs.ms.gov
www.msprojectstart.org

State assisted programs and support group information for people of many abilities. Includes local chapters, referrals, fun and social interaction and support groups.

Dorothy Young, Project Director
Kacee Mott, Administrative Assistant

Missouri

8285 Assistance Technology Project
4731 S Cochise, Suite 114
Independence, MO 64055

816-373-5193
Fax: 816-373-9314
TTY: 816-373-9315
e-mail: matpmo@gni.com
www.doir.state.mo.us/matp/

State assisted programs and support group information for people of many abilities. Includes local chapters, referrals, fun and social interaction and support groups.

8286 Children's Therapy Center
600 E 14th Street
Sedalia, MO 65301

660-826-4400
Fax: 660-826-4420
www.nectas.unc.edu

Services include central directory, representatives of agencies, service providers, families, and coordinators of infant, toddler, and preschool special education programs.

Roger Garlich, Interagency Coordinating Council

8287 Department of Elementary and Secondary Education
PO Box 480
Jefferson City, MO 65102

573-751-2965
Fax: 573-526-4404
e-mail: pgoff@mail.dese.state.mo.us
www.unc.edu

Individuals with Disabilities Education Act requires all states and territories to provide early intervention and preschool special education for children with disabilities and special health care needs. Services include central directory, representatives of agencies, service providers, families, and coordinators of infant, toddler, and preschool special education programs.

Melodie Friedebach, Coordinator

8288 Disabilities Advocacy & Support Network
PO Box 4067
Parker, CO 80134

417-895-7464
Fax: 417-895-7412
TTY: 417-895-7430
e-mail: sdasn@aol.com
www.invisibledisabilities.org

Informational and emotional support to parents who have a child, adolescent, or adult family member with special needs.

Wayne Connell, Founder & President
Steve Tonkin, Vice-President
Rob Germundson, Treasurer

8289 Family Resource Network
Park A Plaza
601 Business Loop 70 W, Suite 2161
Columbia, MO 65203

573-449-8663
e-mail: betty@ece.missouri.edu

Informational and emotional support to parents who have a child, adolescent, or adult family member with special needs.

8290 Missouri Parents Act
8301 State Line Road, Suite 204
Kansas City, MO 64114

816-531-7070
800-743-7634
Fax: 816-531-4777
e-mail: info@ptimpact.org
www.ptimpact.org

Parent Training and Information (PTI) programs help parents to understand their children's specific needs, communicate more effectively with professionals, participate in the educational planning process, and obtain information about relevant programs, services and resources.

Mary Kay Savage, Executive Director
Diana Biere, Associate Director

8291 Parent Act
1 W Armour Boulevard, Suite 301
Kansas City, MO 64111

816-531-7070
Fax: 816-531-4777
e-mail: impactcs@coop.cm.org
www.taalliance.org

Parent Training and Information (PTI) programs help parents to understand their children's specific needs, communicate more effectively with professionals, participate in the educational planning process, and obtain information about relevant programs, services and resources.

8292 Positive Solutions for Life Challenges
Route 3, Box 441
Warswaw, MO 65355

660-438-6990

Informational and emotional support to parents who have a child, adolescent, or adult family member with special needs.

8293 United Services
4140 Old Mill Parkway
Saint Peters, MO 63376

636-926-2700
Fax: 636-447-4919
e-mail: ssalmo@unitedsrvcs.org
www.unitedsrvcs.org

Provides services to children ages infant to five-years-old with special needs. Preschool and daycare onsite. We also offer support groups for siblings and family members, parent library available.

Denise Liebel, President/CEO
Windy Spalding, Chief Operating Officer
Dick Frizzell, CFO

Montana

8294 CO-TEACH/Division of Educational Research and Service
School of Education
University of Montana
Missoula, MT 59812

406-243-5344
Fax: 406-243-2797
e-mail: coteach@selway.umt.edu

Informational and emotional support to parents who have a child, adolescent, or adult family member with special needs.

8295 Developmental Disabilities Program
PO Box 4210
Helena, MT 59604

406-444-5647
Fax: 406-444-0230
e-mail: jspiegle@mt.gov
www.nectas.unc.edu

Individuals with Disabilities Education Act requires all states and territories to provide early intervention and preschool special education for children with disabilities and special health care needs. Services include central directory, representatives of agencies, service providers, families, and coordinators of infant, toddler, and preschool special education programs.

Jan Spiegle, Infant/Toddler Program Coordinator

8296 Division of Special Education
PO Box 202501
Helena, MT 59620
406-444-4429
Fax: 406-444-3924
e-mail: dmccarthy@opi.mt.gov
www.unc.edu

Individuals with Disabilities Education Act requires all states and territories to provide early intervention and preschool special education for children with disabilities and special health care needs. Services include central directory, representatives of agencies, service providers, families, and coordinators of infant, toddler, and preschool special education programs.

Robert Runkel, Director

8297 MonTECH
634 Eddy Avenue, Rural Inst on Disab
Missoula, MT 59812
406-243-5676
800-732-0323
Fax: 406-243-4730
TDD: 800-732-0323
e-mail: montech@selway.umt.edu
www.rudi.montech.umt.edu/

State assisted programs and support group information for people of many abilities. Includes local chapters, referrals, fun and social interaction and support groups.

8298 Parents Let's Unite for Kids
516 N 32nd Street
Billings, MT 59101
406-255-0540
800-222-7585
Fax: 406-255-0523
e-mail: info@pluk.org
www.pluk.org

Parent Training and Information (PTI) programs help parents to understand their children's specific needs, communicate more effectively with professionals, participate in the educational planning process, and obtain information about relevant programs, services and resources.

8299 Quality Life Concepts
215 Smelter Ave. N.E. PO Box 250
Great Falls, MT 59403
406-452-9531
800-761-2680
Fax: 406-453-5930
www.qlc-gtf.org

Informational and emotional support to parents who have a child, adolescent, or adult family member with special needs.

Priscilla Halcro, Chief Executive Officer
Tracy Lane, Business Services Director
Lynn Morley, Community Support Services Director

Nebraska

8300 Assistive Technology Partnership
3901 N 27th Street, Suite 5
Lincoln, NE 68521
402-471-0734
888-806-6287
Fax: 402-471-6052
TDD: 402-471-0734
e-mail: atp@nebraska.gov
www.atp.ne.gov

State assisted programs and support group information for people of many abilities. Includes local chapters, referrals, fun and social interaction and support groups.

David Altman, Technology Specialist
Lauren Rock, Program Director
Leslie Novacek, Director

8301 Individual and Family Support Arc of Lincoln & Lancaster County
645 M Street, Suite 19
Lincoln, NE 68508
402-477-6925
Fax: 402-477-6927

Informational and emotional support to parents who have a child, adolescent, or adult family member with special needs.

8302 Nebraska Parents Center
1941 S 42nd Street, Suite 122
Omaha, NE 68105
402-346-0525
800-284-8520
Fax: 402-346-5253
TDD: 402-346-0525
e-mail: npe@uswest.ne.net
www.neparentcenter.org

Parent Training and Information (PTI) programs help parents to understand their children's specific needs, communicate more effectively with professionals, participate in the educational planning process, and obtain information about relevant programs, services and resources. The Nebrask Parent Center services families statewide. There is no fee for services. Call for additional information.

Glenda Davis, Project Director

8303 Parent Assistance Network
310 W 24th
Kearney, NE 68847
308-237-6025
Fax: 308-237-6014

Informational and emotional support to parents who have a child, adolescent, or adult family member with special needs.

8304 Parent Support Group
123 S Webb Road
Grand Island, NE 68802
308-385-5925
Fax: 308-385-5797
e-mail: msheen@genie.esu10.k12.ne.us

Informational and emotional support to parents who have a child, adolescent, or adult family member with special needs.

8305 Parents Encouraging Parents
NE Department of Education
301 Centennial Mall Street, PO Box 94987
Lincoln, NE 68509
402-471-2471
Fax: 402-471-0117
TTY: 402-471-2471
e-mail: ginny_w@nde4.nde.state.ne.us

Informational and emotional support to parents who have a child, adolescent, or adult family member with special needs.

8306 Special Education Office State Department of Education
301 Centennial Mall South
Lincoln, NE 68509
402-471-9329
Fax: 402-471-6252
e-mail: jan_t@nde4.nde.state.ne.us
www.chasa.org

Individuals with Disabilities Education Act requires all states and territories to provide early intervention and preschool special education for children with disabilities and special health care needs. Services include central directory, representatives of agencies, service providers, families, and coordinators of infant, toddler, and preschool special education programs.

Charlotte Lewis, Part C Co-Coordinator

Nevada

8307 Assistive Technology Collaborative
711 S Stewart Street, Rehab Division
Carson City, NV 89701
775-687-4452
Fax: 775-687-3292
TTY: 702-687-3388
e-mail: pgowins@govmail.state.nv.us
www.state.nv.us.80

State assisted programs and support group information for people of many abilities. Includes local chapters, referrals, fun and social interaction and support groups.

8308 Early Intervention Services Division of Child & Family Services
3987 S McCarren Boulevard
Reno, NV 89502
775-688-2284
Fax: 775-688-2558
e-mail: mkwalter@govmail.state.nv.us
www.nectas.unc.edu

Provides early intervention and preschool special education for children with disabilities and special health care needs. Services include central directory, representatives of agencies, service providers, families, and coordinators of infant, toddler, and preschool special education programs.

Marilyn K Walter, Infant/Toddler Program Coordinator

8309 Educational Equity, Special Education Branch
700 E 5th Street, Suite 113
Carson City, NV 89701

775-687-9171
800-992-0900
Fax: 775-687-9123
e-mail: gdopf@nsn.scs.unr.edu
www.unc.edu

Individuals with Disabilities Education Act requires all states and territories to provide early intervention and preschool special education for children with disabilities and special health care needs. Services include central directory, representatives of agencies, service providers, families, and coordinators of infant, toddler, and preschool special education programs.

Gloria Dopf, Preschool Special Ed. Coordinator

8310 Nevada Parent Network
University of Nevada-Reno
COE, REPC/285
Reno, NV 89557

702-784-4921
800-216-7988
Fax: 702-702-4997
e-mail: cdinnell@scs.unr.edu
www.iser.com/npn-NV.html

Informational and emotional support to parents who have a child, adolescent, or adult family member with special needs.

Cheryl Dinnell, Program Coordinator

8311 Nevada Parents Encouraging Parents (PEP)
2101 S. Jones Blvd., Suite 120
Las Vegas, NV 89146

702-388-8899
800-216-5188
Fax: 702-388-2966
e-mail: pepinfo@nvpep.org
www.nvpep.org

Parent Training and Information (PTI) programs help parents to understand their children's specific needs, communicate more effectively with professionals, participate in the educational planning process, and obtain information about relevant programs, services and resources.

Karen Taycher, Executive Director
Stephanie Vrsnik, Community Development Director
Natalie Filipic, Director of Operations

8312 Parents Encouraging Parents
2101 S. Jones Blvd., Suite 120
Las Vegas, NV 89146

702-388-8899
800-216-5188
Fax: 702-388-2966
e-mail: pepinfo@nvpep.org
www.nvpep.org

Informational and emotional support to parents who have a child, adolescent, or adult family member with special needs.

Karen Taycher, Executive Director
Stephanie Vrsnik, Community Development Director
Natalie Filipic, Director of Operations

New Hampshire

8313 Bureau of Early Learning
101 Pleasant Street
Concord, NH 03301

603-271-3791
Fax: 603-271-1953
e-mail: rlittlefield@ed.state.nh.us
www.education.nh.gov

Individuals with Disabilities Education Act requires all states and territories to provide early intervention and preschool special education for children with disabilities and special health care needs. Services include central directory, representatives of agencies, service providers, families, and coordinators of infant, toddler, and preschool special education programs.

Ruth Littlefield, Preschool Special Ed. Coordinator

8314 Dartmouth-Hitchcock Sleep Disorders Center Dartmouth Medical Center
One Medical Center Drive
Lebanon, NH 03756

603-650-7534
Fax: 603-650-7820
www.dartmouth-hitchcock.org

Rocco R Addante, Director
Glen Greenough MD, Fellowship Director
Joanne MacQuarrie, BS,RPSGT,RRT, Administrator

8315 Division of Special Education
101 Pleasant Street
Concord, NH 03301

603-271-3791
Fax: 603-271-1953
www.education.nh.gov

Individuals with Disabilities Education Act requires all states and territories to provide early intervention and preschool special education for children with disabilities and special health care needs. Services include central directory, representatives of agencies, service providers, families, and coordinators of infant, toddler, and preschool special education programs.

Ruth Littlefield, Preschool Special Ed. Coordinator

8316 Family Center Early Supports & Services
105 Pleasant Street
Concord, NH 03301

603-271-5122
Fax: 603-271-5166
e-mail: cohara@dhhs.state.nh.us
www.familyvoices.org

Services include central directory, representatives of agencies, service providers, families, and coordinators of infant, toddler, and preschool special education programs.

Molly Cole, President
Marcia O'Malley, Vice-President
Lynn Pedraza, Executive Director

8317 High Hopes Foundation of New Hampshire
301 Daniel Webster Hwy., Suite 6
Merrimack, NH 03054

603-529-1010
800-639-6804
Fax: 603-529-0037
e-mail: HighHopeNH@aol.com
www.highhopesfoundation.org

Volunteer organization dedicated to granting wishes of seriously ill New Hampshire children from three through 18 years old.

60+ members

Shaunae Nolet, President
Tom Perkins, Vice President
Dana Wallace, Treasurer

8318 Parent Information Center
PO Box 2405
Concord, NH 03302

603-224-7005
Fax: 603-224-4365
TDD: 603-224-7005
e-mail: mlewis@picnh.org
www.picnh.org

Parent Training and Information (PTI) programs help parents to understand their children's specific needs, communicate more effectively with professionals, participate in the educational planning process, and obtain information about relevant programs, services and resources.

Michelle Lewis, Executive Director
Sylvia Abbott, Administrative Supervisor
Jennifer Cunha, Project Staff

8319 Parent to Parent of New Hampshire
12 Flynn Street
Lebanon, NH 03766

603-448-6393
800-698-5465
Fax: 603-448-6311
www.p2pnh.org

Informational and emotional support to parents who have a child, adolescent, or adult family member with special needs.

Richard Cohen, Executive Director
Judith Iaconianni, Director/Co-founder

8320 Technology Partnership Project Institute on Disability/UAP
The Concord Center
10 West Edge Drive , Suite 101
Durham, NH 03824 603-862-4320
Fax: 603-862-0555
TDD: 603-224-0630
e-mail: institute.disability@unh.edu
iod.unh.edu

State assistive programs funded by the National Institute on Disability and Rehabilitation Research. Includes directories, support group information, training and project information.

New Jersey

8321 Division of Student Services
Riverview Executive Plaza, Building 100
Trenton, NJ 08625 609-633-6833
Fax: 609-984-8422
e-mail: btkach@doh.state.nj.us
www.unc.edu

Individuals with Disabilities Education Act requires all states and territories to provide early intervention and preschool special education for children with disabilities and special health care needs. Services include central directory, representatives of agencies, service providers, families, and coordinators of infant, toddler, and preschool special education programs.

Barbara Tkach, Preschool Special Ed. Coordinator

8322 Early Intervention System
PO Box 364
Trenton, NJ 08625 609-777-7734
Fax: 609-292-3580
e-mail: Terry.Harrison@dob.state.nj.us
www.state.nj-us/health/8hs/eiphome.htm

Individuals with Disabilities Education Act requires all states and territories to provide early intervention and preschool special education for children with disabilities and special health care needs. Services include central directory, representatives of agencies, service providers, families, and coordinators of infant, toddler, and preschool special education programs.

Charles E. Drum, Director & Professor
Jennifer Donahue, Director of Finance
Matthew Gianino, Director of Communications

8323 Family Support Center of New Jersey
Lion's Head Office Park
1 AAA Drive, Suite 203
Trenton, NJ 08691 732-262-8020
800-336-5843
Fax: 609-392-5621
e-mail: FSCNJ@aol.com
www.efnj.com

Informational and emotional support to parents who have a child, adolescent, or adult family member with special needs.

Michael P. Rinaldo, Chairman
Robert L. D'Avanzo, President
Eric B. Geller, M.D., Vice President

8324 New Jersey Self-Help Clearinghouse
375 East McFarlan Street
Dover, NJ 07801 973-989-1122
800-367-6274
Fax: 973-989-1159
TTY: 973-625-9053
e-mail: info@selfhelpgroups.org
www.njgroups.org

The NJ Self-Help Group Clearinghouse provides contacts for over 4,500 New Jersey support groups and over 1,100 national support networks for most illnesses, addictions, disabilities, bereavement, parenting and other stressful life situations. The organization also helps individuals wanting to start a group.

8325 New Jersey Statewide Parent to Parent
2150 Highway 35, Suite 207C
Sea Girt, NJ 08750 800-372-6510
Fax: 973-642-8080
www.spannj.org

Informational and emotional support to parents who have a child, adolescent, or adult family member with special needs.

Malia Corde, Program Coordinator|
Malia Corde, Coordinator
Jeannette Mejias, Bilingual (Spanish) Associate

8326 Statewide Parent Advocacy Network
35 Halsey Street, 4th Floor
Newark, NJ 07102 973-642-8100
800-654-SPAN
Fax: 973-642-8080
e-mail: diana.autin@spannj.org
www.spanadvocacy.org

Parent Training and Information (PTI) programs help parents to understand their children's specific needs, communicate more effectively with professionals, participate in the educational planning process, and obtain information about relevant programs, services and resources.

Diana Autin, Co-Director
Maria Docherty, Co-Director
Carolyn Hayer, Co-Director

New Mexico

8327 EPICS Project-SW Communication Resources
PO Box 788, 2000 Camino del Pueblo
Bernalilo, NM 87004 505-867-3396
800-765-7320
Fax: 505-867-3398
TDD: 505-867-3396
www.disabilityrights.org

Parent Training and Information (PTI) programs help parents to understand their children's specific needs, communicate more effectively with professionals, participate in the educational planning process, and obtain information about relevant programs, services and resources.

8328 Long Term Services Division
PO Box 26110
Santa Fe, NM 87502 505-827-0103
Fax: 505-827-2455
www.nectas.unc.edu

Individuals with Disabilities Education Act requires all states and territories to provide early intervention and preschool special education for children with disabilities and special health care needs. Services include central directory, representatives of agencies, service providers, families, and coordinators of infant, toddler, and preschool special education programs.

Cathy Stevenson, Infant/Toddler Program Coordiantor

8329 Parents Reaching Out
1920 B Columbia Drive SE
Albuquerque, NM 87106 505-247-0192
800-524-5176
Fax: 505-247-1345
TDD: 505-865-3700
e-mail: info@parentsreachingout.org
www.parentsreachingout.org

Provides peer support, technical assistance and information statewide to families in New Mexico who have family member with unique or special needs and professionals who care for them.

Renata Witte, President
Johnny Wilson, Executive Director
Leon Emplit, Director of Operations

8330 Special Education Unit
300 Don Gaspar Avenue
Santa Fe, NM 87501 505-827-6541
Fax: 505-827-6791
e-mail: bpasternack@sde.state.mn.us
www.unc.edu

Individuals with Disabilities Education Act requires all states and territories to provide early intervention and preschool special education for children with disabilities and special health care needs. Services include central directory, representatives of agencies, service providers, families, and coordinators of infant, toddler, and preschool special education programs.

Maria Landazuri, Preschool Special Ed. Coordinator

8331 Technology Assistance Program
435 St Michael's Drive, Building D
Santa Fe, NM 87505
505-954-8539
800-866-2253
Fax: 505-954-8562
TDD: 800-866-2253
e-mail: nmdvrtap@aol.com
www.tap.gcd.state.nm.us

State assisted programs for people of many abilities. Includes local chapters, referrals, fun and social interaction and support groups.

New York

8332 Advocacy Center
590 South Avenue
Rochester, NY 14620
716-546-1700
800-650-4967
Fax: 716-546-7069
e-mail: advocacy@frontiernet.net
www.advocacycenter.com

Parent Training and Information (PTI) programs help parents to understand their children's specific needs, communicate more effectively with professionals, participate in the educational planning process, and obtain information about relevant programs, services and resources.

Stephen G. Schwarz, President
Adam Anolik, Vice President
Paul Visca, Treasurer

8333 Advocates for Children of New York
151 W 30th Street, 5th Floor
New York, NY 10001
212-947-9779
Fax: 212-947-9790
e-mail: info@advocatesforchildren.org
www.advocatesforchildren.org

Parent Training and Information (PTI) programs help parents to understand their children's specific needs, communicate more effectively with professionals, participate in the educational planning process, and obtain information about relevant programs, services and resources.

Jamie A. Levitt, President
Kim Sweet, Executive Director
Matthew Lenaghan, Deputy Director

8334 Aurora of Central New York
518 James Street, Suite 100
Syracuse, NY 13203
315-422-7263
Fax: 315-422-4792
TTY: 315-422-9746
TDD: 315-422-9746
e-mail: auroracny@auroraofcny.org
www.auroraofcny.org

Professional counseling services to assist individuals and their families deal with the trauma of hearing or vision loss.

John McCormick, President
Scott Gucciardi, 1st Vice President
Robert C. Haege, Assistant Treasurer

8335 Early Intervention Program
Corning Tower Room 208, Empire Street Plaza
Albany, NY 12237
518-473-7016
Fax: 518-473-8673
e-mail: dmn02@health.state.ny.us
www.nectas.unc.edu

Individuals with Disabilities Education Act requires all states and territories to provide early intervention and preschool special education for children with disabilities and special health care needs. Services include a central directory, representatives of agencies, service providers, families, and coordinators of infant, toddler, and preschool special education programs.

Donna Noyes, Infant/Toddler Program Coordinator

8336 Friends of Karen
118 Titicus Road, PO Box 190
Purdys, NY 10560
845-277-4547
800-637-2774
www.friendsofkaren.org

Dedicated to helping terminally and catastrophically ill children and their families in the New York metropolitan area only. They provide assistance with payments for physicians, hospitals and medications, help with extra expenses beyond medical bills, provide home nursing services and equipment, supplies for loans, and offers emotional support.

Pam Hervey, President
Bob Goldberg, Vice President
David Rosenberg, Vice President

8337 Marty Lyons Foundation
326 W 48th Street
New York, NY 10036
212-977-9474
877-560-9474
Fax: 212-977-1752
e-mail: mlf_hq@martylyonsfoundation.org
www.martylyonsfoundation.org

Chapters in New Jersey, New York, Massachussets, Connecticut, Maryland, North Carolina, South Carolina, Georgia, Texas, Pennsylvania and Florida provide a special wish to children ages three to seventeen who are terminally ill or have a life-threatening disease.

300 volunteers

Marty Lyons, Chairman
Ken Schroy, Vice Chairman
Richard A. Miller, President

8338 New York Department of Education
1 Commerce Plaza
Albany, NY 12234
518-473-4823
Fax: 518-486-4154
e-mail: mplotzke@mail.nysed.gov

Individuals with Disabilities Education Act requires all states and territories to provide early intervention and preschool special education for children with disabilities and special health care needs. Services include central directory, representatives of agencies, service providers, families, and coordinators of infant, toddler, and preschool special education programs.

Michael Plotzker Vesid, Preschool Special Ed. Coordinator

8339 Parent Network Center
250 Delaware Avenue, Suite 3
Buffalo, NY 14202
716-853-1570
800-724-7408
Fax: 716-853-1574
TDD: 716-853-1573
www.taalliance.org

Parent Training and Information (PTI) programs help parents to understand their children's specific needs, communicate more effectively with professionals, participate in the educational planning process, and obtain information about relevant programs, services and resources.

8340 Parent to Parent of New York State
500 Balltown Road
Schenectady, NY 12304
518-381-4350
800-305-8817
Fax: 518-382-1959
e-mail: parent2par@aol.com
www.parenttoparentnys.org

Informational and emotional support to parents who have a child, adolescent, or adult family member with special needs.

1500 Members

Linda Coull, Vice President
Holly Bartczak, Coordinator
Tina Beauparlant, Parent Advocate

8341 Resources for Children with Special Needs
116 East 16th Street, 5th Floor
New York City, NY 10003   212-667-4650
                                    Fax: 212-254-4070
                              e-mail: info@resourcesnyc.org
                                    www.resourcesnyc.org

Parent Training and Information (PTI) programs help parents to
understand their children's specific needs, communicate more effectively with professionals, participate in the educational planning process, and obtain information about relevant programs,
services and resources.

Ellen Miller-Wachtel, Chair
Shon E. Glusky, President
Stephen Stern, Director of Finance and Administrat

8342 Saint Mary's Healthcare System for Children
One Penn Plaza Suite 2420
New York, NY 10119   212-586-8723
                                    Fax: 212-586-5170
                                    www.nycharities.org

Information and advocacy resources for families and professionals. Includes listings of organizations providing general information and organizations focusing on more specific areas of concern
to families and young adults who have disabilities.

8343 Sinergia/Metropolitan Parent Center
15 W 65th Street, 6th Floor
New York, NY 10023   212-496-1300
                                    Fax: 212-496-5608
                              e-mail: Sinergia@panix.com
                                    www.panic.com/~sinergia

Parent Training and Information (PTI) programs help parents to
understand their children's specific needs, communicate more effectively with professionals, participate in the educational planning process, and obtain information about relevant programs,
services and resources.

8344 TRIAD Project-Advocates for Persons with Disabilities
One Empire State Plaza, Suite 1001
Albany, NY 12223   518-474-2825
                                         800-522-4369
                                    Fax: 518-473-6005
                                    TTY: 518-473-4231
                              e-mail: leffingw@emi.com

State assisted programs and support group information for people
of many abilities. Includes local chapters, referrals, fun and social
interaction and support groups.

8345 Ulster County Social Services
1061 Development Court
Kingston, NY 12401   845-334-5000
                                    Fax: 845-255-3202
                                    www.co.ulster.ny.us

Individuals with Disabilities Education Act requires all states and
territories to provide early intervention and preschool special education for children with disabilities and special health care
needs. Services include central directory, representatives of agencies, service providers, families, and coordinators of infant, toddler, and preschool special education programs.

Thomas Roach, Interagency Coordinating Council
Michael Iapoce, Commissioner

North Carolina

**8346 Assistive Technology Project, Human Resources, Voc. and
Rehab. Services**
1110 Navaho Drive, Suite 101
Raleigh, NC 27609   919-850-2787
                                         800-852-0042
                                    Fax: 919-850-2792
                                    TTY: 919-850-2787
                              e-mail: rickic@mindspring.com
                                    www.ncatp.org

State assisted programs and support group information for people
of many abilities. Includes local chapters, referrals, fun and social
interaction and support groups.

8347 ECAC
907 Barra Row, Suites 102/103
Davidson, NC 28036   704-892-1321
                                    Fax: 704-892-5028
                                    TDD: 704-892-1321
                              e-mail: ecac@ecac.org
                                    www.ecac-parentcenter.org

Parent Training and Information (PTI) programs help parents to
understand their children's specific needs, communicate more effectively with professionals, participate in the educational planning process, and obtain information about relevant programs,
services and resources.

Connie Hawkins, Executive Director
Mary Watson, Director of Exceptional Children Di

8348 Exceptional Children Division
301 N Wilmington Street
Raleigh, NC 27601   919-807-3300
                                    Fax: 919-807-3482
                              e-mail: kbaars@state.nc.us
                                    www.mcpublicschools.org

Individuals with Disabilities Education Act requires all states and
territories to provide early intervention and preschool special education for children with disabilities and special health care
needs. Services include central directory, representatives of agencies, service providers, families, and coordinators of infant, toddler, and preschool special education programs.

Kathy Baars, Preschool Special Ed. Coordinator

8349 Family Support Network of North Carolina
University of North carolina
200 N Greensboro St, Carr Mill Mall, 2nd Fl Ste D9
Carrboro, NC 27510   919-966-2841
                                         800-852-0042
                                    Fax: 919-966-2916
                              e-mail: cdr@med.unc.edu
                                    www.fsnnc.org

Family Support Network of North Carolina promotes and provides support for families with children who have special needs.
Families are in a unique position to offer information and support
to other families. An experienced family member can share the
most practical advice and help a parent navigate the complex service systems. Having support can make it easier for families to
experience the joy and satisfaction that can come from parenting
a child with special needs.

Laura Curtis, Education & Outreach Coordinator
Irene Nathan Zipper, Director

8350 Partnerships for Inclusion
2415 W Vernon Avenue
Kingston, NC 28501   919-559-5156
                              e-mail: msteele@greenvillenc.com
                                    www.nectas.unc.edu

Individuals with Disabilities Education Act requires all states and
territories to provide early intervention and preschool special education for children with disabilities and special health care
needs. Services include central directory, representatives of agencies, service providers, families, and coordinators of infant, toddler, and preschool special education programs.

Sandy Steele, Interagency Coordinating Council

8351 Rockingham County Schools
511 Harrington Highway
Eden, NC 27288   336-627-2615
                                    Fax: 336-627-2660
                              e-mail: speele@greenvillenc.com
                              www.ncpublicschools.org/success/regionalcontacts

Individuals with Disabilities Education Act requires all states and
territories to provide early intervention and preschool special education for children with disabilities and special health care
needs. Services include central directory, representatives of agencies, service providers, families, and coordinators of infant, toddler, and preschool special education programs.

Susan Peele, Interagency Coordinating Council

8352 Developmental Disabilities Unit
1237 W Divide Avenue, Suite 1A
Bismarck, ND 58501
701-328-8936
800-755-8529
Fax: 701-328-8969
e-mail: sobald@nd.gov
www.nectas.unc.edu

Individuals with Disabilities Education Act requires all states and territories to provide early intervention and preschool special education for children with disabilities and special health care needs. Services include central directory, representatives of agencies, service providers, families, and coordinators of infant, toddler, and preschool special education programs.

Debra Balsdon, Infant/Toddler Program Coordinator

8353 Interagency Program Assistive Technology
3240-15th Street South, Suite B
Fargo, ND 58104
701-365-4728
800-895-4728
Fax: 701-365-6242
TDD: 701-265-4807
e-mail: lee@pioneer.state.nd.us
www.ndipat.org

State assisted programs and support group information for people of many abilities. Includes local chapters, referrals, fun and social interaction and support groups.

8354 Special Education Division
600 E Boulevard
Bismarck, ND 58505
701-328-2277
Fax: 701-328-4149
TTY: 701-328-4920
e-mail: dpi@nd.gov
www.dpi.state.nd.us

Individuals with Disabilities Education Act requires all states and territories to provide early intervention and preschool special education for children with disabilities and special health care needs. Services include central directory, representatives of agencies, service providers, families, and coordinators of infant, toddler, and preschool special education programs.

Ann Chase, Child Nutrition, Grant Manager
Jerry Coleman, School Finance, Director
Jim Bosch, Maintenance/Clerk

8355 Bureau of EI Services
246 N High Strees, PO Box 118
Columbus, OH 43215
614-644-8389
Fax: 614-728-9163
e-mail: coser@gw.odh.state.oh.us
www.ohiohelpmegrow.org

Individuals with Disabilities Education Act requires all states and territories to provide early intervention and preschool special education for children with disabilities and special health care needs. Services include central directory, representatives of agencies, service providers, families, and coordinators of infant, toddler, and preschool special education programs.

Cindy Oser, Infant/Toddler Program Coordinator

8356 Celebrating Families of Children & Adults with Special Needs
16 Vassar Drive
Dayton, OH 45406
937-275-0990
800-432-2199
Fax: 937-275-0277
e-mail: families@erinet.com
www.eparent.com

Informational and emotional support to parents who have a child, adolescent, or adult family member with special needs.

Joseph M Valenzano, Jr., President, CEO & Publisher
James P. McGinnis, VP of Operations/CFO
Rick Rader, MD, Editor-in-Chief

8357 Division of Early Childhood Education
65 S Front Street, Room 309
Columbus, OH 43215
614-466-0224
Fax: 614-728-2338
www.dec-sped.org

Individuals with Disabilities Education Act requires all states and territories to provide early intervention and preschool special education for children with disabilities and special health care needs. Services include central directory, representatives of agencies, service providers, families, and coordinators of infant, toddler, and preschool special education programs.

Jane Wiechel, Preschool Special Ed. Coordinator

8358 East Central Regional Office
170 W High Avenue
New Philadelphia, OH 44663
330-364-5567
Fax: 330-343-3038
e-mail: ECE_Greer@ode.ohio.gov@inet
www.nectas.unc.edu

Individuals with Disabilities Education Act requires all states and territories to provide early intervention and preschool special education for children with disabilities and special health care needs. Services include central directory, representatives of agencies, service providers, families, and coordinators of infant, toddler, and preschool special education programs.

Edith Greer, Preschool Special Ed. Coordinator

8359 Family Information Network
143 NW Avenue, Building A
Tallmadge, OH 44278
330-633-2055
Fax: 330-633-2658

Informational and emotional support to parents who have a child, adolescent, or adult family member with special needs.

8360 National Child Advocacy Center
210 Pratt Avenue
Huntaville, AL 35801
256-533-0531
Fax: 256-534-6883
TDD: 513-821-2400
e-mail: CADCCenter@aol.com
www.nationalcac.org

Parent Training and Information (PTI) programs help parents to understand their children's specific needs, communicate more effectively with professionals, participate in the educational planning process, and obtain information about relevant programs, services and resources.

Tim Kauffman, President
Duz Packett, Vice President
Chris Kuffner, Secretary

8361 OCECD
165 W Center Street, Suite 302
Marion, OH 43302
614-382-5452
800-374-2806
Fax: 614-383-6421
e-mail: ocecd@edu.gte.net
www.ocecd.org

Parent Training and Information (PTI) programs help parents to understand their children's specific needs, communicate more effectively with professionals, participate in the educational planning process, and obtain information about relevant programs, services and resources.

Margaret M. Burley, Director

8362 Ohio Protection and Advocacy Organization
5350 Brookpark Avenue
Cleveland, OH 44134
216-398-5501
800-672-1220
Fax: 216-398-5505

Informational and emotional support to parents who have a child, adolescent, or adult family member with special needs.

8363 Operation Liftoff of Ohio
PO Box 1094
Gallipolis, OH 45631
A program for children in Ohio and surrounding states who have a life-threatening illness.

8364 Society for Rehabilitation
9521 Lake Shore Boulevard
Mentor, OH 44060 440-352-8993
Fax: 440-352-6632
e-mail: info@societyhelps.org
www.societyhelps.org

Individuals with Disabilities Education Act requires all states and territories to provide early intervention and preschool special education for children with disabilities and special health care needs. Disability therapy is provided for children and adults.

Richard J Kessler, Executive Director

8365 Train-Ohio Super Computer Center
1224 Kinnear Road
Columbus, OH 43212 614-292-9248
Fax: 614-292-7168
TDD: 614-292-2426
www.osc.edu

State assisted programs and support group information for people of many abilities. Includes local chapters, referrals, fun and social interaction and support groups.

Pankaj Shah, Executive Director
Kevin Wohlever, Director of Supercomputing Operatio
Brian Guilfoos, Client and Technology Support Manag

Oklahoma

8366 Oklahoma ABLE Tech-Wellness Center
1514 W Hall of Fame
Stillwater, OK 74078 405-744-9748
800-257-1705
Fax: 405-744-7670
TTY: 800-257-1705
e-mail: mljwell@okway.okstate.edu
www.okabletech.okstate.edu

State assisted programs and support group information for people of many abilities. Includes local chapters, referrals, fun and social interaction and support groups.

Linda Jaco, Director of Sponsored Programs
Milissa Gofourth, Program Manager
Diana Sargent, Staff Assistant

8367 Parents Reaching Out in Oklahoma
1917 S Harvard Avenue
Oklahoma City, OK 73128 405-681-9710
Fax: 405-685-4006
TDD: 405-681-9710
e-mail: prook@aol.com
www.ucp.org/probase.htm

Parent Training and Information (PTI) programs help parents to understand their children's specific needs, communicate more effectively with professionals, participate in the educational planning process, and obtain information about relevant programs, services and resources.

8368 Special Education Office
2500 N Lincoln Boulevard
Oklahoma City, OK 73105 405-521-3351
Fax: 405-522-2066
TDD: 405-521-4875
e-mail: mark_sharp@mail.sde.state.ok.us
www.ok.gov

Individuals with Disabilities Education Act requires all states and territories to provide early intervention and preschool special education for children with disabilities and special health care needs. Services include central directory, representatives of agencies, service providers, families, and coordinators of infant, toddler, and preschool special education programs.

Joel Robison, Chief of Staff
Mark Sharp, Associate Director
Janet Barresi, State Superintendent of Public Inst

Oregon

8369 Early Childhood CARES Program
1895 E 15th Avenue
Eugene, OR 97403 541-346-2639
Fax: 541-343-5650
e-mail: Judy_Newman@ccmail.uoregon.edu

Individuals with Disabilities Education Act requires all states and territories to provide early intervention and preschool special education for children with disabilities and special health care needs. Services include central directory, representatives of agencies, service providers, families, and coordinators of infant, toddler, and preschool special education programs.

Judy Newman, Interagency Coordinating Council

8370 Early Intervention Programs
255 Capitol Street NE
Salem, OR 97301 503-378-3598
Fax: 503-373-7968
TDD: 503-378-2892
e-mail: steve.johnson@state.or.us
www.unc.edu

Individuals with Disabilities Education Act requires all states and territories to provide early intervention and preschool special education for children with disabilities and special health care needs. Services include central directory, representatives of agencies, service providers, families, and coordinators of infant, toddler, and preschool special education programs.

Steven B. Johnson, Associate Superintendent

8371 Oregon Department of Education
255 Capitol Street NE
Salem, OR 97301 503-947-5747
Fax: 503-378-5156
e-mail: nancy.johnson-dorn@state.or.us
www.ode.state.or.us

Provides early intervention and preschool special education for children with disabilities. Services include central directory, representatives of agencies, service providers, families, and coordinators of infant, toddler, and preschool special education programs.

Nancy Johnson-Dorn, Early Childhood Director
Susan Castillo, State Superintendent of Public Inst

8372 Oregon Parent Training and Information Center
2295 Liberty Street NE
Salem, OR 97303 503-581-8156
888-505-2673
Fax: 503-391-0429
e-mail: orpti@orpti.org
www.orpti.org

Informational and emotional support to parents who have a child, adolescent, or adult family member with special needs.

8373 Technology Access for Life Needs Project
1257 Ferry Street, Se
Salem, OR 97310 503-361-1201
Fax: 503-370-4530
TDD: 503-361-1201
e-mail: ati@orednet.org

State assisted programs and support group information for people of many abilities. Includes local chapters, referrals, fun and social interaction and support groups.

Pennsylvania

8374 Bureau of Special Education
333 Market Street, 7th Floor
Harrisburg, PA 17126 717-783-6788
800-874-2301
Fax: 717-783-6139
TTY: 717-783-8445
TDD: 717-787-7367
e-mail: ebeck@state.pa.us
www.portal.state.pa.us

Conferences

8577 AACAP & CACAP Joint Annual Meeting
American Academy of Child & Adolescent Psychiatry
3615 Wisconsin Avenue NW
Washington, DC 20016   202-966-7300
                                       Fax: 202-966-2891
                              e-mail: clinical@aacap.org
                                          www.aacap.org

The world's largest gathering place for leaders in the field of
child and adolescent psychiatry, children's mental health, and
other allied disciplines.

Martin J. Drell, M.D., President
David R. DeMaso, M.D., Secretary
David R. DeMaso, M.D., Secretary

8578 ADAA Annual Conference
Anxiety Disorders Association of America
8701 Georgia Ave. #412
Silver Spring, MD 20910   240-485-1001
                                       Fax: 240-485-1035
                           e-mail: information@adaa.org
                                           www.adaa.org
April

Alies Muskin, Executive Director
Terence M. Keane, PhD, President
Karen Cassiday, PhD, Secretary

8579 ARC Annual National Convention
The ARC
1825 K Street NW, Suite 1200
Washington, DC 20006   202-534-3700
                                            800-433-5255
                                       Fax: 202-534-3731
                               e-mail: info@thearc.org
                                          www.thearc.org

held in cities throughout the U.S. each fall which attracts nearly
1000 people for educational sessions, business meetings and social events.

Peter V. Berns, Chief Executive Officer
Trudy R. Jacobson, Chief Development & Marketing Offic
Elise McMillan, Secretary

8580 CEC Convention & Expo
Council for Exceptional Children
2900 Crystal Drive, Suite 1000
Arlington, VA 22201   703-243-0446
                                            888-232-7733
                                       Fax: 703-264-9494
                                       TTY: 866-915-5000
                           e-mail: service@cec.sped.org
                                       www.cec.sped.org
April

Bruce Ramirez, Executive Director
Krista Barnes, Assistant Executive Director
Karen Niles, Assistant Executive Director

8581 CLC Annual Conference
Child Life Council
11821 Parklawn Dr., Suite 310
Rockville, MD 20852   301-881-7090
                                            800-252-4515
                                       Fax: 301-881-7092
                          e-mail: CLCadmin@childlife.org
                                          www.childlife.org

The premier educational experience for child life professionals.
The largest gathering of child life specialists of the year, offers
ample opportunities for both formal and informal networking
with peers.
1,000 May

Dennis Reynolds, Executive Director
Amy Bullock Morse, MSEd, CCL, President
Suzanne Graca, MS, CCLS, Secretary

8582 FFCMH Annual Conference
Federation of Families for Childrens Mental Health
9605 Medical Center Drive, Suite 280
Rockville, MD 20850   240-403-1901
                                       Fax: 240-403-1909
                               e-mail: ffcmh@ffcmh.org
                                          www.ffcmh.org

Address the complex issue of trauma; the impact it has on children and families; the promotion of healing and prevention strategies; knowledge about how to address trauma through
resiliency-based interventions, utilizing a familydriven, youth
guided approach; and examples of how family organizations and
the partners they work with are raising awareness and improving
trauma-focused services and supports.

November

Teka Dempson, President
Sherri Luthe, Vice President
Josh Ross, Secretary

8583 Genetic Alliance Annual Conference
Genetic Alliance
4301 Connecticut Avenue NW, Suite 404
Washington, DC 20008   202-966-5557
                                            800-336-4363
                                       Fax: 202-966-8553
                       e-mail: info@geneticalliance.org
                                      www.geneticalliance.org

Consistently inspirational and enables partnership among all
stakeholders: advocates and community leaders, health and industry professionals, policymakers, and academicians.

July

Sharon Terry, President/CEO
Tetyana Murza, Programs/Events Manager

**8584 International Conference On Young Children With Special
Needs & Their Famililies**
Division for Early Childhood
27 Fort Missoula Road, Suite 2
Missoula, MT 59804   406-543-0872
                                       Fax: 406-543-0887
                                       TTY: 703-264-9446
                                e-mail: dec@dec-sped.org
                                          www.dec-sped.org

Attendees from around the world explore the evidence, present
practical strategies, and engage in discussions that will change
the way one thinks about early childhood special education. Topics include: policy, autism, recommended practices, tiered interventions, challenging behavior, personnel development, research,
assessment, cultural diversity and more.

Dr. Leah Weiner, President
Cynthia Wood, Associate Executive Director
Sharon Walsh, Governmental Relations Consultant

8585 Long Term Survivor Conference
Childhood Brain Tumor Foundation
20312 Watkins Meadow Drive
Germantown, MD 20876   301-515-2900
                                            877-217-4166
                                       Fax: 301-540-8367
                     e-mail: cbtf@childhoodbraintumor.org
                                    www.childhoodbraintumor.org

In collaboration with the Children's National Medical Center, includes excellent topics and speakers from the region who shared
their expertise.

Jeanne P. Young, President
Carol Cornman, Vice President
Kiren Day, Vice Pres./ Secretary

8586 NADD Conference & Exhibit Show
National Association for the Dually Diagnosed
132 Fair Street
Kingston, NY 12401   845-331-4336
                                            800-331-5362
                                       Fax: 845-331-4569
                                e-mail: info@thenadd.org
                                          www.thenadd.org

November
Robert J. Fletcher DSW, CEO
Donna McNelis, Ph.D., President
Dan Baker, Ph.d., Vice President

8587 NAMI Convention
National Alliance on Mental Illness
3803 N. Fairfax Dr., Ste. 100
Arlington, VA 22203
703-524-7600
800-950-6264
Fax: 703-524-9094
TDD: 703-516-7227
e-mail: info@nami.org
www.nami.org

The NAMI Convention is packed with information, chances to network, leadership development opportunities, and lots more
July
Keris J,,n Myrick, M.B.A., M.S., Ph, President
Kevin B. Sullivan, First Vice President
Jim Payne, J.D., Second Vice President

Audio Video

8588 A Mind of Your Own
Fanlight Productions
32 Court Street, 21st Floor
Brooklyn, NY 11201
718-488-8900
800-876-1710
Fax: 718-488-8642
e-mail: info@fanlight.com
www.fanlight.com

Learning disabilities can make children feel lonely, confused, hopeless and worthless, even if they know they are smart, but it doesn't have to feel that way. Meet Henry, Matthew, Max and Stephanie, four incredible kids who don't let learning differences hold them back or get them down.

38 minutes DVD or VHS

Nicole Johnson, Publicity Coordinator

8589 Assisting Parents Through the Mourning Process
Hope
55 E 100 N
Logan, UT 84321
435-752-9533
Fax: 435-752-9533

Describes the mourning process experienced by some parents of children with disabilities and ways in which the professional can help them through the process.

20 minutes

8590 CANCER
Rosen Publishing Group
29 E 21st Street
New York, NY 10010
800-237-9932
Fax: 888-436-4643
e-mail: rosenpub@tribeca.ios.com
www.rosenpublishing.com

Interviews with experts and cancer patients reveal the many types, causes, and treatments for cancer. Recommended for grades seven-twelve.

30 Minutes
ISBN: 0-823921-76-0

8591 Disability Awareness
Active Parenting Publishers
1220 Kennestone Circle, Suite 130
Marietta, GA 30066
770-429-0565
Fax: 770-429-0334
e-mail: cservice@activeparenting.com
www.activeparenting.com

Helps viewers think about how they feel when confronted by people with disabilities. Close-captioned with study guide.

19 minutes

Michael H. Popkin, PhD, Founder & President
Virginia Murray, Marketing Manager
Melody Popkin, Manager of Christian Resources

8592 It's Just Part of My Life
National Kidney Foundation
30 E 33rd Street
New York, NY 10016
212-889-2210
800-622-9010
Fax: 212-689-9261
e-mail: info@kidney.org, membership@kidney.org
www.kidney.org

A 15-minute program for adolescent dialysis patients and their families.

Gregory W. Scott, Chairman
Jeffery S. Berns, President
Bruce Skyer, CEO

8593 Kid's Health: TV Late Breaking News Video About Broken Bones and Cast Care
Aquarius Health Care Videos
5 Powderhouse Lane, PO Box 1159
Sherborn, MA 1770
508-651-2963
888-440-2963
Fax: 508-650-4216
e-mail: info@aquariusproductions.com
www.aquariusproductions.com

You probably have lots of questions. How do doctors know if a bone is really broken? What are casts and what do they do? What are some ways to take good care of your cast so you won't need a new one? The Kids Health TV News Tem answer these questions and more in an entertaining format.

Donna Kaufman

8594 Laughter Therapy
PO Box 827
Monterey, CA 93942
408-625-3788

These people can supply tapes of old Candid Camera movies to patients. Maintains a library of 50 topics.

8595 Meeting the Challenge: Parenting Children with Disabilities
Active Parenting Publishers
1220 Kennestone Circle, Suite 130
Marietta, GA 30066
770-429-0565
800-825-0060

Award-winning video for parents of special-needs children. Other parents share their stories.

94 minutes

8596 My Body Is Not Who I Am
Aquarius Health Care Videos
5 Powderhouse Lane, PO Box 1159
Sherborn, MA 1770
508-651-2963
888-440-2963
Fax: 508-650-4216
e-mail: info@aquariusproductions.com
www.aquariusproductions.com

Children host this video and educate themselves and the viewer about disabilities. While profiling adults and children who talk candidly about their disabilites, they learn that people are more alike than different. This video is crafted to foster senitivity toward others and acceptance of people with disabilities. It provides general disability etiquette guidelines that both children and adults can benefit from. The video is fast paced and designed to keep children's attention. Closed caption.

K - 12 25 Minutes

Donna Kaufman

8597 No Fears, No Tears
Fanlight Productions
32 Court Street, 21st Floor
Brooklyn, NY 11201
718-488-8900
800-876-1710
Fax: 718-488-8642
e-mail: info@fanlight.com
www.fanlight.com

Dr. Leora Kuttner explores the pioneer pain management project for children with cancer. The film proves the strenth of the human spirit and mind's ability to ease away excrutiating pain. See No Fears, No Tears - 13 Years Later.

28 minutes DVD
ISBN: 1-572958-73-1

8598 No Fears, No Tears - 13 Years Later
Fanlight Productions
32 Court Street, 21st Floor
Brooklyn, NY 11201   718-488-8900
                                      800-876-1710
                                 Fax: 718-488-8642
                         e-mail: info@fanlight.com
                                  www.fanlight.com

Dr. Leora Kuttner explore the effects of children's pain management therapies 13 years after use. See original No Fears, No Tears. ISBN: DVD: 1-57295-874-X; VHS: 1-572952-77-6

47 minutes DVD or VHS

8599 Not Just a Cancer Patient
Fanlight Productions
32 Court Street, 21st Floor
Brooklyn, NY 11201   718-488-8900
                                      800-876-1710
                                 Fax: 718-488-8642
                         e-mail: info@fanlight.com
                                  www.fanlight.com

Focuses on several articulate teenagers who are undergoing cancer treatment to help caregivers understand the needs and feelings of this very special population.

23 minutes VHS
ISBN: 1-572950-86-2

Nicole Johnson, Publicity Coordinator

8600 Operation Sneek-a-Peek
Aquarius Health Care Videos
5 Powderhouse Lane, PO Box 1159
Sherborn, MA 1770   508-651-2963
                                      888-440-2963
                                 Fax: 508-650-4216
               e-mail: info@aquariusproductions.com
                         www.aquariusproductions.com

Helps children feel more comfortable and safe in a hospital envirnoment. The puppets in the video take the children on an educational, comforting and at times, humorous tour of the hospital operating and recovery rooms. This video eases children's concerns and fears with factual information and truthful demonstrations. Closed captioned.

20 Minutes

Donna Kaufman

8601 Recognizing Children with Special Needs
Aquarius Health Care Videos
5 Powderhouse Lane, PO Box 1159
Sherborn, MA 1770   508-651-2963
                                      888-440-2963
                                 Fax: 508-650-4216
               e-mail: info@aquariusproductions.com
                         www.aquariusproductions.com

A great overview for caregivers of children on how to recognize special needs. Often times it is the little things children do everyday to compensate for, or express, a disability that can be observed by their caregiver. All types of disabilities are addressed, emotional, physical, psychological, and chonic illness. A wonderful tool for teachers, childcare staff, and students who play a vital role in our children's development. Closed captioned.

18 Minutes

Donna Kaufman

8602 Stress Reduction Tapes, Stress Reduction Clinic
University Massachusetts Medical
PO Box 547
Lexington, MA 2420   508-856-2656
                    e-mail: mindfulness@umassmed.edu
                              www.mindfulnesstapes.com

There are two tapes sold separately that are appropriate for preteens or adolescents. Tapes may be ordered from the website.

Jon Kabat-Zinn, PhD, Author

8603 They're Just Kids
Aquarius Health Care Videos
5 Powderhouse Lane, PO Box 1159
Sherborn, MA 1770   508-651-2963
                                      888-440-2963
                                 Fax: 508-650-4216
               e-mail: info@aquariusproductions.com
                         www.aquariusproductions.com

This documentary explores the advantages of the inclusion of disabled children in the classroom, Cub Scouts and other extracurricular activities. Unfortunately, there is a great deal of fear, apprehension and concern regarding mainstreaming. This film is an excellent tool to expedite and ease that integration of children and adults into the community as well as into recreational, social and educational programs. Closed captioned, for schools, parents and those working with disabled children.

27 Minutes

Donna Kaufman

8604 When Parents Can't Fix It
Fanlight Productions
32 Court Street, 21st Floor
Brooklyn, NY 11201   718-488-8900
                                      800-876-1710
                                 Fax: 718-488-8642
                         e-mail: info@fanlight.com
                                  www.fanlight.com

Looks at the stresses and rewards in the lives of five families who are raising children with diabilities. Offers a realistic look and different family strengths and coping styles. ISBN: DVD: 1-57295-876-6; VHS: 1-572952-55-5

58 minutes DVD or VHS

Nicole Johnson, Publicity Coordinator

Web Sites

8605 Adolescent Health On-Line
AMA Plaza, 330 N. Wabash Ave.
Chicago, IL 60611   312-464-4430
                                      800-621-8335
                                   www.ama-assn.org

Includes state-to-state guide to poison control centers, database of pediatrician and hospitals, basic home care instructions and immunizations.

Barbara L. McAneny, MD, Chair
Robert M. Wah, MD, President
Andrew W. Gurman, MD, Speaker

8606 American Academy of Pediatrics
141 Northwest Point Boulevard
Elk Grove Village, IL 60007   847-434-4000
                                      800-433-9016
                                 Fax: 847-434-8000
                                        www.aap.org

The American Academy of Pediatrics and its member pediatricians are committed to the attainment of optimal physical, mental and social health and well-being for all infants, children, adolescents, and young adults.

Sandra Hassink, MD, FAAP, President

8607 American Autoimmune Related Diseases Association
22100 Gratiot Ave.
Eastpointe, MI 48021   586-776-3900
                                      800-598-4668
                                 Fax: 586-776-3903
                                      www.aarda.org

Dedicated to the eradication of autoimmune diseases and the alleviation of suffering and the socio-economic impact of autoimmunity through fostering and facilitating collaboration in the areas of education, public awareness, research and patient services in an effective, ethical and efficient manner.

Betty Diamond, M.D., Chairperson
Virginia T. Ladd, President/ Executive Director
Patricia Barber, Asst. Director

8608 American Board of Pediatrics
111 Silver Cedar Court
Chapel Hill, NC 27514   919-929-0461
                                    Fax: 919-929-9255
                    e-mail: abpeds@abpeds.org, ite@abpeds.org

Is an independent, nonprofit organization whose certificate is recognized throughout the world signifying a high level of physician
competence. It consists of distinguished pediatricians in education, research, and clinical practice, as well as one or more
nonphysicians who have a professional interest in the health and
welfare of children and adolescents.

8609 American College of Medical Genetics
7220 Wisconsin Avenue, Suite 300
Bethesda, MD 20814   301-718-9603
                                    Fax: 301-718-9604
                                e-mail: acmg@acmg.net
                                        www.acmg.net

Provides education, resources and a voice for the medical genetics profession. To make genetic services available to and improve
the health of the public, the ACMG promoted the development
and implementation of methods to diagnose, treat and prevent
genetic disease.

8610 American Society of Pediatric Neurosurgeons
www.aspn.org

                            e-mail: aspnhelp@aspn.org
                                        www.aspn.org

The society is dedicated to the advancement of the subspecialty of
Pediatric Neurosugery and to assure superlative care for children
with neurosurgical disorders. It holds an annual meeting where
recent advances in clinical and basic research into pediatric
neurosurgical disorders are presented and discussed, and sponsors
a journal, Pediatric Neurosurgery.

Alan R. St. Geme III, MD, President
James M. Drake, Secretary
John Ragheb, MD, Treasurer

8611 Archives of Pediatric and Adolescent Medicine
333 Seventh Avenue, 20th Floor
New York, NY 10001   646-674-6300
                                        800-950-2035
                                    Fax: 646-674-6301
                                e-mail: sales@ovid.com
                        www.ovid.com/site/cataloge/journal

It provides a forum for dialogue on a range of scientific, clinical,
and humanistic issues relevant to the care of pediatric patients,
from infancy to young adulthood. The journal's core articles are
original clinical studies and reviews by experts.

**8612 Association for Children with Hand or Arm Deficiency
(REACH)**
Pear idestthemealHomeyBriohlpSctreets and professionals share ex-
periences, information, and support.

8613 Birth Defect Research for Children
976 Lake Baldwin Lane, Suite 104
Orlando, FL 32814   407-895-0802
                                e-mail: staff@birthdefects.org
                                        www.birthdefects.org

Nonprofit organization that provides parents and expectant parents with information about birth defects and support services for
their children, including the National Birth Defect Registry.

8614 Cedars-Sinai Medical Center
8700 Beverly Road
Los Angeles, CA 90048   310-423-3277
                                        800-233-2771
                                        cedars-sinai.edu

Focused on providing the finest healthcare available, resulting in
advances in all areas of healthcare for both children and adult disorders.

Vera S. Guerin, Chair
Marc H. Rapaport, Vice Chair
Thomas M. Priselac, President & CEO

8615 CenterWatch Clinical Trials Listings
10 Winthrop Square, Fifth Floor
Boston, MA 2110   617-948-5100
                                        866-219-3440
                                    Fax: 617-948-5101
                    e-mail: customerservice@centerwatch.com
                                        www.centerwatch.com

CenterWatch is a Boston-based publishing and information services company. We provide information services used by patients, pharmaceutical, biotechnology and medical device
companies, CRO's and research centers involved in clinical
research around the world.

Kenneth A. Getz, Founder & Owner
Joan A. Chambers, COO
Cheryl Appel Rosenfeld, Editor-in-Chief

8616 Council for Exceptional Children
2900 Crystal Drive, Suite 1000
Arlington, VA 22202   888-232-7733
                                    TTY: 866-915-5000
                            e-mail: heidenj@cudahysd.org
                                        www.cec.sped.org

The worldwide mission of The Council for Exceptional Children
is to improve education outcomes for individuals with
exceptionalities. CEC, a nonprofit association, accomplishes its
mission in support of special education professionals and others
working on behalf of individuals with exceptionalities, by advocating for appropriate governmental policies, by setting professional standards, and by providing continuing professional
development.

James P. Heiden, President
Antonis Katsiyannis, President Elect
Sharon Raimondi, Treasurer

8617 CyberPsych
www.cyberpsych.org

CyberPsych presents information about psychoanalysis, psychotherapy, and special topics such as anxiety disorder, the problematic use of alcohol, homophobia, and the traumatic effects of
racism. CyberPsych is a nonprofit network which offers free web
hosting and technical support for internet communication, to
nonprofit groups and individuals.

Carol Lindemann, PHD, Webmaster

8618 Dermatology Foundation
1560 Sherman Ave., Suite 870
Evanston, IL 60201   847-328-2256
                                    Fax: 847-328-0509
                                dermatologyfoundation.org

Committed to advancing dermatologic through research and education. The foundation is a charitable organization that has the
primary service to fund research in skin cancer and other diseases
of the skin, hair, and nails.

Bruce U. Wintroub, MD, Chair
Michael D. Tharp, MD, President
Stuart R. Lessin, MD, Vice President

8619 Easter Seals Disability Services
233 South Wacker Drive, Suite 2400
Chicago, IL 60606   800-221-6827
                                        www.easterseals.com

For more than 80 years, Easter Seals has helped people with disabilities in communities nationwide, from creating the first national voluntary act for children with disabilities in the 1920's to
leading the creation and implementation of the Americans with
Disabilities Act in the 1990's. Easter Seals child development
services build strong foundations for children of all abilities.

Rick Davidson, Chair
Eileen Howard Boone, 1st Vice Chair
Ralph F. Boyd, Jr., 2nd Vice Chair

8620 European Society for Pediatric Urology
www.espu.org

Is a nonprofit society whose main purpose is to promote pediatric
urology, appropriate practice, education as well as exchanges between practitioners involved in the treatment of genitourinary
disorders in children.

Gianantonio Manzoni, President
Guy Bogaert, President-Elect
Serdar Tekgul, Secretary

8621   Federation for Children with Special Needs
529 Main Street, Suite 1M3
Boston, MA 2129

617-236-7210
800-331-0688
Fax: 617-241-0330
e-mail: fcsninfo@fcsn.org
fcsn.org

Mission is to provide information, support, and assistance to parents of children with disabilites, their professional partners, and their communities. We are committed to listening to and learning from families and encouraging full participation in community life by all people, especially those with disabilities.

James F. Whalen, President
Rich Robison, Executive Director
Michael Weiner, Treasurer

8622   GeneTest
481B Edward H. Ross Drive
Elmwood Park, NJ 7407

888-729-1204
Fax: 202-212-6457
e-mail: genetests@genetests.org
www.geneclinics.org

By providing current, authoritative information on genetic testing and its use in diagnosis, management, and genetic couseling, GeneTests promots the appropriate use of genetic services in patient care and personal decision making.

Roberta A. Pagon, MD, Founder & Medical Director
Amar Kamath, Commercial Director
Deb Eunpu, MS, CGC, Program Manager

8623   ICAN (International Child Amputee Network)
PO Box 13812
Tuscon, AZ 85732   child-amputee.net

Is an internet mailing list to provide information and support contacts to children with absent or underdeveloped limbs and their parents.

Sami Madden, President
Mike Holmes, Vice President
Joyce Baughn, Director

8624   International Foundation for Functional Gastrointestinal Disorders
700 W. Virginia St., #201
Milwaukee, WI 53204

414-964-1799
888-964-2001
Fax: 414-964-7176
e-mail: iffgd@iffgd.org
www.iffgd.org

Is a nonprofit education and research organization whoes mission is to inform, assist and support people affected by gastrointestinal disorders.

Nancy J. Norton, President & Director
William Norton, Co-founder & Director
Eleanor Cautley, Vice President & Director

8625   KidsHealth at the AMA
AMA Plaza, 330 N. Wabash Ave.
Chicago, IL 60611

312-464-4430
800-621-8335
www.ama-assn.org

Includes state-to-state guide to poison control centers, database of pediatricians and hospitals, basic home-care instructions and immunizations.

Barbara L. McAneny, MD, Chair
Robert M. Wah, MD, President
Andrew W. Gurman, MD, Speaker

8626   LSUMC Family Medicine Patient Education
lib-sh.lsumc.edu

Offers databases, E-journals, E-books, and a library catalog.

8627   Learning Disabilities Association of Ameri ca
www.ldaamerica.org

Helps families of the affected individual through information and referral to professionals in their area. A membership organization with affiliates across the country.

8628   Low Vision Gateway
www.lowvision.org

Devoted to issues of vision loss, low vision aids, vision rehabilitation and the role of the doctor.

8629   MUMS: National Parent to Parent Network
www.netnet.net/mums

A national parent-to-parent organization for parents or care providers of a child with any disability, rare or not so rare disorder, chromosomal abnormality or health condition. MUM's main purpose is to provide support to parents in the form of a networking system that matches them with other parents whose children have the same or similar condition.

8630   March of Dimes Birth Defects Foundation
1275 Mamaroneck Avenue
White Plains, NY 10605

914-997-4488
www.marchofdimes.org

March of Dimes researchers, volunteers, educators, outreach workers and advocated work together to give all babies a fighting chance against the threats to their health: prematurity, birth defects, low birthweight.

8631   Medical Economics Company
24950 Country Club Drive, Suite 200
North Olmsted, OH 44070   www.medec.com

Full text for non-prescription drugs and the PDR Guide to Drug Interactions.

Georgiann DeCenzo, Executive Vice President
Ken Sylvia, Vice President
Don Berman, Director, Business Development

8632   Medical Matrix: Pediatrics
medmatrix.org/_SPages/Pediatrics.asp

Christoph U. Lehman, MD, Assoc. Professor
Andy Spooner, MD, Pediatrics Dept.

8633   Mental Help Net
P.O. Box 20709
Columbus, OH 43220

614-448-4055
800-232-TALK
e-mail: info@centersite.net, editor@centersite.n
mentalhelp.net

Seeks to advance the state of online mental health communications. We wish to provide the following: to discuss, develop and debate in an open forum the future of the mental health field in America and throughout the world, to help coordinate various componenets of the mental health field.

8634   NADD: National Association for the Dually Diagnosed
132 Fair Street
Kingston, NY 12401

845-331-4336
800-331-5362
Fax: 845-331-4569
e-mail: info@thenadd.org
www.thenadd.org

Nonprofit organization designed to promote the interests of professional and care providers for individuals who have the coexistence of mental illness and mental retardation. NADD provides conferences, educational services and training materials to professionals, parents, concerned citizens and service organizations.

Robert J. Fletcher, DSW, CEO
Michelle Jordan, Office Manager
Lisa Christie, Conference Planner

8635   NIH/National Institute on Disability and Rehabilitative Research (NIDRR)
Department of Education Building, 400 Maryland Ave

Is committed to improving results and outcomes for people with disabilities of all ages. It supports programs that serve millions of children, youth and adults with disablities.

8636 **National Arthritis and Musculoskeletal & Skin Disease Info. Clearinghouse**
Information Clearinghouse, National Institutes of
Bethesda, MD 20892   301-495-4484
                                                                            877-226-4267
                                                                       Fax: 301-718-6366
                                                                       TTY: 301-565-2966
                                                       e-mail: NIAMSinfo@mail.nih.gov
                                                                       www.nih.gov/niams

Supports and provides clinical and public information and research to increase understanding of the many skin diseases and related disorders. Also provides lists and order forms for their resources and materials.

Stephen I. Katz, Director
Robert H. Carter, Deputy Director
Gahan Breithaupt, Assoc. Dir. For Management

8637 **National Association for Visually Handicapped**
111 E 59th St
New York, NY 10022   212-821-9497
                                                                            800-284-4422
                                                       e-mail: kcampbell@lighthouse.org
                                                                            lighthouse.org

Helps to cope with the difficulties of vision impairment.

8638 **National Dissemination Center for Children with Disabilities**
c/o Statewide Parent Advocacy Network, 35 Halsey S

Provides information to the nation on: disabilities in children and youth; programs and services for infants, children, and youth with disabilities; IDEA, the nation's special education law; No Child Left Behind, the nation's general education law; and research-based information on effective practices for children with disabilities.

8639 **National Library Service for the Blind and Physically Handicapped**
1291 Taylor Street, NW
Washington, DC 20542   202-707-5100
                                                                       Fax: 202-707-0712
                                                                       TDD: 202-707-0744
                                                              e-mail: nls@loc.gov
                                                                       www.loc.gov/nls

A free library program of braille and audio materials circulated to eligible borrowers in the United States by postage-free mail.

Karen Keninger, Director
Erica Vaughns, Executive Asst. to the Director
Isabella Marques de Castilla, Deputy Director

8640 **National Newborn Screening and Genetic Resources Center**
3907 Galacia Drive
Austin, TX 78759   512-345-5685
                                                       e-mail: therrell@uthscsa.edu
                                                                       genes-r-us.uthscsa.edu

The mission is to provide a forum for interaction between consumers, health care professionals, researchers, organizations, and policy-makers in-refining and developing public health, newborn screening and geneting programs, and to serve as a national resource center for information and education in the areas of newborn screening and genetics.

Bradford L. Therrell, Jr., Ph.D., Director
Celia Kaye, MD, PhD, Professor & Senior Associate Dean
Louis Bartoshesky, MD, MPH, Pediatrician & Clinical Geneticist

8641 **National Organization of Parents of Blind Children**
200 East Wells Street at Jernigan Place

Is a national membership organization of parents and friends of blind chilren reaching out to each other to give support, encouragement and information. We believe the real problem of blindness is not the loss of eyesight, but the misunderstanding and lack of information which exists. With proper training opportunity, blindness can be reduced to a physical nuisance.

8642 **National Resource Library on Youth With Disabilities**
3 Morrill Hall, 100 Church St. SE
Minneapolis, MN 55455   www.cyfc.umn.edu/NRL/

Brings together comprehensive sources of information related to youth with chrionic or disabling conditions and their families. Topics include psychosocial issues, disability awareness, developmental processes, family, sexuality, education, employment, independent living, cultural issues, gender issues, service delivery, professional issues, advocacy and legal issues, and health issues.

Eric W. Kaler, President
Karen Hanson, Provost
Scott Studham, VP & CIO

8643 **Nuclear Medicine at Children's Hospital, Boston**
www.jpnm.org/contentch.html

8644 **Office of Special Education and Rehabilitative Services**
Department of Education Building, 400 Maryland Ave

Mission is to strengthen the federal commitment to assuring access to equal opportunity for every individual; to supplement and complement the efforts of states, the local school systems and other instrumentalities of the states, the private nonprofit educational research institutions, community-based organizations, parents, and students to improve the quality of education; and to encourage the increased involvement of the public, parents, and students in federal education programs.

8645 **Online Mendelian Inheritance in Man**
www.omim.org

Conducts research on fundamental biomedical problems at the molecular level using mathematical and computational methods, maintains collaborations with several NIH institutes, academia, industry, and other governmental agencies, fosters scientific communication by sponsoring meetings, workshops, and lecture series, and supports training on basic and applied research in computational biology for postdoctoral fellows through the NIH Intramural Research Program.

8646 **PDR - Physicians' Desk Reference**
5 Paragon Drive
Montvale, NJ 7645   888-227-6469
                                                       e-mail: PDRnet@pdr.net
                                                                       www.pdr.net

Robert Carmignani, Sales & Marketing
Kim Marich, Sr. Director, Marketing

8647 **PEDINFO: An index of the Pediatric Internet**
www.pedinfo.org

Collection of links to pediatric information.

8648 **Pediatric Behavior and Development**
www.dbpeds.org

Is an independent web site created to promote better care and outcomes for children and families affected by developmental, learning, and behavioral problems by providing access to clinically relevant information and educational materials for physicians, fellows, resident physicians, and students. The site may also be of interest to psychologists, nurses, nurse practitioners, social workers, therapists, educators, and parents.

8649 **Pediatric Points of Interest**
www.pslgroup.com/dg/20112

Are a collection of updated links for pediatricians, parents and children to medical sources on the internet.

8650 **Planetpsych**
www.planetpsych.com

                                                       e-mail: webmaster@PlanetPsych.com
                                                                       www.planetpsych.com

Planetpsych is an online resource for mental health information.

8651 **Pregnancy and Child Health Resource Center from Mayo Health Oasis**
13400 E. Shea Blvd.
Scottsdale, AZ 85259   480-301-8000
                                                                            800-446-2279
                                                                       www.mayohealth.org

Our mission is to empower people to manage their health. We accomplish this by providing useful and up-to-date information and tools that reflect the expertise and standard of excellence of Mayo Clinic.

Roger W. Harms, MD, Medical Director, Content
Brooks S. Edwards, MD, Founding Medical Director
Philip T. Hagen, Senior Medical Editor

8652 Psych Central
55 Pleasant St., Suite 207
Newburyport, MA 1950   e-mail: sales at psychcentral.com
                               www.psychcentral.com

Offers free informational and educational articles and resources on psychological support and mental health online.

John M. Grohol, Psy.D., CEO & Founder
Gilbert Levin, Ph.D., Member, Advisory Board
Holly R. Counts, Psy.D., Member, Advisory Board

8653 PubMed
National Library of Medicine, Building 38A
Bethesda, MD 20894   888-346-3656
                               e-mail: info@ncbi.nlm.nih.gov
                               www.ncbi.nlm.nih.gov/pubmed/

Creates public databases, conducts research in computational biology, develops software tools for analyzing genome data, and disseminates biomedical information - all for better understanding molecular processes affecting human health and disease.

Christine E. Seidman, M.D., Chair
David J. Lipman, M.D., Executive Secretary

8654 Rare Genetic Diseases in Children (NYU)
550 First Avenue
New York, NY 10016   212-263-7300
                               www.med.nyu.edu/rgdc/homenow.htm

We target issues arising from rare genetic diseases affecting children, and to assist in the endeavor to bring knowledge and hope to those for whom there is, at present, so little.

Kenneth G. Langone, Chair
Laurence D. Fink, Co-Chair
Robert I. Grossman, MD, Dean & CEO

8655 Save Babies Through Screening Foundation
PO Box 42197
Cincinnati, OH 45242   888-454-3383
                               e-mail: email@savebabies.org
                               www.savebabies.org

Is a national nonprofit public charity run by volunteers. Its mission is to improve the lives of babies by working to prevent disabilities and early death resulting from disorders detectable through newborn screening.

Jill Levy-Fisch, President
micki Gartzke, Vice President
Anne Rugari, Treasurer

8656 Society for Adolescent Medicine
111 Deer Lake Road, Suite 100
Deerfield, IL 60015   847-753-5226
                               Fax: 847-480-9282
                               e-mail: info@adolescenthealth.org
                               www.adolescenthealth.org

A multidisciplinary organization of professionals committed to improving the physical and psychosocial health and well-being of all adolescents.

Carol Ford, President
Paula Braverman, Secretary-Treasurer
Michael Resnick, President Elect

8657 Southern Illinois University School of Medicine
PO Box 19639
Springfield, IL 62794   217-545-8000
                               800-342-5748
                               e-mail: admin@siuhealthcare.org
                               www.siumed.edu/peds/index.htm

The mission of SUI School of Medicine is to assist the people of central and southern Illinois in meeting their present and future health care needs through education, clinical service and research.

Paul Castillo, CPA, CFO
Denise A. Gray-Felder, APR, Chief Communication Officer
Quinta Vreede, Chief Administrative Officer

8658 TRIP Database
www.tripdatabase.com

                                          734-615-0863
                                          800-211-8181
                               e-mail: contact@tripdatabase.com
                                          www.tripdatabase.com

The TRIP Database allows users to rapidly and easily identify high quality medical literature from a wide range of sources.

8659 TransWeb
www.transweb.org

Mission is to provide information about donation and transplantation to the general public in order to improve organ and tissue procurement efforts worldwide, to provide transplant patients and families world wide with information specifically dealing with transplant-related issues and concerns and to provide and index sources for transplant-related information available through the internet and otherwise.

8660 Virtual Childrens Hosptial
www.virtualpediatrichospital.org

Is dedicated to helping patients find the highest quality medical information in the world today. We offer patients the tools necessary to make informed treatment decisions within the short timlines dictated by their illness or disease.

8661 WebMD Community Services
my.webmd.com

Provides valuable health information, tools for managing youth health, and support to those who seek information.

Michael Smith, MD, MBA, CPT, Chief Medical Officer
Brunilda Nazario, MD, BC-ADM, Lead Medical Editor
Hansa Bhargava, MD, Medical Editor

Book Publishers

8662 Parental Alienation, DSM-5, and ICD-11
William Bernet, author

Charles C Thomas Publisher
2600 S 1st Street
Springfield, IL 62704   217-789-8980
                                           800-258-8980
                               Fax: 217-789-9130
                               e-mail: books@ccthomas.com
                                          www.ccthomas.com

264 pages
ISBN: 0-398079-44-4

Sue F V Rakow, Co-Author
Carol B Carpenter, Co-Author

Magazines

8663 Childswork Childsplay
135 Dupont Street, PO Box 760
Plainview, NY 11803   800-962-1141
                               Fax: 888-803-3908
                                          www.childswork.com

Full of training tools for children of all ages.

63 pages

8664 Exceptional Parent
209 Harvard Street, Suite 303
Brookline, MA 2146   617-730-5800
                               Fax: 617-730-8742
                                          www.eparent.com

Provides information and support for families, parents, physicians and professionals in the special needs community. Published 11 times monthly plus a special January issue.

Monthly
ISSN: 0046-9157

Joseph M. Valenzano, Jr., President, CEO & Publisher
Rick Rader MD, Editor-in-Chief
Vanessa B. Ira, Contributing Writer / Editor

8665   Future Reflections
National Federation of the Blind
200 East Wells Street at Jernigan Place

National magazine written specifically for parents and educators of blind children. Each issue addresses various topics important to blind children, their families and to school personnel.

Quarterly

8666   Journal of the Academy of Dermatology
American Academy of Dermatology
PO Box 94020
Palatine, IL 60094   847-330-0230
                                        Fax: 847-330-0050

A scientific publication serving the clinical needs of the specialty and providing a wide selection of articles on various topics important to continuing medical education of Academy members and the international dermatologic community.

Monthly

8667   The Deaf-Blind American
American Association of the Deaf-Blind
PO Box 8064
Silver Spring, MD 20907   301-495-4403
                                        Fax: 301-495-4404
                                        TTY: 301-495-4402
                                  e-mail: aadb-info@aadb.org
                                            www.aadb.org

The Deaf-Blind American (DBA), the official quarterly magazine of the AADB, is available only to its members. It contains articles of interest to deaf-blind individuals, their families, and service providers who work with people who are deaf-blind. The DBA is available in large print, Braille, disk and email.

Timothy Jackson, President
Jill Gaus, Vice President
Debby Lieberman, Secretary

Journals

8668   International Journal of Nursing in Intellectual & Developmental Disabilities
Developmental Disabilities Nurses Association
1501 South Loop 288, Suite 104-PMB 381
Denton, TX 76205   800-888-6733
                                        Fax: 844-336-2329
                                  e-mail: ddnahq@aol.com
                                            www.ddna.org

Electronic journal for nurses, individuals, families and others interested in promoting health and nursing supports for individuals with intellectual and developmental disabilities. Provides information and resources, educational strategies and policy development on a variety of clinical topics.

Karen Green McGowan, RN, CDDN, President
Wendy Herbers, RN, CDDN, QDDP, Vice President
Linda Coley, RN, CDDN, Secretary

Newsletters

8669   AADB E-News
American Association of the Deaf-Blind
PO Box 8064
Silver Spring, MD 20907   301-495-4403
                                        Fax: 301-495-4404
                                        TTY: 301-495-4402
                                  e-mail: aadb-info@aadb.org
                                            www.aadb.org

A free newsletter, the AADB E-News is available to anyone during the months when the DBA is not being published. It contains information about the latest events occurring within AADB and in the deaf-blind community. One does not need to be an AADB member to receive the free AADB E-News newsletter.

Timothy Jackson, President
Jill Gaus, Vice President
Debby Lieberman, Secretary

8670   ABDC Newsletter
Association of Birth Defect Children
976 Lake Baldwin Lane, Suite 104
Orlando, FL 32814   407-895-0802
                                        Fax: 407-566-8341
                                  e-mail: staff@birthdefects.org
                                            www.birthdefects.org

Offers updated information on the association activities, events and medical updates. Back issues available.

8 pages Quarterly

8671   BDRC Newsletter
Association of Birth Defect Children
976 Lake Baldwin Lane, Suite 104
Orlando, FL 32814   407-895-0802
                                        Fax: 407-566-8341
                                  e-mail: staff@birthdefects.org
                                            www.birthdefects.org

Offers updated information on the association activities, events and medical updates.

8 pages Quarterly

8672   Child Life Council Newsletter
Child Life Council
11821 Parklawn Drive, Suite 310
Rockville, MD 20852   301-881-7090
                                             800-252-4515
                                        Fax: 301-881-7092
                                  e-mail: CLCadmin@childlife.org
                                            www.childlife.org

The Child Life Council newsletter provides information to promote the well-being of children and families in health care settings. Newsletter is provided to members only.

12 pages Quarterly

Carla Oliver, MSW, CCLS, President
Colleen Maguire, MS, Acting Executive Director
Suku Powers, Dir. Of Development

8673   Children's Hopes and Dreams
Wish Fulfillment Foundation
280 Route 46
Dover, NJ 7801   973-361-7366
                                        Fax: 973-361-6627
                                  e-mail: chdfdover@juno.com
                          childrenscharities.org/childrens_wisheso

Dream Newsletter (describes dreams recently fulfilled, events, request and info about programs) available upon request; at no cost. 4 times per year.

10,000 Members

8674   Connecting
5025 E Washington Street, Suite 204
Phoenix, AZ 85034   602-242-4366
                                             800-237-3007
                                        Fax: 602-242-4306
                                        TDD: 602-242-4366
                                  e-mail: info@raisingspecialkids.org
                                            www.raisingspecialkids.org

Presenting informational and personal articles, calendar of events and news relevant to Arizona families of children with special needs. Subscription is free to families.

Bimonthly

Paula Banahan, President
Blanca Esparza-Pap, Vice President
Joyce Millard Hoie, Executive Director

8675 For Siblings Only
Family Resource Associates
35 Haddon Avenue
Shrewsbury, NJ 7702   732-747-5310
                              Fax: 732-747-1896

Quarterly newsletter for siblings of children with disabilities,
aged four through 10.
S Levine, Editor

8676 Matchmaker
MUMS: National Parent to Parent Network
150 Custer Street
Green Bay, WI 54301   920-336-5333
                                       877-336-5333
                              Fax: 920-339-0995
                         e-mail: mums@netnet.net
                            www.netnet.net/mums/

Matches parents of children with rare disorders. Provides information and advocacy resources for families and professionals. Includes listings of organizations providing general information and
organizations focusing on more specific areas of concern to families and young adults who have disabilities.
Quarterly
Julie Gordon, Director

8677 Newsline
Federation for Children with Special Needs
529 Main Street, Suite 1M3
Boston, MA 2129   617-236-7210
                                       800-331-0688
                              Fax: 617-241-0330
                              TDD: 800-331-0688
                        e-mail: fcsninfo@fcsn.org
                                   www.fcsn.org

Carolyn Romano, Editor
Janet Vohs, Editor
Rich Robison, Executive Director

8678 Orphan Disease Update
National Organization for Rare Disorders
55 Kenosia Avenue
Danbry, CT 6810   203-744-0100
                                       800-999-6673
                              Fax: 203-798-2291
                    e-mail: orphan@rarediseases.org
                               www.rarediseases.org

It provides updates on research, advocacy, and special events, as
well as advice and sources of help for caregivers, Web sites of interest, current clinical trials, and funding opportunities.
16 pages 3/year
Sheldon M. Schuster, Chair
Peter L Saltonstall, President & CEO
Pamela Gavin, COO

8679 PAL News
Parent Professional Advocacy League
529 Main Street, Suite 1M3
Boston, MA 2129   617-236-7210
                                       800-331-0688
                              Fax: 617-241-0330
                        e-mail: fcsninfo@fcsn.org
                                   www.fcsn.org

Offers information on medical and technological updates in the
area of research on birth defects, support groups and family re-
sources for persons with disabled children.
Quarterly
Rich Robison, Executive Director
Sara Miranda, Associate Executive Director
John Sullivan, Associate Executive Director

8680 Sibling Forum
Family Resource Associates
35 Haddon Avenue
Shrewsbury, NJ 7702   732-747-5310
                              Fax: 732-747-1896
                         e-mail: info@frainc.org
                                   www.frainc.org

Quarterly newsletter for siblings of children with disabilities,
aged 10 and up.
Allan Proske, President
Bill Sheeser, Vice President
Sue Levine, Editor

Pamphlets

8681 AAP Education Resource Guide
American Academy of Pediatrics
141 NW Point Boulevard
Elk Grove Village, IL 60007   847-434-4000
                                       800-433-9016
                              Fax: 847-434-8000
                             e-mail: cme@aap.org
                                   www.aap.org

Sandra Hassink, MD, FAAP, President
Benard P. Dreyer, MD, FAAP, President-Elect
?Errol R. Alden, MD, FAAP, Executive Director/CEO

8682 About Children's Eyes
National Association for Visually Handicapped
111 E 59th St
New York, NY 10022   212-821-9497
                                       800-284-4422
                              Fax: 212-727-2931
                  e-mail: kcampbell@lighthouse.org
                                   lighthouse.org

How to identify the child with a visual problem.

8683 About Children's Vision: A Guide for Parents
National Association for Visually Handicapped
111 E 59th St
New York, NY 10022   212-821-9497
                                       800-284-4422
                              Fax: 212-727-2931
                  e-mail: kcampbell@lighthouse.org
                                   lighthouse.org

Offers a better understanding of the normal and possible abnormal development of a child's eyesight.
Eva Cohen, Assistant to the Director

8684 Advanced Cancer: Coping with Advanced Canc er
National Cancer Institute
6116 Executive Blvd, Room 3036A
Bethesda, MD 20892   800-422-6237
                                       800-422-6237
                              TTY: 800-332-8615

Booklet delving into all aspects of everyday living with cancer.
Offers information on coping, how children react, facing the unknown, living wills, additional resources and making treatment
decisions.
30 pages

8685 Amyloidosis and Kidney Disease
Information Clearinghouse
9000 Rockville Pike
Bethesda, MD 20892   301-496-3583
                              Fax: 301-907-8906
                 e-mail: nddic@info.niddk.nih.gov
                                   www.niddk.nih.gov

Griffin P. Rodgers, M.D., M.A.C.P., Director
Kevin Abbott, Program Director
Kristin Abraham, Program Director

8686 Birth Defects: A Brighter Future
March of Dimes Resource Center
1275 Mamaroneck Avenue
White Plains, NY 10605   914-997-4488
                              Fax: 914-997-4763
                              www.marchofdimes.org

8687 Heart Disease, High Blood Pressure, Stroke and Diabetes
Information Clearinghouse
9000 Rockville Pike
Bethesda, MD 20892
301-496-3583
Fax: 301-907-8906
e-mail: nddic@info.niddk.nih.gov
www.niddk.nih.gov

Griffin P. Rodgers, M.D., M.A.C.P., Director
Kevin Abbott, Program Director
Kristin Abraham, Program Director

8688 How to Find Out More About Your Child's Birth Defect or Disability
Association of Birth Defect Children
976 Lake Baldwin Lane, Suite 104
Orlando, FL 32814
407-895-0802
Fax: 407-895-0824
e-mail: staff@birthdefects.org
www.birthdefects.org

An informational fact sheet that encourages parents who have a child with a birth defect or disability to become the expert on the child's disability with some suggestions on how to educate themselves.

8689 Interstitial Cyctitis
Information Clearinghouse
9000 Rockville Pike
Bethesda, MD 20892
301-496-3583
Fax: 301-907-8906
e-mail: ndoc@info.niddk.nih.gov
www.niddk.nih.gov

Griffin P. Rodgers, M.D., M.A.C.P., Director
Kevin Abbott, Program Director
Kristin Abraham, Program Director

8690 Liver Transplantation
American Liver Foundation
1425 Pompton Avenue
Cedar Grove, NJ 7009
973-857-2626
800-223-0179

8691 NPF Benefits of Membership Pamphlets
National Psoriasis Foundation
6600 SW 92nd Avenue, Ste. 300
Portland, OR 97223
503-244-7404
800-723-9166
Fax: 503-245-0626
e-mail: getinfo@psoriasis.org
www.psoriasis.org

Offers all the pamphlets that are published through the foundation for members. Includes NPF 800 number and reply tear-off card.

Krista Kellog, Chair
Pete Redding, Vice Chair
Randy Beranek, President & CEO

8692 New Challenge: Responding to Families
Federation for Children with Special Needs
529 Main Street, Suite 1M3
Boston, MA 2129
617-236-7210
800-331-0688
Fax: 617-241-0330
e-mail: fcsninfo@fcsn.org
www.fcsn.org

Addresses the needs of children with emotional, behavioral and mental disorders and their families.

Rich Robison, Executive Director
Sara Miranda, Associate Executive Director
John Sullivan, Associate Executive Director

8693 Nutrition for Early Chronic Kidney Disease
Information Clearing House
9000 Rockville Pike
Bethesda, MD 20892
301-496-3583
Fax: 301-907-8906
e-mail: nddic@info.niddk.nih.gov
www.niddk.nih.gov

Griffin P. Rodgers, M.D., M.A.C.P., Director
Kevin Abbott, Program Director
Kristin Abraham, Program Director

8694 Nutrition for Later Chronic Disease
Information Clearinghouse
9000 Rockville Pike
Bethesda, MD 20892
301-496-3583
Fax: 301-907-8906
e-mail: nddic@info.niddk.nih.gov
www.niddk.nih.gov

Griffin P. Rodgers, M.D., M.A.C.P., Director
Kevin Abbott, Program Director
Kristin Abraham, Program Director

8695 Pain, Pain Go Away: Helping Children with Pain
Association for the Care of Children's Health
7910 Woodmont Avenue, Suite 300
Bethesda, MD 20814
301-654-6549
800-808-2224
Fax: 301-986-4553

This booklet teaches parents about pain in children.
1993

8696 Proteinuria
Information Clearinghouse
9000 Rockville Pike
Bethesda, MD 20892
301-496-3583
Fax: 301-907-8906
e-mail: nddic@info.niddk.nih.gov
www.niddk.nih.gov

Griffin P. Rodgers, M.D., M.A.C.P., Director
Kevin Abbott, Program Director
Kristin Abraham, Program Director

8697 Renal Tubular Acidosis
Information Clearinghouse
9000 Rockville Pike
Bethesda, MD 20892
301-496-3583
Fax: 301-907-8906
e-mail: nddic@info.niddk.nih.gov
www.niddk.nih.gov

Griffin P. Rodgers, M.D., M.A.C.P., Director
Kevin Abbott, Program Director
Kristin Abraham, Program Director

8698 When Your Child Has a Life-Threatening Illness
Association for the Care of Children's Health
7910 Woodmont Avenue
Bethesda, MD 20814
301-654-6549
Fax: 301-986-4553

A concise, supportive booklet for parents. Sections include initial reactions, hope, communication, other children, impact on marriage, and single parent families.
1983

8699 Wish Fulfillment Organizations
Candlelighters' Childhood Cancer Foundation
7910 Woodmont Avenue, Suite 460
Bethesda, MD 20814
301-657-8401
800-366-2223

A list of groups granting wishes of children with life-threatening, chronic or terminal illnesses, with criteria and contacts.

8700 Young People with Cancer: A Handbook for Parents
National Cancer Institute
BG 9609 MSC 9760, 9609 Medical Center Drive
Bethesda, MD 20892
800-422-6237
TTY: 800-332-8615
www.cancer.gov

Discusses the most common types of childhood cancer, treatments, and side effects and issues that may arise when a child is diagnosed with cancer.

86 pages

Harold Varmus, M.D., Director

8701 Your Kidneys and How They Work
Information Clearinghouse
9000 Rockville Pike
Bethesda, MD 20892

301-496-3583
Fax: 301-907-8906
e-mail: ndoc@info.niddk.nih.gov
www.niddk.nih.gov

Griffin P. Rodgers, M.D., M.A.C.P., Director
Kevin Abbott, Program Director
Kristin Abraham, Program Director

Camps

8702 Camp Brave Eagle
8326 Nabb Rd.
Indianapolis, IN 46260

317-871-0000
www.campbraveeagle.org

Summer camp for children with bleeding disorders and their siblings.

Angel Couch, Program Director
Jennifer Maahs, Pediatric Nurse Practitioner

8703 Camp Horizon
930 E Woodfield Road
Schaumburg, IL 60173

847-240-1280
866-503-7546
Fax: 847-240-1859
e-mail: president@aad.org
www.campdiscovery.org

Camp for children with chronic dermatologic conditions. The camp offers the opportunity to experience summer camp and support each other in a setting of acceptance, love and fun.

Brett M. Coldiron, MD, President
Elise A. Olsen, MD, Vice President
Suzanne M. Olbricht, MD, Secretary-Treasurer

8704 Crotched Mountain School & Rehabilitation Center
One Verney Drive
Greenfield, NH 03047

603-547-3311
Fax: 603-547-3232
e-mail: info@cmf.org
www.cmf.org

Crotched Mountain is a charitable organization with a mission to serve individuals with disabilities and their families, embracing personal choice and development and building communities of mutual support.

William Cossaboon, MS, Director of Education
Jerry Hunter, VP Information Services
Lorrie Rudis, Director of Human Resources

Alabama

8705 Camp ASCCA/Easter Seals
PO Box 21, 5278 Camp Ascca Dr
Jackson's Gap, AL 36861

256-825-9226
800-THE-CAMP
Fax: 256-825-8332
e-mail: info@campascca.org
www.campascca.org

Camp for children and adults with disabilities, ages 6+.

Matt Rickman, Camp Director
John Stephenson, Administrator
Jocelyn Jones, Secretary

8706 Camp Merrimack
3320 Triana Boulevard
Huntsville, AL 35805

256-534-6455
e-mail: ksimari@merrimackhall.com
www.merrimackhall.com

A unique arts half-day camp for children ages 3 through 12; open to children with special needs including Cerebral Palsy, Down Syndrome, autism and others.

Debra Jenkins, Executive Director, Founder
Melissa Reynolds, Program & Operations Dir.
Claire Lindsay, Marketing Manager

8707 Camp Rap A Hope
2701 Airport Blvd
Mobile, AL 36606

251-476-9880
Fax: 251-476-9495
e-mail: info@camprapahope.org
www.camprapahope.org

A week-long summer camp in Alabama that is open to children between the ages of 7 and 17 who have and have ever had cancer.

Sandy Blount, President
Melissa McNichol, Executive Director
Roz Dorsett, Asst. Director

8708 Camp Smile-A-Mile
PO Box 550155
Birmingham, AL 35255

205-323-8427
888-500-7920
e-mail: jennifer.amundsen@campsam.org
www.campsam.org

Camp for children who have or have had cancer. Year round programs are provided for the campers and their family at no cost.

Sam Heide, President
Ryan M. Weiss, Vice President
Fred Elliott, Vice President

Arizona

8709 Camp Abilities Tucson
PO Box 86838
Tucson, AZ 85754

520-770-3204
e-mail: campabilitiestucson@gmail.com
www.campabilitiestucson.org

Comprehensive developmental sports camp for children in middle and high school who are blind, deaf-blind or multiply disabled.

Murry Everson, Camp Director

8710 Camp Civitan
12635 North 42nd Street
Phoenix, AZ 85032

602-953-2944
Fax: 602-953-2946
e-mail: info@campcivitan.org
www.campcivitan.org

A 501c3 non-profit organization, that has been providing multiple ever-changing programs to meet the needs of children and adults who are developmentally disabled.

Jane Armstrong, Director
Rob Adams, Camp Director
Mary Kellogg, Operations

Arkansas

8711 Camp Aldersgate
Med Camps Coordinator
2000 Aldersgate Road
Little Rock, AR 72205

501-225-1444
Fax: 501-225-2019
e-mail: info@campaldersgate.net
www.campaldersgate.net

The camps allow children and youth, ages 6-16, who have various medical conditions and physical disabilities to enjoy traditional camping experiences adapted to their abilities.

Sarah C. Wacaster, CEO
Bill Faggard, COO
Kerri Daniels, Dir. Of Development

California

8712 Ability First
1300 E Green Street
Pasadena, CA 91106
626-396-1010
877-768-4600
Fax: 626-396-1021
e-mail: info@abilityfirst.org
www.abilityfirst.org

Services include residential camping programs, aquatics, lifespan programs and housing.

Steve Brockmeyer, Chair
John Kelly, Vice Chair
Lori Gangemi, President & CEO

8713 Ability First, Camp Paivika
600 Playground Drive
Cedarpines Park, CA 92332
909-338-1102
Fax: 909-338-2502
e-mail: jane.garcia@abilityfirst.org
camppaivika.org

Nonprofit camp owned and operated by Ability First to provide outdoor, recreational camping services for children and adults with physical and/or developmental disabilities. Located in the San Bernadino mountains, the camp has a dining lodge and rec room, four cabins, infirmary, program building and pool that are all fully accessible. Camp is available to rent during winter/spring for up to 80 people.

Kelly Kunsek, Camp Director
Ievgeniia (Jade) Garcia, Camper Services Coordinator
Sonia Ramirez, Marketing Manager

8714 All Nations Camp
1908 Grand Avenue
Nashville, TN 37212
760-249-3822
877-899-2780
Fax: 760-249-4492
e-mail: info@gbod.org
www.gbod.org

Camp for children with disabilities, ages 8 to 18.

Bishop Elaine Stanovsky, President
Eric Park, Vice President
Tim Bias, General Secretary

8715 Camp Alex A. Krem
Camping Unlimited
102 Brook Lane
Boulder Creek, CA 95006
510-222-6662
Fax: 510-223-3046
e-mail: campkrem@campingunlimited.com
www.campingunlimited.com

Camp serves people of all ages and all disabilities. Summer Program: six one- and two-week sessions of residential or outdoor adventure camps. Year-round: weekend outings throughout the year. Vendorized by the California Regional Centers; camperships are available. Member of the American Camping Association.

Mary Farfaglia, Executive Director
Leon Wong, Program Director

8716 Camp Joan Mier
Ability First
11677 E Pacific Coast Highway
Malibu, CA
310-457-9863
Fax: 310-457-6374
www.kidscamps.com

8717 Camp Ronald McDonald at Eagle Lake
1250 Lyman Place
Los Angeles, CA 90029
310-268-8488
Fax: 310-473-3338
rmhcsc.org/camp/

Camp dedicated to creating a positive long-lasting impact on children with cancer and their families by providing, fun-filled, medically supervised year-round camp program.

Edward Lodgen, President
Jodie Lesh, Vice President
Martin Breidsprecher, Chief Executive Officer

8718 Camp Rubber Soul
325A East Redwood Avenue
Fort Bragg, CA 95437
707-962-0906
e-mail: camp@camprubbersoul.org
www.camprubbersoul.org

Summer camp for children and young adults with special needs that is not affiliated with any church, School District or state program.

Rachel Miller, Director
Sayre Statham, Director

8719 Camp-A-Lot
3030 Market Street
San Diego, CA 92102
619-685-1175
800-800-748
Fax: 619-234-3759
e-mail: info@arc-sd.com
www.arc-sd.com

Residential camping program for children and adults, ages 7 and up. San Diego locals offered transportation.

David W. Schneider, President/ CEO
Anthony J. DeSalis, Esq., EVP & COO
Rich Coppa, VP of Infra & Facilities/ CIO

8720 Christian Berets
1317 Oakdale Road, Suite 340
Modesto, CA 95355
209-524-7993
Fax: 209-524-7979
www.christianberets.org

A community-based program for children and adults with developmental disabilities.

James Woodhead, President
Carletta Evans Steele, Treasurer
Kelly Luth, Secretary

8721 Dream Street Foundation
324 South Beverly Drive, Suite 500
Beverly Hills, CA 90212
424-333-1371
Fax: 310-388-0302
e-mail: dreamstreatca@gmail.com
www.dreamstreetfoundation.org

A customized camping program for children with terminal, chronic, and life threatening infirmities. Over 600 children with cancer, AIDS, cystic fibrosis, leukemia, blood disorders and other serious diseases are given the opportunity to enjoy activities.

Patty Grubman, Director

8722 Easter Seal Summer Camp Programs
2645 Pleasant Hill Road
Pleasant Hill, CA
925-689-1777

Offers education, adventure and the experience and enjoyment of living-out-of-doors in a striking and challenging wilderness environment. Serves ages 6 to 60, male and female.

Beverly Mayhall

8723 Gloriana Opera Company
210 N. Corry Street, PO Box 273
Fort Bragg, CA 95437
707-964-7469
Fax: 707-965-9653
e-mail: info@gloriana.org
www.gloriana.org

Since 1977 superlative music theater productions all year long, plus concerts, childrens workshops and classes.

Diane Larson, President
Ana Lucas, Artistic Director

8724 Junior Wheelchair Sports Camp
Santa Barbara Parks and Recreation Department
1819 Farnam St Suite 701
Omaha, NE 68183
402-444-5900
Fax: 402-444-4921
www.ci.omaha.ne.us/parks

This five-day camp is for children 5-19 years old that are physically disabled. Sports instruction in aquatics, tennis, track and field, basketball, archery and new sports activities introduced each year. The camp counselors and instructors are also physically disabled to provide the children with a role model. Fee based on fundraising efforts.

Colorado

8725 Magic of Music and Dance
PO Box M
Aspen, CO 800-5
970-923-0578
Fax: 970-923-7338
www.kidscamps.com

8726 Rocky Mountain Village
Easter Seals Colorado
PO Box 115
Empire, CO 80438
303-569-2333
Fax: 303-569-3857
e-mail: kkoev@eastersealscolorado.org
www.easterseals.com/co/our-programs/camping-recreati

Sessions are conducted for both developmentally and physically disabled children and adults. Activities include swimming, horseback riding, outdoor education, zigline challenge course elements.

Krasimir Koev, Camp Director

Connecticut

8727 Mansfield's Holiday Hill
41 Chaffeeville Road
Mansfield Center, CT 6250
860-423-1375
Fax: 860-456-2444
e-mail: info@holidayrecreation.com
www.holidayrecreation.com/camp

A home not far from home where beautiful fields, forests, facilities and a caring staff support the activities and relationships of our camp families. The camp offers many programs such as: Outdoor Adventure; Tumbling; Dance; Adventure Ropes Course; Swimming; Arts & Crafts; Archery; Tennis and more to thirty boys and girls.

Dudley Hamlin

Florida

8728 Camp Thunderbird
500 E. Colonial Drive
Orlando, FL 32803
407-218-4300
Fax: 407-218-4301
e-mail: campthunderbird@questinc.org
www.questinc.org

Residential summer camping program for children and adults with a developmental disability. Campers enjoy swimming, sports, nature hikes, canoeing, etc. In short, a real summer camp experience provided by people who understand the physical, and behavioral challenges associated with Down syndrome, autism, Cerebral Palsy, and other developmental disabilities. Camp provides the chance to try new things, learn new skills, and focus on can-do with new friends. 6- & 12-day overnights.

Rosa Figueroa, Camp Coordinator

8729 Easter Seals Camp Challenge
31600 Camp Challenge Road
Sorrento, FL
352-383-4711
Fax: 352-383-0744
e-mail: camp@fl.easter-seals.org
www.kidscamps.com

Micheal Currence, Director Camping/Recreation
Melissa Guinta, Summer Camp Director

Hawaii

8730 Camp Erdman YMCA
69-385 Farrington Highway
Waialua, HI
808-637-4615
Fax: 808-637-8874
www.camperdman.net

A specialized youth camp serving the needs of the disabled.

Lance Wihelm, Chair
Steven C. Ai, Vice Chair
Michael A. Pietsch, President & CEO

Illinois

8731 Camp Discovery
American Academy of Dermatology
930 E Woodfield Road
Schaumburg, IL 60173
847-240-1280
866-503-7546
Fax: 847-240-1859
e-mail: jmueller@aad.org
www.aad.org/dermatology-a-to-z/for-kids/camp-discove

A camp for young people with chronic skin conditions. There is no fee and transportation is provided. Three locations: Camp Horizon in Millville, PA, Camp Knutson in Crosslake, MN, and Camp Dermadillo in Burton, TX.

David M Pariser, MD, President
Janine Mueller, Program Coordinator

8732 Easter Seals - Timber Pointe Outdoor Center
507 East Armstrong Avenue
Peoria, IL 61603
309-686-1177
Fax: 309-687-2035
www.easterseals.com/ci/

Handicapable camping for kids.

Brad Halverson, Chair
Don Young, 1st Vice Chair
Wes Blumenshine, 2nd Vice Chair

8733 Jewish Council for Youth Services
JCYS Camp Red Leaf
180 W. Washington Street, Suite 1100
Chicago, IL 60602
312-726-8891
Fax: 312-726-7920
e-mail: jthomason@jcys.org
jcys.org

Overnight summer camp for youth and adults with developmental disabilites. Family Camps, respite weekends, trips, and other special events are offered throughout the year.

Jeffery Heftman, President
Adam Tarantur, President Elect
Jennifer Gartenberg, VP, Programming

8734 Olympia
Southern Illinois University
Mail Code 6519
Carbondale, IL
618-453-1423
Fax: 618-453-1445

Located on 6,500 acres of forests and meadows on the shores of Little Grassy Lake, Olympia Camp is for mentally and physically handicapped children and adults. Among the activities offered are arts and crafts, hay wagon rides, canoeing and swimming.

Craig Dittmar

8735 Summer Wheelchair Sports Camp
University of Illinois
1207 S Oak Street, Division of Rehab Education
Champaign, IL
217-333-4606
Fax: 217-333-0248
TTY: 217-333-1970
www.kidscamps.com

8736 Touch of Nature Environmental Center
Southern Illinois University
Carbondale, IL 62901
618-453-6793
Fax: 618-453-1188
e-mail: webdev@pso.siu.edu
www.pso.siu.edu

Providing a traditional camping experience for non-traditional campers, including recreational and outdoor programs for adults and children with various developmental, mental and physical disabilities as well as learning and behavioral disorders.

Phil Gatton, Director
Dawn Wilson, Administrative Assistant
Tammy Baumharte, Customer Service Specialist

Indiana

8737 Camp Isanogel
7601 W Isanogel Road
Muncie, IN
765-288-1073
Fax: 765-288-3103
e-mail: isanogel@iquest.net
www.isanogelcenter.og

Thirty-two years of programs for special needs of children through adults.

Karen Kovacn, Executive Director
Monica Sauter, Recreation Director

8738 Camp Millhouse
25600 Kelly Road
South Bend, IN
219-287-9833
Fax: 812-358-4381
www.kidscamps.com

8739 Easter Seal Society
4251 S 600 E
Columbus, IN
812-342-0134
www.kidscamps.com

8740 Happiness Bag Incorporated
3833 Union Road
Terre Haute, IN 47802
812-234-8867
Fax: 812-238-0728
www.happinessbag.org

Serves developmentally disabled age 5-adult; day and residential camp program; after school program; scouting; Special Olympic anticipation (basketball, athletics, bowling, softball and aquatics); and a bowling league.

Trudy Rupska, President
Caren Elrod, Vice President
Jodi Moan, Executive Director

8741 Happy Hollow Children's Camp
3049 Happy Hollow Road
Nashville, IN
812-988-4900
Fax: 812-988-7505
e-mail: hhcdir@aol.com
www.happyhollowcamp.net

Accepts disabled campers.

Bernard Schrader, Executive Director

8742 Kiwanis Twin Lakes Camp
15543 12th Road
Plymouth, IN
219-941-2750

Serving the orthopedically handicapped children and young adults.

Iowa

8743 Camp Courageous
PO Box 418
Monticello, IA 52310
319-465-5916
e-mail: info@campcourageous.org
www.campcourageous.org

Over 3,500 disabled campers have attended this recreational and respite care facility. The camp is open 24 hours a day, 365 days a year and operates entirely on donations.

Aly Jonson, Dietary Director
Amanda Brenneman, Assistant Nursing
Amatullah Richard, Communications Director

8744 Camp Courageous of Iowa
PO Box 418
Monticello, IA 52310
319-465-5916
Fax: 319-465-5919
e-mail: info@campcourageous.org
www.campcourageous.com

A year round residential and respite care facility for individuals with special needs. Campers range in age from 3-80 years old. Activities include traditional activities like canoeing, hiking, swimming, nature and crafts plus adventure activities like caving, rock climbing, etc. Campers with disabilities have opportunities to succeed at challenging activities. This feeling of self-worth can transfer to home, work or school environments.

Aly Jonson, Dietary Director
Amanda Brenneman, Assistant Nursing
Amatullah Richard, Communications Director

8745 Camp Tanager
1614 W Mount Vernon Road
Mount Vernon, IA 52314
319-363-0681
Fax: 319-365-6411
www.camptanager.org

Nonprofit camp for children with disabilities.

Robin Butler

8746 Easter Seals Camp Sunnyside
Easter Seals Iowa
233 South Wacker Drive, Suite 2400
Chicago, IL 60606
515-289-1933
800-221-6827
Fax: 515-289-1281
e-mail: essia@netins.net
www.easterseals.com

Each summer from June through August, campers with disabilities ages five and up, take part in one week camping sessions, gaining skills and independence by participating in activities like swimming, horseback riding, canoeing, fishing, camping and more. Financial assistance available.

Brad Halverson, Chair
Don Young, 1st Vice Chair
Wes Blumenshine, 2nd Vice Chair

Kentucky

8747 Bethel Mennonite Camp
2773 Bethel Church Road
Clayhole, KY 41317
606-666-4911
Fax: 606-666-4911
e-mail: grow@bethelcamp.org
www.bethelcamp.org

Roger Voth, Camp Director

8748 Easter Seal Kysoc
2050 Versailles Road
Lexington, KY 40504
859-254-5701
800-233-3260
Fax: 502-732-0783
e-mail: ek1@cardinalhill.org
www.cardinalhill.org

Designed for the fullest camping experience for children or adults with physical disabilities, blind, deaf, behavior disorders, mental retardation, diabetes and multiple handicaps, ages 7 and up.

Gary Payne, President/ CEO
Heide Miller, CCD, CTRS, Director

Jonathon Rondeau, Director
Katrina Johnson, Executive Director

8749 Camp Bon Coeur
405 W. Main St.
Lafeyette, LA 70501
337-233-8437
Fax: 337-233-4160
www.heartcamp.com

8750 Louisiana Lions Camp for Crippled Children
292 L. Beauford Dr.
Anacoco, LA 71403
337-239-0782
800-348-6567
Fax: 337-239-9975
e-mail: lalions@lionscamp.org
www.lionscamp.org

Camp for disabled children.
Raymond Cecil III

8751 Med-Camps of Louisiana
102 Thomas Road Suite 615
West Monroe, LA 71291
318-329-8405
Fax: 318-329-8407
e-mail: info@medcamps.com
www.medcamps.com

8752 Camp Waban
Waban Projects, Inc.
5 Dunaway Drive
Sanford, ME
207-324-7955
Fax: 207-324-6050
www.kidscamps.com

8753 Pine Tree Camp Children - Adults
149 Front Street
Bath, ME 4530
207-443-3341
Fax: 207-443-1070
e-mail: ptcamp@pinetreesociety.org
www.pinetreesociety.org

Paul Jacques, Chair
Dean Paterson, 1st Vice Chair
Penny Plourde, 2nd Vice Chair

8754 Easter Seals Camp Fairlee Manor
22242 Bay Shore Road
Chestertown, MD
410-778-0566
Fax: 410-778-0567
www.kidscamps.com

8755 Kamp-A-Kom-Plish
9035 Ironsides Road
Nanjemoy, MD 20662
301-870-3226
Fax: 301-870-2620
www.kampakomplish.org

8756 The League at Camp Greentop and The Therapeutic Recreation
League: Serving People with Disabilities
1111 E Cold Spring Lane
Baltimore, MD 21239
410-323-0500
Fax: 410-323-3298
TTY: 410-435-4298
e-mail: jrondeau@leagueforpeople.org
www.campgreentop.org

Summer residential camp located in the Catoctin Mountain National Park. Since 1937, Greentop has been serving children and adults with physical, cognitive, emotional and multiple disabilities in a completely accessible camp setting. Campers enjoy a traditional camping program. Medical facilities, staffed with registered nurses 24 hours a day. ACA/MD Youth Camp. Year round travel programs also offered.

8757 Camp Ramah in New England Tikvah Program
39 Bennett Street
Palmer, MA 01609
413-283-9771
Fax: 413-283-6661
e-mail: info@campramahne.org
www.campramahne.org

The Tikvah program is one of the first summer programs for Jewish children with special needs. It continues to grow and evolve as it strives to serve campers with a wide range of special needs including, but not limited to, congitive impairments, autism, cerebral palsy and seizure disorder.

Howard Blas, Tikvah Program Director
Talya Kalender, Director, Camper Care
Benjamin Greene, Director of Education

8758 Camp Ramah in New England (Summer)
39 Bennett Street
Palmer, MA 1069
413-283-9771
Fax: 413-283-6661
www.campramahane.org

8 week sleep-away camp for Jewish adolescents with developmental disabilities. Full camping program includes swimming, Hebrew singing and dancing, sports, arts and crafts, daily services, Kosher food, and Jewish studies classes.

Howard Blas, Director

8759 Camp Ramah in New England (Winter)
35 Highland Circle
Needham Heights, MA
701-449-7090
Fax: 413-283-6661
www.campramahane.org

8 week sleep-away camp for Jewish adolescents with developmental disabilities. Full camping program includes swimming, Hebrew singing and dancing, sports, arts and crafts, daily services, Kosher food, and Jewish studies classes.

Howard Blas, Director

8760 Carroll School Summer Programs
25 Baker Bridge Road
Lincoln, MA 1773
989-879-5199
Fax: 781-259-8852
e-mail: admissions@carrollschool.org
www.carrollschool.org

Academic and recreational programs designed to improve learning skills and build self-confidence. The school is a tutorial program for students not achieving their potential due to poor skills in reading, writing and math. The summer camp complements the summer school offering outdoor activities in a supportive, non-competitive environment.

Sam Foster, Chair
Josh Levy, Co-Vice Chair
Laura Rehnert, Co-Vice Chair

8761 Handi-Kids/King Solomon Foundation
470 Pine Street
Bridgewater, MA
508-697-7557
Fax: 508-697-1529
e-mail: handi7557@aol.com
www.handikids.com

A therapeutic recreational facility in Bridgewater, Massachusetts offering after-school programs, special events, school vacation full-week and summer day camp programs. Every individual is welcome regardless of the severity of a child's disability.

Mary L Gallant, Program Director

8762 Massachusetts Easter Seals Camping Program
484 Main Street
Worcester, MA 1608
800-922-8290
Fax: 508-831-9768
TTY: 800-564-9700
www.kidscamps.com

Michigan

8763 Camp Barakel
PO Box 159
Fairview, MI 48621

989-848-2279
Fax: 979-848-2280
e-mail: info@CampBarakel.org
www.campbarakel.org

Five-day Christian camp experience in mid-August for campers ages 13-55 who are physically disabled, visually impaired, upper trainable mentally impaired or educable mentally impaired, bus transportation provided from locations in Lansing, Flint, Bay City, and Marshall, Michigan.

Lee Brown, Program Director
Mike Alchin, Resident Missionary Staff
Teresa Alchin, Resident Missionary Staff

8764 Camp Fish Tales
2177 Erickson Road
Pinconning, MI 48650

989-879-5199
www.campfishtales.org

Larry Hammond, Chair
Lara Beth Sullivan, Executive Director
Brad Sullivan, Assistant Director

8765 Eric RicStar Winter Music Therapy Summer Camp
4930 S. Hagadorn Rd.
East Lansing, MI 48823

517-353-7661
Fax: 517-355-3292
e-mail: commusic@msu.edu
www.cms.msu.edu

The purpose of this camp is to provide opportunities for musical expression, enjoyment and interaction for all people with special needs and their siblings.

Cindy Edgerton, Director
Judy Winter, Co-Chair

8766 Indian Trails Camp
0-1859 Lake Michigan Drive NW
Grand Rapids, MI

616-677-5251
Fax: 616-677-2955
www.indiantrails-camp.org

Year round residential camping program for children and adults with physical disabilities.

Lynn Gust, Executive Director

Minnesota

8767 Camp Friendship
Friendship Ventures
10509 108th Street NW
Annandale, MN 55302

952-852-0101
800-450-8376
Fax: 952-852-0123
e-mail: fv@friendshipventures.org
truefriends.org

Camp Friendship offers kids, teens, and adults the chance to have the time of their lives. The program focuses on building self-esteem and independence, and practicing social skills; and we nurture each person's strengths and abilities and encourage participation in activies at their own pace. Specially designed for persons with developmental, physical or multiple disabilities, special medical conditions, Down syndrome, autism or other conditions. Weekend camps and longer available.

Jon Salmon, Director of Programs and Services
Mel Kloek, Program Director
Dawn Brenner, Director of Health Care

8768 Camp New Hope
Friendship Ventures
53035 Lake Avenue
McGregor, MN 55760

952-852-0101
800-450-8376
Fax: 952-852-0123
e-mail: fv@friendshipventures.org
truefriends.org

Camp New Hope is a great place for children, teens, and adults to have the time of their lives. The program provides a unique opportunity for having fun, learning skills, boosting confidence, and making friends. Services are specifically designed for persons with developmental, phyisical or multiple disabilities, special medical needs, Down syndrome, autism, or other conditions. Weekend camps and longer available. Other services available throughout the year.

Jon Salmon, Director of Programs and Services
Mel Kloek, Program Director
Dawn Brenner, Director of Health Care

8769 Camp Winnebago
19708 Camp Winnebago Road
Caledonia, MN 55921

507-724-2351
Fax: 507-724-3786
e-mail: director@campwinnebago.org
www.campwinnebago.org

We offer one week summer sessions for children and adults with developmental disabilities. We also do integrated youth sessions to allow friends and siblings to attend with our traditional campers. Respite week-ends are offered monthly throughout the year. Travel vacations are also offered as an option. We also have a campground open to the public.

8-12 pages

Terry Chiglo, President
Eileen Loken, Vice President
Jane Palen, Secretary

8770 Courage Camps
Courage Center
3915 Golden Valley Road
Golden Valley, MN 55422

952-852-0101
800-450-8376
Fax: 952-852-0123
e-mail: camping@mtn.org
truefriends.org

Summer resident camp serving children and adults who have physical or sensory disabilities. Also for children who need the help of a speech clinician. Special sessions include those for children who have been burned, children who have cancer and their siblings, and children who have hemophilia or sickle cell anemia. Offers special outdoor education or leadership sessions for deaf, or physically disabled teens and a sports camp for physically disabled and blind teens.

Jon Salmon, Director of Programs and Services
Mel Kloek, Program Director
Dawn Brenner, Director of Health Care

8771 Courage North
PO Box 1626
Lake George, MN 56458

952-852-0101
800-450-8376
Fax: 952-852-0123
truefriends.org

Jon Salmon, Director of Programs and Services
Mel Kloek, Program Director
Dawn Brenner, Director of Health Care

8772 Eden Wood Center
Friendship Ventures
6350 Indian Chief Road
Eden Prairie, MN

952-852-0101
800-450-8376
Fax: 952-852-0123
e-mail: fv@friendshipventures.org
truefriends.org

Offers resident camp programs for children, teenagers and adults with developmental, physical or multiple disabilities, Down Syndrome, special medical conditions, Williams Syndrome, autism and/or other conditions. Fishing, creative arts, golf, sports and other activities are available. Creative Options Respite Care offers weekend camps year round for children, teenagers and adults. Ventures Travel offers guided vacations for teens and adults with developmental disabilities or other unique needs.

Jon Salmon, Director of Programs and Services
Mel Kloek, Program Director
Dawn Brenner, Director of Health Care

8773 Knutson
523 N 3rd Street
Brainerd, MN
218-828-7610

Provides a camping program for mentally and physically disabled and emotionally disturbed children and adults. Campers must come with an established group that brings its own counselors. Swimming, sailing, archery, nature study and hiking are among the non-competitive activities.

Robert Larson

8774 Search Beyond Adventures
400 S Cedar Lake Road
Minneapolis, MN 800-8
612-374-4845
800-800-800
www.kidscamps.com

Mississippi

8775 Tik-A-Witha
PO Box 126
Van Vleet, MS
662-844-7577
Fax: 662-680-3164
www.kidscamps.com

Missouri

8776 Sidney R. Baer Day Camp
2 Millstone Drive serving campers ages 5-12 years old.
Saint Louis, MO
Astrid Balzer, Special Needs
Andy Brown, Camp Director

Nebraska

8777 Camp Easter Seals
609 N 60th Road
Nebraska City, NE 800-6
402-578-3992
800-800-650
www.kidscamps.com

New Hampshire

8778 Camp Allen
56 Camp Allen Road
Bedford, NH 03110
603-622-8471
Fax: 603-626-4295
e-mail: mary@campallennh.org
www.campallennh.org

A summer camp for individuals with disabilities.

Sebastian Grasso, Chair
Bret Cote, Vice Chair
Mary Constance, Executive Director

8779 Camp Dartmouth-Hitchcock
1 Medical Center Drive
Lebanon, NH
603-650-5597
Fax: 603-650-8980
www.kidscamps.com

8780 Crotched Mountain School & Rehabilitation Center
1 Verney Drive
Greenfield, NH 3047
603-547-3311
800-800-966
Fax: 603-547-3232
e-mail: info@crotchedmountain.org
www.cmf.org

Currently serves children ages 6-22 with multiple-handicaps including: Cerebral Palsy, Spina Bifida, visual and hearing impairments and neurological disabilities, developmental disorders, mental retardation, autism, behavioral and emotional disorders, seizure disorders, spinal cord and head injuries. Member of the National Association of Independent Schools and accredited with the NE Association of Schools and Colleges, Independent Schools of Northern NE.

James W. Varnum, Chair
Donald L. Shumway, President & CEO
Tom Zubricki, CFO

New Jersey

8781 Bancroft Camp
1255 Caldwell Road
Cherry Hill, NJ 8034
856-429-0010
800-774-5516
Fax: 207-729-1603
TTY: 856-428-2697
e-mail: lynn.tomaio@bancroft.org
www.bancroft.org

Has served as a summer camp for children and adults enrolled in Bancroft programs. The camp recognizes the need for individuals with developmental disabilities to vacation with their families. The camp offers a resort program for people wishing to explore the fascinating coast of Maine or to relax in the clean New England air. Accommodations include accessible rustic cabins and bayfront cottages.

Toni Pergolin, MA, CPA, President & CEO
Charles McLister, COO
Thomas J. Burke, MBA, CFO

8782 Camp Chatterbox
200 Portland Rd A-20
Highlands, NJ 7732
908-301-5451
e-mail: campchatterbox@gmail.com
www.campchatterbox.org

Joan Bruno, Ph.D., Director

8783 Camp Oakhurst
111 Monmouth Road
Oakhurst, NJ
908-531-0215
www.kidscamps.com

8784 Cross Roads Outdoor Ministries
29 Pleasant Grove Road
Port Murray, NJ 7865
908-832-7264
Fax: 908-832-6593
e-mail: officemanager@crossroadsretreat.com
www.crossroadsretreat.com

Program for ages 6-15 offers Bible study, worship, swimming, crafts, hiking, canoeing and campfires. Special education program for those with developmental disabilities.

Anthony P. Briggs, Executive Director
Kathy Felch, Office Manager
Kathryn Schaefer, Program Director

New Mexico

8785 Santa Fe Mountain Center
PO Box 449
Tesuque, NM
505-983-6158
Fax: 505-983-0460
e-mail: sky@santafemc.org
www.sf-mc.com

Camp sessions offered to disabled campers from the ages of 1-20.

Juanita Thorne-Connerty, Vice Chair
Seth R. Fullerton, President
Skye Gray, MS, Executive Director

New York

8786 Advocates for Children of New York
151 W 30th Street, 5th Floor
New York, NY 10001
212-947-9779
Fax: 212-947-9790
e-mail: info@advocatesforchildren.org
www.advocatesforchildren.org

Mental Health

Eric F. Grossman, President
Jamie A. Levitt, Vice President
Kim Sweet, Executive Director

8787 Camp Sun 'N Fun
Routes 322 & 555
Williamstown, NJ
856-629-4502
Fax: 856-875-1499
www.kidscamps.com

8788 Freedom Camp
Carr Bldg, 188 Genesee St, Suite 109
Auburn, NY 13021
315-253-5465

A summer day camp for youths with disabilities sponsored by Freedom Recreational Services. Freedom Camp is offered in two-week sessions at Casey Park in Auburn, New York.

Mary Ellen Perry, Executive Director

8789 Gow School Summer Programs
2491 Emery Road, PO Box 85
South Wales, NY 14139
716-652-3450
Fax: 716-652-3457
e-mail: summer@gow.org
www.gow.org

Co-ed summer programs for ages 8-16, offer a balanced blend of morning academics, afternoon/evening traditional camp activities and weekend overnight trips (teen-tours). The primary purpose of these programs is to provide a positive experience while balancing these three elements. Committed to the creation of a positive and enjoyable experience for each participant, by defining and merging the goals of the camp and the school, with those of camper students, their families and educators.

M. Bradley Rogers, Jr., Headmaster
Bekah D Atkinson, Admissions Director

8790 Marist Brothers Mid-Hudson Valley Camp Marist Brothers
1455 Broadway, 9W
Esopus, NY 12429
845-384-6620
Fax: 845-384-6479
e-mail: kids2@esopuscamps.com
www.esopuscamps.com

Individual camps serve different special people: Special Children Camps 1 & 2; Deaf Camp; Young Adult Camp; Sacred Heart Camp; Sr. Pat's Camp; Camp Hope; Molloy Freshman Camp; and Adult Vacation. Cost varies.

Brother Don Nugent, President
Frances Rurley, Coordinator

8791 Oakhurst
853 Broadway
New York, NY
212-253-8680

Accepts children and young adults who are physically handicapped, ages 8-18. The program includes physical therapy, recreational activities and a work program for teenagers.

Marvin Raps

8792 Programs for Children with Special Health Care Needs
Tower Building
Albany, NY
518-474-2084
e-mail: cx104@health.state.ny.us

Claudia Lee, Acting Director

8793 Programs for Infants and Toddlers with Disabilities: Ages Birth Through 2
Box 2000
Albany, NY 12220
518-473-7016
800-698-4543
TTY: 877-898-5849
e-mail: dmn02@health.state.ny.us
www.autismgateway.com/resources_NY.html
Donna M Noyes, PhD, Director

8794 Ramapo Anchorage Camp
PO Box 266, Rt. 52/Salisbury Turnpike

Residential program which serves children, ages 4-16, with a wide range of emotional, behavoral, and learning problems. A one-to-one ratio of counselors-to-campers enables children to build healthy relationships, increase self-esteem and improve learning skills. Character values such as honesty, concern for others, responsibility, and the courage to do one's best are encouraged. Campers demonstrate significant gains in their ability to maintain relationships, control impulses and adjust.

8795 Wagon Road
Children's Aid Society
431 Quaker Road
Chappaqua, NY 10514
914-238-4761
Fax: 914-238-0714
www.childrensaidsociety.org

Provides residential respite services to developmentally disabled children ages 7-18. At its 50 acre campus which is entirely wheelchair accessible, 24 hour RN and MD services are provided.

Phoebe Boyer, President & CEO
William D. Weisberg, PhD, EVP & COO
Dan Lehman, VP & CFO

North Carolina

8796 Camp Winding Gap
Rural Route 1, Box 56
Lake Toxaway, NC
828-966-4520
Fax: 828-883-8720
www.campwindinggap.com

For boys and girls ages 8-16, with facilities for up to 75 campers. A high staff-camper ratio (less than 1 to 3) of carefully selected counselors provides a nurturing family atmosphere. A few children with disabilities are mainstreamed each session. Must be able to handle horseback riding and rugged terrain, this is a ranch type camp in a farm setting with many animals. Program includes regular camp activities.

Ann Hertzberg, Director

8797 Talisman Programs
64 Gap Creek Road
Zirconia, NC 28790
828-669-8639
888-458-8226
Fax: 828-669-2521
e-mail: summer@stonemountainschool.com
www.talismansummercamp.com

Talisman Programs offers summer programs for kids ages 8-17 with ADHD, learning disabilities, high functioning autism, or Aspergers Syndrome. Our high-adventure programs include paddling, hiking, rock climbing, an Alpine Tower, swimming, arts and crafts, and many other activities designed to promote communication and cooperation skills. We focus on building social skills and self esteem in 2 and 3 week programs. One session of academics.

Linda Tatsapaugh, Director

Ohio

8798 Camp Allyn
1414 Lake Allyn Road
Batavia, OH
513-732-0240
Fax: 513-735-1461
e-mail: ssc@one.net
www.steppingstonecenter.org

A camp for children and adults with disabilities.

Dennis Carter, Associated Director

8799 Highbrook Lodge Camp
12944 Aquilla Road
Chardon, OH
216-791-8118
Fax: 216-791-1101
e-mail: mmullin@clevelandsightcenter.org
www.clevelandsightcenter.org

A summer residential camp for blind and disabled children, adults and families.

Mike Mullin, Director

Oregon

8800 Easter Seals Oregon Camping Program
5757 SW Macadam Avenue
Portland, OR 800-5
503-228-5108
Fax: 503-228-1352
e-mail: camp@oregonseals.org
www.kidscamps.com

8801 Mt Hood Kiwanis Camp
9320 SW Barbur Blvd, Suite 165
Portland, OR 97219
503-272-3288
Fax: 503-452-0062
www.kidscamps.com

Pennsylvania

8802 Briarwood Day Camp
1380 Creek Road
Furlong, PA 18925
215-598-7143
Fax: 215-598-9813
e-mail: info@briarwood-camp.com
www.briarwood-camp.com

A comprehensive day camp providing lunch and transportation for children with disabilities.

Ted Levin

8803 Camp Lee Mar
450 Route 590
Lackawaxen, PA
570-685-7188
Fax: 570-685-7590
e-mail: gtour400@aol.com
www.leemar.com

A camp for children with developmental challenges, ages 5-21. Offers a program of academics, speech therapy, vocational training and recreation. The academic program is designed to help each child develop skills in the areas of communication, reading and math. Activities include swimming, boating, team sports, tennis and perceptual motor training.

Ari Segal, MSW, Director
Lynsey Trohoske, BA, Asst. Dir./ Admissions Director
Laura Leibowitz, BA, M.Ed, Asst. Dir./ Academic Coordinator

8804 Camp Yomeca Upper Perkiomen Valley YMCA
476 Pottstown Avenue
Pennsburg, PA 18073
215-679-9622
e-mail: drothenberger@fvymca.org
www.fvymca.org/youth/

The YMCA day camp for children ages 4-18. Small group and camp-wide activities are offered. Streams, woods and trails to explore. Children ages 10-12 also have several overnights offered to them during the summer. Children continue to build upon established skills from earlier years, take on more leadership, challenge and responsibility and strengthen past friendships.

Debbie Rothensberger, Camp Contact; School Age Care Dir

8805 Keystone Community Resources
100 Abington Executive Park
Carks Summit, PA 18411
570-702-8000
Fax: 570-702-8093
e-mail: LCunningham@keycommres.com
www.keycommres.com

Keystone serves both children and adults with developmental disabilities in a variety of residential settings. Support services include 24 hour supervision, on site nursing services, special and therapeutic recreation programs and psychological and psychiatric services.

Robert Fleese, President
Lisa Cunningham, Director Admissions
Ignatz Deutsch, Founder

8806 Variety Club Camp & Development Center
Variety Club
PO Box 609, 2950 Potshop Road

Year-round camping and recreation facility for children with special needs and their families. Includes summer camping, aquatics, weekend retreats and other specialty programs.

South Carolina

8807 Burnt Gin Camp
SC Department of Health and Environmental Control
Box 101106
Columbia, SC
803-898-0455
Fax: 803-898-0613
e-mail: aimonemi@columb60.dhec.state.sc.us
www.scdhec.net/hs/mch/burntgin/hsbgin5.htm

A residental camp for children who have physical disabilities and/or chronic illnesses. Camper/staff ratio is 2:1. Four seven-day sesssions for 7-15 year olds and two six-day sesssions for 16-19 year olds. Limited to residents of South Carolina.

Marie I Aimone, Camp Director

Tennessee

8808 Camp Easter Seal
750 Old Hickory Blvd, #2-260
Brentwood, TN 37027
615-292-6640
Fax: 615-251-0994
www.tn.easter-seals.org

John Pfeiffer, Chair
Chuck Mataya, Vice Chair
Rita Baumgartner, President & CEO

Texas

8809 Children's Association for Maxiumum Potential CAMP
PO Box 27086
San Antonio, TX 78227
210-671-5411
Fax: 210-671-5225
e-mail: campmail@campcamp.org
www.campcamp.org

Overnight camping, day-care, respite and rehabilitation to children with severe medical, physical or mental disabilities. Large medical staff enables nationwide acceptance of children with severe problems.

Mike Zerda, Chair
Susan Osborne, Executive Director
Ben Elble, Camp Director

8810 Hughen Center
2849 9th Avenue
Port Arthur, TX 77642
409-983-6659
Fax: 409-983-6408
www.hughencenter.org/contact_us

The Center provides a therapeutic, educational, and recreational program for children with physical disabilities. Physical and occupational therapy are featured. Day and residential.

Jeff Kuchar, Executive Director

8811 Texas Lions Camp
Lions Clubs of Texas
PO Box 290247
Kerrville, TX 78029
830-896-8500
830-896-8500
Fax: 830-896-3666
e-mail: tlc@ktc.com
www.lionscamp.com

The primary purpose of Texas Lions camp is to provide, without charge, a camp for physically disabled, hearing/vision impaired and diabetic children from the State of Texas, regardless of race, religion, or national origin. Our goal is to create an atmosphere wherein campers will learn the can do philosophy and be allowed to achieve maximum personal growth and self esteem. The camp welcomes boys and girls ages 7-16.

Stephen Mabry, Executive Director
Doug Parker, Business Manager
Steven King, Program/Client Service Director

Utah

8812 Camp Kostopulos
4180 Emigration Canyon Road
Salt Lake City, UT 84108   801-582-0700
                                                   Fax: 801-583-5176
                                                     www.campk.org

One of only a few camps in the Intermountain region that provides recreational opportunities for individuals of all ages with mental or physical disabilities. Activities include fifteen days of swimming, fishing, fieldtrips, nature study, arts and crafts and traditional outdoor adventure games. Five year-round programs offered.

John Miller, Chairman
Rick Lifferth, Vice Chairman
Layne Smith, Vice Chairman

Vermont

8813 Farm and Wilderness Camps
HCR 70, Box 27
Plymouth, VT   802-422-3761
                                                        802-422-3761
                                                   Fax: 802-422-8660
                                                   www.kidscamps.com

Virginia

8814 Camp Baker Services
7600 Beach Road
Chesterfield, VA   804-748-4789
                                                   Fax: 804-796-6889
                        www.veryspecialcamps.com/summer-camps/Camp-Baker-Ser

Year round support services for children and adults with disabilities. Operated by the Richmond Area ARC, programs include: an 8-week summer camp program; weekend congregate respite services; summer day camp (8 wks); spring fling (spring break).

Melissa Wahers, Director
Jolene Loving, Assistant Director
Heather Elliot, Administrative Assistant

8815 Camp Easter Seal East, Camp Easter Seal We st
201 E Main Street
Salem, VA 800-3   540-362-1656
                                                   Fax: 540-563-8928
                                              www.campeasterseal-va.org

Six and 12 day summer camp sessions for children and adults ages 5 and older with physical disabilities, cognitive disabilities, sensory impairments. Therapeutic recreation activities including swimming, fishing, sports, horseback riding, rock climbing, and more. 26 speech therapy camp children with disabilities ages 8-16. 12 day Spina Bifida Self Help Skills Camp.

Deborah Duerk, Director
Devin Brown, Director

8816 Camp Holiday Trails
400 Holiday Trails Lane
Charlottesville, VA 22903   434-977-3781
                                                   Fax: 434-977-8814
                    e-mail: info@campholidaytrails.org, campisgood@c
                                             www.campholidaytrails.org

A nonprofit camp for children with special health needs, various chronic illnesses. Residential, 1 and 2 week sessions are open June - August; camperships are available. Coed 5-17, nationwide and international. Canoeing, swimming, horseback riding, arts and crafts, drama, ropes course, etc. 24-hr. medical supervision by doctor and nursing staff. Air conditioned cabins.

Tina LaRoche, Executive Director

8817 Makemie Woods Camp Conference Center
PO Box 39
Barhamsville, VA 23011   757-566-1496
                                                        800-566-1496
                                                   Fax: 757-566-8803
                                            e-mail: mike@makwoods.org
                                                   www.makwoods.org

Counselors serve as teachers, friends and activity leaders. The individual is important within the small group. No camper is lost in the crowd, but is an integral partner in the group process. Residential Christian Camp and conference center. Summer camp for children 8-18 special camp for children with diabetes.

Michelle Burcher, Director
Beth Martin, Office Assistant

8818 Overlook
RR 1, Box 203
Keezletown, VA   540-269-2267

A Christian life experience for youth and children, located at the base of the scenic Massanutten Mountains.

Ronald Robey

8819 Triangle D Camp for Children
1701 North Beauregard Street
Alexandria, VA 22311   414-248-1330
                                                        800-342-2383

Disabled campers.

Marilyn Caras

West Virginia

8820 Mountain Milestones Stepping Stones
15 Cottage Street
Morgantown, WV 800-9   304-296-0150
                                                        800-800-982
                                                   Fax: 304-296-0194
                                         e-mail: stepping@westco.net
                                                   www.kidscamps.com

A nonprofit organization.

Missy Weimex, Recreation Coordinator

Wisconsin

8821 Camp Joy
W7725 Kettle Moraine Drive
Whitewater, WI 53190   262-473-3132
                                                   Fax: 262-473-0941
                                                     www.campjoy.org

A year round residential camping program for children and adults with mental retardation and physical disabilities. Brochure, video, and application available upon request.

Charlie Hatchett, Camp Director
Todd Hatchett, Program & Promotion
Dannett Smith, JBCF Secretary & Promotion

8822 Timbertop Nature Adventure Camp
1000 Division Street
Stevens Point, WI 54481   715-342-2980
                                                   Fax: 715-342-2987

For children who can benefit from an individualized program of learning in a non-competitive outdoor setting under the skilled leadership of people who understand the environment and the unique potential of these children.

Grant a Wish Foundations

8823 Children's Dream Factory of Maine
400 US Route 1, ATTN: Doris Simard
Falmouth, ME 04105   207-781-3406
                                                        800-639-1492

Grants wishes for chronically or seriously ill children from Maine.

8824 Children's Wish Foundation
8615 Roswell Rd
Atlanta, GA 30350
770-393-WISH
800-323-WISH
Fax: 770-393-0683
www.childrenswish.org

Atlanta-based organization that grants wishes for children with life-threatening illnesses who have not yet reached their 18th birthday. Focuses primarily on children who reside in Florida, but has also granted wishes to children from other parts of the US, Canada, England, and Russia.

8825 Dream Factory
120 W Broadway, Suite 300
Louisville, KY 40202
502-561-3001
800-456-7556
Fax: 502-561-3004
e-mail: dfinfo@dreamfactoryinc.org
www.dreamfactoryinc.org

The Dream Factory grants dreams to children disagnosed with critical or chronic illnesses who are 3 through 18 years of age.

David Zukowski, Director of Program Services
Janice Harris, President
Ralph Coldiron, Vice President

8826 Famous Fone Friends
9101 Sawyer Street
Los Angeles, CA 90035
310-204-5683
e-mail: fonefriends@aol.com
www.famousfonefriends.org

Offers the ability for a sick child's doctor or nurse to arrange for a well-known actor, athlete or other celebrity to call the child.

8827 Freedom's Wings International
324 Charles Street
Coopersberg, PA 18036
800-382-1197
e-mail: rrfucci@earthlink.net
www.freedomswings.org

Freedom's Wings International (FWI) is a non-profit organization run by and for people with physical disabilities. We provide the opportunity for those who are physically challenged to fly in specially adapted sailplanes, either as a passenger or as a member of the flight training program.

8828 Give Kids the World
210 S Bass Road
Kissimmee, FL 34746
407-396-1114
800-995-5437
Fax: 407-396-1207
e-mail: dream@gktw.org
www.gktw.org

Makes dreams come true for children with life-threatening illnesses and their families with a week-long, cost-free fantasy vacation to our 'story book' village located near central Florida's most beloved attractions.

Sarah Jones, Communications Manager

8829 Magic Moments- Children's Hospital of Alabama
2112 11th Aves., Ste 219
Birmingham, AL 35205
205-939-9372
Fax: 205-939-6717
e-mail: info@magicmoments.org
www.magicmoments.org

Grants wishes to children four to nineteen living or being treated in Alabama, who have chronic, life-threatening diseases, or who have severe trauma (burns, spinal cord, head trauma).

8830 Make A Wish Foundation of America
4742 N 24th St, Ste 400
Pheonix, AZ 85016
602-279-9474
800-722-9474
Fax: 602-279-0855
www.wish.org

Information and advocacy resources for families and professionals. Includes listings of organizations providing general information and organizations focusing on more specific areas of concern to families and young adults who have disabilities.

8831 Sunshine Foundation
1041 Mill Creek Drive
Feasterville, PA 19053
215-396-4770
800-767-1976
Fax: 215-396-4774
e-mail: philly@sunshinefoundation.org
www.sunshinefoundation.org

Grants dreams of seriously ill, physically challenged and abused children ages 3-18 whose parents cannot fulfill their request due to the financial strain caused by the child's illness.

Diane Mazzeo, Admin Assistant

8832 Teddi Project
Camp Good Days and Special Times
356 North Midler Avenue
Syracuse, NY 13206
315-434-9477
Fax: 315-434-9590
www.campgooddays.org

Priority given to children from Central Florida and the upstate New York area, especially Buffalo, Rochester, Syracuse, Albany, and Binghamton. Services chronically or terminally ill children ages seven to seventeen.

8833 Thursday's Child
PO Box 95
Mt. Hope, WI 53816
608-988-4234
e-mail: dorothyf@chorus.net

Grants wishes to seriously ill children who live in or are being treated in southwest and south central Wisconsin.

8834 Wish Upon a Star
California Law Enforcement
PO Box 4000
Visalia, CA 93278
559-733-7753
Fax: 559-733-0962
e-mail: info@wishuponastar.org
www.wishuponastar.org

Serves children in the state of California. Nonprofit, law enforcement effort designed to grant wishes of children afflicted with high-risk and terminal illnesses.

Carmen Perez, Executive Director

8835 Wish with Wings
3817 Alamo Ave
Ft. Worth, TX 76107
817-469-9474
Fax: 817-275-6005
e-mail: wish@awishwithwings.org
www.awishwithwings.org

Founded in 1982, grants wishes for children ages three-eighteen years of age who have life threatening diseases. The organization serves children who reside in or are receiving treatment in the state of Texas.

Kim Christian, Executive Director

8836 Wishing Star Foundation
139 S Sherman
Spokane, WA 99202
509-744-3411
Fax: 509-744-3414
e-mail: info@wishingstar.org
www.wishingstar.org

Serves Idaho, eastern and western Washington. Grants wishes to children ages three to twenty-one with life-threatening diseases.

Paula Nordgaarden, Executive Director

8837 Wishing Well Foundation
3000 West Esplanade Ave, Ste 100
Metaine, LA 70002
888-663-9474
www.wishingwellusa.org

Grants wishes to children in the St. Louis area only who are chronically or terminally ill.

Description

Cardiovascular

The cardiovascular system, also known as the circulatory system, consists of the heart and the blood vessels. The functions of the cardiovascular system include the following:

- To maintain the continual flow of blood throughout the body to provide cells with oxygen and vital nutrients

- To assist in the removal of carbon dioxide and other waste products from cells

The Heart

Anatomy

The heart, a hollow, muscular organ the approximate size and shape of a clenched fist, is an efficient pump that maintains the continuous flow of blood through the vessels to all areas of the body. It is located between the lungs in approximately the center of the chest, with its right margin located under the right side of the breastbone (sternum) and the remaining areas pointing toward the left. The "tip" or the lowest point of the heart, known as the apex, rests on the diaphragm and is situated beneath the left nipple.

The heart consists of four chambers and is divided into left and right sides by a thick, fibrous, central partition known as the septum. The upper chambers of the heart are known as atria, and the lower chambers are called ventricles. Each chamber is referred to by its location: i.e., the left and right atria and the left and right ventricles. The atria are smaller and have thinner walls than the ventricles. The walls of the chambers of the heart are composed of specialized cardiac muscle known as the myocardium, and their internal surfaces are lined with a thin layer of smooth membrane tissue called the endocardium.

The heart and the roots of its major blood vessels are surrounded by a membrane (pericardium) that consists of two fibrous layers. The pericardium has a tough outer layer (fibrous pericardium) that surrounds the heart like a loose-fitting bag, providing space for the heart to beat. The inner layer (serous pericardium) consists of an innermost "sheet" (visceral layer) that is attached to the heart and an outermost layer (parietal layer) that lines the inside of the fibrous pericardium. A space between the inner layers contains a thin film of fluid that lubricates the opposing surfaces of the inner membranes, enabling the heart to beat without friction.

Cardiac Function

Contraction of the heart muscle is termed systole, whereas relaxation is known as diastole. The atria and ventricles beat in a precise rhythmic pattern. One cycle of this pattern is known as a heartbeat. As the atria contract, they force blood into the ventricles. Once the ventricles fill with blood, they contract, pumping blood either to the lungs or out to the rest of the body.

The pumping action of the heart also involves the heart valves at the entrance to and exit from the ventricles. These valves control and direct the flow of blood through the heart. Two heart valves separate the atria from the ventricles (atrioventricular valves), preventing the backward flow of blood into the atria during ventricular contraction. The valves include the mitral or bicuspid valve, situated between the left atrium and left ventricle, and the tricuspid valve, located between the right atrium and right ventricle. In addition, two heart valves (semilunar valves) are situated between the two ventricles and the large blood vessels that transport blood away from the heart during ventricular contractions. The aortic semilunar valve, located where the major artery of the body (aorta) arises from the base of the left ventricle, enables blood to flow from the left ventricle into the aorta while preventing the backward flow of blood into the ventricle. The pulmonary semilunar valve, situated where the pulmonary artery arises from the base of the right ventricle, enables blood to flow from the right ventricle to the lungs while preventing the backward flow of blood.

"Oxygen-poor" or deoxygenated blood that has circulated through the body enters the right side of the heart into the right atrium through two large veins (the superior and inferior vena cava). The blood is then pumped through the tricuspid valve into the right ventricle. When the ventricle contracts, blood is pumped through the pulmonary semilunar valve into the pulmonary artery and on to the lungs, where the exchange of oxygen and carbon dioxide occurs. Oxygen-rich blood is returned to the left atrium by way of four pulmonary veins and is pumped through the bicuspid valve into the left ventricle. When the ventricle contracts, blood is pumped through the aortic semilunar valve into the aorta for circulation to the body's tissues.

The heart muscle or myocardium requires an ongoing supply of oxygen and other nutrients to function efficiently; thus, the coronary circulation transports vital oxygen-rich (oxygenated) and nutrient-rich arterial blood to the heart muscle and returns deoxygenated, nutrient-poor blood back to the venous system. Blood is transported to the myocardium by way of the left and right coronary arteries, which are the first branches of the aorta. Once blood is circulated to the myocardium, supplying the heart with oxygen and other nutrients, it passes into the cardiac veins, which then empty into the coronary sinus and into the right atrium.

Each heartbeat, also known as a cardiac cycle, consists of the contraction (systole) and relaxation (diastole) of the atria and ventricles. In order for the heart to pump efficiently, the different areas of the heart and the cardiac muscle fibers must work together in an exact sequence. Precise coordination is achieved through the transmission of electrical impulses originating from the heart's "pacemaker" (the sinoatrial node at the apex of the right atrium). These signals are then relayed to the various areas of the heart via a complex system of fibers (atrioventricular node, bundle of His, and Purkinje fibers). The electrical transmissions are delivered with precision timing to various areas of the heart, resulting in a rhythmic beat.

The Blood Vessels

Blood vessels are like a system of complex tubing of different sizes through which blood flows to various parts of the body. Different types of blood vessels have different purposes. For example:

- Some vessels ensure the movement of blood from one part of the body to another.

- Other much smaller vessels (i.e., the capillaries) facilitate the exchange of certain nutrients and waste products between the blood and the fluid surrounding cells within bodily tissues.

Function

There are several types of blood vessels including arteries, arterioles, capillaries, venules, and veins. The arteries, which carry blood away from the heart, progressively subdivide into smaller and smaller vessels known as arterioles, which control blood flow into the minute vessels known as capillaries. The arterioles help to regulate proper arterial blood distribution and pressure by constricting or expanding as necessary. The thin walls of microscopic capillaries facilitate the exchange of nutrients and waste products between the blood and tissue fluid surrounding the cells. For example, oxygen and glucose move from the blood in the capillaries to the fluid surrounding cells and then into the cells themselves; in contrast, carbon dioxide and other waste products move from the cells into the blood within the capillaries. The oxygen-poor blood then flows from the capillaries into the small blood vessels known as venules. The venules join with other venules and progressively increase in size, becoming larger veins that transport the blood toward the heart.

The systemic circulation also includes a specialized group of vessels known as the hepatic portal circulation, within which blood flow follows a somewhat different route. Veins from certain organs, such as the stomach, intestines, spleen, pancreas, and gallbladder, do not transport blood directly into the inferior vena cava but, rather, into the hepatic portal vein, which carries blood to veins, venules, and capillaries within the liver. Nutrients pass from the blood in the capillaries into liver cells where various toxic substances are filtered from the blood. Hepatic veins carry blood from

the liver and rejoin the systemic circulation via the inferior vena cava.

Structure

Arteries and veins consist of three layers including an outermost layer (tunica adventitia), a middle layer of smooth muscle (involuntary muscle) tissue (tunica media), and an inner lining (tunica intima or endothelium). The middle layer of arteries is thicker than that of veins, enabling the arteries to withstand the pressure of ventricular contractions. In contrast, blood returning to the heart via the veins remains at a relatively low pressure. The passage of blood through the veins is assisted by involuntary muscle that compresses the walls of the veins; in addition, veins have one-way valves that prevent the backward flow of blood.

Capillaries have extremely thin walls and cannot be seen by the naked eye. They consist of only one layer (tunica intima), enabling oxygen and certain wastes to easily pass through them.

Fetal Blood Circulation

Because the developing fetus must obtain nutrients and oxygen from the mother's blood, the fetal circulation differs somewhat from the circulation after birth. During pregnancy, blood vessels carry fetal blood to the placenta, where oxygen and nutrients are exchanged between the fetal and maternal blood supply, and then return blood to the fetus. Two relatively small umbilical arteries carry deoxygenated blood, whereas a larger umbilical vein carries oxygen-rich blood. The fetal circulation also includes vascular channels or openings (e.g., ductus venosus, ductus arteriosus, foramen ovale), enabling most blood to bypass the developing liver and lungs. In most cases, once an infant is born and the pulmonary circulation is established, such vascular channels close and the umbilical blood vessels collapse soon after birth.

Description

Cells

The human body consists of literally trillions of atoms, molecules, and cells that are organized in several "structural levels."

Atoms and molecules. Atoms of oxygen, sodium, nitrogen, and carbon, for example, are the infinitesimal components of the most basic level of living matter of the body. Atoms link to one another to form molecules.

Cells. These are the smallest structural units that are able to live independently. The human body has billions of cells that are functionally integrated to perform the complex, vital tasks necessary for sustaining life. Cells are organized in the following ways:

- Tissues. Bodily tissues are organizations of structurally similar, specialized cells that carry out a common function.

- Organs. The organs of the body are groupings of two or more different types of tissues incorporated into a functional, structural unit to perform certain, specialized functions.

- Bodily systems. These comprise the final level of structural organization within the body. Bodily systems consist of several, interdependent organs that work together to perform integrated functions.

Certain mechanisms enable cells of the body to conduct activities that are vital for ongoing growth and survival. These include the processes of metabolism and homeostasis.

Metabolism

Metabolism refers to all the physical and chemical processes occurring within the body's tissues and includes catabolism and anabolism. Catabolism refers to the breakdown of large, complex substances into simpler, smaller substances, usually resulting in the release of energy. During anabolism, complex substances are built up from simpler substances, usually resulting in consumption of energy. The processes of respiration, circulation, digestion, and excretion, for example, collectively enable the body to provide those substances required for metabolism and remove the byproducts or waste products of metabolism. Abnormal changes in genetic material (mutations) or inherited defective genes may cause inborn errors of metabolism, affecting the body's ability to function properly.

Homeostasis

Homeostasis refers to the processes by which the body maintains a balanced internal environment (equilibrium). In order to maintain homeostasis, the body requires oxygen, water, other nutrients, and regulated atmospheric pressure and body temperature, for example. Because disturbances from the external environment as well as cellular activity continually challenge internal equilibrium, the body has ongoing self-regulating systems (feedback systems) that induce the responses necessary to maintain or restore homeostasis. For example, abnormally decreased levels of oxygen in the blood are counteracted by increased breathing rates that restore normal blood oxygen levels.

Cells

Cells are extremely complex, containing several subcellular structures vital to life. Human cells vary greatly in size and shape and are adapted for their specific functions. However, most cells are similar in structure. They contain fluid material known as cytoplasm surrounded by a thin, outer membrane (plasma membrane). The plasma membrane separates the fluid and specialized structures (organelles) within each cell from the fluid that surrounds and bathes the cells of the body. The cytoplasm of most human cells contains a circular, membrane-bound structure known as the nucleus.

Plasma Membrane

The plasma membrane serves to keep cells intact. In addition, it regulates the entry of oxygen and certain vital nutrients into cells and enables the passage of carbon dioxide and other waste materials out of cells. Certain protein molecules on the surface of the plasma membrane also bind with other protein molecules, activating particular cellular functions.

Cytoplasm

The cytoplasm is essentially the "living matter" of the cell, containing the fluid that comprises the cell's inner environment and the specialized parts known as organelles. The organelles include the following:

- Ribosomes are relatively tiny particles that function as "protein factories." They produce proteins, which are large molecules consisting of combinations of certain chemical "building blocks" (amino acids). Proteins play an essential role in the body. Particular proteins serve as the source of "building materials" for certain tissues and organs of the body (e.g., muscle, skin, blood, etc.). Other protein compounds known as enzymes accelerate the rate of chemical reactions in the body. Proteins also play an essential role in the elimination of waste materials and have many other functions.

- Endoplasmic reticulum (ER) is a complex network of small tubular membranes arranged in complex folds. This network winds throughout the cytoplasm of a cell. Passageways within the endoplasmic reticulum transport proteins and other substances to different areas within a cell. Rough ER has a rough texture due to the presence of ribosomes attached to its outer surface. Carbohydrates, fats, and certain types of proteins are manufactured within smooth ER.

- The Golgi apparatus, which is located near the nucleus, is a system of microscopic, stacked membranous sacs and spaces. Small "bubbles" or sacs (vesicles) from the smooth ER transport newly produced proteins to the Golgi apparatus, where they fuse with the Golgi sacs. The Golgi apparatus then processes and modifies the proteins and packages them into small vesicles. These vesicles break away and eventually fuse with the plasma membrane, at which point they break open and release their contents outside of the cell for transport to other cells.

- Centrioles are typically paired rod-like structures that participate in cell division.

- Mitochondria are tiny organelles that have double membranes and sacs with inner, folded partitions. Known as the "power plants" of the cells, the mitochondria serve as the major source of cellular energy production due to their complex, ongoing chemical reactions.

- Lysosomes are the major digestive units of cells. Enzymes within lysosomes break down (digest) particles of nutrients as well as certain invading particles such as bacteria.

- Cilia are hair-like projections on the surfaces of certain cells that move together in a wave-like manner. For example, cilia within the mucous membranes of the respiratory tract (respiratory mucosa) propel mucus upward and out of the tract.

Nucleus

The nucleus regulates cellular activities by controlling the functions of the organelles and cell reproduction. It is surrounded by a nuclear envelope that encloses a cellular material within the nucleus known as nucleoplasm. Pores within the nuclear envelope's membranes enable the interior of the nucleus to "communicate" with the cell's cytoplasm. The nucleoplasm of the nucleus contains several structures including the nucleolus and chromatin.

The nucleolus regulates the formation of ribosomes within the nucleus. Ribosomes then move through the nuclear envelope to the cell's cytoplasm where they engage in protein production.

Chromatin, the material within the nucleus from which chromosomes are created, consists of thread-like structures comprised of protein and deoxyribonucleic acid (DNA). DNA is the carrier of the genetic code and is described as a "double helix" because of its relatively long, spiraling, lad-

der-like structure. It consists of strands of certain chemical groups that are linked by pairs of substances known as "bases." There are four types of bases including adenine, which always pairs with thymine, and the base cytosine, which always pairs with guanine. Therefore, the sequence of bases on one strand of the helix coincides with the sequence on the other strand, enabling DNA molecules to duplicate before cell division.

Chromosomes

During the division and reproduction of cells, DNA condenses and gradually forms into the rod-like structures known as chromosomes. The DNA of the chromosomes carries the genetic information that controls the ultimate growth, development, and functioning of the body and determines the expression of certain inherited traits, such as blood groups, various physical characteristics (e.g., hair color, eye color, height), etc.

The cell that is produced when an egg (ovum) is fertilized by a sperm is known as a zygote. With the first and each subsequent division of the zygote, chromosomes within the zygote's nucleus are duplicated. Therefore, in most cases, all cells in the human body contain the same chromosomal material. In rare cases, some individuals may have some cells that contain differences in certain genetic material (mosaicism) due to an error in cellular division.

The nuclei of cells (except for ova and sperm) normally contain 46 individual chromosomes, one of each pair from the mother and the other from the father. Chromosome pairs are numbered from 1 to 22 with a 23rd pair consisting of one X chromosome from the mother and an X or a Y chromosome from the father. Males have an X and a Y chromosome and females have two X chromosomes within the 23rd pair. Each chromosome has a long arm designated "q" and a short arm designated "p." Both arms are further divided into numbered bands. Every individual chromosome contains thousands of genes, which are the hereditary units that contain segments of DNA. Genes function within cells by regulating the production of proteins. The 46 human chromosomes collectively contain approximately 100,000 genes that, together, are referred to as the "human genome."

Chromosomal Disorders

In some cases, due to certain abnormalities during cellular division (meiosis or mitosis), individuals may have abnormalities in the structure or number of chromosomes in the nuclei of cells of the body. There may be extra or missing whole chromosomes or chromosomal material within all or some of the body's cells. Because chromosomes contain many genes, the range and severity of associated symptoms and physical findings may vary greatly, depending upon the exact nature and location of the chromosomal abnormality.

RNA

Genes, which are sections of DNA, regulate the production of certain proteins. Ribonucleic acid or RNA is essential in "decoding" the inherited instructions within genes. RNA is similar in structure to one strand of DNA, with some differences-e.g., replacement of the base thymine with uracil. During the formation of RNA, a strand of DNA "unwinds" and a duplicate copy of a gene sequence is created. This copy is known as messenger RNA or mRNA. The mRNA migrates from the nucleus to the cytoplasm, promoting protein production in the ribosomes and endoplasmic reticulum. The ribosomes use information within the mRNA molecule to translate chemical "building blocks" known as amino acids into a properly sequenced protein strand.

Cellular Reproduction: Mitosis

Most cells of the body are replicated or reproduced during a complex process known as mitosis. During mitosis, a single cell divides in order to form two "daughter cells" with chromosomes identical to those within the original cell. The process of mitosis enables the body to produce new cells, to replace cells that have been damaged or lost due to injury or disease, and to replace cells that have aged and no longer function efficiently.

Sometimes mitosis may become uncontrolled, resulting in the development of an abnormal mass of replicating cells known as a neoplasm. Such growths may be noncancerous (benign tumors) or cancerous (malignant).

Cellular Reproduction: Meiosis

Reproductive cells in the male and female sex glands (gonads, including the testes and ovaries) carry out a different form of cell division known as meiosis. During mitosis, one cell division occurs, creating two daughter cells-each of which contains 46 chromosomes. Unlike mitosis, two cellular divisions occur during meiosis, resulting in four daughter cells-each of which contains half of the chromosomes (i.e., 23 chromosomes).

Genetic Mutations

During the processes of mitosis and meiosis, the chromosomes within an original cell and thus its genetic material (DNA) are replicated and passed along to its daughter cells. Sometimes, errors may occur during this replication process, resulting in small changes or mutations in genetic composition. Such genetic mutations are passed along with every subsequent division of the daughter cell. For example, a genetic mutation may occur during the production of a reproductive cell (ovum or sperm). If that cell is eventually involved in fertilization, the resultant zygote and all of its reproduced cells will contain the same genetic error. Thus, every cell of the developing embryo and fetus will contain the identical mutant gene.

Genes function within cells by directing the manufacture of a particular protein. Therefore, mutations of a particular gene may impair the appropriate production of its protein. The effects of a particular gene mutation depend upon the function of its protein within the body. Disorders that result due to such mutations are termed genetic disorders.

Genetic Disorders

Human traits are the result of the interaction of two genes, one received from the mother and one received from the father. There are typically two genes engaged in the regulation of a particular protein. If one such gene changes or mutates and "overrides" the instructions of the normal gene on the other chromosome, the abnormal gene is said to be dominant. If the mutated gene is not expressed and is "masked" by the normal gene on the other chromosome, the mutated gene is termed recessive. In such cases, two copies of the mutated gene are required for possible expression of the disease trait.

Genetic disorders may be classified into unifactorial and multifactorial defects. Unifactorial genetic disorders result due to abnormalities of a single gene or gene pair. Such disorders may be autosomal or X-linked.

In autosomal dominant disorders, the presence of a single copy of the disease gene results in the disorder. The mutated gene "overrides" or dominates the other normal gene. An affected individual may have inherited the disease gene from one of his or her parents, or the disease may arise as a result of an abnormal change (mutation) that occurred randomly, for unknown reasons (sporadically). If an individual with an autosomal dominant disorder has children, all offspring have a 50 percent risk of inheriting the defective gene.

In autosomal recessive disorders, two copies of the same disease gene are necessary for an individual to potentially develop the disorder. If both parents carry a single copy of the disease gene, all offspring have a 25 percent risk of inheriting both disease genes and expressing the disorder. Fifty percent of their children risk being carriers, and 25 percent may receive both normal genes for that trait.

In X-linked disorders, the disease gene is located on the X chromosome. As discussed earlier, females have two X chromosomes, whereas males have one X chromosome from the mother and one Y chromosome from the father. In females, certain disease traits on the X chromosome may be "masked" by the presence of a normal gene on the other X chromosome. In other cases, certain disease traits may not be fully masked by the normal gene; as a result, some females who carry a single copy of such a disease gene (heterozygous carriers) may express some of the symptoms associated with the disorder. In such cases, heterozygous females often have more variable, less severe symptoms than affected males. Because males have only one X chromosome, if they inherit such a disease gene, they generally express the physical characteristics or other findings associated with the disease and are typically more severely affected than females. Males with X-linked disorders transmit the disease gene to their daughters but not to their sons. Females with one copy of such a disease gene have a 50 percent risk of transmitting the gene to their daughters and their sons.

In multifactorial disorders, susceptibility to a disorder is determined by the interaction of several different genes, possibly in association with the involvement of certain environmental factors.

Tissues

As mentioned above, tissues are groups of structurally similar cells that perform a common function. Different tissues within the human body may vary greatly in terms of the size, shape, and specific functioning of their cells.

There are four main types of tissue in the human body including epithelial tissue, connective tissue, muscle tissue, and nervous tissue.

Epithelial tissue or epithelium covers the surfaces of the body, lines most of its hollow structures or cavities, and serves to provide protection and support. In addition, some epithelial tissues permit the absorption of certain nutrients (e.g., oxygen into the blood); help to protect the body against invading microorganisms; or produce and release certain secretions. The cells within epithelial tissue are tightly packed together and contain no blood vessels; however, blood vessels within underlying connective tissue provide epithelial cells with nutrients. Different types of epithelial tissue are categorized based upon cellular shape and thickness.

Connective Tissue

Connective Tissue

The purpose of connective tissue, the most widely distributed tissue of the body, is to bind together and, along with the skeleton, provide a supporting framework to bodily tissues and organs. The shape and arrangement of connective tissue cells and the intercellular substance between such cells differ depending upon the type of connective tissue. There are several major forms of connective tissue in the body including the following:

- Areolar tissue, which consists of cells embedded in webs of loosely arranged fibers, supports and provides form to most internal organs of the body.

- Adipose tissue, which consists of fat cells within a mesh of areolar tissue, serves to insulate the body against heat loss, protect and cushion certain areas of the body, and store fat as a future energy source.

- Fibrous connective tissue, which consists primarily of parallel rows of white collagen fibers, are the cords of strong, dense, flexible tissue that connect muscle to bone (tendons). Collagen is the major structural protein of the body.

- Bone, the hardest connective tissue of the body, provides a supportive framework, assists in movement, and houses bone marrow.

- Cartilage, which has the consistency of firm or gel-like plastic, helps to absorb shock and provides flexibility.

- Blood, interestingly, is considered to be a type of connective tissue. Even though it has a different function in comparison to other connective tissues, it does have an extracellular liquid matrix (plasma). Plasma has several functions including providing a defense against invading microorganisms, repairing damage to blood vessels and tissues through blood clotting, and transporting oxygen, vital nutrients, and waste products.

The purpose of the body's muscle tissue is to enable movement through muscle contraction and relaxation. The nervous tissue of the body includes specialized cells that ensure ongoing, rapid communication between structures of the body and the control of bodily functions necessary to maintain life.

Description

Dermatologic

The dermatologic system includes the skin, the largest organ of the body, and its derivatives, such as the skin glands, the hair, and the nails. The skin, the sheet-like, outermost covering of body tissue, has several vital functions:

- To serve as a sensory organ. The skin's millions of sensory nerve endings (receptors) serve as somatic sense organs, enabling the body to respond to pain, variations in temperature, pressure or touch sensations, and other important changes in the surrounding environment.

- To help protect the human body from the harmful effects of the sun, chemicals, invading microorganisms, injuries, fluid loss, and other hazards.

- To assist in normalizing the body's temperature through the regulation of blood flow close to the body's surface and sweat secretion. For example, when the body is too cold, blood vessels within the skin constrict to help conserve body heat. When the body is too hot, blood vessels within the inner layer of the skin (dermis) widen (dilate) and the sweat glands secrete perspiration to cool the body.

The skin comprises several tissue layers including a thin, outermost layer (epidermis); a thicker, inner layer (dermis); and a thick underlying layer of subcutaneous tissue, which is a loose layer of connective tissue and fat. The subcutaneous tissue helps to insulate the body from extremes in temperature, protects underlying tissues from injury, and serves as a stored energy source.

Epidermis
The epidermis, which serves as the protective outer layer of skin, is made up of tightly packed cells (epithelial cells) that are arranged in layers. The thickness of the epidermis is variable, depending on its function; for example, it is relatively thick on the palms of the hands, yet comparatively thin on the eyelids.

The outermost layer of the epidermis (stratum corneum epidermidis) consists of dead cells that create a tough, protective covering. As the dead cells are sloughed off, they are replaced by new cells that are produced by rapidly dividing cells within the innermost layer of the epidermis (stratum germinativum). As new cells rise upward though cellular layers (strata) and approach the surface, their cytoplasm-i.e., the inner substance of cells other than the nucleus-is replaced by the tough protein keratin. In addition, specialized cells (melanocytes) within the deepest layer of the epidermis produce melanin, a pigment that gives coloration to the skin.

Dermis
The dermis, the innermost layer of skin, consists of connective tissue; lymph vessels, blood vessels, sensory nerve endings (skin receptors), and muscle fibers; as well as other specialized structures, including sweat glands, sebaceous glands, and hair follicles.

The uppermost portion of the dermis contains rows of peg-like projections (dermal papillae) that help bind together the dermal and epidermal layers (dermal-epidermal junction) and form the characteristic grooves and ridges (dermatoglyphic patterns) on the skin of the palms and tips of the fingers. Such ridges, which are unique to each individual, develop before birth.

The deeper portion of the dermis contains a network of fibers including those that provide the skin with the necessary toughness (collagen fibers) as well as elasticity and the ability to stretch (elastic fibers). The number of elastic fibers decreases with advancing age and the level of fat stored within the subcutaneous tissue is also reduced. Consequently, the skin loses its elasticity.

Skin Glands
The sweat glands within the dermis are classified according to their location and type of secretion. These glands include the eccrine and apocrine glands.

The eccrine glands are the most widespread sweat glands in the body. Their function is to produce sweat or perspiration, which helps to eliminate certain waste products (e.g., uric acid, etc.) and to maintain a constant body temperature.

The apocrine glands, larger glands that produce a thicker secretion than that of the eccrine glands, are primarily located under the arms (axilla) and around the genitals. Such glands begin to function during puberty.

The dermis also contains sebaceous glands, tiny glands that open into hair follicles. They produce an oily secretion known as sebum that helps to lubricate the hair and skin and protect the skin from drying. Sebum secretion increases during adolescence (due to increased levels of certain sex hormones); however, it decreases during later adulthood, contributing to skin wrinkling and cracking.

Hair
When epidermal cells grow into the dermis, a small tube called a hair follicle may be formed. The growth of a hair begins from a tiny cluster of cells (hair papilla) at the base of the follicle. New hair replaces any that has been cut or plucked, for example, as long as the hair papilla is alive. The hair itself is a threadlike structure consisting of dead cells filled with keratin. The root is that portion of the hair that remains hidden within the follicle, whereas the shaft is the visible portion of the hair. A particular hair color results

from the amount and specific form of the pigment melanin that has been produced by melanocytes at the base of the hair follicle. The straightness or curliness of the hair depends upon the shape of the hair follicle.

A few areas of the body are hairless, including the palms of the hands, the soles of the feet, and the lips. Most hair on the body is fine and barely visible, with the most visible hair typically including that on the scalp, the eyebrows, and the eyelashes. Coarse hair also typically develops under the arms and in the pubic area during puberty (i.e., in response to the secretion of certain hormones). In addition, most males also develop coarser hair in the facial area, on the trunk, and on the arms and legs.

Skin Receptors

The dermis also has sensory nerve endings (skin receptors) that function as sense organs (i.e., somatic sense organs), transmitting messages to the brain concerning temperature, touch, pressure, and pain. For example, Pacini's corpuscle receptors, which are located deep within the dermis, detect pressure on the surface of the skin. Meissner's corpuscle receptors, which are usually close to the skin's surface, detect light touch sensations. Other skin receptors include those that detect other touch sensations, cold, heat, vibration, or pain.

Nails

The nails are produced when epidermal cells on the ends of the fingers and toes fill with the tough protein keratin. The nail body is the visible portion of the nail, whereas the remainder of the nail, known as the nail root, is hidden by a fold of skin (cuticle). A portion of the nail body that is closest to the root has a white, crescent-shaped area called the lunula. Tissue underneath the nail, known as the nail bed, contains many blood vessels, causing it to appear pinkish in color.

Description

Digestive

The digestive system consists of organs that break down food into small chemical components that ultimately may be used by cells of the body for energy (metabolism), growth, and repair. It includes the alimentary canal or gastrointestinal (GI) tract, which is the long, hollow passageway through which food passes, as well as associated organs, such as glands whose secreted juices help to break down (digest) food. Organs that comprise the GI tract include the mouth, pharynx, esophagus, stomach, small intestine, large intestine, and anus. Associated organs include the tongue, teeth, gallbladder, and digestive glands, such as the salivary glands, pancreas, and liver.

Nutrients

The foods of an individual's diet primarily include water as well as other nutrients necessary for growth and development. These include proteins, which play an essential role in cell repair and replacement; vitamins; carbohydrates, which serve as the primary energy source and assist in the breakdown and metabolism of other nutrients; fats; and minerals. Most minerals and vitamins may be absorbed into the blood circulation from the digestive system with no change in structure. However, other nutrients must be broken down into smaller, simpler (less complex) food molecules. Food is broken down (digested) through physical and chemical processes. Physical breakdown of food materials is performed by the chewing and grinding actions of the teeth, for example. The actions of certain digestive enzymes (i.e., substances that act as catalysts in the breakdown of proteins and other nutrients) as well as other substances (e.g., acids) chemically break down food as it travels through the GI tract. Thus, the nutrients are reduced into smaller molecules that may be absorbed through the lining of the intestinal wall for distribution to body cells.

Layers of the GI Tract

The hollow internal space within the alimentary canal or GI tract is known as the lumen. The walls of the GI tract consist of four layers of tissue, including an outermost covering (serosa); the mucous membrane (mucosa), which produces the mucus that lines the canal; the submucosa, a layer of connective tissue beneath the mucosa; and underlying layers of muscle tissue (muscularis). Regular, rhythmic contractions of involuntary (smooth) muscle within these layers of underlying muscle tissue propel food through the GI tract in a process known as peristalsis.

Mouth

Digestion begins in the mouth. The roof of the mouth, known as the palate, has a hard, bony, front portion (hard palate) and a soft, fleshy area (soft palate) that consists primarily of muscle. The tongue, which forms most of the floor of the mouth, is a flexible, muscular organ that helps manipulate food during chewing. It also contains the microscopic chemical receptors (taste receptors) that produce the nerve impulses necessary for taste (taste buds).

The teeth, which assist in the chewing and grinding of food, are firmly attached to the upper and lower jaws. The gums (gingiva), which consist of a mucous membrane and supporting fibrous tissues, surround the teeth, serving as "shock absorbers" and keeping the teeth tightly set into the jaws. Enclosing the oral cavity are the cheeks and the upper and lower lip. In addition, as with all of the GI tract, the mouth is lined by a mucous membrane. Saliva, a thin, watery fluid that is secreted by the salivary glands and the mucosa of the mouth, assists in the process of swallowing by moistening the oral mucosa; lubricating food; initiating the breakdown of certain food products through its digestive enzymes; and promoting the sense of taste.

Teeth

The teeth are essential for the chewing, tearing, and grinding of food (mastication) as it mixes with saliva. Humans typically have two sets of teeth including the primary (deciduous) teeth and the permanent (secondary) teeth. There are usually 20 primary teeth that erupt between the ages of six months and two to three years. The primary teeth are gradually replaced by the permanent teeth beginning at about six years of age. Adults typically have 32 permanent teeth.

There are four major types of teeth that are classified based upon their shape and location:

- Incisors are chisel shaped and have sharp edges for cutting during mastication. The incisors are the eight front teeth (i.e., four in the upper jaw and four in the lower jaw).

- Canines or cuspids are sharp, pointed teeth that tear or pierce food. The four canines (i.e., two in the upper jaw and two in the lower jaw) are situated next to the incisors.

- Premolars or bicuspids have large, flat surfaces with two grinding "cusps" to assist in the breakdown of food during mastication. The eight premolars are situated next to and in back of the canines. The primary teeth include no premolars.

- Molars or tricuspids also have large, flat surfaces, yet have three grinding "cusps." The 12 molars are located in back of the premolars. The primary teeth typically include only four molars in the upper jaw and four in the lower jaw. Wisdom teeth are typically known as third molars. They usually erupt in the late teens and early twenties.

The interior of each tooth contains living pulp, which includes connective tissue, sensory nerves, and blood and lymphatic vessels. The pulp is surrounded by the dental tissue known as dentin. In addition, each tooth is divided into a crown, neck, and root. The crown, the exposed portion of a tooth, is covered by enamel, the hardest tissue in the human body. The neck, which is the narrow portion of the tooth surrounded by the gums, and the root, which fits into the bony socket of the lower or upper jaw, are covered by the sensitive dental tissue cementum. A fibrous membrane (periodontal membrane) connects the cementum to the jaw and gums.

Salivary Glands

The salivary glands are the three pairs of glands that secrete saliva. Their secretions are released into ducts that empty into the mouth. Because the salivary glands release their secretions into ducts, they are exocrine glands. The salivary glands include the parotid, submandibular, and sublinqual. The parotid glands, the largest of the salivary glands, are located below and in front of the ears at the angle of the jaws. Their ducts open inside the cheeks. The submandibular glands are located toward the back of the mouth, and their ducts open under the tongue. The ducts of the sublingual glands secrete saliva onto the floor of the mouth. Saliva contains digestive enzymes (salivary amylase) that initiate the chemical digestion of certain foods (e.g. carbohydrates).

Pharynx

The pharynx, also known as the throat, is a muscular tube lined with mucous membranes and is part of the digestive and respiratory systems. Food and fluids enter the throat from the mouth and exit via the esophagus. However, air normally enters the pharynx from the nasal cavities and exits via the larynx. (For more information, please see the section entitled The Respiratory System.)

Esophagus

The esophagus is a muscular tube that transports food from the pharynx to the stomach. It is also lined with mucous membrane. The upper portion of the esophagus is encircled by a ring-shaped muscle (sphincter) that opens to allow the passage of food products. A similar muscle (cardiac sphincter) is located where the esophagus joins the stomach. The walls of the esophagus contain strong smooth muscles fibers, and rhythmic wavelike contractions of these involuntary muscles (peristalsis) propel food toward the stomach.

Stomach

The stomach is a hollow, pouch-like organ located in the upper portion of the abdominal cavity. It continues the breakdown of food that began in the mouth. Once food passes through the cardiac sphincter from the esophagus, it is contained in the stomach by contraction of the ring-shaped muscle at the end of the stomach (pyloric sphincter).

The walls of the stomach consist of three layers of smooth muscle and are lined with mucous membrane containing specialized cells that secrete gastric juices. These juices contain hydrochloric acid and digestive enzymes (e.g., rennin, pepsin) that are necessary for the breakdown of proteins. Rhythmic contractions of the stomach's smooth muscle layers mix digesting food with gastric juices, forming a semiliquid mixture known as chyme. Once partially digested food has been mixed into the chyme, relaxation of the pyloric sphincter and contractions of the stomach propel the chyme into the duodenum of the small intestine.

Small Intestine

The small intestine has three sections: the duodenum, jejunum, and the ileum. The function of the small intestine is to continue the breakdown of food products as they travel through the GI tract and to promote the absorption of nutrients into the bloodstream.

As rhythmic contractions of smooth muscles (peristalsis) propel food through the small intestine, digestive juices from the pancreas and bile from the liver are added to partially digested food within the duodenum. In addition, the mucus lining of the small intestine contains tiny glands that secrete intestinal digestive juice. Mucus, the enzymes within the intestinal digestive juice (e.g., maltase, sucrase, lactase, peptidase), and the secretions from the pancreas and liver serve to further break down food into smaller food molecules that may be more easily absorbed.

The mucosa of the small intestine is organized into several circular folds (plicae) covered with minute projections known as villi. Each villus contains finger-like lymphatic vessels (lacteals that absorb fat soluble nutrients (lipids) from the small intestine for transport to the blood circulation. Such fats are absorbed in the form of chyle, a cloudy milky substance containing products of digestion. The villi also contain blood capillaries that absorb certain products of digestion (e.g., amino acids, sugars).

Pancreas

The pancreas, an elongated gland located across the back of the abdomen, functions as both an exocrine and endocrine gland. It primarily consists of exocrine tissues that secrete pancreatic juice into ducts entering the duodenum. Pancreatic juice is an essential digestive juice that contains enzymes (e.g., trypsin, lipase, amylase) necessary for the breakdown of proteins, fats, carbohydrates, and certain acids. The pancreas also contains tiny clumps of endocrine cells (pancreatic islets) that secrete certain hormones, directly into the bloodstream.

The exocrine cells of the pancreas secrete their enzymes into several ducts that combine to form the main pancreatic duct. This duct joins with the common bile duct, which conveys bile from the gallbladder, and then opens into the duodenum. Most of the digestive enzymes secreted by the exocrine cells are activated by enzymes within the duodenum. In addition, exocrine cells of the pancreas secrete sodium bicarbonate, a substance that neutralizes the hydrochloric acid within the stomach's gastric juice as it enters the duodenum.

Liver, Bile Ducts, and Gallbladder

The liver, one of the largest organs of the body, is located within the upper right abdominal cavity. As part of the digestive system, the liver functions as an exocrine gland whose cells secrete the substance known as bile into a network of ducts (bile ducts). Bile, a liquid that consists of waste products, cholesterol, and bile salts, carries waste products from the liver and assists in the digestion and absorption of fats within the small intestine. The bile ducts transport bile from the liver to the gallbladder and on to the uppermost region of the small intestine (duodenum). The gallbladder, a small, muscular sac located under the liver, stores and concentrates bile from the liver. When chyme that contains fats (lipids) enters the duodenum from the stomach, the fats stimulate the secretion of a hormone (cholecystokinin) from the mucous membrane of the duodenum; in turn, the hormone stimulates contraction of the gallbladder, forcing bile into the small intestine.

The liver also has several additional essential functions in the body. These include regulating the blood levels of amino acids, the building blocks of proteins; helping to filter toxic substances from the blood; and producing certain proteins within the fluid portion of the blood (plasma). Such proteins include certain components that play a role in blood clotting (coagulation factors); particular blood proteins (complement system) that, when activated, destroy invading microorganisms; and the protein albumin, which helps to regulate the exchange of water between the bloodstream and bodily tissues. In addition, the liver produces cholesterol and certain proteins that transport fats in the bloodstream to cells throughout the body and processes hemoglobin for use of its iron content. Hemoglobin is the protein that enables red blood cells to transport large amounts of oxygen to cells.

Large Intestine

The large intestine is the organ that forms the lower portion of the GI tract. This organ, which has a larger diameter than the small intestine, consists of several areas. These include a pouch-like area (cecum); the ascending, transverse, descending, and sigmoid colons, the latter of which descends into the pelvic area and terminates in the rectum; and the end of the rectum known as the anal canal, which terminates at the external opening known as the anus. In addition, the appendix, a small, tubular structure, hangs from the cecum. Because the appendix contains lymphatic tissue, it may play a small role in helping to protect the body

against infection; however, it has no known role in the body's digestive system.

As food matter that has not been broken down or absorbed moves through the lower region of the small intestine (ileum), it passes into the large intestine through the ileocecal valve. Bacteria within the large intestine act upon the undigested material, potentially resulting in the release and absorption of additional nutrients. Water, vitamins, fats and minerals are absorbed into the bloodstream through the lining of the large intestine. Remaining undigested material is expelled through the rectum, anal canal, and anus as feces. Swelling (distension) of the rectum typically stimulates the desire to defecate, i.e., empty feces from the rectum. Two ring-shaped muscles (sphincters) usually remain contracted to keep the anus closed except during the process of defecation. The inner anal sphincter consists of involuntary (smooth) muscle, where the outer anal sphincter is composed of voluntary muscle.

Endocrine

Description

Endocrine

The term "endocrine system" is used to describe a group of specialized tissues, glands, and other structures that have the ability to produce and secrete certain complex chemical substances (hormones) into the bloodstream or lymphatic circulation for transport to particular tissues or ogans. These hormones have specific effects on certain bodily functions. Hormones assist in regulating the body's growth; controlling the rate of chemical processes in the body (metabolism); promoting the maturation and function of reproductive organs and the development of secondary sexual characteristics (puberty); and regulating many other bodily activities. Each hormone molecule may eventually combine with (or bind to) a specific area (receptor) on the surface of a cell within its "target organ," triggering the appropriate response. In contrast, exocrine glands are "outwardly secreting glands"-i.e., they secrete certain substances into ducts for emptying into a particular cavity or onto a bodily surface. (For example, the salivary glands of the digestive system secrete saliva via ducts that empty into the mouth.)

The endocrine glands include the pituitary gland, gonads (ovaries and testes), thyroid gland, parathyroid glands, adrenal glands, pancreatic islets, thymus, pineal gland, and placenta.

Pituitary Gland

The pituitary gland, also known as the "master gland," is a relatively small structure located deep in a saddle-shaped cavity in the skull (sella turcica). The gland is connected to a region of the brain known as the hypothalamus by a stalk of nerve fibers (pituitary stalk). The hypothalamus controls the functioning of the pituitary gland through direct nerve stimulation as well as through the actions of certain nerve cells that secrete hormones (hormone-releasing and hormone-inhibiting factors) into the bloodstream for transport directly to the pituitary. Hormone-releasing factors cause the secretion of certain hormones by the pituitary gland, whereas hormone-inhibiting factors inhibit the production and release of such hormones.

The pituitary gland is divided into two main regions: i.e., the anterior pituitary gland (adenohypophysis) and the posterior pituitary gland (neurohypophysis). Each region is responsible for producing different hormones. The anterior lobe of the pituitary gland produces the following hormones, most of which are considered tropic hormones, i.e., hormones that stimulate the growth of another endocrine gland and the secretion of its hormones.

- Prolactin stimulates the growth of the female breasts (mammary glands) during pregnancy and the secretion of milk by the mammary glands after birth.

- Growth hormone serves to stimulate body development.

- Melanocyte-stimulating hormone (MSH) controls the amount of dark brown or black pigment (melanin) produced by certain specialized skin cells (melanocytes).

- Thyroid-stimulating hormone (TSH) stimulates the production of thyroid hormones.

- Adrenocorticotropic hormone (ACTH) stimulates the growth of the outer regions of the adrenal glands (adrenal cortex) and their production of hormones.

- Follicle-stimulating hormone (FSH) and luteinizing hormone (LH), which are known as gonadotropins, stimulate the gonads, i.e., the sex glands (ovaries and testes) within which the reproductive cells (ova and sperm) are produced.

In addition, the posterior region of the pituitary gland releases two hormones:

- Antidiuretic hormone (ADH) decreases urine production by increasing the reabsorption of water from urine into the blood.

- Oxytocin stimulates powerful contractions of involuntary (smooth) muscle within the uterus during labor. This hormone also stimulates the secretion of milk (lactation) by the female mammary glands during breast-feeding.

Gonads

In females, the paired glands, known as the ovaries, produce the female sex cells (ova or eggs), and, in males, the paired structures, called the testes, produce the male sex cells (spermatozoa or sperm). Follicle-stimulating hormone produced by the pituitary gland promotes the growth and maturation of the cavities in the ovaries (follicles) within which the ova develop and mature; in addition, it stimulates the ovarian follicles' production of the female hormone estrogen. In males, FSH promotes the growth and maturation of and production of sperm by the long, coiled tubules (seminiferous tubules) that form the bulk of the testes. In addition, in females, luteinizing hormone produced by the pituitary gland stimulates the maturation of ovarian follicles and their eggs, the follicles' secretion of estrogen, and the monthly release of ova from the follicles (ovulation). LH stimulates the formation of glandular structures (corpus luteum) within the ruptured follicles that secrete the female hormones progesterone and estrogen. In males, LH stimulates the cells located between the seminiferous tubules in the testes to produce and secrete the male sex hormone testosterone.

Thyroid Gland

The horseshoe-shaped thyroid gland consists of two lobes on either side of the windpipe (trachea) that are joined by a narrow region of tissue (isthmus). Tissue within the thyroid gland consists of follicular cells and parafollicular cells. The follicular cells, which comprise most of the thyroid gland, secrete the thyroid hormones thyroxine (T4) and triiodothyronine (T3). Certain amounts of the thyroid hormones are stored as a semifluid material within the follicular cells, from which they are released into the bloodstream as required. The parafollicular cells secrete the hormone calcitonin.

Secretion of the thyroid hormones T4 and T3 is controlled by the pituitary gland. These hormones assist in regulation of the metabolic rate, i.e., chemical activities within cells that release energy from nutrients or consume energy to create certain substances. The thyroid hormones also play a vital role in the normal mental and physical development and growth of infants and children.

Release of the hormone calcitonin occurs independently of the pituitary gland and hypothalamus. This hormone-in coordination with parathyroid hormone released by the parathyroid glands-helps to regulate the concentrations of calcium in the body. Calcium is a mineral that is important for proper functioning of the cells, blood clotting, muscle contraction, nerve impulse transmission, and other vital functions. Most calcium in the body is stored in bones of the skeleton. Calcitonin has the ability to decrease blood levels of calcium. It suppresses resorption of bone by inhibiting the activity of cells that "digests" bone matrix (osteoclasts), releasing calcium and phosphorus into blood.

Parathyroid Glands

The parathyroid glands are the two pairs of small, oval glands on the back of both lobes of the thyroid gland. These glands produce parathyroid hormone, which serves to increase levels of calcium in the blood by stimulating osteoclasts to reabsorb bone mineral, thus liberating calcium into blood.

Adrenal Glands

The adrenal glands are small, triangular organs that curve over the top of each kidney. The outer region (adrenal cortex) and inner region (adrenal medulla) of the glands have different functions.

The secretion of hormones by the adrenal cortex is regulated by hormones produced by the pituitary gland (e.g., adrenocorticotropic hormone [ACTH]). The adrenal cortex consists of three distinct zones of cells. The outer zone secretes hormones known as mineralocorticoids that help to regulate the levels of certain mineral salts (e.g., sodium) in the blood. The main mineralocorticoid, known as aldosterone, assists in maintaining the delicate balance between sodium and potassium-ultimately helping to regulate blood pressure and blood volume.

The middle and inner zones of the adrenal cortex together secrete hormones known as glucocorticoids, such as hydrocortisone. Glucocorticoids help to regulate the body's use of carbohydrates, fats, and proteins; maintain normal blood pressure; produce certain anti-inflammatory effects; and decrease the production of certain white blood cells that produce antibodies (anti-allergic effect). The middle and inner zones of the adrenal cortex also secrete small amounts of sex hormones (androgens) that stimulate the development of male secondary sexual characteristics and the female sexual drive.

The adrenal medulla or inner region of the adrenal glands releases the hormones epinephrine and norepinephrine in response to nerve impulses from sympathetic nerve fibers. The release of such hormones into the bloodstream serves to increase the heart rate, widen the air passages of the lungs, and dilate blood vessels that supply the skeletal muscles of the body.

Pancreatic Islets

The pancreas, an elongated gland that is located across the back of the abdomen, is divided into a head, body, and tail. It primarily consists of exocrine tissue that secretes digestive enzymes necessary for the breakdown of proteins, fats, carbohydrates, and certain acids.

The endocrine tissue of the pancreas, known as pancreatic islets or islets of Langerhans, consists of tiny clumps of cells among the exocrine cells. The alpha cells of the pancreatic islets secrete glucagon, whereas the beta cells secrete insulin. Glucagon promotes a chemical process (glycogenolysis) during which glycogen, a carbohydrate that is stored in the liver, is broken down into glucose and released into the bloodstream. Insulin serves to regulate and stabilize blood glucose levels by promoting the movement of energy-rich glucose into the cells of the body. The secretion of glucagon increases blood glucose levels. In contrast, secretion of insulin decreases levels of glucose in the blood.

Thymus

The thymus, a small lymphoid organ located behind the breastbone (sternum) in the upper portion of the chest, consists of two lobes that join in front of the windpipe (trachea). This organ functions as an essential part of the immune system, beginning its functions at approximately the twelfth week of fetal development until puberty. The thymus serves as a source of certain white blood cells (lymphocytes) before birth. In addition, the organ secretes hormones (e.g., thymosin) that promote the development of specialized lymphocytes, known as T lymphocytes, which defend the body against certain microorganisms (i.e., during cell-mediated immunity.)

Pineal Gland

The pineal gland is a small, cone-shaped gland that is located deep in the brain. It secretes the hormone melatonin, which is thought to play a role in regulating puberty, ovarian cycles, mood, sleep, and the body's "internal clock" (e.g., 24-hour circadian cycle).

Placenta

The placenta, the organ that develops in the uterus during pregnancy, serves to connect the blood supplies of the mother and the developing fetus. It develops from the chorion, i.e., the outermost layer of cells from the fertilized egg (zygote). The placenta produces chorionic gonadotropin hormone, which stimulates the ovaries to produce the female sex hormones estrogen and progesterone. Both of these hormones are necessary for the functioning of the placenta during pregnancy.

Description

Growth and Development

Human growth and development may be encompassed in two broad categories: namely, prenatal growth and postnatal growth.

Prenatal Growth

The prenatal period, which means the "period before birth," begins when the male reproductive cell (sperm) fertilizes the female reproductive cell (egg or ovum). The fertilized egg (zygote) is a single cell containing all the genetic inforrmation (DNA) necessary for the growth and development of a human being. Half of the genetic information (in the form of 23 chromosomes) comes from the egg and half is from the sperm (for a total of 46 chromosomes).

As the zygote begins to travel down the mother's fallopian tube, its single cell immediately begins to divide (in the process called mitosis). (Please see the section entitled Cells for more information.) In approximately three days, the zygote has become a solid mass of cells known as a morula. About a week to 10 days after fertilization, what has become a hollow cellular "ball" (blastocyst) becomes implanted in the lining of the mother's uterus. During the zygote's journey to the uterus for implantation, the ovum supplies nutrients necessary for development of the emmbryo. The "embryonic phase" of development extends from fertilization until the end of the eighth week of pregnancy (gestation).

As the blastocyst continues to develop, its walls form an outer layer of membranes (chorion) that surround and prootect the embryo. In addition, an inner layer of membranes (amnion) forms the amniotic sac, the fluid-filled sac within which the embryo grows and develops, protecting it from injury.

The chorion develops into the placenta, the organ attached to the lining of the uterus that serves to connect the blood supplies of the mother and the developing embryo, enabling the exchange of vital nutrients (including oxygen) and waste products. Blood from the embryo flows through a cord-like structure (umbilical cord) to the placenta and passes into tiny, finger-like blood vessels (chorionic villi) surrounded by maternal blood. The umbilical cord contains three blood vessels: two umbilical arteries that carry oxyygen-poor (deoxygenated) blood and a larger umbilical vein that carries oxygen-rich (oxygenated) blood.

Teratogens and Birth Defects

A thin layer of tissue separates the developing embryo's blood and the mother's blood, thus providing protection from certain harmful substances that may circulate in the mother's bloodstream. However, in some cases, particular substances, such as certain infectious agents or drugs (teratogens), may cross this barrier, potentially interfering with prenatal growth and causing developmental abnormallities. The specific abnormalities that may result depend upon a number of factors, including the stage of developpment during which such exposure occurred, certain genetic influences, the specific teratogen in question, and other ennvironmental factors. Birth defects are abnormalities that are apparent at birth (congenital) or early infancy. Such malforrmations may occur due to prenatal exposure to teratogens, genetic factors, or a combination of both (multifactorial).

As mentioned above, the embryonic stage of development takes place from fertilization until the end of the eighth week of gestation. The fetal stage of development extends from the ninth week of gestation until birth. Pregnancy is usually approximately 39 weeks in duration and is divided into three phases known as trimesters, each of which is about three months in length.

By approximately the third week of gestation, the head of the developing embryo begins to form and the region that will later become the brain and spinal cord (neural crest) starts to develop. At about four weeks, "buds" of tissue have begun to form that will later develop into certain orrgans (e.g., liver, lungs, pancreas, etc.) and into the arms, hands, legs, and feet (limb buds); the neural tube continues to develop; and rudimentary eyes form. By approximately five weeks, all internal organs have begun to develop, the jaws form, and the limb buds continue to grow. And by six weeks, the nose, mouth, and ears are beginning to develop and fingers and toes are becoming apparent.

Early during the first trimester, the growing embryo develops three layers of cells known as primary germ layers: an inner layer (endoderm), a middle layer (mesoderm), and an outer layer (ectoderm). Specific tissues and organs develop from each of these layers. For example, the lining of the lungs, gastrointestional tract, and thyroid arise from the endoderm; the dermis of the skin, the muscles, most bones, the kidneys, and the circulatory system arise from the mesoderm; and the f~ial bones, the brain and spinal cord, the sensory organs such as the eyes and ears, and the epiidermis of the skin arise from the ectoderm. By approxiimately the fourth month of gestation, the internal organs and organ systems are formed and almost mature. Growth and development continues until approximately nine months' gestation, when birth typically occurs.

Labor and Birth

Birth is the process during which the fetus moves from the uterus down through the cervix and passes out through the vagina. During the end of pregnancy, the uterus begins to contract in preparation for birth. The process known as laabor begins when contractions become regular and occur at progressively shorter intervals. In addition, strong uter-

Growth and Development

ine muscular contractions cause the cervix to open and widen (dilate), and the membranes surrounding the amniotic fluid rupture, resulting in the release of the amniotic fluid through the vagina ("breaking of the waters"). The process of labor includes the following stages:

- First stage, which begins with the onset of contractions and ends with full dilation of the cervix

- Second stage, during which the baby exits through the vagina

- Third stage, during which the placenta is expelled through the vagina

Postnatal Growth and Development

The postnatal period, which means "the period after birth," begins at birth and extends until death. The most rapid rate of growth during one's development occurs prenatally during embryonic and fetal development. Although the rate of growth decreases after birth, it remains high during childhood, particularly during the first year of life. Individuals also experience a "growth spurt" at the onset of puberty that progresses until their adult height is obtained.

During the first five months of life, infants grow approximately 30 percent in height and their weight usually doubles. By the age of one year, their height has increased by about 50 percent from birth and their weight has typically tripled. Height and weight are carefully measured and recorded during regular visits to pediatricians to ensure that growth is progressing at a predictable, steady rate. Physicians use measurements known as percentiles to compare the height and weight of infants who are of the same age. If an infant is said to be at the "fiftieth percentile" for weight, 50% of infants weigh more and 50% weigh less. If an infant is at the "tenth percentile" for height, 90% of infants have a higher height and 10% have a lower height. When assessing growth and development, physicians consider the actual percentile as well as changes in percentiles between visits.

Between birth and adolescence, the relative proportions of the head, limbs, and trunk change dramatically. For example, an infant's head tends to be about one quarter of the height of the body; however, an adult's head is approximately one eighth that of the height of the body. In addition, from childhood to adulthood, the trunk tends to become proportionally shorter and the legs proportionally longer.

Different organs have varying rates of growth. For example, the human brain is about one quarter of its adult size at birth. The brain grows primarily during the first year of life and is typically three quarters of its adult size by the age of one year. In contrast, the small lymphoid organ known as the thymus gradually enlarges until puberty, at which time it begins to decrease in size (involution).

Developmental Milestones

Infants and children develop mental, physical, and behavvioral skills in certain stages known as developmental mileestones. Although the particular rate of development may vary from child to child, most children typically acquire such skills at certain ages. The development of these skills depends upon a number of factors including the following:

Genetic factors-e.g., certain developmental patterns, such as developing the ability to speak earlier than otherwise exxpected, may be present in particular families.

Physical factors-e.g., visual or hearing impairment may innterfere with the ability to learn certain skills, potentially neecessitating the use of special supportive techniques or services to ensure that children have the best chance to reach their developmental potential.

Environmental factors-e.g., appropriate levels of stimulaation are important in helping children to develop certain skills, such as receiving regular verbal stimulation to proomote language development.

When infants are born, they primarily communicate any needs (e.g., hunger, thirst, etc.) by crying. In addition, cerrtain essential reflex reactions are typically present at birth. For example, when any objects touch newborns' lips, they usually respond by sucking (sucking reflex). When a side of the mouth is touched, newborns typically move their head toward that side, enabling them to locate the mother's nipple for breast-feeding (rooting reflex). And when newwborns are startled, they stretch their arms and legs forward and out and extend their fingers (startle or Moro's reflex). These reflex reactions gradually fade as infants develop muscle strength and the ability to conduct and coordinate certain voluntary movements. For example, hand-eye coorrdination skills include watching objects, developing the ability to focus, tracking moving objects, and forming an association between seeing and performing certain actions by focusing on hand movements.

Development is typically assessed by evaluating the acquiisition of skills in the areas of vision and fine movement, hearing and speech, locomotion, and social behavior. The following is a description of developmental milestones that are generally acquired during the first year of life:

By approximately one month of age, infants are usually able to:

- Focus on faces

- Bring their hands toward the face (e.g., mouth, eyes)

- Look at objects directly in front of them

- Turn toward familiar voices and respond to other sounds

- Move their head from side to side while lying on their stomach

At about three months, infants are usually able to:

- Track objects that move approximately 180 degrees

- Grasp objects placed in their hands

- Smile at familiar voices (e.g., mother's or father's)

- Make sounds that begin to resemble speech

- Raise their head 45 degrees when lying on their stomach

At approximately five months, infants are usually able to:

- Reach for objects

- Listen carefully to certain voices

- Hold their head steady while upright

- Roll from the stomach to the back

- Spontaneously smile

At about six months, infants are usually able to:

- Reach out for an move objects from one hand to another

- Turn their head to locate sounds

- Laugh, make certain vowel sounds, and babble to toys

- Roll from back to front and vice versa

- Sit with support

- Bear weight on their legs with support

At the age of nine months, infants are usually able to:

- Look for toys that have been hidden

- Grasp for toys that are out of reach

- Manipulate objects with both hands

- Listen to and comprehend certain sounds

- Occasionally utter strings of syllables (e.g., "mama" or "dada")

- Attempt to crawl, sit without support, and pull themselves to a sitting or standing position

- Step on alternative feet with support

By 12 months of age, infants are usually able to:

- Grasp and release objects

- Say several words

- Respond when they hear their names

- Wave good-bye

- Move from their stomach to a sitting position

- Crawl on their hands and knees

- Walk by holding furniture

- Walk without support for a few steps or with one hand held

Description

Hematologic

The blood is a circulating tissue composed of fluid and other formed elements such as red blood cells, white cells, and platelets. The study of the blood, its components, and blood-forming tissues is known as hematology. Blood is pumped by the heart through the body's arteries, veins, and capillaries. The noncellular, fluid portion of the blood is a pale, yellowish liquid known as plasma. The blood has several functions including:

- To serve as a transport system, carrying oxygen and other vital nutrients to body tissues and promoting the exchange and removal of carbon dioxide and other waste products from cells

- To help provide a defense against invading microorganisms, foreign tissue cells, and certain abnormal cells

- To help repair damage to blood vessels and tissues through the process of blood clotting

Blood Plasma
Approximately half of the blood's volume consists of plasma. This liquid, noncellular portion of the blood is approximately 95 percent water. In addition, the blood plasma also contains dissolved sugars (e.g., glucose, etc.), fats, salts, vitamins and minerals, amino acids necessary for the production of cellular proteins, and chemical messengers (such as hormones) that regulate specific cellular activities. Plasma also contains certain plasma proteins including globulins (e.g., antibodies, which are produced in response to a particular foreign protein [antigen]); albumin, which plays an important role in maintaining the balance of pressure from inside and outside the cell, ; and fibrinogen, a protein that is essential for blood clotting. In addition, certain waste products are dissolved in plasma and transported to the kidneys for excretion.

Formed Elements
The formed elements of the blood include red blood cells (erythrocytes), white blood cells (leukocytes), and platelets (thrombocytes). Red blood cells, platelets, and some white blood cells are produced in the bone marrow. However, most white blood cells are produced by lymphatic tissue (e.g., lymph nodes, spleen, thymus).

Red Blood Cells
The red blood cells (RBCs) are mostly rounded, double concave cells with thin centers and thicker edges. A cubic millimeter of blood contains approximately five million red blood cells. The relatively large surface area of the red blood cells because they are concave allows them to absorb and release oxygen molecules, and their shape facilitates

their movement through narrow blood vessels. As mentioned above, red blood cells are produced in the bone marrow, where the rate of their formation is regulated by erythropoietin, a hormone produced by the kidneys. They typically circulate in the blood for approximately four months, at which time they break apart and are removed from the blood by the liver.

The red blood cells perform several essential functions. For example, RBCs transport carbon dioxide from the body's cells to the lungs for release into the environment. Carbon dioxide is a harmful waste product that is generated by normal cellular activities. The red blood cells also carry hemoglobin, an essential protein that contains iron. This red pigmented protein chemically combines (binds) with oxygen, producing oxyhemoglobin, which enables the red blood cells to transport oxygen to cells.

The various blood groups, such as blood types A, B, AB, and O, are classified based upon the presence or absence of certain antigens (or "marker proteins"). Antigens are proteins that stimulate the body to produce antibodies. The red blood cells may have two types of antigens: namely, A and/or B. The different A or B blood types are classified according to whether the red blood cells have both, one or the other, or neither antigen. In individuals with type B blood, for example, the body does not produce antibodies to inactivate or destroy the type B antigen; however, the blood plasma contains anti-A antibodies. In individuals with type A blood, the red blood cells contain type A antigen and the blood plasma has anti-B antibodies. In type O blood, the red blood cells contain neither type A nor type B antigens, whereas the blood plasma has both anti-A and anti-B antibodies. In contrast, in individuals with type AB blood, the red blood cells have both type A and type B antigens, and the blood plasma contains neither anti-A nor anti-B antibodies.

In approximately 85 percent of individuals, red blood cells also contain an antigen called Rh factor. Those with this antigen are said to have Rh-positive blood, whereas those without the antigen have Rh-negative blood.

White Blood Cells
White blood cells (WBCs) are larger than red blood cells; however, they are present in the blood in lower quantities. A cubic millimeter of blood contains approximately 7,500 white blood cells.

The white blood cells include two major categories: granular leukocytes, which have granules in the substance of the cell outside the nucleus (cytoplasm), and nongranular leukocytes. Granular leukocytes include neutrophils, eosinophils, and basophils, and nongranular leukocytes include lymphocytes and monocytes.

Neutrophils and monocytes, which are also known as phagocytes, are responsible for isolating, engulfing, and destroying microorganisms that have invaded the bloodstream. These cells engulf the microorganisms and digest them in a process known as phagocytosis.

Lymphocytes originate in the bone marrow and mature in lymphatic tissue. They become active immune cells in response to the presence of invading microorganisms. Lymphocytes known as B lymphocytes produce specific antibodies to inhibit certain microorganisms, whereas those known as T lymphocytes may actively destroy microorganisms or assist in the functions of the B lymphocytes.

Eosinophils help protect the body from various irritants that may cause allergies and are able to participate in phagocytosis. In addition, white blood cells known as basophils also play a role in allergic reactions and secrete certain chemicals such as heparin, which assists in the prevention of clotting as the blood circulates through the blood vessels (intravascular clotting).

Although granular leukocytes may have a lifespan of only a few days, nongranular leukocytes may survive for over six months. In fact, in some cases, certain individual lymphocytes may remain in the bloodstream for years.

Platelets

Platelets, which are the smallest blood cells, are produced in the bone marrow by specialized cells known as megakaryocytes and typically survive for approximately nine days. A cubic millimeter of blood contains approximately 250,000 platelets.

Platelets usually circulate in the bloodstream in an inactive state. However, when a blood vessel wall is injured, platelets respond through a complex process by clumping at the injury site and sticking to one another. The platelets and damaged tissue cells also release certain chemicals that stimulate blood clotting (coagulation) factors in the blood plasma. Due to a series of complex reactions, known as a cascade, long filaments of fibrin, a fibrous gel, are produced that capture circulating platelets, red blood cells, and white blood cells. Once the damaged blood vessel is "plugged," the filaments contract, forming a solid blood clot.

In some cases, blood clots may form in undamaged blood vessels, potentially blocking vital blood supply to certain tissues and organs. A stationary blood clot is called a thrombus. If a portion of such a clot dislodges and circulates in the bloodstream, it is known as an embolus. Healthy blood vessel walls secrete the chemical prostacyclin, which helps to prevent the unnecessary activation of platelets and clot formation. However, under certain circumstances, emboli travel from their origin to other parts of the body, notably the lungs, heart, and brain.

Measurement of Blood Components

The complete blood count (CBC) is a calculation of the cellular (formed elements) of blood. These calculations are generally determined by specially designed machines that analyze the different components of blood in less than a minute. A major portion of the complete blood count is the measure of the concentration of white blood cells, red blood cells, and platelets in the blood. The complete blood count (also called CBC) is generated by testing a simple blood sample.

White Blood Count (WBC), also called leukocyte count. Normal range varies slightly between laboratories but is generally between 4,300 and 10,800 cells per cubic millimeter (cmm).

Automated white cell differential. A machine generated percentage of the different types of white blood cells, usually split into granulocytes, lymphocytes, monocytes, eosinophils, and basophils.

Red cell count (RBC), also called erythrocyte count. Normal range varies slightly between laboratories but is generally between 4.2 - 5.9 million cells/cmm.

Hemoglobin (Hb). Hemoglobin is the protein molecule within red blood cells that carries oxygen and gives blood its red color. Normal range for hemoglobin is different between the sexes and is approximately 13 - 18 grams per deciliter (g/dl) for men and 12 - 16 g/dl for women.

Platelet count, also called thrombocyte count. Normal range varies slightly between laboratories but is in the range of 150,000 - 400,000 per cubic millimeter.

Immune System

Description

Immune System

The body's immune system consists of specialized proteins, cells, and tissues that function to protect the body against...

- Invading microorganisms (e.g., bacteria, viruses, etc.) that may cause disease

- Foreign tissue cells (such as those that may have been transplanted from a donor)

- Toxins (such as harmful chemicals)

- Cells that have become cancerous

Nonspecific Immunity

Certain mechanisms provide the body with general protection from invading cells and toxins, maintaining "nonspecific immunity." For example, nonspecific immunity is provided by the presence of certain physical barriers that may prevent the entry of invading cells or toxins or expel them-as well as chemical barriers that may destroy invading cells or toxins. Such barriers include certain enzymes within the saliva of the mouth, tears, and sweat; the protective barrier of the skin; the cough reflex; hairs within the nose and the sneeze reflex; the presence of harmless bacteria within the intestines that help to control harmful microorganisms; and secretion of mucus by cells lining certain organs of the respiratory tract.

In addition, tissue injury results in an inflammatory response, which consists of a series of nonspecific immune reactions. During an inflammatory response-which produces characteristic swelling, discomfort, and redness-the blood vessels widen (dilate), increasing the blood supply and enabling certain white blood cells to move from the vessels to the site of injury. For example, invading microorganisms typically encounter white blood cells known as phagocytes, which contain the infection by engulfing and destroying the microbes (phagocytosis). Invading microorganisms may also encounter certain naturally produced substances, such as a group of blood proteins (complement system) that, when activated, serve to destroy such microbes, or interferon, proteins that are produced in response to viral infection.

Specific Immunity

Specific immunity consists of particular defenses against certain invading microorganisms or toxins and includes inborn and acquired immunity. From birth, individuals are immune to certain diseases that affect other animals (inborn immunity). Acquired immunity is obtained when certain protective proteins known as antibodies are passed to a developing fetus via the mother's placenta or to an infant via the mother's breast milk. Acquired immunity also results from casual exposure to certain disease-causing agents and immunization (stimulation of the immune system to provide protection against a particular disease, such as through vaccination).

Humoral or Cellular Immune Responses

Specific immunity, which relies on the actions of the white blood cells known as lymphocytes, includes the humoral- and cell-mediated immune responses.

Humoral Response

A humoral-mediated immune response, also known as an antibody-mediated response, primarily consists of the production of antibodies by cells called B lymphocytes or B cells. B lymphocytes initially arise from primitive cells in the bone marrow known as stem cells. Shortly before and after birth, certain stem cells develop into immature B cells.

When immature B cells recognize a disease-causing agent as foreign (antigen), they develop into activated B cells. Activated B cells rapidly divide into two lines of cells (clones): plasma cells, which secrete large amounts of antibodies into the blood, and memory cells, which are stored within the lymph nodes until they are stimulated by the same antigen that prompted their formation. They then also develop into plasma cells, secreting antibodies into the blood in response to the recognized antigen.

When antibodies are secreted into the blood, they bind to their specific antigens (antibody-antigen complex), making the antigens or the cells on which they are located harmless. Phagocytes then engulf and destroy large numbers of such antibody-antigen complexes. The binding of antibodies and antigens may stimulate the complement system, thereby improving the efficiency of phagocytosis.

Cellular Response

Cell-mediated immunity defends the body against certain microorganisms and possibly cancerous cells through the actions of particular white blood cells known as T lymphocytes or T cells. These cells initially develop within the thymus before birth. They arise from stem cells that migrate from the bone marrow to the thymus, where their development is facilitated by certain hormones. Newly formed T cells then migrate from the thymus to other lymphatic tissues, primarily the lymph nodes.

There are two main types of T lymphocytes involved in cell-mediated immunity including the helper cells and killer cells. Helper cells assist in the recognition of certain antigens and help to activate killer cells. The killer cells bind to cells invaded by viruses or other microbes and destroy them. It is thought that killer cells may function similarly against cancerous cells or foreign tissue cells.

Allergies and Autoimmune Disease

In some cases, humoral- or cell-mediated immune responses may inappropriately occur against the body's own tissues. Such "autoimmunity" may result in hypersensitivity or autoimmune diseases. A hypersensitivity reaction is characterized by an excessive immune response to a substance that the body perceives as foreign (sensitizing antigen). For example, an allergic reaction is a hypersensitive response that occurs upon exposure to previously encountered, usually environmental substances (allergens), such as pollen, dust, or certain foods. Autoimmune diseases may be caused by the production of antibodies against the body's own cells (autoantibodies) and inappropriate cell-mediated immune responses against self antigens (autoantigens). One proposed theory suggests that certain viruses or bacteria may play some role in provoking an abnormal autoimmune reaction. For example, when a foreign protein from an invading bacterium or virus is very similar to one of the body's proteins, the immune system may be unable to distinguish between the invading and the "self" protein, potentially triggering an autoimmune response. It is not known what role genetic, hormonal, or other environmental factors may play in contributing to such a response. Autoimmune diseases may be localized, affecting a particular tissue, or may involve many tissues and organs of the body (systemic).

Infectious Diseases and Vaccination

The purpose of immunization is to induce immunity to provide protection against a certain disease. In response to a vaccine, the body's immune system produces certain immune defenses, such as antibodies or particular white blood cells that should protect against infection upon exposure to the disease-causing organism.

There are two major types of vaccination. In passive vaccination, antibodies obtained from a donor who was previously exposed to the microorganism are introduced into the body, thereby providing short-term protection against the disease-causing organism. In active vaccination, noninfectious portions of bacteria or viruses are introduced into the body, stimulating the production of antibodies against the foreign protein, resulting in longer-term immunity.

Some vaccines are intended for the general population, particularly infants and young children, such as immunization against the infectious diseases diphtheria, pertussis (whooping cough), and tetanus (DPT); measles, mumps, and rubella (German measles); hepatitis B; and polio. The recommended ages for immunization may vary from case to case. A child's pediatrician can recommend an appropriate immunization schedule.

Other vaccines are available for individuals who are at risk for certain infectious diseases due to their work situations (e.g., health care workers); their living situations or age groups (e.g., students living in dormitories, elderly individuals in nursing homes); local outbreaks of dangerous infectious diseases; or travel in certain countries.

Some individuals should not receive certain vaccinations, such as people with deficient immune systems. In individuals who have a fever or a preexisting infection, immunizations should be delayed. In addition, particular vaccines should not be given to young children or pregnant women.

Musculoskeletal

Description

Musculoskeletal

Neuromuscular Activities

The muscles of the body, collectively referred to as the muscular system, consist of bundles of specialized cells that, unlike other cells, have the ability to contract and relax, resulting in movement of body parts and organs. There are two main types of muscles: namely, skeletal muscle and smooth muscle. In addition, the cardiac muscle is a highly specialized muscle that is sometimes referred to as a third muscle type.

Skeletal Muscle

The skeletal muscles, so named because they attach to bones of the skeleton, are the most prominent muscles in the body and typically contribute to approximately 40 to 45 percent of an individual's body weight. These muscles may also be referred to as striated ("cross striped") muscles or called voluntary muscles because their movements are under voluntary control.

Each skeletal muscle consists of groups of threadlike muscle cells, known as muscle fibers, in a highly organized arrangement. Each muscle fiber is made up of slender, striated strands called myofibrils that, in turn, are composed of bunches of microscopic, threadlike structures known as myofilaments. The myofilaments contain minute fibers or threads of proteins known as myosin and actin. The interactions of these proteins are essential for muscle contraction. During voluntary movement, skeletal muscle contracts and the bone to which it is attached (via tendons) moves in response to the contraction.

Neuromuscular Activities and Voluntary Movement:

The brain regulates voluntary movements of skeletal muscles by sending impulses to the nerve fibers that supply the muscle fibers (motor neurons). The area where nerve endings and muscle fibers join is known as the neuromuscular junction. When the brain sends such impulses, nerve endings release a specialized chemical (the neurotransmitter acetylcholine) that serves to stimulate the muscle fibers. A complex series of electrical and chemical processes is initiated resulting in muscle contraction.

When voluntary movements occur, there are coordinated contractions and simultaneous relaxations of several muscles. In other words, as several muscles contract, one muscle is primarily responsible for producing the particular movement (prime mover or agonist) and the others (synergists) contract in order to assist the prime mover in making the movement in question. While such muscles contract, other muscles known as antagonists simultaneously relax, producing movements that oppose those of the prime mover and synergists. Such coordination of skeletal muscle movements helps to ensure smooth rather than jerky motions.

In addition to producing movement, the skeletal muscles also function to maintain posture and to produce body heat. For example, skeletal muscles are typically maintained at a level of slight, continuous contraction (muscle tone). Such muscle tone helps the body to maintain proper posture-i.e., the specific positioning of body parts to support their optimum function, place the least strain on different areas of the body, and maintain proper weight distribution. In addition, muscle fiber contraction creates most of the heat that the body needs to maintain its proper temperature.

Smooth Muscle

Smooth muscle cells have a smooth appearance when viewed under a microscope, lacking the striations of skeletal muscle cells. Rather, they consist of elongated, "spindle-shaped" cells that are typically organized parallel to one another. Also known as involuntary muscles since their movements are not under voluntary control, the smooth muscles help to regulate certain functional movements of internal organs. For example, in the process known as peristalsis, the rhythmic contractions of smooth muscle propel food forward through the digestive tract. Smooth muscle is also located within the blood vessel walls and several other areas of the body.

The actions of the smooth muscles are regulated by the autonomic nervous system, the portion of the nervous system that controls involuntary activities of blood vessels, organs, and other tissues and organ systems. Neurotransmitters released at nerve endings contribute to the series of events that lead to contraction of smooth muscles. As with the skeletal muscles, smooth muscle contractions rely upon the interactions between the myosin and actin filaments. In addition, smooth muscle cell activities may be affected by changes in the chemical composition of the fluid surrounding the cells as well as the release of certain hormones.

Cardiac Muscle

Cardiac muscle, also known as the myocardium, is a special type of striated muscle that is located only in the heart. Like the cells within the skeletal muscles, cardiac muscle cells also have cross striations. In addition, there are dark bands or disks (intercalated disks) at the junctures of adjacent cardiac fibers. These disks enable the fibers to contract as a unit, thereby ensuring the heart's efficiency in pumping blood throughout the circulatory system.

As with the smooth muscles, contraction of cardiac muscle is regulated by the autonomic nervous system. Cardiac muscle activities may also be affected by the release of specific hormones. Electrical impulses that stimulate a regulated, coordinated sequence of contractions originate from the heart's "pacemaker" (sinoatrial node), an area within the upper right chamber of the heart (right atrium).

Description

Nervous System

The nervous system is a complex network of structures that function to...

- obtain information about the body's internal environment and the external environment

- relay and analyze such "data"

- initiate, integrate, and control appropriate responses to this information

The nervous system includes the brain and spinal cord, known as the central nervous system; nerves that extend from the brain and spinal cord to all areas of the body, referred to as the peripheral nervous system; somatic sense organs, which are distributed in almost every area of the body but concentrated primarily in the skin; and special sensory organs, such as the eyes. In addition, the peripheral nervous system is further subdivided into the autonomic nervous system, which includes structures that regulate involuntary functions of the body.

Nervous System Cells

Cells of the nervous system ensure ongoing, rapid communications between different structures of the body and the control of bodily functions necessary to maintain life. There are two main types of cells within the nervous system:

- Nerve cells, also known as neurons, which conduct (transmit) impulses

- Glia, which are the connective tissue cells of the nervous system

Neurons contain a cell body, one or more slender, branching projections (dendrites) that transmit impulses toward the cell body, and a slender extension (axon or nerve fiber) that carries nerve impulses away from the cell body. A whitish, fatty substance known as myelin forms a protective "wrapping" or insulating sheath around certain axons, serving as an electrical insulator and ensuring the efficient conduction of nerve impulses.

There are three types of neurons:

- Sensory neurons (afferent ["toward"] neurons) carry impulses to the brain and spinal cord from all areas of the body.

- Motor neurons (efferent ["away from"] neurons) transmit impulses away from the brain and spinal cord to certain tissues (e.g., muscle or glandular tissues).

- Interneurons (connecting or central neurons) carry impulses from sensory neurons to motor neurons.

Glia hold together and protect neurons. The different types of glia include the following:

- Astrocytes are relatively large cells with thread-like projections. These "branches" connect with blood capillaries and neurons, holding them in proximity to one another. The walls of the capillaries and the projections of the astrocytes are said to form the "blood-brain barrier," which functions to separate systemic blood circulation from the central nervous system. This barrier prevents or slows the passage of certain toxic substances or infectious agents from the blood to the central nervous system.

- Oligodendroglia produce myelin and hold together nerve fibers.

- Microglia are relatively small cells with slender projections. When brain tissue becomes inflamed, these cells migrate toward the affected tissue, surround invading microorganisms or waste products, and digest them (phagocytosis).

Nerves and Nerve Impulses

Nerves consist of one or more bundles of impulse-carrying fibers known as axons that extend from the brain and spinal cord to all areas of the body. Certain nerves transmit impulses from particular receptor organs to the brain and spinal cord (afferent impulses) or from the CNS to certain specialized tissues (efferent impulses). White matter within the central nervous system and peripheral nervous system consists of bundles of axons that are myelinated; in contrast, gray matter of the nervous system primarily includes neuron cell bodies, dendrites, and unmyelinated axons.

The pathways by which nerve impulses are transmitted by neurons are known as neuron pathways. Nerve signals are electrical impulses or waves of electrical disturbances that result due to complex electrochemical changes in a neuron's environment. Such nerve impulses travel from the axon of one neuron (presynaptic neuron) to the dendrite of another neuron (postsynaptic neuron). The junction between two neurons is known as a synapse. As an electrical impulse reaches a synapse, the presynaptic neuron's axon releases small amounts of chemical substances known as neurotransmitters, which bind to certain areas (receptors) of the postsynaptic neuron. Consequently, the electrical impulse is conducted across the synapse to the postsynaptic neuron's dendrite. Thus, neurotransmitters are the chemical substances that enable neurons to communicate with one another.

Central Nervous System

The central nervous system includes the brain and the spinal cord. Bones of the skull enclose the brain, and bones of the spinal column (vertebrae) surround the spinal cord. In addition, a three-layered membrane (meninges) provides additional protection for the brain and spinal cord. The tough, fibrous outermost layer is known as the dura mater. The delicate middle layer, called the arachnoid mater, is separated from the elastic innermost layer (pia mater) by a space (subarachnoid space) that contains cerebrospinal fluid (CSF). This fluid, which acts as a protective "shock absorber," flows through the cavity within the vertebrae containing the spinal cord (spinal canal), the four cavities of the brain (ventricles), and the subarachnoid space.

Brain

The brain controls and regulates the many functions of the central nervous system including muscle control and coordination, sensory reception and response, and speech production as well as elaboration of thought and emotions. It consists of several major regions including the brain stem, diencephalon, cerebellum, and cerebrum.

Brain Stem

The brain stem consists of three structures: the medulla oblongata, pons, and midbrain. All regions of the brain stem serve as "two-lane" conduction "highways," with motor fibers relaying impulses from the brain to the spinal cord, and sensory fibers conducting messages from the spinal cord to other areas of the brain.

The medulla oblongata, a thick extension of the spinal cord, is located above the large opening (foramen magnum) in the bone that forms the back of the skull (occipital bone). It primarily consists of white matter mixed with bits of gray matter (reticular formation). The medulla contains groups of nerve cells (nuclei) of the ninth, eleventh, and twelfth cranial nerves (see below), thereby receiving and sending impulses involved in the sensation of taste and sending messages to muscles involved in swallowing, speech, and movements of the neck, shoulders, and tongue, for example. This region of the brain stem also contains nuclei of the tenth cranial nerve (vagus nerve) and thus receives and relays information concerning the regulation of blood vessel diameter (thus affecting blood pressure), beating of the heart, breathing, and digestion.

The pons and the midbrain both also contain white matter mixed with bits of gray matter. The pons has bundles of nerve fibers that connect with the region of the brain known as the cerebellum. In addition, it contains nuclei of the fifth, sixth, seventh, and eighth cranial nerves, thus relaying messages involved in movement of the eyes, jaws, and muscles of facial expression as well as receiving and transmitting sensory impulses from the face and ears. The midbrain contains nuclei of the third and fourth cranial nerves and therefore relays messages to muscles involved in controlling the reactions of the pupils of the eyes as well as five of the six muscles that move the eyes.

Diencephalon

The diencephalon is the region of the brain located between the midbrain and the cerebrum. It includes the hypothalamus and the thalamus.

The hypothalamus, a relatively small area of the brain, is situated under the thalamus and above the pituitary gland. One of its functions is to regulate the sympathetic nervous system, a division of the autonomic nervous system. The sympathetic nervous system controls certain involuntary activities during times of stress, such as raising blood pressure, increasing the heart rate and the breathing rate, and widening (dilating) the pupils. The hypothalamus is also involved in regulating body temperature, appetite, moods and emotions (such as anger, fear, etc.), and the sleep cycle.

Sleep and the Brain

Sleep is a natural state characterized by reduced consciousness and metabolic activity. During sleep, the brain typically engages in two main cycles, known as REM (rapid eye movement) and NREM (nonrapid eye movement) sleep. NREM sleep, which makes up approximately 80 percent of sleep in adults (and about 50 percent of sleep in infants), consists of four progressively deeper stages of sleep characterized by slow, deep brain waves; muscle relaxation; and regular, reduced autonomic activities (e.g., slowed breathing and heart rate; lowered blood pressure; etc.). Episodes of REM sleep periodically alternate with NREM sleep. REM sleep, which is associated with dreaming, includes increased levels of brain activity, irregular autonomic activities, rapid eye movements, and involuntary muscle jerks. A complete sleep cycle is usually approximately 90 minutes. Most individuals experience approximately four or five sleep cycles each night. It is not completely understood why sleep is a necessity, although most scientists agree that the brain requires regular rest to ensure optimum functioning-and that dreaming may help the brain to sort, manipulate, and store information obtained during waking activities. Many different areas of the brain, including the hypothalamus, are thought to play a role in regulating sleep.

The hypothalamus also controls the functions of the pituitary gland, an endocrine gland also known as the "master gland." The hypothalamus is attached to the pituitary gland by a stalk of nerve fibers known as the pituitary stalk. It regulates the gland's activities through direct nerve stimulation as well as through the actions of certain nerve cells whose axons secrete chemicals (hormone-releasing and hormone-inhibiting factors) into the bloodstream for transport directly to the pituitary. Hormone-releasing factors cause the secretion of certain hormones by the pituitary gland, whereas hormone-inhibiting factors halt the production and release of such hormones. The balance of these factors, via a feedback mechanism, is crucial in maintaining effective function of many of the body's activities.

The thalamus consists of two masses of gray matter located above the hypothalamus. The neurons within the thalamus relay impulses from sense organs of the body to the outer region of the cerebrum (cerebral cortex); transmit motor impulses from the cerebral cortex toward the spinal cord; associate certain sensations with emotions (e.g., unpleasant or pleasant feelings); and play a role in the body's state of responsiveness to sensory stimulation (arousal or alerting mechanisms).

Cerebellum

The cerebellum, a two-lobed, rounded region of the brain, has a "wrinkled" surface and is located under the back portion of the cerebrum and behind the brain stem. The surface (cortex) of the cerebellum contains parallel ridges that are separated by deep fissures. Three stalks of nerve fibers (peduncles) that arise from the inner side of each cerebellar hemisphere link to different areas of the brain stem. Messages between the cerebellum and other regions of the brain travel along these nerve stalks. Through messages transmitted via the brain stem, the cerebellum receives information concerning muscle contraction and relaxation and posture. The cerebellum works in conjunction with the basal ganglia and the thalamus, adjusting messages relayed to muscle groups from a certain area of the cerebrum (motor cortex) in order to maintain normal postures, sustain balance, and produce smooth and coordinated movements.

Cerebrum

The cerebrum is the largest area of the brain and is responsible for voluntary movements, sensory perception, emotions, memory, and comprehensive thought. The cerebrum contains several ridges (gyri) and grooves (sulci or fissures) and one deep groove known as the longitudinal fissure that divides the cerebrum into two halves (cerebral hemispheres). The left cerebral hemisphere controls the right side of the body, whereas the right hemisphere controls the left side of the body due to crossing of nerve fibers in the medulla of the brain stem. A thick band of myelinated nerve fibers known as the corpus callosum joins the lower midportions of and carries messages between the cerebral hemispheres. In addition, each hemisphere contains a fluid-filled cavity known as a ventricle (first and second or lateral ventricles). These ventricles communicate with a third ventricle in the center of the brain, and a fourth ventricle is located between the brain stem and the cerebellum.

Two sulci divide each hemisphere into four lobes that are designated by the bones over them: i.e., frontal, temporal, parietal, and occipital lobes. The surface of the cerebrum, called the cerebral cortex, consists of a thin layer of gray matter, whereas most of the interior of the cerebrum con-

tains bundles of myelinated nerve fibers (white matter) known as tracts. In addition, deep within the white matter of the cerebrum are paired nerve cell clusters of gray matter known as the basal ganglia. Their function includes assisting in the regulation of muscular actions as well as initiating and ceasing movements.

The cerebrum has various areas that are responsible for particular complex functions. These areas include the following:

- Sensory areas, which receive sensory information from somatic sense organs (e.g., in the skin, muscles, internal organs) and special sense organs (e.g., ears, eyes, etc.) and analyze and sort such information

- Motor areas, which transmit messages that control muscles, resulting in movement

- Association areas, which link sensory and motor areas, integrate information received from the various sense organs, and engage in memory storage, recall, recognition, decision making, judgment, comprehensive thought, and the experience of emotions.

Spinal Cord

The spinal cord is housed inside a central canal within the spinal column and extends from the foramen magnum at the base of the skull to the bottom of the first vertebra of the lower back. It is a long, cylindrical structure of nerve tissue and is an extension of the medulla oblongata of the brain stem. As mentioned above, the spinal cord is enclosed and protected by a three-layered membrane (meninges) and is bathed by cerebrospinal fluid.

The inner core of the spinal cord consists of gray matter (i.e., primarily containing nerve cell bodies and dendrites). Its outer portion is composed of columns of white matter that contain bundles of myelinated nerve fibers (spinal tracts). These pathways transmit sensory impulses from the spinal cord to the brain (ascending tracts) and motor impulses from the brain to the spinal cord (descending tracts). Certain ascending tracts transmit impulses that produce sensations of temperature and pain, and certain descending tracts convey impulses that control specific voluntary movements.

Peripheral Nervous System

The peripheral nervous system refers to those nerves outside the central nervous system. This part of the nervous system establishes communications between the brain and spinal cord and outlying (peripheral) parts of the body, such as muscles, glands, and internal organs. Nerves of the peripheral nervous system include the cranial nerves and the spinal nerves.

The cranial nerves are the 12 nerve pairs that arise directly from the brain and emerge through various openings in the skull (foramen). The cranial nerve pairs...

- Carry sensory impulses to the brain that are analyzed, sorted, and integrated, resulting in vision, smell, taste, hearing, and/or balance.

- Transmit motor and/or sensory information to particular areas of the head and neck.

- Convey impulses to glands and organs, resulting in certain involuntary (autonomic) activities.

The cranial nerve pairs include the...
- First cranial nerves or olfactory nerves
- Second cranial nerves or optic nerves
- Third cranial nerves or oculomotor nerves
- Fourth cranial nerves or trochlear nerves
- Fifth cranial nerves or trigeminal nerves
- Sixth cranial nerve or abducens nerves
- Seventh cranial nerves or facial nerves
- Eighth cranial nerves or vestibulocochlear nerves
- Ninth cranial nerves or glossopharyngeal nerves
- Tenth cranial nerves or vagus nerves
- Eleventh cranial nerves or accessory nerves
- Twelfth cranial nerves or hypoglossal nerves

The spinal nerves are the 31 pairs of nerves that emerge from either side of the spinal cord through gaps between adjacent bones (vertebrae) in the spinal column. The nerves are assigned a specific letter and number based upon the level of the spinal column from which they emerge. Eight pairs of spinal nerves are attached to the cervical segments; 12 pairs to the thoracic segments; five pairs to the lumber segments; five pairs to the sacrospinal segments; and one pair to the coccygeal segment. The designation "C2," for example, refers to the pair of spinal nerves attached to the second segment of the cervical region of the spinal cord. The spinal nerves that emerge from the spinal cord branch to form many of the nerves supplying the trunk and limbs. The function of the spinal nerves is to transmit sensory and motor impulses between the spinal cord to those areas of the body that are not supplied (innervated) by the cranial nerve pairs. More specifically, the sensory nerve fibers of the spinal nerves transmit impulses from sensory receptors in muscles, internal organs, and the skin to the spinal cord, whereas the motor nerve fibers convey motor impulses from the spinal cord to glands and muscles.

Autonomic Nervous System

The autonomic nervous system (ANS) is that portion of the peripheral nervous system responsible for regulation of the involuntary functioning of certain tissues and organs. The ANS includes specialized motor neurons that transmit impulses from the brain stem or the spinal cord to involuntary muscle tissue, cardiac muscle tissue, and specialized glan-

dular cells that produce and secrete certain chemical substances (e.g., hormones, enzymes).

The autonomic nervous system includes two groups of motor neurons (preganglionic and postganglionic neurons) and a group of nerve cell bodies (ganglia) located between them. The cell bodies and dendrites of preganglionic neurons are located in gray matter of the brain stem or spinal cord, and their axons extend to a set of ganglia in the peripheral nervous system. Within the ganglia, the endings of preganglionic neuron axons join with cell bodies or dendrites of postganglionic neurons, which, in turn, convey nerve impulses from ganglia to smooth muscle, cardiac muscle, or glandular tissue. The tissues to which postganglionic neurons transmit impulses are known as visceral effectors.

Autonomic Nervous System Neurotransmitters
There are four distinct types of nerve fibers (axons) in the autonomic nervous system that release certain neurotransmitters (i.e., acetylcholine or norepinephrine). The sympathetic and parasympathetic nervous systems work somewhat, although not completely, in opposition to each other (antagonistic), since each division may inhibit certain visceral effectors and activate others.

The autonomic nervous system is further subdivided into the sympathetic and the parasympathetic nervous systems.

Sympathetic Nervous System

The sympathetic nervous system functions to prepare the body for an emergency. When the body is affected by stress, such as occurs during strong emotions (fear, anger) or exercise, sympathetic nerve impulses increase to many of the body's visceral effectors, resulting in what is sometimes called the "fright-or-flight response." During this response, the heart and breathing rates increase; the pupils of the eyes widen (dilate); and secretions of certain glands increase, while those of other glands decrease. In addition, most blood vessels constrict, resulting in raised blood pressure; blood vessels that supply skeletal muscle widen, supplying additional blood; and the digestive process slows due to a reduction in the rate of the wave-like contractions of smooth muscle within the GI tract.

Parasympathetic Nervous System

The parasympathetic nervous system controls most visceral nerve transmission under normal circumstances, thus slowing and steadying certain bodily activities. For example, impulses conducted by parasympathetic neurons tend to increase peristalsis, speeding the digestive process; slow the heart and breathing rates; contract the pupils; and stimulate the salivary glands.

Description

Reproductive

The female reproductive system includes those organs that enable females to produce the specialized reproductive or sex cells (gametes) known as eggs (ova); engage in reproductive activity; provide nourishment to a fertilized ovum (zygote) during embryonic and fetal development; and give birth. The male reproductive system consists of those organs that enable males to produce and store the reproductive cells (gametes) known as sperm, engage in reproductive activity, and fertilize ova with sperm. The production and secretion of certain chemical substances (hormones) by glands of the endocrine system promote the maturation and normal functioning of reproductive organs and the development of secondary sexual characteristics (puberty) in males and females.

Female Reproductive System

The female reproductive system includes several organs, including the ovaries, fallopian tubes, uterus, vagina, and vulva. With the exception of the vulva (external genitalia), the female reproductive organs are located within the pelvic cavity. In addition, the female breasts (mammary glands) are supportive glands of the female reproductive system.

Ovaries

The female reproductive cells are produced in the paired structures known as the ovaries. These small, egg-shaped glands contain cavities known as follicles in which the female sex cells develop and mature (oogenesis). As females reach puberty (i.e., which typically has an onset between approximately nine to 13 years of age), the follicles begin to release eggs (ovulation) on a regular monthly cycle. This cycle is regulated by female sex hormones (estrogen and progesterone) that are also secreted by the ovaries.

The hormone estrogen promotes the development of female secondary sexual characteristics and normal functioning of reproductive organs (i.e., puberty). It promotes the development and maturation of female reproductive organs; development of the breasts; development of female body contours caused by fat deposition in the breasts and hip area, for example; and initiation (menarche) and regulation of the menstrual cycle. The menstrual cycle is the recurring monthly cycle during which the mucous membrane lining of the uterus (endometrium) is shed; begins to regrow, becoming thick and supplied with blood; is maintained in the uterus, and is again shed. The thickening of the endometrium is stimulated by the hormone progesterone in preparation for implantation of a fertilized egg (zygote). If such fertilization does not occur, progesterone and estrogen production decrease, causing the uterine lining and the unfertilized egg to be shed (menstruation). Progesterone also plays an essential role in the normal functioning of the placenta, the organ that nourishes the developing embryo and fetus during pregnancy.

Fallopian Tubes

A funnel-shaped duct, known as a fallopian tube, uterine tube, or oviduct, extends from each ovary to the uterus. Each tube ends in a structure shaped like a funnel whose edge has finger-like projections. When an egg is released from an ovary, it enters the fallopian tube with the assistance of the beating motions of these projections and microscopic hairs (cilia) on their surfaces. These motions help to propel the egg toward the uterus. In addition, the fallopian tubes serve as the passageways within which the male sex cells (sperm) move toward the ovaries.

Uterus

The uterus, a hollow, pear-shaped organ composed almost entirely of muscle (myometrium), is the organ within which a fertilized egg (zygote) becomes implanted and the developing embryo and fetus is nourished and grows during pregnancy. The organ consists of a lower narrow section known as the cervix and an upper portion called the body. The uterus usually lies in the pelvic cavity behind the bladder. However, during pregnancy, the uterus expands in size as the developing fetus grows and may eventually extend to the top of the abdominal cavity. During the end of pregnancy, strong uterine muscular contractions cause the cervix to open and widen (dilate) and expel the fetus through the vagina.

Other Components of the Female Reproductive System

The vagina is the muscular passage that connects the cervix and the external genitalia and is the portion of the female reproductive tract that opens to the exterior of the body. The vulva is the external, visible portion of the external genitalia.

Breasts

The female breasts, which are supportive glands of the female reproductive system, produce milk to nourish infants after birth (lactation). The female breast consists of approximately 15 to 20 divisions or lobes embedded within fatty tissue. Each lobe is comprised of smaller lobules of milk-secreting glandular cells that are organized in grape-like clusters (alveoli). The small ducts that drain the alveoli have their outlet within the nipple. The circular, colored (pigmented) area of skin surrounding the nipple is known as the areola. Due to secretion of the hormones progesterone and estrogen by the placenta and the ovaries during pregnancy, the milk-secreting glandular cells become active, causing the nipple to become enlarged. Before and after birth, the glands initially produce a thin, watery fluid (colostrum) containing antibodies and proteins that help to protect the newborn from certain infections. Another hormone known as prolactin is responsible for the secretion of milk.

Reproductive

Male Reproductive System

The male reproductive system also includes several organs, including the testes, reproductive ducts, seminal vesicles, bulbourethral glands, prostate gland, and penis.

Testes

In males, the gonads, i.e., the sex glands within which the reproductive cells are produced, are the paired oval-shaped structures known as the testes. The male sex cells produced by the testes, known as spermatozoa or sperm, are responsible for fertilizing the female ova. The testes are located in pouch-like structures called the scrotum.

Each testis is surrounded by a tough, fibrous membrane (tunica albuginea) and contains a long, narrow, coiled structure known as a seminiferous tubule. Sperm develop within the walls of the tubules in a process known as spermatogenesis. In addition, cells located between the tubules produce the male sex hormone testosterone. This male hormone and certain hormones produced in the pituitary gland (gonadotropin hormones) are responsible for the development and production of sperm.

As males reach puberty (i.e., which typically has an onset between approximately 12 to 14 years of age), increased secretion of testosterone promotes muscle and bone growth, stimulates the development of male secondary sexual characteristics, and promotes the normal functioning of the reproductive organs. More specifically, it stimulates sperm production; the development and maturation of male reproductive organs (e.g., seminal vesicles, prostate gland); and the development of male characteristics (e.g. deepening of the voice due to enlargement of the larynx and the vocal cords, growth of facial and body hair, etc.).

Reproductive Ducts

Sperm develop within the walls of the seminiferous tubules of the testes and pass through several reproductive ducts: i.e., the epididymis, ductus (vas) deferens, ejaculatory duct, and urethra. The first of these is the epididymis, a tightly coiled tube that runs along the top and behind the testes. The ductus or vas deferens is the muscular, movable tube that enables sperm to pass from the testes and the epididymis. The ductus deferens joins the duct from the seminal vesicles to form the ejaculatory duct. This duct enables sperm to empty into the urethra, the tube that passes along the length of the penis and carries sperm to the exterior of the body. In males, the urethra also serves as the passageway through which urine is excreted from the body.

Other Components of the Male Reproductive System

Semen (seminal fluid) is a fluid consisting of sperm as well as the secretions of certain supportive sex glands of the male reproductive tract. Such glands include the seminal vesicles, the prostate gland, and the bulbourethral glands.

Semen serves to protect sperm from the acidic environment within the female reproductive tract.

The seminal vesicles, a pair of pouch-like glands, produce the largest portion of the semen's volume. The secretions of the seminal vesicles contain the sugar fructose, which provides a source of energy promoting the mobility of the sperm. The prostate gland, the chestnut-shaped organ under the bladder and in front of the rectum, secretes a thin fluid that forms a portion of the semen's volume and helps sperm to maintain their mobility. The bulbourethral glands, also known as Cowper's glands, are two relatively small, pea-shaped organs located below the prostate gland. The glands produce mucus-like fluids that form a small portion of the semen's volume. In addition, such secretions help to lubricate the end of the urethra. The penis is the portion of the male genitalia through which semen and urine pass.

Description

Respiratory

The respiratory system, comprising the air passages from the nose, throat, bronchial tubes, and lungs, is responsible for filtering the air that enters the body, supplying oxygen to the body, and removing carbon dioxide from the blood. This process is known as respiration. Certain organs of the respiratory (pulmonary) system also influence speech and help to produce the sense of smell (olfaction).

The organs of the respiratory system are often classified into the upper and lower respiratory tract. The upper respiratory tract, which consists of organs that are located outside the actual chest cavity (thorax), includes the nose, pharynx, and larynx. The organs within the lower respiratory tract are located primarily within the thorax and include the trachea, the bronchial tree, and the lungs.

Nose
The nose functions as the uppermost portion of the respiratory tract. This hollow passage, which connects the naval cavities and the upper portion of the throat (nasopharynx), serves to filter, warm, and moisten the air entering the respiratory tract. Mucous membranes (respiratory mucosa) covered by microscopic hairs (cilia) line the entire nasal passage-as well as most passageways of the respiratory tract. Located within the nasal mucosa are specialized nerve receptors necessary for the sense of smell.

During inspiration, air enters the respiratory tract through the nostrils (external nares). Small hairs within the nostrils trap foreign particles, such as dust, pollen, or microorganisms, thus protecting against infection and allergic responses. Filtered air passes into the nasal cavities, which have moist surfaces due to mucus production. The nasal cavities are divided by a structure made of cartilage (nasal septum). Bones surrounding the nose contain hollow, air-filled cavities (paranasal sinuses) that affect the resonance of sound (e.g., during speech). In addition, these mucous-membrane lined cavities, which drain into the nasal cavities, assist in producing mucus for the respiratory tract.

As air passes through the nasal cavities, it is warmed, humidified, and filtered by three thin, mucosa-covered structures (conchae). Mucus on the surface of the conchae and other organs of the respiratory tract flows toward the nasopharynx due to the beating action of the cilia, thereby helping to move trapped foreign particles out of the respiratory tract.

Pharynx
The pharyx, also known as the throat, is a muscular tube lined with mucous membranes. The throat is part of both the respiratory and digestive systems and is divided into three regions: an uppermost portion (nasopharynx) that serves as an air passage; an area of the throat behind the mouth (oropharynx) that is a passage for food and air; and a lower segment (laryngopharynx) that functions as a passage for food only. Air normally enters the pharynx from the nasal cavities (although it may sometimes enter through the mouth) and exits via the larynx. However, food enters the pharynx from the mouth and continues through the digestive system via the esophagus.

The eustachian or auditory tubes also open into the nasopharynx, connecting the middle ears and the throat. In addition, the masses of lymphoid tissue that serve as the "front line" against invading microorganisms (tonsils) are located under the mucous membranes at the back of the pharynx.

Larynx
The larynx, also known as the voice box, connects the pharynx with the trachea. It consists of several areas of fibrous, flexible connective tissue (cartilage) and is also lined with mucous membranes. The larynx is responsible for producing the voice and preventing food from entering the airway during swallowing.

The opening of the larynx is partially covered by a "lid-like" flap of cartilage known as the epiglottis. This structure normally remains open, maintaining the larynx as part of the airway. However, when swallowing occurs, the epiglottis closes, sealing off the opening of the larynx and preventing food from passing into the larynx and the trachea. In addition, two strong, fibrous sheets of tissue known as the vocal cords stretch across the interior of the larynx. Passage of air over the vocal cords results in vibrations that help to create speech.

Trachea
The trachea, also known as the windpipe, extends from the larynx to an area behind the upper breastbone (sternum), where it then divides to form the two bronchi. The windpipe is a tube-like structure composed of elastic and fibrous tissues, smooth (involuntary) muscle, and rings of cartilage that help to keep the trachea open (patent). As with other organs of the respiratory tract, the trachea is also lined with mucous membranes (respiratory mucosa) covered by cilia. The secreted mucus helps to trap tiny foreign particles remaining in the inhaled air of the trachea, and the beating action of the cilia propels the mucus upward toward the pharynx and out of the respiratory tract.

Bronchial Tree
Because the numerous air passages of the lungs resemble an upside-down, tree-like structure, the bronchi and their branching airways are known as the bronchial tree. The trachea branches to form the main bronchi (primary bronchi) of the left and right lungs. Both of the primary bronchi then branch into smaller bronchi (secondary bronchi). The bron-

chi walls consist of three layers including an outer layer of fibrous, dense tissue; a middle layer of smooth muscle; and an inner layer of mucous membranes. In addition, the walls of the primary and secondary bronchi, like the trachea, are kept open by rings of cartilage, allowing the passage of air.

The bronchi divide into progressively smaller airways that eventually branch into tiny passages known as bronchioles. The walls of the bronchioles include only smooth muscle. The bronchioles then branch into microscopic tubes known as alveolar ducts that lead to the alveolar sacs. The walls of the alveolar sacs consist of many microscopic, grape-like structures called alveoli. The alveoli lie in contact with microscopic blood vessels (capillaries). The exchange of oxygen and carbon dioxide takes place across the thin walls of the alveoli, i.e., oxygen moves from the alveoli to the blood while carbon dioxide moves from the blood to the alveoli.

Lungs

The lungs, which are spongy, elastic organs located in the chest cavity, are divided into lobes: the left lung has two lobes, whereas the right lung has three. The narrow, rounded, upper area of each lung is known as the apex, and the broad, concave, lower portion of each lung that rests on the diaphragm is referred to as the base. In addition, a thin, moist, two-layered membrane known as the pleura lines the outside of the lungs and the inside of the chest cavity. A small amount of fluid separates the two layers of the pleura, serving as a lubricant as the lungs contract and expand during respiration.

The act of breathing (pulmonary ventilation) consists of two phases: inspiration and expiration. During inspiration, the chest and lungs expand, and air is drawn into the lungs. During expiration, the chest and lungs contract and air is forced out of the lungs.

Pulmonary Circulation

Pulmonary circulation refers to the movement of blood through vessels between the heart and the lungs for the removal of carbon dioxide and the addition of oxygen (oxygenation) to the blood. When the right lower chamber of the heart (ventricle) contracts, "oxygen-poor" (deoxygenated) blood is pumped to the lungs via the pulmonary artery. From there, the blood flows through the capillaries that lie in contact with the air-filled alveoli. Oxygen moves across the thin walls of the alveoli into the blood, whereas carbon dioxide is transported by the blood to the alveoli. Carbon dioxide exits the lungs during expiration. Oxygenated blood is returned to the left upper chamber of the heart (atrium) via four pulmonary veins and is propelled into the left ventricle. When the left ventricle contracts, the blood is pumped into the major artery of the body (aorta) for circulation to the body's tissues. In addition, the blood that nourishes the lungs themselves is supplied by the bronchial arteries.

Description

Sensory Organs

Certain specialized components of the nervous system, known as sense organs, are able to recognize specific stimuli in the external environment that affect the body, such as light, sound, temperature, or pressure. When the specialized microscopic structures that comprise the sensory organs (sensory receptors) recognize certain stimuli, they produce nervous impulses that are sent to the brain, the spinal cord, or both. The sense organs may be classified into two general categories: the somatic sense organs and the special sense organs.

Special Sense Organs

Sensory receptors for the special senses of hearing, vision, smell, and taste, are collected in the special sense organs, including the eyes (i.e., in the retinas), the ears (within the hearing apparatus), the nose (smell receptors), and the tongue (taste receptors). Sensory information received by these special sense organs travels to the brain via the cranial nerves, the 12 nerve pairs that arise from the brain and emerge through various openings in the skull. Most sensory information is transmitted to the sensory cortex of the brain.

Ears, Hearing, and Balance

The ear is the special sensory organ involved in hearing and balance. It consists of three major parts including

- external ear
- middle ear
- inner ear

The External Ear

The external ear includes the visible portion of the ear (pinna or auricle) and the external auditory canal. The pinna consists of folds of cartilage and skin surrounding the opening of the auditory canal, which is the tube that extends into the lower cranium bone (temporal bone) and ends at the partition between the external and middle ear (eardrum or tympanic membrane). The skin of the auditory canal contains specialized glands (ceruminous glands) that produce cerumen, a waxy substance that traps dust and other foreign bodies. Sound waves pass through the auditory canal and strike the eardrum, causing it to vibrate.

The Middle Ear

The middle ear, a tiny cavity between the eardrum and the inner ear, contains three minute, movable bones (ossicles) that conduct sound to the inner ear. The names of the bones essentially describe their shapes: i.e., the malleus (hammer), incus (anvil), and stapes (stirrup). When the eardrum vibrates in response to sound waves, the vibrations are transmitted and amplified by the three ear bones. The stapes' movement against a membrane-covered opening to the inner ear results in movement of the fluid within the inner ear.

The eustachian or auditory tube connects the middle ear to the uppermost region of the throat (nasopharynx). Although the eustachian tube is usually closed at rest, it opens due to muscle contractions associated with swallowing or yawning. The eustachian tube is shorter in infants and young children than in older children and adults. As a result, when an upper respiratory tract infection occurs, infants and young children have an increased likelihood of experiencing the backward flow of secretions from the nasopharynx into the middle ear space and associated infection of the middle ear (otitis media).

The Inner Ear

The inner ear contains a maze of complex, winding passages (known as the labyrinth) deep within the temporal bone. The major parts of the inner ear include the organ of hearing, known as the cochlea, and the organ of balance, the semicircular canals.

The cochlea, a hollow, coiled passage that resembles a snail's shell, contains the organ of Corti and thick fluid. The organ of Corti has tiny cells with hair-like extensions projecting into the fluid. Vibrations transmitted to the inner ear cause the fluid and the hair-like extensions to vibrate. As a result, the hair cells are stimulated to generate nerve impulses that are transmitted by the vestibulocochlear nerve (acoustic nerve or eighth cranial nerve) to the brain.

The three semicircular canals are fluid-filled tubes containing specialized hair cells that respond to movement of the fluid. When movements of the head cause fluid movement within a canal, the cells initiate nerve impulses to the brain via the vestibulocochlear nerve, resulting in necessary adjustments to maintain balance.

The Eyes and Vision

The eye is a specialized sensory organ that is actually part of the central nervous system. It focuses light waves to create an image on the nerve-rich membrane at the back of the eye (retina). The retina, in turn, converts the image into nerve impulses that are transmitted to the brain via the optic nerve (second cranial nerve).

Anatomy and Function of the Eye

The eye is embedded in pads of fat within the bony socket in the skull. Movements of the eye are regulated by a network of six muscles, each of which moves the eye in a particular direction or directions.

The outermost layer of the eye, known as the sclera, is a tough, fibrous tissue that includes the "white" of the eye and the cornea, which is the front, circular, transparent area that serves as the eye's primary lens. A flexible mucous membrane, the conjunctiva, covers the sclera and lines the eyelid; in addition, the conjunctiva contains several glands that secrete tears and mucus. The eyelid consists of a thin layer of skin over muscle that covers a thin plate of connective tissue (tarsal plate). The edge of the eyelid contains a row of strong protective hairs known as eyelashes as well as several glands (meibomian glands) that produce an oily secretion known as sebum. The combined actions of the tear-secreting and mucus-producing glands of the conjunctiva and the meibomian glands of the eyelid produce an essential tear film that protects the conjunctiva and cornea from damage due to drying. The eyelid spreads the tear film over the cornea during the blink reflex, helping to ensure clear vision. Moreover, the eyelid further protects the eye by closing quickly as an involuntary reaction (reflex action) to the approach of any foreign object.

The middle layer of the eye, known as the choroid, includes two involuntary muscles: the iris and the ciliary muscle. The iris, the pigmented area visible through the cornea, is a circular muscle with a hole in its center known as the pupil, which controls the amount of light entering the eye. When certain fibers in the iris contract, the pupil widens, allowing in additional light; in contrast, when other iris fibers contract, the pupil constricts, allowing in less light. The lens of the eye, which is behind the pupil, is held in place by the ciliary muscle, a circular muscle that changes the shape of the lens to make appropriate adjustments in focus. For example, the ciliary muscle contracts when the eye focuses on near objects and relaxes when the eye views distant objects.

The hollow main cavity of the eye is filled with fluids that help to ensure the proper shape of the eyeball and assist in bending light rays that fall on the retina. The fluids include the thin, watery fluid in front of the lens (aqueous humor) and the jelly-like fluid behind the lens (vitreous humor).

The retina, the innermost layer of the eye, is a complex nerve-rich membrane upon which images created by the cornea and the lens fall. More specifically, as light passes through the cornea, the pupil, the aqueous humor, the lens, and the vitreous humor, it is bent (refracted) so that it is properly focused on the retina, which contains millions of tiny nerve cells that respond to light (photoreceptors). Such nerve cells are named based upon their shapes: i.e., rods and cones. Rods are stimulated by dim light and are necessary for night vision. Cones are stimulated by brighter light and are the receptors for daytime vision. Three different types of cones respond to the colors red, blue, or green. The rods and cones convert images formed on the retina into nerve impulses that are transmitted by the optic nerve (second cranial nerve) to the brain.

The Nose and the Smell Receptors

In addition to serving as the uppermost region of the respiratory tract, the nose also functions as the special sensory organ involved in the sense of smell (olfaction). The chemical receptors necessary for olfaction are specialized nerve cell endings located in a small area of mucous membrane (nasal mucosa) lining the nasal cavities. The olfactory cells have specialized, microscopic hairs (cilia) that are stimulated by different chemicals. In response to such chemicals, the cilia generate nerve impulses that pass through the olfactory nerve (first cranial nerve) to the smell centers of the brain.

The Tongue and the Taste Receptors

The tongue is the muscular, flexible organ in the floor of the mouth. This organ-which also plays an essential role in producing speech, breaking down food during chewing (mastication), and swallowing - functions as a specialized sensory organ involved in taste.

There are approximately 10,000 microscopic chemical receptors known as taste buds that produce the nerve impulses required for taste. Although most are located on the tongue, there are also some taste buds on the roof of the mouth (palate) and the back of the throat. The taste buds surround the bases of nipple-shaped elevations (papillae) that cover the surface of the tone and other tissues. Specialized cells within the taste buds (gustatory cells) generate nerve impulses in response to dissolved chemicals within saliva. Most of these impulses pass through the facial nerve (seventh cranial nerve) and the glossopharyngeal nerve (ninth cranial nerve) to the taste center of the brain. Stimulation of the taste buds results in four types of taste sensations including sour, sweet, bitter, and salty. Other taste sensations or "flavors" result due to the combined stimulation of taste and olfactory receptors.

Description

Urologic

The urinary system, which consists of the two kidneys, the ureters, the bladder, and the urethra, filters waste products from the blood, returns essential nutrients back into the blood, and produces and excretes urine.

The Kidneys

The kidneys, which are located at the back of the abdominal cavity, are situated on either side of the spinal column above the waistline. The right kidney lies beneath the liver. The left kidney, which is usually slightly higher than the right, is located below the spleen.

The primary functions of the kidneys are to regulate the delicate balance of electrolytes including sodium and potassium; control the acid-base balance of the body (i.e., ensuring that the blood and other bodily fluids are neither too acidic nor alkaline); and filter soluble wastes from the blood and eliminate these waste products. More specifically, the purpose of the kidneys includes the following:

- To filter certain waste products (e.g., urea, ammonia) and excessive sodium and water from the blood

- To reabsorb particular substances and return them to the blood

- To regulate the levels of certain substances in the blood and maintain the appropriate balance between water and salt content in the body (i.e., by filtration, reabsorption, and secretion)

- To regulate blood pressure and the production and release of red blood cells. For example, cells of the juxtaglomerular apparatus of the kidneys secrete a hormone (renin) that results in the constriction of blood vessels, thereby raising blood pressure. In addition, the kidneys produce erythropoietin, a hormone that assists in stimulating and regulating the production and release of red blood cells (erythrocytes) from the bone marrow. An increase in the number of circulating red blood cells boosts the body's capacity to carry oxygen to its tissues and organs.

Urine Production and Excretion

The kidneys each contain approximately one million nephrons, the filtering units of the kidneys. Each nephron consists of two primary components, the renal corpuscle and the renal tubule, both of which are further divided into additional regions.

The top of each nephron consists of a cup-shaped structure known as Bowman's capsule. Within Bowman's capsule is a network of tiny capillaries known as a glomerulus. Together, the two structures are known as the renal corpuscle.

As blood flows through the kidneys, the fluid portion of the blood is filtered by minute pores in the blood vessels of the glomerulus and the inner layer of Bowman's capsule. The fluid then moves into the region between the inner and outer layers of Bowman's capsule and enters into the first portion of the renal tubule (proximal convoluted tubule), where most filtered substances (e.g., most of the water, glucose, and sodium) are reabsorbed into the blood via capillaries around the tubules (peritubular capillaries). Next, as fluid moves into the loop of Henle, sodium and other electrolytes are pumped out. As the fluid passes through the next portion of the renal tubule (distal convoluted tubule), additional sodium is removed in exchange for potassium. Diluted fluid from distal convoluted tubules then passes into a collecting tubule, where fluid may continue to pass through the urinary tract as dilute urine or be returned to the blood to ensure appropriate water content in the body.

Urine then drains from the collecting tubules into central collecting areas (renal pelvis) of each kidney, which are the upper portions of the ureters. The ureters are narrow muscular tubes lined by mucous membranes. Contractions of the ureters' muscular walls move small quantities of urine into the bladder, a hollow organ that gradually expands as the volume of urine increases. As the bladder nears its capacity, nerve signals are transmitted to the brain to signal that urination is necessary. When urination occurs, the circular muscle (sphincter) between the bladder and the urethra opens, allowing urine to pass out of the body. Contractions of the bladder create pressure that forces urine into the urethra and out its external opening (urinary meatus).

Administration for Children & Families-Child Abuse and Neglect Prevention, 5644
Administration on DevelopmentalDisabilities, 7824
Adolescent Health On-Line, 8605
Adolescent Idiopathic Scoliosis-Prevalence ,Natural History, Treatments, 6509
Adolescents with Down Syndrome, 2730
Adoptive Families of America, 7870
Adriene Resource Center for Blind Children, 1875, 2022, 5252, 6177
Adult Brain Tumor Support Group, 1254
Adult Down Syndrome Center of LutheranGeneral Hospital, 2683
Adult GHD Educational Convention, 10, 332, 1812
Advanced Cancer: Coping with Advanced Cancer, 8684
Adventure Learning Center Camp Programs, 1803, 7764
Adventures of Maxx, 4057
Advocacy Center, 8332
Advocate Lutheran General Children'sHospital, Pediatric Research, 2684
Advocates Across America, 7871
Advocates for Children of New York, 8333, 8786
Advocates for Deaf & Hard of HearingYouth, 7872
Advocates for Justice and Education, 8160
Advocure NF2, 6749
African American Collaborative Obesity Research Network, 5305
After Sudden Infant Death Syndrome, 7101
After the Diagnosis...The Next Steps, 7411
After the Tears: Parents Talk AboutRaising a Child with a Disability, 1515
Agency for Health Care Research, 7825
Agency for Healthcare Research and Quality, 2439
Aggression and Violence Throughout theLife Span, 1791, 7734
Aging with Autism, 715
Agoraphobics in Motion, 5561
Air Support America, 403
Al Capone Does My Shirts: A Novel, 910
Alabama Department of RehabilitationServices, 3989
Alabama Head Injury Foundation, 3365
Alabama Institute for the Deaf & Blind, 1826, 1971, 3553, 5202, 6118
Alabama/Northwest Florida Chapter of Crohns Colitis Foundation of America, 2146
Alandra's Lilacs, 3729
Alaska Chapter of Asthma and Allergy Foundation of America, 428
Alaska Department of Education, 8085
Albany Library for the Blind and PhysicalHandicapped, 1846, 1992, 5223, 6148
Albany Medical College Pediatric Pulmonary& Cystic Fibrosis Center, 2308
Albany New York Regional ComprehensiveHemophilia Treatment Center, 3992
Albinism, 173
Alcohol, Tobacco and Other Drugs May Harmthe Unborn, 3157
Aleh Foundation, 2637, 2721
Alert, 570
Alex's Journey: The Story of a Child witha Brain Tumor, 1269
Alex: The Life of a ChildRutledge Press, 2361
Alexander Graham Bell Association for theDeaf and Hard of Hearing, 3480, 7873
Alexandria Library Talking Book Service, 1885, 2032, 5262, 6187
Alexis Foundation - Premature Infants andChildren, 5897
All About Amblyopia (Lazy Eye), 4472
All About Vision, 4473
All About Vision.Com, 4474
All Ages Support Group, 1166
All Children Have Different Eyes, 4485
All Kids By TwoHealth Services Agency, 5954
All Kinds of Friends, Even Green!, 6875
All Kinds of Minds, 647
All Nations Camp, 8714
All of Us Together, 3730
Alleghenies United Cerebral Palsy, 1474
Allen County Public Library, 8475
Allergy & Asthma Issues, 457, 6345
Allergy & Asthma Network Mothers of Asthmatics, 404, 466
Allergy & Asthma Today, 484
Allergy Control Begins at Home: House Dust Allergy, 458
Allergy Web, 7658
Allergy and Asthma Medical Group and Research Center, 6322
Allergy and Asthma Support Group of Central New Jersey, 6319
Allergy and Pulmonary Medicine, 434
Alliance Brochure, 575
Alliance for Assistive Service andTechnology (FAAST), 8166

Alliance for Eating Disorder Awarenes, 2838
Alliance for Eating Disorders Awareness, 2905
Alliance for Technology Access (ATA), 7874, 8449
Alliance for a Healthier Generation, 5306
Alliance of Genetic Support Groups, 3254
Aloha Special Technology Access Center, 8468
Alone in the Mainstream: A Deaf Women Remembers Public School, 3731
Alopecia Areata, 197
Alpha Omega International Dental Fraternity, 2397
Alpha-1-Antitrypsin Deficiency, 209
AlphaNet, Inc., 210
Alphabet Soup: A Recipe for Understanding& Treating ADD, 648
Alphabet of Animal Signs, 3732
Alternative Approaches, 6046
Amblyopia, 4493
Ambulatory Pediatric Association, 7875
AmeriFace, 1683, 2115, 3033, 4578
AmeriFace Newsletter, 1702, 3049
America's Special Kidz, 344
American Academy for Cerebral Palsy andDevelopmental Medicine, 1381, 1500, 1503
American Academy of Allergy, Asthma & Immunology, 6312
American Academy of Allergy, Asthma &Immunology, 405
American Academy of Allergy, Asthma and Immunology, 467
American Academy of Audiology, 3481, 5473, 7876
American Academy of Child & AdolescentPsychiatry, 7321, 7331, 7354, 7422
American Academy of Child and AdolescentPsychiatry, 1670, 5419, 5422, 7668, 7877
American Academy of Cosmetic Dentistry, 2398
American Academy of Dental Hygiene, 2399
American Academy of Dental Practice Administration, 2400
American Academy of Dermatology, 198
American Academy of Dermatology (AAD), 3919, 4417, 5738, 6026, 7194, 7203, 7239, 7878
American Academy of Esthetic Dentistry, 2401
American Academy of Family Physicians, 2097, 7669
American Academy of HIV Medicine, 3285
American Academy of Neurology, 4747, 4753
American Academy of Neurology: TouretteSyndrome, 7423
American Academy of Orthopaedic Surgeons, 6485
American Academy of Otolaryngology Head and Neck Surgery, 1010
American Academy of Otolaryngology-Headand Neck Surgery, 1004
American Academy of Pediatric DentistryFoundation, 2402, 2433
American Academy of Pediatrics, 5, 22, 65, 124, 175, 199, 211, 223, 234, 248, 258, 283, 294, 301, 311, 327, 345, 406, 500, 588, 602
American Academy of Periodontology, 2404
American Academy of Sleep Medicine, 4881, 5096, 5126, 6671, 6678, 6698
American Academy of Somnology, 5112, 5135, 6675, 6703
American Action Fund for Blind Childrenand Adults, 1834, 1980, 3555, 5211, 6136
American Amputee Foundation, 7880
American Annals of the Deaf, 3862
American Anorexia Bulimia Association of Philadelphia, 5337
American Asperger's Association, 346
American Association for Cancer Research, 1083
American Association for Dental Research, 2405
American Association for Leisureand Recreation, 7881
American Association for Marriage and Family Therapy, 347
American Association for Pediatric Opthalmology, 1891, 1903, 2639, 3142
American Association for Respiratory Care, 407, 5926
American Association for Thoracic Surgery, 5927
American Association for the Study ofLiver Diseases, 1016
American Association of Children'sResidential Centers (AACRC), 7882
American Association of ClinicalEndocrinologists, 2228, 4347, 4354
American Association of Diabetes Educators, 2553
American Association of Endodontists, 2406
American Association of Neurological Surgeons, 1084
American Association of Oral and Maxillofacial Surgeons, 2407
American Association of Orthodontics, 2408
American Association of Orthodontists, 2409
American Association of People with Disabilities, 4677
American Association of Public Health Dentistry, 2410
American Association of Sleep Technologists, 5097
American Association of Suicidology, 2441
American Association of the Deaf-Blind, 3483, 7883
American Association on Health and Disabilities, 4678

D

G

T

V

W

Y

Z

Alabama

ARC of Morgan County, 8079
Alabama Department of Rehabilitation Services, 3989
Alabama Head Injury Foundation, 3365
Alabama Institute for the Deaf & Blind, 1826, 1971, 3553, 5202, 6118
Alabama/Northwest Florida Chapter of Crohn s Colitis Foundation of
   America, 2146
Autism Society of Alabama, 776
Autism Society of North Alabama, 777
Birmingham Support Group, 502
Camp ASCCA/Easter Seals, 8705
Camp Merrimack, 984, 1540, 2767, 8706
Camp Rap A Hope, 8707
Camp Shocco for the Deaf, 3903
Camp Smile-A-Mile, 8708
Down Syndrome Clinic, Children's Hospital of Alabama, 2679
Early Intervention Program, 8080
Gregory Fleming James Cystic Fibrosis Cent er, 2247
Mobile Association for the Blind, 1893, 1977, 2043, 5208, 5269, 6133
National Child Advocacy Center, 8360
Pediatric Brain Tumor Support Group, 1124
Sickle Cell Foundation of Greater Montgomery, 6629
Special Education Action Committee Huntsville Outreach Office, 8082
Special Education Services, 8083
Spina Bifida Association of Alabama, 6814
Statewide Technology Access & Response System for Alabamians with
   Disabilities, 8084
United Cerebral Palsy of Alabama, 1395
United Cerebral Palsy of Greater Birmingham, 1396
United Cerebral Palsy of Huntsville & Tennessee Valley, 1397
United Cerebral Palsy of Mobile, 1398
United Cerebral Palsy of Northwest Alabama, 1399
United Cerebral Palsy of West Alabama, 1400
University of Alabama - Birmingham Arthrit is Clinical Intervention
   Program, 6444
University of Alabama Speech and Hearing Center, 3554

Alaska

Alaska Chapter of Asthma and Allergy Found ation of America, 428
Alaska Department of Education, 8085
Assistive Technologies of Alaska, 8086
Camp Kushtaka, 2609
Maternal, Child & Family Health, Early Intervention/Infant Learning
   Program, 8087
PARENTS, 8088
Rid Alaska of Child Abuse, 5669
SIDS Information & Counseling Program Alaska Department of Health,
   6994
Turner's Syndrome Society of Alaska, 7557
United Cerebral Palsy of Alaska/PARENTS, 1401
University of Alaska, Fairbanks, 8573

Arizona

Arizona Ataxia Support Group, 503
Arizona Camp Sunrise, 114, 167, 1297, 3122, 5180, 7804
Arizona Chapter of Crohn's & Colitis Foundation of America, 2147
Arizona Early Intervention Program/ Department of Economic Security,
   8089
Arizona Sleep Disorders Center, 4889
Arizona Spina Bifida Association, 6815
Arizona Technology Access Program Institute for Human Development,
   8090
Autism Society of America Greater Phoenix Chapter, 778
Autism Society of America Northern Arizona Chapter, 779
Autism Society of America Pima County Chapter, 780
Blake Foundation Children's Achievement Center, 8091
Brain Injury Association of Arizona, 3366
Brain Tumor Support Group at NovaCare Rehabilitation Institute of
   Tucson, 1125
Brain Tumor Support Group at Phoenix, 1126
Camp Abilities Tucson, 8709
Camp Civitan, 1931, 2083, 3899, 8710
Camp Shane Arizona, 5350

Children's Center for Neurodevelopmental Studies, 864
Crisis Nursery, 5670
Cystic Fibrosis Center: Phoenix Children's Hospital, 2248
Division of Special Education State Department of Education, 8092
Families of SMA - Arizona Chapter, 6917
Injury Prevention Center, 4228
Maricopa Co Childhood Immunization Program, 5951
Mayo Clinic Scleroderma Service, 6445
Mayo Comprehensive Hemophilia Center, 4020
National Center for Neurogenic Communicati on Disorders, 6781
Neurofibromatosis, Inc - Arizona Chapter, 5013
Office of Women's & Children's Health, 6995
Phoenix Center for Cancer and Blood Disorders, 4029
Pilot Parents of Southern Arizona, 8093
Prader-Willi Syndrome Arizona Association, 5818
Raising Special Kids, 8094
Southwest Chapter of Crohn's & Colitis Foundation of America, 2170
Special Needs Center/Phoenix Public Library, 8443
Steele Children's Research Center, 4038
Technology Access Center of Tucson, 8444
The Arizona Partnership for Immunization, 5952
Tourette Syndrome Association - Arizona Chapter, 7378
Turner's Syndrome Society of Arizona, 7558
United Cerebral Palsy of Central Arizona, 1402
United Cerebral Palsy of Southern Arizona, 1403

Arkansas

Arkansas Department of Health - SIDS Information & Counseling Program,
   6996
Arkansas Department of Health Div. of Comm Diseases/Immunizations,
   5953
Arkansas Disability Coalition, 8096
Arkansas Disability Coalition Parent Train ing and Information Center,
   8097
Arkansas Easter Seals Technology Resource Center, 8445
Arkansas Regional Library for the Blind and Physically Handicapped, 1833,
   1979, 5210, 6135
Arkansas Rehabilitation Research and Training Center for Deaf Persons,
   3569
Autism Society of America Arkansas Chapter, 781
Brain Injury Association of Arkansas, 3367
Camp Aldersgate, 8711
Camp Funshine, 2379
Children's Tumor Foundation-Arkansas Chapt er, 5014
Crowley Ridge Regional Library, 8446
DD Services, Department of Human Services, 8098
Educational Services for the Visually Impaired, 1832, 1978, 5209, 6134,
   8447
Epilepsy Education Association of Arkansas, 6532
FOCUS, 8099
Family-2-Family Health Information Center of Arkansas, 8100
Hemophilia Center of Arkansas, 3944, 4006
Increasing Capabilities Access Network, 8101
Library for the Blind and Handicapped, Southwest, 8448
Parent to Parent Arc of Arkansas, 8102
Special Education Section State Department of Education, 8103
United Cerebral Palsy of Central Arkansas, 1404

California

ARC Family Resource Project, 8104
Ability First, 8712
Ability First, Camp Paivika, 8713
All Kids By Two Health Services Agency, 5954
Allergy and Asthma Medical Group and Resea rch Center, 6322
American Action Fund for Blind Children and Adults, 1980, 3555, 5211,
   6136
American Association for Pediatric Ophthalmology and Strabismus, 1891
Assistive Technology Center Simi Valley Hospital, 8450
Ataxia Telangiectasia Medical Research Foundation, 553
Autism Research Institute, 862
Autism Society of America Coachella Valley, 782
Autism Society of America Greater Long Beach/South Bay Chapter, 783
Autism Society of America Inland Empire Chapter, 784
Autism Society of America Los Angeles Chapter, 785

San Fernando Valley Support Group, 510
San Francisco Brain Tumor Support Group, 1140
San Francisco Public Library for the Blind and Print Disabled, 1840, 1986, 5217, 6142
San Gabriel/Pomona Parents' Place, 8126
Santa Barbara Brain Tumor Support Group, 1141
Santa Cruz County Brain Tumor Support Group, 1142
Santa Rosa Brain Tumor Support Group, 1143
Scleroderma Research Foundation, 6446
Sickle Cell Disease Foundation of California, 6630
South Bay Brain Tumor Support Group, 1144
South Central Los Angeles Regional Center for Devlopmentally Disabled Persons, 8127
Southern California Pediatric Brain Tumor Network, 1145
Special Connections Family Resource Center, 8128
Special Education Division State Department of Education, 8129
Stanford CF Center, 2260
Stanford University Center for Narcolepsy, 4891
Starlight Children's Foundation, 8130
Support Group for Caregivers of Brain Tumor Patients, 1146
Support Group for Parents of Children with Brain Tumors, 1147
Support for Families of Children with Disabilities, 8131
Team Advocates for Special Kids, Anaheim, 8132
Team Advocates for Special Kids, San Diego, 8133
Team of Advocates for Special Kids, 8570
Tourette Syndrome Association - Southern California Chapter, 7380
Turner's Syndrome Society Central And Northern, 7559
Turner's Syndrome Society of Southern California, 7560
UC Berkeley School of Social Welfare, 5136, 5586, 8572
UCD Hemophilia Treatment Center, 4040
UCSD Hemophilia Treatment Center, 4041
USC - Neonatology Research Units, 7077
United Cerebral Palsy of Central California, 1405
United Cerebral Palsy of Greater Sacramento, 1406
United Cerebral Palsy of Los Angeles, Ventura and Santa Barbara Counties, 1407
United Cerebral Palsy of Orange County, 1408
United Cerebral Palsy of San Diego County, 1409
United Cerebral Palsy of San Joaquin, Calaveras & Amador Counties, 1410
United Cerebral Palsy of San Luis Obispo, 1411
United Cerebral Palsy of Santa Clara & San Mateo Counties, 1412
United Cerebral Palsy of Stanislaus County Stanislaus, 1413
United Cerebral Palsy of the Golden State, 1414
United Cerebral Palsy of the Inland Empire, 1415
United Cerebral Palsy of the North Bay, 1416
University of California, San Francisco Dermatology Drug Research, 1578, 1584, 3002, 3008, 5628, 5634
University of Southern California Comprehensive Sickle Cell Center, 6646
Variety Audio, 1841, 1987, 5218, 6143
Vital Options, 1148
Warmline Family Resource Center, 8134
Wellness Community San Francisco/East Bay, 1149
Wellspring Camps, 5355
West Los Angeles Brain Tumor Support Group, 1150

Colorado

Assistive Technology Partners, 8135
Autism Society of America Larimer County Chapter, 796
Autism Society of America Pikes Peak Chapter, 797
Autism Society of America: Colorado Chapter, 798
Autism Society of American Boulder County Chapter, 799
Brain Injury Association of Colorado, 3370
Brain Tumor Patient & Family Support Group, 1151
Brain Tumor Patient/Family Group, 1152
Breckenridge Outdoor Education Center, 1930
Cardiac Kids/Association of Volunteers, 4311
Children's Hospital: Academic Pediatric Surgery Department, 1739
Children's Tumor Foundation - Colorado Cha pter, 5017
Colorado Consortium of Intensive Care Nurseries United Parents (UP), 8136
Colorado Dept. of Public Heand & Environme nt: Immunization Program, DCEED-IMM-A3, 5958
Colorado SIDS Program, 7000
Colorado Support Group, 511
Delta/Montrose Parent to Parent, 8137
Denver Children's Hospital, 2261

Denver Early Childhood Connections, 8138
Denver Sarcoidosis Awareness Support Group, 6355
Disabilities Advocacy & Support Network, 8288
Disability Connection and RAFT, Larimer County's Early Childhood Connection, 8139
Effective Parent Project, 8140
El Groupo Vida, 8141
Help Parent Support Group Hope & Education for Loving Parents, 8142
Hemophilia Society of Colorado, 3949
Little People of America - Front Range Chapter, 3240, 5442
Magic of Music and Dance, 8725
Mile High Down Syndrome Association, 2663
Mountain States Regional Genetics Services Network, 512
National Jewish Center for Immunology and Respiratory Medicine, 446
National Jewish Health, 440
National Jewish Medical & Research Center, 447, 5748, 6373
Oasis, 8143
PEAK Parent Center, 8144
Parent Support Group of Littleton & Auora, 8145
Parents Supporting Parents of Eagle County, 8146
Parents Supporting Parents of Garfield and Pitkin County, 8147
Parents of Asthmatic/Allergic Children, In c., 430, 6317
Prader-Willi Colorado Association, 5820
Prevention Initiatives State Department of Education, 8148
Region VIII Office Program Consultants for Maternal and Child Health, 7001
Resources for Young Children and Families, 8149
Rocky Mountain Chapter of Crohn's & Colitis Foundation of America, 2151
Rocky Mountain Village, 8726
Speech, Language, & Hearing Center University of Colorado, 6957
Speech, Language, and Hearing Center, 6782
Spina Bifida Association of Colorado, 6819
TIES, The Children's Hospital, 8569
Tourette Syndrome Association - Rocky Mountain Region, 7381, 7392, 7393, 7407
Turner's Syndrome Society of Rocky Mountain, 7561
Wilderness on Wheels Foundation, 8150

Connecticut

A.J. Pappanikou Center for Developmental D isabilities, 8151
Assistive Technology Project, 8152
Autism Society of America Connecticut Chapter, 800
Brain Injury Association of Connecticut, 3371
Brain Tumor Support Group, 1153, 1154
CPAC, 8153
Central Connecticut Chapter of Crohn's & Colitis Foundation of America, 2152
Connecticut Brain Tumor Support Group (Adult), 1155
Connecticut Down Syndrome Congress, 2664
Connecticut Lead Poisoning Prevention Program, 4497
Department of Mental Retardation, 8154
Families of SMA - Connecticut Chapter, 6919
Gaylord Hospital Sleep Medicine, 4892
Hemlocks Easter Seals Recreation, 1731, 6521
Hole in the Wall Gang Camp, 3351, 4093
Mansfield's Holiday Hill, 8727
Marvelwood Summer, 2803
Northern Connecticut Affiliate Chapter of Crohn's & Colitis Foundation of America, 2154
Parent to Parent Network of Connecticut the Family Center, 8155
Parents Association of Connecticut Childre n with Visual Impairments (PACVI), 6276
Prader-Willi Connecticut Association, 5821
Region 1 of the National Association for Parents of the Visually Impaired, 6121
Spina Bifida Association of Connecticut, 6820
State Department of Education, 8156
Sudden Infant Death Syndrome (SIDS) Network, 7067
TBI Support Group for Families & Survivors, 3372
Tourette Syndrome Association - Connecticut Chapter, 7382
Turner's Syndrome Society of Connecticut, 7562
United Cerebral Palsy of Eastern Connecticut, 1417
United Cerebral Palsy of Greater Hartford, 1418
United Cerebral Palsy of Southern Connecticut, 1419
University of Connecticut Health Center, 2262

Yale Pediatric Hematology/Oncology Research Center, 4051
Yale University Cystic Fibrosis Research Center, 2263
Yale University, Behavioral Medicine Clinic, 2482
Yale University, Ribicoff Research Facilities, 2483

Delaware

Autism Society of Delaware, 801
Brain Injury Association of Delaware, 3373
Children's Beach House, 3905
Delaware Assisstive Technology Initiative (DATI), 8157
Delaware Division of Libraries for the Blind and Physically Handicapped, 1579, 3003, 5629
Department of Public Instruction, 8158
Parent Information Center of Delaware, 8159
Pediatric Brain Tumor Support Group, 1156
Prader-Willi Delaware Association, 5822
SIDS Information & Counseling - Division of Public Health, 7002
Turner's Syndrome Society of Philadelphia, 7583
United Cerebral Palsy of Delaware, 1420

District of Columbia

Advocates for Justice and Education, 8160
Autism Society of America District of Columbia Chapter, 802
Brain Injury Association of Washington DC, 3374
Brain Research Center, 1260
Center for Auditory and Speech Sciences-Gallaudet University, 3557
Child Welfare Information Gateway, 5680
Children's National Medical Center, 95, 155, 6323
Commission of Public Health Immunization Program, 5959
Council of Families with Visual Impairment, 1842, 1988, 5219, 6144
Counseling and Research Center for SIDS, 7064
DC Arc, 8161
DC-EIP Services, 8162
Department of Health Division of Immunization, 5960
District of Columbia Public Library/ Librarian for the Deaf Community, 3558
Division of Community Health Nursing, 7003
Georgetown University, 6447
Georgetown University Child Development Center, 8163, 8454, 8558
Georgetown University Sleep Disorders Center, 4893
HEATH Resource Center, 8455
Hemophilia Program at Children's National Medical Center, 4010
Howard University Center for Sickle Cell Disease, 6647
Lab School of Washington Summer Program, 707, 995, 4543
Laurent Clerc National Deaf Education Center-Gallaudet Universty, 3559
National Center for Education in Maternal and Child Health, 5906
National Technical Assistance Center for Children's Mental Health, 1776, 7699
Partnership for Assistive Technology, 8165
Scottish Rite Centers for Childhood Langua ge Disorders, 6779
Spina Bifida Association Pittsburgh, 6852
Spina Bifida Association of Arkansas, 6816
Spina Bifida Association of Greater Bay Ar ea, 6817
Spina Bifida Association of Greater Fox Valley, 6862
Spina Bifida Association of Greater San Di ego, 6818
Spina Bifida Association of Northern Indiana, 6828
Spina Bifida Assisstion of Southeast Florida, 6823
Spina Bifida Association of Tennessee, 6855
Talking Books - National Library Service, 4469
Technical Assistance Partnership for Child and Family Mental Health, 1779, 7702
United Cerebral Palsy of Washington DC & Northern Virginia, 1421
United Cerebral Palsy of Washington DC & Northern Virginia, 1492
Volta Bureau Library, 3560
Washington DC Metropolitan Area Support Group, 1157

Florida

Alliance for Assistive Service and Technology (FAAST), 8166
Alliance for Eating Disorders Awareness, 2905
American SIDS Institute, 7068
Angels in the Sun Brain Tumor Support Group, 1158
Ataxia Telangiectasia Children's Project, 552
Autism Society of America Broward Chapter, 803

Autism Society of America Emerald Coast Chapter, 804
Autism Society of America Florida Chapter, 805
Autism Society of America Jacksonville Chapter, 806
Autism Society of America Panhandle Chapter, 808
Autism Society of Greater Orlando, 809
Brain Injury Association of Florida, 3375
Brain Tumor Support Group, 1159
Brain Tumor Support Group at Miami, 1160
Brain Tumor Support Group at St. Petersburg, 1161
Brain Tumor Support Group at Tampa, 1162
Broward County Support Group, 513
CF & Pediatric Pulmonary Disease Center, 2264
Camp Boggy Creek, 6905
Camp Thunderbird, 8728
Cancer Support Group for Children, 1163
Center for Independence Technology and Education, (CITE), 8456
Child and Family Connections, 8191
Children's Medical Services Program Florida SIDS Program, 7004
Children's Tumor Foundation - Florida Chap ter, 5018
Clearwater, FL Support Group, 514
Coconut Creek Eating Disorders Support Group, 2887
Comprehensive Pediatric Hemophilia Treatment Center, 4000
Cystic Fibrosis Center - All Children's Hospital, 2265
Developmental Center, 703, 990, 4539
Dyslexia Research Institute, 2783
Early Intervention Unit, Division of Children's Medical Services, 8167
Easter Seals Camp Challenge, 8729
Epilepsy Association of the Big Bend, 6534
Epilepsy Foundation of Florida, 6535
Family Network on Disabilities, 8168
Family/Community Support Group of the Brain Injury Association of Florida, 3376
Florida Bureau of Braille and Talking Book Library Services, 1843, 1989, 5220, 6145
Florida Camp for Children and Youth, 2615
Florida Chapter of Crohn's & Colitis Found ation of America, 2155
Florida Department of Education, 8169
Florida Department of Health Immunization Program, 5961
Florida Epilepsy Services Providers Associ ation, 6536
Florida Families of Children with Visual I mpairments, 6277
Florida Hemophilia Association, 3950
Florida Ophthalmic Institute, 2039
Florida School-Deaf and Blind Summer Camp, 1934, 2085, 3909, 5300, 6226
Florida's Collaboration for Young Children and their Families Head State, 8170
Frontier Travel Camp, 395
Gold Coast Down Syndrome Organization, 2665
Goodwill Industries-Suncoast, 2666
Goodwill Industries-Suncoast: Choices for Work Program, 3377
Hemophilia Foundation of Greater Florida, 3951
Hydrocephalus Family Support Group of Central Florida, 4230
Kris' Camp, 994
Miami Children's Hospital, Division of Pulmonology, 2266
Miami Comprehensive Hemophilia Center, 4021
NE Florida Support Group, 515
National Ophthalmic Research Institute, 2045
Neurofibromatosis Center at North Broward Medical Center, 5043
New Heights (formerly Cerebral Palsy of No rtheast Florida), 1422
PWSA Florida Chapter, 5823
Pediatric Heart Foundation, 4312
Prader-Willi Alliance of New York, 5843
Pulmonary Wellness Program, 2267
Renfrew Center of Miami, 2888
Research & Training Center for Children's Mental Health at University of South FL, 1777, 7700
Research and Training Center for Children' Mental Health, 8566
Scleroderma Foundation Southeast Florida Chapter, 6435
Shriners Hospital for Children, 6474
South Florida Brain Tumor Association Lynn Regional Cancer Center, 1164
Spina Bifida Association of Central Florid a, 6821
Spina Bifida Association of Jacksonville N emours Childrens Clinic, 6822
Spina Bifida Association of Tampa Bay, 6824
Suncoast Residential Training Center/Developmental Services Program, 1624
Talking Book Library, Jacksonville Public Library, 1844, 1990, 5221, 6146

Georgia

Hawaii

Idaho

Illinois

Indiana

Iowa

ARC of East Central Iowa Pilot Parents, 8218
Blank Children's Hospital: Department of P ulmonology, 2277
Brain Injury Association of Iowa, 3384
Brain Tumor Support Group, 1181
Bureau of Children, Family, and Community Services, 8219
Camp Courageous, 8743
Camp Courageous of Iowa, 8744
Camp Tanager, 8745
Children's Tumor Foundation - Iowa Chapter, 5025
Des Moines YMCA Camp, 119, 171, 496, 1302, 2380, 2612
Family & Educator Connection - Cedar Falls /Waterloo Region, 8220
Family & Educator Connection - Clear Lake/ Mason City Region, 8221
Family & Educator Connection - Marshalltow n Region, 8222
Hemophilia Treatment Center at the University of Iowa, 4011
Iowa Department of Public Health Bureau of Immunization, 5965
Iowa Library for the Blind and Physically Handicapped, 1856, 2002, 5233, 6158
Iowa Program for Assistive Technology, 8223
Iowa SIDS Program, 7013
Iowa's System of EI Services, 8224
Mercy Sleep Laboratory, 4940
PWSA of Iowa, 5829
Parent Educator Connection, 8225
Parent Educator Connection Program, 8226
Prevent Child Abuse Iowa, 5675
Quad Cities Brain Tumor Support Group, 1182
Spina Bifida Association of Iowa, 6829
The Link, 816
The University of Iowa Libraries, 6320
Turner's Syndrome Society of Iowa/New Found Friends, 7566
University of Iowa - Wendell Johnson Speech and Hearing Clinic, 3914, 6802, 6966
University of Iowa Birth Defects and Genetic Disorders Unit, 1811, 1857, 1948, 1959, 2003, 8574
University of Iowa Hospitals & Clinics, 2278

Kansas

Assistive Technology for Kansas Project, 8227
Autism Society of Kansas, 817
Brain Injury Association of Kansas & Greater Kansas City, 3385
CKLS Headquarters, 2004
Camp Discovery American Diabetes Association, 2605
Department of Health & Environment, 8228
Families Together, 8229
Families Together/Parent to Parent of KS, 8230
Great Plains Region-Helen Keller National Center, 6125
Headstrong Brain Tumor Support Group, 1183
Heart to Heart, 4313, 4331, 4333, 4335
Kansas Department of Health & Environment Bureau of Family Health, 7014
Kansas Department of Health & Environment Immunization Program, 5966
Kansas State Library, 8480
Kansas University Medical Center: Departme nt of Pulmonology, 2279
Manhattan Public Library, 8481
Neurofibromatosis, Inc - Kansas & Central Plains, 5026
Prenatal Diagnostic and Genetic Center, 8482, 8564
Services for the Visually Disabled, 1859, 2005, 5235, 6160
Solution Outreach Center at OCCK, Inc., 8483
South Central Kansas Library System, 8484
Special Education Administration Kansas St ate Department of Education, 8231
United Cerebral Palsy of Kansas, 1442
University of Kansas Center for Research on Learning, 4518
Via Christi Specialty Clinics: Cystic Fibr osis, Adult and Pediatrics, 2280
Wesley Medical Research Institutes, 8485, 8576
Wichita Public Library, 8486

Kentucky

AbleData, 3547
Assistive Technology Services Network, 8232
Autism Society of America Bluegrass Chapter, 818
Bethel Mennonite Camp, 8747
Bluegrass Technology Center, 8487
Brain Injury Association of Kentucky, 3386
Brain Injury Support Group, 1184
College of Education - Western Kentucky University, 8233
Division of Preschool Services, 8234
Easter Seal Kysoc, 2614, 3907, 4724, 8748
EnTech: Enabling Technologies of Kentuckiana, 8488
Infant-Toddler Program, Division of Mental Retardation, 8235
Kentucky Chapter of Crohn's & Colitis Foundation of America, 2161
Kentucky Department of Human Resources Bureau of Health Services, 7015
Kentucky Hemophilia Foundation, 3957
Kentucky Library for the Blind and Physically Handicapped, 1860, 2006, 5236, 6161
Life Adventure Center, 1804, 7765
Louisville Talking Book Library, 8489
Northern Kentucky Talking Book Library, 8490
PWSA of Kentucky, 5831
Special Parent Involvement Network, 8236
Spina Bifida Association of Kentucky, 6830
Turner's Syndrome Society of Kentucky, 7567
University of Kentucky: Pediatric Pulmonar y Medicine, 2281
Western Kentucky Assistive Technology Consortium, 8491

Louisiana

Autism Society of Louisiana, 819
Brain Injury Association of Louisiana, 3387
Brain Injury Support And Education Group, 1185
Brain Injury Support Group, 1186
Camp Bon Coeur, 8749
Division of Special Populations, 8237
Families Helping Families of Greater New Orleans, 8238
LA Lions Camp Pelican, 2381
Louisiana Assistive Technology Access Network, 8239
Louisiana Chapter, 524
Louisiana Comprehensive Hemophilia Care Center, 4018
Louisiana Hemophilia Foundation, 3958
Louisiana Lions Camp for Crippled Children, 8750
Louisiana State Library, 8492
Louisiana State University Genetics Section of Pediatrics, 8493, 8561
Louisiana State University Health Sciences Center, 2282
Louisiana Support Group, 525
Louisiana/Mississippi Chapter of Crohn's & Colitis Foundation of America, 2162
Louisiana/Mississippi Chapter of Crohn's & Colitis Foundation of America, 2167
Med-Camps of Louisiana, 8751
NE Louisiana Sickle Cell Anemia Foundation, 6633
Preschool Programs - Division of Special Populations, 8240
Project PROMPT, 8241
Public Health Services of Louisiana, 7016
Spina Bifida Association of Greater New Orleans, 6831
Tlane Cancer Center, 1187
Tulane University Clinical Immunology Section, 449
Tulane University, US-Japan Biomedical Research Laboratories, 3428
Turner's Syndrome Society of Gulf Coast, 7568
United Cerebral Palsy of Baton Rouge McMains Children's Developmental Center, 1443
United Cerebral Palsy of Greater New Orleans, 1444

Maine

Autism Society of Maine, 820
Bangor Public Library, 8494
Brain Tumor Support Group of Maine, 1188
CDC Lincoln County, 8242
Camp Waban, 8752
Cary Library, 8495
Central Maine Medical Center, 2283
Child Department Services, 8243
Child Department Services, Department of Education, 8244
Consumer Information and Technology Training Exchange (Maine CITE), 8245
Department of Human Services, 7017
Eastern Maine Medical Center: Cystic Fibrosis Center, 2284

Jackson Laboratory, 3249
Lewiston Public Library, 8496
Maine Dept. of Human Services: Bureau of Health Immunization Program, 5967
Maine Hemophilia and Thrombosis Center, 4019
Maine State Library, 8497
Maine Support, 526
Open Support Group-All Kinds of Cancer Care of Maine, 1189
Pediatric Cystic Fibrosis Center, 2285
Pine Tree Camp Children - Adults, 8753
Portland Public Library, 8499
Sleep Laboratory, Maine Medical Center, 4941
Special Needs Parent Info Network, 8246
United Cerebral Palsy of Northeastern Maine, 1445
University of Maine, Conley Speech and Hearing Center, 3562
Waterville Public Library, 8500
York County Parent Awareness, 8247

Maryland

ARC Family Connection Parent to Parent Program, 8248
American Action Fund for Blind Children and Adults, 1834
Autism Society of America Baltimore Chesapeake Chapter, 821
Behavioral and Developmental Pediatrics Division, University of Maryland, 2687
Bell's Palsy Research Foundation, 1008
Brain Injury Association of Maryland, 3389
Center for Eating Disorders, 2890
Center for Infant & Child Loss, 7018
Center for Research for Mothers & Children, 7070
Chesapeake Chapter, 528
Cooley's Anemia Foundation-Capital Area (DC, VA, MD), 7259
Dept. of Health & Mental Hygiene-Immunizat ion, 5968
Developmental Pediatrics School of Medicine, University of Maryland, 8249
East Central Region-Helen Keller National Center, 1829, 6130
Easter Seals Camp Fairlee Manor, 8754
Epilepsy Research Laboratory, Department o f Neurology, 6546
Hemophilia Foundation of Maryland, 3959
International Center for Skeletal Dysplasia Registry, 2988
John Hopkins Arthritis Center, 444
John Hopkins Children's Hospital, 2286
Johns Hopkins Arthritis Center, 445
Johns Hopkins Brain Tumor Education Group, 1191
Johns Hopkins Department of Orthopaedics Surgery, 6472
Johns Hopkins Division of Allergy and Clin ical Immunology, 6325
Johns Hopkins University Sleep Disorders Center, 4899
Kamp-A-Kom-Plish, 8755
Kennedy Krieger Institute, 4752
Kennedy Krieger Institute, Down Syndrome Clinic, 2688
Learning Independence Through Computers, 8501
MD Infant/Toddler/Preschool Services Division, 8250
Maryland Infant and Toddlers Program Family Support Network, 8251
Maryland SIDS Information & Counseling Program, 7019
Maryland State Library for the Blind and Physically Handicapped, 1861, 2007, 5237, 6162
Maryland-Greater Washington, DC Chapter As thma and Allergy Foundation of America, 431
Maryland/South Delaware Chapter of Crohn's & Colitis Foundation of America, 2163
NAD Youth Leadership Camp, 3912
NIH/National Institute of Child Health and Human Development, 5907
NIH/National Institute of Mental Health Eating Disorders Program, 5908
NIH/National Library of Medicine (NLM), 9
NIH/Osteoporosis and Related Bone Diseases National Resource Center, 5450
National Diabetes Information Clearinghouse, 2559
National Digestive Diseases Information Clearinghouse, 30, 268, 1755, 1947, 2191, 2246
National Rehabilitation Information Center, 1497, 3079
Neurofibromatosis, Inc - MidAtlantic, 5027
PWSA of Maryland, Virginia & DC, 5833
Parents Place of Maryland, 8252
Parents of Children with Down Syndrome Arc of Montgomery County, 2671
Partners in Intensive Care, 8253
Patient Recruitment & Public Liaison Office Clinical Center, 7774

Prince George's County Memorial Library Talking Book Center, 1862, 2008, 5238, 6163
Raven Rock Lutheran Camp, 4726
Sarcoidosis Awareness Network, 6358
Sickle Cell Disease Association of America - Connecticut Chapter, 6631
Sickle Cell Disease Association of the Piedmont, 6637
Spina Bifida Association of Chesapeake-Pot omac, 6832
Spinal Muscular Atrophy Project, 6925
Sudden Infant Death Syndrome Institute of The University of Maryland, 7076
Technology Assistance Program Maryland Rehabilitation Center, 8254
The League at Camp Greentop and The Therapeutic Recreation, 8756
Tourette Syndrome Association of Greater Washington, 7388
Turner's Syndrome Society of Maryland, 7569
Turner's Syndrome Society of National Capitol Area, 7592
United Cerebral Palsy of Central Maryland, 1446
United Cerebral Palsy of Prince Georges & Montgomery Counties, 1447
United Cerebral Palsy of Southern Maryland, 1448
University of Maryland Medical Center, 4942

Massachusetts

Association of Gastrointestinal Motility Disorders, 2906
Asthma & Allergy Foundation of America New England Chapter, 432
Autism Research Foundation, 861
Autism Society of America Massachusetts Chapter, 822
Baystate Medical Center, 2287
Berkshire Center, 4516
Boston Children's Hospital Dept. of Otolaryngology & Communication, 3568
Boston Hemophilia Center, 3994
Braille and Talking Book Library Perkins School for the Blind, 1863, 2009, 5239, 6164
Brain Center Brain Tumor Support Group, 1192
Brain Injury Association of Massachusetts, 3390
Brain Tumor Support Group, 1193
Brain Tumor Support Group at Burlington, 1194
Brain Tumor Support Group at Worcester, 1195
Brain Tumor Survivor Support Group, 1196
Brigham and Women's Hospital, Asthma and Allergic Disease Research Center, 442
Bureau of Early Childhood Programs, 8255
Bureau of Family Health Services-Alabama Child Death Review, 6993
CKLS Headquarters, 1858, 5234, 6159
Camp Joslin, 2607
Camp Ramah in New England (Summer), 8758
Camp Ramah in New England (Winter), 8759
Camp Ramah in New England Tikvah Program, 987, 1542, 6618, 8757
Carroll Center for the Blind, 2010, 4517, 5240, 6165
Carroll School Summer Programs, 8760
Center for Digestive Disorders, 7623
Center for Interdisciplinary Research on Immunologic Diseases, 443
Children's Happiness Foundation, 8256
Children's Hospital Boston, 2288
Children's Tumor Foundation - Northern New England, 5028
Clara Barton Camp, 2611
Community Sickle Cell Support Group, 6634
Cooley's Anemia Foundation-Massachusetts Chapter, 7260
Developmental Medicine Center, 3320
Down Syndrome Program, Children's Hospital Boston, 2689
Eagle Hill School - Summer Program, 704, 991, 4540
Early Intervention Services, 8257
Eaton-Peabody Laboratory of Auditory Physiology, 3563
Education Development Center - EDC, 8258
Family Ties at Massachusetts Department of Public Health, 8259
Federation for Children with Special Needs, 8260
Greater Boston Arc Parent Support, 8261
Handi-Kids/King Solomon Foundation, 8761
Hard of Hearing Advocates, 3551
Harold Goodglass Aphasia Research Center, 3429
Heart to Heart Fund, 4318
Hemophilia Center of the New England Medical Center, 4009
Joslin Diabetes Center, 2561
Kingsmont, 5353
Landmark School, 2802
Massachusetts Assistive Technology Partnership, 8262

Massachusetts Association for Parents of t he Visually Impaired (MAPVI), 6278
Massachusetts Chapter of SIDS Alliance, 7020
Massachusetts Down Syndrome Congress (MDSC), 2672
Massachusetts Easter Seals Camping Program, 8762
Massachusetts Eating Disorder Association (MEDA), 2891
Massachusetts General Hospital, 2289
Massachusetts Sudden Infant Death Syndrome, 7071
Massachusetts, New England Hemophilia Association, 3960
National Association for Parents of the Visually Impaired, 1827, 1972, 5203, 6119, 6123
National Birth Defects Center, 8263
National Temporal Bone, Hearing and Balanc e Pathology Resource Registry, 3570
New England Chapter of Crohn's & Colitis Foundation of America, 2164
New England Region-Helen Keller National Center, 6127
New England Regional Genetics Group, 527, 8498, 8562
New England Support Group, 529
Option Institute: Son Rise Program, 823
Parent Education/Support Group, 1197
Pediatric Clinical Trials International, 2699
Pediatric Pulmonary Unit, 7074
Prader-Willi Association of New England (Maine, Mass, RI, NH, VT), 5832, 5834
Region I Office Program Consultants For Maternal and Child Health, 7021
Resources for Rehabilitation, 8502
Sleep Disorders Center, 6676
Sleep Disorders Unit, Beth Israel Hospital, 4900
Spina Bifida Association of Massachusetts, 6833
Talking Book Library at Worcester Public Library, 8503
Tourette Syndrome Association of Massachusetts, 7389
Tufts New England Medical Center Floating Hospital for Children, 2290
Turner's Syndrome Society of New England, 7570
United Cerebral Palsy of Berkshire County, 1449
United Cerebral Palsy of MetroBoston, 1450
Worcester Public Library, 8504

Michigan

Adventure Learning Center Camp Programs, 1803, 7764
Anchor Point Camp, 391, 977, 4532
Apnea Identification Program, 7022
Autism Society of Michigan, 824
Big Crystal Camp, 979
Bioengineering Center of Wayne State University, 3430
Brain Injury Association of Michigan, 3391, 3423
Brain Tumor Networking Club, 1198
Brain Tumor Support Group at Ann Arbor, 1200
Brain Tumor Support Group for Patients & F amilies: University of Michigan Med Ctr, 1201
Burger School for the Autistic, 853
Butterworth Hospital, Cystic Fibrosis Center, 2291
CAUSE, 8264
Camp Barakel, 8763
Camp Barefoot, 3471
Camp Catch-A-Rainbow, 116, 168, 1298, 3123, 7805
Camp Fish Tales, 8764
Camp O' Fair Winds, 4537
Camp Tushmehata, 1932
Center for Sleep Science at University of Michigan, 4901
Central Michigan University Summer Clinics, 3904, 6800
Children's Hospital of Michigan Cystic Fibrosis Care, Teaching & Resource, 2292
Children's Tumor Foundation - Michigan Cha pter, 5030
Cystic Fibrosis Center/Pediatric Pulmonary and Sleep Medicine, 2293
Detroit Michigian Ataxia Support Group, 530
Downtown Detroit Subregional Library for the Blind and Handicapped, 1864, 2011, 5241, 6166
Early on Michigan, 8265
Eastern Michigan Hemophilia Center, 4002
Eric RicStar Winter Music Therapy Summer Camp, 1547, 8765
Families at Heart, 4319
Family Support Network of Michigan Parent Participation Program-MDCH, 8266
Frederick Douglas Branch for Specialized Services and Physically Handicapped, 8505
Genesee County Health Department, 7023

Glaucoma Laser Trabeculoplasty Study, 2041
Hemophilia Foundation of Michigan, 3961
Indian Trails Camp, 8766
Kalamazoo Center for Medical Studies, 2294
Kalamazoo Comprehensive Hemophilia Treatment Center, 4017
Kent County Health Department, 7024
Kent County Library for the Blind, 1865, 2012, 5242, 6167
Library of Michigan Service for the Blind, 1866, 2013, 5243, 6168
Livingston County CMH Services, 8267
Macomb Library for the Blind and Physically Handicapped, 1867, 2014, 5244, 6169
Michigan Chapter of Allergy and Asthma Foundation of America, 433
Michigan Chapter of Crohn's & Colitis Foundation of America, 2165
Michigan State University Comprehensive Center for Bleeding Disorders, 4022
Mideastern Michigan Library Co-op, 1868, 2015, 5245, 6170
Muskegon County Library for the Blind, 1869, 2016, 5246, 6171
Northern Regional Bleeding Disorder Center, 4025
Oakland County Health Division - SIDS Project, 7025
PWSA of Michigan, 5835
Parents are Experts, 8269
Regional Hemophilia Program, 4031
Rehabilitation Institute of Michigan, 3392, 3431
SIDS LEAD - Children's Special Health Care Services, 7026
SIDS Nursing Intervention Program, 7027
SW Michican Spina Bifida & Hydrocephalus Association, 4232
Sarcoidosis Awareness Foundation, 6359
Sarcoidosis Resource Support Group, 6360
Sarcoidosis Support - Beaumont, 6361
Seeking Techniques Advancing Research in Shunts (STARS), 4243
Spectrum Brain Tumor Support Group, 1202
Spectrum Health Research, 4037
Spina Bifida Association of Upper Peninsula Michigan, 6834
Spina Bifida Association of West Michigan, 6835
TECH 2000 Project-Michigan Disability Rights Coalition, 8270
Turner's Syndrome Society of Southeastern Michigan, 7571
Turner's Syndrome Society of West Michigan, 7572
United Cerebral Palsy Michigan, 1451
United Cerebral Palsy of Metropolitan Detroit, 1452
University Center for the Development of L anguage & Literacy, 6783
University of Michigan Adult Hemophilia and Cougulation Disorders Program, 4045
University of Michigan, Cystic Fibrosis Center, 2295
University of Michigan, Kresge Hearing Research Institute, 3571
Upper Peninsula Library for the Blind Physically Handicapped, 1870, 2017, 5247, 6172
Washtenaw County Library, 1871, 2018, 5248, 6173
Washtenaw County Library for the Blind and Physically Disabled, 1872, 2019, 5249, 6174
Wayne County Regional Library for the Blind, 1873, 2020, 5250, 6175
West Michigan Cancer Center Support Group, 1203

Minnesota

ARC Suburban, 8271
Abbott Northwestern Brain Tumor Support Group at Abbott Northwestern Hospital, 1204
Autism Society of America Manasota Chapter, 807
Autism Society of Minnesota, 825
Brain Injury Association of Minnesota, 3393
Brain Injury Support Group at Abbott Northwestern Hospital, 1205
Brain Tumor Support Group at Duluth, 1206
Brain Tumor Support Group at Robbinside, 1207
Brain Tumor Support Group at United Hospital, 1208
Camp Buckskin, 700, 980, 4534
Camp Friendship, 981, 2764, 8767
Camp New Hope, 985, 2768, 8768
Camp Winnebago, 8769
Center for Sleep Diagnostics, 4902
Courage Camps, 8770
Courage North, 8771
Department of Children, Family, & Learning, 8272
Down Syndrome Association of Minnesota, 2673
Down Syndrome Clinic of Minneapolis Children's Medical Center, 2690
Eden Wood Center, 2770, 7783, 8772
Family to Family Network ARC of Hennepin County, 8273
Groves Academy, 705, 992, 4541

Hemophilia Foundation of Minnesota and the Dakotas, 3962

Hemophilia and Thrombosis Center at the University of Minnesota Medical Center, 4013

Interagency Early Intervention Project, 8274

Knutson, 8773

Mayo Clinic and Foundation, 4827

Minneapolis, MN Support Group, 531

Minnesota Cystic Fibrosis Center, 2296

Minnesota Library for the Blind & Physically Handicapped, 1874, 2021, 5251, 6176

Minnesota Sudden Infant Death Center, 7028

Minnesota/Dakotas Chapter of Crohn's & Colitis Foundation of America, 2166

Non-Malignant Brain Tumor Support Group, 1209

PACER Center, 8506

PWSA Chapter - Minnesota, 5836

Parents For Heart of Minnesota, 4320

Parents for Parents, 8275

Pilot Parents in Anoka and Ramsey Counties, 8276

Pilot Parents of Northeast Minnesota, 8277

Search Beyond Adventures, 8774

Spina Bifida Association of Minnesota, 6836

Star Center for Family Health, 8507

Tourette Syndrome Association - Minnesota Chapter, 7390

Turner's Syndrome Society of Minnesota, 7573

United Cerebral Palsy of Central Minnesota, 1453

United Cerebral Palsy of Minnesota, 1454

Vinland Center, 8278

Voyageur Outward Bound School, 8279

Wilderness Inquiry, 8280

Mississippi

Autism Society of Mississippi, 826

Brain Injury Association of Mississippi, 3394

First Steps Program, 8281

Mississippi Chapter, 532

Mississippi Dept. of Health Bureau of Preventative Health Immunization, 5969

Mississippi Hemophilia Foundation, 3963

Mississippi State Department of Health and Child Health Services, 7029

Office of Special Education, 8268, 8282

Parent Partners, 8283

Project Start, 8284

Spina Bifida Association of Mississippi, 6837

Tik-A-Witha, 8775

University of Mississippi Medical Center, 2297, 2431

Missouri

AMOR - A Cancer Support Group for Patients & Their Families, 1210

Adriene Resource Center for Blind Children, 1875, 2022, 5252, 6177

Allergy and Pulmonary Medicine, 434

Assemblies of God National Center for the Blind, 1876, 2023, 5253, 6178

Assistance Technology Project, 8285

Asthma and Allergy Foundation of America - Saint Louis Chapter, 436

Asthma and Allergy Foundation of America Greater Kansas City Chapter, 435

Autism Society of America Gateway Chapter, 827

Brain Cancer Support Group at Mid-America Cancer Center, 1211

Brain Injury Association of Missouri, 3395

Brain Tumor Support Group, 1199, 1212

Brain Tumor Support Group of Greater St Louis, 1213

Central Institute for the Deaf, 3572

Central Missouri Area Support Group, 533

Children's Mercy Hospital, Down Syndrome Clinic, 2691

Children's Mercy Hospital, University of Missouri, 2298

Children's Therapy Center, 8286

Children's Tumor Foundation - Missouri Cha pter, 5031

Council for Extended Care of Mentally Retarded Citizens, 4722

Cystic Fibrosis, Pediatric Pulmonary and Pediatric Gastrointestinal Center, 2299

Department of Elementary and Secondary Education, 8287

Down's Syndrome Medical Clinic, 2692

EDI, 2613

Family Resource Network, 8289

Gateway Hemophilia Association of Missouri, 3964

Heart to Heart - St. Louis, 4321

Hickory Hill, 2617

Hydrocephalus Support Group, 4231, 4233

Judevine Center for Autism, 854

Kansas City, Missouri Support Group, 534

Mid-America Chapter of Crohn's & Colitis F oundation of America, 2160

Missouri Parents Act, 8290

PWSA Missouri Chapter, 5837

Parent Act, 8291

Pediatric Epilepsy Center, 6547

Positive Solutions for Life Challenges, 8292

Prader-Willi Syndrome Advocates, 5830

Region VII Office Program Consultants for Maternal and Child Health, 7030

SIDS Resources, 7031

Saint Louis Chapter of Crohn's & Colitis Foundation of America, 2168

Sidney R. Baer Day Camp, 8776

Spina Bifida Association of Greater Saint Louis, 6838

Springfield Area Support Group, 535

Tourette Syndrome Association - Greater Missouri Chapter, 7391

Turner's Syndrome Society of St. Louis/ West Illinois, 7574

United Cerebral Palsy of Greater Kansas City, 1441, 1455

United Cerebral Palsy of Greater St. Louis, 1456

United Cerebral Palsy of Northwest Missouri, 1457

United Services, 8293

University of Missouri-Columbia Cystic Fibrosis Center, 2300

Washington University Cystic Fibrosis Center, 2301

Whitney Library for the Blind, 8509

Wolfner Memorial Library for the Blind, 1877, 2024, 5254, 6179

Montana

Big Sky Kids Cancer Camp, 115

Brain Injury Association of Montana, 3396

CO-TEACH/Division of Educational Research and Service, 8294

Charles Campbell Children's Camp, 1544

Developmental Disabilities Program, 8295

Division of Special Education, 8296

MonTECH, 8297

Montana Department of Health & Environmental Sciences, 7032

Montana State Library, 8510

Parents Let's Unite for Kids, 8298

Quality Life Concepts, 8299

Nebraska

Assistive Technology Partnership, 8300

Autism Society of Nebraska, 828

Boys Town National Research Hospital, 6784

Brain Tumor Support Group at the Nebraska Medical Center, 1214

Camp Easter Seals, 8777

Camp Kindle, 3349

Floyd Rogers, 2616

Individual and Family Support Arc of Lincoln & Lancaster County, 8301

Iowa Chapter of Crohn's Colitis Foundation of America, 2159

Junior Wheelchair Sports Camp, 8724

Lied Learning and Technology Center for Ch ildhood Deafness and Vision Disorders, 3573

National Camps for Blind Children, 1936, 2087, 5301, 6227

Nebraska Chapter of the National Hemophilia Foundation, 3965

Nebraska Dept. of Health Immunization Prog ram, 5970

Nebraska Library Commission Talking Book & Braille Services, 1878, 2025, 5255, 6180

Nebraska Parents Center, 8302

Nebraska Regional Hemophilia Center, 4023

Nebraska SIDS Foundation, 7033

North Platte Public Library, 8511

PWSA of Nebraska, 5839

Parent Assistance Network, 8303

Parent Support Group, 8304

Special Education Office State Department of Education, 8306

Spina Bifida Association of Nebraska, 6839

United Cerebral Palsy of Nebraska, 1458

University of Nebraska at Omaha Pediatric Pulmonary/Cystic Fibrosis Center, 2302

University of Nebraska, Lincoln Barkley Memorial Center, 3564

Nevada

American Academy of Somnology, 5112, 5135, 6675, 6703
Assistive Technology Collaborative, 8307
Autism Society of Northern Nevada Chapter, 829
Camp Lotsafun, 983
Children's Lung Specialists, 2303
Children's Tumor Foundation - Nevada, 5032
Early Intervention Services Division of Child & Family Services, 8308
Educational Equity, Special Education Branch, 8309
Hemophilia and Thrombosis Center of Nevada, 4014
Las Vegas-Clark County Library District, 8512
Nevada Parent Network, 8310
Nevada Parents Encouraging Parents (PEP), 8311
Nevada State Division of Health, Maternal & Child Health, 7034
Nevada State Health Division Bureau of Com munity Health - Immunization Program, 5971
Nevada State Library and Archives, 8513
Parents Encouraging Parents, 8305, 8312
Scleroderma Foundation Nevada Chapter, 6437
Southern Nevada 'Grey Matters' Valley Hospital Medical Center, 1215
University of Nevada - Department of Speec h-Language Pathology, 6785

New Hampshire

Angels of Hope, 1216
Autism Society of New Hampshire, 830
Brain Injury Association of Maine, 3388
Brain Injury Association of New Hampshire, 3397
Bureau of Early Learning, 8313
Camp Allen, 8778
Camp Dartmouth-Hitchcock, 8779
Crotched Mountain School & Rehabilitation Center, 988, 1545, 3473, 4723, 6620, 8704
Dartmouth-Hitchcock Sleep Disorders Center Dartmouth Medical Center, 4903, 8314
Division of Special Education, 8315
Families with Heart, 4322
Family Center Early Supports & Services, 8316
Hemophilia and Coagulation Programs, 4012
High Hopes Foundation of New Hampshire, 8317
Medical Genetics Clinic, 2693
NH Dept. of Health & Human Services Immunization Program, 5972
New England Retinoblastoma Support Group (NERSG), 6279
New Hampshire Cystic Fibrosis Care and Teaching Center, 2304
New Hampshire SIDS Program, 7035
New Hampshire State Library, 8514
Parent Information Center, 8318
Parent to Parent of New Hampshire, 8319
Sleep/Wake Disorders Center, Hampstead Hospital, 4904
Technology Partnership Project Institute on Disability/UAP, 8320
Turner's Syndrome Society of Northern New England, 7576
Windsor Mountain Camp, 3915

New Jersey

Bancroft Camp, 8781
Blood Research Institute of Saint Michael's Medical Center, 3993
Brain Injury Association of New Jersey, 3398
Brain Tumor Support Group at Plainfield Muhlenberg Medical Center, Neuroscience, 1218
CJ Foundation for SIDS, 7069
CRI Worldwide Pediatric Center for Excellence, 1756
Camp Chatterbox, 8782
Camp Merry Heart/Easter Seals Easter Seal Society, 1300, 1541
Camp Oakhurst, 6906, 8783
Camp Sun 'N Fun, 8787
Camp Vacamas, 495, 6668
Center for Enabling Technology, 8515
Cerebral Palsy Center Summer Program, 1543
Cross Roads Outdoor Ministries, 8784
Division of Student Services, 8321
Early Intervention System, 8322
Eating Disorders Association of New Jersey, 2892

Epilepsy Foundation New Jersey, 6537
Family Support Center of New Jersey, 8323
Hydrocephalus Group - Children's Hospital of New Jersey, 4234
Monmouth Medical Center, Cystic Fibrosis & Pediatric Pulmonary Center, 2305
National Sarcoidosis Resource Center, 6371
New Image Camps, 5354
New Jersey Camp Jaycee, 4725
New Jersey Center for Outreach & Services for the Autism Community (COSAC), 831
New Jersey Center for Outreach and Service s for the Autism Community (COSAC), 855
New Jersey Chapter of Crohn's & Colitis Foundation of America, 2169
New Jersey Department of Health - Child Health Program, 7036
New Jersey Department of Health Immunizations Program, 5973
New Jersey Institute of Technology Center for Biomedical Engineering, 3250
New Jersey Medical School, 2306
New Jersey SIDS Resource Center, 7037
New Jersey Self-Help Clearinghouse, 8324
New Jersey State Library Talking Book and Braille Center, 1879, 2026, 5256, 6181
New Jersey Statewide Parent to Parent, 8325
Newark Sleep Disorders Center, 4905
PWSA - New Jersey Chapter, 5841
Parent Project for Muscular Dystrophy Research, 4830
Renfrew Center of Northern New Jersey, 2893
Round Lake Camp, 709, 997
Sarcoidosis Support Resource Central New J ersey, 6362
Scleroderma Foundation New Jersey Chapter, 6438
Spina Bifida Association of the Tri-State Region, 6840
Statewide Parent Advocacy Network, 8326
Tourette Syndrome Association of New Jersey, 7394
Turner's Syndrome Society of New Jersey, 7577
US Rowing Assocation, 8217
United Cerebral Palsy Research and Educational Foundation, 1499
United Cerebral Palsy of Hudson County, 1459
United Cerebral Palsy of Northern, Central & Southern New Jersey, 1460
Young Hearts, 4323

New Mexico

Brain Injury Association of New Mexico, 3399
Computer Access Center, 8554
EPICS Project-SW Communication Resources, 8327
Long Term Services Division, 8328
NM Alliance for the Neurologically Impaired, 1219
New Mexico Autism Society, 832
New Mexico Department of Health Immunization Program, 5974
New Mexico State Library for the Blind and Physically Handicapped, 1880, 2027, 5257, 6182
Parents Reaching Out, 8329
People Living Through Cancer, 1220
Region 5 of the National Association for Parents of the Visually Impaired, 6128
Santa Fe Mountain Center, 8785
Sickle Cell Council of New Mexico, Inc., 6635
Special Education Unit, 8330
Technology Assistance Program, 8331
Ted R. Montoya Hemophilia Program, 4039
University of New Mexico School of Medicine, 2307

New York

Advocacy Center, 8332
Advocates for Children of New York, 8333, 8786
Albany Medical College Pediatric Pulmonary & Cystic Fibrosis Center, 2308
Albany New York Regional Comprehensive Hemophilia Treatment Center, 3992
American Foundation for AIDS Research, 3318
Arlene R Gordon Research Institute, 6193
Armond V. Mascia CF Center, 2309
Aspire of WNY, 1461
Association for Research of Childhood Cancer, 8551
Aurora of Central New York, 8334
Autism Speaks, 863

Support for Parents of Children with Brain Tumors, Siblings and Young Adults, 1227
Syracuse University, Institute for Sensory Research, 3576
TRIAD Project-Advocates for Persons with Disabilities, 8344
Techspress Resource Center for Independent Living, 8520
Tourette Syndrome Association - Greater New York State Chapter, 7397
Tourette Syndrome Association - Greater Rochester and Finger Lakes Area, 7396
Tourette Syndrome Association - Hudson Valley Chapter, 7398
Tourette Syndrome Association - Long Island Chapter, 7399
Tourette Syndrome Association - New Mexico Chapter, 7395
Tri-State Support Group, 539
Turner's Syndrome Society of Central New York, 7578
Turner's Syndrome Society of Upstate New York, 7579
UCP of Greater Suffolk, 1465
Ulster County Social Services, 8345
United Cerebral Palsy of Nassau County, 1466
United Cerebral Palsy of New York City, 1467
United Health Services Blood Disorder Center, 4043
Unity Sleep Disorders Clinic Unity Health System, 4915
University of Rochester Medical Center, 2317
Upstate/Northeast New York Chapter of Croh n's & Colitis Foundation of America, 2176
VISIONS/Vacation Camp for the Blind, 1938, 2089, 5302, 6228
WNY Brain Tumor Support Group, 1228
Wagon Road, 8795
Wallace Memorial Library, 3565
Washington Leukemia and Lymphoma Society Alaska Chapter, 8427
Westchester Center for Eating Disorders, 2898
Western New York Chapter of Crohn's & Colitis Foundation of America, 2177
Western New York SIDS Center, 7041
Winthrop-University Hospital Sleep Disorders Center, 4916

North Carolina

Assistive Technology Project, Human Resources, Voc. and Rehab. Services, 8346
Autism Society of North Carolina, 835, 858
Brain Injury Association of North Carolina, 3403
Brain Tumor Support Group of the Carolinas and Virginia Cancer Services, 1229
Camp Shining Stars, 5352
Camp Winding Gap, 8796
Carolina Computer Access Center, 8521
Carolinas Chapter of Crohn's & Colitis Foundation of America, 2178
Communications Disorders Clinic, 6787
Duke Brain Tumor Support Group, 1230
Duke Pediatric Brain Tumor Family Support Program, 1231
Duke University Comprehensive Epilepsy Cen ter, 6549
Duke University Comprehensive Sickle Cell Center, 6650
Duke University Medical Center/ CF Center, 2318
Duke University School of Medicine Pediatr ic and Allergy Immunology, 6324
ECAC, 8347
Eastern North Carolina Chapter (SCDAA), 6636
Exceptional Children Division, 8348
Family Support Network of North Carolina, 8349
Giddings School Special Education Division, 8164
Hemophila Foundation of North Carolina, 3969
Herpes Resource Center, 4147, 4964
Leukemia & Lymphoma Society-Western NC Chapter, 82, 142
Lipomyelomeningocele Family Support, 4236
North Carolina Library for the Blind, 1882, 2029, 5259, 6184
North Carolina SIDS Information and Counseling Program, 7042
North Carolina Speech, Hearing and Languag e Association, 6772
PWSA of North Carolina, 5844
Partnerships for Inclusion, 8350
Pediatric Rheumatoid Clinic, 4392
Prevent Child Abuse North Carolina, 5678
Rockingham County Schools, 8351
Sarcoidosis Support Group, 6364
Sickle Cell Regional Network, 6638
South Carolina Chapter of Crohn's & Colitis Foundation of America, 2185
Spina Bifida Association of North Carolina, 6845
Talisman Programs, 8797
Talisman Summer Camps, 1805, 7766

Turner's Syndrome Society of North Carolina, 7580
UNC CF Center, 2319
United Cerebral Palsy of North Carolina, 1468
University of North Carolina Sarcoidosis Support Group, 6365
University of North Carolina at Chapel Hill, Brain Research Center, 868
Western North Carolina Brain Tumor Support Group, 1232

North Dakota

Brain Injury Association of North Dakota, 3404
Children's Hospital Merit Care Down Syndrome Service, 2696
Developmental Disabilities Unit, 8352
Interagency Program Assistive Technology, 8353
North Dakota Comprehensive Hemophilia and Thrombosis Treatment Center, 4024
North Dakota SIDS Management Program, 7043
Saint Alexius Medical Center/CF Center, 2320
Special Education Division, 8354

Ohio

American Council of Blind Parents, 1883, 2030, 5260, 6185
Autism Society of Greater Cincinatti, 836
Autism Society of Ohio Tri-County Chapter, 837
Beech Brook, 978, 4533
Bethesda Oak Hospital, Sleep Disorders Center, 4917
Blick Clinic for Developmental Disabilities, 8522
Brain Injury Association of Ohio, 3405
Brain Tumor Support Group, 1233
Bureau of EI Services, 8355
CMTA Chapter - Ohio, 1551
Camp Allyn, 8798
Camp Catch-A-Rainbow, 5181
Camp Emanuel, 3900
Camp Nuhop, 701, 986, 4536
Case Western Research University, Bolton Brush Growth Study Center, 3248
Case Western Reserve University Cystic Fibrosis Center, 2321
Celebrating Families of Children & Adults with Special Needs, 8356
Center for Sleep & Wake Disorders, Miami Valley Hospital, 4918
Central Ohio Brain Tumor Support Group, 1234
Central Ohio Chapter of Crohn's & Colitis Foundation of America, 2179
Central Ohio Chapter of the National Hemophilia Foundation, 3970
Children's Tumor Foundation - Ohio, 5033
Cincinnati Digestive Diseases Research Development Center, 1758
Cleveland Brain Tumor Patient Network - Adult and Pediatric, 1235
Cleveland Clinic, 4237
Cleveland Clinic Foundation, Sleep Disorders Center, 4919
Cleveland Hearing and Speech Center, 6773
Cleveland Public Library, 8523
Clinical Research Center, Pediatrics, 1020
Columbus Children's Hospital, Cystic Fibrosis Center, 2322
Comprehensive Sickle Cell Center, 6651
Division of Early Childhood Education, 8357
Down Syndrome Clinic, Rainbow Babies and Children's Hospital, 2697
East Central Regional Office, 8358
Family Information Network, 8359
Fragile X Alliance of Ohio, 3186
Hemophilia and Thrombosis Center: Division of Blood Disease Center, 4015
Highbrook Lodge Camp, 1935, 2086, 8799
Jane and Richard Thomas Center for Down Syndrome, 2698
Kettering Medical Center, Sleep Disorders Center, 4920
Leukemia Society of America - Central Ohio Chapter, 83, 143
Leukemia Society of America - Northern Ohio Chapter, 84, 144
Leukemia Society of America - Southern Ohio Chapter, 85, 145
Lewis H. Walker, MD, Cystic Fibrosis Center, 2323
Miami Valley Downs Syndrome Association, 2675
NW Ohio Sleep Disorders Center, 4921
Northeast Ohio Chapter of Crohn's & Colitis Foundation of America, 2180
Northern Ohio Chapter of the National Hemophilia Foundation, 3971
Northwest Ohio Hemophilia Foundation, 3972
Northwest Ohio Hemophilia Treatment Center, 4026
OCECD, 8361
Ohio Department of Health Immunization Program, 5976
Ohio Protection and Advocacy Organization, 8362

Rhode Island

South Carolina

South Dakota

Tennessee

Children's Tumor Foundation - Tennessee Af filiate, 5037
Down Syndrome Association of Middle Tennessee, 2676
East Tennessee Comprehensive Hemophilia Center, 4001
East Tennessee Technology Access Center, 8535
Families of SMA - Tennessee Chapter, 6922
First Regional Hemophilia Center, 4005
Leukemia & Lymphoma Society, Tennessee Chapter, 89, 149
Memphis Cystic Fibrosis Center, 2335
Memphis Regional Brain Tumor Survivors Group, 1247
Memphis State University, Center for the Communicatively Impaired, 6777
Middle Tennessee Sarcoidosis Support Group, 6368
Neuroscience Institute, University of Tenn essee Health Science Center, 6550
Office of Special Education, State Department of Education, 8398
PWSA - Tennessee, 5851
Pediatric Pulmonary Medicine, 2336
STEP (Support & Training for Exceptional Parents), 8399
Saint Jude Children's Research Hospital, 8536
Sarcoidosis Center, 6372
Sarcoidosis Patient Forum, 6369
Sarcoidosis Research Institute, 6374
Technology Access Center, 8508
Technology Access Center of Middle Tennessee, 8400
Tennesse Hemophilia & Bleeding Disorders Foundation, 3980
Tennessee Chapter of Crohn's & Colitis Foundation of America, 2186
Tennessee Department of Health Immunization, 5981
Tennessee SIDS Program, 7053
Tennessee Saving Little Hearts, 4330
Turner's Syndrome Society of Mid-South, 7586
Turner's Syndrome Society of Tennessee, 7587
United Cerebral Palsy of Middle Tennessee, 1486
United Cerebral Palsy of the Mid-South, 1487
University of Memphis Neuropsychology Lab, 3439
University of Tennessee Hemophilia Clinic, 4046
Vanderbilt Hemostasis-Thrombosis Clinic, 4048

Texas

Arizona HeartLight, 4310
Asthma and Allergy Foundation of America - North Texas Chapter, 439
Ataxia Telangiectasia Project, 554
Autism Society of America Greater Austin Chapter, 845
Baylor College of Medicine, 4832
Baylor College of Medicine Birth Defects Center, 8537, 8552
Baylor Comprehensive Epilepsy Center, 6551
Baylor Sleep Wellness Center, 4944
Benign Essential Blepharospasm Research Foundation, 2814
Brain Injury Association of Texas, 3414
Brain Injury Research Center of the Institute for Rehabilitation & Research, 3440
Brain Tumor Support Group at Dallas, 1248
Brain Tumor Support Group at Plano, 1249
CF Center, Pulmonary Section, 2337
Callier Center for Communication Disorders, 6778
Center for Cancer and Blood Disorders, 6652
Center for Cancer and Blood Disorders at Children's Medical Center in Dallas, 3996
Central Texas Brain Tumor Support Group, 1250
Charis Hills, 394
Children's Association for Maxiumum Potential CAMP, 8809
Children's Cancer Research Institute, 5070, 8553
Cook-Ft. Worth Medical Center, CF Center, 2338
Cooley's Anemia Foundation - Texas, 7267
Cystic Fibrosis Care, Teaching and Research Center, 2339
Cystic Fibrosis-Lung Disease Center Santa Rosa Children's Hospital, 2340
Dallas Academy, 702, 989, 4538
Department of Assistive and Rehabilitation Services, 8401
Down Syndrome Guild of Dallas, 2677
Down Syndrome Specialty Clinic, 2705
HOPE (Helping Oncology Parents Endure) Brain Tumor Foundation of the Southwest, 1251
Harris County Health Department, 7054
Hill School of Fort Worth, 706, 993, 4542
Houston Area Brain Tumor Network, 1252
Houston Ear Research Foundation, 3580
Houston Support Group, 548

Houston-Gulf Coast/South Texas Chapter of Crohn's & Colitis Foundation of America, 2187
Hughen Center, 8810
Hydrocephalus Association of N Texas, 4239
International Pemphigus Foundation: Housto n Support Group, 5536
Leukemia Society of America - North Texas Chapter, 90, 150
Leukemia Society of America - South/West Texas Chapter, 91, 151
Leukemia Society of America - Texas Gulf Coast Chapter, 92, 152
Lone Star Chapter of the National Hemophilia Foundation, 3981
Menninger Child & Family Program, 1775, 7698
North Texas Chapter of Crohn's & Colitis Foundation of America, 2188
North Texas SIDS Information And Counseling Program, 7055
North Texas Support Group, 549
Office of the Dean, University of Texas at Austin, 8402
Parent Case Management, 8403
Partners Resource Network, 8404
Project PODER, 8405
Region VI Office Program Consultants For Maternal and Child Health, 7056
Scleroderma Foundation Texas Bluebonnet Ch apter, 6441
Sickle Cell Association of Austin - Marc Thomas Chapter, 6642
Sickle Cell Association of the Texas Gulf Coast, 6643
Sleep Disorders Center for Children, 4936
Sleep Medicine Associates of Texas, 4937
South Central Region-Helen Keller National Center, 8406
South Texas Comprehensive Hemophilia and Thrombophilia Treatment Center, 4036
Southwest Human Development, 8095
Southwest SIDS Research Institute, 7075
Southwestern Comprehensive Sickle Cell Cen ter, 6653
Spina Bifida Association of Houston-Gulf Coast, 6856
Spina Bifida Association of North Texas, 6857
Spina Bifida Association of Texas, 6858
Sweeney, 2620
Texas Assistive Technology Partnership, 8408
Texas Association on Mental Retardation, 2678
Texas Central Chapter of the National Hemophilia Foundation, 3982
Texas Department oF Health Immunization Division, 5982
Texas Department of Health - SIDS Information and Counseling Program, 7057
Texas Heart to Heart, 4332
Texas Lions Camp, 1937, 2088, 3913, 8811
Texas Perinatal Association, 5904
Texas Prader-Willi Syndrome Association, 5852
Texas State Library, 8538
Tri-Services Military CF Center, 2341
Turner's Syndrome Society Resource Center, 7595
Turner's Syndrome Society of Houston, 7588
Turner's Syndrome Society of North Texas, 7589
Turner's Syndrome Society of San Antonio, 7590
UT Southwestern Medical Center at Dallas: Hematology-Oncology Research, 4042
United Cerebral Palsy of Greater Houston, 1488
United Cerebral Palsy of Metropolitan Dallas, 1489
United Cerebral Palsy of Texas, 1490
Univ. of Texas-Southwestern Med. Ctr. at D allas - Clinical Ctr. for Liver Disease, 1021
University of Texas Department of Hematology Research, 4047
University of Texas Medical Branch at Galveston, Clinical Research Center, 4945
University of Texas Sleep/Wake Disorders Center, 4938
University of Texas Southwestern Medical Center/Asthma & Allergic Diseases, 450
University of Texas, Mental Health Clinical Research Center, 2481
Vitamin C Foundation, 6013

Utah

Baby Watch Early Intervention Program, 8409
Brain Injury Association of Utah, 3415
Camp Kostopulos, 8812
Children's Tumor Foundation - Utah Chapter, 5038
Computer Center for Citizens with Disabilities, 8410
Early Intervention Research Institute, Developmental Center, 8557
Heart of the Matter, 4316
Prader-Willi Utah Association, 5853
Primary Children's Medical Center, 8565

Special Education Services Unit, 8411
Spina Bifida Association of Utah, 6859
Tourette Syndrome Association - Utah Chapter, 7405
Turner's Syndrome Society of Salt Lake City, 7591
US Disabled Ski Team, 8412
United Cerebral Palsy of Utah, 1491
University of Utah, 4833
University of Utah Intermountain Cystic Fibrosis Center, 2342
Utah Center for Assistive Technology, 8413
Utah Chapter of the National Hemophilia Foundation, 3983
Utah Department of Health, 5983, 7058
Utah Parent Center, 8414
Utah State Library Commission, 8539
Utah Support Group National Ataxia Foundation, 550

Vermont

Assistive Technology Project, 8415
Autism Society of Vermont, 846
Brain Injury Association of Vermont, 3416
Camp Akeela, 392
Center on Disabilities and Community Inclusion, 8416
Family, Infant, and Toddler Project, 8417
Farm and Wilderness Camps, 8813
Medical Center Hospital of Vermont, 2343
Special Education Unit, 8418
Thorpe Camp, 4727
Vermont Department oF Health State Immunication Program, 5984
Vermont Department of Health - SIDS Information and Counseling
   Program, 7059
Vermont Department of Libraries Special Service Unit, 8540
Vermont Parent Information Center, 8419
Vermont Regional Hemophilia Center, 4049

Virginia

Alexandria Library Talking Book Service, 1885, 2032, 5262, 6187
American Diabetes Association, 2604
Arlington County Department of Libraries, 8541
Autism Society of America Northern Virginia Chapter, 847
Brain Injury Association of Virginia, 3417
Brain Tumor Support Group, 1253
Camp Baker Services, 8814
Camp Easter Seal East, Camp Easter Seal We st, 8815
Camp Fantastic, 117, 169, 1299
Camp Holiday Trails, 8816
Childhelp Children's Center of Virginia, 5679
Children's Tumor Foundation - MidAtlantic Region Chapter, 5039
Cystic Fibrosis Center/University of Virginia Health System, 2344
Cystic Fibrosis Program of the Medical College of Virginia, 2345
Division for Research (CEC-DR), 8555
Division for the Visually Handicapped, 1886, 2033, 5263, 6188
Division on Visual Impairments, 1887, 2034, 5264, 6189
ERIC Clearinghouse on Disabilities and Gifted Education, 8542
Eastern Virginia Medical Center, 2346
Fairfax County Public Library, 8543
Families Empowered and Supporting Treatmen t of Eating Disorders, 2907
Hemophilia Association of the Capital Area, 3984
Infant & Toddler Program, 8420
Leukemia Society of America - National Capital Area Chapter, 93, 153
Makemie Woods Camp Conference Center, 2619, 8817
National Sudden Infant Death Syndrome Research Center, 7072
National Sudden Infant Death Syndrome Resource Center, 7066
Newport News Public Library System, 8544
Oakland School & Camp, 4545
Office of Special Education, Virginia, 8421
Overlook, 8818
PWSA of Maryland, Virginia & DC, 5854
Parent Educational Advocacy Training Cente r, 8422
Precious Hearts, 4334
Roanoke City Public Library System, 8545
Sarcoidosis Support Group, 6370
Scleroderma Foundation Greater Washington DC Chapter, 6442
Spina Bifida Association of the Roanoke Valley, 6860
Tidewater Center for Technology Access, 8423
Triangle D Camp for Children, 8819

Trisomy 18 Foundation, 7409, 7498
United Virginia Chapter of the National Hemophilia Foundation, 3985
University of Virginia General Clinical Research Center, 451
Virginia Assistive Technology System, 8424
Virginia Beach Public Library, 8546
Virginia Commonwealth University Department of Neurosurgery Research,
   3441
Virginia Department of Health Bureau of Immunization, 5985
Virginia SIDS Program - Virginia Department of Health, 7060
Virginia State Library for the Visually and Physically Handicapped, 1888,
   2035, 5265, 6190

Washington

Adult Brain Tumor Support Group, 1254
Autism Society of Washington, 848
Bleeding Disorders Foundation of Washington, 3986
Brain Injury Association of Washington, 3418
Brain Tumor Support Group University of Washington Medical Center,
   1255
Children's Tumor Foundation - Washington C hapter, 5040
Epilepsy Foundation Northwest, 6542
Evergreen Spina Bifida Association, 6861
Head Injury Hotline, 3419
Healing Hearts, 4327
Hemophilia Foundation of Washington, 3987
Hydrocephalus Support Group of Seattle, 4240
Infant Toddler Early Intervention Program, 8425
National Foundation for Ectodermal Dysplasias- Regional Office, 2987
National Wilms Tumor Study, 7796
Northwestern Region-Helen Keller National Center, 1831, 5207, 6132
Office of the Superintendent of Public Instruction, 8426
Prader-Willi Northwest Association, 5817, 5825, 5838
Puget Sound Blood Center, 4030
Region X Office Program Consultants for Maternal and Child Health, 7061
SIDS Northwest Regional Center, 7062
Scleroderma Foundation Evergreen Chapter, 6443
Seattle Area Support Group, 551
Tourette Syndrome Association - Washington and Oregon Chapter, 7402,
   7406
Turner's Syndrome Society of Inland Northwest, 7593
United Cerebral Palsy of South Puget Sound, 1493
University of Washington CF Center, 2347
University of Washington Department of Spe ech & Hearing Sciences, 6780
University of Washington Speech and Hearin g Clinic, 6788
University of Washington: Experimental Education Unit, 2706
Washington Library for the Blind and Physically Handicapped, 1889, 2036,
   5266, 6191
Washington PAVE, 8428
Washington State Chapter of Crohn's & Colitis Foundation of America,
   2189
Washington State Department of Health Immunization Program, 5986

West Virginia

Autism Services Center, 859
Autism Society of West Virginia, 849
Autism Training Center, 860
Brain Injury Association of West Virginia, 3420
Cabell County Public Library, 8547
Early Intervention Program, 8429
Kanawha County Public Library, 8548
Mountain Milestones Stepping Stones, 8820
Mountaineer Spina Bifida Camp, 6907
Office of Special Education Administration, 8430
West Virginia Assistive Technology System, 8431
West Virginia Department of Health and Human Services, 7063
West Virginia Library Commission, 8549
West Virginia Parent Training and Information, 8432
West Virginia School for the Blind, 1890, 2037, 5267, 6192
West Virginia University Cystic Fibrosis Center, 2348
West Virginia University Mountain State Cystic Fibrosis Center, 2349

Wisconsin

Autism Society of Wisconsin, 850

Wyoming

Disorder & Related Term Index

K

KFS, 4447
Kanner's syndrome, 711
Kasabach-merritt syndrome, 3917
Kawasaki Disease, 4408
Kawasaki disease, 4408
Keloids, 4415
Kernicterus, 4422
Kidney tumor, 7784
Kleeblattschadel deformity, 2114
Klinefelter Syndrome, 4434
Klippel-Feil Syndrome, 4447
Klippel-Feil syndrome Type I, 4447
Klippel-Feil syndrome Type II, 4447
Klippel-Feil syndrome Type III, 4447
Kostmann's disease, 5080
Krabbe disease, 4563
Kugelberg-Welander disease, 6908
Kyphosis, 6466

L

LCH, 4175
LCPD, 4553
LDD, 4501
Lactose intolerance, 4783
Landouzy-Dejerine disease, 4819
Landry's paralysis, 3272
Langerhans cell histiocytosis, 4175
Language, 6747
Laron syndrome, 3228
Lazy eye, 4457
Lead exposure, 4494
Lead poisoning, 4494
Lead toxicity, 4494
Learning disability, 2771, 4501
Learning disorder, 4501
Leber congenital retinal amaurosis, 6248
Left heart obstruction, 280
Legg-Calve-Perthes Disease, 4553
Lens opacities, 1818
Letterer-Siwe disease, 4175
Leukemia, 62
Leukodystrophies, 4563
Limb-girdle muscular dystrophy, 4819
Linear scleroderma, 6428
Lissencephaly, 4576
Liver, inflammation of, 4095
Localized tetanus, 5921
Loss of hair, 197
Lupus, 7130
Lyme Disease, 4599
Lymphangiomas, 3917
Lymphatic System, 8845
Lymphatic malformations, 3917
Lymphoma, Hodgkin's, 4186
Lysosomal storage disorders, 4797

M

MAS, 4653
MCNS, 4990
MFS, 4643
ML, 4797
MLNS, 4408
MPS, 4807
MSUD, 4632
Macrocephalia, 4624
Macrocephaly, 4216, 4624
Macrocephaly, benign familial, 4624
Major depressive disorder, 2437
Male Turner syndrome, 5184
Malocclusion, 2390
Manic-depressive disorder, 1030
Manic-depressive illness, 1030

Manic-depressive psychosis, 1030
Manifest deviation, 6936
Maple Syrup Urine Disease, 4632
Marfan Syndrome, 4643
Marfan syndrome, infantile, 4643
Marfan syndrome, neonatal, 4643
Marie-Strumpell spondylitis, 246
Marker X Syndrome, 3177
Martin-Bell Syndrome, 3177
Maternal phenylketonuria, 5543
McCune-Albright Syndrome, 4653
Measles, 5921, 6967
Meckel-Gruber syndrome, 3031
Meconium aspiration syndrome, 6229
Medulloblastoma, 1077
Megacolon, aganglionic, 4156
Megacolon, congenital aganglionic, 4156
Megalencephaly, 4624
Megalocephaly, 4624
Meningitis, 4664
Meningitis, bacterial, 4664
Meningitis, chronic, 4664
Meningitis, neonatal, 4664
Meningitis, viral, 4664
Meningocele, 6803
Meningomyelocele, 6803
Mental deficiency, 4674
Mental retardation, 4674
Mesiodens, 2390
Metachromatic leukodystrophy, 4563
Methionine, 4200
Methylcobalamin defect, 4200
Methylenetetrahydrofolate reductase, 4200
Microcephalia, 4728
Microcephalism, 4728
Microcephaly, 4728
Microdontia, 4737
Microdontism, 4737
Microencephaly, 4728
Middle ear, inflammation of, 5471
Migraine headaches, 4745
Migraine with aura, 4745
Migraine without aura, 4745
Mild (intermediate) MSUD, 4632
Milk Protein Allergy/Lactose Intolerance, 4783
Miller-Dieker lissencephaly syndrome, 4576
Miller-Fisher syndrome, 3272
Minimal change nephrotic syndrome, 4990
Mixed cerebral palsy, 1377
Mixed hearing loss, 3475
Mixed hemangiomas, 3917
Mood disturbance, 2437
Morbilli, 5921
Morphea, 6428
Movement disorders, 1668, 2804
Mucocutaneous lymph node syndrome, 4408
Mucolipidoses, 4797
Mucopolysaccharidoses, 4807
Mucoviscidosis, 2239
Mumps, 5921
Muscular Dystrophies, 4819
Muscular System, 8846
Muscular dystrophy, 4819
Mycobacterium africanum, 7509
Mycobacterium bovis, 7509
Mycobacterium tuberculosis, 7509
Myelocele (Myelomeningocele, Meningomyelocele), 6803
Myelomeningocele, 299, 6803
Myopia (Nearsightedness), 6110

N

NB, 5062
NF, 5005
NF1, 5005
NF2, 5005
NHL, 5163

NS, 5184
Narcolepsy, 4878
Natal teeth, 2390
Nearsightedness, 6110
Neonatal Herpes Simplex, 4959
Neonatal Jaundice, 4973
Neonatal conjunctivitis, 2091
Neonatal herpes simplex, 4959
Neonatal jaundice, 4973
Neonatal meningitis, 4664
Neonatal opthalmia, 2091
Neonatal or infantile Marfan syndrome, 4643
Neonatal pemphigus vulgaris, 5520
Neonatal tetanus, 5921
Nephroblastoma, 7784
Nephrotic Syndrome, 4990
Nervous System, 8847
Neural tube defect, 221, 3031
Neuroblastoma, 5062
Neurocardiogenic syncope, 7112
Neurofibromatosis, 5005
Neurofibromatosis type I, 5005
Neurofibromatosis type I (von Recklinghausen disease) (NF1), 5005
Neurofibromatosis type II, 5005
Neurofibromatosis type II (NF2), 5005
Neuromuscular scoliosis, 6466
Neutropenia, 5080
Neutropenia, chronic, 5080
Neutropenia, cyclic, 5080
Neutropenia, transient, 5080
Nevi, strawberry, 3917
Newborn respiratory distress, 6229
Night terrors, 5122, 6695
Nightmares, 5092
Nine-day measles, 5921
Nocturnal enuresis, 5148
Noise Induced Hearing Loss, 3475
Non-Allergic Rhinitis, 6311
Non-Hodgkin's Lymphoma, 5163
Non-Hodgkin's lymphoma, Burkitt's type, 5163
Non-Hodgkin's lymphoma, SNCC type, 5163
Non-Hodgkin's lymphoma, large cell type, 5163
Non-Hodgkin's lymphoma, lymphoblastic type, 5163
Non-Hodgkin's lymphoma, small noncleaved cell (SNC), 5163
Non-allergic rhinitis, 6311
Non-communicating hydrocephalus, 4216
Non-obstructive hydrocephalus, 4216
Noninfectious conjunctivitis, 2091
Nonparalytic strabismus, 6936
Nontropical sprue, 1335
Noonan Syndrome, 5184
Noonan syndrome, 5184
Norman-Roberts lissencephaly syndrome, 4576
Nystagmus, 5195
Nystagmus, acquired, 5195
Nystagmus, congenital, 5195
Nystagmus, convergent, 5195
Nystagmus, jerky, 5195
Nystagmus, pendular, 5195

O

OCD, 5356
ODD, 5418
OI, 5431
OPCA, 498
OPCA of neonatal onset, 498
OSA, 6669
Obesity, 5303
Obsessive-compulsive disorder, 5356
Obsessive-compulsive neurosis, 5356
Obstructive hydrocephalus, 4216
Obstructive sleep apnea, 6669
Occult tension hydrocephalus, 4216
Ocular albinism, 173

Grey House Publishing

Grey House Publishing

2015 Title List
Visit www.GreyHouse.com for Product Information, Table of Contents, and Sample Pages.

General Reference
An African Biographical Dictionary
America's College Museums
American Environmental Leaders: From Colonial Times to the Present
Encyclopedia of African-American Writing
Encyclopedia of Constitutional Amendments
Encyclopedia of Gun Control & Gun Rights
An Encyclopedia of Human Rights in the United States
Encyclopedia of Invasions & Conquests
Encyclopedia of Prisoners of War & Internment
Encyclopedia of Religion & Law in America
Encyclopedia of Rural America
Encyclopedia of the Continental Congress
Encyclopedia of the United States Cabinet, 1789-2010
Encyclopedia of War Journalism
Encyclopedia of Warrior Peoples & Fighting Groups
The Environmental Debate: A Documentary History
The Evolution Wars: A Guide to the Debates
From Suffrage to the Senate: America's Political Women
Global Terror & Political Risk Assessment
Media & Communications 1900-2020
Nations of the World
Political Corruption in America
Privacy Rights in the Digital Era
The Religious Right: A Reference Handbook
Speakers of the House of Representatives, 1789-2009
This is Who We Were: 1880-1900
This is Who We Were: A Companion to the 1940 Census
This is Who We Were: In the 1910s
This is Who We Were: In the 1920s
This is Who We Were: In the 1940s
This is Who We Were: In the 1950s
This is Who We Were: In the 1960s
This is Who We Were: In the 1970s
U.S. Land & Natural Resource Policy
The Value of a Dollar 1600-1865: Colonial Era to the Civil War
The Value of a Dollar: 1860-2014
Working Americans 1770-1869 Vol. IX: Revolutionary War to the Civil War
Working Americans 1880-1999 Vol. I: The Working Class
Working Americans 1880-1999 Vol. II: The Middle Class
Working Americans 1880-1999 Vol. III: The Upper Class
Working Americans 1880-1999 Vol. IV: Their Children
Working Americans 1880-2015 Vol. V: Americans At War
Working Americans 1880-2005 Vol. VI: Women at Work
Working Americans 1880-2006 Vol. VII: Social Movements
Working Americans 1880-2007 Vol. VIII: Immigrants
Working Americans 1880-2009 Vol. X: Sports & Recreation
Working Americans 1880-2010 Vol. XI: Inventors & Entrepreneurs
Working Americans 1880-2011 Vol. XII: Our History through Music
Working Americans 1880-2012 Vol. XIII: Education & Educators
World Cultural Leaders of the 20th & 21st Centuries

Education Information
Charter School Movement
Comparative Guide to American Elementary & Secondary Schools
Complete Learning Disabilities Directory
Educators Resource Directory
Special Education: A Reference Book for Policy and Curriculum Development

Health Information
Comparative Guide to American Hospitals
Complete Directory for Pediatric Disorders
Complete Directory for People with Chronic Illness
Complete Directory for People with Disabilities
Complete Mental Health Directory
Diabetes in America: Analysis of an Epidemic
Directory of Drug & Alcohol Residential Rehab Facilities
Directory of Health Care Group Purchasing Organizations
Directory of Hospital Personnel
HMO/PPO Directory
Medical Device Register
Older Americans Information Directory

Business Information
Complete Television, Radio & Cable Industry Directory
Directory of Business Information Resources
Directory of Mail Order Catalogs
Directory of Venture Capital & Private Equity Firms
Environmental Resource Handbook
Food & Beverage Market Place
Grey House Homeland Security Directory
Grey House Performing Arts Directory
Grey House Safety & Security Directory
Grey House Transportation Security Directory
Hudson's Washington News Media Contacts Directory
New York State Directory
Rauch Market Research Guides
Sports Market Place Directory

Statistics & Demographics
American Tally
America's Top-Rated Cities
America's Top-Rated Smaller Cities
America's Top-Rated Small Towns & Cities
Ancestry & Ethnicity in America
The Asian Databook
Comparative Guide to American Suburbs
The Hispanic Databook
Profiles of America
"Profiles of" Series – State Handbooks
Weather America

Financial Ratings Series
TheStreet Ratings' Guide to Bond & Money Market Mutual Funds
TheStreet Ratings' Guide to Common Stocks
TheStreet Ratings' Guide to Exchange-Traded Funds
TheStreet Ratings' Guide to Stock Mutual Funds
TheStreet Ratings' Ultimate Guided Tour of Stock Investing
Weiss Ratings' Consumer Guides
Weiss Ratings' Guide to Banks
Weiss Ratings' Guide to Credit Unions
Weiss Ratings' Guide to Health Insurers
Weiss Ratings' Guide to Life & Annuity Insurers
Weiss Ratings' Guide to Property & Casualty Insurers

Bowker's Books In Print® Titles
American Book Publishing Record® Annual
American Book Publishing Record® Monthly
Books In Print®
Books In Print® Supplement
Books Out Loud™
Bowker's Complete Video Directory™
Children's Books In Print®
El-Hi Textbooks & Serials In Print®
Forthcoming Books®
Large Print Books & Serials™
Law Books & Serials In Print™
Medical & Health Care Books In Print™
Publishers, Distributors & Wholesalers of the US™
Subject Guide to Books In Print®
Subject Guide to Children's Books In Print®

Canadian General Reference
Associations Canada
Canadian Almanac & Directory
Canadian Environmental Resource Guide
Canadian Parliamentary Guide
Canadian Venture Capital & Private Equity Firms
Financial Services Canada
Governments Canada
Health Guide Canada
The History of Canada
Libraries Canada
Major Canadian Cities

2015 Title List

Visit www.SalemPress.com for Product Information, Table of Contents, and Sample Pages.

Science, Careers & Mathematics

Ancient Creatures: Unearthed
Applied Science
Applied Science: Engineering & Mathematics
Applied Science: Science & Medicine
Applied Science: Technology
Biomes and Ecosystems
Careers in Business
Careers in Chemistry
Careers in Communications & Media
Careers in Environment & Conservation
Careers in Healthcare
Careers in Hospitality & Tourism
Careers in Human Services
Careers in Law, Criminal Justice & Emergency Services
Careers in Physics
Careers in Technology Services & Repair
Computer Technology Innovators
Contemporary Biographies in Business
Contemporary Biographies in Chemistry
Contemporary Biographies in Communications & Media
Contemporary Biographies in Environment & Conservation
Contemporary Biographies in Healthcare
Contemporary Biographies in Hospitality & Tourism
Contemporary Biographies in Law & Criminal Justice
Contemporary Biographies in Physics
Earth Science
Earth Science: Earth Materials & Resources
Earth Science: Earth's Surface and History
Earth Science: Physics & Chemistry of the Earth
Earth Science: Weather, Water & Atmosphere
Encyclopedia of Energy
Encyclopedia of Environmental Issues
Encyclopedia of Environmental Issues: Atmosphere and Air Pollution
Encyclopedia of Environmental Issues: Ecology and Ecosystems
Encyclopedia of Environmental Issues: Energy and Energy Use
Encyclopedia of Environmental Issues: Policy and Activism
Encyclopedia of Environmental Issues: Preservation/Wilderness Issues
Encyclopedia of Environmental Issues: Water and Water Pollution
Encyclopedia of Global Resources
Encyclopedia of Global Warming
Encyclopedia of Mathematics & Society
Encyclopedia of Mathematics & Society: Engineering, Tech, Medicine
Encyclopedia of Mathematics & Society: Great Mathematicians
Encyclopedia of Mathematics & Society: Math & Social Sciences
Encyclopedia of Mathematics & Society: Math Development/Concepts
Encyclopedia of Mathematics & Society: Math in Culture & Society
Encyclopedia of Mathematics & Society: Space, Science, Environment
Encyclopedia of the Ancient World
Forensic Science
Geography Basics
Internet Innovators
Inventions and Inventors
Magill's Encyclopedia of Science: Animal Life
Magill's Encyclopedia of Science: Plant life
Notable Natural Disasters
Principles of Chemistry
Science and Scientists
Solar System
Solar System: Great Astronomers
Solar System: Study of the Universe
Solar System: The Inner Planets
Solar System: The Moon and Other Small Bodies
Solar System: The Outer Planets
Solar System: The Sun and Other Stars
World Geography

Literature

American Ethnic Writers
Classics of Science Fiction & Fantasy Literature
Critical Insights: Authors
Critical Insights: New Literary Collection Bundles
Critical Insights: Themes
Critical Insights: Works
Critical Survey of Drama
Critical Survey of Graphic Novels: Heroes & Super Heroes
Critical Survey of Graphic Novels: History, Theme & Technique
Critical Survey of Graphic Novels: Independents/Underground Classics
Critical Survey of Graphic Novels: Manga
Critical Survey of Long Fiction
Critical Survey of Mystery & Detective Fiction
Critical Survey of Mythology and Folklore: Heroes and Heroines
Critical Survey of Mythology and Folklore: Love, Sexuality & Desire
Critical Survey of Mythology and Folklore: World Mythology
Critical Survey of Poetry
Critical Survey of Poetry: American Poets
Critical Survey of Poetry: British, Irish & Commonwealth Poets
Critical Survey of Poetry: Cumulative Index
Critical Survey of Poetry: European Poets
Critical Survey of Poetry: Topical Essays
Critical Survey of Poetry: World Poets
Critical Survey of Shakespeare's Sonnets
Critical Survey of Short Fiction
Critical Survey of Short Fiction: American Writers
Critical Survey of Short Fiction: British, Irish, Commonwealth Writers
Critical Survey of Short Fiction: Cumulative Index
Critical Survey of Short Fiction: European Writers
Critical Survey of Short Fiction: Topical Essays
Critical Survey of Short Fiction: World Writers
Cyclopedia of Literary Characters
Holocaust Literature
Introduction to Literary Context: American Poetry of the 20th Century
Introduction to Literary Context: American Post-Modernist Novels
Introduction to Literary Context: American Short Fiction
Introduction to Literary Context: English Literature
Introduction to Literary Context: Plays
Introduction to Literary Context: World Literature
Magill's Literary Annual 2015
Magill's Survey of American Literature
Magill's Survey of World Literature
Masterplots
Masterplots II: African American Literature
Masterplots II: American Fiction Series
Masterplots II: British & Commonwealth Fiction Series
Masterplots II: Christian Literature
Masterplots II: Drama Series
Masterplots II: Juvenile & Young Adult Literature, Supplement
Masterplots II: Nonfiction Series
Masterplots II: Poetry Series
Masterplots II: Short Story Series
Masterplots II: Women's Literature Series
Notable African American Writers
Notable American Novelists
Notable Playwrights
Notable Poets
Recommended Reading: 500 Classics Reviewed
Short Story Writers

Grey House Publishing | Salem Press | H.W. Wilson | 4919 Route, 22 PO Box 56, Amenia NY 12501-0056

2015 Title List

Visit www.SalemPress.com for Product Information, Table of Contents, and Sample Pages.

History and Social Science

The 2000s in America
50 States
African American History
Agriculture in History
American First Ladies
American Heroes
American Indian Culture
American Indian History
American Indian Tribes
American Presidents
American Villains
America's Historic Sites
Ancient Greece
The Bill of Rights
The Civil Rights Movement
The Cold War
Countries, Peoples & Cultures
Countries, Peoples & Cultures: Central & South America
Countries, Peoples & Cultures: Central, South & Southeast Asia
Countries, Peoples & Cultures: East & South Africa
Countries, Peoples & Cultures: East Asia & the Pacific
Countries, Peoples & Cultures: Eastern Europe
Countries, Peoples & Cultures: Middle East & North Africa
Countries, Peoples & Cultures: North America & the Caribbean
Countries, Peoples & Cultures: West & Central Africa
Countries, Peoples & Cultures: Western Europe
Defining Documents: American Revolution (1754-1805)
Defining Documents: Civil War (1860-1865)
Defining Documents: Emergence of Modern America (1868-1918)
Defining Documents: Exploration & Colonial America (1492-1755)
Defining Documents: Manifest Destiny (1803-1860)
Defining Documents: Post-War 1940s (1945-1949)
Defining Documents: Reconstruction (1865-1880)
Defining Documents: The 1920s
Defining Documents: The 1930s
Defining Documents: The American West (1836-1900)
Defining Documents: The Ancient World (2700 B.C.E.-50 C.E.)
Defining Documents: The Middle Ages (524-1431)
Defining Documents: World War I
Defining Documents: World War II (1939-1946)
The Eighties in America
Encyclopedia of American Immigration
Encyclopedia of Flight
Encyclopedia of the Ancient World
The Fifties in America
The Forties in America
Great Athletes
Great Athletes: Baseball
Great Athletes: Basketball
Great Athletes: Boxing & Soccer
Great Athletes: Cumulative Index
Great Athletes: Football
Great Athletes: Golf & Tennis
Great Athletes: Olympics
Great Athletes: Racing & Individual Sports
Great Events from History: 17th Century
Great Events from History: 18th Century
Great Events from History: 19th Century
Great Events from History: 20th Century (1901-1940)
Great Events from History: 20th Century (1941-1970)
Great Events from History: 20th Century (1971-2000)
Great Events from History: Ancient World
Great Events from History: Cumulative Indexes
Great Events from History: Gay, Lesbian, Bisexual, Transgender Events
Great Events from History: Middle Ages
Great Events from History: Modern Scandals
Great Events from History: Renaissance & Early Modern Era

Great Lives from History: 17th Century
Great Lives from History: 18th Century
Great Lives from History: 19th Century
Great Lives from History: 20th Century
Great Lives from History: African Americans
Great Lives from History: Ancient World
Great Lives from History: Asian & Pacific Islander Americans
Great Lives from History: Cumulative Indexes
Great Lives from History: Incredibly Wealthy
Great Lives from History: Inventors & Inventions
Great Lives from History: Jewish Americans
Great Lives from History: Latinos
Great Lives from History: Middle Ages
Great Lives from History: Notorious Lives
Great Lives from History: Renaissance & Early Modern Era
Great Lives from History: Scientists & Science
Historical Encyclopedia of American Business
Immigration in U.S. History
Magill's Guide to Military History
Milestone Documents in African American History
Milestone Documents in American History
Milestone Documents in World History
Milestone Documents of American Leaders
Milestone Documents of World Religions
Musicians & Composers 20th Century
The Nineties in America
The Seventies in America
The Sixties in America
Survey of American Industry and Careers
The Thirties in America
The Twenties in America
United States at War
U.S.A. in Space
U.S. Court Cases
U.S. Government Leaders
U.S. Laws, Acts, and Treaties
U.S. Legal System
U.S. Supreme Court
Weapons and Warfare
World Conflicts: Asia and the Middle East

Health

Addictions & Substance Abuse
Adolescent Health
Cancer
Complementary & Alternative Medicine
Genetics & Inherited Conditions
Health Issues
Infectious Diseases & Conditions
Magill's Medical Guide
Psychology & Behavioral Health
Psychology Basics

Current Biography
Current Biography Cumulative Index 1946-2013
Current Biography Monthly Magazine
Current Biography Yearbook: 2003
Current Biography Yearbook: 2004
Current Biography Yearbook: 2005
Current Biography Yearbook: 2006
Current Biography Yearbook: 2007
Current Biography Yearbook: 2008
Current Biography Yearbook: 2009
Current Biography Yearbook: 2010
Current Biography Yearbook: 2011
Current Biography Yearbook: 2012
Current Biography Yearbook: 2013
Current Biography Yearbook: 2014
Current Biography Yearbook: 2015

Core Collections
Children's Core Collection
Fiction Core Collection
Middle & Junior High School Core
Public Library Core Collection: Nonfiction
Senior High Core Collection

The Reference Shelf
Aging in America
American Military Presence Overseas
The Arab Spring
The Brain
The Business of Food
Conspiracy Theories
The Digital Age
Dinosaurs
Embracing New Paradigms in Education
Faith & Science
Families: Traditional and New Structures
The Future of U.S. Economic Relations: Mexico, Cuba, and Venezuela
Global Climate Change
Graphic Novels and Comic Books
Immigration in the U.S.
Internet Safety
Marijuana Reform
The News and its Future
The Paranormal
Politics of the Ocean
Reality Television
Representative American Speeches: 2008-2009
Representative American Speeches: 2009-2010
Representative American Speeches: 2010-2011
Representative American Speeches: 2011-2012
Representative American Speeches: 2012-2013
Representative American Speeches: 2013-2014
Representative American Speeches: 2014-2015
Revisiting Gender
Robotics
Russia
Social Networking
Social Services for the Poor
Space Exploration & Development
Sports in America
The Supreme Court
The Transformation of American Cities
U.S. Infrastructure
U.S. National Debate Topic: Surveillance
U.S. National Debate Topic: The Ocean
U.S. National Debate Topic: Transportation Infrastructure
Whistleblowers

Readers' Guide
Abridged Readers' Guide to Periodical Literature
Readers' Guide to Periodical Literature

Indexes
Index to Legal Periodicals & Books
Short Story Index
Book Review Digest

Sears List
Sears List of Subject Headings
Sears: Lista de Encabezamientos de Materia

Facts About Series
Facts About American Immigration
Facts About China
Facts About the 20th Century
Facts About the Presidents
Facts About the World's Languages

Nobel Prize Winners
Nobel Prize Winners: 1901-1986
Nobel Prize Winners: 1987-1991
Nobel Prize Winners: 1992-1996
Nobel Prize Winners: 1997-2001

World Authors
World Authors: 1995-2000
World Authors: 2000-2005

Famous First Facts
Famous First Facts
Famous First Facts About American Politics
Famous First Facts About Sports
Famous First Facts About the Environment
Famous First Facts: International Edition

American Book of Days
The American Book of Days
The International Book of Days

Junior Authors & Illustrators
Tenth Book of Junior Authors & Illustrations

Monographs
The Barnhart Dictionary of Etymology
Celebrate the World
Guide to the Ancient World
Indexing from A to Z
The Poetry Break
Radical Change: Books for Youth in a Digital Age

Wilson Chronology
Wilson Chronology of Asia and the Pacific
Wilson Chronology of Human Rights
Wilson Chronology of Ideas
Wilson Chronology of the Arts
Wilson Chronology of the World's Religions
Wilson Chronology of Women's Achievements

Grey House Publishing | Salem Press | H.W. Wilson | 4919 Route, 22 PO Box 56, Amenia NY 12501-0056